FOOD, NUTRITION AND DIET THERAPY

MARIE V. KRAUSE, B.S., M.S., R.D.

Formerly Dietitian in Charge of Nutrition Clinic and Associate Director of
Education, Department of Nutrition, New York Hospital.
Therapeutic Dietitian and Instructor in Dietetics, Mount Sinai Hospital,
Philadelphia, Pa. Therapeutic Dietitian and First Assistant to Instructor in
Nutrition, Department of Medicine, University of Chicago Clinics.

MARTHA A. HUNSCHER, B.S., M.Ed., R.D., M.R.S.H.

Formerly Assistant Professor of Nutrition, School of Nursing, University of Pennsylvania,
Philadelphia, Pennsylvania.
Director, Food Clinic, Pennsylvania Hospital, Philadelphia, Pennsylvania.
Chief, Nutrition Clinic, North End Clinic, Detroit, Michigan.

Fifth Edition — Illustrated

W. B. SAUNDERS COMPANY   PHILADELPHIA   LONDON   TORONTO

W. B. Saunders Company: West Washington Square
Philadelphia, Pa. 19105

12 Dyott Street
London, WC1A 1DB

833 Oxford Street
Toronto 18, Ontario

Food, Nutrition and Diet Therapy   ISBN   0-7216-5512-2

Print No.:   9   8   7   6   5   4   3   2

PREFACE

Good nutrition and the maintenance thereof is basic to health. A knowledge of nutrition as a science and its application become an integral part of the education of health professionals, particularly nurses.

The science of nutrition and diet therapy is presented at a level of sophistication that will meet the needs of students presently entering nursing and other health professions. The organization of the contents of this edition lends itself to the various methods of incorporating nutrition in curricula of the health professions.

Health care is no longer confined to the treatment of illness at the bedside in the hospital environment. Health professionals and consumers of health care services are concerned with the mental and social well-being of individuals as well as the physical well-being. Discussions throughout this text relate to and deal with the *individual* as a member of a community, i.e., his uniqueness in terms of nutritional needs, life style and goals; in terms of the meaning of food and eating; in terms of his stage of growth and development in the life cycle; and particularly in terms of the meaning of change in behavior needed to improve dietary habits and the process through which learning takes place.

Attention is focused on the recognition and significance of dealing with problems of nutrition in underdeveloped nations as well as in the United States. Malnutrition adversely affects the life, development, and health of more people in the world than does any single disease. Metabolic diseases which can be controlled to some extent by nutritional management are also of major concern. Since many more people today survive to face the infirmities of later years, emphasis in the field of nutrition as well as in the field of medicine has shifted from acute to degenerative diseases and from treatment to prevention; this text reflects this shift.

In this edition, Part One includes the nutritional needs of individuals in the life cycle in order that the student may better understand the particular needs in each stage of life and the role of normal nutrition throughout the life cycle. In the chapter discussing pregnancy and lactation, emphasis in this revision has been shifted from diet in pregnancy to diet in preparation for pregnancy, because life experiences, including nutrition, greatly influence reproductive efficiency. The chapters on infancy, childhood and adolescence illustrate how the fulfillment of nutritional needs correlates with growth and development.

Many chapters have been reorganized and charts, tables and new figures have been added. Chapter 7 on Digestion, Absorption and Cell Metabolism is expanded to discuss and illustrate the common metabolic pathway of energy release from protein, fat and carbohydrate. Chapter 6 now includes a discussion of nucleoproteins.

Part Two, Diet Therapy, discusses nutritional management during illness, including diseases of infancy and childhood. The chapters on nutrition in maternal and child health have been moved to Part One where they are considered along with other topics in normal nutrition. The content on diet therapy has been upgraded and expanded, particularly in the areas of ulcer management, hyperlipidemia and malabsorption. Although many frank deficiency diseases such as scurvy, rickets and beriberi are no longer widespread, they do occur as the result of a primary disease which produces secondary nutritional deficiency. Information on the nutritional deficiency diseases therefore continues to be included. Prevention, diagnosis and treatment are apt to be overlooked if these deficiency diseases are not borne in mind.

Emphasis is placed on the need to understand that the dietary modifications are based on the nutritional needs of the individual and the medical findings. In order to meet these goals of therapy strong emphasis is placed on the individual's particular dietary pattern and life style and the learning process through which change in behavior occurs.

The section on Foods, Part Three, is drastically revised. It is organized around pertinent information on four groups of foods and seasonings in normal and therapeutic regimens. This section serves as a general reference and includes additional suggested readings. It is not intended for organized classroom study.

New tables have been added to the Appendix and some have been deleted. The tables on minerals and monosaccharides and disaccharides are new.

Grateful appreciation is extended to students, colleagues and patients, who have been instructive for many years. Special appreciation is given to Audrey L. Kocher, R.D., who reviewed the manuscript and assisted in many ways to make the revision of this edition possible. Particular acknowledgment is made to Catherine Rose, Ph.D., and Lauretta Pierce, Ph.D., R.N., who critically evaluated certain sections of this revised edition. Sincere appreciation is directed to Barbara Sosiak, R.N., Dorothy Warren, Alice Kennedy, Ruth Floeck and Mary Dawson, R.N.; to Martha M. Hunscher and Anne W. Hunscher, R.N.; and to Lisa A., William H., Jr., and Karen B. Hunscher for their valuable contributions and assistance. Particular acknowledgment and appreciation is offered to the W. B. Saunders Company and to all the staff, especially Diane Q. Forti, who cooperated in the preparation of this revised edition. The writing of this text has benefited from the inspiration and encouragement of Garfield G. Duncan, M.D., and the late Frances Stern.

The addition of a co-author for this fifth edition has resulted in the incorporation in the text of new and, in some cases, different interpretations and viewpoints. The knowledge of nutrition and its application progresses so very rapidly that the reader interested in a thorough study of a specific subject must rely on current literature to keep abreast of new developments in the field of nutrition and nutrition education.

MARTHA A. HUNSCHER
MARIE V. KRAUSE

CONTENTS

Part Three   *Foods*

Part One
NORMAL NUTRITION AND FOODS

This section of the book deals with the information relative to normal nutrition and the foods that supply it. Special emphasis is given to the principles of optimum nutrition and their application to the life cycle; appreciation of the importance of nutrition in providing and maintaining health; background and knowledge for the application of nutrition to the student's personal needs; and principles of learning and application for teaching nutrition. Stress is placed on selection of foods required to meet the physiological and psychological needs of an individual and to conform to his socioeconomic background.

Chapter 1
NUTRITION AND HEALTH

The volume of scientific knowledge in nutrition is in the process of translation into action with a speed unparalleled in history. Much progress has been made to date in the understanding of foods and their relation to health. Most people concern themselves with food several times daily, and there is undoubtedly no practice or habit which can influence the health of an individual as much as the decisions that are made with regard to the kinds and amount of foods consumed. The body is made up of many materials. These can be supplied by a wide variety of foods to insure good health. The body is, broadly speaking, the product of its nutrition. You are what you eat. Therefore, it is important that daily decision-making on this important aspect of health be properly guided and not conditioned by pseudoscientific or faddist influences.

NUTRITION

Good nutrition is necessary for good health, and concern with food is important if certain illnesses are to be prevented. What is *nutrition*? It has different meanings. Many people identify it with that portion of nutrition that arouses their own interest. To some nutritionists, the subject is only biochemistry. To nurses, dietitians and physicians, nutrition may mean meals for the sick in terms of calories, protein, carbohydrate, fat, minerals and vitamins. To the layman, it represents food or it may mean a "special diet." By one definition, nutrition is "the combination of processes by which the living organism receives and utilizes the materials (food) necessary for the maintenance of its functions and for the growth and renewal of its components"[1]

Sir Harold Himsworth proposed that "nutrition is the analysis of the effect of food and its constituents on the living organism."[2] The science of nutrition is a young and dynamic biological science. It is based on the fundamental principles of chemistry and biology, biochemistry, microbiology, anatomy and physiology. The practice of nutrition is dependent upon the application of the principles of many sciences and the correlation of many disciplines, some of which include agriculture, food technology, anthropology, psychology, sociology, economics, religion and communications.

Nutrition, in the concept of this book, is food and its relationship to the well-being of the human body. It includes (1) the metabolism of foods, (2) the nutritive value of foods, (3) the qualitative and quantitative requirements of food at different age and developmental levels to meet physiological changes and to meet activity needs, and (4) the selection and eating of foods at different economic, social and cultural levels and for psychological reasons. The science and practice of nutrition exist for and attempt to contribute to the advance of populations throughout the world toward longer and more secure living, relatively free of disease and retarded mental and physical development. The food we eat and do not eat has much to do with health.

NUTRITIONAL STATUS

Sometimes the term nutrition is used to refer to the nutritional status of an individual. "The condition of the body resulting from the utilization of the essential nutrients available to the body"[1] is termed the *nutritional status*. It may be good, fair or poor, depending on the intake of dietary essentials, on the relative need for them, and on the body's ability to utilize them.

Good nutritional status is noted when man

[1]Turner, D.: Handbook of Diet Therapy. 5th ed. Chicago, University of Chicago Press, 1970.

[2]Himsworth, H.: What nutrition really means. Nutrition Today, 3:18, No. 3, September, 1968.

benefits from the intake of a well-balanced dietary. *Optimum* nutrition means that the essential nutrients, namely carbohydrates, proteins, fats, minerals, vitamins and water, are supplied and utilized to maintain health and well-being at the highest possible level. In good nutritional status a reserve of many of the nutrients is provided.

Good nutrition is essential for normal organ development and function; for normal reproduction, growth and maintenance; for optimum activity and working efficiency; for resistance to infection; and for the ability to repair bodily damage or injury. *Poor* nutritional status exists when man is deprived of an adequate amount of the essential nutrients over an extended period of time. This is relative, because the body stores of some nutrients last longer than others. Demands may go up at times, and intake, being constant, may become inadequate.

Nutritional deficiencies result whenever inadequate amounts of essential nutrients are provided to tissues which require them for normal functioning. The deficiency may be primary or secondary. A primary deficiency may occur when the dietary is lacking in a particular nutrient or nutrients. Scurvy is due to a lack of ascorbic acid in the dietary. An adequate amount of the vitamin will correct the condition. According to Jolliffe,[3] a nutritional deficiency disease may occur as a result of conditioning factors in persons consuming diets considered adequate. If the deficiency is caused by bodily states that interfere with digestion, absorption, or utilization of essential nutrients, or by stress factors that increase the requirements for or cause destruction of or abnormal excretion of nutrients, it is referred to as a secondary deficiency.

Pernicious anemia, which is caused by a deficiency of vitamin B_{12}, is considered a secondary deficiency because individuals with this disorder cannot absorb vitamin B_{12}, even though it may be present in the food ingested. The absorption depends on the presence of an intrinsic factor, a mucoprotein enzyme secreted in the stomach.

A clear distinction between primary and secondary malnutrition in population surveys is important. False conclusions can be drawn when the conditioning factors associated with secondary malnutrition are not recognized. All examples of malnutrition are not caused by dietary inadequacies.

The first step in evaluating a person's nutritional status is to obtain a dietary history. (See page 19.) A history of a previously inadequate diet is often the first clue to a nutritional deficiency influencing the disease process. The correlation of the information found in the dietary history, medical history, physical examination and appropriate laboratory tests is used to determine the nutritional status of an individual or group.

Table 1–1 illustrates various clinical findings, which are grouped with the deficiencies or syndromes which they suggest. Many of these clinical findings are related more or less to deficiencies of one or more of the vitamins. Although these signs are important, their presence in tabular form does not indicate that vitamin deficiencies in nutrition are all important. Other serious forms of malnutrition[4] are as prevalent, but their clinical signs do not lend themselves as readily to tabulation. Less than normal weight and height for a certain age, for example, are important clinical indicators for calorie and protein undernutrition. These findings will be discussed in detail in subsequent chapters.

APPLIED NUTRITION

The objective of *applied nutrition* is to adapt the principles of the science of nutrition to meet the needs of an individual or group.

Dietetics is the science and art of utilizing food and the fundamental knowledge of nutrition and metabolism in the various conditions of health and disease. The science consists of a knowledge of food composition and dietary constituency needed in different states of health and disease, and the art consists of knowing how to plan and prepare the necessary foods, at the various economic levels, and how to offer them in such a pleasing and attractive form (keeping in mind individual or racial eating habits) that the individual, well or ill, will be persuaded to eat the foods and adhere to the dietary program. If the individual is ill and has little appetite, or if he has well-established food habits, the task of fulfilling the dietary prescribed may be too difficult. This calls for knowledge of the relationship of the disease process to appetite and the ability to apply the principles of the teaching and learning processes in order to implement a therapeutic change in the food habits of an individual.

Diet therapy is the use of food as a factor in aiding recovery from illness, relating the art and science of nutrition to the symptoms of the disease.

The dietary regimens are *classified* according to nutrients, fiber, texture and consistency, qualitative and quantitative restrictions,

[3]Jolliffe, N. (ed.): Clinical Nutrition. 2nd ed. New York, Harper & Bros., 1962.

[4]Malnutrition can mean either *under-* or *over*nutrition. The prefix "mal" means bad.

TABLE 1–1   CLINICAL FINDINGS AND SUGGESTED DEFICIENCY
OR SYNDROME

FINDINGS	SUGGESTED DEFICIENCY OR SYNDROME
General	
Underweight (T)*	Calories, protein, calcium, phosphorus, vitamins
Underheight	Iron, folic acid, vitamin B_{12}, ascorbic acid, thiamin, B complex
Pallor (T)	
Hair	
Dry, staring hair, usually with pediculi (N)	Unknown
Skin	
Perifolliculosis (N)	Ascorbic acid, unknown
Follicular hyperkeratosis	Vitamin A, unknown
Xerosis (N)	Vitamin A, unknown
Dermatitis of pellagra (N)	Niacin
Erythematous	
Intertriginous	
Hyperkeratotic	
Ichthyotic	
Dyssebacea, especially in nasolabial folds, external canthi, behind ears and in body folds (N)	Riboflavin, unknown
Intertrigo (N)	Niacin, riboflavin, unknown
Acne (T)	
Acne vulgaris	Unknown, riboflavin, pyridoxine, vitamin A
Acne rosacea	Unknown, riboflavin
Acne varioliformis	Unknown
Palmar erythema	Unknown, B complex, riboflavin, amino acids
Spider telangiectasis	Unknown
Suborbital pigmentation (T)	Unknown
Hemorrhagic manifestations (N)	Ascorbic acid, vitamin K, unknown
Eyes	
Bitot's spots	Vitamin A
Corneal vascularity	Unknown, riboflavin
Circumcorneal injection	Unknown, riboflavin
Rosacea keratitis	Unknown, riboflavin
Follicular conjunctivitis	Vitamin A, unknown
Scarlet conjunctivitis (T)	Niacin
Blepharitis (T)	Unknown, vitamin A, riboflavin
Canthi fissures (T)	Riboflavin, unknown
Night blindness	Vitamin A
Photophobia (T)	Vitamin A, riboflavin
Lips	
Cheilosis	Riboflavin, B complex, pyridoxine
Chapping (N)	Unknown
Increase in vertical fissuring	
Atrophic cheilosis	
Angular stomatitis (N)	Riboflavin, B complex, iron
Angular fissures (N)	Riboflavin, B complex, iron
La perleche (N)	Riboflavin, B complex, iron
Tongue	
Scarlet red glossitis (N)	Niacin, folic acid, vitamin B_{12}, protein
Beefy red glossitis (N)	Niacin, B complex, folic acid, vitamin B_{12}, protein
Magenta glossitis (N)	B complex, riboflavin
Chronic glossitis of malnutrition (N)	Niacin, folic acid, vitamin B_{12}, B complex, protein, unknown
Edema of the tongue (N)	Niacin, unknown
Oral Mucous Membranes	
Scarlet stomatitis (N)	Niacin
Lichen planus	Unknown
Leukoplakia	Unknown
Teeth and Gums	
Caries (N)	Unknown
Malocclusion (T)	Vitamin D, unknown
Scorbutic gums (N)	Vitamin C
Gingivitis	Vitamin C, unknown
Skeletal	
Rachitic deformities (N)	Vitamin D, calcium, phosphorus
Osteomalacia	Vitamin D, calcium, phosphorus
Nervous	
Nutritional polyneuropathy	Thiamin, B complex
Retrobulbar neuritis	Thiamin, unknown
Central ophthalmoplegia	Thiamin
Encephalopathic states	Thiamin, niacin, B complex, unknown
Combined system disease	B complex, vitamin B_{12}
Organic reactive psychoses	Thiamin, niacin, B complex, unknown
Circulatory	
Beriberi heart disease	Thiamin
Edema (T)	Protein, thiamin, famine
Endocrine	
Simple goiter	Iodine

From Jolliffe, N. (ed.): Clinical Nutrition. 2nd ed. New York, Harper & Brothers, 1962.
*Teachers (T) or nurses (N) may be instructed to detect appearance of these signs.

and management programs, or a combination of these factors. The high protein, high vitamin, high calorie regimen is an example of a diet concerned with nutrients. Low residue and high residue modifications are examples of diets classified according to fiber. The soft diet and liquid diet are types of dietaries prescribed for texture and consistency. Restricted or quantitative designations are the diabetic diet, the 1000 kcalorie dietary and the 500 mg. sodium diet. A diet given in consecutive stages for treatment of gastric ulcer is considered a type of therapeutic management program. All diets overlap in some respects. The goal is to modify the customary dietary pattern of an individual as little as possible for the therapy indicated. The therapy may well be, quite simply, an adequate diet.

HISTORY

Man has always been concerned about food, along with the two other factors basic to living, namely, shelter and clothing. He apparently began his life as a carnivorous animal; he was a hunter of game and a fisherman. Only at the end of the Stone Age did he begin to cultivate grains for food and add berries and honey to his staple, meat.

Archeological evidence reveals that the development of communities, towns and cities came through the settling of groups of people to cultivate foods. Learned men of ancient times offered theories about the health values of specific foods. Some of their wisdom is recorded in historical philosophical treatises and in chapters of the Bible.

During the eighteenth century when scientific discoveries were changing concepts and causing intellectual ferment, the French chemist Antoine Laurent Lavoisier recognized the relationship of the process of respiration (intake of oxygen and output of carbon dioxide) to the metabolism of food. He had discovered the role of oxygen in combustion and investigated the relation of the burning flame to the metabolism of organic foods. Lavoisier is called the "father of nutrition." He, with the physicist Laplace, used guinea pigs for the first quantitative studies on respiration, and animals have continued to play a major role in nutritional studies. These early investigations were followed by concentrated interest in the energy value or calorie value of foods, particularly the carbohydrates, fats and proteins.

In 1896 W. O. Atwater, who has been called "the father of American nutrition," published the first extensive table of food values ever published in this country. At that time, only proteins and calories were generally considered to be of nutritional importance. It was not until 20 years later that E. V. McCollum, one of the principal early workers in the field of accessory food factors, popularized the concept of "protective foods"—those primarily useful for their content of vitamins and minerals. Shortly after World War I, this resulted in a marked increase in the consumption of leafy vegetables, citrus fruit and milk.

At the same time, Graham Lusk was exerting his far-reaching influence on dietary habits. An expert on calorie needs, it was he who first secured popular acceptance of the fact that adolescents required as much food as did adults. Space does not permit a comprehensive listing of all the other nutritionists who have contributed to our knowledge of the science of nutrition during the past century. Many men, ideas and equipment, along with the sciences of chemistry, physiology, biology and medicine, have contributed to the development of the science of nutrition. Some of the various pathways that have been used to accrue present knowledge in this field are summarized in Figure 1–1.

An abundance of reading material on the history of nutrition is available for exploration by the interested student. Not only is it pleasant reading, but it is essential to present and future knowledge.[5, 6, 7]

NATIONAL AND INTERNATIONAL NUTRITIONAL PROGRESS

In the history of nutrition science, one major trend is outstanding: the application has become ever broader. It remained for the twentieth century and the days of World War I to bring the modern concept. Prior to this, available knowledge was used mainly for the prevention and alleviation of dietary deficiency diseases in the individual or in small groups. The next step, an organized health approach, was planned distribution of preventive foods, such as butter, iodized salt and cod liver oil. Meanwhile, the isolation of vitamins progressed; and just before World War II, it became practical to improve staple foods with synthetic nutrients as a means of attacking deficiency diseases in large populations. Vitamin D was added to milk, vitamin A to margarine. White flour and bread were enriched with thiamin, riboflavin, niacin and iron. Nationwide control of specific dietary

[5]Todhunter, E. N.: J. Am. Dietet. A., *41*:328 and 335, 1962; 44:100, 1964; 46:120, 1965; Elvehjem, C. A.: J. Am. Dietet. A., 38:236, 1961.
[6]McCollum, E. V.: A History of Nutrition. Boston, Houghton Mifflin Co., 1957.
[7]Lowenberg, M. E., et al.: Food and Man. New York, John Wiley & Sons, Inc., 1968.

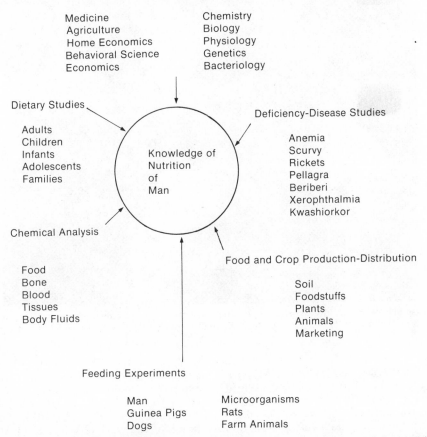

Contributing Fields:

Medicine
Agriculture
Home Economics
Behavioral Science
Economics

Chemistry
Biology
Physiology
Genetics
Bacteriology

Dietary Studies

Adults
Children
Infants
Adolescents
Families

Knowledge of
Nutrition
of
Man

Deficiency-Disease Studies

Anemia
Scurvy
Rickets
Pellagra
Beriberi
Xerophthalmia
Kwashiorkor

Chemical Analysis

Food
Bone
Blood
Tissues
Body Fluids

Food and Crop Production-Distribution

Soil
Foodstuffs
Plants
Animals
Marketing

Feeding Experiments

Man
Guinea Pigs
Dogs

Microorganisms
Rats
Farm Animals

Figure 1–1 Methods and areas of investigations that lead to the development of the science of nutrition. (After Lowenberg, M. E.: Food and Man. New York, John Wiley & Sons, Inc., 1967.)

diseases was now feasible, and a program was launched. Better nutrition education, a national school lunch program, improvements in agriculture practices, advances in food handling, preservation and distribution were included in the program.

INTERNATIONAL NUTRITION AGENCIES

The League of Nations planted the seeds for international cooperation in nutrition by publication of a document entitled "The Relation of Nutrition to Health, Agriculture, and Economic Policy." This famous report drew attention to the connections between food and health. Although World War II prevented the cooperative plans of the League of Nations from being put into full-scale use, a series of notable events insofar as nutrition was concerned took place in the United States during this period. In 1940, the Food and Nutrition Board of the National Research Council was established and accepted the

responsibility to study nutrition on a worldwide scale. This organization drew on the substantial material on nutrition published by the League of Nations and published the first recommended daily dietary allowances in 1941. These allowances have been updated and revised approximately every five years, the most recent revision being published in 1968.[8] These recommended goals can be used in planning and in evaluating food supplies for healthy people from the nutritional point of view and are discussed in detail in Chapter 11. In 1952 the amounts of nutrients adjusted to cover the additional requirements created by disease and injury as outlined by the Committee on Therapeutic Nutrition were published.[9]

---

[8]Food and Nutrition Board: Recommended Dietary Allowances. 7th revised edition. Washington, D.C., National Academy of Sciences, National Research Council, Pub. No. 1694, 1968.
[9]Pollack, H., and Halpern, S. L.: Therapeutic Nutrition. Washington, D.C., National Research Council, Pub. No. 234, 1952.

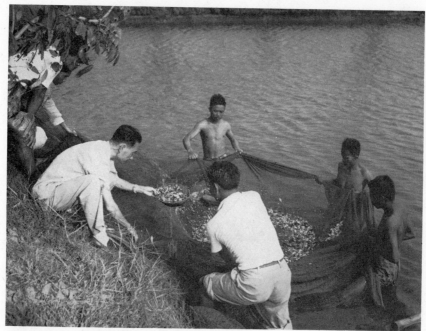

Figure 1–2   Dr. Shao Wen-ling, FAO fisheries expert, giving fish culture instruction in Thailand. This education resulted in adding much needed protein to the diet. (Courtesy of the Food and Agriculture Organization of the United Nations.)

After World War II, the Food and Agricultural Organization (FAO) and the World Health Organizations (WHO) were created as divisions of the United Nations. FAO is dedicated to raising world-wide levels of nutrition and standards of living by securing improvement in the efficiency of production and distribution of food and agricultural products (Fig. 1–2). To tackle this huge task from different angles, many sub-units of FAO were created, such as the Divisions of Nutrition, Economics, Forestry, Fisheries and Agriculture. As an example of a broad effort that one way or another involves all these specialties, one can point to the FAO-sponsored development of fish-farming. Dr. Shao Wen-ling, FAO's Chinese authority on fish-farming, helped to develop fish-farming projects in Thailand, Burma, Indonesia and Ceylon. The king of the cultivatable fishes is the common carp. Several varieties of this fish are reared in ponds, particularly in Southeast Asia, and make significant contributions to the protein content of the national dietaries. Such FAO experts as Dr. Wen-ling (seen in action in Fig. 1–2) are sent into a country for a given period of time. There they establish centers for fish culture and train local personnel so that when they leave the country the work continues.

The World Health Organization (WHO) is the medically oriented unit of the United Nations. The Nutrition Division of WHO concerns itself primarily with the medical aspects of malnutrition as part of an overall effort to raise levels of nutrition throughout the world (Fig. 1–3). As might be expected, much of the work of WHO and FAO overlaps. Indeed, it has been customary during the past few years for these two organizations to convene joint committees to prepare authoritative reports on some pressing nutrition subjects, such as nutritional requirements.

Still another subdivision of the United Nations is the United Nations Children's Fund. This was originally called the United Nations International Children's Emergency Fund (UNICEF) and is still known by these initials. UNICEF is principally a supply agency and has been active in bringing relief to children of the "have-not" nations through food distribution programs using surplus foods from the "have" nations. In recent years this agency has been primarily concerned with eradication of widespread protein malnutrition and was awarded a Nobel Prize in 1965 for its great contributions to child health. Another United Nations Organization subdivision that sometimes works tangentially in nutrition is the United Nations Educational Scientific and Cultural Organization (UNESCO).

The International Education and Health Act of 1966, the Foreign Aid Program and the Food for Freedom Program were set up to include combating malnutrition as a major

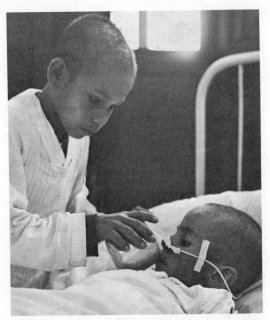

Figure 1–3 General Hospital, Guatemala City, Guatemala. Two victims of malnutrition – one recovering, the other one with a long way to go. There is almost a daily arrival of malnutrition cases at hospitals in Central America where, either because of ignorance or insufficiency, children's diets are often found to be extremely low in protein, vitamin A, and riboflavin. Eggs, meat and citrus juices are not considered foods for children. The task of nutrition education undertaken by the Institute of Nutrition of Central America and Panama is a tremendous one when it is realized that these people have used the same low nutritive value foods for generations, have seen the ravages of resulting disease without determining the cause, and have made little change in their eating habits. (Photo by Maxine Rude. Courtesy of the World Health Organization.)

objective in their programs. The efforts of these United States programs are closely coordinated with FAO, WHO and UNICEF. Together they give hope for a better tomorrow for the world's children.

To this list of international agencies should be added the names of the Nutrition Program of the Bureau of Disease Prevention and Environmental Control and Agency for International Development, both U.S. government agencies. Variously known in the past as the "Interdepartmental Committee for Nutrition in National Development (ICNND)" and the "Nutrition Section of the Office of International Research," this agency once had nutritional responsibilities principally at the international level. Its nutrition survey programs in more than 25 countries serve as models of excellence and its introduction of nutrition into long-range government planning will continue to bear fruit for years to come.

UNITED STATES NUTRITION AGENCIES

The principal agencies of the federal government of the United States involved in public health nutrition programs are the Department of Health, Education and Welfare and the Department of Agriculture. In the former department, the agencies dealing primarily with public health nutrition are the Public Health Service, the Children's Bureau and the Food and Drug Administration.

The Public Health Service provides some nutrition services for native Indians and the general population and also trains qualified candidates in public health nutrition. The Division of Medical Care Administration, concerned principally with Medicare, also deals with public health nutrition.

The National Institutes of Health not only has a program of nutrition research in its facilities in Bethesda, Maryland, but supports nutrition research through its grants program.

The Children's Bureau is principally a service agency concerned with the practical aspects of maternal and child care.

The Nutrition and Consumer Research Institute of the U.S. Department of Agriculture (USDA) coordinates nutrition services available to the public through federal, state, and other agencies. This organization works through the research and education programs of the State Land Grant Universities. The Agricultural Research Services also conduct research in their laboratories in Beltsville, Maryland, and cooperate with State Experiment Stations research programs. The standard food composition tables result largely from the food analysis data compiled and assembled by the USDA laboratories. Of great importance are the dietary surveys of the household consumption of foods in the United States performed by the USDA. The results of these studies are published every 10 years and show trends in nutrient consumption in the United States. The Food and Drug Administration has a division of nutrition that is assigned the responsibility of insuring the safety of the national food supply. To this end it has developed analytical methods, established food standards and examined the safety of food additives. Its activity best known to the public is its constant campaign against food faddism and nutrition quackery.

PRIVATE NUTRITION GROUPS

In addition to these international and federal agencies, numerous private organizations devote some or all of their energies to nutrition – both basic and applied. Among these are three professional organizations, members of which have carried on research and teaching in all aspects of nutrition. These are the American Home Economics Association (1909), the American Dietetic Association (1917) and the American Institute of Nutrition (1933).

The Nutrition Foundation (1941) is supported by food and related industries. This organization makes funds available for nutrition research. Also, it summarizes and interprets current research in nutrition through the monthly publication, Nutrition Reviews.

The Council on Foods and Nutrition of the American Medical Association (A.M.A.) is an extremely active organization whose primary purpose is the dissemination of sound nutrition information to physicians. To this end it publishes scholarly articles on nutrition in the Journal of the American Medical Association and sponsors nutrition conferences and the like. For the lay public, nutrition articles appear in Today's Health, a monthly family magazine published by the A.M.A. The Council is also particularly effective in combating the nutritional misinformation dispensed by health food lecturers, food faddists and pseudo-health writers.

WORLD NUTRITION PROBLEMS

In 1960, FAO intensified its efforts to resolve the nutrition problems by launching a 5-year Freedom from Hunger Campaign to dramatize the world's need for food. Attention was focused on information concerning research and national action programs. The United States, Canada and Australia, among other nations, contributed a great deal of financial and technical help and material toward providing food and other services to developing countries.

In May, 1966, FAO issued a statement to the effect that more babies were born in 1965 than the world can feed. Consequences of this situation, which usually means insufficient calories and protein, are far-reaching. Severe shortage of protein lowers resistance of infants and young children to most infective agents, results in the syndromes of kwashiorkor and marasmus and causes physical and mental retardation.

Iron deficiency affects millions of people in the world, augmenting the degree of anemia already caused by intestinal and blood parasites. Low levels of calcium intake, especially in children and pregnant and lactating women, and of iodine are causes for concern. In practically every nutrition survey made, vitamin A deficiency has been found in some groups of the child population. Populations which use corn as the staple food often develop pellagra. Beriberi results when polished rice constitutes 80 to 90 per cent of their diet. Ascorbic acid deficiencies occur in such countries as Ethiopia, Libya, Iran, Turkey and Chile.

The widespread suffering from undernutrition, especially in the underdeveloped countries, shows that a large segment of the world's population has not yet escaped the fear of malnutrition and hunger. The effective application of the spectacular developments in agriculture, animal husbandry, and food science and technology is needed to increase food production in the developing countries. However, without limitation of the present rate of increase of the population, these efforts can achieve only limited success in combating malnutrition.

In 1969 a White House Conference on Food, Nutrition and Health was held to explore what needed to be done in the United States (1) to improve the nutrition of the most vulnerable groups of people—the very poor, pregnant and nursing mothers, children and adolescents, and the aging; (2) to develop new technologies of food production, processing and packaging; (3) to improve nutrition teaching in the schools—from Head Start to nursing and medical schools; (4) to improve Federal programs that affect nutrition such as food stamp, commodity distribution and school lunch programs. Surveys indicate considerable malnutrition (both undernutrition and overnutrition), anemia and degenerative disease in the United States.

Assistance is needed in areas where the problem of nutrition is of crucial importance for the development of individuals to their highest potential, mentally and emotionally as well as physically. How to make enough food of the right kind available to all people everywhere and how to teach all people of the world to choose and enjoy foods for nutritive value is a great challenge. It is best to begin with the food resources to which people are accustomed. Patience and tact are essential in order to introduce new habits to people—individually or in groups.

PREVENTIVE MEDICINE AND NUTRITION

In the last half century medical care, public health and scientific research have brought about dramatic progress in the betterment of health. Perhaps nothing is more indicative of this improvement than the increase in longevity. In 1900 the average span of life in the United States was about 49 years. Today the figure is over 70.

Much of this progress has been due to the

control of preventable diseases, particularly those affecting the young, and nutrition has played a large part. Malnutrition adversely affects the life, development and health of more people in the world than any disease. It kills millions of infants and small children, especially in the technically underdeveloped areas (Fig. 1–2). More and more attention is being focused on preventive medicine or productive health than on curative measures. Prevention is far more effective than therapy, for what can be prevented does not need to be treated. The World Health Organization defines health as "a state of complete physical, mental, and social well-being, and not merely the absence of disease infirmity."[10] Nutrition is one of the most important environmental factors affecting the state of an individual's or nation's health.

Sufficient activity, rest, recreation and sleep contribute to health. Eating the correct proportion and assortment of foods each day is the contribution of nutrition to health.

A dietary *inadequate in calories* has been demonstrated to bring about an impairment of physical efficiency, and production output diminishes in direct proportion to the caloric insufficiency. Muscle strength and muscle endurance are diminished in prolonged semistarvation.

Vitamin deficiency impairs physical fitness, affects mental well-being, and will also affect the capacity for work.

Protein deficiency brings about muscular weakness, easy fatigability and, as a result, impaired work performance.

A controlled study, as well as observation during and following World War II, demonstrated clearly that poorly fed people are affected mentally as well as physically. Changes of personality and outlook were observed. As a result of inadequate nutrition, people become irritable, morose, depressed, and lacking in initiative and ambition. Sufficient kinds and amounts of food prevent or correct these changes. The nurse can do much in her daily contact with patients and the public to apply her knowledge of nutrition. When the meals are served, a word of wisdom at the bedside is usually more helpful than a planned lecture.

NUTRITION IN INDUSTRY

Studies of industrial workers in various sections of the United States reveal that many people consume inadequate diets with resulting poor nutritional status. Poor nutrition is costly in both time and money to industry. Poorly nourished workers frequently show more fatigue, are less efficient and more accident prone and have a higher absenteeism record due to illness than workers whose food habits are good.

Various nutrition education programs have been tried and have been successful. Nutrition posters, exhibits, folders, company publications, newsletters and films that emphasize the importance of food selection and good nutrition to productive health are effective educational material. The industrial nurse has opportunities to help workers improve their dietary patterns.

FOOD HABITS

Food habits have been with us a long time. They are as old as yesterday, as contemporary as today, as modern as tomorrow. Food habits are the response of individuals or groups to social and cultural pressures, selecting, consuming, and utilizing portions of the available food supply.[11]

HISTORY   Food habits, the foodways of cultures, are influenced by social organization. Through the study of habits of primitive tribes, it was found that the role of food was related to the social status as well as to the physical status of the members of the tribe. During pregnancy women received favorite foods, the implication being that a prospective warrior might be born. Children were well fed, either from the milk of the mother's breasts or from the milk of animals. The aged were nourished because they were the ones who could provide wisdom to the younger generation. However, in some tribes the aged were allowed to die if they interfered with the activities of, or did not fulfill a useful function in, the tribe. The strong, superior individuals helped to evolve a caste system. Those who did not make the upper grade of leadership were assigned to perform the necessary chores, to take care of the soil, crops and animals.

Today's social structure of rural and urban groupings has developed from yesterday's primitive tribes. In this country, since the beginning of the twentieth century, changes have occurred in social organization, with movement from rural to urban and metropolitan areas where factories are located. From the traditional slow pace of rural living, families have moved to city life where the tempo is accelerated by competitiveness. With the increasing urbanization in the United States during the past generation, breakfast and lunch have become skimpier and dinner larger. Except for rural areas

---

[10]World Health Organization – What It Is, What It Does, How It Works. Leaflet. Switzerland, Geneva, 1956.

[11] Manual for the Study of Food Habits. Washington, D.C., National Research Council, Bull. No. 111.

where dinner is usually served at the noon meal, supper is rarely heard of. Authorities have questioned the advisability of the large dinner at night, which is usually followed by little or no physical activity.

Urban food supply includes variety of food and variety in food service, while the characteristics of rural food supply are home-grown products which are home-processed, home-cooked, and home-served. However, present shipping and shopping centers throughout the country give urban and rural dwellers equal opportunities of choice in most sections of the United States. Ready to eat foods are available and utilized in both the urban and rural areas, thus replacing many of the home-prepared foods.

DEVELOPMENT OF FOOD HABITS   The American dietary is continually changing. Changes in food habits are motivated by moral dictation, social desirability, scientific sanction or forced changes which are stimulated by physical circumstances, such as pressure for time, crop failures, or lowering of economic status of individuals, groups or nations, which may follow as the result of war. The most notable changes are those which have resulted from improvement in transportation. At the beginning of the twentieth century, the United States was largely agricultural and a considerable proportion of the food was grown by the consumer or his neighbors. With the present elaborate system of transportation, perishable foods are available the year round, as compared to the previous marked seasonal variations in the diet. Refrigeration, automated processing and packaging conspire to defy seasons and banish spoilage. Technological advancements have made it possible for innumerable new items to appear on grocery shelves and, ultimately, on the family table.

Changes in food habits are also motivated by the bodily state of individuals during pregnancy, illness, increased age and obesity. An illness which imposes dietary restrictions or an unpleasant experience with food may result in a lifelong dislike for some particular food or foods. Food used as a punishment for children may result in a permanent dislike of the food the child is forced to eat.

Attitudes toward foods are influenced by the geographical location. Groups residing along the seacoast where fish is available like to eat fish, while inland groups eat available grains and the flesh of animals.

The baby is taught to eat foods which the mother likes and which the mother had been taught to eat by her mother. If the mother likes sweetened cereal, the baby will establish a habit of eating sweetened cereal. (See page 269, eating habits and the psychology of infant and child feeding.) The growing child is influenced by the environment and habits of the family group (see page 283, adolescent food habits), the social group, the school group and, later, the work or professional group. If there is an intermarriage of cultures, an adjustment or blending of the eating habits of the wedded nationalities occurs. The offspring from this intermarriage are influenced by the food habits of each parent.

Each nationality has characteristic food plans. The food plans started with available foods which served as the basic core. For example, cereal or rice is the basic core of the food plan of Orientals, while meat is the principal core of the Eskimo's food plan. A mixture of food is the basis of our food plan. Characteristic beverages, supplementary foods, and ceremonial or festival foods are added to the food plans. (Consult food plans of different nationalities in Chapter 13).

Food also has social and ceremonial significances. Many business transactions are conducted at the dining table in a club or restaurant. To maintain social position, women's clubs hold their meetings at a luncheon in a desirable hotel. Holidays are celebrated with special meals. Religious festivities are designated with feasts or banquets, and decisive moments in life, such as christenings, weddings, and funerals, are honored with serving of special food. Orthodox Jews observe dietary laws (page 205, and Catholics observe fast days during Lent (page 205).

Food habits are largely established during early childhood and can be changed later only by gradual introduction of new foods and new ideas. The enlarged dietary of many Americans shows that new food will be accepted. Europeans and others came to America with their national foods. Now many people, and not only in large urban centers, enjoy Italian spaghetti, Chinese specialties, German sauerkraut and many others.

Poor food habits account for a large number of the nutritional deficiencies which are prevalent today. The persons who either skip breakfast or eat an inadequate one (see Omitting a Meal, Chap. 11), those who are grossly overweight, and poorly nourished teen-age girls are groups who have acquired poor food habits. They fail to regulate the intake of food energy to body needs. Good food habits are basic to sound body structure. Studies in the United States reveal that many Americans have low nutritional standards, and poor food habits through the years ultimately take a toll. A poor diet is the first step toward poor nutrition. To improve the nutritional status and health of the masses, better food habits are needed. The nurse can set a good example as one way to foster good food habits. The changes an individual will make in his dietary depend on the motivation he himself develops. The nurse is in a position to identify that motivation and to determine whether the individual's dietary provides the essential nutrients (see Dietary History, page 19). In this way, the nurse identifies the group of foods supplying the nutrients that the individual must include or restrict in order to improve his dietary. Thus the individual may adhere to his customary pattern and be encouraged to select foods providing the necessary nutrients from those known to him.

FOOD FADS, FALLACIES AND QUACKERY

Many cults and fads have developed from food habits. There are always faddists who insist there is some magic quality in some peculiar kind of food or diet. Examples are the all-vegetable diet, or use of large amounts of seaweed or of blackstrap molasses. Various fad diets have caught the fancy of the overweight populace who try to lose poundage by "not counting calories," consuming extra protein foods, or adhering to formula diet routines. Some people associate the consumption of meat with masculinity, virility, and aggression. There are the self-styled "experts"–food quacks–who have a smattering of knowledge or are promoting some patented product they want to sell. Food faddists and food quacks are closely related. The psychosomatic manifestations of food dislikes are numerous, adding to food fallacies and symbolism.

The mere fact that a diet sounds extraordinary is no reason for condemning it if it is adequate in nutrients. In fact various native diets may sound strange to an American but provide nutrients which meet standards as well as or better than the pattern to which he is accustomed. The type of fad diet which is not recommended is one which is inadequate in nutrients or recommends replacing wholesome foods with expensive so-called "health foods."

Television and radio advertising are often misleading. Facts of minor importance are built up to suit advertising purposes. The same is true of popular or unreliable literature. The information may not necessarily be harmful but may lead to use of the fad food, which is expensive, at the sacrifice of relatively inexpensive, basic foods that are needed.

The promotion of the use of vitamin concentrates has been overworked in the field of advertising. There is a definite need for

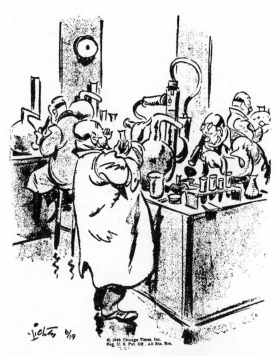

Figure 1–4   "I've worked on vitamins for years and I've discovered that the three most important elements necessary to life are breakfast, lunch and dinner!" (Courtesy of George Lichty and the Chicago Sun-Times Syndicate.)

these products, but they should be taken under the advice of a physician, not because they are recommended on the radio or television. It is the general consensus that the natural foodstuffs rich in the various vitamins are the best source. In other words, plan an adequate daily dietary. The American people have been made exceedingly "diet-conscious." "Diet" usually means a specific hard-to-follow regimen. Clever advertising through the radio, television, the press, drug store windows, and the mails has done much to convince the public that it needs to buy, at high prices, products which actually could be supplied from ordinary foodstuffs at little additional cost. This is especially true regarding the vitamins. (See Fig. 1–4.)

The Food and Drug Administration is especially concerned about the promotion of "food supplements" as cure-alls for conditions which require medical attention. In 1958 the Food and Drug Administration[12] outlined the following four basic "myths" of nutrition used by practically all food-fad promoters:

MYTH NO. 1   Most disease is due to faulty diet. It is implied that it is virtually impossible for the average person to obtain

---

[12] Food Facts vs. Food Fallacies. Washington, D.C., Food and Drug Administration, 1958.

an adequate dietary without use of a food supplement. False claims for prevention or cure of many serious diseases are made in favor of the preparation being promoted.

MYTH NO. 2   Soil depletion causes malnutrition. It is claimed that crops grown on poor soil or where chemical fertilizers are used are nutritionally inferior. The true story is that genetic make-up of the seed, not soil fertility, primarily affects the nutritional composition of a food.[13] The *quantity* may be reduced on poor soil but there will be very little if any effect on the *quality.*

MYTH NO. 3   Foods are overprocessed. The faddists claim that much nutritive value is lost in processed foods such as white flour, milled cereals, canned foods, and even pasteurized milk. This is very much exaggerated.

MYTH NO. 4   Subclinical deficiencies are a constant danger. It is claimed that anyone with a tired feeling, an ache or a pain in any part of the body is using a faulty diet and needs a supplement of some kind. This is an especially appealing argument for the hypochondriac who is looking for just such a "cure." Diseases caused by dietary deficiencies are relatively rare in the United States, and the food supply is unsurpassed in volume, variety and nutritional value. Any normal person will experience occasional worn-out, dragged-down feelings. If such feelings persist, the advice of a competent physician should be sought, not that of a food quack.

Certain food superstitions have been brought down through the ages with no basis of truth. For example, one will hear that "milk products and fish cannot be eaten at the same meal"; that "fish and celery are brain foods"; that "whole wheat bread is low in calories"; that "honey has no calories"; that "tomato juice makes acid"; that "starch and protein cannot be eaten together," and many other "facts" equally as ridiculous.

COMBATING FOOD FADDISM   The most effective means of combating food faddism and misinformation is through nutrition education. A nutritionally informed population will not succumb to false propaganda. The nurse has many opportunities to clarify the information and to present sound facts, as well as to set an example through good food attitudes and food habits, including weight control. The American Medical Association, the American Dietetic Association, and other related groups have extensive programs and available material to combat food fallacies and quackery.

[13] Janssen, W. F.: Food quackery—a law enforcement problem. J. Am. Dietet. A., 36:110, 1960.

THE CARE AND FEEDING OF PATIENTS

While the nurse does not plan menus or prepare foods served to patients in the hospital or in the home, assistance in meeting their nutritional needs is given by her in many ways. The nurse devises ways and means of feeding those who have to be fed and encourages those who need encouragement to consume an adequate amount and kind of food. It is important for the nurse to know whether the patient eats the food served and how much he eats. The nurse consults members of the team concerning the nutritional welfare of the patients and takes the necessary steps to revise the dietary regimen or improve the problems presented. The nurse implements the knowledge of nutrition principles and understandings of the eating practices of people in the nursing care that is given to patients in the hospital or in the home.

A patient's eating habits are influenced largely by his economic status, food idiosyncrasies, nationality or ethnic group, religion and social environment. During his hospitalization, especially if it is prolonged, the nurse has an opportunity to assist the person to improve his customary dietary where indicated. Many patients utilize their hospitalization as a learning experience and are motivated to make changes in their food habits. Often times, individuals on the regular dietary of the hospital offer as much of a challenge for teaching as those on therapeutic regimens. The extent to which they will adjust to or adopt the change in their customary pattern will depend largely on how they perceive the task. An individual may find the choice of food and the regimen unsatisfactory, and if the nurse has not explored with him his usual selections, he will not have benefited by his hospitalization from a nutritional viewpoint.

To change deep-seated food habits is usually a slow process. Extensive changes must be made as gradually as possible, with complete understanding on the part of the patient as to why the change is being made. In certain circumstances, while giving a bath or delivering the food tray, the nurse has an excellent opportunity to teach good food habits. She can discuss or make suggestions to guide the patient toward good habits.

NUTRITION RELATED TO TOTAL NURSING CARE

Nutrition is considered one of the important medical sciences and has an important place in the nursing education program. Research in some phase of nutrition is being carried on in many colleges and universities throughout the world, and the practical application of the science of nutrition plays a vital part in the attainment and maintenance of good health, as well as in the treatment of disease. It is a comparatively new science. Thus, many of the concepts and much of the knowledge gained so far must be considered as subject to modification when still more knowledge is obtained. The nutrition picture is constantly changing. Progress lies in research, investigation, and new knowledge.

The study of nutrition fulfills the twofold purpose of education: (1) it provides knowledge useful in personal living, and (2) it provides knowledge useful for professional practice. It is the responsibility of every student of health to apply personally the principles of nutrition and to pass on to others the knowledge gained in order to keep a far-reaching nutritional improvement program alive. The person with his family or group presents individual needs and they differ with each individual. This uniqueness makes nursing interesting. The type of nutritional assistance needed offers a challenge in good nursing care.

PROBLEMS AND SUGGESTED TOPICS FOR DISCUSSION

1. What do the following terms mean: nutrition, optimum nutrition, dietetics, science of nutrition, nutritional status, health, diet, diet therapy, and applied nutrition? Explain the difference between food and nutrition.
2. How are nutrition and health related?
3. Explain the importance of food habits. How are food habits developed? Analyze your food habits, and decide which ones need to be improved.
4. From the list of references select those pertaining to the history of nutrition and prepare a short report on some historical event in nutrition.
5. Either as a member of a committee, or individually, prepare a report of a food plan of a nationality or culture. If possible, arrange a field trip to visit some community centers or eating places of different nationalities.
6. List at least ten "food fads and fallacies," and state what is wrong with each one.
7. Analyze the community where you live and describe an example in which a community agency has fostered improved nutrition.
8. Explain how nutrition becomes an aspect of total nursing care.

SUGGESTED ADDITIONAL READING REFERENCES

Arrington, L. R.: Foods of the Bible. J. Am. Dietet. A., 35:816, 1959.

Beeuwkes, A. M. Characteristics of the self-styled scientist. J. Am. Dietet. A., 32:627, 1956.

Bell, J. N.: Let 'em eat hay. Today's Health, Sept., 1958.

Bengoa, J. M.: Nutrition activities of the World Health Organization. J. Am. Dietet. A., 55:228, 1969.

Bogert, L. J.: Nutrition and Physical Fitness. 8th ed. Philadelphia, W. B. Saunders Company, 1966, Chapters 1 and 16.

Bruch, H.: The allure of food cults and nutrition quackery. J. Am. Dietet. A., 57:316, 1970.

Cassel, J.: Social and cultural implications of food and food habits. Amer. J. Pub. Health, 47:732, 1957.

Food and Agriculture Organization: Nutrition and Working Efficiency. Pamphlet. Rome, 1962.

Food and Agriculture Organization: World Food Problems. No. 2: Man and Hunger. Pamphlet. Rome, 1957.

Food Facts Talk Back. Chicago, American Dietetic Association, 1957.

Food Facts vs. Food Fallacies. Washington, D.C., Food and Drug Administration, 1958.

Holt, L. E.: Perspective in nutrition – Nutrition in a changing world. Am. J. Clin. Med., 11:543, 1962.

King, C. G.: America's role in world nutrition. Review of Nutrition Research. New York, Borden, Inc., 30: No. 1, 1, 1969.

– – –: Notes on history of nutrition in America. J. Am. Dietet. A.: 56:188, 1970.

Lowenberg, M. E., et al.: Food and Man. New York, John Wiley & Sons, Inc., 1968.

Manual for the Study of Food Habits. Washington, D.C., National Research Council, Bulletin No. 111.

McCollum, E. V.: A History of Nutrition: The Sequence of Ideas in Nutrition Investigations. Boston, Houghton Mifflin Company, 1957.

McHenry, E. W.: Foods Without Fads. Philadelphia, J. B. Lippincott, 1960.

Mead, M.: Food Habits Research: Problems of the 1960's. Washington, D.C., National Academy of Sciences – National Research Council Publication 1225, 1964.

Moore, H. B.: The meaning of food. Am. J. Clin. Nutrition, 5:77, 1957.

National Academy of Science: Role of Nutrition in International Programs. Pamphlet. Washington, D.C., National Research Council, 1961.

Paddock, W., and Paddock, P.: Famine – 1975. America's decision: Who will survive? Boston, Little, Brown and Company, 1967.

Recommended Dietary Allowances. Washington, D.C., National Academy of Sciences, National Research Council, Publ. No. 1694, 1968.

Schaefer, A. E., et al.: Are we well fed? Nutrition Today, 4:2, Spring, 1969.

Sledge, M., and Coston, H. M.: From pots and pans to patients. Nursing Outlook, 4:30, 1956.

Stiebeling, H. K.: Our share in better world nutrition. J. Am. Dietet. A., 45:315, 1964.

Stiebeling, H. K.: Improved use of nutritional knowledge – Progress and problems. J. Am. Dietet. A., 45:321, 1964.

Swaminathan, M.: Nutrition and the world food problem. Review of Nutrition Research, New York, Borden Inc., 28:No. 1, 1, 1967.

Todhunter, E. N.: The evolution of nutrition concepts – perspectives and new horizons. J. Am. Dietet. A., 46:120, 1965.

Todhunter, E. N., and Weigley, E. S.: Essays on History of Nutrition and Dietetics. Chicago, J. Am. Dietet. A., 1967.

Travelbee: Interpersonal Aspects of Nursing. Philadelphia, F. A. Davis Company, 1966.

Chapter 2
TEACHING NUTRITION

Nutrition has rapidly become a complicated highly specialized science, with every indication that it will continue to grow. To interpret the findings of nutrition research into practical everyday working knowledge is indeed a tremendous undertaking and challenge. It might be well to review methods of teaching, since much misinformation about foods and diets prevails. Until sound knowledge is applied, the teaching-learning processes are not fully effective. The needs and interests of the individual or group determine appropriate educational programs. Active participation by the individual or group in a problem solving approach is essential to making the subject interesting and personal. Group projects, such as one for weight control, may be one way to arouse and sustain interest and stimulate action for change in improper eating habits.

TEACHING NUTRITION AROUND THE WORLD

Interpreting nutrition to all peoples of the world calls for high specialization and concentrated effort. As was pointed out in Chapter 1, the combined efforts of FAO, WHO and UNESCO are directed toward setting up stations and nutrition education programs in all parts of the world to foster better diets and, as a result, better health (Fig. 11-1). Scientific knowledge in the field of nutrition is increasing so rapidly it is difficult to keep abreast of it, yet there is a great lag between the discoveries of research and their practical application.

Food is generally plentiful in the United States. The average citizen can buy more calories than he can consume. However, intelligent application of the knowledge of food and nutrition is needed to prevent malnutrition and chronic disorders and to rehabilitate disabilities resulting from poor nutritional status. Educational efforts directed toward developing programs that stimulate desirable food habits and modify poor ones are needed.

Food in every culture and to every individual has a basic meaning. (See Chapter 13, Geographic and Cultural Dietary Variations.) One must understand these meanings in order to plan and execute sound nutritional education approaches. Changes in cultural food patterns take place only when people are involved and convinced that proposed changes will further the attainment of some goal. The World Health Organization has recognized this factor and is sending cultural anthropologists into the field to assist in learning and understanding the role of food in particular societies, the attitude toward food and toward change in food habits. The ways people are motivated to improve or change food habits are many and varied. Any improvement of nutritional status can be attained only through the nutrition education program suitable to the needs of the group or individual.

NUTRITION EDUCATION

All people, regardless of their level of education, income, social or economic status or geographic location, need nutrition education. Man has no instinct nor does he inherit knowledge that will guide him to choose those foods which meet the nutritional needs of the body. Each generation learns what foods to select and why and how foods affect health.

The function of nutrition education is to make it possible for everyone to learn and to use nutrition information through individual responsibility and action. The greatest job in nutrition education is to look at the problems through the eyes of the people who need to learn. Educators are concerned with helping people to understand how to select foods to meet nutrient and energy needs. Individuals who evaluate knowledge and are motivated to apply it will implement the changes necessary to improve their dietary habits. There are many, however, who may not realize their need to change.

Concepts which summarized all the nutrition knowledge that is applicable to food for people for health were developed by a subcommittee of the Interagency Committee on Nutrition Education in 1964 and in simple terms, as represented here, reflect the research findings that constitute our knowledge of nutrition needed for wise food selection.

1. Nutrition is the food you eat and how the body uses it. We eat food to live, to grow, to keep healthy and well and to get energy for work and play.

2. Food is made up of different nutrients needed for growth and health. All nutrients needed by the body are available through food. Many kinds and combinations of food can lead to a well-balanced diet. No food by itself, has all the nutrients needed for full growth and health. Each nutrient has specific uses in the body. Most nutrients do their best work in the body when teamed with other nutrients.

3. All persons throughout their lives, have need of the same nutrients but in varying amounts. The amounts of nutrients needed are influenced by age, sex, size, activity and state of health. Suggestions for the kinds and amounts of food needed are made by scientists.

4. The way food is handled influences the amount of nutrients in food, its safety, appearance and taste. Handling means everything that happens to food while it is being grown, processed, stored and prepared for eating.

One observes that these basic concepts do not imply that nutrition is eating what you don't like because it is good for you; there is a need for a variety of foods; there is an interdependence between the nutrients and the foods that supply them; the best source of the nutrients is food. The useful tool for obtaining the nutrients is the daily food guide (basic food group); the daily allowances (Recommended Dietary Allowances) are the quantitative amounts of nutrient needs of healthy people differing in age, sex, size and activity, and the directions for the selection, care and preparation of foods based on research combine procedures that ensure safety, maximize eating quality and minimize loss of nutritive value.[1]

The effectiveness of nutrition education reflects the degree to which provision is made for the application of basic learning principles. Any change in behavior of people depends upon the emphasis placed on the individual as a member of a family unit. He must be helped to determine or clarify his goals and to become personally involved in attaining them. Fleming[2] lists the following factors that are forces important in the teaching-learning processes.

1. Learning takes place more readily when emphasis is placed on the individual. Each individual is a unique individual with different hereditary, social and home background. The purposes of different individuals differ yet must be recognized. The individual should participate in planning ways of accomplishing his goals.

2. Learning tends to occur as emphasis is placed on the learner's perception of tasks to be accomplished. Each individual has his own perception of the task. The learner's perception of a task often differs from that of the teacher. The leader facilitates learning through creating a readiness for the fulfillment of important tasks. All teachers (or a team representing different subjects or fields) should coordinate their efforts.

3. Learning is facilitated as emphasis is placed on human relation factors. As emphasis is given to feelings, anxieties, concerns, questions, problems of the learner, a setting is being created for growth. Belongingness and security are basic to maximum learning. Permissive leadership fosters learning.

4. Learning is facilitated as the learner is involved in an active way. Learning is an active process. Leadership should help students clarify goals, plan, experience, try out, manipulate, explore. As learners assume responsibility growth is extended.

5. Learning is facilitated as emphasis is placed on the wise use of materials and resources. The use of a variety of appropriate materials contributes to the effectiveness of learning. The teacher is but one resource, there are many "people," "places," and "things" in the local environment which, if carefully used, contribute to the learning operation.

Briefly, when helping people to improve their nutritional habits, it is important to begin with the person's interest and his point of view rather than with the teacher's knowl-

[1]Leverton, R. M.: Development of basic nutrition concepts for use in nutrition education: Proceedings of Nutrition Education Conference. U.S. Department of Agriculture, Pub. No. 1075, February 20–22, 1967.

[2]Fleming, R. S.: Principles of learning. Proceedings of Nutrition Education Conference, U.S. Department of Agriculture, Miscel. Pub. 745, April 1–3, 1957, p. 17.

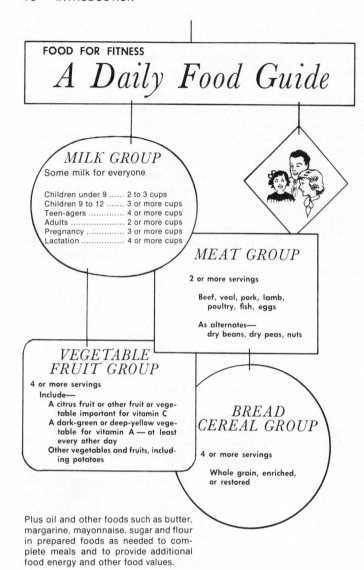

FOOD FOR FITNESS

A Daily Food Guide

MILK GROUP
Some milk for everyone

Children under 9	2 to 3 cups
Children 9 to 12	3 or more cups
Teen-agers	4 or more cups
Adults	2 or more cups
Pregnancy	3 or more cups
Lactation	4 or more cups

MEAT GROUP

2 or more servings

Beef, veal, pork, lamb,
poultry, fish, eggs

As alternates—
dry beans, dry peas, nuts

VEGETABLE FRUIT GROUP

4 or more servings
Include—
A citrus fruit or other fruit or vegetable important for vitamin C
A dark-green or deep-yellow vegetable for vitamin A — at least
every other day
Other vegetables and fruits, including potatoes

BREAD CEREAL GROUP

4 or more servings

Whole grain, enriched,
or restored

Plus oil and other foods such as butter,
margarine, mayonnaise, sugar and flour
in prepared foods as needed to complete meals and to provide additional
food energy and other food values.

Figure 2–1 The "Basic Four Food Groups" Dietary Pattern. Modified from Leaflet No. 424, Institute of Home Economics, U.S. Department of Agriculture, Washington, D.C.

edge of nutrition. Begin with their present dietary practices and modify these only as much as necessary to achieve good nutrition. When the approach is centered on people rather than the diet the teaching is more effective. Food habits are ingrained, and it is not human nature to make sudden changes. Pick up the good points in each individual's diet and build from what he is eating rather than change the entire food pattern.

PATTERN FOR APPLICATION OF DIETARY ALLOWANCES

In nutrition interpretation, one must be able to take the scientific facts which result from research and put these facts into terms that are understood and can be applied to everyday use.

The Bureau of Human Nutrition and Home Economics, United States Department of Agriculture,[3] interpreted the Recommended Daily Dietary Allowances into the "Basic Seven Food Groups." Although this was first published as far back as World War II, it is still sound and an excellent aid in teaching nutrition and evaluating dietary patterns.

In response to many requests for more simple grouping of foods to use in nutrition education programs, the Institute of Home Economics, United States Department of

[3]National Food Guide. Washington, D.C., U.S. Department of Agriculture, Leaflet No. 288, Reviewed March, 1957.

Agriculture,[4] interpreted the Recommended Daily Dietary Allowances (pp. 161–162) into four groups. These four groups of food form the foundation of an adequate diet. The number of servings in each are suggested in Figure 2–1 and Table 11–3. These foods are rich sources of the essential food elements and are called the "protective foods." More of these foods, and additional foods such as butter, margarine, oil, sugar, desserts that supply calories and added nutrients, will be used as needed to round out meals for growth, for activity and for desirable weight. By following such a pattern it is not difficult to plan meals to meet the body needs for nutrients. Meal planning will be discussed in Chapter 11, An Adequate Diet.

The choice of teaching devices depends upon the needs of the group or individual. Some are suitable for one purpose, some for another. Cultural, regional and seasonal differences in food supplies, variations in nutritive needs and economic problems determine the choice to make and procedure to use. Our daily food intakes must meet the body's nutritional needs. These nutrients and their relation to body needs and health are developed in the chapters which follow.

THE DIETARY HISTORY

Any desired dietary change of an individual (or group) begins with the person's customary food intake and food habits. An evaluation of the present habits indicates to the teacher and learner where the necessary changes are needed to improve nutrition. This approach helps the person to identify areas in which changes should be made and gives him an opportunity to make some evaluations of his own.

In a hospital or clinic situation, the nurse has access to personal information about the individual, all of which is related to the food intake and food habits. His name, age, sex, occupation, marital status and ethnic group, economic status, present weight, pertinent laboratory findings, diagnosis (determined or probable) and physicians dietary order are a matter of record.

The interviewer (nurse) asks the patient to recall usual foods eaten on a typical day. A notation is made by the nurse while the person is supplying the information or the person may write it himself. In this way, both the nurse and patient can be looking at and

thinking about his dietary pattern objectively while it is recorded as shown in the following example:

10:00 A.M.:	Coffee
	Doughnut
Noon Meal:	Sandwich
	cheese
	egg
	hamburger
	Coke
Evening Meal:	Meat, fish, chicken
	Potatoes or grits
	Vegetables
	Bread
	Cake
	Jello
Late Evening:	Crackers
	Cookies
	Coke

The nurse accepts this pattern and proceeds to determine the number of cups of coffee, slices of bread as well as what and how much is in and on coffee, bread, potatoes, sandwich; the place and time food is eaten; who prepares the food and the number for whom the food is prepared or the number in the family; the kinds and amounts of meat, vegetables, and desserts eaten; the kinds and amounts of food eaten between meals or for snacks and noting the time of day they are eaten. If the weekend pattern differs from that of the typical day, notation of the differences are made.

The person becomes involved in giving information and is usually interested in knowing how his diet rates. He looks to the nurse for an evaluation. The nurse determines the adequacy of the food pattern, points out the positive practices and designates the areas which are in need of improvement. In the example given above, milk, vegetables and fruit seem to be the foods which the nurse would try to stimulate the person to think about. When given an opportunity the person usually suggests what foods and how much of them he is willing to include on a daily basis. The nurse may need to explore further with the person the way he believes that he could implement the changes in his dietary. Together the nurse and patient formulate the revised dietary pattern.

The above presentation illustrates briefly a practical method which the nurse may use to obtain the dietary pattern of an individual and utilize it to improve nutrition. Some interviewers may prefer to score the person's dietary pattern or have the person do it himself. An example of a score card is shown in Table 2–1. From this exercise the nurse and patient learn where the low scores in the diet occur. Further discussion relating to the kind of meals, time of meals and other pertinent

---

[4] Page, L., and Phipard, E. F.: Essentials of an Adequate Diet. . . . Facts for Nutrition Programs. Washington, D.C., U.S. Department of Agriculture, Home Economics Research Report No. 3, Agricultural Research Service, November, 1957.

TABLE 2–1   FOOD SELECTION SCORE CARD

Score your diet for each day and determine your average score for the week. If your final score is between 85 and 100, your food selection standard has been good. A score of from 75 to 85 indicates a fair standard. A score below 75 indicates a low standard.

MAXIMUM SCORE FOR EACH FOOD GROUP	CREDITS	COLUMNS FOR DAILY CHECK						
20	Milk Group: Milk (including foods prepared with milk as cheese and ice cream) Adults: 1 glass, 10; 1½ glasses, 15; 2 glasses, 20 Children: 1 glass, 5; 1½ glasses, 10; 2 glasses, 15; 4 glasses, 20							
35	Vegetable – Fruit Group: Vegetables: 1 serving, 5; 2 servings, 10; 3 servings, 15 Potatoes may be included as one of the above servings If dark green or deep-yellow vegetable is included, extra credit, 5 Fruits: 1 serving, 5; 2 servings, 10 If citrus fruit or raw vegetables or canned tomatoes are included, extra credit, 5							
15	Bread – Cereal Group: Bread – dark whole grain, enriched or restored Cereals – dark whole grain, enriched or restored 2 servings of either, 10; 4 servings of either, 15							
25	Meat Group: Eggs, Meat, Cheese, Fish, Poultry, Dry Peas, Dry Beans, and Nuts 1 serving of any one of above, 10 1 serving of any two above, 20 If liver (beef, lamb, pork, or calf's) or kidney is used, extra credit, 5							
5	Water (total liquid including coffee, tea, or other beverage): Adults: 6 glasses, 2½; 8 glasses, 5 Children: 4 glasses, 2; 6 glasses, 5							
100	Final Score							

information is needed to help improve the dietary pattern and food habits.

A brief statement of the interviewer's evaluation of the patient's dietary and how the problem was handled or resolved should be recorded in the nurses' notes or patient's chart or referred to the dietitian or nutritionist for further instruction as indicated.

Obviously these methods serve only to determine the individual's present dietary pattern and to show the teacher and learner what the needs are and where to place the emphasis to obtain better nutrition. Detailed forms and specific procedures are available and well documented for use in nutritional surveys of population and research activities where accuracy of the nutrients ingested is required.

TEACHING TECHNIQUES

There is no one way or method to teach nutrition. The method must be adapted to the individual or group needs. Telling, in-forming, going-over-a-list, and showing are not effective ways of learning. The problem-solving approach is effective because it involves the learner. People are interested in what change means to them. The teaching-learning process may occur at the bedside, or, if the patient is ambulatory, the environment of a nutrition clinic or a classroom would offer an atmosphere free of distractions and interruptions (see Fig. 2–2).

Obtaining the dietary pattern requires a personal approach, respect and consideration for the person. Through use of words, action and attitude the person becomes aware of the interviewer's concern about the resolution of his dietary problem. Rapport is achieved when the person has attained confidence in the interviewer. Allowing the person to talk about what food means to him, gives the interviewer some hints on how to begin the dietary evaluation. The person responds with interest to the request. "Tell me what foods you regularly eat." The person proceeds

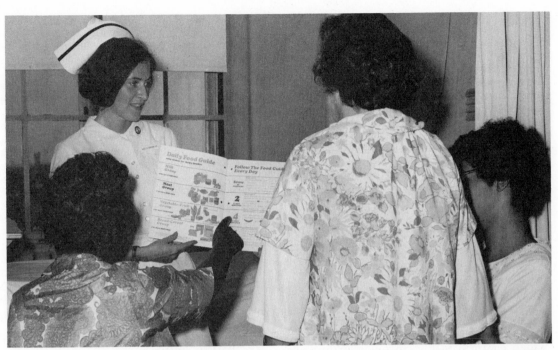

Figure 2–2   Some of the best opportunities for teaching occur during discussions with small groups of patients. Here the nurse is discussing the selection of well-balanced meals. (Courtesy of Graduate Hospital of the University of Pennsylvania. Photo by Paul Axler.)

(sometimes hesitates) to give the necessary information on a personal basis and concern. The interviewer accepts the program conveyed and begins the evaluation when the person is ready. In the sample dietary pattern given (p. 19), the interviewer would briefly review the positive aspects of the person's dietary and follow with "I did not hear you mention milk." Following the person's explanation or rationalization, the question "How could you use milk" would bring further suggestions and give the interviewer some idea of what and how other suggestions could be offered. It opens a discussion about the nutrients in milk that would benefit him. The use of vegetables could be approached in a similar manner. Thus the person would have some part in planning the changes needed to improve his dietary. The person is likely to try it and adopt the dietary he, himself, had a part in revising.

Not all patients change behavior. They can show signs of being aware and interested in a change or changes and may appear to understand the changes recommended but may not necessarily be motivated to change. What motivates a person to adopt the changes is an individual matter. One thing is certain—it is the learner who must go through the process and adopt the change.

"Timing" is exceedingly important. There may be days when no learning can take place, and other days when the patient is eager to learn. Effective points can be put across through conversation rather than lecturing. For example, if the hospitalized patient is not drinking milk, instead of admonishing with the remark, "Milk is good," the nurse can say, "Here is some valuable protein food which your body tissues need for repair to get well." When the patient rejects the food tray because unfamiliar foods are on it, the nurse can say, "The food on this tray was selected expecially to help you get well." Pointing to the various items on the tray she can say, "Here is protein food which your body tissues need for repair. Here are some vitamins, and here are some minerals. This bread provides calories." Sharing facts about nutrition with a patient helps him to feel that he is important, an essential part of his feeling of well-being. At this point perhaps the patient is ready to talk about what he likes to eat, what he considers a good meal. This is an opening to look at the patient's present dietary pattern. It serves as the basis for teaching the normal and therapeutic nutrition. In both instances all essential nutrients and calories for energy are needed by each individual. The therapeutic regimens are modifications of the normal, depending upon the characteristics of the therapy for the disease process.

The person should be given a written copy of the plan discussed, especially if there are many changes in his customary pattern. In the case of a normal diet often the person himself would write the program that he plans to adopt and be given appropriate supplementary visual aids. It is meaningful when the nurse approves the plan and addresses herself to his needs. If the person's dietary management is related to a therapeutic condition he should have a written copy of the plan which he has helped develop along with appropriate supplementary materials. More than one opportunity should be granted a person to discuss such an important topic as the changes required in his dietary pattern. Such an interview should take place before the day of discharge from the hospital.

Follow up interviews to answer questions or to adjust the pattern to meet changing needs are encouraged. Circumstances (economics, social, psychological, seasonal) alter conditions, and adjustments in the dietary pattern are necessary.

Giving a patient a standardized printed diet sheet and expecting him to follow it per se is an unrealistic and unsound practice. The person tends to choose foods from the list which conform to his customary pattern or discard other recommendations for dietary treatment. If such a practice prevails, the patient should be given an opportunity to indicate the pattern he will choose and an evaluation made. It is important that the person and interviewer tailor the plan of therapy to fit the person's needs and life style.

There are times when the nurse may have group discussions with patients especially those served regular (normal) diets. (See Figure 2–2). These individuals are usually neglected diet-wise. Other reference is made such as "He's on a house diet"—meaning he needs no dietary attention. No referral is made to a dietitian or nutritionist (hospital, clinic or home). The nurse is the only one who has any knowledge of this aspect of the patient's treatment. As a part of nursing care the nurse (nurse's aide or assistant) may plan to gather two or three together to talk about what an adequate diet means to the group.

Nurses have many opportunities to give sound nutrition facts and dietary practices while giving bedside care, during the bath and when the trays are served at mealtime. Other opportunities are available in the outpatient clinics, in the home and in the community. The role of the nurse as a member of the team teaching nutrition is a vital one. Nursing includes meeting the nutritional needs of patients. Meeting these needs on an individual basis is vital to the complete care of patients.

NUTRITION CLINIC

The nutrition clinic in outpatient departments of hospitals provides an educational program for people. Physicians refer those patients who need counseling for specific conditions in which the dietary management is an important part of the therapy. Nurses, social workers and dental hygienists also refer people for counseling. A careful dietary history is taken by the nutritionists. The teaching is based on these findings much the

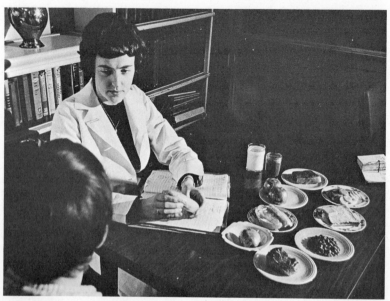

Figure 2–3   Patients needing dietary adjustment and/or help with meal planning, food marketing and selection can be referred to a nutrition clinic for advice. (Courtesy of the Frances Stern Food Clinic at the Boston Dispensary, a unit of the Tufts-New England Medical Center, Boston.)

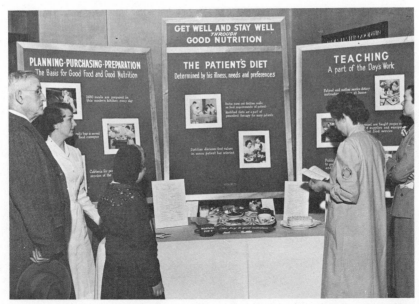

Figure 2-4 Visual aids are employed to put across nutrition facts.

same way as has been explained. The dietary history, the dietary plan of the patient and follow-up notations are recorded in the patient's record, thus sharing and promoting continuity of care. Food models, leaflets, posters and other visual aids are widely used to help people learn about nutrition and how to plan an adequate diet for themselves. In Figure 2-3 the nutritionist is using the food models to help the patient visualize the size of serving of food under discussion. Exhibits of actual foods or models, posters and films are used in the waiting rooms of clinics to stimulate interest in nutrition facts and to provide an opportunity to learn about foods in general (Fig. 2-4). Sometimes cooking classes are conducted in an endeavor to introduce a discussion on food and preparation. The focus of the group could be on weight control, fashion, snacks, or a concern of the group. The nursing student participates in this learning experience by interviewing patients and planning exhibits.

PRENATAL AND POSTPARTUM CLINIC

In the prenatal clinic the teaching of patients centers around the nutritional needs during pregnancy. The diet during pregnancy is a normal diet for the individual mother with additional nutrients during the second half to provide for the nutritional needs of the fetus. Counseling begins with the patient's dietary pattern and focuses on the areas needing improvement. The time spent in "going over" the standardized diet sheets frequently distributed in clinics could be

used more appropriately on the individual's dietary practices to help where changes are necessary.

During the postpartum period opportunities for teaching are many and varied. Weight control, adequate diet and eating habits, breast feeding, and infant feeding are areas to be considered. This is the time to emphasize good nutrition and eating habits for the family beginning with the new baby. It is a time to review the dietary problems manifested during pregnancy and to stress the importance of good nutritional status prior to conception.

WELL BABY CLINIC

The mother in the Well Baby Clinic is concerned with the progress of the child and is ready to learn about the foods the child should have. She is eager to discuss the problems she encounters. These are important clues for the nurse to observe and incorporate in her plan of teaching. The mother is the "gatekeeper" in Kurt Levins "channel theory" of why people eat what they eat. She determines largely what and how food comes to the table and as a mother she is likely to modify and change food habits in the desired direction.

PRESCHOOL NUTRITION PROGRAMS

The Head Start Nutrition and Food Program in Child Development Centers under the auspices of the Office of Economic Opportunity brings children and food together in a good emotional and physical environ-

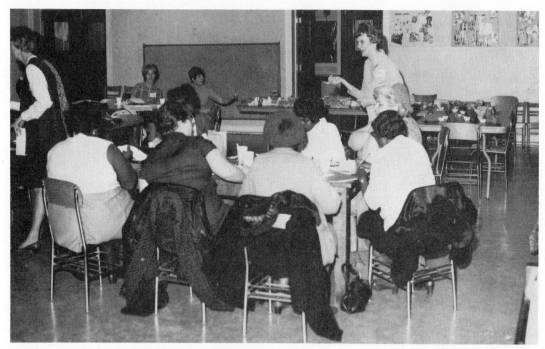

Figure 2-5   Health aides gain interest and skills in nutrition as they set their own goals and learn by doing at a training session coordinated by Maryland State Department of Health nutritionists. (Courtesy of Division of Nutrition.)

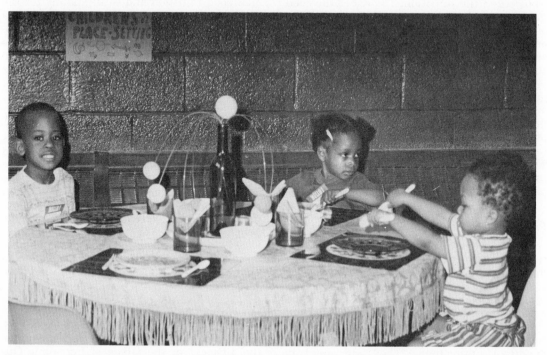

Figure 2-6   Children demonstrate effectiveness of nutrition education activities developed by participants at a nutrition workshop for staff and parents from Head Start centers in Baltimore city. (Courtesy of Division of Nutrition, Maryland State Department of Health, Baltimore, Maryland.)

ment. The emphasis is "to establish sound nutritional practices by providing food to program participants as well as educating families in the selection and preparation of food in the home." Children attending the Center are given food at snack time and at lunch, and in some instances breakfast is served.

Parents participate actively in the program by developing policies and working in the Centers. Opportunities to interview and counsel parents, to feed the children and to train staff and health aides in developing sound attitudes toward nutrition and good food practices are many and varied. The program draws heavily on the professional skills of persons in nutrition, health, education, psychology, social work and recreation. Nonprofessionals play an important role in working with the children and parents. In Figure 2–5 the health aides are shown in a training session where they gain knowledge and skill in nutrition education. Figure 2–6 shows the children demonstrating the effectiveness of nutrition education activities.

SCHOOL LUNCH PROGRAMS

A type of food service is available to public school children in the United States, provided by local school districts or subsidized by the National School Lunch Act. If the child is fed inadequately at home, the school lunch program offers an opportunity to provide at least one sufficiently nutritious meal five days a week and to teach facts about food. The School Nurse has an important role in the nutrition education program of the school system. The nurse is in a position to know where emphasis is needed through findings of physical and dental examinations, discussions on health, office visits of students and contact with parents.

The child may carry a packed lunch from home and supplement it with a hot beverage, hot dish, or soup at school, or the entire meal may be prepared and served as part of the school lunch program. The National School Lunch program encourages schoolchildren to eat more nutritious lunches. It carries out the National School Lunch Act of June 4, 1946, which authorized federal aid to school lunch programs in the form of a state grant-in-aid program, providing for both cash and food assistance. (See Fig. 2–7.) The federal government has subsidized many school lunch programs which provide nourishment for children at an economical cost or at no cost for those who cannot afford to pay. Surplus food commodities have been allotted to the school lunch program of participating schools and technical assistance provided.

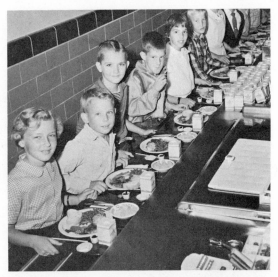

Figure 2–7   Hot, nutritious lunches are made possible with the aid of the National School Lunch Program. (Courtesy of Agricultural Marketing Service, U.S. Department of Agriculture.)

Major responsibility for program operations rests with the state and local governments. Applications for subsidy must come from the school district. Hearings before the Senate Committee on Nutrition and Human Needs has shown that many eligible school districts have not applied for assistance. The standards set by the Department of Agriculture are expressed in terms of the food groups that make up a well-balanced lunch, called the "Type A" Lunch. (See Fig. 2–8).

THE "TYPE "A" LUNCH   Lunches served under the National School Lunch Program, in order to be eligible for reimbursement, must contain as a minimum:[5]

1. One-half pint of fluid whole milk as a beverage.
2. Two ounces (edible portion as served) of lean meat, poultry, or fish; or two ounces of cheese; or one egg; or one-half cup of cooked dry beans or peas; or four tablespoons of peanut butter; or an equivalent quantity of any combination of the above-listed foods. To be counted in meeting this requirement, these foods must be served in a main dish, or in a main dish and one other menu item.
3. A three-fourths cup serving consisting of two or more vegetables or fruits or or both. Full-strength vegetable or fruit juice may be counted to meet not more than one-fourth cup of this requirement. An ascorbic acid-rich food should be

[5] National School Lunch Program. U.S. Department of Agriculture, Bulletin PA-19, Revised June, 1959.

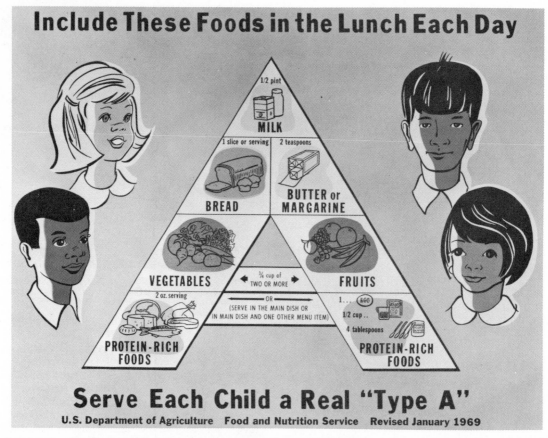

Figure 2–8   The National School Lunch Program's plan for a well-balanced lunch expressed as the "Type A" Lunch. (Courtesy of the U.S. Dept. of Agriculture, Agricultural Marketing Service.)

served daily and a vitamin A-rich food at least twice a week. Several sources of iron should be included each day.

4. One serving whole-grain or enriched bread; or muffins, cornbread, biscuits or roll made of enriched or whole-grain flour.

5. Two teaspoons butter or fortified margarine used as a spread, as a seasoning or in food preparation.

6. Other foods to round out meals and supply energy.

Part of the cost of milk to schools, non-profit child care centers, Head Start programs and summer camps is subsidized under the Special Milk Program, U.S. Department of Agriculture.

If these foods are included in the lunch, in general, one-third of the daily dietary needs for children aged 10 to 12 years or about one-fourth of the total nutritive needs for the week (five days) will be met. Larger portions are served to older children.

The idea of serving lunches to school-children is not new. As early as 1849 France operated some school lunch programs and was one of the first countries to provide school lunches on a national scale. In 1904 the English Parliament authorized the installation of facilities for preparing and serving food as part of the standard school equipment. The first record of an organized school feeding program in the United States was in 1853, when the Children's Aid Society of New York opened a vocational school for poor children and served meals. The program has grown, and today serving food in school has become a generally accepted part of the American school system; yet there are many schools without a food preparation unit in the school system. More work needs to be done to provide opportunity for children to obtain an adequate lunch at school.

Some of the objectives of the school lunch program are provision of (1) nutritious food in sufficient quantities, (2) time to enjoy the lunch, (3) a pleasant eating place and (4) improvement of food habits of the child, indirectly his parents and his family.

The school lunch program offers an opportunity for children to participate in the planning of menus and to learn about the nutrients in food as they relate to good nutrition and healthy bodies. Various aspects of the application of nutrition principles attract interest in many class discussions in social studies, mathematics, biology, English, art, science. Field trips to local plants, markets, and farms utilize community resources. The school lunchroom should be the laboratory in which the principles learned in the classroom are put into action.

The school lunch program is potentially one of society's most useful tools for the promotion of better health and the inculcation of good nutritional habits. The availability of confections and carbonated beverages on school premises may tempt children to spend lunch money for them and lead to poor food habits. The high energy value and constant availability are likely to affect children's appetites for regular meals. Also, the nutritional yield is greatly inferior to that of milk, fruit, and other basic foods. The Council on Foods and Nutrition of the American Medical Association[6] opposes the sale and distribution of these foods in school lunchrooms.

One state educational program has centered on food for better nutrition, food and eating habits, solving of lunchroom problems, suggested activities for the classroom, making and keeping the lunchroom attractive, sanitary standards, a social atmosphere, setting the table, and table manners.

NUTRITION IN THE HEALTH EDUCATION CURRICULUM

A dynamic nutrition education program that begins in early childhood and continues through the elementary and secondary schools can help young children to acquire positive attitudes toward food. Also it can help older children to assume responsibility for their own food selection and prepare them for adult and parental responsibility. As future citizens in a democracy, children must develop acceptable nutritional practices and a sense of social consciousness to enable them to participate intelligently in the adoption of public policy affecting the nutrition of people.

— White House Conference on Food, Nutrition and Health, 1969

TEACHING AIDS

Charts, posters, pictures, pamphlets and slides help a great deal in teaching patients; some excellent ones are available. Practical

and accurate graphic presentation is particularly useful if there are linguistic difficulties. Copies of Figure 2–1 (discussed in Chapter 11, An Adequate Diet) are available from the U.S. Department of Agriculture office at small cost. This can be used on a personal basis as a guide for individuals or groups. Many of the commercial food companies have good posters and colorful material which are adapted from reliable sources. These, of course, should be used with discretion in reference to advertising. At the end of this chapter is a list of sources of health education material on nutrition, available free or at small cost. Wax or paper food models are also good visual aid material to use. If you do not have any, make some![7]

The *size* of a serving may be demonstrated, using either a model or actual food. (See Fig. 2–3.) Also, a demonstration of standard household measures most frequently used, as the cup, tablespoon and teaspoon, will help fix in the patient's mind units of measurement.

PROBLEMS AND SUGGESTED TOPICS FOR DISCUSSION

1. Obtain a dietary history from a patient. Score the diet using Table 2–1.
2. How would you go about teaching a patient receiving a normal diet?
3. Keep a personal record of food consumed during a three-day period. Compare it with the basic food groups.
4. Visit the nutrition clinic and the well baby and prenatal clinics in the hospital and report observations.
5. Prepare some form of teaching aid, either individually or in group work, which will be useful in teaching patients nutrition facts.
6. What is meant by the "Type A" school lunch? Plan a week's menus for packed lunches for a boy aged 11 years to carry from home. How does it compare with the lunch served at school?
7. What are the objections to the sale of confections and carbonated beverages on school premises?
8. List reasons for providing a good school lunch. In what way can a school nurse aid in bringing about the improvement of food habits of schoolchildren?

SOURCES OF NUTRITION AND HEALTH EDUCATION MATERIAL

American Can Company, Home Economics Section, 100 Park Avenue, New York, New York 10017.
American Dietetic Association, 620 North Michigan Avenue, Chicago, Illinois 60611.
American Institute of Baking, 400 East Ontario Street, Chicago, Illinois.
American National Red Cross, Washington, D.C.
Borden's Company, 350 Madison Avenue, New York, New York.
California Fruit Growers Exchange, Educational Department, Los Angeles, California.
Campbell Soup Company, 375 Memorial Avenue, Camden, New Jersey, 08101.

[6] J.A.M.A., *180*:1118, 1962.

[7] Schild, D. T.: Make your own visual aids! J. Am. Dietet. A., *37*:581, 1960.

Cereal Institute, Inc., 135 South LaSalle Street, Chicago, Illinois.

Children's Bureau, Department of Health, Education, and Welfare, Washington, D.C.

Evaporated Milk Association, 228 North LaSalle Street, Chicago, Illinois.

General Foods Corporation, 250 Park Avenue, New York, New York 10017.

General Mills, Inc., Ed. Section, Dept. of Public Services, 400 Second Avenue South, Minneapolis, Minnesota.

Gerber Products, Department of Nutrition, Fremont, Michigan.

H. J. Heinz Company, P. O. Box 5, Pittsburgh, Pennsylvania.

Institute of American Poultry, 110 North Franklin Street, Chicago, Illinois.

Merck and Company, Rahway, New Jersey.

Metropolitan Life Insurance Company, 1 Madison Avenue, New York, New York.

National Dairy Council, 111 North Canal Street, Chicago, Illinois.

National Live Stock and Meat Board, 36 South Wabash Avenue, Chicago, Illinois 60603.

National Research Council, 2101 Constitution Avenue, Washington, D.C.

Pet Milk Company, Home Economics Department, St. Louis, Missouri.

Poultry and Egg National Board, 250 West 57th Street, New York, New York 10019.

U.S. Department of Agriculture, Institute of Home Economics, Washington, D. C.

Wheat Flour Institute, 309 West Jackson Boulevard, Chicago, Illinois.

SUGGESTED ADDITIONAL READING REFERENCES

Aldrich, C. K.: Prescribing a diet is not enough. J. Am. Dietet. A., 33:785, 1957.

Babcock, C.: Attitudes and the use of food. J. Am. Dietet. A., 38:546, 1961.

Beeuwkes, A. M.: Teaching nutrition – Progress and problems. J. Am. Dietet. A., 35:797, 1959.

Bergevin, P.: Telling vs. teaching – Learning by participation. J. Am. Dietet. A., 33:781, 1957.

Burke, B. S.: The dietary history as a tool in research, J. Am. Dietet. A., 23:1041, 1947.

Cassel, J.: Social and cultural implications of food and food habits. Am. J. Pub. Health, 47:732, 1957.

Craig, D. G.: Guiding the change process in people. J. Am. Dietet. A., 58:22, 1971.

Davis, A. J.: The skills of communication. Am. J. Nurs., 63:66, 1963.

Hearings Before the Select Committee on Nutrition and Human Needs of the United States Senate, Part 2, National School Lunch Program, Washington, D.C., March 23, 1970.

Hill, M. M.: A conceptual approach to nutrition education. J. Am. Dietet. A., 49:20, 1966.

Jones, R. J.: Nutrition education in medical practice. Nutr. Rev., 21:193, 1963.

King, C. G.: Research and educational progress in nutrition. J. Am. Dietet. A., 42:199, 1963.

Kintzer, F. C.: Approaches to teaching adults. J. Am. Dietet. A., 50:475, 1967.

Knudson, A. L., and Newton, M. E.: Behavioral factors in nutrition education. J. Am. Dietet. A., 37:222 and 226, 1960.

Lewin, K.: Forces behind food habits and methods of change. Committee on Food Habits. The Problem of Changing Food Habits. National Research Council, 1943.

Mann, G. V.: Nutrition education – U.S.A. Food and Nutrition News National Live Stock and Meat Board, Chicago, 41: November, 1969.

Morgan, A. F.: Dietary records and nutritional status. National Live Stock and Meat Board Food and Nutrition News, 33(No. 9):1, 1962.

Morris, E.: How does a nurse teach nutrition to patients? Am. J. Nursing, 60:67, 1960.

Myers, M. L.: The ambulatory clinic in community and public health nutrition. J. Am. Dietet. A., 59:48, 1971.

Neihoff, A.: Changing food habits, J. Nutr. Educ., No. 1, 1:10, Summer, 1969.

Niemeyer, K. A.: Nutrition education is behavioral change. J. Nutr. Educ., 3:No. 1, Summer, 1971.

Pattison, M., Barbour, H., and Eppright, E.: Teaching Nutrition. Ames, Iowa, Iowa State College Press, 1963.

Proceedings of Nutrition Education Conference, April 1–3, 1957, Washington, D.C. U.S. Department of Agriculture, Miscel. Pub. 745, Nov., 1957.

Proceedings of Nutrition Education Conference, January 29–31, 1962. Washington, D.C., U.S. Department of Agriculture, Miscel. Publ. No. 913.

Proceedings of Nutrition Education Conference, February 20–22, 1967. Washington, D.C., U.S. Department of Agriculture, Miscel. Pub. No. 1075.

Reams, A.: Education of the patient. J. Home Econ., 51:207, 1959.

Review: The effects of a balanced lunch program on the growth and nutritional status of school children. Nutr. Rev., 23:35, 1965.

Roth, A.: The teenage clinic. J. Am. Dietet. A., 36:27, 1960.

Schild, D. T.: Make your own visual aids! J. Am. Dietet. A., 37:581, 1960.

Sipple, H. L.: Problems and progress in nutrition education. J. Am. Dietet. A., 59:19, 1971.

Sliepcevich, E. M., and Creswell, W. H.: A conceptual approach to health education: complications for nutritive education. Am. J. Pub. Health, 58:684, 1968.

Stefferud, A. (ed.): Food: The Yearbook of Agriculture, 1959, U.S. Department of Agriculture, pages 631–701.

Vargas, J. S.: Teaching is changing behavior. J. Am. Dietet. Assoc., 58:512, 1971.

Vaughn, M. E.: An agency nutritionist looks at home health care under Medicare. J. Am. Dietet. A., 51:146, 1967.

Young, C. M.: Teaching the patient means reaching the patient. J. Am. Dietet. A., 33:42, 1957.

Young, C. M.: The interview itself: J. Am. Dietet. A., 35:677, 1959.

Young, C. M.: Interviewing the patient. Am. J. Clin. Nutr., 8:523, 1960.

INTRODUCTION

Foods constitute all the solid and liquid materials taken into the digestive tract that are utilized to maintain and build body tissues, regulate body processes, and supply heat, thereby sustaining life.

Foods are composed of various compounds, both organic and inorganic, so that any food is a chemical compound or mixture of chemical compounds. These compounds and elements of which foods are composed are proteins, lipids, carbohydrates, minerals, vitamins and water, and can be grouped as organic and inorganic compounds and elements.

Organic Compounds. Proteins, lipids, carbohydrates, vitamins.

Inorganic Elements. Water, and minerals: calcium, phosphorus, sodium, potassium, sulfur, chlorine, iron, iodine, copper, magnesium, manganese, cobalt, zinc and others.

The constituents in food are known as nutrients. All the nutrients essential for the normal functioning of the body depend on the wise selection of foods. If food is not properly chosen, there will be an inadequacy of one or more of the essential nutrients. An essential nutrient is one that must be provided as such to the body by food. It cannot be synthesized by the body. The nutrients that must be supplied in food and are essential for growth and normal functioning of the body are as follows:

Proteins as sources of amino acids such as:
    isoleucine
    leucine
    lysine
    methionine
    phenylalanine
    threonine
    tryptophan
    valine

Minerals such as:
    calcium
    phosphorus
    iron
    sodium
    potassium
    iodine
    magnesium
    sulphur
    chlorine
    manganese
    copper
    zinc
    cobalt
    molybdenum

Carbohydrate as source of:
    glucose
Fat as source of:
    linoleic acid

Fat-soluble Vitamins such as:
    A
    D
    E
    K

Water-soluble Vitamins such as:
    thiamin
    riboflavin
    niacin
    pyridoxine

All the food constituents enumerated above and their specific functions in human nutrition will be more fully discussed in later chapters under their respective headings.

METABOLISM

Metabolism comes from a Greek word, "metaballein," meaning to change or alter.

29

Broadly speaking, metabolism may be defined as tissue change. It is the chemical process of transforming foods into complex tissue elements and of transforming complex body substances into simple ones, along with the production of heat and energy. The two main phases of metabolism are (1) *anabolism,* the synthesis of cellular materials for growth, maintenance and repair of body tissues and (2) *catabolism,* the breaking down of cellular materials into simpler constituents for energy production or excretion.

The anabolic processes are the chemical changes whereby simple substances are combined to form more complex substances with the net result that new cellular materials are produced and energy is stored. The catabolic processes are concerned with the breaking down of the complex substances which results in the release of energy and a wearing out and using up of cellular materials. These processes occur constantly and simultaneously in the body. When anabolism exceeds catabolism, growth occurs. If catabolism exceeds anabolism, the breakdown is faster than the building up processes, making the body lose substance and weight. In health, a balance is maintained between these two constantly operating opposing processes so that body weight and tissue substance are maintained, or added to if desired.

The amount of food consumed can have a profound effect on whether anabolism or catabolism will predominate in a given situation. The person who consumes less food than he requires loses weight because the catabolic state predominates. The person who consumes more food than required and gains adipose tissue is in an anabolic state.

Some factors that increase anabolism are increase in the supply of raw materials (food) to the body plant, rest, and certain endocrine secretions such as insulin and some adrenal and sex hormones (for example, at adolescence increased secretions of sex hormones stimulate growth). Some factors that increase catabolism are fever, bacterial toxins, fractures, burns and certain endocrine secretions (for example, thyroxine and cortisone).

Chapter 3
ENERGY

Energy is defined as the capacity to do work or to produce a change in matter. When used in nutrition, energy deals mostly with the chemical energy locked in foodstuffs by reason of the chemical bonding present in the nutrients.

The ultimate source of all energy in living organisms is derived from the kinetic energy of the sun. Plants transform heat and light, through the action of chlorophyll with sunlight (photosynthesis), into energy which is stored as potential chemical bond energy within different foodstuffs, principally as carbohydrates, proteins and fats. (See Chapter 4, Fig. 4–1.) This chemical energy is used by animals which are unable to use the energy of the sun directly.

The comparisons often drawn between a steam engine and the human body, while useful, may be misleading. The steam engine relies upon the combustion of fuel to yield heat to generate steam to perform work required. Although foods undergo combustion in the body and eventually yield heat, that heat is not productive. It is largely a by-product of metabolism generated by the mechanical activity of muscles (mechanical energy). It is useful in that it does maintain body temperature. The chemical energy available from foods is used for muscular work (kinetic energy), for brain and nerve activity (electrical energy) and in synthesis of body tissue (chemical energy). Man's source of energy is released by the metabolism of food and it must be supplied regularly to meet the energy needs for the body's survival.

The foods from which energy is available (carbohydrate, fat and protein) are converted in the body to glucose, fatty acids and amino acids before they reach the cell. Within the cell these nutrients react with oxygen to form carbon dioxide and water. This over-all reaction proceeds through a long series of steps, the rates of reaction controlled by various enzymes. The energy produced is used to form adenosine triphosphate (ATP). ATP is a nucleotide composed of adenine (nitrogen base), ribose (pentose sugar) and three phosphate radicals. The last two phosphate radicals in this compound are attached through an "energy-rich bond." These bonds contain several times the energy of other chemical bonds and are very labile. ATP can release its energy instantly for mechanical work (muscle contraction), transport of material through cell walls and syntheses of chemical compounds. In the reaction ADP (adenosine diphosphate) is formed, which can be phosphorylated to ATP by the oxidative reactions. This process is continuous. ATP has been referred to as the energy currency of the cell for it can be spent and remade again and again.[1] (See Fig. 3–1.)

The rapid chemical changes are brought about by the action of enzymes, coenzymes and hormones. They control biologic oxidation of the cells. Every cell synthesizes the thousands of enzymes required for its metabolic processes. They are proteins of high molecular weight. Those enzymes concerned with metabolism of the cell are usually retained within the cell and are called endoenzymes. Those enzymes which are released by the cell and catalyze reactions in the environment of the cell are called exoenzymes. These are the digestive enzymes, a small group but very important to nutrition. They are liberated by special cells in the salivary glands, liver and pancreas and pass into the digestive tract where they reduce foodstuffs to simpler, readily absorbed compounds.

Enzymes show a great deal of specificity in that each enzyme is so constructed that it will

[1]Guyton, A. C.: Textbook of Medical Physiology. 4th ed. Philadelphia, W. B. Saunders Company, 1971, p. 23.

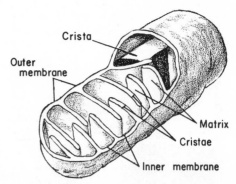

Figure 3–2   Structure of a mitochondrion. (Redrawn from DeRobertis, Nowinski, and Saez: Cell Biology. 5th ed. W. B. Saunders Company, 1970).

catalyze only one particular reaction. The compound being acted on by an enzyme is called the enzyme's "substrate." It is thought that the enzyme and its substrate fit together like lock and key during the catalytic process. The enzyme and substrate must fit together or the reaction will not take place. They first combine in a complex, then break apart, producing the new reaction products and the original enzyme. Evidence suggests that the enzyme attaches to its substrate at two points on the substrate surface. This attachment places a strain upon the substrate molecule, so that it becomes reactive; the enzyme breaks away unchanged and is ready to repeat the process.

Some enzymes (pepsin, for example) consist entirely of protein while others may contain a non-protein portion. The protein part is called the apoenzyme and the non-protein part is called a coenzyme. Coenzymes are usually small, organic molecules (of which the B vitamins are a part) and almost always contain a phosphate group. The reactions involved in cellular oxidation and formation of ATP require a series of enzymes with their coenzymes to effect the combination of hydrogen with oxygen to form water. These with all the other enzymes of the oxidative process are believed to be arranged in an orderly fashion on the inner surface of the mitochondria (Fig. 3–2), thus facilitating rapid procession of the chemical reactions.

Hormones, which are secretions of the endocrine glands, act as chemical messengers in energy production to initiate or control enzyme action. Thyroxine from the thyroid gland controls the body's metabolic rate; production of thyroxine, in turn, is controlled by thyrotropic hormone from the anterior pituitary gland. Steroid hormones regulate the ability of the cell to synthesize enzymes. Insulin secreted by the pancreas gland controls the rate of glucose utilization in the tissues.

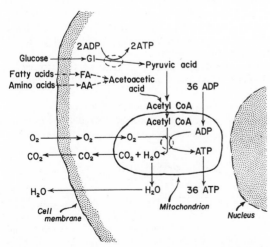

Figure 3–1   Formation of adenosine triphosphate in the cell, showing that most of the ATP is formed in the mitochondria. (From Guyton, A. C.: Textbook of Medical Physiology. 4th Ed. W. B. Saunders Co., 1971.)

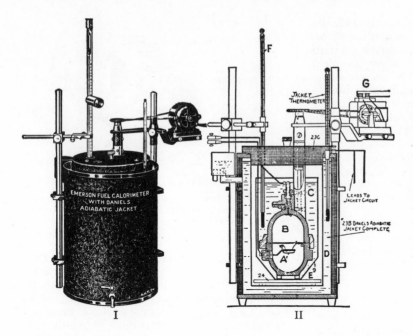

Figure 3–3   Bomb calorimeter as seen from the outside (I) and in longitudinal section (II). The water in the inner chamber (C) changes in temperature when the food in the food pan (A) is burned. The water in the outer chamber (D) acts as insulation, with the intervening air in the air space (E). The amount of heat produced is measured at F by the change in temperature of a measured amount of water. B is an oxygen chamber, and G is an electric motor for stirring the water.

THE CALORIE

The unit of energy commonly used in human nutrition is the *kilogram* calorie (kcalorie). The *calorie* is the standard unit for measure of heat. Since heat is one result of energy generated by the body, the calorie can serve as a measure of energy production. One kcalorie is the heat energy required to raise the temperature of 1 kilogram of water 1 degree Centigrade.

MEASUREMENT

The total caloric content (total energy) available from a food can be measured by means of a device called a bomb calorimeter. (See Fig. 3–3.) This consists of a closed steel container in which the food is burned while the container is immersed in a known volume of water. The weighed food sample is burned in an oxygen atmosphere by igniting it with an electric spark. The rise in temperature of the water after ignition of food can be used to calculate the calories generated. Each food has a specific caloric value; that is, a given amount of food will yield a certain number of calories when metabolized, and the caloric yield depends on the composition of the food in terms of protein, fat and carbohydrate.

The amount of heat produced per gram of purified samples of protein, fat and carbohydrate burned in the bomb calorimeter is as follows:

1 gm. of protein	5.65 kcalories
1 gm. of fat	9.45 kcalories
1 gm. of carbohydrate	4.10 kcalories

In the body some food is not completely digested and absorbed. Since the body is not completely efficient in this process, the extent to which the ingested nutrient is available to the cells is of importance. Normally about 98 per cent of the carbohydrate, 95 per cent of the fat and 92 per cent of the protein is absorbed. However, there is a rather large variation in the digestibility of proteins.

As far as utilization by the cells is concerned the calorie yield of carbohydrate and fat in the body is the same as in the bomb calorimeter because they are completely oxidized to carbon dioxide and water. This is not true of the proteins. The amino group of the amino acids is not oxidized in the body as it is in the bomb but is excreted in the urine, chiefly as urea, with smaller amounts of creatinine, uric acid and other compounds.

The potential energy value of the energy-yielding nutrients in food is summarized in Table 3–1.

The approximate caloric values 4, 9, 4 per gram of protein, fat and carbohydrate respectively can be used for all practical purposes to

TABLE 3–1   POTENTIAL ENERGY VALUE OF NUTRIENTS IN FOOD

	KILOCALORIES PER GRAM		
	Protein	*Fat*	*Carbohydrate*
Bomb calorimeter	5.65	9.45	4.10
Energy lost from combustion lost in urine	1.30	0	0
Net energy value	4.35	9.45	4.10
Approximate energy value	4.00	9.00	4.00

estimate the caloric values of foods in the average American mixed diet.

CALCULATION OF FOOD VALUE   The energy value of one tablespoon of oil (14 grams of fat) is approximately 126 kcalories (14 × 9). Most foods, however, are complex and contain protein, fat and carbohydrate. For example, 2 eggs (100 grams) contain approximately:

13% protein or 13 × 4	=	52 kcalories
12% fat or 12 × 9	=	108 kcalories
1% carbohydrate or 1 × 4 =		4 kcalories
Total		164 kcalories

Research in food values has repeatedly demonstrated that the composition of foods is variable because of factors beyond control, such as climate, soil, variety, degree of maturity, storage, methods of handling and analyzing.

More precise calorie values of foods based on analysis of samples reported by chemists may be found in The Agriculture Handbook, No. 8, 1963 revision, and Bulletin (Home and Garden), No. 72, 1970, published by the United States Department of Agriculture (see Appendix). These tables are useful in calculating the specific nutritive value of each food. The values in Handbook No. 8 are given for 100-gram portions of food and those in Bulletin No. 72 are listed for average servings of foods. From such tables of caloric values of foods (see Appendix, Tables 1, 2, and 3), the approximate caloric value of any diet can be calculated.

THE JOULE

The International Organization for Standardization (ISO) recommended the adoption of the joule (J.) as the preferred unit for energy measurements in all branches of science. The recommendation was adopted by the National Bureau of Standards in the United States in 1964.

The nutritional kilocalorie (thermochemical calorie) is the heat of combusion of benzoic acid. It is expressed in joules per gram mole. In terms of thermochemical calories per mole the joule is divided by 4.184. This is the conversion factor recommended by the Committee on Nomenclature, International Union of Nutritional Sciences. The Committee on Nomenclature of the American Institute of Nutrition in 1970 recommended that replacement of the kilocalorie (kcal.) by the kilojoule (kJ.) be effected as soon as the mechanics of the transition can be established.[2] The conversion factor 4.184 is used in Table

TABLE 3–2   ENERGY ALLOWANCES FOR ADULTS 22 YEARS OF AGE

BODY WEIGHT (in kg.)	WOMEN		MEN	
	kcal.	kJ.	kcal.	kJ.
40	1,550	6,500	——	——
45	1,700	7,100		
50	1,800	7,500	2,200	9,200
55	1,950	8,200	2,350	9,800
60	2,000	8,400	2,500	10,500
65	2,050	8,600	2,650	11,100
70	2,200	9,200	2,800	11,700
75	2,300	9,600	2,950	12,300
80	——	——	3,050	12,800
85	——	——	3,200	13,400
90	——	——	3,350	14,000

From Harper, A. E.: Remarks on the joule. J. Am. Diet. Assoc. 57:417, 1970.

3–2. The final values have been rounded off after conversion to the closest 50 kcal.

The figures of 4 kcal. per gram of carbohydrate and of protein and 9 kcal. per gram of fat are generally accepted for practical use. These values, converted from kilocalories to kilojoules and rounded off, would be 17 kJ. per gram for carbohydrate and for protein and 38 kJ. per gram for fat.[3]

MEASUREMENT OF HEAT PRODUCED BY THE BODY

The amount of heat produced by the body can be measured by direct or indirect methods.

DIRECT CALORIMETRY   In the direct method a human subject is placed in a special calorimeter, and the amount of heat produced is measured. This method is very expensive, and there are few such large calorimeters available.

INDIRECT CALORIMETRY   The indirect method is a much simpler technique whereby the rate of metabolism is measured by determining with a respiration apparatus, the oxygen consumption or carbon dioxide production of the body in a given period of time. These determinations are then converted into calories of heat produced per square meter of body surface per hour and expressed as caloric expenditure. This method is much more widely used and has the added advantage of mobility and low equipment cost.

This method may be applied when the body is lying at rest or engaged in various activities. To determine the caloric expenditure for various activities, the subject would carry the respirator apparatus with him. (See Figure 3–4.)

[2] Ames, S. R.: The joule—unit of energy. J. Am. Dietet. A., 57:415, 1970.

[3] Harper, A. E.: Remarks on the joule. J. Amer. Dietet. A., 57:416, 1970.

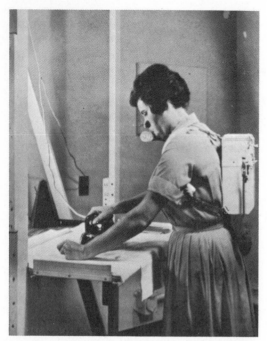

Figure 3–4   Subject standing at a work table ironing and wearing a respirometer, which measures the caloric expenditure. (Courtesy of U.S. Department of Agriculture, Office of Information.)

BASAL METABOLISM

The basal metabolism is the minimum amount of energy needed by the body at rest in the fasting state. It indicates the amount of energy needed to sustain the life processes: respiration, cellular metabolism, circulation, glandular activity and the maintenance of body temperature. It is usually measured by indirect calorimetry, with a tank type respiration apparatus, with the body at complete physical and mental rest, relaxed, but not asleep, at least 12 hours after the last meal and several hours after any strenuous exercise or activity in a comfortable temperature and environment. It is frequently referred to as the basal metabolism test and is used as an aid to diagnosis, particularly in endocrine disorders. The determinations are expressed as a percentage above or below the standard metabolic rate for the body surface of the patient (determined from standard tables based on heights and weights). For example, if a basal metabolism rate (BMR) is reported as "plus 25," it means that, based on his height, weight and body surface, the patient produced heat at a rate 25 per cent above the average rate predicted from the standard tables.

Measurement of protein-bound iodine (PBI), a much simpler test, is used frequently to determine the level of metabolism. The major portion of the PBI is contributed by thyroxine,

so it is a measure of the level of thyroxine produced. Only a small quantity of blood is needed for the test. Normally PBI levels are 4 to 8 micrograms per 100 ml. of blood. This test is used mainly for diagnostic purposes. It must be interpreted with caution, since some radiopaque drugs used in x-ray contain iodine.

FACTORS THAT AFFECT THE BASAL METABOLIC RATE   It is generally accepted that a variation of from 10 to 15 per cent above or below the normal metabolic rate per square meter of body surface at each age for each sex is within normal limits. Factors that influence the basal metabolic rate are outlined below.

Surface Area   The greater the body surface or skin area, the greater will be the amount of heat loss and, in turn, the greater the necessary heat produced by the body. It is surprising to find that a tall thin person has a larger surface area than a short stout individual of the same weight and, consequently, a higher basal metabolism. Muscle tissue requires more oxygen than does adipose tissue.

Sex   Women, in general, have a metabolism about 5 to 10 per cent lower than men even when of the same weight and height. This may be accounted for by a difference in body composition between the male and female. Generally speaking, women have a little more fat and less muscular development than men. The reason for the difference in basal metabolic rate may revolve around the effects of the male and female hormones on metabolism. During pregnancy and lactation, the adult female has an increased metabolism due to increases in muscle development of the uterus, placenta and fetus; respiration rate, cardiac work, activity of the mammary gland, and milk production of the female. During menstruation metabolism increases somewhat.

Age   The metabolic rate is highest during the periods of rapid growth, chiefly during the first and second years, and reaches a lesser peak through the ages of puberty and adolescence in both sexes. The BMR declines slowly with increasing age during the adult life probably due to lower muscle tone from lessened activity. (See Fig. 3–5.)

Body Composition   A large proportion of inactive adipose tissue lowers the basal metabolic rate. Athletes with greater muscular development show about a 5 per cent increase in basal metabolism over nonathletic individuals. The muscular tissues consume relatively large amounts of oxygen per unit of weight.

Endocrine Glands   The secretions of the endocrine glands are the principal regulators

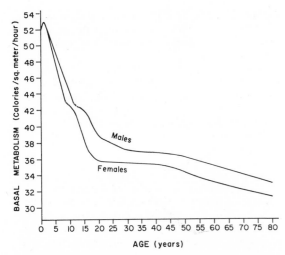

Figure 3–5   Normal basal metabolic rates for each sex at different ages. (From Guyton, A. C.: *Textbook of Medical Physiology.* 4th ed. W. B. Saunders Company, 1971.)

of the metabolic rate. When the supply of thyroxine is inadequate, the basal metabolism may fall to as little as 30 to 50 per cent of the normal rate. If it is hyperactive, the basal metabolic rate may increase to almost twice the normal amount.

The male sex hormones increase the basal metabolic rate about 10 to 15 per cent and the female sex hormones a little less. (See Fig. 3–5.)

The growth hormone can increase the BMR as much as 15 to 20 per cent, resulting from the stimulation of cellular metabolism.

Stimulation of the sympathetic nervous system increases cellular activity by the release of the hormone epinephrine which acts directly to cause glycogenolysis. Other hormones, adrenalin, cortisol and insulin may influence metabolic rate.

State of Nutrition   In marked undernourishment or starvation conditions, an individual will demonstrate a lowered metabolism, often as much as 50 per cent below normal. This decrease in metabolism has been found to be due, almost completely, to the decrease in mass of active tissue.

Sleep   During sleep the metabolic rate falls approximately 10 to 15 per cent below that of waking levels. This drop is due to muscular relaxation and decreased activity of the sympathetic nervous system. This usually amounts to 40 to 80 kcalories less per day, depending upon the number of hours of sleep, the degree of relaxation and the size of the body.

Climate   Differences in metabolic rates have been noted between individuals living in the tropical regions and those living in cold regions. Those living in the tropics exhibit as much as 10 to 20 per cent lower metabolic

rates than those in cold climates. This is largely a result of the increased secretion of thyroxine in cold climates and decreased secretion in hot climates. The incidence of hyperthyroidism tends to be greater in the colder areas than in the tropical areas.[4]

Fever   Infections or fevers increase the BMR about 7 per cent for each degree rise in body temperature above 98.6° F.

TOTAL ENERGY REQUIREMENT

The energy requirement of an individual takes precedence over all other needs. Many individuals throughout the world are not meeting their requirements to supply the total energy needs of their bodies. The minimum calorie needs must be met first and other specific nutrients can be acquired later.

The three factors that determine the total energy requirement of an adult are the basal metabolism, the physical activity and the specific dynamic action of food. In addition to these factors the growth increment during childhood must be considered.

BASAL ENERGY REQUIREMENT   The basal metabolic needs (involuntary activity) provide approximately 50 per cent to 70 per cent of the total daily caloric requirements for many individuals, especially those engaged in sedentary or moderately active activities. The standard allowance for individuals of average build (height and weight) is 1 kcalorie per kilogram of body weight. For a young adult male whose ideal weight is 70 kilograms, the basal requirement would be 1680 kcalories. For a young adult female whose ideal weight is 58 kilograms, the basal requirement would be approximately 1400 kcalories. The ideal or desired weight for height and age is used in determining the energy requirement instead of actual weight because the present weight of an individual may be abnormal—overweight or underweight. (See Table 13 in Appendix for women, and Tables 14 and 15 for children.)

No person could exist for very long if he received only sufficient calories to cover his basal metabolic needs. The ordinary activities of life which require moving about and the various form of muscular activity and the ingestion of food increase the energy needs of the body.

PHYSICAL ACTIVITY   In addition to basal needs, physical activity is the greatest single factor influencing the energy needs of an individual. Often the kind and intensity of the work or exercise is the factor of concern in determining the total energy requirement. The more vigorous the physical work, the

---

[4]Guyton, A. C.: Textbook of Medical Physiology. 4th ed. Philadelphia, W. B. Saunders Company, 1971, p. 828.

greater the calorie cost. A man doing heavy work (i.e., a miner) may need 4800 or more kcalories per day, while an individual of the same body build and age and height living in the same climate but doing sedentary work (i.e., a bank clerk) may require only 2500 kcalories. In general the food intake should meet the energy output except in individuals who need to gain or lose weight. Modern living with its many labor-saving devices and electronic equipment is conducive to more rest and less activity. A discussion of overweight and underweight is given in Chapter 29.

Mental work does not affect appreciably the energy requirement. Fatigue after studying results not from the mental work but from the physical activities or muscle tension that accompany the study habits.

In highly emotional states the physical activity expended in restlessness, muscle tension and aggravated motions of the body expend energy. The metabolic rate is affected mostly by stress. The adrenal glands which secrete more adrenalin in turn increase the rates of most body processes and energy is required.

The state of health may have a marked effect on physical activity. Such physiological and psychological stresses as fatigue, tension and lack of sleep may influence the total caloric requirement.

Other Factors

A very low environmental temperature or a very high environmental temperature may increase slightly the caloric needs. These additional calories are required to cover the work cost of maintaining body temperature at 37.5° C. Nature, however, regulates heat loss very effectively in the various climates by enabling human beings to shiver or sweat as the temperature dictates.

The following list illustrates the calories per hour utilized in various activities:

TABLE 3-3 ENERGY COST OF ACTIVITIES EXCLUSIVE OF BASAL METABOLISM AND INFLUENCE OF FOOD

ACTIVITY	CAL. PER KG. PER HR.	ACTIVITY	CAL. PER KG. PER HR.
Bicycling (century run)	7.6	Organ playing (30% to 40% of energy hand work)	1.5
Bicycling (moderate speed)	2.5	Painting furniture	1.5
Bookbinding	0.8	Paring potatoes	0.6
Boxing	11.4	Playing ping pong	4.4
Carpentry (heavy)	2.3	Piano playing (Mendelssohn's Songs)	0.8
Cello playing	1.3		
Crocheting	0.4	Piano playing (Beethoven's *Appasionata*)	1.4
Dancing, foxtrot	3.8		
Dancing, waltz	3.0	Piano playing (Liszt's *Tarantella*)	2.0
Dishwashing	1.0	Reading aloud	0.4
Dressing and undressing	0.7	Rowing in race	16.0
Driving automobile	0.9	Running	7.0
Eating	0.4	Sawing wood	5.7
Fencing	7.3	Sewing, hand	0.4
Horseback riding, walk	1.4	Sewing, foot-driven machine	0.6
Horseback riding, trot	4.3	Sewing, motor-driven machine	0.4
Horseback riding, gallop	6.7	Shoemaking	1.0
Ironing (5 lb. iron)	1.0	Singing in loud voice	0.8
Knitting sweater	0.7	Sitting quietly	0.4
Laundry, light	1.3	Skating	3.5
Lying still, awake	0.1		

(From Taylor, C. M. and McLeod, G.: Roses' Laboratory Handbook of Dietetics. 5th ed. New York, The Macmillan Company, 1949, p. 18.)

TABLE 3–4   ADJUSTMENT OF KCALORIC ALLOWANCES FOR ADULT INDIVIDUALS OF VARIOUS BODY WEIGHTS AND AGES

IDEAL BODY WEIGHT			KCALORIC ALLOWANCE		
	kg.	lb.	22 years	45 years	65 years
MEN	50	110	2,200	2,000	1,850
	55	121	2,350	2,100	1,950
	60	132	2,500	2,300	2,100
	65	143	2,650	2,400	2,200
	70*	154	2,800	2,600	2,400
	75	165	2,950	2,700	2,500
	80	176	3,050	2,800	2,600
	85	187	3,200	2,950	2,700
	90	198	3,350	3,100	2,800
	95	209	3,500	3,200	2,900
	100	220	3,700	3,400	3,100
WOMEN	40	88	1,550	1,450	1,300
	45	99	1,700	1,550	1,450
	50	110	1,800	1,650	1,500
	55	121	1,950	1,800	1,650
	58*	128	2,000	1,850	1,700
	60	132	2,050	1,900	1,700
	65	143	2,200	2,000	1,850
	70	154	2,300	2,100	1,950

*Reference man and woman. Adapted from National Research Council, Recommended Dietary Allowances. 7th ed. Washington, D.C., Pub. No. 1694, 1968, p. 5.

Individual energy expenditure varies considerably in performing a given piece of work or activity. Most people have characteristic habits of motion or twitches. One person will sit quietly relaxed while another will unconsciously be making many habitual motions. The same is true in performing a task. One person will be very efficient and make few motions while another individual will expend much more energy making many unnecessary motions. If these two individuals are eating the same number of calories, the efficient one is more apt to store calories not used or needed. Each individual has a characteristic capacity to utilize and store calories, as well as all chemical elements from ingested foodstuffs.

With increased age and decreased activity people need to adjust their eating habits and caloric intake to maintain the desired weight. It has been proposed by The Food and Nutrition Board National Research Council (see Table 3–4) that kcalorie allowances be reduced by 5 per cent between ages 22 and 35, by 3 per cent per decade between ages 35 and 55 and by 5 per cent per decade from 55 to 75. After 75 years of age 7 per cent decrement is recommended.

SPECIFIC DYNAMIC ACTION OF FOOD All foods give a stimulus to metabolism but not all foods have the same effect on metabolism. Carbohydrate or fat increases the heat production by about 5 per cent of the total calories consumed. If the food intake is composed solely of protein, the increase may be as much as 30 per cent. In a maintenance diet, about 6 per cent of the total food calories should be added and 6 to 8 per cent for a liberal mixed diet. If the food intake is very high in protein, about 15 per cent should be added.[5] Approximately 10 per cent is the usual estimated rise in metabolism after meals for a person on an average mixed diet.

GROWTH In the growing child, energy must be provided over and above that required for the basal metabolic rate and for physical activity. This additional energy is required to cover the cost of increasing body weight and height. Growing infants may store as much as 12 to 15 per cent of the energy value of their food intake in the form of new tissue. As a child becomes older, the rate of growth diminishes and the caloric requirement for growth is reduced. (See Table 11–1.) There are wide variations in the physical activity of children. The kcaloric allowances in the Table are proposed as average and approximate amounts for feeding groups. The needs of an individual child are governed by his growth and eating patterns. (See Chapters 16 and 17.)

Additional calories are required to meet the energy costs of pregnancy and lactation. (See Chapter 15.)

ESTIMATION OF DAILY ENERGY REQUIREMENT OF AN ADULT The total daily energy requirement is commonly estimated by adding together the requirement for basal metabolism, physical or muscular activity and the specific dynamic action (SDA) of food.

The method used depends on the degree of accuracy desired. For research purposes the individual has a basal metabolism test to determine the basal needs. The energy cost of the daily activities is determined by the respirometer which the individual carries around with him (Fig. 3–4). The results of all activities added together would give the total energy requirement. Another method involves estimating the basal metabolism requirements from surface area measurements and the activity needs from accurate records of all energy (kcalories) expended in activities during the waking hours plus the additional factor of the effect of food in metabolism (SDA). See Table 3–3 to determine the approximate energy cost of activities during the day.

A less precise procedure but accurate enough for many purposes is as follows:

1. Determine the ideal or desired weight in kilograms of the individual.

[5]Cantarow, A., and Trumper, M.: Clinical Biochemistry. 6th ed. Philadelphia, W. B. Saunders Company, 1962, p. 365.

2. Determine basal needs:

   male = 1.0 kcalorie/kilo of ideal body wt./hour × 24

   female = 0.9 kcalorie/kilo of ideal body wt./hour × 24

3. Subtract 0.1 kcalorie/kilo of ideal body wt./hours of sleep.
4. Add activity increment.
5. Add specific dynamic action (10 per cent of basal needs plus activity increment).
6. Sum equals the approximate daily calorie requirement.

A short method[6] for estimating the activity increment utilizes the following estimations.

Activity	Kcal./day	
	Men	Women
Sedentary or light	225	225
Moderate work	750	500
Heavy work	1500	1000
Very heavy work	2500	——

Activities may be classified as sedentary or light, moderate, heavy and very heavy work. The sedentary person expends very few work calories daily. He may spend most of his time sitting, reading and talking. The person who engages in light physical activity sits, walks and stands. The person who exercises moderately may stand, walk, do housework, gardening or carpentry and spends little time sitting. The person with strenuous or heavy work is constantly active. His least strenuous exercise is standing and walking. He may participate actively in outdoor games, skating, swimming, tennis, and so on for significant lengths of time and engage in work activities involving considerable expenditure of energy (i.e., a lumberman).

RECOMMENDED CALORIE ALLOWANCES

The calorie recommendations for adults, revised in 1968 by the Food and Nutrition Board, National Academy of Sciences–National Research Council, are based on the degree of activity of a reference man and woman, both aged 22, living in a temperate climate and weighing 70 and 58 kilograms, respectively. (Weight gained after this age is likely to be adipose tissue.) The physical activity of these individuals is considered to be "light" with occupations that could be described neither as sedentary nor as hard as heavy physical labor. The man could be employed as a delivery man, a painter or a labor-atory worker. The woman could be an active homemaker or a saleswoman in a shop. Thus the daily kcaloric allowances for the reference man and woman are 2800 and 2000 respectively. These are lower calorie allowances than were recommended in the previous standards (1958 and 1963), based on changes in the American way of life, new research information and concern for the large segment of the population which is now overweight. As previously stated the report recommends a decrease in calories needed for each decade after the age of 22.

It is understood that calorie allowances must be adjusted to meet the specific needs of an individual and to maintain body weight at the desired level.

The daily allowances for infants and children, different age groups, and for pregnancy and lactation are listed in the table of Recommended Dietary Allowances (Chap. 11). In order to better understand the use of the material, it is strongly advised that every student read and become familiar with the scientific basis for the allowances as revised in 1968.[7]

The calorie allowance for pregnancy, lactation, infants, and children will be discussed in Chapter 16, Nutrition in Pregnancy and Lactation; Chapter 17, Nutrition in Infancy; and Chapter 18, Nutrition in Childhood and Adolescence.

CHOICE OF FOODS TO PROVIDE ENERGY

After the number of calories needed for daily activity is determined, the raw materials to provide the calories are supplied in the form of food in various proportions of proteins, fats, and carbohydrates, and the auxiliary materials, water, vitamins, and minerals needed under various circumstances of daily life or disease. A great variety of common foods are available for supplying the necessary minerals and vitamins in addition to furnishing fuel. In this country there is an abundance of food and food products for the majority of the population, and the problem is one of wise selection based on nutrition education, rather than availability, whereas in many parts of the world there are extreme calorie shortages.

Overweight in this country from the standpoint of overconsumption of calories is of growing concern to all individuals interested in the health of the people. The weight problem in a great majority of people is largely due to imbalances between food calorie in-

---

[6]Burton, B. (ed.): Heinz Handbook of Nutrition. 2nd ed. New York, McGraw-Hill Book Company, Inc., 1965.

[7]Recommended Dietary Allowances. Washington, D.C., National Academy of Sciences–National Research Council, Publication 1694, 1968.

take and calorie expenditure, both of which are subject to the individual's control. Studies of energy metabolism in humans make it apparent that of the many individuals whose weight is substantially different from the desired weight for their builds, it is rare that these abnormalities can be attributed to major endocrine disorders or differences in digestion or metabolic efficiencies. Overweight and underweight are discussed in Chapter 29.

People's ideas about the caloric value of specific foods are often incorrect. For example, there are approximately 60 kcalories in an average slice of bread—slightly *less* than in a medium apple. A cup of whole milk contains about 170 kcalories, and one small scoop (1/8 qt.) of orange water ice contains approximately the same.

A common rule in building a suitable diet is to include first the necessary protective foods, then complete the calorie allowance by adding any foods desired. This procedure will be discussed in detail in Chapter 11, An Adequate Diet, and Chapter 19, Therapeutic Diets. (See Fig. 2–1, The Basic Four Food Groups, p. 18.)

PROBLEMS AND SUGGESTED TOPICS FOR DISCUSSION

1. What does "calorie" in nutrition mean? How is it used?
2. (a) Consult food composition tables for the calorie values of food and list those which have 500 kcalories per serving, 200 kcalories per serving, 100 kcalories per serving, and 50 kcalories per serving. (b) On the basis of the protein, fat and carbohydrate value, determine the energy value (kcalories) of:
    23 gm. whole wheat bread
    244 gm. whole milk
    190 gm. grapefruit sections
    150 gm. raw tomato
3. What is meant by basal metabolism, energy metabolism and total metabolism?
4. List the foods you have consumed during one 24-hour period and compute the total calorie value. Compare with the calorie allowance recommended by the Food and Nutrition Board of the National Research Council.

SUGGESTED ADDITIONAL READING REFERENCES

Bogert, L. J.: Nutrition and Physical Fitness. 8th ed. Philadelphia, W. B. Saunders Company, 1966, Chapters 3 and 4.

Burton, B. R. (ed.): The Heinz Handbook of Nutrition. 2nd ed. New York, McGraw-Hill Book Co., Inc., 1965, Chapter 6, Calorie requirements.

Calorie Requirements. Washington, D.C., FAO of the United Nations. FAO Nutrition Studies, No. 15, Rome, 1956.

Food: The Yearbook of Agriculture, 1959. United States Department of Agriculture, pp. 39–56.

Guyton, A. C.: Textbook of Medical Physiology. 4th ed. Philadelphia, W. B. Saunders Company, 1971.

Keys, A.: Energy requirements of adults. J.A.M.A., *142*:33, 1950.

Konishi, F.: Food energy equivalents of various activities. J. Am. Dietet. A., *46*:186, 1965.

Leichsenring, J. M., and Wilson, E. D.: Food composition table for short method of dietary analysis (3rd revision). J. Am. Dietet. A., November, 1965.

McMasters, V.: History of food composition tables of the world. J. Am. Dietet. A., *43*:442, 1963.

Moore, T.: The calories versus the joule. J. Am. Dietet. A., *59*:327, 1971.

Nutritive Value of Foods. United States Department of Agriculture, Home and Garden Bulletin No. 72, 1970.

Olson, R. E.: The two-carbon chain in metabolism. J.A.M.A., *183*:471, 1963.

Review: Variability in metabolic rate. Nutr. Rev., 25:12, 1967.

Symposium on energy balance. Am. J. Clin. Nutr., 8:527, 1960.

The Nutrition Foundation, Inc.: Present Knowledge in Nutrition. 3rd ed. 1967. Chapter 2. Present knowledge of calories.

Watt, B. K., and Merrill, A. L.: Composition of Food: Raw, Processed and Prepared. U.S. Department of Agriculture, Agriculture Handbook Number 8, revised, 1963.

Wohl, M. G., and Goodhart, R. S. (ed.): Modern Nutrition in Health and Disease. 4th ed. Philadelphia, Lea & Febiger, 1968, Chapter 1, Body Weight, Body Composition and Calorie Status; Chapter 3, The Hormonal Control of Metabolism.

Wu Leung, W. T.: Problems in compiling food composition data. J. Am. Dietet. A., *40*:19, 1962.

Chapter 4
CARBOHYDRATES

CARBOHYDRATES AROUND THE WORLD

Carbohydrates furnish most of the energy which is needed to move, perform work, and live; they are the starches and sugars. In the form of grains they furnish the major source of food for the people of the world. However, the consumption of carbohydrates throughout the world is highly variable. In America about 50 to 60 per cent of the diet is composed of them, and an even higher proportion is used in other countries. In the Orient, for example, where rice is a dietary staple, a higher proportion of calories is provided by carbohydrates. In the tropics carbohydrates may furnish as much as 90 per cent of the energy. See Chapter 13, Geographic and Cultural Dietary Variations, for grains used in the various countries. They are the cheapest, most easily obtainable, and most readily digested form of fuel. Since many of the foods which are high in carbohydrate content, such as bread, cereals, potatoes and other root vegetables are relatively inexpensive, the proportion of carbohydrates in the diet is greater at the lower economic levels. The chief sources of carbohydrates are grains, vegetables, fruits, syrups and sugars. That grains supply only carbohydrates is a popular misconception. Grains also supply a major portion of the protein for much of the world's population.

DEFINITION AND COMPOSITION

Carbohydrates are an important group of organic compounds that are composed of the three elements of carbon, hydrogen and oxygen. In their simplest form the general formula is $C_nH_{2n}O_n$. The hydrogen and oxygen are present in the same proportion as in water, H_2O, and there is one molecule of water for each carbon. This gives the term carbohydrate but this simple relationship gives no indication of their structure. More accurately the carbohydrates are defined as polyhydroxy aldehydes and ketones. They vary from simple sugars containing from three to seven carbon atoms to very complex polymers. Only the hexoses (6-carbon sugars) and pentoses (5-carbon sugars) and polymers built up from them play important roles in nutrition.

PHOTOSYNTHESIS   Plants store carbohydrates as their chief source of energy. Water, minerals and nitrogen in the soil are taken by the plant roots, trunk and branches to the leaves. The leaves absorb carbon dioxide (CO_2) from the air. The energy of sunlight acting on water (H_2O) and carbon dioxide in the presence of chlorophyll (the

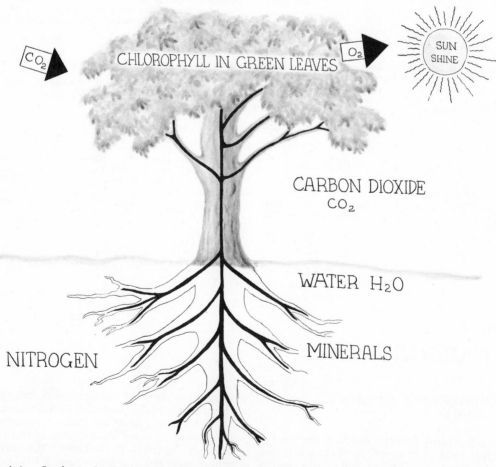

Figure 4–1   Synthesis of carbohydrates in plant life. Light from the sun is harnessed by the green chlorophyll of plant leaves. Cells in green leaves utilize this energy in synthesizing carbohydrates from the carbon dioxide in the air and the water in the soil. Carbohydrates are the chief form in which plants store potential energy.

green coloring matter of leaves) enables the leaves to make sugar and release oxygen (O_2).

$$CO_2 + H_2O \xrightarrow[\text{plant enzymes}]{\underset{\text{chlorophyll}}{\text{sunlight}}} \text{Carbohydrate (CH}_2\text{O)} + O_2$$

This process is photosynthesis (Fig. 4–1). It involves the hydration of carbon dioxide to yield carbohydrate, and is nature's first step in the manufacture of all foods. The carbohydrate made in the leaves will be used in the growth of the plant (or tree) and be stored in its leaves, stems, roots, seeds, pods and fruits. Thus, it can be said that the sun furnishes the energy for all living matter. To recover the locked-in energy of sunlight, the carbohydrate in plants is burned in the body and yields carbon dioxide and water. Not all the potential energy in sunlight is captured by photosynthesis.

CLASSIFICATION

Carbohydrates are classified as monosaccharides, disaccharides, oligosaccharides and polysaccharides. Monosaccharides (the simple sugars) cannot be hydrolyzed to a simpler form. Disaccharides may be hydrolyzed to give 2 molecules of the same or different monosaccharides. Oligosaccharides yield 3 to 10 monosaccharide units and polysaccharides more than 10 units—up to 10,000 or more.

MONOSACCHARIDES The principal monosaccharides which occur free in foods are glucose, an aldohexose, and fructose, a ketohexose. They may exist in either an open-chain or a ring structure, as shown below. When they are linked together as di- or polysaccharides they are held in the cyclic form. Galactose and mannose, two other aldohexoses which occur in bound form in food, have the same structure as glucose except for the orientation of the hydroxyl groups around the carbon atoms.

Glucose (dextrose, grape sugar) is abundant in fruits, sweet corn, corn syrup, certain roots and honey. Glucose is the principal product formed by hydrolysis of more complex carbohydrates in the process of digestion. It is the form of sugar normally found in the blood stream. Glucose is oxidized in the cells to give energy and is stored in the liver and muscles as *glycogen*, a complex carbohydrate known as "animal starch." The central nervous system can utilize only glucose as a major source of fuel. Glucose is only about three-fifths as sweet as cane sugar. It is the best form of sugar to use when an immediate supply of sugar is needed, for it requires no changes in order to be utilized. It is relatively

Glucose   *Fructose*   *Glucose* / *Fructose*

TABLE 4–1   COMPARATIVE SWEETNESS
OF THE COMMON SUGARS AS
COMPARED TO SUCROSE (TABLE SUGAR)

Sucrose	100
Fructose	110–175
Glucose	75
Galactose	35–70
Lactose	15–30

inexpensive and may be added to liquid foods to increase carbohydrate intake without seriously affecting the flavor of the food since it has only a limited sweetness.

Sorbitol and mannitol, hexahydric alcohols derived from glucose and mannose respectively have a sweetening power similar to glucose (Table 4–1). Sorbitol is absorbed slowly and it serves to keep blood sugar levels high following a meal. It has been used in weight reduction as an aid to delay the onset of hunger sensations. It has the same calorie value as glucose and is found in many fruits and vegetables.

Mannitol is poorly digested and yields about one-half the calories per gram as glucose. It has been added to some foods for use as a drying agent. Pineapples, olives, asparagus, sweet potatoes and carrots contain some mannitol.

Fructose (levulose, fruit sugar) is found together with glucose and sucrose in honey and fruit. It is the sweetest of the sugars.

Galactose is not found free in nature but is produced from lactose (milk sugar) by hydrolysis in the digestive process. It is found in combination in nerve tissue.

Mannose is not found free in foods but is derived from mannosans which are found in manna and some legumes. (See Table 4–2.)

Several pentoses (5 carbon sugars) occur in bound form in food. Ribose and deoxyribose are derived from the nucleic acids of meat. They are essential components of nucleic acids and some coenzymes but are not essential nutrients since they can be synthesized in the body. Arabinose and xylose are constituents of the pentosans in fruits.

DISACCHARIDES   Disaccharides or double sugars are exemplified by sucrose (cane or beet sugar), maltose (malt sugar) and lactose (milk sugar). Each of the three double sugars is made up of two hexose molecules:

Sucrose = glucose and fructose
Maltose = glucose and glucose
Lactose = glucose and galactose

They are hydrolyzed by digestive enzymes to the constituent monosaccharides before absorption into the body.

Sucrose is ordinary table sugar. It is found mainly in sugar cane, sugar beets, molasses, maple syrup and maple sugar. When sucrose is hydrolyzed a 50:50 mixture of glucose and fructose forms. This mixture is called invert sugar. Sucrose is a very inexpensive and common form of sugar in the diet. Purified it is a white crystalline, quite soluble, sweet material.

Maltose or malt sugar does not occur free in nature. It is a so-called "derived" sugar, since it is a product of the digestion of starch by diastase, a plant enzyme obtained from sprouting grain. (This occurs in the manufacture of beer.) Maltose is formed during digestion by the action of enzymes called anylases. The reaction begins with salivary amylase; other amylases are present in the intestine. Another enzyme *maltase* in the intestine hydrolyzes maltose to two molecules of glucose in which form it is absorbed. Maltose is not readily fermented by bacteria in the colon. Because fermentation frequently leads to diarrhea, this property makes maltose useful in combination with dextrin in infant formulas.

Lactose is the principal sugar found in milk; 4 to 6 per cent in cow's milk and 5 to 8 per cent in human milk. It is not found in plants and is limited almost exclusively to the mammary glands of lactating animals. It is less soluble than the other common disaccharides and is only about one-sixth as sweet as sucrose. It yields glucose and galactose upon hydrolysis. It is digested more slowly than the other disaccharides. Some individuals have a deficiency of the enzyme *lactase* which hydrolyzes lactose. Under such circumstances, some of this sugar passes into the the large intestine where it is fermented by intestinal bacteria and may have a laxative action. An excess amount may cause diarrhea. Because it is less sweet than sucrose, it is often used to increase the calorie content of a liquid feeding without making it taste too sweet. However, it is difficult to dissolve and therefore not very practical. In the process of making cheese, some of the lactose in milk is converted to lactic and other acids which contribute to the flavor. Lactose is obtained commercially as a by-product of the manufacture of cheese and may be made from skim milk powder.

POLYSACCHARIDES   The chief polysaccharides of interest in nutrition—starch, dextrin, cellulose, glycogen—are built up completely of glucose units. Other important plant and animal structures contain other monosaccharides. In some cases several different monosaccharides are combined in the polysaccharide molecule. As a group, polysaccharides are far less soluble and more stable than the monosaccharides. Starch and glycogen are completely digestible; other polysaccharides are partially or completely indigestible.

Starch occurs in two forms, namely, amy-

TABLE 4–2   TYPES, SOURCES AND END PRODUCTS OF THE CARBOHYDRATES

CARBOHYDRATES	APPROXIMATE PERCENTAGE OF TOTAL CARBOHYDRATE INTAKE*	CHIEF FOOD SOURCES	END-PRODUCTS OF DIGESTION	REMARKS
Polysaccharides:				
a) Indigestible..........	3			
1. Celluloses and hemicelluloses		Stalks and leaves of vegetables; outer covering of seeds	0	May be partially split to glucose by bacterial action in large bowel
2. Pectins..........	2	Fruits	0	Chemical hydrolysis yields galactose and arabinose
b) Partially digestible..........				
1. Inulin..........		Jerusalem artichokes, onions, garlic	Fructose	
2. Galactogens..........		Snails	Galactose	Digestion incomplete; further splitting by bacteria may occur in large bowel
3. Mannosans..........		Legumes	Mannose	
4. Raffinose..........		Sugar beets	Glucose, fructose, and galactose	
5. Pentosans..........		Fruits and gums	Pentoses	
c) Digestible:				
1. Starch and dextrins..........	50	Grains; vegetables (especially tubers and legumes)	Glucose	The most important group quantitatively. Usually accompanied by some maltose
2. Glycogen..........	Negligible	Meat products and sea food	Glucose	
Disaccharides:				
1. Sucrose..........	25	Cane and beet sugars; molasses; maple syrup	Glucose and fructose	
2. Lactose..........	10	Milk and milk products	Glucose and galactose	
3. Maltose..........	Negligible	Malt products	Glucose	
Monosaccharides:				
a) Hexoses:				
1. Glucose..........	5	Fruits; honey; corn syrup	Glucose	In fruits and vegetables the contents of glucose and fructose depend on species, ripeness, and state of preservation
2. Fructose..........	5	Fruits; honey	Fructose	
3. Galactose..........	0	0	Galactose	These monosaccharides do not occur in free form in foods; see under lactose and mannosans
4. Mannose..........	0	0	Mannose	
b) Pentoses:				
1. Ribose..........	0	0	Ribose	These monosaccharides do not occur in free form in foods.
2. Xylose..........	0	0	Xylose	They are derived from pentosans of fruits and from the nucleic acids of meat products and sea food
3. Arabinose..........	0	0	Arabinose	
Carbohydrate derivatives:				
1. Ethyl alcohol..........	Variable	Fermented liquors	Absorbed as such	These substances are the products of natural or induced carbohydrate breakdown
2. Lactic acid..........	Negligible	Milk and milk products		
3. Malic acid..........	Negligible	Fruits		
4. Citric acid..........	Negligible	Fruits		

*Calculated from the average dietary of the middle-income group in the United States.

(From Duncan, G. G. (ed.): Diseases of Metabolism. 5th ed. Philadelphia, W. B. Saunders Company, 1964, p. 106.)

lose (long straight-chain glucose units) and amylopectin (branched arrangement of glucose units). It is found in grains, roots, vegetables and legumes. Starches are encased within the plant cells by cellulose walls in the form of granules of varying sizes and shapes and are typical for each starch. The composition of each starch differs, but all contain both amylose and amylopectin. Starches are insoluble in cold water and must be cooked. Cooking causes the granules to swell and the mixture to thicken or gel. Amylopectin in the starch granules participates in this process. Cooking softens and ruptures the cell to make the starch available for the enzymatic digestive processes in the intestine.

Dextrins are the intermediate products in the hydrolysis of starch to maltose and finally to glucose. This is accomplished by the action of dry heat (toasting of bread) or by enzymes during digestion. Dextrin is more soluble and sweeter than the original starch.

Glycogen is a polysaccharide branched very much like amylopectin. Figure 4–2 illustrates the structure of glycogen. It is a very large molecule with a molecular weight from one million to four million. Glycogen is the form of carbohydrate stored in man and animals. Normally about 3/4 pound or 340 grams of glycogen is stored in liver and muscle. Muscle glycogen is used directly for energy. Liver glycogen may be converted to glucose and carried by the blood to the tissues for their use. Very little glycogen is found in food. The small amounts in meat and seafood are largely converted to lactic acid at the time the animals are slaughtered. Since the amount stored at any time is very small, a constant supply of carbohydrate should be available. It is the prime, quickest and greatest source of body energy. Most of the carbohydrates consumed daily are in excess of the immediate energy needs and limited storage capacity. They are quickly converted into fats and stored in the adipose tissues.

Cellulose and *hemicellulose* are the cellular framework of plants. Cellulose resembles starch in that it is made up of many glucose molecules. The molecules are unbranched and resemble amylose. It is not soluble in ordinary solvents. The angle of attachment between the glucose molecules of starch and cellulose is different. Whereas starch is readily digested by humans, cellulose is not. Humans do not have the enzyme needed to make the hydrolysis of cellulose rapid enough to be of any use. An economic process for the conversion of cellulose to a carbohydrate form utilizable for energy production has not been developed. Ruminants can make use of cellulose, since it is digested by bacteria in the rumen.

The principal function of cellulose in human nutrition is to furnish indigestible "bulk" which promotes efficient intestinal function. This is commonly referred to as "roughage"

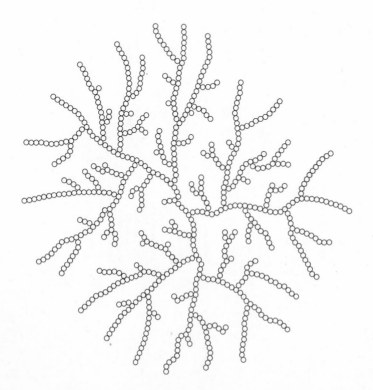

Figure 4–2   The structure of glycogen. (From McGilvery, R. W.: Biochemistry: A Functional Approach. W. B. Saunders Company, 1970.)

in the diet. Cellulose occurs in fruit, vegetable pulp and skin, stalks and leaves and the outer coverings of grains, nuts and legumes.

Hemicelluloses differ chemically from cellulose in that they may consist of hexoses, pentoses and acid forms of these compounds. They are also readily broken down by dilute acid. Pectin and agar-agar are typical hemicelluloses. Pectin is made up of units of a derivative of galactose whereas agar is composed of galactose units. These compounds are not energy sources because they are not hydrolyzed in the gut to yield simple sugars. Their nutritional function resides in the fact that they absorb water, form a gel and increase bulk which gives them a laxative property. Pectins, found in partially ripe fruit and fruit seeds and commercial preparations, liquid or powder, are widely used for making jelly. Agar-agar is extracted from a seaweed. It is used as a thickening agent.

Additional types of insoluble carbohydrates occurring in the cell walls of plants are lignin, algin and gums. These are used in food processing to give body and smooth consistency or to serve as a stabilizer to the product. Inulin, a polysaccharide, composed of fructose units is found in onions, garlic, artichokes and mushrooms. It has little dietary significance.

Methyl cellulose, a synthetic product, is used commercially in low-calorie food products.

OTHER POLYSACCHARIDES[1, 2]   The mucopolysaccharides occur in combination with protein in body secretions and structures and are responsible for the viscosity of body mucous secretions. They are not found in significant quantity in food. Some of the common mucopolysaccharides are hyaluronic acids, present in the fluid lubricating the joints of the body skeleton; chrondroitin sulfate, found in cornea, cartilage, skin, aorta and heart valves; heparin, present as a naturally occurring anticoagulant in blood; and keratosulphate, present in hard structures such as nails.

Table 4-2 summarizes briefly the types, sources and end products of carbohydrates. It also indicates the particular carbohydrates in the American diet and the quantitative importance of each carbohydrate to the total intake.

The increasing awareness that specific carbohydrates play roles in metabolic processes not previously suspected, prompted the preparation of a table of both the simple as well as the more complex sugars found in foods.[3] Such a table would be useful in comparing the intake of specific carbohydrates in dietaries.

FUNCTION OF CARBOHYDRATES IN THE BODY

The body tissues require a constant daily supply of carbohydrate in the form of glucose in all metabolic reactions. Comparatively little is stored. The amount of glycogen stored in the liver is approximately 110 gm. and in the muscles about 225 gm. and there is about 10 gm. of glucose in the blood. For some individuals, the supply available from the storage depots would be insufficient for one day's need.

1. The principal function of carbohydrate is to serve as a major source of energy for the body. It must be supplied regularly and at frequent intervals in order to meet the energy needs of the body. Each gram of carbohydrate yields approximately 4 kcalories regardless of the source—monosaccharide, disaccharide or polysaccharide.

2. Carbohydrates exert a protein-sparing action. If insufficient carbohydrates are available in the diet, the body will convert protein to glucose in order to supply energy. The energy needs of the body take precedence over all other needs. It has been found that for optimum utilization of amino acids for protein formation, carbohydrates must be supplied simultaneously with the essential amino acids. Protein utilization seems to be favorably affected by the presence of carbohydrates in the same meal, and nitrogen balance is improved.

3. The presence of carbohydrates is necessary for normal fat metabolism. If there is insufficient carbohydrate larger amounts of fat are used for energy than the body is equipped to handle and oxidation is incomplete. There is an accumulation of acidic intermediate products (the ketone bodies) and acidosis results.

4. In the liver glucuronic acid, a metabolite of glucose, has an important function in combining with chemical and bacterial toxins as well as some normal metabolites, converting them into a form in which they may be excreted.

5. Glucose as such has a specific influence; it is indispensable for the maintenance of the functional integrity of the nerve tissue and is the sole source of energy for the brain. Thus a constant supply of glucose from the blood is

[1] Pike, R. L., and Brown, M. L.: Nutrition: An Integrated Approach. John Wiley & Sons, 1967, p. 14.
[2] Guthrie, H. A.: Introductory Nutrition. 2nd ed. St. Louis, C. V. Mosby Company, 1971.

[3] Hardinge, M. G., et al.: Carbohydrates in foods. J. Am. Dietet. A., 46:197, 1965.

essential for the proper functioning of these tissues. Any lack of glucose or the oxygen for its oxidation may cause irreversible damage to the brain.

6. Lactose remains in the intestines longer than the other disaccharides and thus encourages the growth of beneficial bacteria, resulting in a laxative action. One of the functions of these bacteria is believed to be the synthesis of certain vitamins (B-complex vitamins and vitamin K).

7. As previously described, cellulose and the closely related insoluble, indigestible carbohydrates aid in normal elimination. They stimulate the peristaltic movements of the gastrointestinal tract and absorb water to give bulk to the intestinal contents.

8. Carbohydrates or products derived from them, serve as precursors to such compounds as nucleic acids and connective tissue matrix and galactosides of nerve tissue.

9. Foods which we tend to think of primarily for their carbohydrate content (e.g., cereals) also supply significant quantities of protein, minerals, and B-vitamins.

METABOLISM OF CARBOHYDRATES

The digestion, absorption and metabolic breakdown of carbohydrates are discussed in Chapter 7. Figure 4–3 briefly summarizes and reviews the digestion products of carbohydrates in the gastrointestinal tract, and their subsequent fate, demonstrating the interrelations among carbohydrates.

Carbohydrates are absorbed through the intestinal mucosa as monosaccharides, primarily glucose with minor quantities of other sugars. Much of the glucose is used for immediate energy needs, part is stored as glycogen in liver and muscle and the rest is converted to and stored as fat.

The utilization of glucose for energy involves a complex series of reactions (each one catalyzed by its specific enzyme) in which the energy is released, part of it as heat and part in the form of ATP (adenosine triphosphate), a special "high energy phosphate" which can be used as needed for muscular work, synthetic processes and other needs of the body. The first step in glucose metabolism is conversion of glucose to glucose-6-phosphate. From this point it may be broken down anaerobically to two 3-carbon units with release of a small amount of energy and then via an active 2-carbon unit, called acetyl coenzyme A, to carbon dioxide and water with liberation of a much larger amount of energy. These reactions occur in all tissues. Refer to discussion on cell metabolism in Chapter 7.

Glycogen synthesis (glycogenesis) also starts by way of glucose-6-phosphate which one may envision as sitting astride the crossroads of carbohydrate metabolism. Figure 4–4 gives an abbreviated schematic outline of these reactions.

Fructose and galactose are converted to glucose in the liver. Some individuals lack the specific enzymes required for one or the other of these transformations. Mild to severe abnormalities in metabolism may result. (See Figure 4–4.) The amount of glucose available is not limited to that supplied by the carbohydrates in the food. Glucose may be synthesized from amino acids, from protein and from the glycerol portion of fat. This process is known as gluconeogenesis. It is linked to the level of glucose in the blood and is under hormonal control. Refer to the discussion on cell metabolism in Chapter 7.

The blood sugar is held at a remarkably constant level, 70 to 100 mg. per 100 ml. under fasting conditions. Some of the factors which influence the level of blood sugar are listed in Table 4–3. After a meal the sugar level in-

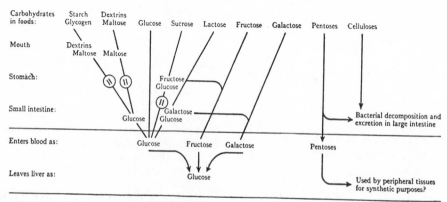

Figure 4–3   Products of carbohydrate digestion at various levels of the gastrointestinal tract, and subsequent fate. The ringed "ditto" signs indicate that the same products as at the preceding level continue to appear. (From Duncan, G. G. [ed.]: Diseases of Metabolism. 5th ed. W. B. Saunders Company, 1964.)

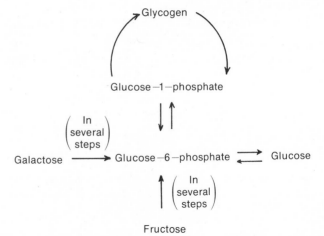

Figure 4–4   Summary of the overall process of glycogen formation and hydrolysis. Glycogen synthesis involves uridine diphosphate (UDP) and uridine triphosphate (UTP) as well as ADP and ATP.

creases but returns to the normal level as the glucose is utilized and stored. As glucose in the blood is taken up by the tissues, liver glycogen is continually converted to glucose (glycogenolysis) and diffuses into the blood. (See Figure 4–4.) Muscle glycogen is used only for energy and cannot be returned to the blood as glucose. If fasting is prolonged, gluconeogenesis occurs and amino acids and glycerol are converted to glucose.

A battery of hormones is involved in the regulation of these reactions. Insulin, produced by the beta cells of the islets of Langerhans in the pancreas, promotes the uptake and oxidation of glucose by cells. Its liberation is enhanced by a high blood glucose level and it immediately works to return the latter to a normal level. Insulin also promotes the storage of glucose as glycogen in the liver and muscle.

Glucagon, produced by the alpha cells of the islets of Langerhans has an effect exactly opposite to that of insulin. It causes a rise in the amount of sugar in the blood by increasing glycogenolysis and gluconeogenesis. Thus, insulin and glucagon may be considered to be antagonists, and it is at least in part

through their opposing efforts that carbohydrate metabolism is maintained at a steady state.

The pituitary gland also secretes substances that are antagonistic to the action of insulin. Epinephrine, a hormone derived from the amino acid tyrosine and produced by the adrenal medulla gland, tends to favor the breakdown of liver glycogen to yield blood glucose (glycogenolysis), thereby raising the blood sugar. The secretion of epinephrine is increased during anger or fear and the increased formation of glucose which follows presumably serves as a source of extra energy to permit the body to respond more rapidly to the crisis.

Certain steroid hormones elaborated by the adrenal cortex also influence blood glucose levels by stimulating gluconeogenesis. These hormones apparently reduce the utilization of glucose by the tissues and also increase the rate at which protein is converted into glucose. The net result of these two actions is to increase blood glucose, i.e., these steroid hormones counteract the action of insulin.

When the blood glucose concentration is severely decreased, thyroxine secretion by

TABLE 4–3   FACTORS INFLUENCING THE LEVEL OF BLOOD SUGAR

	FACTORS THAT LOWER BLOOD SUGAR	FACTORS THAT INCREASE BLOOD SUGAR
DIETARY	Prolonged undernutrition Decreased absorption of glucose Increased exercise Liver damage Kidney abnormalities (Renal glycosuria)	Excessive carbohydrate intake Increased absorption of glucose Reduced exercise Liver damage Hyperactivity of anterior pituitary Hyperactivity of adrenal cortex
HORMONES	Anterior pituitary deficiency Hypothyroidism Adrenal insufficiency Insulin	Diabetes mellitus Epinephrine Anesthesia Toxemias Head injuries Fright and anger

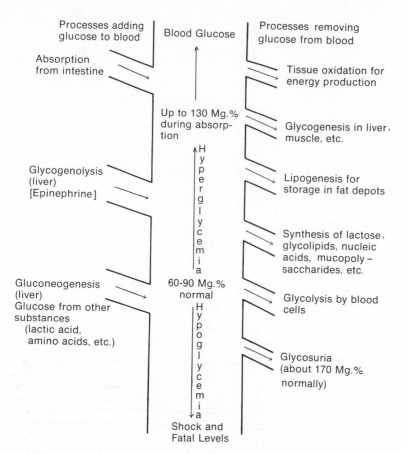

Figure 4–5   Blood glucose maintenance. (Adapted from West, E. S., et al.: Textbook of Biochemistry. 4th ed., The Macmillan Company, 1966.)

the thyroid gland is increased. It stimulates gluconeogenesis and the blood glucose concentration rises.

The growth hormone and adrenocorticotropic hormones elaborated by the anterior pituitary gland also raise the blood glucose level by acting as insulin antagonists.

For a summary of the processes adding glucose to the blood and the process of removing glucose from the blood refer to Figure 4–5.

METABOLISM OF ETHYL ALCOHOL (ETHANOL)[4]   Ethyl alcohol yields approximately 7.0 kcal./gm., when completely metabolized. It is rapidly absorbed from the stomach and small intestine; uniformly distributed throughout the body water; and rapidly oxidized with little or none stored. Small amounts are lost into the urine and into the respired air by diffusion.

In the liver, ethyl alcohol is converted to acetaldehyde, and then to acetyl-CoA which,

as has been discussed, may readily be utilized for energy.

Experimental animals fed appreciable amounts of ethanol will grow about as efficiently as animals fed isocaloric quantities of carbohydrate or fat, if the protein, vitamin, essential amino acids and fatty acid requirements are met. Apparently, a high ethanol diet can provide the major portion of the calorie needs of an individual; however, such a diet would be inadequate in all other respects.

This has been of necessity a very brief outline of carbohydrate metabolism. (The details of this very complex subject are presented in biochemistry texts listed at the end of this chapter.) Common abnormalities of carbohydrate metabolism are presented in Part 2 of this volume.

DAILY DIETARY ALLOWANCE

The body can utilize protein or fat for energy if carbohydrate is limited. However, if fat is serving as the main source of energy, intermediates in the oxidative process are

[4]Food and Nutrition Board: Recommended Dietary Allowances. 7th ed. Washington, D.C., National Research Council, National Academy of Sciences, Pub. No. 1694, 1968, p. 17.

formed faster than they can be completely oxidized. Accumulation of these products causes acidosis. Utilization of protein for energy is wasteful. Protein foods are expensive and the part burned for energy cannot be used for building body proteins. Approximately 58 per cent of the amino acids in the body proteins and approximately 10 per cent of the fat can be converted to glucose.

Adequate nutrition is possible at extremes of either high or low carbohydrate intake, provided that the calories and essential nutritional needs of the body are met. An active adult consumes about 50 per cent (300 to 400 gm.) of his daily calories in carbohydrates. According to the Food and Nutrition Board of the National Research Council in the 1968 revision, "A precise minimal requirement for carbohydrate is difficult to assess. Adaptation to diets very low in carbohydrates is possible, but, in individuals accustomed to normal diets, at least 100 gm. of carbohydrates per day appear to be needed to avoid ketosis, excessive protein breakdown and other undesirable metabolic responses."[5]

TRENDS OF CARBOHYDRATE INTAKE IN THE AMERICAN DIET

During the past 60 years, the changes in the quantity and kinds of carbohydrate consumed by Americans have been significant. The total carbohydrate intake has decreased by almost 25 per cent but the consumption of sugars and syrups has increased by 25 per cent.[6] The amount of carbohydrate has dropped from 492 gm. per person per day to

374 gm., a total decrease of 118 gm. daily. (See Table 4–4.)

The decreased consumption of flour, cereals and potato products has accounted for the decline. (See Figure 4–6.) Approximately two-thirds of the carbohydrate was provided by starch and one-third by sugars at the beginning of the century. Both forms of carbohydrate contributed about equally to the total amount by 1957–1959. The portion of the total carbohydrate supplied by sugars has increased steadily and the consumption of the starch containing foods has decreased. During this period of increasing consumption of sugars the incidence of coronary heart disease increased. Some investigators have attempted to relate these changes in the dietary to the increase in coronary heart disease.[7]

COMMON SOURCES OF STARCHES AND SUGARS

The groups of food providing appreciable amounts of carbohydrate in the dietary are (1) grains, (2) fruits, (3) vegetables, (4) milk, and (5) the concentrated sweets. (See Table 4–5.) Most of these foods provide other nutrients as well as carbohydrate.

Refined sugar, syrups and cornstarch are examples of pure carbohydrates and many of the sweets such as candy, honey, jellies, molasses and soft drinks contain little, if any, other nutrients. These are referred to as "empty calories" because they contribute nothing except calories to the dietary of an individual. An excessive intake of these empty calories tends to reduce the intake of the health-protecting foods, largely by taking away one's appetite for them.

Most carbohydrate foods contain more than one nutrient. For example, the whole grains, wheat, corn, rice and to a lesser degree oats, rye, barley, buckwheat and millet, contain in addition to starch varying amounts of proteins (incomplete), minerals and vitamins.

The carbohydrates in fruits are principally the monosaccharides, glucose and fructose (sucrose if sweetened). They contribute vitamins, minerals, cellulose, hemicellulose and water, in varying amounts. (Fruits such as avocados and olives contain considerable fat.)

Vegetables have a varying amount of glucose. The leafy vegetables are high in water and cellulose content and many contribute minerals and vitamins. The root tubers and seed variety (potatoes, beets, carrots,

[5]Food and Nutrition Board: Recommended Dietary Allowances. 7th ed. Washington, D.C., National Research Council, National Academy of Sciences, Pub. No. 1694, 1968, p. 10.

[6]Ibid., p. 9.

TABLE 4–4 CARBOHYDRATE AVAILABLE PER PERSON PER DAY AND PER CENT FURNISHED BY STARCH AND SUGARS

YEAR	GRAMS CARBOHYDRATE	PER CENT STARCH[1]	PER CENT SUGARS[2]	PER CENT OF TOTAL KCALORIES
1909–1913	492	68.3	31.7	56.2
1925–1929	476	58.7	41.3	54.4
1935–1939	436	56.8	43.2	52.8
1947–1949	403	52.4	47.6	49.4
1957–1959	374	49.6	50.4	47.3
1965	374	48.8	51.2	47.0

[1]Grains and starch vegetables.
[2]Fruits and sugar.
(Adapted from Friend, B.: Nutrients in United States food supply. Am. J. Clin. Nutr. 20:911 and 912, 1967.)

[7]Antar, M. A., et al.: Changes in retail market food supplies in the United States in the last seventy years in relation to the incidence of coronary heart disease with special reference to dietary carbohydrate and essential fatty acids. Am. J. Clin. Nutr., 14:169, 1964.

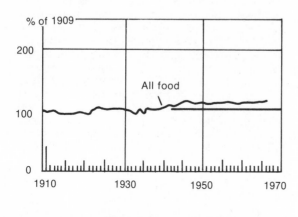

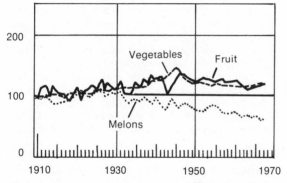

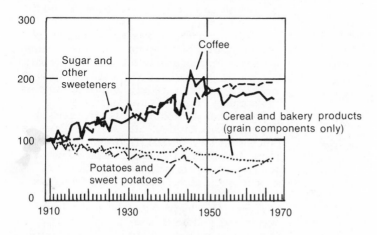

Figure 4–6 Trends in carbohydrate consumption per capita in the United States. (Adapted from Ford Agricultural Economics Report No. 138, U. S. Department of Agriculture, Economic Research Service, 1968.)

TABLE 4–5   CARBOHYDRATE CONTENT* OF SOME TYPICAL FOODS

SUGAR	CARBO-HYDRATE (PER CENT)	STARCH	CARBO-HYDRATE (PER CENT)
Concentrated Sweets		*Grain Products*	
Sugar: Cane, beet, powdered	99.5	Starches: Corn, tapioca, arrowroot	88–86
brown, maple	96–90	Cereals (dry): Corn, wheat, oat, bran	85–68
Candies	95–70	Flour: Corn, wheat-sifted	80–70
Honey (extracted)	82	Popcorn (popped)	77
Syrup: Table blends, molasses	75–55	Cookies: Plain, assorted	71
Jams, jellies, marmalades	70	Crackers, saltines	72
Carbonated, sweetened beverages	10–12	Cakes: Plain, without icing	56
Fruits		Bread: White, rye, whole wheat	52–48
Prunes, apricots, figs, (cooked, unsweet)	31–12	Macaroni, spaghetti noodles, rice (cooked)	30–23
Bananas, grapes, cherries, apples, pears	23–15	Cereals (cooked): Oat, wheat, grits	16–10
Fresh: Pineapples, grapefruits, oranges,		*Vegetables*	
apricots, strawberries	14–8	Boiled: Corn, white and sweet potatoes, lima,	
Milk		dried beans, peas	26–15
Skim	6	Beets, carrots, onions, tomatoes	7–5
Whole	5	Leafy: Lettuce, asparagus, cabbage, greens,	
		spinach	4–3

*From Composition of Foods, Agriculture Handbook No. 8. Agricultural Research Science, U.S. Department of Agriculture, Washington, D.C.

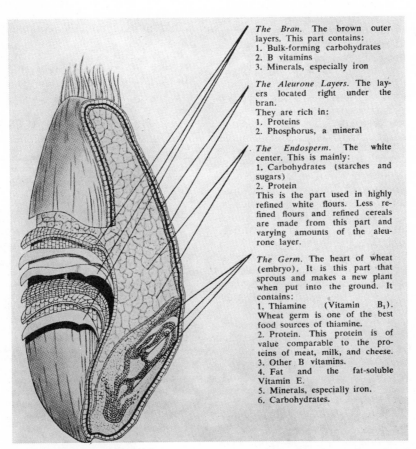

The Bran. The brown outer layers. This part contains:
1. Bulk-forming carbohydrates
2. B vitamins
3. Minerals, especially iron

The Aleurone Layers. The layers located right under the bran.
They are rich in:
1. Proteins
2. Phosphorus, a mineral

The Endosperm. The white center. This is mainly:
1. Carbohydrates (starches and sugars)
2. Protein
This is the part used in highly refined white flours. Less refined flours and refined cereals are made from this part and varying amounts of the aleurone layer.

The Germ. The heart of wheat (embryo). It is this part that sprouts and makes a new plant when put into the ground. It contains:
1. Thiamine (Vitamin B_1). Wheat germ is one of the best food sources of thiamine.
2. Protein. This protein is of value comparable to the proteins of meat, milk, and cheese.
3. Other B vitamins.
4. Fat and the fat-soluble Vitamin E.
5. Minerals, especially iron.
6. Carbohydrates.

Figure 4–7   Whole wheat. This diagram shows the structure, composition and nutritive values of a whole wheat grain. (Courtesy of the Ralston Purina Company.)

turnips, peas, beans) have a higher starch content. They, too, contribute some protein, minerals, and vitamins, water and cellulose, in varying amounts. Legumes (dry beans, dry peas, soybeans, nuts) contain appreciable amounts of protein as well as minerals and vitamins. Soybeans and nuts contribute good quality protein and fat.

Milk, though generally listed with the protein foods, supplies the disaccharide, lactose. It is the only animal food contributing appreciable quantities of carbohydrate in the dietary. The glycogen in meat is usually broken down before the meat reaches the market.

THE ENRICHMENT OF BREAD, FLOUR AND CEREALS

Because the American diet was considered to be short in certain essential nutrients, the Food and Nutrition Council of the American Medical Association, and the Food and Nutrition Board of the National Research Council approved several staple foods as carriers of additional nutrients. They have issued statements regarding the addition of specific nutrients to foods from time to time, and in 1953 issued a joint statement to serve as a valuable guide. This will be more fully discussed in Chapter 12, Food Economics, and Chapter 41, Bread-Cereal Group.

Among the common staple foods selected or approved as carriers of added nutrients are bread, flour and cereals. The highly refined grains are more resistant to spoilage, but have become deprived of the most protective elements, such as essential amino acids (proteins), vitamins and minerals.

When the whole grain is used, minerals and vitamins are present in appreciable amounts. When the bran layers and germ (see Figure 4-7) are removed by the process of refining, most of the thiamin, riboflavin, niacin and iron are lost. Since people have become accustomed to, and prefer, the refined products, enrichment to replace the elements removed in the milling process has been accepted as the best solution.

The results of the enrichment of bread is seen in Table 4-6. Bread and flour enrichment is mandatory in more than 30 states (also Puerto Rico, Canada and other countries). It is widely practiced in those states without legal requirements. Almost 90 per cent of the white bread sold in the United States is enriched.[8] There also are federal standards for the enrichment of rice and corn grits. Nutrition scientists are in general agreement that

this improvement in the nutritive quality of food has made a significant contribution to the improvement of nutrition and health (see Table, 41-1, p. 000. See also Chapter 12, Food Economics, and Chapter 41, Bread-Cereal Group, for additional description and discussion of grain products, and their use in the diet.

TABLE 4-6   COMPARISON OF THREE B-VITAMINS AND IRON IN WHEAT BREAD (POUND LOAVES)

BREAD	THIAMIN (mg.)	RIBOFLAVIN (mg.)	NIACIN (mg.)	IRON (mg.)
Whole wheat made with 2% non-fat dry milk	1.17	0.56	12.9	10.4
White enriched* with 3 to 4% non-fat dry milk	1.13	0.95	10.8	11.3
White unenriched with 3 to 4% non-fat dry milk	0.31	0.39	5.0	3.2

*Enriched bread may also furnish, as an optional ingredient, added vitamin D in such quantity that each pound of the finished bread will contain not less than 150 U.S.P. units and not more than 750 U.S.P. units of vitamin D. It may also contain as an optional ingredient added harmless calcium salts in such quantity that each pound of the finished bread will contain not less than 300 milligrams and not more than 500 milligrams of calcium. (From Bread Standards, Federal Security Agency, Food and Drug Administration as issued in the Federal Register, May 15, 1952.)
(From Composition of Foods, Agriculture Handbook No. 8. Agricultural Research Science, U. S. Department of Agriculture, Washington, D.C.)

PROBLEMS AND SUGGESTED TOPICS FOR DISCUSSION

1. List the most popular carbohydrate foods.
2. List the amounts of the various carbohydrate foods you consume during a period of 24 hours and a period of 3 days.
3. Evaluate the list of carbohydrate foods. Classify them into "sugars" and "starches." List the monosaccharides.
4. What per cent of the daily dietary should be normally consumed in the form of carbohydrate foods? When might it be increased? Decreased?
5. Keep a record of your diet for one day. Calculate the carbohydrate and calorie content. What percentage of the calories were derived from carbohydrates? What percentage of the carbohydrate calories were derived from fruits, vegetables, breadstuffs and cereal foods? What percentage of the carbohydrate calories were derived from sugars, candy, soft drinks, cake and pie? List any changes you could make in carbohydrate content to improve your diet, and give reasons.
6. Why do you like to eat carbohydrate foods?
7. What factors tend to raise and to lower the blood sugar? What is the form of carbohydrate in the circulating blood? What is the normal concentration?
8. List the functions of carbohydrates in the body. What becomes of the carbohydrate eaten in excess of the body's daily need for energy?

SUGGESTED ADDITIONAL READING REFERENCES

Antar, M. A., et al.: Changes in retail market food supplies in the United States in the last seventy years in relation

---

[8] Parman, G. K.: Vitaminization of food outside the United States. Ann. N.Y. Acad. Sci., 98:607, 1962.

to the incidence of coronary heart disease with special reference to dietary carbohydrate and essential fatty acids. Am. J. Clin. Nutr. *14*:169, 1964.

Bogert, L. J.: Nutrition and Physical Fitness. 8th ed. Philadelphia, W. B. Saunders Company, 1966.

Duncan, G. G. (ed.): Diseases of Metabolism. 5th ed. Philadelphia, W. B. Saunders Company, 1964, Chapter 2, Carbohydrate Metabolism.

Friend, B.: Nutrients in United States Food Supply. Am. J. Clin. Nutr., *20*:907, 1967.

Green, D. E.: The Mitochondrion.: Sci. Am., *210*:63, 1964.

Guyton, A. C.: Textbook of Medical Physiology. 4th ed. Philadelphia, W. B. Saunders Company, 1971.

Hardinge, M. G., Swarner, J. B., and Crooks, H.: Carbohydrates in foods. Am. J. Dietet. A. *46*:197, 1965.

Harper, H. A.: Review of Physiological Chemistry, 12th ed., Canada, Lange Medical Publications, 1969.

Holum, J. R.: Principles of Physical, Organic and Biological Chemistry. New York, John Wiley & Sons, 1969.

Mazur, A., and Harrow, B.: Textbook of Biochemistry. 10th ed. Philadelphia, W. B. Saunders Company, 1971.

McGilvery, R. W.: Biochemistry: A Functional Approach. Philadelphia, W. B. Saunders Company, 1970.

Recommended Dietary Allowances. 7th ed. Food and Nutrition Board, National Research Council, Washington, D.C.: Pub. No. 1694, 1968.

Review: Carbohydrate intake and respiratory quotient. Nutr. Rev., 22:104, 1964.

Review: Metabolic interrelationships of dietary carbohydrate and fat. Nutr. Rev., 22:216, 1964.

Review: The role of carbohydrates in the diet. Nutr. Rev., 22:102, 1964.

The Nutrition Foundation Inc.: Present Knowledge in Nutrition 3rd ed. 1967, Chapter 3, Present Knowledge of Carbohydrate.

Wohl, M. G., and Goodhart, R. S.: Modern Nutrition in Health and Disease. 4th ed. Philadelphia, Lea & Febiger, 1968, The Role of Carbohydrates in the Diet.

Chapter 5
LIPIDS

The term lipid, which is often used interchangeably with the term fat, was created to include a heterogeneous group of compounds related actually, or potentially, to the fatty acids. They have in common the properties of being (1) insoluble in water, (2) soluble in organic solvents such as ether and chloroform and (3) utilizable by living organisms. The group thus includes the ordinary fats and oils, waxes and related compounds. The principal foods contributing fat to the diet are butter, margarine, lard, vegetable oil, salad dressing, the visible fat of meat, the skin of chicken and the invisible fat found in cream, homogenized milk, milk products, egg yolk, meat, fish, nuts, olives, avocados and in whole-grain cereals.

CLASSIFICATION AND COMPOSITION

The principal groups of lipids important in nutrition are listed and classified in Table 5–1.

Most natural fats are composed of about 98 to 99 per cent triglycerides. The 1 or 2 per cent remaining include traces of mono- and diglycerides, free fatty acids, phospholipids and unsaponifiable matter containing sterols.[1]

---

[1]Report: Dietary Fat and Human Health. Food and Nutrition Board, Washington, D.C., National Academy of Sciences, National Research Council, Pub. No. 1147, 1966.

TABLE 5–1   CLASSIFICATION OF LIPIDS IMPORTANT TO NUTRITION

I. *Simple Lipids*
  A. Fatty Acids
  B. Neutral fats: Mono-, di-, triglycerides (esters of fatty acids and glycerol)
  C. Waxes (esters of fatty acids with high molecular weight alcohols)
    1. Sterol esters
    2. Nonsterol esters

II. *Compound Lipids*
  A. Phospholipids: Compounds of fatty acids, phosphoric acid and nitrogenous base
    1. Phosphoglycerides
      a. Lecithin
      b. Cephalin
      c. Sphingomyelins
  B. Glycolipids: Compounds of fatty acid combined with carbohydrate and a nitrogenous base
      a. Cerebrosides
      b. Gangliosides
  C. Lipoproteins: Lipids in combination with protein

III. *Derived Lipids*
  A. Fatty Acid: Mono- and diglycerides
  B. Glycerol: Water-soluble component of triglycerides and interconvertible with carbohydrate
  C. Sterols
    1. Cholesterol, ergosterol
    2. Steroid hormones
    3. Vitamin D
    4. Bile salts
  D. Fat-soluble vitamins
    1. Vitamin A
    2. Vitamin E
    3. Vitamin K
    4. Coenzyme Q (ubiquinone)

TRIGLYCERIDES

Like carbohydrates, triglycerides (the main component of ordinary fats and oils) are com-

```
        H                                    H
        |                                    |
    H —C —OH                            H —C —OOC —R₁
        |                                    |
   HO —C —H          R —COOH           R₂ —COO —C —H
        |                                    |
    H —C —OH                            H —C —OOC —R₃
        |                                    |
        H                                    H


       Glycerol           Fatty Acid          Triglyceride
```

posed of carbon, hydrogen and oxygen. Structurally they are esters of a trihydric alcohol, glycerol and fatty acids. These are a series of straight chains containing an even number of carbon atoms, ranging from 4 to 30 carbons.

FATTY ACIDS   The diversity of natural fats depends on the variety of fatty acids which make up its triglycerides. The hydrocarbon chain (represented by R in the formula) may be either saturated or unsaturated (i.e., have one or more double bonds). The whole series of saturated fatty acids has been found in natural fats. The only unsaturated fatty acids which occur in large amount contain 18 carbons; there are small amounts of 16 and 20 carbon acids.

The biochemist uses the systematic chemical nomenclature for the fatty acids. The nutritionist generally uses the older, common names, many of which were derived from the fat from which an acid was isolated (butyric, butter; linoleic, linseed oil). A convenient shorthand gives the number of carbon atoms and the number of double bonds; for example, linoleic acid may be designated as $C_{18:2}$.

The physical properties of the fatty acids are related to their chemical structure. Short chain acids or long chain acids with one or more double bonds are liquid; longer chain saturated acids are solid, and those with 16 or more carbons very hard. The properties of the triglycerides are related to the nature of their fatty acids. Solid fats such as mutton tallow contain large amounts of palmitic ($C_{16:0}$) and stearic ($C_{18:0}$) acids. Oils (an oil is a fat which is liquid at room temperature) usually have a high proportion of oleic ($C_{18:1}$) and linoleic acids ($C_{18:2}$).

SATURATED AND UNSATURATED FATTY ACIDS   When fatty acids contain as many hydrogen atoms as the carbon chain can hold, they are called saturated fatty acids.

The *iodine number* is a measure of the degree of unsaturation of a lipid. Double bonds are reactive and 2 atoms of iodine will attach to the molecule at each double bond. The iodine number is defined as the number of grams of iodine which will add to 100 grams of fat. Animal fats have low iodine numbers (25 to 40); vegetable oils have high numbers (90 to more than 200). For safflower oil, which consists largely of linoleic acid, the number is 181. The iodine number gives only limited information, since it indicates only the total number of double bonds and not their distribution between mono- (one double bond) and polyunsaturated acids (two or more double bonds). Olive oil and peanut oil have the same iodine number (90) but peanut oil has twice as much polyunsaturated acid. In view of the importance attached to the polyunsaturated fatty acids in the dietary, this is a significant difference.

Complete separation and identification of the fatty acids in a fat was an almost impossible task using the older chemical proce-

$CH_3(CH_2)_{16}COOH$ Stearic Acid (Saturated)

$CH_3(CH_2)_7CH=CH(CH_2)_7COOH$ Oleic Acid (Mono-unsaturated)

$CH_3(CH_2)_4CH=CHCH_2CH=CH(CH_2)_7COOH$ Linoleic Acid (Polyunsaturated)

$CH_3CH_2CH=CHCH_2CH=CH—CH_2—CH=CH(CH_2)_7COOH$ Linolenic Acid (Polyunsaturated)

18 Carbon Acids

dures. By means of gas-liquid chromatography it is now possible to get a complete profile. At least 60 different fatty acids have been found in butter fat.

CHARACTERISTICS OF ANIMAL AND VEGETABLE FATS There is considerable species variation in fats from animal sources. The major components of the fats of land animals are palmitic, stearic and oleic acids, with smaller amounts of linoleic acid and traces of arachidonic acid ($C_{20:4}$). The fat of the herbivorous animals (beef and mutton tallow) is harder (more saturated) than pork and poultry fats. The degree of unsaturation of pork and chicken fat may vary, depending on the diet. Fish have softer fat than land animals and fatty acids with 20 and 22 carbons predominate. The flavors of all meats are distinguished from each other by the flavor of their respective fats. Dairy fats have a high percentage of short chain acids (6 to 10 carbons) which give them their characteristic flavor and relatively low melting point.

Vegetable oils are predominantly unsaturated. About 85 per cent of the fatty acid of the common food oils is oleic and linoleic, although the proportions of the two vary widely, from 15 per cent linoleic in olive oil to 75 per cent in safflower oil. An exception is coconut oil. It is almost completely saturated but has a low melting point because of a high content of medium chain fatty acids (8 to 12 carbons). Table 5–2 lists the analysis of some fats of animal and plant origin.

In 1965, the total amount of fat available in

America per capita per day was 145 grams. Of this total, 37 per cent was provided by the saturated fatty acids.[2] Approximately 41 per cent of the total fat in the American diet is provided by the monounsaturated fatty acid, oleic acid. Oleic acid is found abundantly in both animal (except fish) and vegetable fats. Appreciable amounts are contained in olive oil and bacon. Linoleic acid accounts for approximately 13 per cent of the total fat in the American diet. Americans ingest linoleic acid in the form of vegetable oil such as corn oil, soybean oil, cottonseed oil, safflower oil and peanut oil.

REACTIONS OF FATS Enzymes of the digestive tract act as catalysts for the hydrolysis of triglycerides to their component fatty acids and glycerol. If the fat is hydrolyzed with alkali (saponification), salts of the fatty acids are formed. These salts are soaps. Formation of insoluble soaps in the intestinal tract may be of concern in some abnormal conditions characterized by poor fat absorption.

High temperature (to the smoking point) causes decomposition of fat and the formation of acrolein from the glycerol portion. Acrolein is irritating to the intestinal mucosa.

Hydrogenation Unsaturated fatty acids may add hydrogen to the double bonds in the same manner as they add iodine in determination of the iodine number to form the saturated acid. So oleic acid, linoleic acid and linolenic acid, when completely hydrogenated, become stearic acid. Vegetable oils may be converted to solid fats by hydrogenation. Complete hydrogenation would produce a very hard and unpalatable fat. When the process is controlled, fat of any desired consistency can be prepared, and commercially hydrogenated vegetable oils such as Crisco and Spry are creamy solids at room temperature, similar to lard and butter fat, and are used extensively for cooking.

Margarine is made by hydrogenating oils also but with additional processing to produce a product that will melt readily and simulate butter. It is emulsified with milk (about 17 per cent by weight) that has been cultured with a microorganism to add flavor. A yellow vegetable dye and vitamins A and D are added to give the margarine the appearance and nutritive value of butter.

A serious disadvantage of hydrogenation is that it lowers the polyunsaturated fatty acid content of the fat and may form some trans-isomers of the unsaturated acids. A product

TABLE 5–2   DISTRIBUTION OF SATURATED AND UNSATURATED FATTY ACIDS IN SOME COMMON FOOD FATS*

| | GRAMS PER 100 GM. OF TOTAL FAT | | |
	Saturated	Unsaturated	Linoleic Acid
Animal fats			
Beef fat	48	47	9
Butter	55	39	3
Lamb or mutton fat	56	40	3
Pork fat (lard)	38	57	10
Vegetable fats			
Corn oil	10	84	53
Cottonseed oil	25	71	50
Margarine (regular)	17–22	56–72	7–15
Margarine (special)	14–28	40–76	22–34
Peanut oil	18	76	29
Shortening, hydrogenated vegetable oils	23	72	7
Soybean oil	15	80	52

*(From Bogert, L. J., et al.: Nutrition and Physical Fitness. 8th ed. Philadelphia, W. B. Saunders Company, 1966, p. 35. Figures selected from U.S. Department of Agriculture: Home Economics Research Report No. 7, 1959, and from American Medical Association Council on Foods and Nutrition: Composition of Certain Margarines. J.A.M.A., 170:719, 1962.)

[2]Friend, B.: Nutrients in United States food supply. A review of trends 1909–1913 to 1965. Am. J. Clin. Nutr., 20:911, 1967.

of the same consistency but of higher linoleic acid content may be prepared by mixing a portion of almost completely hydrogenated fat with some of the original oil. This procedure is used for some margarines. Table 5–2 shows the distribution of saturated and unsaturated fatty acids in some common natural and hydrogenated food fats.

Rancidity   When fats and oils are exposed to warm, moist air over a period of time, chemical changes occur which produce unpalatable flavors and disagreeable odors. Hydrolysis of butter fat in the presence of oxygen, airborne bacteria and heat releases butyric acid and other products with very strong taste. The oxygen of the air can attack the double bonds of the polyunsaturated fatty acids, forming peroxides which may be toxic in large amount. Rancid fat has a toxic effect on rats given low-fat diets.

The oxidative process destroys vitamin A and vitamin E. Vitamin E is present in rather large amount in vegetable fats. It is an antioxidant and protects against rancidity but in the process is, itself, inactivated. Fortification of fats or fatty foods with antioxidants extends the storage time and protects essential nutrients. Precautions should be taken to lessen the danger of rancidity by storage of fat-containing foods at low temperature and limiting the storage time of susceptible foods such as butter and lard.

FUNCTIONS OF TRIGLYCERIDES IN THE BODY

ENERGY   Fats serve as a concentrated source of energy. Each gram of fat supplies 9 kcalories, which is more than twice the amount of energy supplied by each gram of carbohydrate. The main source of this energy is the fatty acids which supply 40 to 50 carbon atoms for oxidation as compared with 3 from glycerol. Because of the high energy density and low solubility of fats, they are used as a store of energy. Not only ingested fat but carbohydrate and amino acids not immediately used by the tissues are converted to fat and stored in the adipose tissue. Up to two-thirds of the total energy of the cells may be supplied by triglyceride rather than carbohydrate. Fat spares protein for tissue synthesis.

OTHER FUNCTIONS   Adipose tissue helps to hold the body organs and nerves in position and to protect them against traumatic injury and shock. The subcutaneous layer of fat insulates the body, which serves to preserve body heat and maintain body temperature. Fats aid in transport and absorption of the fat-soluble vitamins. Fats spare thiamin. In the stomach they depress gastric secretions; they slow the emptying time of the stomach, providing a pleasant feeling of satiety after a meal. Fats also retard the rapid development of hunger which occurs after a carbohydrate meal. Fats add to the palatability of food as well as to the flavor of the diet.

ESSENTIAL FATTY ACID (EFA)   Three polyunsaturated fatty acids, namely, linoleic, linolenic and arachidonic acids, are necessary for growth. They have important roles in fat transport and metabolism and in maintaining the function and integrity of cellular membranes. They also are a part of the fatty acids of cholesterol esters and phospholipids in plasma lipoproteins and mitochondrial lipoproteins.[3] Fatty acids with EFA activity are also precursors of a group of compounds, prostaglandins, which participate in the regulation of blood pressure, heart rate, lipolysis and the central nervous system.[4] In the presence of a dietary source of linoleic acid (along with Vitamin B_6) the body can synthesize arachidonic and linolenic acids, but no conversion of the other acids to linoleic acid occurs. Linoleic acid was shown to be a dietary essential for infants by Hansen, Wiese and associates,[5] who found that linoleic acid would prevent or cure a characteristic dermatitis (eczema) observed in infants fed a fat-free diet (Fig. 5–1). Only linoleic acid is considered to be an essential component of human dietaries.

EFA deficiency in animals produces not only poor growth and dermatitis but a poor reproductive capacity, lowered efficiency of energy utilization, decreased resistance to certain stresses such as x-ray and ultraviolet light, impairment of lipid transport and changes in the polyunsaturated fatty acid content of tissues.

The dietary requirement of linoleic acid for infants has been estimated to be between 1 and 3 per cent of the total calories.[6] The requirement for the adult is relatively low. The minimum human requirement would appear to be near 2 per cent of the calorie intake.[7] The tissue storage of linoleic acid in the adult with the average dietary is high. An excess amount in the diet may be harmful. Excessive

[3]Report: Dietary fat and human health. Washington, D.C., National Academy of Sciences, National Research Council, Pub. No. 1147, 1966.

[4]Dairy Council Digest: Current research on dietary fatty acids, National Dairy Council, Chicago, 41: No. 3, May-June, 1970.

[5]Hansen, A. E., and Wiese, H.: Role of linoleic acid in infant nutrition. J. Nutr., 52:367, 1954, and Pediatrics, 31:171, 1963.

[6]Report: Dietary fat and human health: National Academy of Sciences, National Research Council, Pub. No. 1147, 1966, p. 22.

[7]Daily Dietary Allowances: National Academy of Sciences, Pub. No. 1694, 1968, p. 12.

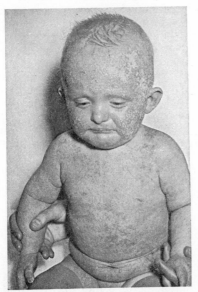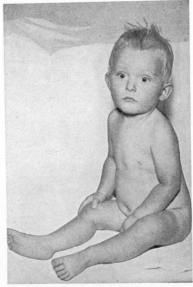

Figure 5–1   Certain fatty acids, found in fats of low melting point, must be furnished in the food. Skin troubles result when these essential fatty acids (linoleic and arachidonic acids) are lacking. Left, 6-month-old infant with very resistant eczema since 2½ months of age. Right, same child 6 months later, after lard had been included in the diet. (Courtesy of Dr. A. E. Hansen.)

amounts of polyunsaturated fatty acids have been observed to reduce the vitamin E level in animal tissues to a dangerously low level, resulting in encephalomalacia in chicks, creatinuria in rats and sterility in male chicks.[8] Vegetable oils supplying the linoleic content in a diet high in the EFA have a natural vitamin E content, which serves as a lipid antioxidant.

LIPIDS WITH SPECIAL FUNCTIONS

PHOSPHOLIPIDS Any lipid containing phosphorus is included in this classification. They are the next largest lipid component of the body after the triglycerides. Phospholipids are formed in essentially all cells of the body, although a greater portion that enter the blood are formed in the liver cells and the intestinal mucosa. Phospholipids have a strong affinity for both water-soluble and fat-soluble substances in the molecule. The phospholipids function in maintaining the structural integrity of the cells rather than as fat stores. Large concentrations of phospholipids are found in combination with protein in cell membranes where they act as a liaison between fat-soluble and water-soluble substances that facilitate the passage of fat in and out of the cell. They act as carriers in the active transport systems through the cell membrane. Despite the loss of body fat that occurs in extreme starvation the phospholipid content remains fairly constant, thus maintaining the integrity of tissue cells.

The lecithins contain glycerol and fatty acids as well as phosphoric acid and the nitrogen-containing base choline. They are the most widely distributed of the phospholipids. Traces are present in liver and egg yolk and in raw vegetable oils such as corn oil. Lecithin is added to food products such as cheese, margarine and confections to aid in emulsification.

Phospholipids such as cephalins (which are similar in structure to lecithins), lipontols (which contain inositol, a compound with vitamin-like activity) and sphingomyelins (which contain no glycerol but a complex amino alcohol) are found in rather high concentrations in nerve tissue. A cephalin is needed to form thromboplastin for the blood clotting process. Sphingomyelin is found in the brain and other nerve tissue as a component of the myelin sheath. This substance acts as an insulator around the nerve fibers. Egg yolk and liver are good sources of these phospholipids.

As a rule, the invisible and not the visible fat of both plant and animal tissue contains appreciable amounts of phospholipids. The amount in oils, lard and butter is small owing to the processing which removes most of the phospholipids.

GLYCOLIPIDS The glycolipids include the cerebrosides and gangliosides. They con-

---

[8]Roels, O. A.: Present knowledge of vitamin E. Present Knowledge of Nutrition. 3rd ed. New York, The Nutrition Foundation, Inc., 1967, p. 87.

tain the base sphingosine and fatty acids with 22 and 24 carbons. The carbohydrate component of the cerebrosides is galactose; the gangliosides contain, in addition, glucose and a complex compound containing an amino sugar. Structurally both the cerebrosides and gangliosides are components of nerve tissue and certain cell membranes, where they play a role in fat transport.

LIPOPROTEINS Lipoproteins are formed primarily in the liver and are found in cell and organelle membranes (mitochondria and lysosomes). Lipoproteins are combinations of triglycerides, phospholipids and cholesterol with protein. Lipids are insoluble in water and to effect their transport and activity in an aqueous medium they are combined with protein complex. Lipoproteins are classified as (1) chylomicrons, very low density lipoproteins (formed in the chyle as lipids are absorbed) which consist of a core of triglyceride coated with phospholipid and protein; (2) high density lipoproteins (alpha lipoproteins), which contain high concentrations of protein and low concentrations of triglycerides; and (3) non-esterified fatty acid, which occurs in combination with serum protein.

HYDROCARBONS Mention should be made here of the term "oil," a confusing word that may refer to fats in a liquid state, or to other substances which have the same properties but have no relation to fats. So sulfuric acid was called oil of vitriol and hydrocarbons from petroleum, mineral oil. Motor oil is a hydrocarbon, and many hydrocarbon oils are physically like fats when cool (petroleum jelly, for example). Hydrocarbons have no nutritive value and are not metabolized or absorbed by the body. Some are used for specific purposes in medicine, such as mineral oil for its laxative and lubricating qualities in the bowel. Because the fat-soluble vitamins are readily absorbed in mineral oil and the latter is not absorbed, its administration may reduce the absorption of the fat-soluble vitamin. Thus, it should not be used regularly and always with caution.

CHOLESTEROL

Cholesterol is a member of the large group of compounds called steroids. They all have

the same complex ring structure. The "-ol" ending indicates that cholesterol is an alcohol. Cholesterol is found only in animal tissues. Somewhat similar sterols are found in plants. Ergosterol, a yeast sterol, is converted to vitamin D_2 on exposure to ultraviolet light. Cholesterol is found not only as the free alcohol but also in combination with fatty acids as esters. It is an essential constituent of all cells of the body. It is a component of the structural membranes of all cells and is a major component of brain and nerve cells. It is the chief component of gallstones. It is found abundantly in organ meats, dairy products, egg yolk and all animal fat. See Appendix Table 4 for cholesterol content of foods. Not only is cholesterol present in foods consumed (exogenous cholesterol), but it also can be synthesized in the cell (endogenous cholesterol).

FUNCTION The structural function of cholesterol is not entirely understood. It is, however, a key intermediate in the biosynthesis of a number of other important steroids. These include the bile acids, adrenocortical hormones, estrogens, androgens and progesterone. The bile acids are compounds with a detergent-like action necessary for the proper absorption of fats from the intestines. The adrenocortical hormones help control the sodium-potassium stores of the body and the rates of metabolism of carbohydrate and nitrogen compounds. This group of steroids includes aldosterone, corticosterone and cortisone. The sex hormones, estrogens, androgens and progesterone, also participate in the development of typical secondary sex characteristics of the female and male. Cholesterol is converted by the intestinal mucosa to 7-dehydrocholesterol, the provitamin of vitamin D. This transformation is also effected by skin and other tissues. The provitamin, when irradiated with ultraviolet light, usually through exposure of the body to sunlight, is transformed into active vitamin D_3. Cholesterol in the skin along with other lipids makes the skin resistant to the action of many chemical agents and to the absorption of water-soluble substances. Cholesterol and other lipids are highly inert to acids and certain solvents, which serves to prevent penetration into the body. Water evaporation from the skin is prevented by the presence of cholesterol and other lipids. Abnormal deposits of cholesterol in the tissues are associated with several conditions, including atherosclerosis, hypertension and diabetes.

METABOLISM The main site of cholesterol synthesis is in the liver cells but it can also be synthesized in almost all other tissues. The liver is also a storage depot for cholesterol absorbed from the intestine. The rate of endogenous cholesterol synthesis is variable. It has been estimated to vary between 0.5 gm. and 2 gm. per day.[9] The enterohepatic cholesterol pool has been estimated to be about 2000 mg. (2 gm.).

The complex ring structure of cholesterol can be completely synthesized in the body from a simple two-carbon unit, acetate, through the active form acetyl-coenzyme A. Cholesterol is on the pathway of synthesis of yet more complicated structures such as the steroid hormones and the bile acids.

Cholesterol esters are hydrolyzed in the intestinal tract but the cholesterol is largely re-esterified during the process of absorption. It is incorporated into the chylomicrons formed in the intestinal wall and transported via the lymphatic circulation to the liver. In the blood, cholesterol is present free and esterified with fatty acids as part of the lipoprotein complex.

The principal products of cholesterol breakdown are the bile acids which are formed in the liver and are delivered into the small intestine in the bile secretions. About 80 per cent of the cholesterol metabolized is converted to bile acids. Both bile acids and cholesterol are continually reabsorbed from the intestine, pass again into the liver and are re-excreted in the bile. This is known as the enterohepatic cycle. The liver is also responsible for regulating the rate of loss of cholesterol from the body. Cholesterol is excreted as such or as a cholic acid derivative in the bile. Little cholic acid is excreted in the feces. Some cholesterol enters the intestinal tract by direct excretion across the intestinal mucosa as well as via the bile. In the lumen of the intestine a portion is hydrogenated to coprosterol by intestinal organisms. Coprosterol cannot be absorbed and is excreted in the feces. Very little cholesterol is excreted in the urine; some is lost by way of the skin.

The physiological and metabolic relationships among body fat, cholesterol, phospholipids, unsaturated fatty acids and atherosclerosis are complex and not completely understood, but are the object of much present-day medical research.

Dietary Sources   Cholesterol occurs in largest amounts in egg yolk, liver, kidney, sweetbreads, brains, fish roe, and oysters. Cholesterol is also present in smaller amount in the fat of meat, whole milk, cream, ice cream, cheese, and butter. Foods that are low in cholesterol or contain no cholesterol are fruits, vegetables, cereals, breadstuffs, syrup,

egg white, low-fat fish, very lean meats, soup stock made without fat, and skim milk. However, it must be pointed out that the amount synthesized and metabolized daily by the body itself is far greater than the amount usually consumed in the diet. It has been estimated that in humans receiving 0.5 to 0.8 gm. of cholesterol in the diet (exogenous), 1.0 to 1.5 gm is synthesized:

EXOGENOUS CHOLESTEROL

1 egg	275 mg.
4 oz. meat	100 mg.
1 pt. milk, whole	50 mg.
2 tbsp. butter	75 mg.
Total	500 mg.

The level of cholesterol in the blood is not significantly influenced by the amount present in foods. If protective foods such as eggs, milk and organ meats are omitted from the diet to control the cholesterol level of the blood, one may be denying the body needed protein, minerals and vitamins. It is important that the nurse understand the limitations of diet in the lowering of blood cholesterol so that she can intelligently answer the numerous questions of her patients.

REGULATION OF DIETARY FATS AND BLOOD CHOLESTEROL LEVELS

The dietary fat intake has been shown to have an effect on the serum cholesterol level of individuals. Populations (United States, Great Britain, Finland) consuming diets high in fat usually have relatively high serum cholesterol levels. Populations (Japan, Italy) with a low fat intake usually have relatively low serum cholesterol levels.

The total concentration of cholesterol in the blood plasma is highly variable, averaging about 200 mg. per 100 ml. (range between 150 and 250 mg. per 100 ml.) in the adult, of which amount 30 per cent is in the free form and the remainder in the form of cholesterol esters. The liver is primarily responsible for the maintenance of plasma cholesterol level as well as the ester-free cholesterol ratio. The blood cholesterol levels probably reflect the difference between the rate of synthesis and the rate of destruction. The dietary factors[10] that affect the plasma concentration of cholesterol may be summarized as follows:

[9]Report: Dietary fat and human health, Washington, D.C., National Research Council, Pub. No. 1147, 1966, p. 19.

[10]Guyton, A. C.: Textbook of Medical Physiology. 4th ed. Philadelphia, W. B. Saunders Company, 1971, p. 809.

1. A high intake of dietary cholesterol normally increases the blood cholesterol level a few milligrams per 100 ml. The liver normally compensates for the high exogenous intake of cholesterol by synthesizing smaller quantities of endogenous cholesterol.

2. A dietary containing only saturated fat (butter, coconut oil, fat of meat) increases the blood cholesterol level as much as 40 to 50 mg. per 100 ml. A high fat consumption presumably increases fat deposition in the liver which in turn increases the rate of fat metabolism and supplies increased amounts of acetyl-CoA in the liver cells for the manufacture of cholesterol. A decrease, therefore, in the amount of saturated fats rather than of cholesterol is indicated.

3. A dietary intake of the polyunsaturated fats such as corn oil, cottonseed oil and safflower oil effectively lowers serum cholesterol levels.

Other factors such as the lack of thyroxine and an excess secretion of the thyroid hormone decrease the blood cholesterol levels. Estrogens decrease serum cholesterol and androgens increase serum cholesterol. How this occurs is unknown. In diabetes mellitus the blood cholesterol level rises, probably because of the increase in the mobilization of lipids. The blood cholesterol level rises along with blood triglyceride and phospholipid levels in renal retention diseases, resulting from a diminished removal of lipoproteins from the blood.

Claims for hydrogenated vegetable oils must be reviewed with the knowledge that hydrogenation converts polyunsaturated fatty acids into monounsaturated or completely saturated compounds. A product may be derived from 100 per cent vegetable oil, but when it is hydrogenated, it loses most, or all, of its polyunsaturated qualities. Vegetable oil is converted to solid margarine in two ways. In one method, a measured amount of saturated or hydrogenated fat is mixed with pure oil. The resulting loss of polyunsaturated fatty acids is by dilution. In the other method, direct hydrogenation is used. This process significantly reduces polyunsaturated fatty acid content. See Table 5–3 for characteristics of various margarines.

In 1964 the Food and Drug Administration moved to prohibit manufacturers from branding vegetable oil products as "polyunsaturated." The action was taken following a consumer survey on public understanding of current labeling of such products. The survey revealed that label terms such as "polyunsaturated," "unsaturated," "low in cholesterol," and similar statements mislead many people to believe that these foods will reduce blood cholesterol and thus be effective in treating or preventing heart and artery diseases. It is believed they play no significant part in reducing blood cholesterol unless the diet is changed in other respects; even this is still experimental theory. Cholesterol is further discussed under diseases of the gallbladder and in relation to atherosclerosis. Diets with modified cholesterol and fat content appear on page 363. Also, see Appendix Tables 1, 4, and 5 for cholesterol and fatty acid content of foods.

METABOLISM AND STORAGE OF FAT

Almost all the lipids of the diet are absorbed into the lymph from the intestinal mucosa. Only the medium chain fatty acids are absorbed directly into the portal blood. The lipids are carried in the lymph as chylomicrons, droplets of fat with cholesterol and phospholipids with a small amount of protein adsorbed to their outer surface. The droplets are large enough to make the plasma appear milky. They empty into the venous blood at the thoracic duct and are carried to the liver.

In the liver lipids may be metabolized or converted to alpha- and beta-lipoproteins in which form they are carried in the blood to the tissues for immediate use for energy or special functions or to the adipose tissue for storage.

The principal stores of body fat are found in three places: (1) subcutaneous tissue—50 per cent, (2) abdominal cavity, around the internal organs—45 per cent, (3) intramuscular tissue —5 per cent. The fat present in adipose tissue appears mostly as triglyceride. In the fat cells are modified fibroblasts which store up to 95 per cent of their volume as triglycerides

TABLE 5–3   CHARACTERISTICS OF MARGARINES

TYPE OF MARGARINE	IODINE NO.	EFA* (PERCENTAGE)
Hydrogenated cottonseed-soybean oil	95.7	27.7
Hydrogenated corn oil	82.9	14.5
Hydrogenated soybean, liquid corn oil	94.8	3.17
Liquid and hydrogenated soy-cotton oil	114.5	47.6
Safflower, hydrogenated soybean oil	125.1	66.4
Liquid cottonseed and soybean oil	97.7	40.9
Canadian (hydrogenated rapeseed oil)	77.2	3.0

*EFA = Essential fatty acid.
(From Sgoutas, D. S., and Kummerow, F.: Incorporation of trans-fatty acids into tissue lipids. Am. J. Clin. Nutr., 23:1112, 1970.)

in liquid form. Fat storage is not static. Adipose tissue contains considerable amounts of lipases, the enzymes which catalyze the hydrolysis of fats to fatty acids and glycerol and the reverse synthetic reaction. There is rapid exchange between the non-esterified fatty acids of the plasma and the adipose tissue lipid.

The first step in catabolism of triglyceride is hydrolysis to glycerol and fatty acid. The non-esterified fatty acid is bound to serum albumin—it is not a component of lipoproteins. Although a great deal of fatty acid is transported in this form, its level in the plasma remains low, since it is picked up by the tissues very rapidly. As the first stage in oxidation of fatty acids they are broken down stepwise into two-carbon units complexed with Coenzyme A. This complex is also an intermediate metabolite in glucose metabolism and from this point fatty acids and glucose are oxidized by the same pathway. Glycerol also, after activation, may be converted to an intermediate of glucose oxidation. These steps will be discussed in detail in a later chapter.

Almost all tissues can utilize fatty acids for energy. Contrary to earlier opinion they form a large portion of the energy for muscular tissue even when glucose is available. Glycerol can be oxidized in only a few tissues; most of it is carried to the liver.

The liver is a major center of lipid metabolism and is largely responsible for regulation of lipid levels in the body. Among its important functions are (1) synthesis of triglycerides from carbohydrate and, to a smaller extent, from protein; (2) synthesis of other lipids such as phospholipids and cholesterol from triglycerides; and (3) desaturation of fatty acids (oleic acid is the predominant acid in human adipose tissue). A primary function is degradation of triglycerides for use as energy. Even under normal conditions the liver produces more acetyl-CoA than it can oxidize completely. Two molecules of acetyl-CoA condense to form acetoacetic acid.

$$2 \text{ CH}_3\text{CO CoA H}_2\text{O} \xrightleftharpoons[\text{Other Cells}]{\text{Liver Cells}}$$
Acetyl-CoA

$$\begin{array}{ll} \text{CH}_3\text{COCH}_2\text{COOH} & 2 \text{ H CoA} \\ \text{Acetoacetic Acid} & \text{Coenzyme A} \end{array}$$

The acetoacetic acid diffuses through the liver cell membranes and is carried to peripheral tissues where it is converted again to acetyl-CoA and oxidized. When the body is relying almost entirely on fat for energy, as in diabetes mellitus or prolonged starvation, large quantities of triglyceride appear in the liver and the production of acetoacetic acids far outstrips the ability of the peripheral tissues to oxidize it and the level in the blood rises. Part of the acetoacetic acid is converted to beta-hydroxybutyric acid and acetone—the three compounds being known collectively as the ketone bodies. Two of the ketone bodies are strongly acidic and must be carried in the blood and excreted in the urine in combination with base (sodium ion). This reduces the available base in the body and the condition, if unchecked, leads to a lowering of the pH of body fluids (acidosis) which may be fatal. In diabetic acidosis carbohydrate metabolism returns to normal when insulin and glucose are given and the breakdown of fat is slowed to a normal pace.

HORMONAL CONTROL OF FAT METABOLISM The hormones secreted by the endocrine glands which have marked effects on carbohydrate metabolism also affect fat metabolism. They are

(1) Insulin, which in insufficient amount decreases fat synthesis and increases fat mobilization and utilization. Excessive insulin inhibits fat utilization and increases fat synthesis.

(2) Thyroxine, which increases mobilization of fats caused indirectly by the increased rate of energy metabolism regulated by this hormone.

(3) Glucocorticoids, which increase the rate of fat mobilization. Lack of or absence of glucocorticoids depresses fat mobilization and utilization.

(4) Adrenocorticoids (growth hormone), which increase fat mobilization.

(5) Epinephrine, which increases the rate of fat mobilization by releasing free fatty acids from fat cells for metabolism. Figure 5–2 shows in simple fashion the various excursions fat can take in the body.

CHANGES IN FAT CONSUMPTION

Fats supply roughly 41 per cent of the total calories available for consumption in the retail market in the United States.[11, 12] Fat consumed from animal and vegetable sources has increased from 125 to 145 gm. per person per day (Table 5–4) from the period of 1909–1912 to 1965.[13] The consumption of vegetable fat during the same period has increased from 17.0 to 34.1 per cent. During the period from

[11]U.S. Department of Agriculture, Economic Research Service: U.S. Food Consumption: Sources of Data and Trends. Washington, D.C., Statist. Bull. No. 364, 1965.

[12]U.S. Department of Agriculture: National Food Situation, 122:31, 1967.

[13]Friend, B.: Nutrients in United States food supply, A review of trends 1909–13 to 1965. Am. J. Clin. Nutr., 20:907, 1967.

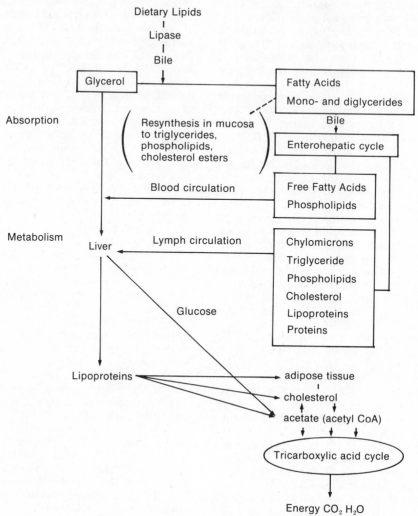

Figure 5–2   Brief summary of fat metabolism.

TABLE 5–4   FAT AVAILABLE PER PERSON PER DAY, AND SOURCES OF FAT

| | | ANIMAL SOURCES | | | | | VEGETABLE SOURCES | | | | |
YEAR	FAT, g	% Meat, Poultry, Fish	% Eggs	% Dairy Products, Excluding Butter	% Butter and Lard[a]	% Total[b]	% Other Fats and Oils[c]	% Dry Beans, Peas, Nuts, Soya Products	% Flour and Cereal Products	% Other Foods	% Total[b]
1909–1913	125	37.4	3.8	14.9	27.0	83.1	9.8	11.9	3.8	1.5	17.0
1925–1929	135	32.9	3.8	15.3	26.2	78.2	14.0	22.8	2.9	2.9	21.8
1935–1939	133	29.9	3.5	15.8	24.1	73.3	18.4	33.3	2.5	2.6	26.8
1947–1949	141	33.5	4.3	17.3	19.5	74.6	17.8	33.4	1.9	2.4	25.6
1957–1959	143	33.0	4.0	16.5	17.1	70.6	22.3	33.2	1.5	2.3	29.3
1965	145	33.6	3.4	14.6	14.4	66.0	26.7	33.7	1.5	2.2	34.1

[a]Includes small amounts of edible beef fats.
[b]Components may not add to total due to rounding.
[c]Includes margarine and shortening minus lard used in their manufacture, salad and cooking oils.
(Adapted from Friend, B.: Nutrients in U. S. food supply. A review of trends 1909–1913 to 1965. Am. J. Clin. Nutr., 20:910, 1967.)

TABLE 5–5   FATTY ACIDS AVAILABLE, PER PERSON PER DAY, AND PER CENT OF TOTAL CALORIES

YEAR	FATTY ACIDS			KCALORIES FURNISHED BY FATTY ACIDS			RATIO OF POLYUNSATURATED TO SATURATED FATTY ACIDS
	Total Saturated, g	Oleic Acid, g	Linoleic, Acid, g	% Total Saturated	% Oleic Acid	% Linoleic Acid	
1909–1913	50.3	51.5	10.7	12.9	13.3	2.7	0.20
1925–1929	53.3	55.2	12.5	13.7	14.2	3.2	0.23
1935–1939	52.9	54.5	12.7	14.4	14.8	3.5	0.24
1947–1949	54.4	58.0	14.8	15.0	16.0	4.1	0.27
1957–1959	54.7	58.2	16.6	15.6	16.6	4.7	0.30
1965	53.9	58.8	19.1	15.2	16.6	5.4	0.35

(Adapted from Friend, B.: Nutrients in U. S. food supply. A review of trends 1909–1913 to 1965. Am. J. Clin. Nutr., 20:911, 1967.)

1947 to 1965 the proportion of total fat available from animal sources has decreased from approximately 75 to 66 per cent and that from vegetable sources has increased from approximately 26 to 34 per cent. Although the American diet contained more fat in 1965, the saturated fatty acid content decreased from 40 to 37 per cent during the 55-year period.[14] The consumption of oleic acid remains about the same at 41 per cent of the total fat, and linoleic acid has increased from 8 to 13 per cent of the total fat during this period of study.[15] For the 18-year period from 1947 there was practically no change in the quantity of saturated fatty acids in marketed foods but the polyunsaturated fatty acid content was increased (Table 5–5).[16] The ratio of polyunsaturated (linoleic acid) to saturated fatty acids progressively increased from 0.27 in 1947 to 0.35 in 1965. It should be pointed out that wastage, cooking and other losses were not considered in the survey, so that the actual fat ingested is less than that available for consumption.

The trend toward a higher proportion of the calorie intake in the form of fat has been accompanied by a shift in dietary sources of food fats. Consumption of corn, cottonseed and soybean oils in salad and cooking; the trend toward the substitution of margarines for butter; and the increase in poultry consumption are in part reducing the consumption of foods that may be higher in saturated fatty acids.

According to a recent survey[17] about two-fifths of the calories from fat available per person per day comes from the visible fats such as butter and lard, margarine, and salad and cooking oils. Approximately three-fifths of the fat calories are supplied by the so-called invisible fats in foods such as meat, eggs, dairy products excluding butter, nuts, leg-

[14]Friend, B.: Nutrients in United States food supply. A review of trends 1909–1913 to 1965. Am. J. Clin. Nutr., 20:907, 1967.
[15]Ibid.
[16]Ibid.

[17]Friend, B.: Nutrients in United States food supply. A review of trends 1909–1913 to 1965. Am. J. Clin. Nutr., 20:907, 1967.

TABLE 5–6   SOURCES OF FAT IN THE FATS AND OILS GROUP, PER PERSON PER DAY[a]

YEAR	ANIMAL SOURCES								VEGETABLE SOURCES			
	Butter, g	Lard				Edible Beef Fats			Total, g[c]	Marga-rine, g	Short-ening, g	Salad and Cooking Oils, g	Total, g[c]
		Direct Use,[b] g	Indirect Use		Total, g[c]	Short-ening, g	Marga-rine, g	Total, g[c]					
			Short-ening, g	Marga-rine, g									
1909–1913	17.7	14.7	0.0	0.2	14.9	0.8	0.4	1.2	33.8	0.8	9.6	1.9	12.3
1925–1929	18.1	15.7	0.1	0.2	16.1	0.6	0.5	1.1	35.3	1.7	11.2	6.0	18.9
1935–1939	17.1	13.7	[d]	0.0	13.7	1.1	0.1	1.2	32.0	2.8	13.6	8.1	24.5
1947–1949	10.6	15.4	1.0	0.0	16.4	0.4	0.1	0.5	27.5	5.5	10.6	9.1	25.2
1957–1959	8.2	11.5	2.9	0.1	14.5	1.6	0.1	1.8	24.5	8.7	9.7	13.5	31.9
1965	6.5	8.0	3.1	0.5	11.6	2.6	0.1	2.7	20.8	9.5	11.6	17.6	38.7

[a]Quantities are given in terms of grams to facilitate use of data.
[b]Use of lard as lard.
[c]Components may not add to total due to rounding.
[d]0.05 g or less.
(Adapted from Friend, B.: Nutrients in U. S. food supply. A review of trends 1909–1913 to 1965. Am. J. Clin. Nutr., 20:911, 1967.)

umes and cereals (Table 5–6). Approximately two-thirds of the fat is from animal sources and one-third is of vegetable origin.

RECOMMENDED ALLOWANCE OF FATS IN THE DIET

The average American adult eats about 110 pounds of fat yearly, receiving perhaps 41 per cent of his total calories as fat. This includes both visible and invisible fats, a distinction of convenience. Fats are popular because of their flavor and satiety value. But their cost is greater than the cost of carbohydrates.

Americans consume more fat than is necessary and probably more than is good for them. The requirement of the human for the essential fatty acid has been estimated to be approximately 2 per cent of the calorie intake (infants, 1 to 3 per cent) of the diet. It is the consensus among nutritionists that the average diet should contain at least 25 per cent of its calories as fat. The precise amount of fat in the diets of the general public becomes less meaningful in the light of results published by Albrink and others which show that a decrease in dietary fat is usually accompanied by an increase in carbohydrate, which may correlate with a rise in blood triglycerides.[18]

Recently, dietary fat has become a very controversial topic. Emphasis has been placed on the possible ill effect of an excess intake of fat per se or excess intake of cholesterol and the saturated fatty acids. The high fat diet consumed in America is generally rich in saturated fatty acids, though this component still amounts to less than half of the total fat. However, it is certainly premature to recommend that all saturated fats be eliminated from the diet, even if this were possible.

The American Medical Association Council on Foods and Nutrition[19] expresses concern over possible harm resulting from severe reduction (0 to 15 per cent of total calories) of dietary fat, both in quantity and in proportion to other nutrients. Prolonged low fat regimens may lead to deficiencies of the essential polyunsaturated fatty acid. Since dietary fat is the carrier of the four fat-soluble vitamins (A, D, E, and K) and carotene, deficiencies in those nutrients may develop during prolonged periods of fat restriction.

Although the precise role of dietary fat in the pathogenesis of coronary atherosclerosis has not been determined, most authorities currently advocate some dietary restriction of total fat, saturated fatty acids, cholesterol and sucrose for the prevention of coronary artery disease. This is further discussed in Chapter 30, Cardiovascular Diseases.

As information on amounts of these factors present in different foods has become available, use has been made of the findings in prescribing and planning diets. See Appendix, Tables 1, 4, and 5 for fatty acid and cholesterol content of foods.

COOKING AND DIGESTIBILITY OF FATS

Cooking by the usual methods has no appreciable effect on the essential fatty acid. However, heating fat at very high temperatures burns the fat, resulting in the decomposition of the fat and the production of the substance acrolein. Acrolein may be very irritating to the nasal passages and to the gastrointestinal mucosa. Properly fried foods should have no adverse effect on normal digestion, but improperly fried foods do involve more effort on the part of the digestive system and therefore should never be served to the sick.

Digestibility of food fats varies to some degree and, of course, the hydrocarbon materials are not digestible or absorbable, as mentioned previously. Contrary to popular opinion, most fats are highly digestible; over 95 per cent of ingested fats is normally absorbed and utilized in the body. The absorption rate of fats varies, depending largely upon the melting point of the fat. Fats which are liquid at body temperature are more rapidly absorbed than the solid fats. The rate of absorption is markedly enhanced by the presence of phospholipids and is also influenced by the quantity and type of mixture of fats eaten. The more rapidly absorbed fat is more quickly available to the tissues for energy. However, the more slowly absorbed fats remain in the intestines longer, thus extending the satiety period and producing much lower fluctuations in blood lipid levels following a meal. Sherman[20] suggests that these fats offer likelihood of overtaxing the lipid transport system of the blood with solid fats, which may be of significance in connecction with the currently much discussed development of atherosclerosis.

---

[18]Mead, J. E.: Present knowledge of fat. In: Present Knowledge in Nutrition. 3rd ed. New York, The Nutrition Foundation, Inc., 1967, p. 16.

[19]J.A.M.A., *181*:411, 1962.

---

[20]Sherman, W. C.: Foods and nutrition news. National Live Stock and Meat Board, 33(No. 2):3, 1961.

PROBLEMS AND SUGGESTED TOPICS FOR DISCUSSION

1. List the amount of the various fat foods you consume during a period of 24 hours. Calculate the percentage of total calories that were derived from fat.
2. Classify the fats in your diet for 1 day into "invisible" and "visible" fat foods; saturated and unsaturated.
3. What percentage of the daily dietary in the United States is consumed in the form of fat foods? What does this mean in terms of fat intake?
4. Why do you like to eat fat foods?
5. How do you obtain essential fatty acid in your diet?
6. Explain what is meant by saturated fat, unsaturated fat and hydrogenation. Explain their importance in nutrition and health.
7. Explain the metabolism and storage of fats in the body after absorption.
8. What is ketosis? Under what conditions does it occur?
9. Are fats a cheap or expensive source of energy? Explain.
10. What are the functions of fats in the body?
11. Survey the literature and report on the most recent research on human fat requirements in relation to cholesterol, saturated and unsaturated fats.
12. Evaluate the fats in your usual diet. How can your diet be improved?

SUGGESTED ADDITIONAL READING REFERENCES

Brown, H. B.: Fashioning a practical vegetable-oil food pattern. J. Am. Dietet. A., 38:536, 1961.

Burton, B. T. (ed.): The Heinz Handbook of Nutrition. 2nd ed. New York, McGraw-Hill Book Company, Inc., 1965, Chapter 9.

Calvy, G. L., et al.: Serum lipids and enzymes. J.A.M.A., 183:1, 1963.

Cantarow, A., and Trumper, M.: Clinical Biochemistry. 6th ed. Philadelphia, W. B. Saunders Company, 1962, pp. 71–102.

Dairy Council Digest: Current research on dietary fatty acids. National Dairy Council, Chicago, 41:No. 3, May-June, 1970.

Duncan, G. G. (ed.): Diseases of Metabolism. 5th ed. Philadelphia, W. B. Saunders Company, 1964, Chapter 3, Lipid Metabolism.

Ende, N.: Starvation studies with special reference to cholesterol. Am. J. Clin. Nutr., 11:270, 1962.

Food: The Yearbook of Agriculture. Washington, D.C., United States Department of Agriculture, 1959, pp. 74–87.

Friend, B.: Nutrients in United States food supplies. A review of trends 1909–1913 to 1965. Am. J. Clin. Nutr., 20:907, 1967.

Gorman, J. C., and Moore, M. E.: Fatty acids in vegetarian diets. J. Am. Dietet. A., 50:372, 1967.

Green, J. G., et al.: Use of fat-modified foods for serum cholesterol reduction. J.A.M.A., 183:5, 1963.

Guyton, A. C.: Textbook of Medical Physiology. 4th ed. Philadelphia, W. B. Saunders Company, 1971.

Hansen, A. E., et al.: Role of linoleic acid in infant nutrition. Pediatrics, 31:171, 1963.

Hayes, O. B., and Rose, G.: Supplementary food composition table. J. Am. Dietet. A., 33:26, 1957.

Holman, R. T.: How essential are fatty acids? J.A.M.A., 178:930, 1961.

Kinsell, L. W., et al.: Dietary considerations with regard to type of fat. Am. J. Clin. Nutr., 15:198, 1964.

Macdonald, I.: Interrelationships between the influences of dietary carbohydrates and fats on fasting serum lipids. Am. J. Clin. Nutr., 20:345, 1967.

Mazur, A., and Harrow, B.: Textbook of Biochemistry. 10th ed. Philadelphia, W. B. Saunders Company, 1971.

McOsker, D. E., et al.: The influence of partially hydrogenated dietary fats on serum cholesterol levels. J.A.M.A., 180:380, 1962.

Morse, E. H., et al.: Effect of two fats on blood lipids in young men. J. Am. Dietet. A., 46:193, 1965.

Perkins, R., Wright, I. S., and Gatzi, B. W.: Safflower oil-pyridoxine and corn oil-pyridoxine emulsions. J.A.M.A., 169:1731, 1959.

Report. Council on Foods and Nutrition, A.M.A.: The regulation of dietary fat. J.A.M.A., 181:139, 1962.

Report: Dietary Fat and Human Health. A Report of the Food and Nutrition Board, National Academy of Sciences–National Research Council, Pub. No. 1147, 1966.

Report. Household Food Consumption Survey 1955, Report No. 10. Washington, D.C., United States Department of Agriculture.

Review. Body fat and adipose tissue. Nutr. Rev., 22:99, 1964.

Review. Council report on dietary fat regulation. Nutr. Rev., 21:36, 1963.

Review. Diet and human depot fat. Nutr. Rev., 21:4, 1963.

Review. Fat and cholesterol in the diet. Nutr. Rev., 23:3, 1965.

Roehm, R. R., and Mayfield, H. L.: Effect of dietary fat on cholesterol. Metabolism, 40:417, 1962.

Sgoutas, D., and Kummerow, F. A.: Incorporation of trans-fatty acids into tissue lipids. Am. J. Clin. Nutr., 23:1111, 1970.

Sherman, W. C.: Fat in nutrition. National Live Stock and Meat Board Food and Nutrition News, 33(No. 2):3; (No. 3):3, 1961; (No. 4):3, 1962.

Steiner, A., Howard, E. J., and Akgun, S.: Importance of dietary cholesterol in man. J.A.M.A., 181:186, 1962.

The Nutrition Foundation Inc.: Present Knowledge in Nutrition. 3rd ed. New York, 99 Park Avenue, 1967. Chapter 4. Present Knowledge of Fat.

Underwood, B. A., et al.: Fatty acid absorption and metabolism in protein-calorie malnutrition. Am. J. Clin. Nutr., 20:226, 1967.

Wilcox, E. B., and Galloway, L. S.: Serum cholesterol and different dietary fats. J. Am. Dietet. A., 38:227, 1961.

Wohl, M. G., and Goodhart, R. S. (ed.): Modern Nutrition in Health and Disease. 4th ed. Philadelphia, Lea & Febiger, 1968, Chapter 8, The Absorption, Digestion and Metabolism of Fats and of Related Lipids.

Chapter 6
PROTEINS
AND
AMINO
ACIDS

DEFINITION AND IMPORTANCE

Protein derived its name more than a century ago from a Greek word meaning "of first importance." It was the first substance recognized as a vital part of living tissue. Proteins, the key components of all living organisms, are nitrogen-containing compounds which yield amino acids on hydrolysis. Proteins are the fundamental structural compounds of the cell, antibodies, enzymes and many of the hormones. They are essential constituents of the nucleus and protoplasm of every cell and they are almost the sole form in which man can replace nitrogen. Proteins are the most abundant of the organic compounds in the body. Most of the protein is found in muscle tissue; the remainder is distributed in soft tissues, bones, teeth, blood and other body fluids. Since proteins serve such important and essential functions in the body, and since certain indispensable protein components can be obtained solely through dietary intake, it is obvious that the quality and amounts of protein in the daily diet and a knowledge of protein sources and of protein metabolism are matters of considerable moment to those interested in dietetics and medical sciences.

THE COMPOSITION AND NATURE OF PROTEINS

Proteins, like fats and carbohydrates, contain carbon, hydrogen and oxygen but, in addition, they also contain about 16 per cent *nitrogen* along with sulfur and sometimes other elements such as phosphorus, iron and cobalt. The structural units of protein are the amino acids. They are united in long chains in various geometric structures and chemical combinations to form specific proteins, all of which are very large and complex molecules, each with its own physiological specificity. Despite their structural complexity proteins can be hydrolyzed (broken down) into their amino acid constituent by enzymes or by boiling with acids and alkalis under certain conditions. Pure dry proteins are fairly stable, but under the conditions in which they are found in foods they tend to decompose at room temperatures, aided by bacterial action, and may form products that are toxic to the body; thus, the necessity for keeping protein foods such as eggs, fish, fowl, meat and milk refrigerated.

Plants obtain their nitrogen from the nitrates and ammonia in the soil, and from them synthesize their protein. Animals, in turn, obtain their nitrogen and protein from protein foods (plants and other animals). Animal metabolism, excretion and death finally return the nitrogen to the soil. This continuing process is known as the "nitrogen cycle."

AMINO ACIDS

Twenty-three amino acids have been recognized as constituents of protein. They are all alpha-amino carboxylic acids: that is, they have a basic amino group and an acid carboxylic group attached to the same carbon atom.

$$
\begin{array}{c}
H \\
| \\
R-C-COOH \\
| \\
NH_2
\end{array}
$$

They are differentiated by the remainder of the molecule (R), as illustrated above.

66

$$\underset{\text{Alanine}}{\underset{\underset{\displaystyle CH_3}{|}}{\underset{\displaystyle H_2N-CH}{|}}\overset{\displaystyle O}{\underset{\displaystyle C}{\|}}-\boxed{OH \quad H}} \quad \underset{\text{Serine}}{\overset{\displaystyle H \quad COOH}{\underset{\underset{\displaystyle CH_2OH}{|}}{N-CH}}} \quad \xrightarrow{H_2O} \quad \underset{\text{Alanyl-serine}}{\overset{\displaystyle O \quad H \quad COOH}{\underset{\underset{\displaystyle CH_3}{|}}{\underset{\displaystyle H_2N-CH \quad CH_2OH}{|}}}}$$

Formation of a Dipeptide

Amino acids, because they have both an acidic and basic group, have a buffer capacity. Depending on pH they can form salts with either acids or bases.

STRUCTURE OF PROTEINS   Amino acids join together to form proteins by means of the peptide link: the carboxylic carbon of one acid attaches to the nitrogen of another acid (a molecule of water being formed at the same time). The resulting compound has a free carboxyl group at one end and a free amino group at the other, so that the chain can continue to be built up from both ends.

Proteins vary in size from relatively small polypeptides such as ACTH with a molecular weight of 3200 (23 amino acid units) to very complex molecules with several hundred thousand amino acid units. The polypeptide chains take the form of a helix. Several chains may be linked together (usually through the S–S link of cystine). In addition, the entire chain may be wound upon itself into a globular or other form—the whole being held rigid by interatomic forces such as hydrogen bonds. The structure of a protein may thus be considered at three levels: the primary structure is the number, kind, and order of the amino acid chains; the secondary structure is the helical form; and the tertiary structure is the spatial arrangement. It is because of the almost infinite possibilities of variation offered by these structures that there are millions (or more) of different proteins with specific properties and biological functions.

Studies on the shape of protein molecules indicate that there are two general types: globular proteins, with a length:width ratio less than 10, and fibrous proteins with a ratio greater than 10. The fibrous proteins are used in the formation of structural elements. They may have several helical peptide chains twisted together to form a stiff rod. They are characterized by low solubility and high mechanical strength. Collagen of connective tissue, keratin of hair and myosin of muscle tissue are examples of fibrous protein.

Globular proteins are found in the extracellular fluid of plants and animals, and in conjugated form constitute most intracellular enzymes. They are very soluble and are easily denatured.[1] Some globular proteins of interest in nutrition are caseinogen in milk, egg albumin, the albumins and globulins of blood plasma, and hemoglobin.

ESSENTIAL AMINO ACIDS   There are eight amino acids which are classfied as essential, since they must be supplied in the food. Body synthesis is lacking or so limited as to be unable to meet metabolic needs. They are valine, lysine, threonine, leucine, isoleucine, tryptophan, phenylalanine and methionine. Two other amino acids, arginine and histidine, are required by children during periods of growth. Without an adequate supply of the essential amino acids, protein cannot be synthesized or body tissue maintained. (See Figure 6–1.)

The other amino acids which can be syn-

---

[1] Agents and conditions that do not hydrolyze peptide bonds may destroy the biological nature and activity of the protein. These are heat, air, ultraviolet radiations, alcohol, strong acids or bases, detergents, salts of heavy metals, alkaloidal reagents such as tannic acid and violent shaking. The protein usually coagulates after denaturation.

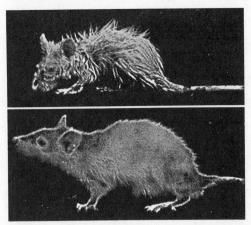

Figure 6–1   Effects of lack of one of the essential amino acids. The upper photograph shows a rat on the 28th day of valine deprivation. The lower photograph shows the same animal after valine had been administered for 25 days. (Courtesy of Rose and Eppstein and the Journal of Biological Chemistry.)

TABLE 6–1   ESSENTIAL AMINO ACIDS

ESSENTIAL AMINO ACIDS	MINIMUM REQUIREMENTS			RECOMMENDED DAILY INTAKE (in gm.)	AVERAGE AMERICAN DIET (in gm.)‡
	Infants (gm. per kilogram)*	Adult, female (gm. per day)**	Adult, male (gm. per day)†		
Tryptophan	0.022	0.157	0.25	0.5	0.9
Threonine	0.087	0.350	0.50	1.0	2.8
Isoleucine	0.126	0.450	0.70	1.4	4.2
Leucine	0.150	0.620	1.10	2.2	6.5
Lysine	0.103	0.500	0.80	1.6	4.0
Methionine	0.045[1]	0.350[1]	1.10[3]	2.2	3.0
Phenylalanine	0.090[2]	0.220[2]	1.10[4]	2.2	4.1
Valine	0.105	0.650	0.80	1.6	4.2
Histidine	0.034	—	—	—	—

[1]In presence of adequate cystine.
[2]In presence of adequate tyrosine.
[3]Cystine replaces part of methionine allowance (about one-sixth).
[4]Tyrosine replaces part of phenylalanine allowance (about one-half).

*Holt, L. E., et al.: Protein and amino acid requirements in early life. New York, New York University Press, 1960.
** Food and Nutrition Board. Committee in Amino Acids: Evaluation of protein nutrition. Washington, D.C., National Academy of Science, National Research Council, Pub. No. 711, 1959.
†Rose, W. C., et al.: The amino acid requirements of man. J. Biol. Chem., 217:987, 1955.
‡Bogert, L. J., et al.: Nutrition and Physical Fitness. 8th ed. Philadelphia, W. B. Saunders Company, 1966, p. 115.

thesized by the body in adequate amounts for normal function are termed non-essential. This is not to suggest that these amino acids are not essential constituents of the proteins but that the tissues can make their own supply from carbohydrate, fat and other amino acids. The minimum daily requirements of the essential amino acids for the infant and the adult are listed in Table 6–1. The minimum requirement for the adult female is somewhat lower than that for the adult male.

SPECIAL FUNCTIONS OF AMINO ACIDS Although virtually all the amino acids have certain unique functions in the body, a few are worth singling out. Tryptophan is a precursor of the vitamin niacin. Tryptophan is also a precursor of serotonin, a potent vasoconstrictor found in serum, and it is active in stimulating gastrointestinal activity. Methionine is a principal donor of methyl groups for the synthesis of various compounds such as choline and creatine. Phenylalanine is a precursor of tyrosine and together they lead to the formation of thyroxine and epinephrine. Arginine, ornithine and citrulline, all nonessential amino acids, are specifically involved in the synthesis of urea in the liver. Glycine, the simplest and perhaps most ubiquitous of the amino acids, combines with many toxic substances and converts them to harmless forms which are then excreted. Glycine is also used in the synthesis of the porphyrin nucleus of hemoglobin and is a constituent of one of the bile acids (glycocholic acid). Histidine is essential for the synthesis of histamine which causes vasodilatation in the circulatory system. Epinephrine, synthesized from tyrosine, has a methyl group from methionine. Creatine, synthesized from arginine, glycine and methionine, combines with

phosphate to form creatine phosphate. Creatine phosphate is an important reservoir of high energy phosphate in the cell. Glutamine formed from glutamic acid and asparagin formed from aspartic acid have important roles as reservoirs of amino groups throughout the body. In addition, hippuric acid, nicotinic acid, ornithine, pantothenic acid, purines and taurine are all derived from amino acids.[2] These few examples illustrate some of the important intracellular substances synthesized from amino acids.

CLASSIFICATION OF PROTEINS

It is difficult to devise a consistent system for classification of the multitude of proteins. The following system is based partly on solubility and characteristic physical properties and partly on chemical composition. They are grouped as simple proteins, conjugated proteins and derived proteins.

Simple proteins are those which yield only amino acids upon hydrolysis. They include

Albumins – soluble in water, coagulated by heat.

Globulins – insoluble in water, soluble in dilute salt solution, coagulated by heat.

Glutelins – insoluble in neutral solvents but soluble in dilute acids and alkalis, coagulated by heat.

Prolamins – soluble in 70 to 80 per cent alcohol, insoluble in absolute alcohol, water and salt solutions.

Albuminoids – insoluble in all neutral

[2]Guyton, A. C.: Textbook of Medical Physiology. 4th ed. Philadelphia, W. B. Saunders Company, 1971, p. 296.

solvents and in dilute acids and alkalis (the fibrous proteins).

Histones and Protamines – basic polypeptides, soluble in water, not coagulable by heat. They are found in nuclei of cells.

Conjugated proteins or proteids are combinations of simple proteins and some other non-protein substance, called a prosthetic group, attached to the molecule. They perform functions which neither constituent could properly perform by itself. These include

Nucleoproteins – combinations of simple proteins and nucleic acid. Deoxyribose nucleoproteins are the principal constituents of the genes, and ribose nucleoproteins are necessary for the synthesis of proteins in cytoplasm.

Mucoproteins and Glycoproteins – combination of a protein and large quantities of complex polysaccharides such as mucin found in secretions from gastric mucous membranes.

Lipoproteins – compounds of a protein and a triglyceride or other lipid such as phospholipid or cholesterol found in cell and organelle membranes.

Phosphoproteins – phosphoric acid joined in ester linkage to protein found in casein of milk.

Chromoproteins – compounds of proteins and a non-protein pigment found in flavoproteins, hemoglobin and cytochromes.

Metalloproteins – compounds of metals (copper, magnesium, zinc, iron) attached to protein found in ferritin, hemosiderin, transferrin.

Derived proteins are products formed in the various stages of hydrolysis of the protein molecule. For example, proteoses are formed early in the hydrolysis process while peptones, polypeptides and peptides are products that form near the final stages of protein breakdown.

NITROGEN BALANCE

To determine the extent of protein utilization, the nitrogen balance is studied. The amount of nitrogen is an accurate index of the amount of protein involved. Most proteins contain about 16 per cent nitrogen and this fact is utilized in determining the amount of protein in foods or body substances. The nitrogen content is determined chemically and this figure, multiplied by 6.25, gives the amount of protein present in the substance. Thus, if the amount of nitrogen that goes into the body in food and the amount that leaves the body in the excreta are determined, what has been used by the body can be calculated. If the nitrogen intake and the nitrogen output are equal, the individual is in *nitrogen balance or equilibrium.* Should the intake of nitrogen be greater than the amount excreted in the urine and feces, the individual is in a state of *positive balance;* that is, the build up (anabolism) or synthesis of tissue proteins is greater than the breakdown (catabolic) activities. There is a net gain of protein in the body. Should the excretion of nitrogen be more than that consumed, a state of negative balance exists; that is, the rate of protein breakdown is exceeding the rate of protein synthesis or there is a greater protein utilization than protein intake.

An adult may be maintained in nitrogen and protein equilibrium, or put into positive nitrogen balance (more intake of nitrogen than output in a given period of time) by feeding him mixtures of pure essential amino acids. In other words, protein itself is dispensable, if necessary, so long as the essential amino acids are provided in correct amount and proportion. This fact is utilized medically in parenteral feeding with protein hydrolysate or amino acid mixtures if the patient cannot ingest food. It is necessary, however, to supply adequate calories, vitamins and minerals in these feedings for tissue synthesis to take place.

The Committee on Therapeutic Nutrition, Food and Nutrition Board, National Research Council[3] compiled results to show that "when a mixture of only essential amino acids serves as the sole source of dietary nitrogen, it does not support growth at a rate commensurate with that of intact proteins in a diet of equicaloric and equal nitrogen content. The superiority of a diet containing all of the protein components may indicate that the synthesis of the nonessential amino acids, in addition to the formation of tissue structures, presents too great a burden upon the chemical resources of the cell. When tissue growth or tissue repletion is proceeding at a rapid pace, nonessential amino acids may become limiting factors in the anabolic processes."

BIOLOGICAL VALUE OF PROTEINS AND MUTUAL SUPPLEMENTATION

COMPLETE AND INCOMPLETE PROTEINS
Proteins that contain all the essential amino acids in sufficient quantity and in the right ratio to maintain nitrogen equilibrium and

---

[3]Pollack, H., and Halpern, S. L.: Therapeutic Nutrition. Washington, D.C., National Research Council, Pub. No. 234, 1952, p. 4.

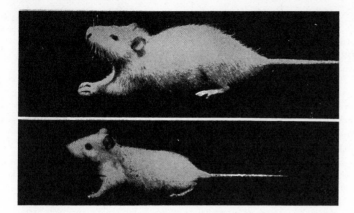

Figure 6–2   Stunting of growth due to feeding an incomplete protein as sole source of protein in the diet. Contrast between two rats of same age kept on diets alike except for the protein, which was a complete protein (casein from milk) in the case of A, and an incomplete protein in the case of B (gliadin from wheat). (From experiments by Osborne and Mendel, Connecticut Agricultural Experimental Station; pictures reproduced by courtesy of Yale University Press.)

permit growth of the young are known as complete proteins. Such proteins are ovalbumin, the main protein of egg, and casein, the principal protein in milk. Other complete proteins are meat, fish and poultry. Proteins that do not supply all the essential amino acids in appropriate amounts to maintain nitrogen equilibrium and growth are incomplete proteins. (See Figure 6–2.) The proteins in vegetables and grains are classified as incomplete proteins. We also refer to the "biological value" of proteins and the biological value is high or low depending upon the completeness with which a protein supplies the essential amino acids. Foods of high protein value are largely of animal origin. Most grain and vegetable proteins are incomplete proteins and thus are of only fair or low biological value.

The incompleteness of proteins may be partial or total. A partially incomplete protein will sustain life but, lacking sufficient amounts of amino acids, will not support normal growth. These are found in legumes, (dried beans and peas, peanuts), nuts and grains. A food protein lacking an essential amino acid will not support life or growth.

Zein, in corn, and gelatin, an animal protein, are examples of totally incomplete proteins. Plant foods generally contain an insufficient quantity of lysine, methionine, threonine and tryptophan. (See Table 6–2.) The amino acids which mutual supplemented plant foods do contribute, however, are important and should be made use of by feeding simultaneously with small amounts of a complete protein food, or by providing a correct mixture of several plant foods which will give all the amino acids in appropriate amounts, or by adding synthetic amino acids to foods to make a complete protein. The distribution of the essential amino acids in eggs and human milk (see Table 6–3) have been recommended by the Joint Committee of FAO/WHO for use as the ideal reference pattern[4] in the appraisal of food combinations which supply a complete protein. The distribution of the essential amino acids found in the proteins of cow's milk is also shown in Table 6–3. The amount of protein, 6 to 7 gm., is provided by a 50-gm.

---

[4] Joint FAO/WHO Expert Group: Protein requirements. Technical Report 301, World Health Organization, Geneva, Switzerland, 1965.

TABLE 6–2   ESSENTIAL AMINO ACIDS SUPPLIED BY BREAD AND MILK
(4 slices (100 gm.) of Bread and 2 cups (480 gm.) of Milk)

ESSENTIAL AMINO ACIDS	BREAD (white)– 4 slices yield 8.5 gm. protein	MILK (whole or skim) –2 cups yield 16.8 gm. protein	TOTAL	ADULT MINIMUM* DAILY NEEDS (male)
		Amounts in Grams		
Tryptophan	0.091	0.235	0.326	0.25
Threonine	0.282	0.773	1.055	0.50
Isoleucine	0.429	1.070	1.449	0.70
Leucine	0.668	1.651	2.319	1.10
Lysine	0.225	1.306	1.531	0.80
Methionine	0.142	0.413	0.704**	1.10
Phenylalanine	0.465	0.716	1.181	1.10
Valine	0.435	1.152	1.587	0.80

*Minimum is approximately one-half the recommended daily amount for an adult, as shown in Table 6–1.
**Cystine (0.149 gm.) supplied by the casein in milk, spares methionine.
See also Appendix Table 6, Amino Acid Content of Foods.

TABLE 6–3   PROTEINS OF EGG, HUMAN MILK AND COW'S MILK
(6 to 7 gm. Protein)

ESSENTIAL AMINO ACIDS	EGG (50 gm. yield 6.4 gm. protein)	HUMAN MILK (480 gm. yield 6.7 gm. protein)	COW'S MILK (200 gm. yield 7 gm. protein)
	Amount in Grams		
Tryptophan	0.105	0.110	0.098
Threonine	0.318	0.298	0.322
Isoleucine	0.425	0.360	0.669
Leucine	0.563	0.595	0.688
Lysine	0.409	0.432	0.544
Methionine	0.200	0.134	0.172
Phenylalanine	0.369	0.288	0.340
Valine	0.475	0.412	0.480
Arginine	0.420	0.264	0.256
Histidine	0.153	0.144	0.184

Adapted from Table 2 compiled by M. L. Orr and B. K. Watt in "Amino Acid Content of Foods." Home Economics Research Report No. 4, reviewed and approved for printing December, 1968. U.S. Department of Agriculture. See also Appendix Table 6, Amino Acid Content of Foods.

egg (12.8 per cent of protein), by 480 gm. of human milk (1.4 per cent protein), or by 200 gm. of cow's milk (3.5 per cent protein).

Many people tend to ingest a mixture of foods in a meal and the combination of proteins, complete and incomplete, in sufficient quality and quantity, are apt to supplement one another to provide all the essential amino acids. The minimum requirement for the adult male, for example, is readily obtained in four slices of bread and one pint of milk (Table 6–2).

When the use of a complete protein is restricted, mixtures of a carbohydrate with a small amount of a complete protein will supply the essential amino acids. Examples of this supplementation are cereal with milk; macaroni and cheese; rice, beans and sofrito (meat or fish sauce). Small amounts of fish meal or skim milk may be added to vegetable or carbohydrate mixtures to provide the essential amino acids. In areas where animal protein is scarce or unavailable, plant proteins may be combined according to the reference pattern of the amino acids in egg to form a complete protein. This mixture, referred to as mutual supplementation, supplies all the essential amino acids. One of the first of these products, Incaparina, was developed by the Institute of Nutrition in Central America and Panama. It consists of a mixture of ground maize, sorghum, cottonseed flour, torula yeast and vitamin A.[5] Suitable products have been developed in other countries to meet the protein needs, especially of infants and children. Enrichment of grains and legumes with amino acids (lysine to bread; methionine to legumes) in which they are insufficiently supplied, provide a good source of protein for many people.

[5] Scrimshaw, N. S., and Bressani, R.: Vegetable protein mixtures for human consumption. Fed. Proc., 20:80, 1961.

METABOLISM OF PROTEINS

The processes of digestion and absorption of proteins are discussed in Chapter 7. All proteins must be broken down into amino acids by digestion before absorption and use by the body. Absorption through the intestinal lumen is an active process, not simple diffusion; it requires energy (ATP), pyridoxal phosphate (B_6) and manganese ion. The amino acids are carried in the portal vein to the liver and then into the general circulation. Amino acids which are constantly being formed by breakdown of tissue proteins and non-essential amino acids synthesized in the body contribute to the circulating pool.

The fundamental and most interesting use of the amino acid is as a building block for the body proteins. Each cell in the body has the capacity to synthesize an enormous number of specific proteins. For the synthesis of a protein all the essential amino acids must be available from the blood stream at the same time. Protein synthesis is not a step-wise process. Complete peptides are laid down in a short period of time and there is no provision for storage of incomplete sections. The non-essential amino acids must either be supplied as such or there must be suitable precursors, including amino groups from other amino acids, so that they can be synthesized. The synthesis of the characteristic proteins of each cell is controlled by the genetic material, deoxyribose nucleic acid (DNA) in the nucleus. DNA is used as a template for the synthesis of ribose nucleic acid (RNA) which carries the information to the cytoplasm where the proteins are synthesized. DNA and RNA are composed of nucleotide units consisting of ribose (or deoxyribose), phosphoric acid and one of the four cyclic nitrogenous bases (a purine or pyrimidine). (See Figure 6–3, Building Blocks of DNA.) They are

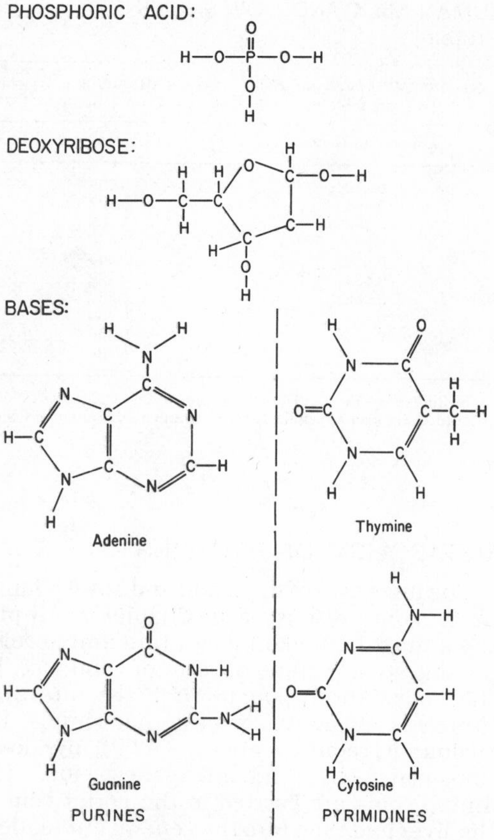

PHOSPHORIC ACID:

DEOXYRIBOSE:

BASES:

Adenine

Thymine

Guanine

Cytosine

PURINES

PYRIMIDINES

Figure 6–3   The basic building blocks of DNA. (From Guyton, A. C.: Textbook of Medical Physiology. 4th ed. W. B. Saunders Company, 1971.)

strung together in long chains of pentose and phosphoric acid alternately with the purines and pyrimidine molecules as branches. DNA is a double-stranded molecule, the two chains in the form of a double helix held together by hydrogen bonds linking a purine and a pyrimidine. It may have a molecular weight of two billion, with a million or more bases arranged in a continuous line. RNA (of which there are several types) is a single strand. It is the sequence of the bases along the chain which specifies the arrangement of amino acids in the protein, each amino acid being defined by a set of three bases. In the cytoplasm are other RNA molecules, relatively small, one for each amino acid. These t (transfer) RNA's direct the amino acids to the appropriate position along the m (messenger) RNA so that the peptide chain can be synthesized. Major steps in this intricate process are shown in Figure 6–4. Of course, among the proteins which must be synthesized are the enzymes needed to catalyze the synthesis. Energy for synthesis is supplied by ATP, itself a nucleotide.

There is no large reserve of free amino acids in the body and any amount above that needed for synthesis of tissue protein and the varied non-protein nitrogen-containing compounds is oxidized, providing high-energy phosphate. Adults of constant weight excrete each day an amount of nitrogen equivalent to that in the protein eaten. The amino group is detached from the amino acid before oxidation of the remaining portion of the molecule. Most of the amino nitrogen is converted to urea in the liver and excreted in the urine. The liver is the main location for deamination and other early steps in amino acid metabolism (including synthesis of non-essential amino acids). The carbon skeletons are converted into some of the same intermediates formed during glucose and fatty acid catabolism. These can be carried to the peripheral tissues where they are needed for oxidation to produce high-energy phosphate. These fragments can also be used in synthetic processes to make glucose or fats. The mechanisms of these reactions will be further discussed in Chapter 7.

Under certain conditions it is possible for about 46 per cent of the protein to be converted into fatty acids. Other amino acids may form glucose, which can be used immediately for energy or stored as fat. About 58 per cent of the protein consumed can be converted into glucose. Others are utilized for the formation of specific substances such as bile salts, enzymes, certain hormones, and glutathione. (Glutathione is an important sulfur-containing polypeptide

Figure 6–4   Schematic summary of protein synthesis. *Top, step 1.* A molecule of DNA in the nucleus unfolds, and one of its strands is used as a template to direct the formation of messenger RNA from nucleoside triphosphates, which lose inorganic pyrophosphate (PP$_i$) as they attach to the growing RNA chain. The completed mRNA moves to the cytoplasm *(bottom)*, where it binds ribosomes into a polysome, and acts as a template for protein synthesis.
The following steps are shown on separate ribosomes for clarity, but in fact they are repeated in sequence on each ribosome. The successive ribosomes grow longer and longer peptide chains as they move down the molecule of mRNA.
Step 2.   Meanwhile, amino acids are combined with specific molecules of transfer RNA (tRNA) in the cytoplasm by a reaction that also involves the cleavage of adenosine triphosphate (ATP) into adenosine monophosphate (AMP) and PP$_i$.
Step 3.   The tRNA molecules, carrying the amino acids in the form of aminoacyl groups, diffuse to the polysome, where the growing peptide chain is on another molecule of tRNA already attached. The incoming tRNA, which bears the next group required for the growing peptide (in this case a leucyl residue), has the proper configuration to complex with mRNA on the ribosome.

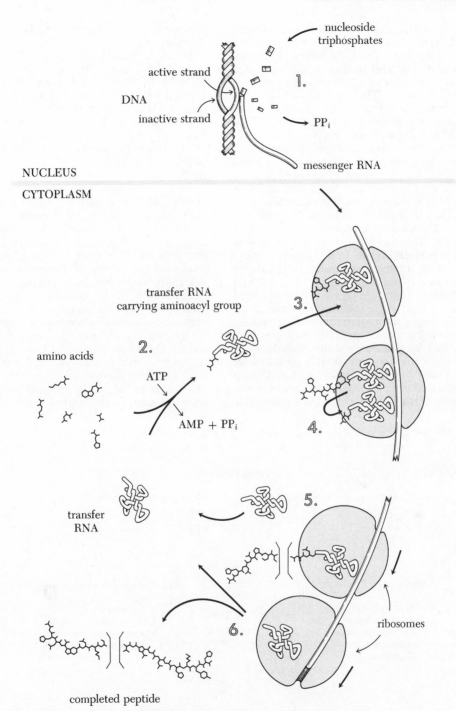

nucleoside triphosphates

active strand

DNA

inactive strand

1.

PP_i

messenger RNA

NUCLEUS

CYTOPLASM

transfer RNA
carrying aminoacyl group

3.

amino acids

2.

ATP

AMP + PP_i

4.

transfer
RNA

5.

ribosomes

6.

completed peptide

Step 4.   When the proper tRNA is in place, the peptide chain is transferred onto the amino group of the new residue brought in by tRNA, so that the chain is now one residue longer.

Step 5.   When the transfer of the previous step is completed, the previously bound tRNA no longer carries a peptide chain and is free to dissociate from the ribosome, returning to the mixed pool of tRNA in the soluble cytoplasm, where it is available for transport of another molecule of its specific amino acid. The ribosome now moves along the mRNA molecule to the position where the placement of the next amino acid will be directed.

Step 6.   Steps 3, 4 and 5 are repeated. As each amino acid residue adds to the peptide chain, the ribosome moves down the mRNA molecule. When a ribosome has reached the end of the molecule, the peptide is completed and is detached into the soluble cytoplasm. The ribosome itself can then move free of the mRNA and be available for attachment to the beginning of yet another molecule of mRNA (not shown). (From McGilvery, R. W.: Biochemistry—A Functional Approach. W. B. Saunders Company, 1970.)

which functions in the biological system of oxidation.) Since most types of proteins of the body are regularly being built up and torn down, the amino acids used for protein synthesis also are eventually replaced and metabolized. The nitrogen from the protein must be excreted in the urine. Besides urea, the major excretory products are uric acid and creatinine. Uric acid is the end-product of the metabolism of purines, important components of the nucleic acids (vide infra). Disturbed metabolism of purines and uric acid is found in gout, discussed in Chapter 28. Creatinine is the excretion form of creatine, present in all muscle tissue and creatine phosphate, a store of high-energy phosphate. The amount of urea excreted is related to protein intake. Creatinine excretion is related to muscle mass and is relatively constant in any individual.

Metabolism of proteins is sometimes divided into two types: (1) *exogenous* metabolism, which includes the metabolism of all protein ingested in excess of essential body requirements, and is obviously quite variable; (2) *endogenous* metabolism, which includes all the necessary protein buildup and breakdown processes that are essential to life and growth and repair of the body. Creatinine excretion is

regarded as a measure of the endogenous metabolism.

There is practically no storage of amino acids in the body. They are constantly being utilized to form other compounds and reformed by breakdown and ingestion of protein, with the excess being excreted as previously mentioned. As with fats and carbohydrates, there exists a state of dynamic equilibrium for amino acids, with constant buildup, breakdown, and interchange, and there exists a metabolic pool of amino acids at any given time in this state of dynamic equilibrium that may be called upon by the body for any appropriate need. Figure 6–5 summarizes the anabolic and catabolic reactions of amino acids. The direction taken depends on the supply of amino acids in the food and the needs of the body. Regulation is largely under hormone control.

Hormones have anabolic and catabolic effects on protein metabolism. The growth hormone stimulates protein synthesis, thus increasing tissue concentration. This occurs during the growth periods. Insulin also stimulates protein synthesis by accelerating amino acid transport across the cell membrane. Lack of insulin reduces protein synthesis. Insulin and the gonad-stimulating hormones, espe-

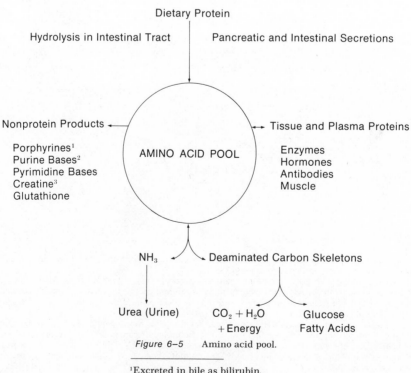

Figure 6–5   Amino acid pool.

[1]Excreted in bile as bilirubin.
[2]Excreted in urine as uric acid.
[3]Excreted in urine as creatinine.

cially testosterone, stimulate protein synthesis during growth periods. The glucocorticoids stimulate gluconeogenesis and ketogenesis from proteins.[6] Thyroxine indirectly affects protein metabolism by increasing the rate of metabolism in all cells. Thyroxine causes degradation of proteins to be used for energy when the intake of carbohydrate and fats is insufficient for energy. Thyroxine may increase the rate of protein synthesis when there is an excess of amino acids in the presence of adequate carbohydrate and fat for energy. A deficiency of thyroxine causes retarded growth during the growth periods because of lack of protein synthesis.

FUNCTIONS OF PROTEINS IN THE BODY

Dietary proteins furnish the amino acids for synthesis of tissue protein and other special metabolic functions. A concise summary of the numerous functions of proteins would be as follows:

1. Proteins are used in repairing worn-out body tissue proteins (anabolism) resulting from the continued "wear and tear" (catabolism) going on in the body. This is a function provided only by protein. No other nutrients can do it because the amino acid building blocks of tissue are available only from protein.

2. Proteins are used to build new tissue (anabolism) by supplying the necessary amino acid building blocks. This is the reason for an increased protein need during periods of rapid growth, as in infancy, childhood and pregnancy.

3. Proteins are a source of heat and energy. They supply 4 kcalories per gram of protein, the same as does a carbohydrate, but in a more expensive fashion than a carbohydrate. Protein is not only a more expensive source of energy to buy and eat, but it will be remembered that protein has a greater specific dynamic action than carbohydrate, which adds to the total energy expended by the body. (Specific dynamic action of food may be defined as the stimulus given to metabolism which is exhibited to a notable degree by protein and to a lesser degree by carbohydrate and fat.) Also, one of the end products of protein metabolism is nitrogen, which has to be excreted by the body, a function that involves a cost in work by the body. Carbohydrate, on the other hand, is cheap to obtain and burns completely to carbon dioxide and water.

4. Proteins contribute to numerous essential body secretions and fluids. Enzymes are proteins. Some hormones have protein or amino acid components. Mucus and milk are largely protein. Sperm are largely protein, as is the fluid in which sperm are contained. Sweat, bile, and urine are about the only protein-free body fluids.

5. Proteins are important in the maintenance of normal osmotic relations among the various body fluids. The plasma proteins of the blood play the vital role in these relations. Indeed, one of the main signs of hypoproteinemia is the appearance of edema (excessive tissue fluid) as a result of loss of osmotic balance.

6. Proteins play a large role in the resistance of the body to disease. Antibodies to specific disease are found in part of the plasma globulin, specifically in what is known as the gamma globulin fraction of plasma.

7. Dietary proteins furnish the amino acids for a variety of metabolic functions. They are components or precursors of many nonprotein nitrogen-containing substances. Some of these have been discussed (p. 68).

RECOMMENDED PROTEIN AND AMINO ACID ALLOWANCES

The daily recommended allowances (RDA) for the 70-kg. reference man and 58-kg. reference woman is approximately 0.9 gm. of protein per kg. of body weight per day.[7] This amounts to 65 gm. and 55 gm. per day for the reference man and woman respectively (see Table 11–1, p. 158), or approximately 10 per cent of the total daily calories. These recommendations are based on the amount of protein needed to compensate for the nitrogen lost in urine and feces by individuals adjusted to a protein-free diet; the amount to compensate for skin, sweat, hair and nail losses; and the amount necessary for the increase in body mass during normal growth.

Nitrogen losses are used to estimate the amount of ideal protein required. If the protein provides both the exact amount of nitrogen lost from the body and the precise mixture of amino acids needed, additional nitrogen will not be excreted. Nitrogen balance would be attained. Such a protein would be a "reference protein," one which would produce one gram of tissue for each gram consumed, thus having a biological value of 100. A whole egg and human milk would be an example (Table 6–3). They have been designated by the Joint Committee FAO/WHO as the reference pattern.

The minimum requirement of protein

---

[6]Guyton, A. C.: Textbook of Medical Physiology. 4th ed. Philadelphia, W. B. Saunders Company, 1971, p. 818.

[7]Food and Nutrition Board: Daily Recommended Allowances. Washington, D.C., National Research Council, Pub. No. 1694, 1968.

needed to maintain nitrogen balance has been determined to be about 0.35 gm. per kg. of body weight daily. An allowance of 1.5 times the minimum to cover individual differences as a safety factor is recommended. The minimum requirements for the adult would be 0.350 to 0.525 gm. per kg. of body weight, when the biological value of the protein is 100. When the biological value of the customary diet scores 70, the daily allowance ranges from 0.50 to 0.75 grams of protein per kg. of body weight. In the 1968 Report of the Food and Nutrition Board,[8] 20 mg. of ideal protein (N × 6.25) per basal kcal. is used as the maintenance protein requirement for children and adults. An allowance of 10.5 gm. (30 per cent) for individual variabilities within a large population is used. For a 70-kg. reference man, this is 45.5 gm. per day of ideal protein. Applying the 70 per cent utilization value for protein for the customary diet, the RDA becomes 65 gm. per day for the reference man. This amount allows for intake of some proteins of low biological value. It is good nutritional practice to include at least one-third of the protein intake from complete protein foods. The efficiency of various proteins in meeting the requirements is dependent upon their quality.

It is not necessary to be too concerned about the proportions of different amino acids when the supply of protein is generous and comes from a mixture of ordinary foods. However, in parts of the world where protein of high quality and calories are scarce, the proportion or ratio of the amino acids may be of utmost significance.[9] (See Fig. 6–6.) The tryptophan requirement has been assigned the value of 1, since it is the essential amino acid present in lowest amount in the "ideal protein," and the amounts of the other acids are expressed as multiples of this. Thus, there should be 2 times as much phenylalanine and threonine as there is tryptophan; 3 times as much isoleucine, lysine and valine; and 3.4 times as much leucine for a protein to match the "ideal protein." Examples of good combinations are cereal and milk; bread and eggs; bread and milk. (See Table 6–2.)

If the fat and carbohydrate in a diet are supplied in adequate amounts to meet energy requirements, there can be nitrogen equilibrium even when the intake of protein is very low. They will "spare" the proteins. Unless sufficient calories are available in the diet for energy needs, an increased amount of protein is metabolized to compensate for

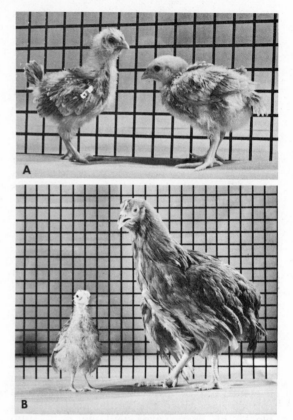

Figure 6–6   Effect of amino acid, tryptophan, on growth and health. (A), Week-old chicks. Chick at left to be fed a tryptophan-free diet. Chick at right will continue eating standard feed. (B), Same chicks at 9 weeks of age. The chick at left on tryptophan-free diet remains at approximately his week-old size. There are some changes in appearance, however, because most of the feathers, the beak and the eyes developed at normal rate. When tryptophan is restored to the diet, the chick will immediately begin to grow and mature, reaching maturation without ill effects. (Courtesy, Monsanto Chemical Company's Agricultural Experiment Farm, St. Louis, Missouri.)

the dietary inadequacy. The practical implication is that proteins and amino acids should not be ingested by themselves. Protein is an expensive source of calories and during its catabolism yields nitrogen compounds which must be excreted by the kidney. The requirements for the essential amino acids is also "spared" by the dietary content of the nonessential amino acids, since they need not be deaminated to supply amino groups for non-essential amino acids. A low protein intake, continued over a length of time, may place the organism in a precarious position, however.

The general belief has been that an inadequate protein intake compels the body to call upon "reserve" or body "store" of proteins in order to supply the necessary amino acids to meet situations of privation or stress. The depletion of the store is speeded up if the pro-

[8]Food and Nutrition Board: Daily Recommended Allowances. Washington, D.C., National Research Council, Pub. No. 1694, 1968, p. 18.

[9]Christensen, H. N.: Transport of amino acids. Nutr. Rev., 21:101, 1963.

tein stores are also called upon to act as a source of energy. However, Holt et al.[10] have questioned the concept of a protein "store" or "reserve" ready to meet the needs of privation and stress. After a critical examination of the literature and a review of some animal experiments, they conclude that there is no virtue in feeding protein beyond the minimum adequate quantity. These authors believe there is no value in consuming extra proteins in anticipation of privation and stress but that time for eating extra protein is during the untoward event and especially during convalescence, not before. The general trend at present is, however, toward a generous protein allowance for all ages.

Any condition of health or disease that imposes an increased nitrogen requirement upon the body (growth, pregnancy, lactation, burns, fever, hyperthyroidism) must be met by increased protein intake if destruction of tissue and of plasma protein (negative nitrogen balance) is to be avoided.

Protein allowances should be based upon ideal body weight—what the person should weigh, not what he does weigh.

Refer to Table 11-1, page 158, for the allowances of protein recommended by the Food and Nutrition Board of the National Research Council. The recommended allowances assume adequate calorie intake.

EFFECT OF GROWTH   During growth the need for protein is greater than at any other time in a person's life. (See Fig. 6-7.) Thus, infants and children need relatively more than the adult allowance because they accumulate new tissue of high protein con-

tent. Recommended allowances for children are 2.2 gm. per kg. of body weight for the infant; 1.8 gm. per kg. of body weight for the 1-year-old; 1.2 gm. later in childhood and 1.0 gm. in adolescence. (see Chapters 16 and 17.)

EFFECT OF PREGNANCY AND LACTATION   Because pregnancy represents another form of rapid growth, the mother has an additional need for protein. The Food and Nutrition Board of the National Research Council (NRC) suggests than an additional 10 grams is needed daily over and above the normal allowance of 0.9 gm. per kg. of body weight. Lactation imposes an additional protein burden on the body inasmuch as 12 to 15 gm. of protein may be secreted daily in the breast milk. The NRC recommends an intake of an additional 20 gm. of protein above the normal allowance during lactation.

EFFECT OF AGE   The protein allowance of 0.9 gm. per kg. of body weight is maintained throughout adult life. However, a higher proportion of protein in the diet is required to achieve this level when the total calorie consumption is decreased with age. Proteins are essential in spite of the fact that the stomach secretes less acid and pepsin with age. Commonly we see older people who lose their zest for eating, or who, living alone, do not care to prepare well-balanced meals, or who have too little money for food. These people show the signs of dietary deficiencies, most commonly of proteins and vitamins. This is discussed in more detail in Chapter 18, Nutrition and Aging.

EFFECT OF EXERCISE   The amount of physical work or exercise done is not of prime importance in determining protein allowance. Heavy work will require more expenditure of energy than light work will, but protein needs

[10]Holt, L. E., Jr., et al.: The concept of protein stores and its implication in diet. J.A.M.A., *181*:699, 1962.

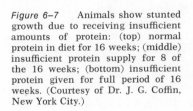

Figure 6-7   Animals show stunted growth due to receiving insufficient amounts of protein: (top) normal protein in diet for 16 weeks; (middle) insufficient protein supply for 8 of the 16 weeks; (bottom) insufficient protein given for full period of 16 weeks. (Courtesy of Dr. J. G. Coffin, New York City.)

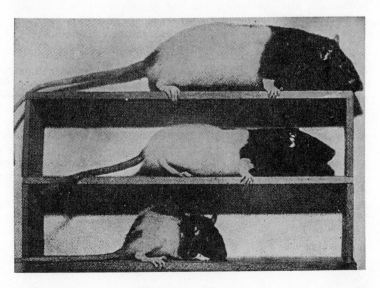

will not be increased, provided the calorie requirement is satisfied. During the period when a person is getting into "top physical condition," additional protein may be helpful in building up protein reserves to aid muscle growth during the time in which muscle development is accelerated. During the training period when an athlete increases his total muscle mass, extra protein is required.[11] The actual protein needs of the athlete are little different from those of the non-athlete, provided the calorie requirements are satisfied. The same is true for the sedentary individual who undertakes work requiring the use of muscles for strenuous and continuous work.

Most people doing heavy work seem to prefer high protein intakes, perhaps because of the sense of well-being and vigor produced by high protein diets as well as the pleasant way of receiving the additional calories needed.

EFFECT OF ILLNESS AND SURGERY
Any physical illness increases protein breakdown in the body. Indeed, merely staying in bed and decreasing food intake for several days will put a person into negative nitrogen balance. It is important therefore that these factors be considered in diet planning for the ill and convalescent. Surgery is frequently preceded by a poor or precarious protein balance that should, when time permits, be corrected before surgical procedures are undertaken, for the surgery itself contributes to establishing or continuing a negative nitrogen balance and such a balance retards wound healing and convalescence. (See Chapter 26, Diets in Surgery and Surgical Conditions.)

If the loss of protein is sudden, as occurs in hemorrhage following surgery, or loss of blood plasma in burns, the patient will manifest shock. If the protein deficiency is gradual and prolonged, the following clinical signs of protein malnutrition may occur: loss of weight, skin changes (from soft, moist, pliable character to dry, scaly), reduced resistance to infection, impaired healing, hepatic insufficiency, nutritional edema, and changes in concentration of hemoglobin and plasma protein.

Protein malnutrition is best prevented through the consumption of sufficient protein foods of high biologic value. In fact, the period of convalescence of the patient is shortened if protein deficiency does not develop, an important economic factor in the care of the sick. However, if the patient already has a protein deficiency, it should not be aggravated by inadequate dietary care. Instead, the backlog

of poor nutrition needs to be improved along with the curing of the disease.

LOW AND HIGH PROTEIN INTAKE
The adult apparently can, if necessary, get along on protein intakes as low as 30 to 40 gm. daily, depending upon the quality of protein ingested. Concidentally, on such a low protein intake the urinary nitrogen output falls drastically, which indicates an adaptation process going on within the body to compensate for the low protein intake. If the protein in the diet is suddenly decreased, a negative nitrogen balance will exist for a few days. Eventually, equilibrium is reestablished at a lower level, unless the decreased intake of protein is below the critical point. Real protein deficiency is accompanied by edema, retardation of growth, wasting of body tissues, weakness, and loss of vigor. On the other side of the scale, people on very high intakes of protein have been studied and found to have tolerated them without apparent harm. The normal kidney can handle large amounts of nitrogenous waste without difficulty. There is, however, one important condition in which a high protein intake is harmful, that is, chronic kidney disease with nitrogen retention. The damaged kidney cannot excrete nitrogenous wastes, and giving excess protein only adds to the burden of a kidney that cannot do its normal work. Consequently, nitrogen retention is increased. However, in chronic kidney disease accompanied by low blood proteins (due to loss through the injured kidney) and no excessive nitrogen retention, a high protein intake is indicated to make up for the urinary loss of protein. These conditions of disease and diet will be dealt with in more detail in Part Two.

PROTEINS AROUND THE WORLD

Intake of protein below the recommended allowance is found in many parts of the world. Protein malnutrition is the most widespread, serious nutritional problem in the underdeveloped areas and is particularly serious in its effect on infants and children. Severe protein deficiency may lead to death. The chronic form leads more often to grossly retarded physical growth and development. Mental development, learning and behavior may be impaired as well. This deficiency results in an increased susceptibility to acute and chronic infections. Kwashiorkor, a disease observed in infants and children when protein intake, especially animal protein, is severely restricted, is a major public health problem in

---

[11]Van Itallie, T.: If only we knew. Nutrition Today. 3:3, No. 2, 1968.

underdeveloped parts of the world. (See Ch. 34). As stated previously, the adult apparently can establish nitrogen equilibria at various levels of protein intake.

Food sources of good protein are very scarce in many parts of the world. Some peoples lack protein because there is a scarcity of animals, or they have an aversion to or religious scruples against consuming eggs or meat. In other countries there are possibilities for production of the desired protein, but the quality is not good, or information on food is lacking. More information is needed by the masses on food values. The various divisions of the United Nations are attempting to supply this. Any new foods that are to find wide acceptance must be integrated into existing diets; they must be compatible with existing customs and food habits. A solution for one country may not be applicable in another country of different climate, geography, economic resources, social patterns and eating habits. Nutritional inprovement of people or population groups takes place only if and when a better diet is actually consumed.

In a number of the technically underdeveloped areas and countries, efforts to develop vegetable sources of protein have been, to a great extent, stimulated and aided by WHO, FAO, and UNICEF. In French West Africa and the Belgian Congo, peanut flour is being explored as a source of protein for child feeding. Soya and sunflower seed press cakes are being used in Uganda. In Japan, research is being conducted on soya products prepared by traditional fermentation methods. Fish flour plants and ponds for raising fish have been set up to provide a low-cost source of animal protein in a number of countries (Fig. 1–2). Surplus skin milk has been made available in various countries through UNICEF for a number of years.

Worldwide endeavor to develop protein-rich foods of low cost has been the most important new attempt to prevent protein malnutrition. In India, the Belgian Congo and other parts of Africa and Central America, inexpensive mixtures of vegetable origin with a high protein content of good biological value have been contrived to be used as a dietary supplement, especially for children. Experience has shown that the vegetable mixtures can be fed indefinitely as the staple food if supplemented with sources of ascorbic acid and additional calories. They are to be produced commercially, will be low in cost, and will be promoted among low-income groups. An excellent example of a properly selected mixture from available plant protein sources, developed by the Institute of Nutrition of Central America and Panama—and named Incaparina—contains corn, sorghum,

cottonseed meal, yeast, and vitamin A and is used to combat protein deficiency in young children. (See Chap. 34.)

In Peru a food supplement was developed, made of cottonseed flour and quinua flour (Peruvita). Quinua is a locally grown cereal and its flour contains about 14 per cent high-quality protein. Thus, Peruvita is rich in protein and can be added to foods such as stews, soups, and gravies; can be used in cookies; or can be mixed with other cereals. According to reports, it is widely accepted.

African children whose diets had been enriched with "meat powder"—a flour made entirely from meat—proved to be taller and healthier than control groups. The meat powder contains 74 per cent crude protein, is yellowish-brown in color, and has an agreeable cooked-meat odor and meat-gravy flavor. While it can be used by itself, it can also easily be added to the carbohydrate foods eaten extensively in Africa, e.g., cassava, maize, and potatoes. It is considered a better supplement for children than milk powder (and is also more acceptable) because of the richer iron and protein content. A mixture of 40 parts dry skim milk and 60 parts meat powder, called Nyamaziwa, is on the market and selling well.

In the United States, during World War II, a mixture providing 50 per cent protein known as MPF (Multi-Purpose Food), was compounded from toasted soy grits, calcium carbonate, vitamin C, niacin, riboflavin, vitamin B_6, thiamin, vitamin A and vitamin D, vitamin B_{12} and potassium iodide. It is precooked and can be sprinkled over ready-to-eat cereal or used in milk over cereal. More recently, a cereal product with 20 per cent protein content containing sorghum, corn, wheat, soy meal and non-fat dry milk was developed by the State Department of Agriculture and Economic Development of Nebraska. From the laboratory there is a new kind of food called Single Cell Protein (SCP). It may become human food in a few years. It is a tasteless, odorless mass of edible microorganisms (yeasts, bacteria and fungi) that are treated and dried. It is fed presently to animals. Other new high-protein foods called meat analogues also are on the market for consumer consumption. They include vegetable proteins such as spun soybean fiber. These products contain 40 to 60 per cent protein of good biological value and are able to imitate with varying degrees of acceptance, ground beef, diced chicken, ham, bacon, scallops and turkey. Alfalfa extract and cultured algae offer some promise. A most exotic new protein source under consideration is that harvested from unicellular organisms grown on petroleum products.

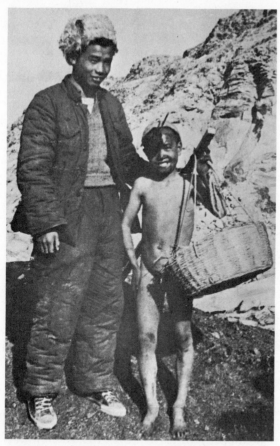

Figure 6–8   Two Asian boys of the same age. The boy on the right worked in a mine and received ordinary protein-poor local food. The other boy spent four years in a boarding school where he was well fed. (Photo courtesy of FAO.)

There is an increase in the use of synthetic essential amino acids to improve the quality of the proteins of cereals and other vegetable sources. For an example, lysine added to wheat flour dramatically improves the quality of wheat protein. A new strain of corn "opaque-2" has been developed at Purdue University. It contains higher amounts of lysine and tryptophan (essential amino acids) than found in ordinary strains of corn. Its nutritive value approaches that of milk protein in feeding trials and there is much optimism concerning its potential impact in the corn-consuming countries of the world. Work is under way to develop soybean varieties containing larger amounts of methionine and wheat and sorghum containing more lysine.

There is evidence that stature is influenced by the kind and amount of protein, as well as by heredity (Fig. 6–8). Orientals, who depend largely on a vegetable diet, are relatively short as contrasted with native New Zea-landers, who are renowned meat-eaters and who are tall and have large physiques. Statistics[12] point out a remarkable increase in the stature of Japanese youth during the past decades, which is most marked in children born since the period of postwar shortages. Evidence, direct and indirect, indicates better nutrition has contributed to increased growth rate. From changes in average nutrient intake during the past decade, it is concluded that protein or nutrients associated with protein mush have played a major role. Total protein consumption in Japan has increased 10 per cent in the past decades with intake of animal protein almost doubled.

TRENDS OF PROTEIN INTAKE IN THE AMERICAN DIET

According to the estimate of per capita consumption, by Consumer and Food Economics Research Division Agricultural Research Science, Department of Agriculture[13] protein decreased from 102 gm. in the 1909 to 1913 period to a low of 90 gm. per day in the 1935 to 1939 period. The figure for 1965 was 96 gm. The type of protein shifted from 56 per cent animal protein in the 1935 to 1939 period to 68 per cent in 1965, while vegetable protein decreased from 44 per cent to 32 per cent during this period. It is interesting to find that flour and cereal products contributed 36 per cent of the total protein available for consumption in the 1909 to 1913 period, but only 19 per cent in 1965. As these foods decreased in importance as sources of protein, dairy products, eggs, meat, poultry and fish increased in importance by contributing more of the total protein in the diet. Per capita consumption of eggs decreased from 7.1 per cent to 5.8 per cent of the animal sources of protein during 1947–49 and 1965 respectively. The distribution of the proteins contributed by major food groups has changed little in the last few years. In general, the North American diet provides protein in generous amounts, about two-thirds from animal source and one-third from plants. Most families eat regularly a combination of animal and plant proteins.

FOOD SOURCES OF PROTEIN

The importance of taking into consideration the *quality* of protein has been mentioned previously. (See page 69.) Generally speak-

[12]Mitchell, H. S.: Nutrition in relation to stature. J. Am. Dietet. A., 40:521, 1962.
[13]Friend, B.: Nutrients in United States food supply. Am. J. Clin. Nutr., 20:910, 1967.

TABLE 6–4   PROTEINS AVAILABLE IN COMMON FOODS

FOOD	CHIEF PROTEINS PRESENT	COMPLEMENT OF ESSENTIAL AMINO ACIDS	AVERAGE SERVING Grams of Proteins	Approximate Measure	WEIGHT GRAMS
Milk, whole	Casein and lact-albumin	Complete	9 gm.	1 glass (8 oz.)	244
Meat, lean	Albumin and myosin	Complete	22 gm.	2.5 oz.	72
Cheese, uncreamed cottage	Casein and lact-albumin	Complete	5 gm.	1 oz.	28
Egg	Ovalbumin and ovovitellin	Complete	6 gm.	1 egg	50
Navy beans	Phaesolin	Incomplete	7.5 gm.	½ cup	128
Peas, small, green	Legumin	Incomplete	4 gm.	½ cup	80
Corn, canned	Glutelin	Incomplete	2.5 gm.	½ cup	128
	Zein	Incomplete			
Bread	Gliadin	Incomplete	2 gm.	1 slice	23
Soy beans	Glycinin	Complete	3 gm.	½ cup	54
	Legumelin	Incomplete			
Dry, nonfat milk	Casein and lact-albumin	Complete	¼ cup (17.5 gm.) provides 6+ grams of protein. A good source of protein supplement for diets.		

ing, animal proteins are of good biological value, while most plant proteins are of fair or poor biological value. However, the eating of various protein foods, each containing some of the essential amino acids, may, in additive fashion, supply all the essential amino acids, although the total quantity of the poor quality proteins ingested must necessarily be much larger than the amount of good quality protein that would provide the same necessary nutrients.

The better the protein, the more essential amino acids it contains. The animal proteins, such as meat, poultry, fish, eggs, milk (skim, dried and whole) and milk products (cheese), head the list. Plant products richest in protein include soybeans, peanuts, cereals (especially wheat), peas, beans and lentils.

Table 6–4 shows the kinds of protein in various common foods, their biological value and the amounts of protein available in the average serving of foods.

AVAILABILITY OF AMINO ACIDS FROM FOOD PROTEIN   The availability of the essential amino acids in some foodstuffs was determined by Kuiken and Lyman.[14] They found that all the essential amino acids in roast beef are completely available, and that those of wheat and peanut butter are relatively high. Research has demonstrated that the protein in milk, eggs and meat is completely absorbed, yielding 95 to 100 per cent of their nutritive value.

In view of the recent knowledge concerning interrelationships between amino acids, hormones, enzymes, vitamins and calories, a demand for more information concerning the amino acid composition of foods has de-

veloped. The Home Economics Research Report No. 4, U.S. Department of Agriculture booklet entitled "Amino Acid Content of Foods," by M. L. Orr and B. K. Watt, was published in 1957, reviewed and approved for reprinting in 1968. It contains data on 18 amino acids, both in terms of amino acids per gram of total nitrogen (202 food items) and in terms of amino acids in 100-gram foods (316 food items). Table 6–6 in the Appendix is taken from this pamphlet, which includes the average amount of amino acids per 100-gram foods for the essential amino acids necessary for growth; it can be used to calculate the amino acid content of foods.

EFFECT OF PROCESSING OF PROTEIN FOODS   Processing of foods alters the nutritive value of protein.[15] Overheating, particularly in the absence of water (dry heat, frying), may either destroy certain essential amino acids such as lysine, which is heat labile, or alter them by tying them up in new chemical linkages so that the protein becomes resistant to digestive enzymes, or the release of individual amino acids in the intestinal tract is retarded. On the other hand, processing may have a favorable effect on protein foods by increasing the digestibility or increasing the liberation of individual amino acids. For example, dry heat decreases the availability of lysine in cereals, but cooking in the presence of water increases the nutritive value and digestibility of navy beans. High, dry heat exerts a deleterious effect on the nutritive value of wheat and oat protein. Similarly, toasting reduces the nutritive value of bread. Marked heat will decrease the avail-

[14]Kuiken, K. A., and Lyman, C. L.: Availability of amino acids in some foods. J. Nutrition, 36:359, 1948.

[15]Melnick, D.: The influence of heat processing on the functional and nutritive properties of protein. Food Technol., 3:57, 1949.

ability of protein in soybeans, while mild heat is favorable. It appears that the proteins of meat are not greatly diminished in nutritive value, if at all, by the ordinary cooking methods. However, severe heat treatment (such as autoclaving or pressure cooking) may lessen the nutritive value of meat proteins. Heat appears to reduce the nutritive value of milk used in cooking. On the other hand, the heat treatment involved in preparing evaporated or dried milk not only fails to decrease the nutritive value but enhances the digestibility and utilization of protein.

In general, low temperature cooking (300 to 350° F.) produces a tender, desirable result, while high temperature (400° F. plus) produces a tough, dry product. This will be discussed in more detail in Part Four.

PROBLEMS AND SUGGESTED TOPICS FOR DISCUSSION

1. List the most popular protein foods. Classify as to *complete* and *incomplete protein*.
2. What is meant by the "essential amino acids"? Name them. What are the physiological functions of amino acids?
3. Give examples of specific functions of four of the amino acids.
4. List the amounts of various protein foods you consume during a period of 24 hours and a period of 3 days; calculate the protein content.
5. Evaluate the list of protein foods. Classify them into animal and vegetable-grain proteins. Which ones have high biological value? What percentage of your diet is protein? Was the total amount of protein consumed in 24 hours equally distributed between the three meals? Make suggestions for improving your protein intake.
6. Give five reasons why you eat protein foods.
7. (a) Compare the protein content of rare and welldone beef. Explain.
   (b) Compare the protein content of cooked and uncooked oatmeal. Explain.
   (c) Cook an egg for 3 minutes in water below the boiling point and compare the texture with an egg which has been cooked in *boiling* water for 3 minutes. Explain.
8. Plan a basic dietary pattern of protein foods you require daily. Divide into three meals, keeping in mind the recent findings as to quality and quantity.
9. How is the need for good protein being met throughout the world?
10. What is the trend in protein consumption in the United States?
11. What is meant by a negative nitrogen balance? When might this occur? Describe two kinds of diets most likely to maintain nitrogen balance or equilibrium.
12. Using the ratio pattern for essential amino acids in Table 6 in the Appendix, determine the balance of amino acids in your food intake for one day. Is your diet properly balanced in essential amino acids? If not, show how it can be corrected.
13. Why are proteins considered to be a wasteful source of energy?
14. What effect does cooking have on protein foods? Explain and give examples.
15. Take a nutrition history of a patient on a normal diet. Plan a diet for the patient to follow when discharged from the hospital, keeping in mind the food budget, protein allowance, biological value of proteins, balance of essential amino acids, and any environmental factors involved.

SUGGESTED ADDITIONAL READING REFERENCES

Allison, J. B., and Wannemacher, R. W., Jr.: The concept and significance of labile and over-all protein reserves of the body. Am. J. Clin. Nutr. 16:445, 1965.

Brock, J. F.: Dietary protein in relation to man's health. Fed. Proc., 20:61, 1961. (Fifth Int. Congress of Nutrition.)

Burton, B. T. (ed.): The Heinz Handbook of Nutrition. 2nd ed. New York, McGraw-Hill Book Company, Inc., 1965, Chapter 7.

Christensen, H. N.: Transport of amino acids. Nutr. Rev., 21:97, 1963.

Duncan, G. G. (ed.): Diseases of Metabolism. 5th ed. Philadelphia, W. B. Saunders Company, 1964, Chapter 1, Protein Metabolism.

Food and Agriculture Organization of the United Nations: Protein Requirement Study No. 16, Rome 1957.

Food and Nutrition Board: Recommended Daily Allowances. Washington, D.C. National Academy of Sciences Pub. 1694, 1968.

Guyton, A. C.: Textbook of Medical Physiology. Philadelphia. 4th ed. W. B. Saunders Company, 1971.

Halac, E., Jr.: Studies of the relation between protein intake and resistance to protein deprivation. Am. J. Clin. Nutr., 11:514, 1962.

Harper, H. A.: Review of Physiological Chemistry. 12th ed. Canade, Lange Medical Publications, 1969.

Hartman, R. H., and Rice, E. E.: Supplementary relationships of proteins. J. Am. Diet. A., 35:34, 1958.

Holt, L. E., et al.: The concept of protein stores and its implication in diet. J.A.M.A., 181:699, 1962.

Howe, E. E., et al.: Amino acid supplementation of cereal grains as related to the world food supply. Am. J. Clin. Nutr. 16:315, 1965.

Howe, E. E., et al.: Amino acid supplementation of protein concentrates as related to the world protein supply. Am. J. Clin. Nutr., 16:321, 1965.

Leverton, R. M.: Food, The Yearbook of Agriculture, 1959. Washington, D.C., United States Department of Agriculture, Proteins, pp. 57–63; Amino acids pp. 64–87.

Lowenberg, M. E., et al.: Food and Man. New York, John Wiley & Sons, Inc., 1968.

Mazur, A., and Harrow, B.: Textbook of Biochemistry. 10th ed. Philadelphia, W. B. Saunders Company, 1971.

McGilvery, R. W.: Biochemistry: A Functional Approach. Philadelphia, W. B. Saunders Company, 1970.

Milner, P.: Protein food problems in developing countries. Food Tech., 16:51, 1962.

Mitchell, H. S.: Protein limitation and human growth. J. Am. Dietet. A., 44:165, 1964.

Nutrition Foundation, Inc.: Present Knowledge of Nutrition. 3rd ed. New York, 1967, Chapter 4, Present knowledge of protein.

Review: Caloric intake and protein metabolism. Nutr. Rev., 21:147, 1963.

Review: Evaluation of a peanut-soybean mixture. Nutr. Rev., 23:75, 1965.

Review: Evaluation of the FAO amino acid reference pattern. Nutr. Rev., 21:101, 1963.

Review: Protein and amino acid requirements. Nutr. Rev., 20:235, 1962.

Review: The concept of protein stores. Nutr. Rev., 21:45, 1963.

Review: Transport of dietary nitrogen. Nutr. Rev., 21:47, 1963.

Sanchez, A., et al.: Nutritive value of selected proteins and protein combinations. I. The biological value of proteins singly and in meal patterns with varying fat composition. II. Biological value predictability. Am. J. Clin. Nutr., 13:243; 13:250, 1963.

Sherman, W. C.: Protein in nutrition. National Live Stock and Meat Board Food and Nutrition News, 33(No. 5): 3;(No. 6):3, 1962.

Tuttle, S. G., et al.: Study of the essential amino acid

requirements of men over fifty. Metabolism, 6:564, 1957.

Watson, I. D.: The Double Helix: A Personal Account of the Structure of DNA. New York, Academic Press, 1968.

Watts, J. H.: Evaluation of protein in selected American diets, J. Am. Dietet. A., 46:116, 1965.

Williams, H. H.: Amino acid requirements. J. Am. Dietet. A., 35:929, 1959.

Wohl, M. G., and Goodhart, R. S. (ed.): Modern Nutrition in Health and Disease. 4th ed. Philadelphia, Lea & Febiger, 1968, Chapter 6, The Proteins and Amino Acids.

Chapter 7

DIGESTION, ABSORPTION AND CELL METABOLISM

Most of the major nutrients in foods are bound in large molecules which cannot be absorbed from the intestine because of size or because they are not water-soluble. The reduction of these large molecules into smaller, readily absorbed units and conversion of the insoluble molecules into soluble forms is the work of the digestive tract.

The digestive system extends from the mouth to the anus. (See Figure 7-1.) It consists of the alimentary canal and the exocrine and endocrine functions of its appendage organs, e.g., the liver and biliary tree and the pancreas.

FUNCTIONS   The functions of the digestive system include: (1) the receipt, maceration and transport of ingested substances and waste products; (2) secretion of acid, mucus, digestive enzymes, bile and other materials; (3) digestion of ingested foodstuffs; (4) absorption; (5) storage of waste products; (6) excretion; and (7) certain ancillary functions.

Mouth   The mouth receives food into the oral cavity, reduces it in size by chewing and mixes it with saliva, mucus and the digestive enzyme ptyalin (salivary amylase).

Esophagus   The esophagus functions to transport food and liquids from the oral cavity and pharynx to the stomach.

Stomach   The stomach and first portion of duodenum participate in the storage, digestion, and transport of ingested materials. The stomach secretes hydrochloric acid; the inactive protease pepsinogen; gastric lipase; mucus; and the gastrointestinal hormone gastrin. Absorption occurs in limited degree.

Small Intestine   The small intestine func-tions to secrete and to participate in digestion, absorption, and transport of ingested materials. It consists of the duodenum, jejunum and ileum. The duodenum receives the secretions of the large accessory glands of digestion—the pancreas and the liver. The small intestine functions to absorb the end-products of digestion of carbohydrates, proteins and fats. It secretes the enzymes lactase, sucrase, maltase and isomaltase and its epithelial cells contain carboxypeptidase, aminopeptidase, dipeptidases and small quantities of enteric lipase. The gastrointestinal hormones secretin and enterogastrone are formed in the wall of the duodenum.

Large Intestine and Rectum   The large intestine and rectum absorb water, electrolytes, and—in reduced amounts—some of the final products of digestion. It also provides a temporary storage for waste products which serve as a medium for bacterial synthesis of some nutritional factors.

Anus   The anus functions to control defecation. Power for this function is provided by the propulsive contractions of the colon and rectum which are normally coordinated with the involuntary and voluntary portions of the anal sphincter.

Pancreas   The pancreas functions to produce secretions required for the digestion and absorption of food. Enzymes excreted include pancreatic lipase, pancreatic amylase, procarboxypeptidase, trypsin and chymotrypsin (in their respective inactive forms, trypsinogen and chymotrypsinogen). Under the influence of secretin, the pancreas se-

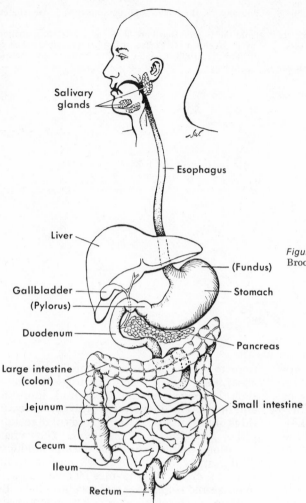

Salivary glands

Esophagus

Liver

(Fundus)

Gallbladder

Stomach

(Pylorus)

Duodenum

Pancreas

Large intestine (colon)

Jejunum

Small intestine

Cecum

Ileum

Rectum

Figure 7–1   The digestive system. (Modified from Brooks: Basic Facts of General Chemistry.)

cretes fluid containing large amounts of the bicarbonate ion. Important endocrine secretions of the pancreas are insulin and glucagon.

Liver and Biliary Tract   The major functions of the liver include the metabolism of protein, carbohydrate and lipid; the conjugation and detoxification of hormones and drugs; and the synthesis of proteins. In addition, the metabolism of bile pigments and bile salts takes place within the liver, and these products, important in the digestive process, are dumped into the duodenum through the biliary tract.

Each of these function will be discussed in more detail.

DIGESTION AND ABSORPTION

Digestion and absorption do not take place one step at a time as isolated functions. They are continuous processes with many mechanical and chemical reactions taking place simultaneously; a defect in one phase hampers the other phase.

Normally 92 to 97 per cent of the mixed American dietary is digested and absorbed. Foods are prepared for ingestion in a variety of ways and combinations; processing methods and cooking may begin a slight breakdown of complex compounds such as starch and collagen before they are eaten. Water, monosaccharides and inorganic ions are usually absorbed in their original form. The di- and polysaccharides, lipids and proteins must be converted to their simple constituents before they are absorbed.

It is assumed that knowledge in this subject has been acquired elsewhere. However, a briew review is included for the purpose of integration. For additional details, it is recommended that the reader consult a textbook on physiology[1] or biochemistry.[2]

DIGESTION

Digestion is a series of physical and chemical changes by which food, taken into the body, is broken down and hydrolyzed in preparation for absorption from the intestinal tract into the blood stream. These changes take place in the digestive tract, which includes the mouth, pharynx, esophagus, stomach, small intestine and large intestine. The teeth, tongue and salivary glands are accessory structures associated with the mouth. The liver, gallbladder and pancreas are important accessory structures of the digestive system. (See Fig. 7–1).

The physical changes in food are brought about by grinding, crushing and mixing of the food with the digestive juices and propulsion of the mass through the digestive tract. The propulsive force of the gastrointestinal tract resides in the circular and longitudinal smooth muscles contained in it walls. These muscles churn and push the food mass (chyme) along the digestive tract in rhythmic waves (peristalsis) toward the anus. During the propulsion of the chyme through the gut, it is mixed at appropriate times with the digestive juices which begin their chemical changes of food. The active materials in the digestive juices which cause this chemical breakdown are enzymes, both endoenzymes and exoenzymes.

DIGESTION IN THE MOUTH
In the mouth the teeth function to grind and crush the food into small particles. Simultaneously, the food mass is moistened and lubricated by saliva secreted by three pairs of glands; the parotid, submillary and sublingual.

These three pairs of glands produce about 1.5 liters of saliva daily. There are two types of saliva. One type is watery and serves to dissolve dry foods and the other contains mucus, a protein that makes particles of food stick together and lubricates the mass for easier swallowing. Saliva also contains the enzyme salivary amylase (ptyalin) which begins the digestion of starch in the mouth. The masticated food mass, now known as the bolus, passes back to the pharynx under voluntary control but from there on and through the esophagus the process of swallowing is involuntary. Peristalsis then moves the food rapidly into the stomach.

DIGESTION IN THE STOMACH
There is a mixing and propulsion of the food particles with gastric secretions in wave-like contractions. The churning and mixing waves are usually described as going from the fundus to the antrum of the pylorus. The food remains in the upper part of the stomach (fundus) for $1/2$ to 2 hours while salivary digestion of starch proceeds, and slowly moves downward in small portions. In the process of gastric digestion the food becomes semiliquid, and contains approximately 50 per cent water.

Active chemical digestion begins in the middle portion of the stomach. An average of 2000 to 2500 ml. of gastric juice is secreted daily, and contains the enzymes, mucus and hydrochloric acid necessary for digestion. Foodstuffs, when taken alone, leave the stomach in the following order: carbohydrate first, protein next, then fat, which takes the longest. But when carbohydrate, protein and fat are mixed, they all take longer. The stomach normally is emptied in 1 to 4 hours, depending upon the amount and kinds of foods eaten.

DIGESTION OF THE SMALL INTESTINE
The small intestine is divided into three sections: the duodenum, the jejunum and the ileum. (See Fig. 7–1.) The well-liquefied mass (chyme) slowly moves through the exit valve (pylorus) at the junction of the stomach and duodenum into the duodenum where it mixes with duodenal juices, bile (produced by the liver and stored in the gallbladder until needed), and the secretions from the pancreas.

The valves (sphincters), guarding the entrance to and the exit from the stomach, prevent backflow of the mixture from the duodenum into the stomach and from the stomach into the pharynx. These structures open and close at the proper time; but because the nervous system influences their behavior, they become too energetic during emotional upsets. When the exit pyloric valve tightens or goes into spasms, pain is excruciating. Irritation from nearby ulcers also may alter the performance of this structure. Mild exercise is advantageous to the digestive process but violent exercise inhibits it; fluids speed it along. In general, the average meal will arrive in the duodenum 2 or 3 hours after ingestion. Most of the digestion process is completed rapidly in the duodenum. The remainder of the small intestine (jejunum and ileum) functions principally in the absorption of nutrients.

ABSORPTION

ABSORPTION FROM THE SMALL INTESTINE
The remarkable structural feature of the small intestine is its tremendous absorptive area. The inner lining of the intes-

[1]Guyton, A. C.: Textbook of Medical Physiology. 4th ed. Philadelphia, W. B. Saunders Company, 1971.

[2]McGilvery, R. W.: Biochemistry—A Functional Approach. Philadelphia, W. B. Saunders Company, 1970, and Mazur, A. and Harrow, B.: Textbook of Biochemistry. 10th ed. Philadelphia, W. B. Saunders Company, 1971.

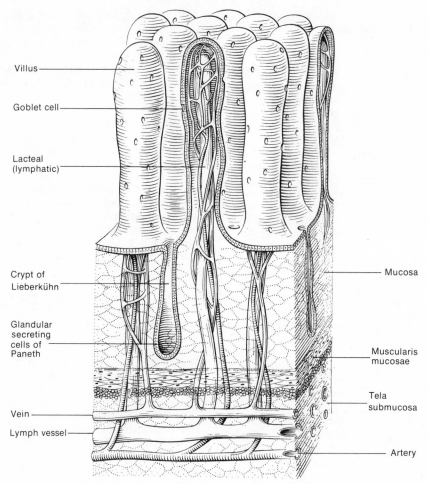

Villus

Goblet cell

Lacteal
(lymphatic)

Crypt of
Lieberkühn

Glandular
secreting
cells of
Paneth

Vein

Lymph vessel

Mucosa

Muscularis
mucosae

Tela
submucosa

Artery

Figure 7–2   Diagram of villi of human intestine showing their structure and blood and lymph vessels. (From Villee and Dethier: Biological Principles and Processes, W. B. Saunders Company, 1970.)

tine, the mucosa, is in immediate contact with the products of digestion. The mucosa is made up of columnar epithelial cells which are heaped up into folds called villi. The epithelial cells which make up the villi are covered with thousands of tiny projections called microvilli. The convoluted villi and their microvilli give the intestine an enormous absorptive surface which rests on a supporting structure called the lamina propia. The lamina propia is composed of connective tissue in which are suspended the blood and lymph vessels. These vessels receive the absorbed nutrients from the mucosal cells. Figure 7–3 schematically represents a villous absorptive cell.

THE MECHANISM OF ABSORPTION   Absorption is an extremely complex process and all its ramifications are not completely understood. It is not a question of diffusion of the nutrients through the mucosal cells into the blood stream for transport to other parts of

the body. Diffusion does occur in some instances but other more intricate processes are also involved, to explain how large amounts of nutrients constantly enter and leave the cell. Physiologists and biochemists discuss current absorption theory in terms of pores, carriers, pumps and pinocytosis. (These mechanisms, though not proven fact, may apply equally to other tissues as well—liver, muscle, kidney, etc.).

Pores   The presence of a layer of lipoprotein in the wall of the microvilli, makes the cell relatively impervious to water and water-soluble substances. It is postulated that these lipoprotein cell membranes are perforated by thousands of tiny pores which permit water, certain electrolytes and very small water-soluble molecules to enter the cell.

Carriers   Water molecules and other inorganic ions are sufficiently small to gain access to the inside of the epithelial cells through the pores. Amino acids, simple sugars

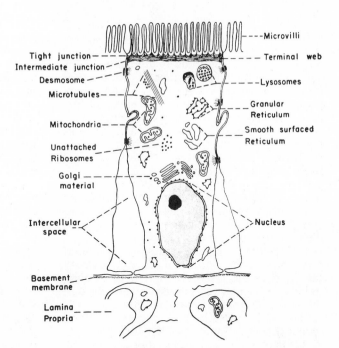

Microvilli

Terminal web

Lysosomes

Granular
Reticulum

Smooth surfaced
Reticulum

Tight junction
Intermediate junction
Desmosome
Microtubules

Mitochondria

Unattached
Ribosomes

Golgi
material

Intercellular
space

Nucleus

Basement
membrane

Lamina
Propria

Figure 7–3   Schematic diagram of a villous absorptive cell. (From Trier, J. S.: Structure of the mucosa of the small intestine as it relates to intestinal function. Fed. Proc., 26:1392, 1967.)

and fats have molecules larger than water molecules and therefore cannot pass easily through small pores. It is proposed that these relatively large fat-insoluble substances are escorted across the cell membranes by a carrier, an agent that shuttles back and forth like a ferry. At one side of the membrane it combines with the material needing transport, shuttles it across the cell membrane and then releases it to the interior of the cell. In so doing, it is then free to return for another load. It is apparent that there are specific carriers for specific substances. Sugars and amino acids are thought to have specific carriers which aid in their transport into cells. Presumably, the transported substance sits in a "special chair" on the carrier similar to substrates which have specific sites of attachment on enzymes. The best known carrier is that responsible for the absorption of vitamin B_{12}. A carrier protein called intrinsic factor is produced by the lining of the stomach. This specialized protein joins with vitamin B_{12} in the intestine and according to the carrier system provides for its absorption.

Pumps   In the process of diffusion, small molecules in greater concentration on one side of a semi-permeable membrane will move across the membrane until equivalent concentrations are found on both sides of the membrane. No work is required in this process. Sodium, however, requires energy in order to move from the intestinal lumen into the mucosa cell even if the sodium concentration within the cell is far greater than that in the lumen, and a pump is required.

These pumps are operated by cellular energy derived mostly from carbohydrate breakdown and act to rapidly move certain nutrients into the cells and thence to the blood supply. The absorption of glucose, sodium, amino acids, calcium, iron and vitamin B_{12}, undoubtedly, require both carriers and a pump.

Pinocytosis   Pinocytosis has been described by Ingelfinger[3] as a "drinking in" of a small drop of intestinal contents by the epithelial cell membrane. In this way, large particles such as whole proteins may be absorbed in small quantity. Even though it is doubtful that much nutrient is normally absorbed via pinocytosis, allergic reactions to foods which result from foreign proteins somehow finding their way across the gastrointestinal tract into the blood stream are probably the result of pinocytosis.

ABSORPTION FROM THE LARGE INTESTINE   The large intestine is approximately five feet long and consists of the cecum, colon and rectum. (See Figure 7–1). It is the site of the absorption of water, salts and some of the vitamins leaving the mass in a semi-solid state. In the large intestine the sodium ion is actively absorbed by the mucosa; because of the electrical potential thus created across the membrane, chloride and other negative ions as well as water move out of the colon into the intestinal fluids. The large intestine also serves to permit bacteria to reduce materials resistant to the previous digestive processes.

---

[3]Ingelfinger, F. J.: Gastrointestinal absorption. Nutrition Today, 2:2, 1967.

Normally, almost everything of nutritional value has been utilized and the waste is composed mostly of cellulose (and a number of other polysaccharides and related substances such as pectins and pentosans) and other indigestible products. The feces contain some water, dead mucosal cells and bacteria, the non-absorbed remains of the digestive processes, inorganic matter and fat, which comes from the unabsorbed fatty acids from the diet, fat formed by bacterial action and fat found in the sloughed epithelial cells.

Digestion and absorption do not always proceed in an orderly fashion. An irritant such as an infection may increase the rate of peristalsis causing the intestinal contents to pass through the intestinal tract rapidly (diarrhea). If the condition becomes chronic, a considerable loss of body water and electrolytes may result, causing dehydration and electrolyte imbalance. When the contents pass through too slowly so that a large amount of water is removed, the feces become excessively hard (constipation). Some of the diseases and disturbances will be discussed in Chapter 23, Diet in Gastric Diseases, and Chapter 24, Diet in Intestinal Diseases.

THE DIGESTIVE ENZYMES—THEIR RELATION TO DIGESTION AND ABSORPTION

The digestive enzymes are both exoenzymes and endoenzymes. Those enzymes concerned with metabolism of the cell are usually retained within the cell and are called endoenzymes. Those enzymes which are released by the cell and catalyze reactions in the environment of the cell are called exoenzymes. The latter are synthesized within specialized cells in the liver and pancreas, extruded and then delivered into the lumen of the intestine where they exert their catalytic action. The former enzymes are localized in the lipoprotein membranes of the mucosal cells and attach their substrates as they enter the cell. A discussion of the digestive enzymes is best considered in terms of the nutrient being digested.

CARBOHYDRATE DIGESTION AND ABSORPTION   In the mouth, the enzyme salivary amylase (ptyalin) which is neutral or slightly alkaline starts the digestive action on starch, hydrolyzing it to dextrins and maltose. Approximately 1500 ml. (3 pints) of saliva is secreted daily. The activity of amylase continues in the stomach until the hydrochloric acid destroys the ptyalin or salivary amylase activity. If the digestible carbohydrates remained in the stomach long enough, the acid hydrolysis could reduce much of it to the monosaccharide stage. How-

ever, the stomach usually empties itself before this can take place, and carbohydrate digestion takes place almost entirely in the small intestine, with the greatest activity in the duodenum. Amylase from the pancreas breaks the starches into dextrins and maltose, and maltase from the intestinal juice changes maltose to glucose. This breakdown occurs on the surfaces of the epithelial cells lining the intestines. These outer cell membranes contain the endoenzymes sucrase, lactase and maltase which act on sucrose, lactose and maltose, respectively. The resulting monosaccharides (hexoses) pass through the mucosal cell and are actively absorbed into the blood stream and delivered via the portal vein to the liver. In passing through the mucosal cell to the blood stream, specific carriers are apparently employed and the process requires energy. From the liver, glucose is transported to the tissues as needed; some glucose is stored in the liver and muscles as glycogen until needed. It is of interest that the pancreatic hormone, insulin, necessary for the proper utilization of glucose seems to exert its biochemical effect by promoting the transport of glucose into cells. Fructose may be converted to glucose before it passes from

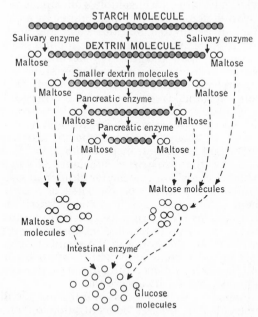

Figure 7–4   Breakdown of starch molecule to glucose. Gradual breaking down of large starch molecules by enzymes in digestion. The disaccharide maltose is split off by enzymes in the saliva and pancreatic juice, with smaller and smaller dextrin molecules formed as intermediate products, until the starch has been completely reduced to maltose. An intestinal enzyme then acts on the maltose molecules, splitting them into molecules of the monosaccharide, or simple sugar, glucose. (From Bogert, L. J., et al.: Nutrition and Physical Fitness, W. B. Saunders Company, 1966.)

the intestinal cell to the blood stream by diffusion or may be converted to glucose in the liver. It is probable that galactose is actively transported. Glucose is the principal carbohydrate used by the body and is the sugar normally found in the blood. The nerve cells of the body depend entirely upon glucose as a source of energy, since they are unable to use other energy-yielding nutrients (Fig. 7–4).

Some forms of carbohydrate cannot be digested by man. Cellulose, hemicellulose, and lignin are excreted in the feces unchanged. Neither salivary amylase or pancreatic amylase has the ability to split the cellulose bond. The termite, cow and other lower animals, however, can digest cellulose with ease.

FAT DIGESTION AND ABSORPTION   Fat digestion starts in the stomach with the action of gastric lipase, but it is only able to break naturally occurring emulsified fat into fatty acids and glycerol. It is unable to attack the larger molecules of unemulsified fat. However, the presence of fat in the diet causes food to be retained in the stomach for an extended period. If a considerable amount of fat is eaten with a meal the hormone enterogastrone, which inhibits gastric secretion and

motility, is released from the intestinal mucosa cell. Food may remain in the stomach as much as four hours or longer before being discharged to the small intestines, which gives a prolonged feeling of satiety. In the small intestine bile acts on the larger fat molecules to break them into smaller fat particles and digestion continues with the aid of pancreatic lipase and, to a less extent, intestinal lipase. This enzyme usually splits off two of the three fatty acids from triglycerides. These resulting free fatty acids and monoglycerides are emulsified by liver bile which pours into the duodenum along with enzymes from the pancreas. Complexes of bile salt, fatty acids and monosaccharides attach themselves to the surface of the microvilli and the lipid part of the complex enters the cell. The bile salts are then released from their lipid components and re-enter the lumen of the gut. Most of the bile salts are actively reabsorbed in the lower part of the small intestine and are recycled back to the liver to enter the gut at the duodenum.

The finding that short chain fatty acids are absorbed quite differently than long chain fatty acids is of clinical usefulness. There are individuals who cannot efficiently absorb the

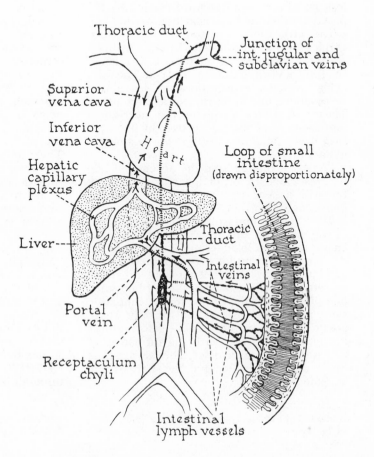

Figure 7–5   Routes by which the absorbed foods reach the blood of the general circulation. Intestinal veins converging to form, in part, the portal vein, which enters the liver and by repeated branchings assists in the formation of the hepatic capillary plexus; the hepatic veins carrying blood from the liver discharging it into the inferior vena cava; the intestinal lymph vessels converging to discharge their contents, chyle, into the receptaculum chyli, the lower expanded part of the thoracic duct; the thoracic duct discharging lymph and chyle into the blood at the junction of the internal jugular and subclavian veins. (Modified scheme after Bachman.)

usual types of dietary fat because they lack the means for transporting triglycerides out of their intestinal epithelial cells into the lymphatics. The medium chain triglycerides enter the blood stream with ease because they are not synthesized into triglycerides in the mucosal cells.

The longer chain fatty acids are absorbed into the mucosal cell with the aid of bile salts and phospholipids where they are reassembled on the glycerol molecule to form triglycerides again. With the assistance of beta-lipoprotein, the fat particles (chyle) pass into the lacteals. This chyle is transported by the lymph vessels to the thoracic duct which empties at the junction of the left internal jugular and left subclavian veins. (See Figure 7–5.) The triglycerides in the form of chylomicrons enter the blood stream and are carried to the liver and adipose tissue for metabolism and storage. Cholesterol and fat-soluble vitamins are absorbed with triglycerides.[4] Under normal conditions about 60 to 70 per cent of ingested fat is absorbed via lymph vessels. The remainder enters the small intestinal capillaries and is transported to the liver via the portal circulation. Fatty acids with 12 carbons or more are re-esterified to triglycerides prior to transportation as chylomicrons in the lymph, whereas fatty acids with 10 carbons or less go directly into and are carried by the portal vein without esterification to the liver.

The utilization of medium chain triglycerides C_8 and C_{10} is assisted by rapid hydrolysis of the triglycerides and rapid absorption of the fatty acids into the mucosal cell. The fatty acids without re-esterification leave the mycosal cell and enter the portal circulation. These properties facilitate the nutritional management of disorders caused by impaired hydrolysis and absorption of customary dietary fats.

Increased motility and the absence of bile decreases absorption of fat, and undigested fat will appear in the feces—a condition known as steatorrhea.

Bile is a secretion from the liver which aids in the digestion and absorption of fats. It is stored in the gallbladder until called into the duodenum by stimulus of food in the stomach and duodenum. About 2 pints (1 liter) are secreted daily. Bile is composed of bile salts, bile pigments (which color feces), inorganic salts, mucin, cholesterol and lecithin. There are no enzymes in bile. The bile salts promote the emulsion of fats with the formation of tiny water-soluble particles. The fats are thus made more accessible for digestion by the enzyme lipase.

In addition, bile salts combine with fatty acids and monoglycerides and produce water-soluble complexes which are easily absorbed. (See Chapter 25 for a more detailed discussion of the liver and gallbladder.)

PROTEIN DIGESTION AND ABSORPTION Protein must be broken down to its constituents, the amino acids, to leave the cells in the lining of the intestine and pass through the capillary wall into the intracellular spaces and through the cell membrane into the cell. This involves breaking the peptide linkages that join the amino acids. Protein digestion begins in the stomach where the acid medium of the gastric contents begins to reduce the protein in amino acids (rennin curdles milk protein—this function seems to be more important in infants than in adults). The curd formed is in better condition to be acted upon by pepsin, which breaks the protein down into simpler molecules, proteoses and peptones. Hydrochloric acid in the stomach activates pepsinogen to pepsin.

From the stomach, the partially digested protein (peptones, peptides, amino acids) moves into the duodenum where the proteolytic enzymes trypsin and chymotrypsin split the peptide chains into smaller fragments. Intestinal juice is alkaline in reaction and is produced in the intestinal mucosa. It contains enterokinase, an enzyme which transforms inactive pancreatic trypsinogen into active trypsin. Trypsin, in turn, activates the other pancreatic proteolytic enzymes. Pancreatic trypsin, chymotrypsin and carboxypolypeptidase break down intact protein and continue the breakdown started in the stomach until simple peptides and amino acids are formed. In the intestinal juice the proteolytic peptidases act on polypeptides and dipeptides, changing them to amino acids. These amino acids are actively absorbed from the lumen of the small intestine into the mucosal cells, enter the blood stream and are then sent to the liver via the portal vein. There they are released into general circulation and carried to the various tissues and cells or built into new protein as demanded by the body. Some amino acids may remain in the epithelial cell to be used in the synthesis of intestinal enzymes and new cells.

It has been reported[5] that the absorption of amino acids through the intestinal mucosa stimulates the release of insulin. See Table 7–1 for a summary of digestion and absorption and Figure 7–5 for routes by which the absorbed foods reach the blood.

OTHER   NUTRIENTS   The   vitamins, minerals and fluids are being absorbed simul-

[4]Mead, J. F.: Present knowledge of fat. Nutr. Rev., 24:33, 1966.

[5]Review: Amino acid transport and insulin release. Nutr. Rev., 25:41, 1967.

TABLE 7–1 SUMMARY OF ENZYMATIC DIGESTION AND ABSORPTION

SOURCE	SECRETION	ENZYME	SUBSTRATE	PRODUCTS FROM ACTION	ABSORBED
Salivary glands in mouth	Saliva	Ptyalin (salivary amylase)	Starch	Starts breakdown of polysaccharides to disaccharide (dextrins and maltose), a very minor part of digestion.	
Gastric mucosa in stomach	Gastric juice	Rennin	Casein of milk	Curdles milk protein (calcium caseinate) and prepares it for pepsin action.	
	Gastric juice	Pepsin (gastric protease)	Proteins	Proteose and peptone. Acts only in presence of HCl.	
	Gastric juice	Lipase	Emulsified fats	Fatty acids and glycerol (small amounts)	
Pancreas	Pancreatic juice	Trypsin (protease)	Proteins	Proteoses, peptones, and polypeptides	
Pancreas	Pancreatic juice	Chymotrypsin	Proteoses and peptones	Dipeptides	
Pancreas	Pancreatic juice	Steapsin (lipase)	Fats	Simple glycerides, fatty acids and → glycerol	Mostly in lymph Small amounts in blood
Pancreas	Pancreatic juice	Amylopsin (amylase)	Starch and dextrins	Starch → dextrin → maltose Dextrin → maltose	
Pancreas	Pancreatic juice	Carboxypeptidase	Polypeptides	Amino Acids	Amino acids in blood to liver
Intestinal mucosa	Intestinal juice	Erepsin (3 peptidases — carboxypeptidase, aminopeptidase, and dipeptidase)	Peptones, polypeptides, and depeptides	Proteose → peptone Peptone → amino acids	Amino acids in blood to liver
Intestinal mucosa	Intestinal juice	Enterokinase	Trypsinogen	Trypsin	
Intestinal mucosa	Intestinal juice	Sucrase	Sucrose (table sugar)	Glucose and fructose	Galactose, fructose, and glucose in blood to liver
Intestinal mucosa	Intestinal juice	Maltase	Maltose	Glucose	
Intestinal mucosa	Intestinal juice	Lactase	Lactose	Glucose and galactose	
Intestinal mucosa	Intestinal juice	Steapsin (lipase)	Fats (small amount)	Fatty acid and → glycerol	Lymph and blood

There are no digestive enzymes in the large intestine. Digestion and absorption of food are completed by the time the colon is reached. Only water, salts, and vitamins are absorbed thereafter.

taneously through the intestinal mucosa. Each day about 8 liters of fluid from the body pass back and forth across the membrane of the gut to keep the nutrients in solution.

HORMONAL CONTROL OF DIGESTION In addition to the few enzymes mentioned, a variety of hormones are involved in the complex process of food transport of digestion and absorption. Gastrin, secreted by the gastric mucosa, responds to the stimulus of distention of the pylorus and the presence of protein derivatives. In turn, gastrin stimulates secretion of hydrochloric acid by the gastric glands and promotes digestion by providing an acid environment to activate pepsin and enhance its action.

Musosa of the small intestines secrete enterogastrone under the stimulus of the presence of fats or acid chyme in the duodenum. This hormone inhibits gastric secretion and motility of the stomach which explains the tendency of a high-fat meal to remain in the stomach longer than a low-fat meal. Fat in the duodenum also stimulates the

secretion of cholecystokinin by the intestinal mucosa. This hormone stimulates contractions of the gallbladder, causing the delivery of bile into the duodenum. The presence of polypeptides and acid chyme in the duodenum results in the secretion of the enzyme secretin and pancreozymin by the intestinal mucosa. These enzymes stimulate the secretion of alkaline enzyme-rich solutions by the pancreas.

FACTORS AFFECTING DIGESTION

The term *digestibility* has several meanings. Atwater used the term to mean the proportion of food material actually digested. The most common interpretation, especially by laymen, is to refer to the rapidity rather than to the completeness of digestion. Who has not heard someone say, "I cannot digest that"? What he really means is that the food remains in the alimentary tract for a long period of time, yet in the end may be as completely

TABLE 7–2   PER CENT DIGESTIBILITY OF NUTRIENTS

FOOD GROUP	PROTEIN	FAT	CARBO-HYDRATE
	Per Cent	Per Cent	Per Cent
Animal Foods	97	95	98
Cereals	85	90	98
Legumes, dried	78	90	97
Sugars and starches			98
Vegetables	83	90	95
Fruits	85	90	90
Vegetable foods	84	90	97
Total food*	92	95	97

*Weighted by consumption statistics based on a survey of 185 dietaries.

From Merrill, A. L., and Watts, B. K.: Energy Value of Foods—Basis and Derivation. Washington, D.C., U.S. Department of Agriculture, Handbook No. 74, 1955.

digested and absorbed as food digested in much less time.

Atwater assembled results of many digestive experiments on men in which the apparent digestibility of a food was studied. It was found that over 90 per cent of the food in a mixed diet is utilized. The average coefficients of apparent digestibility (availability as Atwater used the term) for the nutrients in different food groups and for nutrients in a mixed diet are shown in Table 7–2.

PSYCHOLOGICAL FACTORS Sight, smell and taste of food or even the thought of food increases secretions of saliva and the stomach juices, and increases muscular activity of the gastrointestinal tract. The term "the sight of food makes my mouth water" applies to the psychic factor of digestion. Attractive food presentation in happy surroundings enhances digestion; unattractive food or unfamiliar tastes of food, served under emotional stress, retards digestion. Anger, fear, fright and worry have a depressing effect on the secretions and may delay digestion. Anger and fear produce an immediate effect in slowing down the process of digestion and worry tends to produce a delayed effect. Emotions stimulate the hypothalamus, which activates the portion of the autonomic nervous system to depress secretions, inhibit peristalsis and increase the tone of the sphincters. The propulsion of food through the gastrointestinal tract is slowed considerably. These are important points to remember when assisting individuals with dietary problems. The appearance of the food served, the combinations and the tastes of food along with the existing emotional stresses have an impact on the digestion of food.

MECHANICAL FACTORS These are the physical changes brought about by the grinding, crushing and mixing of the food that occur in the gastrointestinal tract. They facilitate the mixing of the food with the digestive juices and propel the mass through the digestive tract. Movements in the stomach are weak and shallow in the fundic wall and are strong and vigorous in the pyloric region. In the intestines the chyme is propelled caudally by waves of rhythmic contractions (peristalsis), mixed, and brought into contact with the intestinal mucosa containing layers of circular and longitudinal muscles which produce segmentation movements. Some of the reduction of food can be done before it enters the body. Foods prepared to have a fine consistency, such as mashed foods, purées and liquids, are frequently served patients who require easily swallowed and readily digested foods. Cellulose present in vegetables slows digestion and may increase putrefaction in the colon.

Abuses in the quantity or combination of foods may cause the digestive system to rebel and bring about digestive disorders or distress. Small, frequent meals may be more easily tolerated than three large meals, an important factor to remember when feeding the sick.

In general, properly cooked foods are more digestible than raw foods. Proper cooking of meat, for example, loosens the connective tissue, aids chewing and makes the meat more accessible to the digestive juices. Bolting of food has the result of introducing large chunks into the stomach, bypassing the benefit of mastication to break it down. It is an added tax on the digestive system.

CHEMICAL FACTORS These apply to the chemical reactions between food and the secretions of the digestive system. Fatty and improperly fried foods will retard the flow of digestive juices, while meat extracts, for example, will stimulate digestion.

Some foods agree with many people and disagree with others. Personal idiosyncrasy or an allergy may account for this. It has been suggested that there are people who are peculiarly sensitive to some chemical substances or to its physical state. For example, why do some people have distress from drinking orange juice? Although orange juice is considered a very easily digested food, there are those in good physical condition who claim it causes genuine distress, especially if ice cold and ingested when the stomach is empty.

BACTERIAL ACTION The gastrointestinal tract is essentially sterile at birth, but implantation of various microorganisms soon takes place. *Lactobacillus* is the first organism to appear and is the chief component of the flora until solid foods are ingested. Next, the *coli* gradually become predominant. The primary intestinal flora appears to be *anaerobic,* with the *bacteroides* group most frequent. Lactobacilli are also present in the stools of most persons on an ordinary mixed diet.

Normally, there is very little bacterial action in the stomach as the hydrochloric acid acts as a germicidal agent. However, in conditions in which there is decreased secretion of hydrochloric acid, resistance to bacterial action (both fermentative and putrefactive) is lowered.

Bacterial action is most intense in the large intestine. Although dietary intake alters the fecal flora, the response varies markedly in degree from time to time, and from individual to individual. (1) Gases (hydrogen, carbon dioxide, ammonia, methane), (2) acids (lactic, acetic, etc.), and (3) various toxic substances (indole, phenol, etc.) are formed. The ingestion of carbohydrate, in general, leads to increased fermentation in the large intestine; protein yields increased putrefaction. If large amounts of carbohydrate or protein reach the large intestine as a result of faulty absorption in the small intestine, bacterial action may give rise to the formation of excessive gas and also of certain toxic substances. The colon also contains great numbers of bacteria which grow on the waste products and help generate compounds which account for the odor of the feces. The brown color of feces is caused by stercobilin and urobilin, derivatives of bilirubin.

Intestinal flora plays a much more important role in nutrition than was previously considered. Some of the intestinal organisms have the ability to synthesize a number of the vitamins of the B-complex (especially biotin, folic acid and B_{12}) and vitamin K. In addition, they contribute toward maintaining the intestines in a healthy condition. The organic acids produced help to check the growth of some of the less desirable bacteria. They also increase the solubility, and therefore the absorption, of calcium.

CELL METABOLISM

The absorbed nutrients including water and electrolytes are carried in the blood stream to the cells. The complex chemical changes for converting the nutrients in carbohydrate, fat

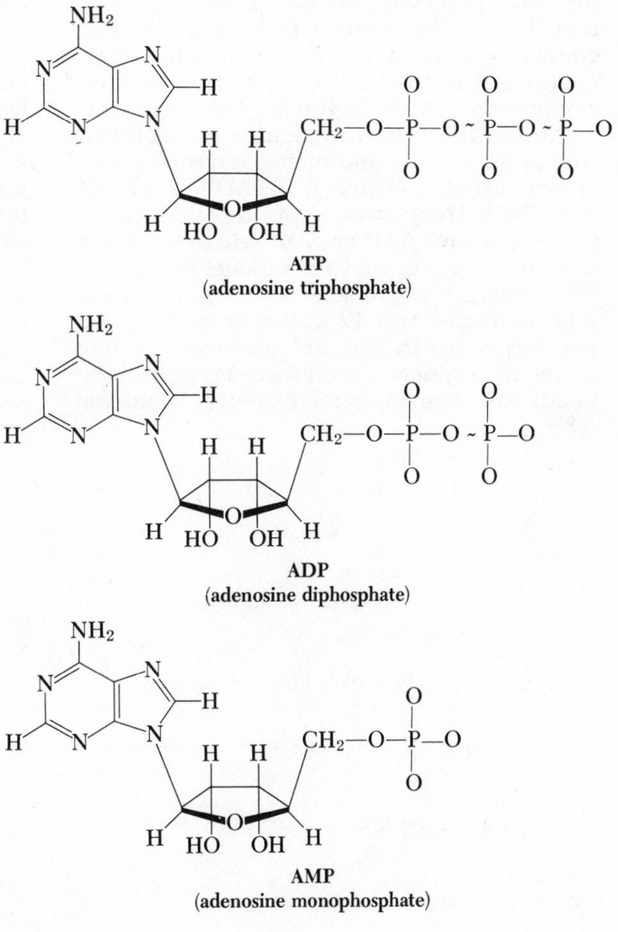

Figure 7–6   High energy bonds of adenine nucleotides. (Adapted from McGilvery, R. W.: Biochemistry–A Functional Approach, W. B. Saunders Company, 1970.)

ATP
(adenosine triphosphate)

ADP
(adenosine diphosphate)

AMP
(adenosine monophosphate)

and protein foods into energy (catabolism) and the synthesis of new molecules (anabolism) are continuous and proceed simultaneously. The metabolism of glucose, fats and amino acids is regulated and controlled by cellular enzymes, their coenzymes (many of which are the B vitamins), other co-factors and hormones. The end-products of glucose, fat and amino acids are the same, namely, carbon dioxide and water. In addition to carbon dioxide and water, the end-products of amino acid metabolism are the nitrogenous wastes in the urine.

In earlier chapters the general metabolism of the carbohydrates, fats and proteins has been described. The present discussion will consider the nutrition of the individual cells, the intricate biochemical pathway by which the chemical energy of the foods is made available to the cells as needed, and the steps by which the three major nutrients enter this pathway. The same preliminary steps are needed whether the nutrients are used immediately for energy or are transformed for utilization or storage.

ADENINE NUCLEOTIDES   The source of energy for the body is the oxidation of foods. This energy must be in a utilizable form and for many processes, notably muscle contraction, it must be immediately available. The energy is trapped in certain organic phosphates and is released very rapidly when the compounds are hydrolyzed. The most important of these are the adenine nucleotides: adenosine tri-, di-, and monoadenosine phosphates, usually written ATP, ADP and AMP (Fig. 7–6). Hydrolysis of the terminal phosphate group of ATP or ADP releases a large amount of energy and the linkage is called a "high-energy phosphate bond" ($\sim$). When ATP is hydrolyzed, 12 kcalories are released per molecule. In the full oxidation of one molecule of glucose 38 high-energy phosphate bonds are formed, a total of 456 kcalories.

Thus about 70 per cent of the total energy of the glucose (646 kcalories) is made available for muscular work or other vital activity. This is very efficient transfer for any thermodynamic process.

A heavy demand for energy can outstrip the capacity of a muscle to regenerate ATP by complete oxidation of glucose or fatty acid. There are two mechanisms by which this need can be met. One is the storage of part of the high-energy phosphate as creatine phosphate. The other is by glycolysis, the conversion of glucose to lactic acid,[6] which will be discussed in the next section.

GLUCOSE   The complete oxidation of glucose may be divided into two stages: anaerobic and aerobic. The first converts one molecule of glucose into two molecules of pyruvic acid. This conversion requires 10 successive steps, each with its specific enzyme and its own requirements for cofactors. In the process 2 molecules of ATP are used and 4 are produced, a net gain of 2 molecules of ATP available for immediate use. Figure 7–7 gives an abbreviated outline of this pathway. There is no involvement of oxygen in the series of reactions. If there is heavy demand for muscular work and there is insufficient oxygen to continue with the aerobic pathway, the anaerobic reaction may go one step further with reduction of pyruvic acid to lactic acid. The lactic acid will diffuse out of the cells and its level in the blood stream will rise. The lactic acid can again be converted to glucose (largely in the liver). The steps indicated in the diagram can all occur in the reverse direction, but in a few cases the reverse reaction is catalyzed by a different enzyme.

The second stage of carbohydrate metabolism which cannot take place without the

---

[6] It is convenient to use the term "lactic acid," but it must be remembered that at body pH the acids formed in metabolism do not exist as the free acid but as organic anions.

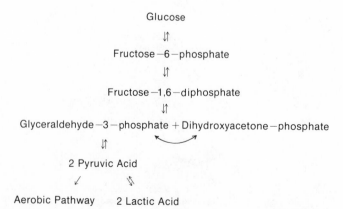

Glucose

$\Updownarrow$

Fructose –6–phosphate

$\Updownarrow$

Fructose –1,6–diphosphate

$\Updownarrow$

Glyceraldehyde –3–phosphate + Dihydroxyacetone –phosphate

$\Updownarrow$

2 Pyruvic Acid

Aerobic Pathway   2 Lactic Acid

Figure 7–7   Embden-Meyerhof anaerobic pathway.

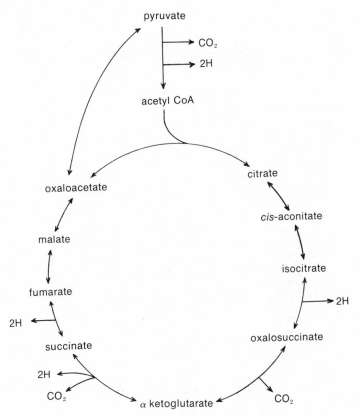

Figure 7–8   Krebs cycle.

presence of molecular oxygen is variously referred to as the aerobic cycle, Krebs cycle and the tricarboxylic or citric acid cycle (because of the formation of citric and several related 6-carbon acids with 3 COOH groups). Pyruvic acid may be regarded as the starting point of the cycle. It was early recognized that the first step involved oxidative decarboxylation of pyruvic acid with formation of CO_2 and acetic acid. The acetic acid was in some active form; the nature of this acid form was elusive but was finally identified as a combination of acetic acid with a derivative of pantothenic acid. The coenzyme was called Coenzyme A and the active molecule acetyl-CoA. In another reaction pyruvic acid may combine with a molecule of CO_2 to form oxaloacetic acid.

Figure 7–8 shows the cycle with oxaloacetic acid combining with acetyl-CoA to form citric acid. By a further series of steps 2 atoms of carbon are oxidized to CO_2 and oxaloacetic acid formed. The net result is the oxidation of the active acetyl unit and the reformation of oxaloacetic acid, which consequently is needed only in catalytic amounts.

Several steps in the cycle involve dehydrogenation. These steps cannot occur without simultaneous oxidation of the hydrogen to water. This is brought about through what is called the *respiratory or electron chain*, a series of steps involving alternate oxidation and reduction of a sequence of coenzymes, culminating in the combination of hydrogen with molecular oxygen (Fig. 7–9). Most of the

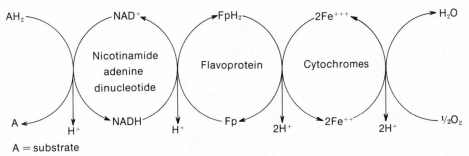

Figure 7–9   Respiratory chain.

capture of energy as ATP occurs during this phase. Oxidation of hydrogen and phosphorylation are *coupled*. The two must occur together and ADP is essential for the operation of the respiratory chain. Recent studies of cell structure at the molecular level have shown that these enzyme systems and others are not randomly dispersed in the cell but are arranged in an orderly fashion for carrying out the reaction in production-line fashion. (See Figure 3–2.)

It is of interest to note here the role of the vitamins in tissue metabolism. Thiamin pyrophosphate is the coenzyme for decarboxylation of pyruvic acid. Coenzyme-A is a derivative of pantothenic acid. Riboflavin and nicotinic acid are constitutents of coenzymes of the respiratory chain. The role of vitamin E is less clear but it also appears to be involved in electron transport in conjunction with the cytochromes.

FATS   The first step in utilization of fat in the body is hydrolysis to fatty acids and glycerol. This takes place largely in the adiposte tissue. Glycerol, in certain tissues (notably liver and kidney), forms glycerophosphate which can be oxidized to CO_2 and water or converted to glucose. Fatty acids are taken into the tissues, most of which have the capacity to oxidize them. As early as 1905 Knoop proposed that fatty acids were metabolized by beta-oxidation (the beta carbon is the second from the carboxyl carbon). The chain was shortened by two carbons at a time, forming in each step acetic acid and a shorter fatty acid. This is still recognized as the major pathway of fatty acid oxidation and the mechanisms have been worked out (Fig. 7–10). The fatty acid forms an active complex with Coenzyme-A, this initial step being supplied with energy by ATP. As each acetyl-CoA molecule is formed it is oxidized via the citric acid cycle.

AMINO ACIDS   It is impossible in a brief

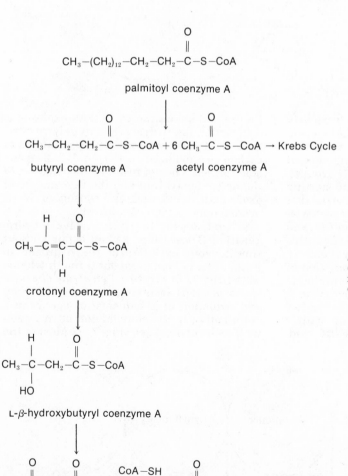

Figure 7–10   Beta-oxidation of fatty acids. (Adapted from McGilvery, R. W.: Biochemistry–a Functional Approach, W. B. Saunders Company, 1970.)

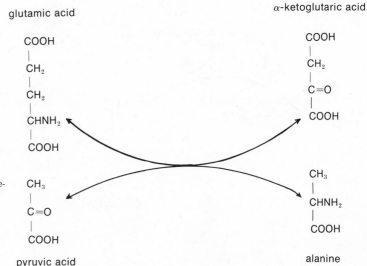

Figure 7–11   Transamination and deamination.

summary to show the catabolic pathways for all the amino acids. Important common steps may be illustrated. One of these steps is removal of the amino group. This occurs largely in the liver and usually involves oxidation with the formation of a keto acid. This may occur as oxidative deamination or, in many cases, as transamination, with exchange of an amino group and a keto group between two acids (Figure 7–11). The keto acids (and ketoglutaric and pyruvic acid) resulting from these reactions are members of the aerobic cycle. Either directly, as in these two cases, or after a longer series of preliminary reactions, the carbon skeleton of the amino acid can enter the citric acid cycle for complete oxidation.

The amino group of the amino acids is released as ammonia (chiefly as ammonium ion at body pH) and is used in synthetic processes or carried to the liver for conversion to urea, the form in which most of it is excreted. Ammonia is very toxic and so it is transported in combination with glutamic acid, as glutamine. Most tissues are rich in the enzyme which catalyzes synthesis of glutamine. The liver and kidney, where ammonia will be used, have a large amount of the enzyme which catalyzes the hydrolysis. Glutamine plays an active role in many metabolic processes such as formation of purines, pyrimidines and amino sugars as well as in synthesis of proteins.

Synthesis of urea occurs through a process sometimes referred to as the ornithine cycle which is presented in condensed form in Figure 7–12. Carbon dioxide and NH_3 (with energy from ATP) combine with ornithine through a series of steps to form arginine. The arginine is hydrolyzed to yield urea and ornithine. Thus an ornithine molecule is used over and over in the formation of arginine.

COMMON METABOLIC PATHWAY Figure 7–13 is an integration of the metabolic pathways which have been described. It shows how carbohydrate, fat and protein may be utilized for energy by a common pathway; how carbohydrate may be converted to fat for storage or to cholesterol via acetyl-CoA; how some amino acids may be converted to glucose and some to fat and how some of the nonessential amino acids are synthesized. It

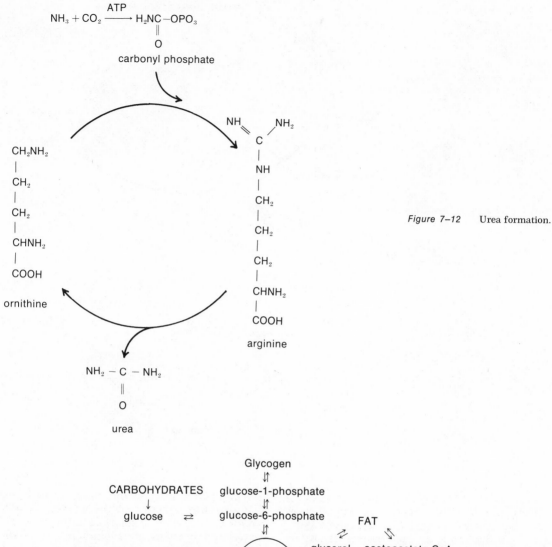

Figure 7–12   Urea formation.

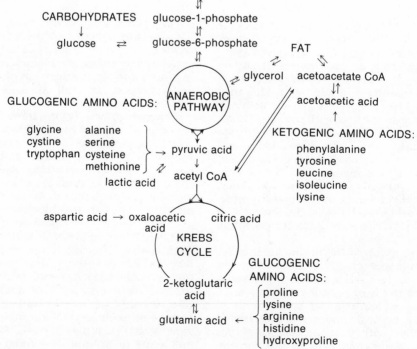

Figure 7–13   Metabolic integration of carbohydrate, fat and protein.

should be noted that the step from pyruvic acid to acetyl-CoA is not reversible, so fatty acids cannot be used for net gain of carbohydrate. It is by these interrelationships, and only a few of many have been shown, that the body can function smoothly under a variety of dietary and metabolic conditions.

The processes of anabolism and catabolism are continuous and proceed simultaneously. A food intake in excess of body energy needs results in storage of glycogen and fat. When the food intake is inadequate to meet the energy needs of the body, body stores of glycogen and fat and, lastly, the tissue amino acids are oxidized. The composition of the body remains remarkably constant but study with nutrients tagged with radioactive elements shows that there is constant exchange even in such tissues as bone or fat. Thus there is a state of dynamic equilibrium, constancy in the face of continuous change.

PROBLEMS AND SUGGESTED TOPICS FOR DISCUSSION

1. Describe what is meant by digestion; absorption; enzyme. Describe the physical or mechanical factors of the alimentary canal; explain how they aid digestion and absorption.
2. Chart the digestive course of fruit juice, egg, toast, butter and milk.
3. What role does attractive food service play in digestion? Suggest some ways to make food service more attractive.
4. Describe the functions of the enzymes in digestion, mentioning the enzymes of the stomach, the small intestine and the pancreas; the material acted upon (substrate); and products of the action.
5. Describe the function of bile.
6. Compare the rate of digestion and absorption of carbohydrate, protein and fat. Explain.
7. List all the factors that affect *your* food digestion in one day.

SUGGESTED ADDITIONAL READING REFERENCES

Bogert, L. J.: Nutrition and Physical Fitness. 8th ed. Philadelphia, W. B. Saunders Company, 1966, Chapter 18, Digestion and Absorption of Food.

Cantrow, A., and Trumper, M.: Clinical Biochemistry. 6th ed. Philadelphia, W. B. Saunders Company, 1962.

Clifton, J. A.: Intestinal absorption and malabsorption. J. Am. Dietet. A., 39:449, 1961.

Daniels, B. T., et al.: Changing concepts of common bile duct anatomy and physiology. J.A.M.A., 178:394, 1961.

Danielsson, H.: Influence of bile acids on digestion and absorption of lipids. Am. J. Clin. Nutr., 12:214, 1963.

Dragstedt, L. R.: Why does not the stomach digest itself? J.A.M.A., 177:758, 1961.

Duncan, G. G. (ed.): Diseases of Metabolism. 5th ed. Philadelphia, W. B. Saunders Company, 1964, pp. 25–27; 105–109; 191–201.

Guyton, A. C.: Textbook of Medial Physiology. 4th ed. Philadelphia, W. B. Saunders Company, 1971.

Harkins, R. W., and Sarett, H. P.: Medium-chain triglycerides. J.A.M.A. 203:272, 1968.

Ingelfinger, F. J.: Gastrointestinal absorption: Nutrition Today. 2:2, 1967.

King, B. G., and Showers, M. J.: Human Anatomy and Physiology. 6th ed. Philadelphia, W. B. Saunders Company, 1969.

Mazur, A., and Harrow, B.: Textbook of Biochemistry. 10th ed. Philadelphia, W. B. Saunders Company, 1971.

McGilvery, R. W.: Biochemistry—A Functional Approach. Philadelphia, W. B. Saunders Company, 1970.

Miller, D., and Crane, R. K.: The digestion of carbohydrates in the small intestine. Am. J. Clin. Nutr., 12:220, 1963.

Review. Digestion and absorption of disaccharides in man. Nutr. Rev., 20:203, 1962.

Wohl, M. G., and Goodhart, R. S.: Modern Nutrition in Health and Disease. 4th ed. Philadelphia, Lea & Febiger, 1968.

Chapter 8
THE MINERALS

DEFINITION   By the term *"minerals"* we mean the elements in their simple inorganic form. In nutrition they are commonly referred to as *mineral elements* or *inorganic nutrients.*

MINERAL COMPOSITION OF THE BODY

There are many mineral elements. Approximately 17 have been proved essential in nutrition. Analysis of mineral ash shows the presence of more than 20. The minerals of the body include: calcium, phosphorus, potassium, sulfur, sodium, chlorine, magnesium, iron, zinc, selenium, manganese, copper, iodine, molybdenum, cobalt, chromium, fluorine, and traces of vanadium, barium, bromine, strontium, gold, silver, nickel, aluminum, tin, bismuth, gallium, silicon, arsenic and others. They exist in the body and in food in organic and inorganic combinations.

TABLE 8-1   MINERAL ELEMENTS OF THE ADULT BODY

CLASSIFICATION	ELEMENTS	PER CENT OF BODY WEIGHT
Essential for Nutrition		
1. Macronutrients	Calcium	1.5-2.2
	Phosphorus	0.8-1.2
	Potassium	0.35
	Sulfur	0.25
	Sodium	0.15
	Chlorine	0.15
	Magnesium	0.05
2. Micronutrients	Iron	0.004
	Zinc	0.002
	Selenium	0.0003
	Manganese	0.0002
	Copper	0.00015
	Iodine	0.00004
	Molybdenum	trace
	Cobalt	trace
	Fluorine	trace
	Chromium	trace
3. Others (Function not known. Present in traces only.)		
	Strontium	
	Bromine	
	Vanadium	
	Gold	
	Silver	
	Nickel	
	Tin	
	Aluminum	
	Bismuth	
	Arsenic	
	Boron	
	Oxygen	65
	Carbon	18
	Hydrogen	10
	Nitrogen	3

Adapted from Sherman, H. C.: Chemistry of Food and Nutrition. 8th ed. New York, The Macmillan Company, 1952, p. 227.

The human body contains minerals in relatively small amounts and, in view of their great importance, the amounts seem minimal indeed. Only about 4 per cent of man's weight is in the form of minerals. For a man weighing 150 pounds this would mean about 6 pounds of minerals, and most of this amount is in the bones.

Table 8-1 shows the mineral composition of the body.

CLASSIFICATION

The minerals are found in the body and in food chiefly in the form of the positively charged and negatively charged ions of salts. Metals form positive ions (cations); nonmetals form negative ions (anions). Among the positive ions are sodium, potassium and calcium. Non-metals forming anions include chlorine, sulfur (as sulfate) and phosphorus (as phosphate). Typical salts are sodium chloride and calcium phosphate. In bones and teeth the minerals are found as the fixed salts, primarily of calcium and phosphorus. In solution the salts dissociate and in body fluids

we find Na^+, K^+, Ca^{++}, Cl^- and $H_2PO_4^{--}$ rather than fixed compounds.

The minerals also enter into organic compounds such as phosphoproteins, phospholipids and hemoglobin. The hormone thyroxine is an amino acid containing four atoms of iodine. Phosphorus has been shown previously to occur in carbohydrates, fats and proteins; and sulfur has been shown to be an integral part of some amino acids and enzymes.

The essential minerals for nutrition are classified as macronutrient elements (> 0.005 per cent body weight) and micronutrient elements (< 0.005 per cent body weight). The minerals in these categories are listed in Table 8-1.

FUNCTION

Mineral elements have many essential roles, both in their ionic forms in solution in body fluids and as constituents of essential compounds. The balance of mineral ions in body fluids regulates the metabolism of many enzymes, maintains acid-base balance and osmotic pressure, facilitates membrane transfer of essential compounds, maintains nerve and muscular irritability and in some cases are building constituents of body tissue. Indirectly many minerals are involved in the growth process. Other minerals have no known function as yet. A few of the trace elements may be mere contaminants in the body.

Although the various minerals will be discussed individually, it must be remembered that their actions in the body occur in interrelated patterns and no one element can function, be deficient, or be overabundant in the body without affecting others.

REQUIREMENTS

The mineral elements which are needed by the body in what may be regarded as substantial amounts are calcium, phosphorus, iron, sulfur, magnesium, sodium, potassium, and chlorine. In addition, the body needs minute (trace) amounts of iodine, copper, cobalt, manganese, zinc, selenium, molybdenum and probably fluorine and some others.

Of the minerals known to be needed by the human body, all must be supplied in the diet. Calcium, iron and iodine are the 3 elements most frequently insufficient in the diet, especially in the underdeveloped countries. Youmans[1] lists zinc, iron, copper, magnesium and

[1]Some Inorganic Elements in Human Nutrition. Symposium I. Chicago, American Medical Association Council on Food and Nutrition, 1955.

potassium as among the minerals that are most frequently involved in disturbances of metabolism.

The Food and Nutrition Board of the National Research Council has established recommended intakes for calcium, phosphorus, iodine and iron. Specific allowances are not yet established for the other minerals. To summarize our present knowledge of mineral requirement, it is suggested that a varied or mixed diet of animal and vegetable products which meet the energy and protein needs will also furnish adequate minerals. As a rule when the calcium, iron and iodine needs of the body are met, the rest of the minerals will be supplied.

SOURCES

The body is supplied with minerals mainly in the form of mineral salts, found mixed or combined with carbohydrate, fat and protein in the natural foods. An exception is sodium chloride, "table salt," which is used in large amounts as a condiment. The "empty calorie" foods such as sugar, pure fats and cornstarch contain few or no mineral elements (or vitamins). These foods are practically electrolyte-free. The mineral content of a food is determined by burning and analysis of the ash.

CALCIUM AND PHOSPHORUS

Calcium and phosphorus are usually associated together because they are so closely related in the body. They are discussed separately to emphasize their independent roles as well as their association in the way they function together in the body. The normal metabolism of calcium and phosphorus is maintained by a number of physiological mechanisms.

CALCIUM

Body need for calcium occurs throughout life, but especially during childhood, pregnancy and lactation. It is the mineral frequently found to be low in the dietary.

Calcium is the most abundant mineral in the body. It makes up about 1.5 to 2.0 per cent of the body weight and 39 per cent of the total minerals present; 99 per cent of it is in the hard tissues, bones and teeth. Thus an adult male has about 1200 grams of calcium and the adult female 1000 grams. The 1 per cent not contained in bones and teeth is present in the blood, extracellular fluids and within the cells of soft tissues where it regulates many important metabolic functions.

In the bones, calcium occurs in the form of salts, hydroxyapatite, composed of calcium phosphate and calcium carbonate arranged in a characteristic crystal structure around a framework of softer protein material (organic matrix). The hydroxyapatite serves to provide strength and rigidity to the soft matrix. Many other ions are also present in this crystal complex including fluoride, hydroxyl, magnesium and sodium. Blood and lymph vessels, nerves and bone marrow pass through the matrix and between the crystal structures. The mineral ions diffuse into the extracellular fluid, bathing the crystals and permitting deposition of new mineral or its absorption from bones.

The same type of crystals are present in the enamel and dentin of teeth. However, the crystals are larger. Recent data suggest that the size of the apatite crystals depends in part upon fluoride. The larger size of the crystals thus formed may explain increased resistance of teeth to erosion when adequate fluoride is present. It may account for the relative inactivity of the minerals of mature teeth in body metabolism (i.e., the calcium or phosphate is not readily available during periods of deprivation).

In the skeleton, calcium exists in two forms: (1) a stable component, the calcium of the apatite crystal and (2) a non-stable component, calcium attached to the surface of the crystal. The non-stable calcium is more or less in equilibrium with that in the extracellular fluids. The latter may be considered to be a reserve which may be built up when the dietary provides an adequate intake of calcium. This reserve is stored especially in the trabeculae, the ends of the long bones. It may be called upon in times of stress to meet the body's increased need (growth, pregnancy, lactation) if calcium is not supplied in adequate amounts by the food intake. If there is no reserve, the calcium must be drawn from the bone substance itself, which must be broken down before calcium is liberated. This results in a deficiency in the bone structure following prolonged inadequate intake. As it is with most components in the body, bone is constantly made and broken down. Depending upon physiological state or age of the individual, one aspect of the process may predominate. In children, for example, bone synthesis is greater than the destruction of bone. At the other end of the age spectrum, bone breakdown may predominate with a decrease in the absolute amount of bone present. In the normal adult there is a balance of these processes; a constant mobilization of calcium from and to the bones and to and from the body fluids, maintaining dynamic equilibrium.

FUNCTION   In addition to the major function of calcium to build and maintain bones and teeth, the remaining 1 per cent of the body's calcium is found in the body fluids and soft tissues. This calcium, present principally in ionic form has important metabolic functions. It is essential for the activity of certain enzymes, notably adenosine triphosphatase in the release of energy for muscular contraction.

In the blood clotting process, calcium must be present to initiate the changes needed for the formation of the clot, fibrin. The ionized calcium stimulates the release of thromboplastin from the blood platelets. Thromboplastin catalyzes the conversion of prothrombin to thrombin. Thrombin aids in the polymerization of fibrinogen to fibrin.

In the control of the passage of fluids to cell walls, calcium controls the permeability of the cell membrane to various nutrients. It regulates the uptake of nutrients by the cell. It is closely bound to lecithin in the cell membrane.

In normal nerve transmission and regulation of the heartbeat, calcium is required. Calcium ion concentrations together with correct amounts of sodium, potassium and magnesium maintain muscle tone and control muscle irritability.

ABSORPTION AND UTILIZATION   Calcium absorption in humans is very inefficient. Usually only 20 to 30 per cent of the ingested calcium is absorbed and sometimes it is as low as 10 per cent. About 70 per cent is unabsorbed and is excreted in the feces. Calcium is absorbed in the duodenum in an acid medium, and its absorption ceases in the lower part of the intestinal tract when the food content becomes alkaline. Calcium is absorbed by active transport requiring energy. The amount absorbed depends largely upon the nature of the diet, for unless it is present in a water-soluble form in the intestine and is not precipitated by another dietary constituent, it will not be absorbed.

Many factors influence the actual amount of calcium absorbed. The body absorbs calcium more effectively when in need. The greater the need and the smaller the dietary supply the more efficient the absorption. During periods of rapid growth, the absorption of calcium is increased. The factors favoring calcium absorption are as follows:

Vitamin D   This is required for the efficient absorption of calcium. In the presence of vitamin D, more calcium is absorbed before the food reaches the colon and absorption ceases. It increases the permeability of the intestinal membrane to calcium. Vitamin D activates the active transport system causing some absorption.

Acidity of Gastric Juices   Calcium is made soluble by acids. The hydrochloric acid secreted in the stomach provides the acid medium of the contents of the digestive tract in the small intestine.

Lactose   In the presence of lactose, calcium absorption is improved. A relatively high ratio of lactose to calcium to form a sugar-calcium complex in the intestine keeps the calcium in the form in which it can be transported to and across the intestinal mucosa. The lactose-calcium complex also prevents the precipitation of calcium in an insoluble complex as the contents of the intestinal tract change from acid to alkaline.

Fat   Fat content in moderate amounts, moving slowly through the digestive tract, tends to facilitate calcium absorption.

Protein Intake   When the intake of protein is high, a greater percentage of calcium is absorbed than when the intake of protein is low. The action of certain amino acids upon intestinal pH and upon the formation of the soluble complex with calcium facilitates calcium absorption.

On the other hand, there are many factors which depress the absorption of calcium:

Vitamin D Deficiency   Lack of or insufficient amount of vitamin D decreases or prevents the absorption of calcium and thus it is not available to the body.

Fats   An excessive intake of dietary fats or poor absorption of fats results in an excess of free fatty acids which unite with calcium to form insoluble soaps. The calcium soaps are excreted in the feces.

Oxalic Acid   The calcium content and availability in some fruits and vegetables depend upon the oxalic acid they contain. Oxalic acid combines in the digestive tract with calcium to form an insoluble compound, calcium oxalate. The calcium is not absorbed. Rhubarb, spinach, chard and beet greens contain oxalic acid in appreciable amounts.

Phytic Acid   Phytic acid, a phosphorus-containing compound found principally in the outer husks of cereal grains (especially oatmeal) combines with calcium to form calcium phytate which is insoluble and is not absorbed from the intestines.

Alkaline Medium   In an alkaline medium, calcium (and phosphorus) will form insoluble and non-absorbable calcium phosphate.

Gastrointestinal Motility   When the food passes through the intestinal tract too rapidly, calcium absorption is decreased.

Immobilization   Lack of exercise, lack of weight-bearing on the legs causes a decrease in the ability to absorb calcium.

Stress   Emotional instability may influence the efficiency of calcium absorption. Mental stress tends to decrease absorption and increase excretion of calcium. Under distress, emotional or physical, a higher intake of calcium is required to maintain calcium equilibrium.

CALCIUM-PHOSPHORUS RATIO   The ratio of calcium to phosphorus in the dietary is important in the absorption of both elements. Adults require an intake of phosphorus in the ratio of $1\frac{1}{2}$ to 1 of calcium. The ratio in the dietary of children and of females during pregnancy and lactation is 1 to 1. An excess of either one in the dietary causes poor absorption of both and increased excretion of one or the other.

Calcium is transported by the blood to the fluids bathing the tissues of the body and to the cells and is used wherever needed. Most of the calcium is used in the bones. The calcium in the bone is in equilibrium with calcium in the blood. The parathyroid hormone, parathormone, and calcitonin, secreted chiefly by the thyroid gland, keep the blood calcium at a normal concentration of about 10 mg. per 100 ml. of blood serum. When it falls below this level, parathormone transfers exchangeable calcium from the bone into the blood. At the same time the parathyroid causes the kidney to reabsorb calcium which normally might be excreted in the urine and it stimulates more absorption of calcium from the intestines. When the blood calcium level is above normal, calcitonin acts to lower it and calcium is thus excreted by the kidney.

EXCRETION   Normally, most of the calcium (65 to 75 per cent) is excreted in the feces and the rest in the urine. Some is excreted in the perspiration, which may become significant in environmental and physiological conditions producing active sweating.[2] Most of the calcium in the feces is unabsorbed food calcium, which is variable. Despite wide variation in calcium intake, under normal conditions the amount excreted in the urine remains rather constant at about 100–150 mg./day.

DIETARY SOURCES   Calcium is assimilated better from some foods than from others. The calcium in milk is assimilated readily. Milk and milk products are the best sources of calcium. Dark green leafy vegetables such as kale, turnip greens, mustard greens and broccoli, and sardines, clams and oysters are good sources of calcium. It is difficult to have an adequate intake of calcium without milk or milk products. Eight ounces of milk (whole or non-fat) daily would supply about 288 to 298 mg. of calcium. Along with something from the bread-cereal, vegetable-fruit and meat groups in the amounts suggested (page 18) approximately three-fourths of the recommended daily amounts of calcium would be provided for an adult.

Infants can easily meet the calcium intake requirement of milk, since this is their chief food. Children can best meet the requirement by including the amount of milk recommended for each age group (Table 17–1), or its equivalent, daily. Appendix Table 7 shows the foods high in calcium content.

RECOMMENDED DIETARY ALLOWANCE Most of the data regarding calcium requirements for man have been obtained from calcium balance studies. (A controversy exists regarding the interpretation of the data and the use of the balance studies as a basis for requirements.) These studies measure the intake and output of calcium over periods of time. To determine the minimum calcium requirement, the calcium intake is reduced until the person can no longer remain in balance (i.e., his excretion becomes greater than his intake). It is evident from these studies that man, if given time to adjust to changes in levels, can remain in calcium balance over a very wide range of calcium intakes.

The 1968 revision of Recommended Dietary Allowances of the National Research Council states that the normal adult male and female should receive 800 mg. of calcium daily. This amount covers basic needs and allows for a margin of safety. These allowances are greater than those recommended by the FAO/WHO Expert Group.[3] This report concludes that intakes of 400 to 500 mg. per day would represent a suggested practical allowance for adults. They feel that this level can more readily be achieved by a larger segment of the world's population. Sources of calcium are limited in the national food supply of many countries.

The Food and Nutrition Board, National Research Council justify their allowance of 800 mg. on the basis that calcium losses in metabolism amount to approximately 320 mg. per day. Since only 20–30 per cent of the dietary calcium is absorbed, 800 mg. would be required to maintain balance. Food sources of calcium are readily available to the population of the United States. Cognizance was also taken of the relatively high prevalence of osteoporosis in older persons and the possibility that minimal or moderate inadequacy in calcium intake over a period of years may contribute to the occurrence or accentuation of this disease.

The need for calcium is increased during pregnancy and lactation. The calcium needed by the fetus must be provided by the mother.

[2]Consolazio, C. F., et al.: Relationship between calcium in sweat, calcium balance, and calcium requirements. J. Nutr., 78:78–88, 1962.

[3]WHO Technical Report Series No. 230:Calcium requirement. Geneva, 1962.

An increase in calcium is needed for the calcification of fetal bones and teeth and for the storage of calcium by the mother to meet the demands of lactation. The National Research Council has recommended an additional 400 mg. of calcium daily to meet the demands of the fetus and mother. Indications are that the pregnant woman may absorb up to 40 per cent of dietary calcium, depending on the need.

The amount needed by the lactating mother is 500 mg. daily over normal requirements in order to provide adequate calcium in milk without causing depletion of the mother's calcium reserve or decrease in milk production.

During these periods of increased dietary needs for calcium the growing fetus or nursing child will satisfy his need for calcium at the mother's expense. If her dietary intake is deficient, presumably the mother will lose bone calcium.

The calcium requirement of the infant is not precisely known. A breast-fed infant receives about 60 mg. of calcium per kilo body weight and retains about two-thirds of this amount. An infant fed a standard cow's milk formula receives about three times this amount of calcium per kilo body weight, and retains 35 per cent to 50 per cent. The National Research Council states that their recommended calcium intakes are from 0.4 to 0.6 grams per day in infants up to one year of age and are based on the infant fed cow's milk formula.

It is assumed that the calcium needs of the breast-fed infant have been met even though calcium intake is considerably less than that obtained on a cow's milk diet.

Children from ages 1 to 10 years need 0.7 to 1.0 grams of calcium daily. From 10 to 18 years of age the recommendation for males is 1.2 to 1.4 grams and for the female 1.2 to 1.3 grams of calcium daily.

Obviously an adequate intake of calcium is not enough. The conditions influencing the absorption and metabolism of calcium must be considered and the nutrients involved must be provided in the daily food intake.

CALCIUM DEFICIENCIES   These aspects will be considered in more detail in Chapter 34. Suffice it to state here that calcium deficiency in children may lead to *rickets* with retarded growth or, more likely, continued body growth, but with abnormal development of bones resulting in bowed legs and other bone deformities. (See Figs. 8–1 and 34–15). Deficiency of calcium in adults may result in osteomalacia (sometimes referred to as adult rickets), a failure to mineralize the bone matrix, resulting in a reduction in the mineral content of the bone. Usually, rickets and osteomalacia are associated with a concurrent lack of vitamin D and imbalance in calcium-phosphorus intake. In scurvy, the lack of ascorbic acid prevents the formation of bone matrix and normal mineralization does not occur.

Osteoporosis develops when the dietary intake of calcium is low over an extended period of time or when dietary needs are abnormally high because of poor absorption. Bone resorption occurs at an accelerated rate to maintain normal calcium blood levels. The bone is of normal composition but a reduced amount of bone is present.

Extremely low levels of calcium in the blood may increase the irritability of nerve fibers and nerve centers and result in muscle spasms such as leg cramps. This condition is known as tetany. It sometimes occurs in pregnant women who have received too little calcium in their diets or who have received too much phosphorus. (The latter is responsible for hastening the excretion of calcium during pregnancy.) The rise in serum phosphorus causes a compensatory decrease in serum calcium. It sometimes occurs in newborn infants fed undiluted cow's milk, which contains more phosphorus than calcium. The kidneys of the infants cannot clear the phosphate.

Calcium rigor occurs when the calcium levels are well above normal causing tonic contractions of the muscle. Both of these conditions are due to abnormal functioning of the parathyroid.

A high intake of calcium and the presence of a high intake of vitamin D such as may occur in children is a potential source of hypercalcemia (elevated blood calcium lev-

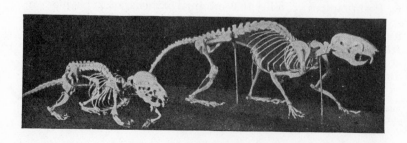

Figure 8–1   Skeletons of twin albino rats showing influence of calcium content of the diet on the growth and character of the bones. The rat fed a diet adequate in calcium (right) attained full growth and had strong bones; the one on the left received a diet deficient in calcium; its growth was stunted and bones were soft, brittle and more or less deformed. (Courtesy of Sherman and Macleod and the Journal of Biological Chemistry.)

els). This may lead to widespread excessive calcification not only in bone but in the soft tissues such as kidneys.

PHOSPHORUS

The metabolism of phosphorus is intimately related to that of calcium. It is second to calcium in abundance forming 22 per cent of the total minerals. Most of it (about 80 per cent) is in the form of insoluble calcium phosphate (apatite) crystals that give strength and rigidity to the bones and teeth. The remaining phosphorus is distributed in every cell of the body and in the extracellular fluid in combination with carbohydrates, lipids, proteins and a variety of other compounds.

FUNCTION   Phosphorus has numerous functions in the body beyond its important part in the structure of bones and teeth; more than any other mineral element. It is an essential component of the nucleic acids. Phosphorylation is the first step in the metabolism of glucose and in many other phases of the metabolic processes. ATP and creatine phosphate serve to store the energy liberated by oxidation. Many of the B vitamins function as coenzymes only when in combination with phosphate. Phosphorus is a member of certain conjugated proteins of which casein in milk is a good example. Phospholipids are important in the structure of cell membranes. The phosphate buffer system is important particularly in intracellular fluid where its concentration is much higher than in extracellular fluid and in the tubular fluids of the kidney.

ABSORPTION   Normally, about 70 per cent of the phosphorus ingested in foods is absorbed. Most favorable absorption takes place when calcium and phosphorus are ingested in approximately equal amounts. As with calcium, the presence of vitamin D increases absorption. Simple phosphates such as calcium phosphate or potassium sodium phosphate are absorbed as such in the small intestine. In the digestion of phosphoprotein and nucleoprotein, phosphate is split off and absorbed. The factors that aid or deter the absorption of calcium act essentially in the same manner with regard to the absorption of phosphate. Phosphorus present as phytic acid in some cereals and flour is not well absorbed and may depress absorption of calcium and iron.

DIETARY SOURCES   Meat, poultry, fish and eggs are excellent sources of phosphorus. Milk and milk products are good sources, as are nuts and legumes. Cereals are good sources but the availability of the phosphorus (especially in bran) is somewhat doubtful due to the phytic acid, as explained previously. Table 8–2 shows the phosphorus content of average servings of various foods. Note that the good sources of protein are also good sources of phosphorus.

RECOMMENDED DIETARY ALLOWANCE The Food and Nutrition Board recommends that the daily intake of phosphorus at least equal that of calcium for all age groups except the young infant. The phosphorus allowances for young infants to one year of age are slightly less than those for calcium. (See Table 11–1.) Because phosphorus is so liberally distributed in foods, there is little possibility of a dietary inadequacy if the food intake contains adequate protein and calcium.

TABLE 8–2   PHOSPHORUS CONTENT OF FOODS

FOOD	AVERAGE SERVING		
	APPROXIMATE MEASURE	WEIGHT GRAMS	MILLIGRAMS OF PHOSPHORUS*
Peanuts, roasted, with skins	²/₃ cup	100	407
Turkey, roasted, flesh only	3¹/₃ oz.	100	251
Fish (halibut, broiled)	3¹/₃ oz.	100	248
Pork loin, broiled, med. fat	3¹/₃ oz.	100	268
Milk, nonfat (skim), fluid	1 glass (8 oz.)	246	232
Milk, whole, fluid	1 glass (8 oz.)	244	227
Chicken, roasted	3¹/₃ oz.	100	220
Loin lamb chop, broiled	3¹/₃ oz.	100	179
Beef, hamburger, cooked (regular ground)	3¹/₃ oz.	100	194
Oysters, raw	6 oysters	100	143
Cheese, cheddar	1 oz.	30	143
Peas, cooked	²/₃ cup	100	99
Egg, poached	1 medium	50	101
Wheat cereal, flakes	1 cup	25	77
Sweet corn, cooked	²/₃ cup	100	89
Spinach, cooked	½ cup packed	100	38
Bread, white, enriched, 4 per cent, nonfat milk solids	1 slice	23	22

*Agriculture Handbook Number 8, United States Department of Agriculture, 1963.

IRON

Iron is present in the body in relatively small amounts, 3 to 5 grams. Normally an adult male has 40 to 50 mg. of iron per kilogram of body weight and the female 35 to 50 mg. per kilogram of body weight. Sixty to 70 per cent is classified as essential and 30 to 40 per cent as storage or non-essential. Most of the essential iron is in the red blood cells (hemoglobin). Approximately 5 per cent of the essential iron is in muscles (myoglobin), and a small amount (less than 1 per cent) is found in the body cells as a constituent of certain enzymes that catalyze oxidation-reduction processes in the cell. Approximately 20 per cent is stored in the liver, bone marrow and spleen as ferritin and hemosiderin. It is present in the transport form, bound to protein (transferrin), in the blood plasma.

FUNCTIONS   Iron plays an essential role in the body in transport of oxygen from the lungs to the tissues and in the processes of cellular respiration. The first of these functions is accomplished by hemoglobin in the erythrocytes. Hemoglobin is a metalloprotein with heme, an iron-porphyrin attached to the protein moiety. The iron combines with oxygen in the lungs where the concentration is high and releases it in the tissues where it is needed. Myoglobin and the cytochromes are also heme-containing proteins. Myoglobin, within the muscle cell, has a function similar to that of hemoglobin. The cytochromes do not combine with oxygen but function in the respiratory chain in transfer of electrons through alternate oxidation and reduction of the iron ($Fe^{++} \rightleftarrows Fe^{+++}$). The enzymes catalase and peroxidase have a heme component.

In fetal life the red blood cells or erythrocytes are manufactured principally in the liver and in the spleen. In the adult they are formed chiefly in the bone marrow. The red blood cells begin as immature cells (erythroblasts). As they mature in the bone marrow the porphyrin ring of heme is synthesized from simple units (glycine and intermediates of the Krebs cycle) and combined with the globin. The presence of copper is essential for the synthesis of hemoglobin. The average life span of the red blood cell is about 120 days. As the cells age they become more fragile and rupture; they are disintegrated in the reticulo-endothelial system. The iron is released from the porphyrin and returned to the stores to be used again. The iron-free porphyrin is converted to bilirubin and carried to the liver for excretion in the bile. Virtually all the iron released is taken up by transferrin molecules. These return most of the iron to the bone marrow, for production of new blood cells. The destruction of red blood cells may occur more rapidly in the presence of ascorbic acid and vitamin E deficiencies.

ABSORPTION   Inorganic forms of iron ($FeSO_4$) are readily absorbed by the mucosa of the small intestine. The ferrous (Fe^{++}) salts appear to be more readily absorbed than are the ferric (Fe^{+++}) salts. The greatest absorption occurs in the upper duodenum. The rate of iron absorption seems to be controlled by the intestinal mucosa in response to the body's requirement for iron. The iron is attached to the plasma protein, transferrin, and carried to the storage depots where it combines with apoferritin to form ferritin. Normally about 30 per cent of the transferrin is combined with iron. As the apoferritin stores become saturated, the amount of iron remaining attached to the transferrin increases and there is less absorbed from the mucosal cells. As the level of ferritin in the mucosa increases, it is exfoliated and excreted in the feces. If there is need for iron these processes are reversed. Greater absorption takes place when there is an increased rate of blood formation as needed in pregnancy, during growth and as a result of loss of blood. Childred may absorb iron at a rate twice that of adults.

It is estimated that only 5 to 15 per cent of the iron in food is absorbed by normal adults. From 2 to 10 per cent of iron in vegetables and from 10 to 30 per cent of iron in animal protein can be absorbed. Animal protein improves iron absorption. Ascorbic acid enhances iron absorption by helping to reduce ferric to ferrous iron. The degree of gastric acidity influences solubility and availability of the iron in food. The presence of an adequate amount of calcium helps to bind and remove phosphate, oxalate and phytate that otherwise would combine with iron and inhibit its absorption.

The lack of hydrochloric acid in the stomach; the administration of alkalis; a high intake of cellulose; the presence of insoluble iron complexes such as phytates, oxalates and phosphates; increased intestinal motility and steatorrhea interfere with iron absorption.

When abnormally large amounts of iron are present as a result of long-term ingestion of extremely high amounts or excessive blood transfusions, the apoferritin becomes saturated and hemosiderin appears in large quantities. It is similar to ferritin but contains more iron and is very insoluble. Also some individuals with a genetic defect absorb more than an ordinary amount of iron and develop this iron storage condition which is called hemosiderosis.

STORAGE   Approximately 1000 mg. of iron is stored in the body at any one time as ferritin and hemosiderin. Approximately 30

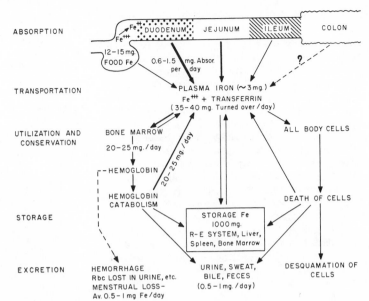

ABSORPTION

TRANSPORTATION

UTILIZATION AND
CONSERVATION

STORAGE

EXCRETION

Figure 8–2   Schematic outline of iron metabolism in adults. (From Moore, C. V., Wohl, M. G., and Goodhart, R. S., (eds.): Modern Nutrition in Health and Disease. 3rd ed. Lea and Febiger, 1964.)

per cent is in the liver and 30 per cent in the bone marrow and the rest is in the spleen and muscles. About 20 mg. of iron is used daily in hemoglobin synthesis. Iron is used very conservatively in the body. Approximately 90 per cent is conserved and used over and over again.

EXCRETION   Only very small amounts of iron are normally excreted from the body. The bulk of the iron lost in the feces consists of that not absorbed from food intake. The body iron stores which are lost in the feces appear largely in the form of exfoliated cells from the gastrointestinal epithelium. Some iron is lost from the excretion of bile and from normal exfoliation of the cells of the skin and from bleeding. Virtually no iron is excreted in the urine and sweat.

The normal male loses about 1.0 mg. of iron daily. In the female, there is the additional loss of iron accompanying menstruation which averages about 0.5 mg. per day. Wide variations exist among individuals and menstrual losses of over 1.4 mg. per day have been reported in about 5 per cent of normal women.

METABOLISM   Figure 8–2 is a schematic outline of the essential steps in the metabolism of iron in adults.

DIETARY SOURCES   By far the best source of dietary iron is liver, with oysters, shellfish, kidney, heart, lean meat and tongue as second choices. Leafy green vegetables are the best plant source. Some other foods that add iron are egg yolks, meat in general, dried peas and beans, dried fruits, dark molasses, whole grain and enriched breads and cereals. Milk is practically devoid of iron. Foods high

in iron content are shown in Appendix Table 8.

The size of average food servings and the availability to the body of the iron present in foods must be taken into account when thinking of sources of dietary iron. For example, only half or less of the iron in whole cereals and some green leaves is available in utilizable form, and raisins, though popularly thought to be a good source of iron, really are not because of the relatively small size of the average serving, even though percentagewise their iron content may be good.

Iron fortification of cereals, flours and bread has added significantly to the total iron intake. However, according to the Recommended Daily Allowance, an adequate iron intake cannot be met by ingestion of ordinary food products. An otherwise adequate diet contains no more than 6 mg. of iron per 1000 kcalories. For the adult female population in accord with the recommended calorie allowances, iron fortification of more foods is indicated or an iron supplement is required.

RECOMMENDED DIETARY ALLOWANCE A sufficient quantity of iron is needed in the diet to prevent the development of anemia. Recommendations of the Food and Nutrition Board of the National Research Council are for a daily intake of 10 mg. of iron for men and older women. Eighteen mg. per day are required by women during the child-bearing years. This amount is required to cover menstrual losses and the demands for pregnancy and lactation.

The infant is born with a reserve supply of iron and is apparently unable to utilize additional iron over and above that furnished by reduction of its hemoglobin mass shortly following birth and by maternal milk. The recommended allowance for a normal term infant is based on an average need of 1.5 mg. per kg. per day during the first year of life. The need for iron to support rapid growth becomes apparent at approximately 3 months of age. The recommended allowance for the period of 3 to 12 months is 10 to 15 mg.; for children 1 to 3 years it is 15 mg.; for children ages 3 to 12 years it is 10 mg. The daily need for boys ages 12 to 18 years is 18 mg. and for girls ages 10 through the child-bearing years is 18 mg. Iron requirements during adolescence are enhanced because of the growth spurt which occurs. The Food and Nutrition Board allowance for iron is intended to afford a sufficient margin. Iron needs vary with age and situations so that individuals with iron intake below the recommended allowances are not necessarily in a deficiency state. When the iron reserves have been depleted evidence of deficiency occurs.

IRON DEFICIENCIES   A deficiency of iron has been cited as the commonest of all deficiency diseases in humans. Iron deficiency manifests itself by the development of an *iron deficiency anemia* (hypochromic anemia), which is corrected by giving diets rich in iron and by providing iron supplements in the form of ferrous sulfate or ferrous gluconate. Iron deficiency anemia is usually caused by blood loss through illness, injury or hemorrhage and is aggravated by a poorly balanced diet that is often deficient in dietary iron, protein and vitamin B-complex. However, iron deficiency anemia may develop on a purely nutritional basis as a result of an inadequate diet or faulty absorption. See Chapters 31 and 34 for discussion of the anemias.

SULFUR

Sulfur occurs principally as a constituent of the amino acids, cystine, cysteine and methionine. It is present in all proteins but is most prevalent in the keratin of skin and hair and in insulin, the hormone which regulates carbohydrate metabolism. Glutathione, a tripeptide containing cysteine, is important in cellular reactions involving the sulfur amino acids in protein. Sulfur exists in a reduced form $(-SH)$ in cysteine and in an oxidized form $(-S-S-)$ as the double molecule, cystine. This is important in the specific configuration of some proteins and in the activity of some enzymes. Sulfur also occurs in carbohydrates such as heparin, an anticoagulant found in liver and some other tissues, and chondroitin sulfate in bone and cartilage. Two vitamins, thiamin and biotin, contain sulfur.

MAGNESIUM

Magnesium, an essential nutrient, comprises about 0.7 per cent (20 to 25 gm.) of total body minerals and 70 per cent of this is found in the bones combined with calcium and phosphorus in the complex hydroxyapatite salts. The remaining 30 per cent is found in the soft tissues and body fluids. Most of the magnesium occurs inside the cells and relatively little appears in the extracellular fluid.

Within the cell the magnesium ion has an important function as an activator for enzymes of carbohydrate metabolism (particularly those concerned in oxidative phosphorylation) and of amino acid metabolism. It plays a role in neuromuscular contraction.

ABSORPTION   The rate of absorption of magnesium ranges from 24 per cent to 85 per cent. The rest is excreted mainly in the feces. The kidney conserves magnesium efficiently. The factors that increase the absorption of magnesium from the upper intestine are similar to those governing calcium absorption but vitamin D has no effect on magnesium absorption. The factors that decrease calcium absorption inhibit magnesium absorption.

FUNCTIONS   Magnesium and calcium, having similar functions, may antagonize each other. An excess amount of magnesium will inhibit bone calcification. Conversely, an excessive amount of calcium may induce signs typical of magnesium deficiency.

Magnesium deficiency is clinically manifested by nervous irritability and in some instances convulsions. The tetany seen in magnesium deficiency is very similar to that seen in hypocalcemia. Such symptoms of magnesium deficiencies are seen primarily in alcoholics.[4] Low serum magnesium levels have been observed in various clinical conditions including alcoholism, diabetes, kwashiorkor, malabsorption syndromes, neuromuscular conditions in some cases associated with parathyroid diseases and in individuals maintained for long periods of time post-operatively on magnesium-free fluids or restricted dietary regimens.[5] Deficiency is likely to occur in situations of insufficient intake and excessive loss.

It is of interest that rats and monkeys fed diets of low magnesium content are considerably more susceptible to atherosclerosis induced by cholesterol feeding.[6] It has also

[4]Syndromes of magnesium depletion and retention in man. Nutr. Rev., *18*:72 and 101, 1960.

[5]National Academy of Sciences: Recommended Daily Allowance. 7th ed. Washington, D.C., 1968, p. 60.

[6]Nakamura, M., et al.: The effect of dietary magnesium and thyroxine on progression and regression of cardiovascular lipid deposition in the rat. J. Nutr. *71*:347–355, 1960.

been shown that diets high in magnesium are partially effective in preventing the deposition of oxalate stones in the kidneys of rats deficient in vitamin B_6.[7]

The daily requirement of magnesium based on balance studies recommended by the National Research Council (1968 revision) is 350 mg. per day for adult males and 300 mg. per day for adult females. The recommended allowances for children have been based on the magnesium content of human milk (4 mg. per 100 ml.) and cow's milk (12 mg. per 100 ml.). (See Table 5 in Composition of Foods, Agriculture Handbook, No. 8.)

The ordinary diet is generally believed to provide adequate amounts of magnesium, since it occurs abundantly in foods, particularly nuts, legumes, cereal grains, and dark green vegetables, where it is an essential constituent of chlorophyll. Other sources are seafood, cocoa and chocolate. However, since high calcium, protein and vitamin D intakes, and alcohol all function to increase the requirement (particularly in those on low magnesium intake), the widespread assumption that the average daily intake is adequate has been questioned.[8]

SODIUM, CHLORINE AND POTASSIUM

These three elements are indispensable dietary constituents, so intimately related in the body that it is most convenient to discuss them together. Sodium constitutes 2 per cent, potassium 5 per cent, and chlorine 3 per cent of the total mineral content of the body. They are distributed ubiquitously throughout all body fluids and tissues, but sodium and chloride are primarily extracellular elements, while potassium is mainly an intracellular element. Sodium, potassium, and chloride are concerned in at least four important physiological functions of the body:

1. Maintenance of normal water balance and distribution.
2. Maintenance of normal osmotic equilibrium.
3. Maintenance of normal acid-base balance.
4. Maintenance of normal muscular irritability.

All three elements are readily absorbed through the intestinal tract and are excreted through the urine, feces and sweat. These minerals are widely found in nature and in the ordinary diet. In a healthy person there is little chance of an occurrence of deficiency.

Hormonal control of sodium, potassium, and chloride is mediated through the adrenal cortex hormones and hormones of the anterior pituitary gland. An example of this important regulatory function is seen in Addison's disease, in which there is a decreased secretion of the adrenal cortex hormones with consequent sodium chloride loss and potassium retention by the body, causing weakness, muscle cramps, weight loss and other symptoms. The symptoms can be dramatically alleviated by giving sodium chloride alone or with adrenal cortex extract.

SODIUM CHLORIDE

Historically, the need for salt has been known ever since man and animals started living on this planet. The carnivora do not have an urge for salt, because animal foods and milk contain sufficient salt, but the herbivorous animals and agricultural peoples demand salt because of the lack in cereals, grains, fruits and vegetables. The usual intake of sodium chloride is 6 to 18 gm. daily,[9] of which approximately 40 per cent is sodium and 60 per cent is chloride. This includes sodium chloride contained in foods, as well as that added as table salt. Infants receiving much of their caloric intake from commercially prepared and processed foods may have an intake higher than that of an adult.[10]

LOW SALT SYNDROME   Deficiency of sodium chloride occurs mainly during hot weather or as a result of heavy work in a hot climate when excessive sweating takes place and great quantities of water are ingested without providing extra salt to compensate for that lost. Whenever more than 4 liters of water are consumed, extra sodium chloride should be provided. The simple provision of extra salt in food or in salt tablets will prevent or correct this condition. Fifteen to 20 gm. daily, or even more, may be needed until acclimatization to heat is established.

Adrenal cortical insufficiency, or certain conditions arising after marked vomiting and diarrhea, after burns, after surgical procedures with marked loss of blood, and after long-term and overly vigorous treatment of heart failure or kidney disease with very low salt (sodium) diets, are some instances which may produce the "low salt syndrome." Clinical signs of salt depletion are anorexia, nausea, vomiting, headache, lassitude, muscular

[7]Gershoff, S. N., and Andrus, S. B.: Dietary magnesium, calcium and vitamin B_6, and experimental nephropathies in rats: Calcium oxalate calculi, apatite nephrocalcinosis. J. Nutr., 73:308, 1968.

[8]Seelig, M. S.: The requirement of magnesium by the normal adult. Am. J. Clin. Nutr., 14:342, 1964.

[9]Dahl, L. K.: Salt intake and salt need. New Eng. J. Med., 258:1122–1205, 1958.

[10]Payan, F. A., et al.: Infant feeding practices. Am. J. Dis. Child, 111:370, 1966.

weakness developing into painful leg and abdominal cramps, alterations in appearance (sunken eyes, hollow cheeks, wrinkled skin) and, in severe cases, mental confusion. Resultant circulatory changes will manifest signs of "shock."

SODIUM

Sodium is readily absorbed in the intestine and carried by the blood to the kidneys, where it is filtered out and returned to the blood in the amounts needed to maintain blood levels required by the body. About 90 to 95 per cent is excreted in the urine and the rest is lost in perspiration and in the feces. Normally the quantity of sodium excreted daily equals the amount ingested, so that a state of sodium balance prevails. Aldosterone, a mineralocorticoid, controls the regulation of sodium balance. When blood sodium levels rise, the thirst receptors in the hypothalamus stimulate the thirst sensation. When blood levels are low, the excretion of sodium through the urine decreases. The levels of sodium in the urine reflect the dietary intake.

Daily requirements for sodium are not known. Deficiencies are rarely encountered under normal conditions. The body functions on a wide range of intakes through the mechanisms it has to conserve or excrete sodium. The sodium intake of Americans has been estimated to be 3 to 7 gm. per day (6 to 18 gm. of sodium chloride). The National Research Council recommends under normal circumstances a sodium chloride intake of 1 gm. per kilogram of water.

In addition to salt (sodium chloride) used in cooking, processing and as seasoning, sodium is present in all foods in varying amounts. (See Table 8–3.) Generally more sodium is present in the protein foods than in vegetables and grains. Fruits contain little or no sodium. The salt added to these foods in the preparation could be many times that found naturally in foods. The sodium content of the water supply varies considerably. In some areas of the country, the amount of sodium in water is of a sufficient quantity to be of significance in the total daily intake.[11, 12]

One of the problems of clinical medicine is the provision of palatable, diversified, sodium-restricted diets. It is frequently necessary to restrict sodium intake in order to control the over-retention of body water in various pathological states.

[11] White, J. M., et al.: Sodium ion in drinking water. Part I. J. Am. Diet. Assoc., 50:32, 1967.

[12] Cooper, G. R., and Heap, B.: Sodium ion in drinking water. Part II. J. Am. Diet. Assoc., 50:37, 1967.

CHLORINE

Chlorine is widely distributed throughout the body as chloride. It is the principal anion of the extracellular fluids. Together with sodium it helps to maintain water balance and osmotic pressure. The highest concentration is in the cerebrospinal fluid and in the gastric and pancreatic juices of the gastrointestinal tract. In the gastric juice, chloride is secreted as hydrochloric acid which is necessary to maintain normal acidity of the stomach. Chloride is present in relatively small amounts in the alkaline pancreatic juice. Along with phosphate and sulfate, chloride helps to maintain acid-base balance in the body fluids. Chloride ions participate in the chloride-bicarbonate shift by having the ability to move in and out of the red blood cells and blood plasma, to maintain osmotic equilibrium in face of the changing levels of carbon dioxide as bicarbonate in the plasma and red blood cells.

Chloride is almost completely absorbed in the intestine and excreted by the kidney. Most of the chloride ingested in the diet occurs as sodium chloride. The amount in food and added table salt provides approximately 3 to 9 gm. daily. Whenever there are excessive losses of sodium, as in vomiting, diarrhea and in profuse sweating, there are losses of chloride ions.

POTASSIUM

Potassium constitutes 5 per cent of the total mineral content of the body. It is the major cation of the intracellular fluid with a small amount in the extracellular fluid. Potassium with sodium is involved in the maintenance of normal water balance, osmotic equilibrium and acid-base balance. It is important with calcium in the regulation of neuromuscular activity. Any considerable increase or decrease of potassium in the extracellular fluid may be regarded as evidence of serious disturbances in muscle biochemistry, since the change in the extracellular fluid occurs late in the process.

Potassium is readily absorbed from the small intestine. It is excreted mainly in the urine. Very little is lost in the feces. The kidney maintains normal serum levels through its ability to filter, reabsorb, secrete and excrete potassium. The adrenal cortex hormone, aldosterone, influences potassium excretion. It conserves sodium and ionized potassium is excreted in place of ionized sodium by means of the exchange mechanism in the renal tubule.

Potassium level in muscle is related to muscle mass; therefore if muscle is being

TABLE 8–3   MINERAL ELEMENTS IN HUMAN NUTRITION
(Known or Believed to be Essential)

MINERAL	LOCATION IN BODY AND SOME BIOLOGICAL FUNCTIONS	ESTIMATED DAILY REQUIREMENT FOR ADULT	FOOD SOURCES	COMMENTS ON LIKELIHOOD OF A DEFICIENCY
I. Macrominerals				
Calcium	99% in bones and teeth. Ionic calcium in body fluids essential for ion transport across cell membranes. Calcium is also bound to protein, citrate or inorganic acids.	Recommended Dietary Allowance: 800 mg.	Milk and milk products; sardines, clams, oysters, kale, turnip greens, mustard greens, broccoli.	Dietary surveys indicate that many diets do not meet Recommended Dietary Allowances for calcium. Since bone serves as a homeostatic mechanism to maintain calcium level in blood, many essential functions are maintained, regardless of diet. Long-term dietary deficiency is probably one of the factors responsible for making osteoporosis (bone-thinning) a significant clinical problem.
Phosphorus	About 80% in inorganic phase of bones and teeth. Phosphorus is a component of every cell and of highly important metabolites, including DNA, RNA, ATP (high energy compound), phospholipids. Important to pH regulation.	In ordinary diets, phosphorus intake of adults is approx. 1½ times that of calcium. On an intake of 800 mg. calcium, phosphorus intake is approx. 1200 mg.	Cheese, egg yolk, milk, meat, fish, poultry, whole-grain cereals, legumes, nuts.	Dietary inadequacy not likely to occur if protein and calcium intake is adequate. However, increased need for phosphorus is postulated with diet leading to acid urine and during prolonged therapy with certain antacids.
Magnesium	About 50% in bone. Remaining 50% is almost entirely inside body cells with only about 1% in extracellular fluid. Ionic Mg functions as an activator of many enzymes and must influence almost all processes.	120 mg./1000 kcal. in average diets (200 to 300 mg./day).	Whole-grain cereals, nuts, meat, milk, green vegetables, legumes.	Dietary inadequacy considered unlikely, but conditioned deficiency is often seen in clinical medicine, associated with surgery, malabsorption, loss of body fluids, certain hormone and renal diseases, etc. Magnesium deficiency has a profound effect on other minerals.
Sodium	30 to 45% in bone. Major cation of extracellular fluid and only a small amount is inside cell. Regulates body fluid osmolarity, pH and body fluid volume.	About 10 gm. NaCl/day usual intake in U.S. Average diet 2 to 6 gm.	Common table salt, seafoods, animal foods, milk, eggs. Abundant in most foods except fruit.	Dietary inadequacy probably never occurs, although low blood sodium requires treatment in certain clinical disorders. Evidence is accumulating that requirements increase during pregnancy. Sodium restriction is practiced in certain cardiovascular disorders.
Chlorine	Major anion of extracellular fluid, functioning in combination with sodium; serves as a buffer, enzyme activator; component of gastric hydrochloric acid. Mostly present in extracellular fluid; less than 15% inside cells.	(Included under Sodium.)	Common table salt, seafoods, milk, meat, eggs.	In most cases, dietary intake is of little significance except in presence of vomiting, diarrhea or profuse sweating.

TABLE 8–3   (*Continued*)

MINERAL	LOCATION IN BODY AND SOME BIOLOGICAL FUNCTIONS	ESTIMATED DAILY REQUIREMENT FOR ADULT	FOOD SOURCES	COMMENTS ON LIKELIHOOD OF A DEFICIENCY
I. Macrominerals				
Potassium	Major cation of intracellular fluid, with only small amounts in extracellular fluid. Functions in regulating pH and osmolarity, cell membrane transfer. Ion is necessary for carbohydrate and protein metabolism.	Usual diet in U.S. contains from 0.8 to 1.5 gm. potassium/1000 kcal. Average diet 2 to 4 gm.	Fruits, milk, meat, cereals, vegetables legumes.	Dietary inadequacy unlikely, but conditioned deficiency may be found in kidney disease, diabetic acidosis, excessive vomiting or diarrhea, hyperfunction of adrenal cortex, etc. Potassium excess may be a problem in renal failure and severe acidosis.
Sulfur	Bulk of dietary sulfur is present in sulfur-containing amino acids needed for synthesis of essential metabolites; functions in oxidation-reduction reactions. Sulfur also functions in thiamin, biotin, and as inorganic sulfur.	Need for sulfur is satisfied by estimated daily requirements for essential sulfur-containing amino acids and vitamins.	Protein foods (meat, fish, poultry, eggs, milk, cheese, legumes, nuts).	Dietary intake is chiefly from sulfur-containing amino acids and adequacy is related to protein intake.
Iron	About 70% is in hemoglobin; about 26% stored in liver, spleen and bone. Iron is component of hemoglobin and myoglobin, important in oxygen transfer; also present in serum transferrin and certain enzymes. Almost none in ionic form.	Recommended Dietary Allowance: 10 mg. for adult man; 18 mg. for woman during childbearing years.	Liver, meat, egg yolk, legumes, whole or enriched grains, dark green vegetables, dark molasses, shrimp, oysters.	Iron-deficiency anemia occurs in women in reproductive years and in infants and preschool children. May be associated in some cases with unusual blood loss, parasites, malabsorption.
II. Microminerals				
Zinc	Present in most tissues, with higher amounts in liver, voluntary muscle, and bone. Constituent of essential enzymes and insulin. May be of importance in nucleic acid metabolism.	Daily intake estimated as 10 to 15 mg. Possibility of higher requirements in adolescent boys.	Milk, liver, shellfish, herring, wheat bran (widely distributed).	Zinc deficiency has been demonstrated in Iran and Egypt in certain patients whose diet is also inadequate in protein and iron. Possibility of dietary inadequacy in this country considered remote, but conditioned deficiency may be seen in systemic childhood illnesses; and in patients who are nutritionally depleted or have been subjected to severe stress such as surgery.
Copper	Found in all body tissues; larger amounts in liver, brain, heart and kidney. Constituent of enzymes; of ceruloplasm and erythrocuprein in blood. May be integral part of DNA or RNA molecule.	Daily intake of 2 mg. appears to maintain balance; ordinary diets provide 2 to 5 mg./day.	Liver, shellfish, whole grains, cherries, legumes, kidney, poultry, oysters, chocolate, nuts.	No evidence that specific deficiencies of copper occur in the human.

TABLE 8–3   (Continued)

MINERAL	LOCATION IN BODY AND SOME BIOLOGICAL FUNCTIONS	ESTIMATED DAILY REQUIREMENT FOR ADULT	FOOD SOURCES	COMMENTS ON LIKELIHOOD OF A DEFICIENCY
II. Microminerals				
Iodine	Constituent of thyroxine and related compounds synthesized by thyroid gland. Thyroxine functions in control of reactions involving cellular energy.	100 to 150μg.	Iodized table salt, seafoods, water and vegetables in non-goitrous regions.	Iodization of table salt is recommended especially in areas where food is low in iodine. Certain foods contain goitrogens which may accentuate effect of low dietary iodine.
Manganese	Highest concentration is in bone, also relatively high concentrations in pituitary, liver, pancreas and gastrointestinal tissue. Constituent of essential enzyme systems; rich in mitochondria of liver cells.	3 to 9 mg. For children: 0.2 mg./kg.	Beet greens, blueberries, whole grains, nuts, legumes, fruit, tea.	Unlikely that deficiency occurs in humans.
Fluorine	Present in bone. In optimal amounts in water and diet, reduces dental caries and may minimize bone loss. This effect appears to be due to its combination with bone crystal to form a more stable compound.	Essentiality not established, but appears to be necessary for optimal health of bones and teeth.	Drinking water (1 ppm. Fl), tea, coffee, rice, soybeans, spinach, gelatin, onions, lettuce.	In areas where fluorine content of water is low, fluoridation of water (1 ppm.) has been found beneficial in reducing incidence of dental caries. (Excess may be toxic.)
Molybdenum	Constituent of essential enzyme (xanthine oxidase) and of flavoproteins.	Little quantitative evidence of requirement.	Legumes, cereal grains, dark green leafy vegetables, organs.	No information.
Cobalt	Constituent of cyanocobalamin (vitamin B$_{12}$), occurring bound to protein in foods of animal origin. Essential to normal function of all cells, particularly cells of bone marrow, nervous system and gastrointestinal system.	3–5 μg. vitamin B$_{12}$.	Liver, kidney, oysters, clams, poultry, milk, variable in vegetables and grains—depends upon cobalt content of soil).	Primary dietary inadequacy is rare except when no animal products are consumed. Deficiency may be found in such conditions as lack of gastric intrinsic factor, gastrectomy, and malabsorption syndromes.
Selenium	Associated with fat metabolism, component of "Factor 3" with vitamin E to prevent fatty liver.	Minute amounts.	Grains, onions, meats, milk, vegetables: variable—depends upon selenium content of soil.	No known deficiency disease seen in man.
Chromium	Associated with glucose metabolism.	Ordinary intake 80 to 100 μg., approx. 2 to 5 μg. are absorbed.	Corn oil, clams, whole-grain cereals, meats, drinking water: variable.	Deficiency found in severe malnutrition, diabetes and cardiovascular diseases.

Adapted from Dairy Council Digest 39, No. 5, September–October, 1968.

formed, an adequate supply of potassium is essential; the same applies to glycogen storage.

A potassium deficiency is not likely to happen in healthy individuals. Potassium is widely distributed in foods. No requirement has been established.[13] The average intake is estimated to range from 0.8 to 1.5 gm. of potassium per 1000 kcalories (2 to 4 gm. for 2000 kcalorie dietary). An adequate intake of milk, meats, cereals, vegetables and fruits will provide ample potassium (see Table 9 in Appendix).

Excessive loss of extracellular fluid may result in potassium deficiency. The loss may be due to vomiting, diarrhea, excessive diuresis or prolonged malnutrition. These are conditions in which potassium from the intracellular fluid is transferred to the extracellular fluid. The serum potassium level is low and ionized potassium excretion is increased. In hypokalemia cardiac failure can result from depletion of ionized potassium in heart muscle. Diabetic acidosis requires replacement of potassium when insulin and glucose are given.[14]

Intravenous feedings may lack sufficient potassium. Certain diuretics and adrenal cortical hormones may cause potassium depletion if efforts are not made to replace potassium in the diet.[15]

In hyperkalemia, the serum level is elevated resulting from kidney failure to clear ionized potassium. The symptoms are mental confusion, numbness of extremities, poor respiration and weakening of heart action.

TRACE ELEMENTS OR MICRONUTRIENTS

The essential micronutrients, besides iron discussed on p. 106, comprising less than 0.005 per cent body weight are copper, cobalt, manganese, iodine, zinc, molybdenum, fluorine, chromium and selenium. Some have important or even essential parts to play in the bodily economy while others as yet have no known function or may even be contaminants. They are most frequently associated with enzyme systems. Copper, cobalt, fluorine, manganese, iodine, and zinc are needed for normal tissue functioning, but the amounts required are very small and are supplied by the average mixed diet. Generally,

the trace minerals are toxic when intake levels only slightly exceed the normal functional levels.

COPPER

Although copper is not a part of the hemoglobin molecule, it is involved in promoting the maturation of red blood cells and the formation of hemoglobin and influences iron absorption. It helps to maintain the myelin sheath surrounding nerve fibers. A number of copper-containing proteins and enzymes have been identified. They include ceruloplasmin, erythrocuprein, hepatocuprein, cytochrome C-oxidase, tyrosinase, monoamine oxidase, ascorbic acid oxidase and others which are associated with the oxidation-reduction enzymes in the body. Cytochrome oxidase is a member of the respiratory chain. Tyrosinase functions in the formation of melamia pigments. Copper is present in butyryl Coenzyme A dehydrogenase, an important enzyme in fatty acid catabolism, but does not seem to be essential to its activity. Mahler and his associates of Wisconsin proved that copper controls the oxidation of fatty acids (fatty acid Coenzyme A dehydrogenase). Here it is combined with iron and riboflavin to function with the vitamin, pantothenic acid, at one end of the reaction chain, and with the cytochrome system at the other, where oxygen enters the cycle.

The body of an adult contains from 75 to 150 mg. of copper. It is found in all tissues, but the highest concentration is in the liver, kidneys, heart, and brain. Bones and muscles have lower concentrations but because of their greater mass, they contain over 50 per cent of the total copper in the body. Copper is absorbed from the upper portion of the small intestines and is stored chiefly in the liver. About 93 per cent of serum copper is bound to ceruloplasmin. Excretion is primarily via the bile. Small amounts are present in urine, sweat and menstrual flow. Unabsorbed copper is found in the feces. There is no danger of deficiency in ordinary diets because of the minute amounts needed and the relatively abundant supply. Foods high in copper content include liver (highest), kidney, oysters, chocolate, nuts, dried legumes, cereals, dried fruits, poultry, shellfish, and animal tissues. Milk is poor in copper and iron. The adult requirement is about 2 mg. daily, and the average person ingests 2.5 to 5.0 mg. per day. Infants and children require approximately 0.05 to 0.1 mg. per kg. of body weight per day. With preadolescent girls daily intake of 1.3 mg. was satisfactory.[16]

[13]Food and Nutrition Board: Recommended Daily Allowances. Washington, D.C., National Research Council, National Academy of Science, Pub. No. 1694, 1968, p. 64.

[14]Seftel, H. C.: Early and intensive potassium replacement in diabetic acidosis. Diabetes, 15:694, 1966.

[15]Krehl, W. A.: Sodium — A most extraordinary dietary essential. Nutrition Today., 1:20, 1966.

[16]Engel, R. W., et al.: J. Nutr. 92:197, 1967.

In general, the requirement for copper is about one-tenth that for iron.

Copper deficiency is extremely rare in man. Low blood levels of copper, hypocupremia, have been noted in children with iron-deficiency anemia and edema, kwashiorkor, and the nephrotic syndrome.[17]

In Wilson's disease, a rare hereditary condition, the body continues to absorb copper and large amounts are stored. Ceruloplasmin, which regulates the level of plasma copper and prevents accumulation of toxic levels, is not produced in normal amounts.

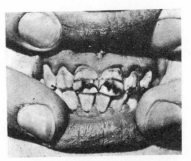

Figure 8–3   Mottled enamel caused by excess fluorine in water. (Fluorine and Dental Health Pub. No. 19. Am. Assoc. for the Advancement of Science, Washington, D.C., 1942.)

COBALT

Cobalt is a component of vitamin B_{12} and as such is an essential nutrient. This is the only known biological function of cobalt. The vitamin is essential for maturation of red blood cells and normal functioning of all cells. Deficiency of the vitamin is responsible for the symptoms of pernicious anemia. This represents a genetic defect rather than a dietary inadequacy: failure of the gastric mucosa to form a mucoprotein necessary for absorption of vitamin B_{12}. Cobalt is poorly absorbed and most of it passes through the intestinal tract unabsorbed. Of that absorbed, most of it is excreted in the urine and small amounts in the bile. The cobalt retained in the body is found mostly in the liver and some in the spleen, kidneys and pancreas. About 1 μg. per 100 ml. is found in blood plasma. The dietary requirement of cobalt is very low; less than 1 μg. per day. Neither animals nor higher plants can synthesize vitamin B_{12}. Plants do not need it and the content is very low. The ultimate source for animals is microorganisms which do synthesize it. Humans get it from animal foods. Strict vegetarians are known to become deficient. The best food sources, however, are liver, kidney, oysters, clams, meat and milk.

High intake of inorganic cobalt in animal diets has been shown to produce polycythemia (overproduction of red blood cells) and hyperplasia of bone marrow. In view of the levels of cobalt required this should be regarded as a pharmacological rather than a physiological effect.

FLUORINE

Fluorine is normally present in small amounts in most plant and animal tissue, with greatest concentration in bones and teeth. It is necessary in the proper formation of tooth enamel and confers maximal resistance to dental caries. Deficiency of it causes poor teeth and subsequent excessive dental caries. Surveys reveal that the quantity of fluorine ingested in food is a relatively unimportant variable, with seafoods, tea, bone meal, spinach, soybeans and gelatin ranking highest; of greatest import is the variable quantity ingested in drinking water. An average daily diet will provide 0.25 to 0.35 mg. of fluorine. In addition, the average adult may ingest 1.0 to 1.5 mg. from drinking and cooking water containing 1 ppm. of fluorine. Dental fluorosis may occur at fluoride concentrations of 2 to 8 ppm., osteosclerosis at 8 to 20 ppm. Higher levels depress growth and may cause death. (See Fig. 8–3.) There are areas in this country where fluorine supplies in water are high and tooth mottling is endemic, and other areas where fluorine is deficient and the incidence of dental decay is quite high. Extensive surveys in a variety of communities and cities have led to the finding that 1 part per million parts of drinking water is the best level for fluorine, and some communities in which the content is low have added this amount to their water supplies in an effort to reduce the incidence of dental caries among the young. This practice is recognized as an important public health measure of special benefit to children. (See Dental Caries in Chapter 34.) Studies have demonstrated that the hydroxyapatite crystals in bone are larger and more perfectly formed when the fluoride content of the diet is high.[18] Bone containing fluoride is more stable and more resistant to degeneration.

MANGANESE

Manganese, an essential element, plays a role in activating numerous enzymes. Bone phosphatase and blood phosphatase require

[17]Cordano, A., et al.: Copper deficiency in infancy. Pediatrics, 34:324, 1964, and Hypocupremia neutropenia in copper deficiency. Blood, 28:280, 1966.

[18]Hegsted, D. M., et al.: Fluoride protects against bone loss. J.A.M.A., 200:31, 1967.

manganese for their action. It is part of the molecular structure of arginase, which is essential for urea formation. Manganese is an activator of carboxylase, cholinesterase muscle adenosine triphosphatase and other enzymes. It is poorly absorbed, especially in the presence of large amounts of calcium and phosphorus, and is excreted via the intestinal tract in the feces. It is believed that the mechanisms of manganese and iron absorption are similar.[19] It is present in all human tissues. The highest concentration is in the bone, liver, pancreas and pituitary. The gastrointestinal tissue also contains considerable amounts.

The total amount in the body is about 20 mg. and the average daily mixed diet contains approximately 4 mg., which is within the amount (3 to 9 mg.) estimated to be required for an adult. Children may require 0.2 to 0.3 mg. per kilogram of body weight.[20]

Dependent upon the soil content of manganese, the richest sources are blueberries, wheat bran, dried legumes, nuts, lettuce, beet tops and pineapple. Animal tissue, seafood and dairy products are poor sources. A deficiency in humans is not apt to occur. Manganese toxicity has been found in miners as a result of prolonged exposure to dust with absorption of manganese through the respiratory tract. The excess accumulates in the liver and central nervous system. Symptoms resemble those found in Parkinson's and Wilson's diseases.

IODINE

Iodine, an essential element, is an integral part of the thyroid gland hormones, thyroxine and triiodothyronine. Its function as a constituent of thyroxine and other compounds synthesized by the thyroid gland is apparently the only role of iodine in the human body. The body normally contains 20 to 30 mg. of iodine. About 60 per cent of it is in the thyroid gland and the rest is widely diffused throughout all tissues, especially in ovaries, muscles and blood.

Iodides are readily absorbed and excreted (chiefly in the urine). Iodides absorbed from the intestinal tract are rapidly transported via the blood stream to the thyroid gland where they are oxidized to iodine and incorporated into the tyrosine molecules of thyroglobulin, converting them to thyroxine and triiodothyronine. Action of a proteolytic enzyme breaks down thyroglobulin and re-

leases thyroxine into the plasma. Within the plasma all but a very small portion of the thyroxine is carried bound to protein. It may be that the small amount of free thyroxine is the active hormone.

On demand, when the blood hormone level is low, the pituitary gland secretes the thyroid-stimulating hormone (TSH), which stimulates the thyroid to increase the production and release of the hormones. Thyroid cells increase in size and the gland becomes hypertrophied under conditions of iodine deficiency. The condition is known as simple goiter. Hyperfunction of the gland results in a toxic goiter.

Administration of a given amount of radioactive iodine is used at present as a test of thyroid function.

RECOMMENDED DIETARY ALLOWANCES
The National Research Council (1968) has suggested that an intake of 1 μg. of iodine per kilogram of body weight is sufficient for most adults. Growing children, especially girls, and pregnant or lactating women may need more.

DIETARY SOURCES   Iodine occurs in extremely variable amounts in foods and drinking water. Seafoods, such as clams, lobsters, oysters, sardines and other sea fish, are rich sources of iodine. The iodine content of cows' milk and eggs is determined by the iodides available in the diets of the cows and chickens, and the iodides in vegetables depend upon the iodine in the soil in which they are grown.

The best way to obtain an adequate intake of iodine is to use iodized salt (1 part potassium iodide to 10,000 parts of salt) in the cooking of food. Because only about 50 per cent of the table salt sold in the United States is iodized, the Food and Nutrition Board (1968) has recommended federal legislation making the iodization of salt mandatory. (Mandatory salt iodization has been adopted by many nations.) In the meantime, the importance of iodized salt should be emphasized. Other methods of increasing iodine intake (adding iodine to water supply and to tablets) have been tried in the low iodine areas and were found impractical.

An active antithyroid substance, goitrin, found in cabbage, rutabagas, turnips and peanuts, interferes with iodine utilization and has been found experimentally to produce goiters. It is doubtful that humans consume enough to affect thyroid activity. Cooking prevents the action of goitrin.

GOITER   It has been established that a lack of iodine intake is associated with the development of a type of thyroid gland dysfunction known as colloid, endemic or simple goiter. This condition formerly was especially

[19]Samstead, H. H.: Present knowledge of the minerals. Present Knowledge in Nutrition. 3rd ed. New York, The Nutrition Foundation, Inc., 1967, p. 122.
[20]Cheek, D. B.: Human Growth, Energy and Intelligence. Lea & Febiger, 1968, p. 424.

prevalent in the geographical areas of this country known as the "goiter belt," where iodine was lacking in the water and soils. The goiter belt includes the Great Lakes regions, Wisconsin, Nebraska, the Dakotas, Colorado, Montana, Utah, Oregon and Washington. Nowadays, with the rapid transportation of food, the regular use of iodized salt (0.5 to 1.0 part iodine per 10,000 parts of salt),[21] iodized fertilizers, and even the addition of iodine to drinking water, the problem of colloid goiter in the goiter belt has largely diminished. It is still, however, one of the most prevalent nutritional diseases in the underdeveloped countries and in those regions remote from the sea. (See Chap. 34.) A relationship to cretinism associated with endemic goiter has been established. Other environmental dietary goitrogens and genetic factors play a role in the development of goiter.[22]

ZINC

Zinc is essential for growth and gonadal development in man. It is found in many body tissues and foods. The human body contains approximately 2.2 gm., which is about one half the amount of iron in an adult. The liver, pancreas, kidney, bone and voluntary muscles have the largest concentration. Tissues with high concentration include the various parts of the eye (lens, retina, cornea and iris), prostate gland and spermatozoa, skin, hair, fingernails and toenails. Most of the zinc in the blood is present in the cells with higher concentration in the white cells.

Zinc is readily absorbed in the upper small intestine and the major routes of excretion are through the pancreas and intestinal secretions. Urinary excretion is very small. It is present in sweat and the amount excreted in hot climates may be significant.

Zinc has a variety of functions. The most important function is that of a coenzyme. It is a component of carbonic anhydrase, carboxypeptidase, lactic dehydrogenase, alcohol dehydrogenase, alkaline phosphatase and other metalloenzymes. Carbonic anhydrase converts carbon dioxide to carbonic acid in the cells and blood plasma and releases carbion dioxide from carbonic acid in the lungs. Carboxypeptidase participates in removing the carboxyl group from peptides to form amino acids. Lactic dehydrogenase is essential for the lactic acid and pyruvic acid interconversion in the glycolytic pathway for glucose oxidation.

Zinc, along with iron, calcium, magnesium and manganese, participates in ribonucleic acid (RNA) metabolism. Its role is not understood. As an integral part of the RNA molecule it is thought to help maintain the stability of the molecular configuration.

Zinc is associated with the hormone insulin which is necessary for carbohydrate metabolism. Apparently it is not a part of the insulin molecule but may hold it in the pancreas until needed. The relationship of the role of zinc in stimulating wound healing has been observed.[23]

The best dietary source of zinc is found in animal products. Phytate found in whole grains binds zinc and decreases the availability of zinc. In the presence of phytate, excess calcium depresses the absorption of zinc.[24]

Dietary deficiency of zinc impairs growth. A pilot experiment involving boys aged 12 to 14 years whose height was below the third percentile of the Iowa growth standards showed that zinc deficiency is an important etiological factor in growth retardation and delayed sexual maturation among boys living in rural southern Iran.[25]

Illnesses in which both the serum and erythrocyte levels of zinc decrease include cirrhosis of the liver, hepatitis, nephrosis, malabsorption syndrome, chronic infectious diseases, myocardial infarction, hypothryoidism, male dwarfism and hypogonadism.

Evidence of increased urinary zinc excretion and decreased body stores is apparent in alcoholic liver cirrhosis, lead poisoning and acute rheumatic fever.

The average daily diet is thought to contain 10 to 15 mg. of zinc. It is estimated that an intake of 6 mg. zinc daily will meet the requirement in our mixed North American diet.[26] The richest sources are oysters, herring, whole grains, meats, milk and egg yolk. (Phytic acid and high calcium intake depresses the absorption of zinc.)

MOLYBDENUM

Molybdenum has been shown to be an integral part of two enzymes—xanthine oxidase and aldehyde oxidase, a flavoprotein. Xanthine oxidase is involved in the formation of uric acid from the purine xanthine and is important in the mobilization of ferritin iron

[21] Federal Register. 37:15746, Dec. 14, 1966.

[22] Nutrition Foundation, Inc.: Present Knowledge in Nutrition. 3rd ed. New York, 1967, p. 121.

[23] Hoekstra, W.G.: Present knowledge of zinc in nutrition. In: Present Knowledge of Nutrition. 3rd ed. New York, Nutrition Foundation, Inc., 1967, p. 141.

[24] O'Dell, B. L.: Effect of dietary components upon zinc availability. Am. J. Clin. Nutr., 22:1315, 1969.

[25] Ronaghy, H., et al.: Controlled zinc supplementation for malnourished school boys: A pilot experiment. Am. J. Clin. Nutr., 22:1279, 1969.

[26] Sandstead, H. H.: Zinc: A metal to grow on. Nutrition Today, 3:12, 1968.

from liver reserves. Aldehyde oxidase functions as a catalyst in the oxidation of aldehydes.

Molybdenum is found in minute amounts in the body, is readily absorbed from the gastrointestinal tract and is excreted mainly in the urine. The daily requirement is not known. It is widely distributed in commonly used foods such as legumes, whole-grain cereals, dark green leafy vegetables, milk and liver.

SELENIUM

Selenium is found in minute amounts in the body. It has been shown in animals that the activity of cystine in preventing liver necrosis is attributed to traces of selenium present in cystine. The actions of selenium and vitamin E in animals are interrelated in preventing tissue damage. The antioxidant role of selenium related to vitamin E has been noted.

The selenium content of foods is dependent on the amount present in the soil in which they are grown. Grains and onions usually have greater concentrations of selenium than do vegetables. Meats and milk contain traces of selenium. Selenium may be lost from foods by washing, cooking and storage.[27]

It has been observed that low selenium areas are also usually low fluoride areas and have high dental caries rates. Evidence is forthcoming, however, to associate nutrient levels of selenium with causes of dental caries. Only a few isolated instances of selenium toxicity have been reported in humans living in areas where the selenium content of soil is high.[28]

CHROMIUM

Evidence that trivalent chromium is a required trace nutrient for man is increasing. There are about twenty parts of chromium per one billion parts of blood and somewhat more in other organs. Certain proteins in the cell can concentrate chromium in much higher amounts. Chromium is present at birth and concentrations are higher during early childhood, with a steady decline in some tissues with age. It is believed that the intake of this mineral is not sufficient to maintain chromium tissue concentration throughout life.

In experimental animals, chromium stimulates the activity of enzymes involved in energy metabolism and in glucose metabolism. It also stimulates the synthesis of fatty acids and cholesterol in the liver. Chromium deficient diets fed to rats result in growth retardation and a syndrome similar to diabetes mellitus.[29, 30]

Dr. Walter Mertz and co-workers by means of animal experiments discovered the biological importance of chromium and isolated the glucose tolerance factor (GTF) required for the efficient utilization of glucose in cereal grains, potatoes, rice, corns, honey and other foods which have a high starch or sugar content. Chromium is believed to be found in food in organic (the GTF type) and inorganic combination. Most of the GTF type is absorbed but only a small percentage of the inorganic chromium is absorbed. The GTF chromium in the experimental animals is the physiological co-factor that assists insulin in moving glucose through the membrane into the cell. It is stored in the tissues and released into the blood stream following the ingestion of glucose. When it is deficient, the effectiveness of insulin is decreased, resulting in the inability to tolerate normal amounts of glucose. It appears from preliminary experiments that poor glucose tolerance in some adult diabetics, middle-aged and elderly people and in malnourished children with chromium deficiency can be improved by a daily supplement of chromium. It is postulated that some individuals in this group with impaired glucose tolerance who did not respond to chromium supplement could not synthesize enough GTF. Further investigations of the prevalence of chromium deficiency and the glucose tolerance factor in man are needed.[31]

The daily chromium intake of humans is estimated to range from 80 to 100 micrograms. The average person probably does not absorb more than 2 to 5 μg. The dietary sources of chromium include corn oil (highest), clams, whole-grain cereals and meats. Fruits and vegetables contain trace amounts. Drinking water may supply very little, up to 10 μg. per liter, depending upon the area.[32]

ADDITIONAL TRACE ELEMENTS

In addition to the above, other minerals may have specific essential physiological functions. Research and interest is ever

[27] Frost, D. V.: Selenium, a dramatic entree to nutrition. Nat'l. Live Stock and Meat Board. Food and Nutrition News, 39:No. 2, 1967.

[28] Frost, Ibid.

[29] Shroeder, H. A., et al.: Abnormal trace metals in man: Chromium. J. Chron. Dis., 15:941, 1962.

[30] Schwarz, K., and Mertz, W.: Chromium III and the glucose tolerance factor. Arch Biochem. Biophys. 85:292, 1959.

[31] Mertz, W., et al.: Some aspects of glucose metabolism of chromium-deficient rats raised in a strictly controlled environment. J. Nutr. 86:107, 1965, and Agricultural Research. United States Department of Agriculture, Dec., 1970, p. 3.

[32] Shroeder, loc. cit.

growing. *Vanadium* may function in cholesterol metabolism. At a level of 100 to 125 mg. per day, vanadium has been shown to inhibit the synthesis of cholesterol.[33] High levels of cadmium in kidneys were found in patients with high blood pressure.[34] The role of cadmium in hypertension has not been identified. There are no known functions or needs for *aluminum, arsenic, boron, bromine, nickel* and *silicon*, although these elements are found in animal and plant tissues. They seem to be harmless for man in their naturally occurring concentrations.

PROBLEMS AND SUGGESTED TOPICS FOR DISCUSSION

1. Keep a record of your food intake for 24 hours and evaluate the intake for food high in iron and calcium. Make suggestions for improvement in selection.
2. Plan a diet for yourself, omitting milk and milk products, and check for adequacy of calcium.
3. What is the importance to the body of (a) calcium, (b) iron, (c) potassium, (d) sodium, (e) sulfur, (f) magnesium?
4. Survey the literature and report on a mineral now under investigation for its importance to human nutrition.

SUGGESTED ADDITIONAL READING REFERENCES

GENERAL BIBLIOGRAPHY

Cantarow, A., and Trumper, M.: Clinical Biochemistry. 6th ed. Philadelphia, W. B. Saunders Company, 1962. Chapters 6–11, 13 and 14.
Davis, G. K.: Excess minerals in the diet. J. Am. Dietet. A., 51:46, 1967.
Duncan, G. G. (ed.): Diseases of Metabolism. 5th ed. Philadelphia, W. B. Saunders Company, 1964. Chapter 4, Mineral Metabolism.
Food and Nutrition Board: Recommended Dietary Allowances. 7th ed. Washington, D.C., National Research Council. National Academy of Sciences, Pub. No. 1694, 1968.
Mazur, A., and Harrow, B.: Textbook of Biochemistry. 10th ed. Philadelphia, W. B. Saunders Company, 1966.
McGilvery, R. W.: Biochemistry: A Functional Approach. Philadelphia, W. B. Saunders Company, 1970.
Nutrition Foundation, Inc.: Present Knowledge of Nutrition. 3rd ed. New York, 1967.
Pike, R. L., and Brown, M. L.: Nutrition: An Integrated Approach. New York, John Wiley & Sons, Inc., 1967.
Tipton, I. H.: Trace elements in human nutrition—a need for standards. J. Am. Clin. Nutr., 23:141, 1970.
Vallee, B. L.: Clinical significance of trace elements. Mod. Med., Feb. 18, 1963, p. 111.
Wohl, M. G., and Goodhart, R. S.: Modern Nutrition in Health and Disease. 4th ed. Philadelphia, Lea & Febiger, 1968. Chapters 10, 11 and 12.

CALCIUM AND PHOSPHORUS

Ebel, J. G., et al.: Vitamin D induced calcium building protein of intestinal mucosa. Am. J. Clin. Nutr., 22:431, 1969.

---

[33]Dimond, E. G., et al.: Vanadium excretion, toxicity and lipid effect in man. Am. J. Clin. Nutr., 12:49, 1963.
[34]Schroeder, H. A.: Cadmium as a factor in hypertension. J. Chron. Dis., 18:647, 1965.

Greenwald, E., et al.: Effect of lactose on calcium metabolism in man. J. Nutr., 79:531, 1963.
Hegsted, D. M.: Nutrition, bone and calcified tissue. J. Am. Dietet. A., 50:105, 1967.
Hegsted, D. M.: Present knowledge of calcium, phosphorus and magnesium. Nutr. Rev., 26:65, 1968.
Holemans, K. C., and Meyer, B. J.: A quantitative relationship between the absorption of calcium and phosphorus. Am. J. Clin. Nutr., 12:30, 1963.
Lutwak, L.: Osteoporosis-A mineral deficiency disease? J. Am. Dietet. A., 44:173, 1964.
Symposium on Human Calcium Requirements. J.A.M.A., 185:588, 1963.
WHO Technical Report Series No. 230: Calcium requirement. Geneva, 1962.

IRON

Brown, E. B.: The absorption of iron. Am. J. Clin. Nutr., 12:205, 1963.
Crosby, W. H.: Intestinal response to the body's requirement for iron. J.A.M.A., 208:347, No. 2, 1969.
Elwood, P. D., and Waters, W. E.: The vital distinction. (Iron deficiency). Nutrition Today, 4:14, No. 2, 1969.
Finch, C. A.: Iron metabolism. Nutrition Today., 4:2, No. 2, 1969.
Iron Deficiency in the United States. A report of the Committee on Iron Deficiency, Council on Foods and Nutrition. J.A.M.A., 203:119, 1968.
Mendel, G. A.: Iron metabolism and etiology of iron-storage diseases. An interpretive formulation. J.A.M.A., 189:45, 1964.
Review: Iron storage in bone marrow. Nutr. Rev., 21:329, 1963.
Scott, D. E., and Pritchard, J. A.: Iron deficiency in healthy young college women. J.A.M.A., 199:897, 1967.

MAGNESIUM

Briscoe, A. M., and Ragan, C.: Effect of magnesium or calcium metabolism in man. Am. J. Clin. Nutr., 19:296, 1966.
Hunt, S. McC., and Schafield, F. A.: Magnesium balance and protein intake level in adult human female. Am. J. Clin. Nutr., 22:367, 1969.
Manalo, R., et al.: A simple method for estimating dietary magnesium. Am. J. Clin. Nutr., 20:627, 1967.
Review: magnesium deficiency. Nutr. Rev., 20:335, 1962.
Seelig, M. S.: The requirement of magnesium by the normal adult. Am. J. Clin. Nutr., 14:342, 1964.
Wacker, W. E. C.: Magnesium metabolism. J. Am. Dietet. A., 44:362, 1964.

SODIUM, CHLORIDE AND POTASSIUM

Cooper, G. R., and Heap, B.: Sodium ion in drinking water. II. Importance, problems, and potential applications of sodium-ion-restricted therapy. J. Am. Dietet. A., 50:37, 1967.
Krehl, W. A.: Sodium—a most extraordinary dietary essential. Nutrition Today, 1:16, 1966.
Krehl, W. A.: The potassium depletion syndrome. Nutrition Today, 1:20, 1966.
White, J. M., et al.: Sodium ion in drinking water. I. Properties, analysis, and occurrence. J. Am. Dietet. A., 50:32, 1967.

COPPER

Cartwright, G. E., and Wintrobe, M. M.: Copper metabolism in normal subjects. Am. J. Clin. Nutr., 14:224, 1964.
Copper cooking utensils. J.A.M.A., 200:426, 1967.
Cordana, A., and Graham, G. G.: Copper deficiency com-

plicating chronic intestinal malabsorption. Pediatrics, 38:596, 1966.

Dowdy, R. P.: Copper metabolism. Am. J. Clin. Nutr., 22:887, 1969.

Report: Preventing Wilson's disease sequelae. J.A.M.A., 200:41, 1967.

FLUORINE

Report: Fluoride protects against bone loss. J.A.M.A., 200:31, 1967.

Review: Metabolism of fluorides. Nutr. Rev., 19:259, 1961.

Waldbott, G. L.: Fluoride in food. Am. J. Clin. Nutr., 12:455, 1963.

MANGANESE

Sherman, W. C.: Manganese. National Live Stock and Meat Board. Food and Nutrition News, 36: No. 8, 1965.

ZINC

Hoekstra, W. G.: Present knowledge of zinc in nutrition. In: Present Knowledge of Nutrition. 3rd ed. New York, Nutrition Foundation, Inc., 1967, p. 141.

Leuche, R. W.: The significance of zinc in nutrition. Borden's Review of Nutrition Research. 26:45, 1965.

Mann, G. V.: Sulphur metabolism. National Live Stock and Meat Board Food and Nutrition News, 34: No. 10, 1960.

Prasad, A. S.: Nutritional metabolic role of zinc. Fed. Proc., 26:172, 1967.

Ronaghy, H., et al.: Controlled zinc supplementation for malnourished school boys: A pilot experiment. Am. J. Clin. Nutr., 22:1279, 1969.

Sandstead, H. H.: Zinc: A metal to grow on. Nutrition Today, 3:12, 1968.

Sandstead, H. H., et al.: Human zinc deficiency, endocrine manifestations and responses to treatment. Am. J. Clin. Nutr., 20:422, 1967.

Sullivan, J. F., and Lankford, H. G.: Zinc metabolism and alcoholism. Am. J. Clin. Nutr., 17:57, 1965.

Symposium: Zinc metabolism. Am. J. Clin. Nutr., 22:1215 and 1279, 1969.

OTHER MINERAL ELEMENTS

Dimond, E. G.: Vanadium excretion, toxicity and lipid effect in man. Am. J. Clin. Nutr., 12:49, 1963.

Frost, D. V.: Selenium, a dramatic entree to nutrition. National Live Stock and Meat Board. Food and Nutrition News, 38: Nos. 2 and 3, 1967.

Glinsman, W. H., et al.: Plasma chromium after glucose administration. Science, 152:1243, 1966.

Levander, O. A.: Present knowledge of selenium. In: Present Knowledge in Nutrition, 3rd ed. New York, Nutrition Foundation, Inc., 1967, p. 138.

Mertz, W.: Chromium in our food. National Live Stock and Meat Board Food and Nutrition News, 38: No. 3, 1966.

Review: Intestinal absorption of chromium. 25:76, 1967.

Review: Trivalent chromium in human nutrition. Nutr. Rev., 25:50, 1967.

Schroeder, H. A., et al.: Abnormal trace metals in man: Chromium. J. Chron. Dis., 15:941, 1962.

Schwartz, K., and Murtz, W.: Chromium III and the glucose tolerance factor. Arch. Biochem. Biophys., 85:292, 1959.

Chapter 9
VITAMINS

DEFINITION   *Vitamins* are a group of unrelated organic compounds needed only in minute quantities in the diet but essential for specific metabolic reactions within the cell and necessary for normal growth and maintenance of health. Many act as coenzymes or a prosthetic group of enzymes responsible for promoting essential chemical reactions. They are often called "accessory food factors" in view of the fact that they do not supply calories nor contribute appreciably to body mass. Animals fed on pure mixtures of carbohydrate, fat, protein, water, and minerals fail to grow properly and thrive because, as is now known, they lack vitamins. Vitamins vary widely in chemical structure and in their body functions. Some are relatively simple while others are quite complex. With a few exceptions the body cannot synthesize vitamins; they must be supplied in the diet or in addition to the diet. Certain vitamins (K, thiamin, folacin and B_{12}) to some extent may be formed by microorganisms in the intestinal tract, and it is known that vitamins A, choline and niacin can be formed if their precursors are supplied.

FUNCTION   Vitamins have different functions in various animal species. For the most part, this discussion will be restricted to the functions known for man and to the effects of deficiencies in man. Vitamins regulate metabolism, help convert fat and carbohydrate into energy, and assist in forming bones and tissues. Although a great deal is known about the vitamins, investigations continue to determine their biochemical structures and functions.

HISTORY   Vitamin investigation began with the search for the unknown accessory dietary factors which would prevent or cure the classic deficiency diseases. People have died or have lived miserable existences in poor health because of vitamin deficiencies, and the solutions of such medical riddles as pellagra, scurvy, rickets, night blindness, and hemorrhagic disease of the newborn, to name a few, through the elucidation of the etiologic role of vitamin deficiencies in these diseases, are among the brightest chapters in medical and nutritional history.

With the possible exception of scurvy, the classic deficiency diseases have largely disappeared in the United States. They do, however, exist in a number of the underdeveloped countries, either through a scarcity of food or ignorance of the basic food principles. The reader is urged to consult treatises on the development of vitamin knowledge for stimulating and interesting reading on vitamin history.[1,2,3,4]

While history cites evidence as far back as the Egyptians that indicates a knowledge of vitamins, the modern story dates back only to the close of the nineteenth century. Eijkman in 1897 described a disease in chickens and pigeons, resembling beriberi in man. He induced this disease by feeding milled rice exclusively. The symptoms could be cured by feeding the rice polishings. This recognition of the importance of other factors, besides carbohydrate, fat and protein, to promote healthy nutrition stimulated investigations by many workers and led to the modern concept of vitamins. Today approximately 20 vitamins are known or believed to be important to human well-being, and the existence of several more has been postulated.

NOMENCLATURE The term "vitamine," meaning a vital amine, was introduced by Funk (a polish chemist working at the Lister Institute in London) in 1912 to designate the accessory food factors necessary to life. The final "e" has been dropped, since the chemical nature of these various substances has been proved and most of them are not amines.

The vitamins were originally named by letter or by their function. For example, vitamin B was commonly called the antineuritic or antiberiberi vitamin because it was found to be definitely useful in preventing the onset of these conditions. When it was found that the semi-purified materials contained several active substances, additional letters or numerical subscripts were used to identify the newly discovered vitamins. This led to some confusion. As each vitamin was isolated in pure form and its chemical structure determined specific names were assigned. At present the names are generally related to the chemical structure. The original names of some of the vitamins are still in use. See Table 9–1 for the current nomenclature of the original vitamins.

CLASSIFICATION It is convenient to divide the vitamins into two groups on the basis of solubility: (1) the fat-soluble vitamins A, D, E and K, which are found in foods in association with lipids, and (2) the water-soluble vitamins B-complex and C. Vitamins may also be classified according to their physiological effects.

RECOMMENDED DAILY DIETARY ALLOWANCES Much work has been done to determine requirements of vitamins for the various age groups and in circumstances of additional needs such as pregnancy and lactation. The National Research Council's Food and Nutrition Board has established desirable levels, as revised in 1968, for those vitamins whose requirements are known to be essential to healthy man. These are intended to apply to persons whose physical activity is considered "light" (neither sedentary nor heavy physical activity) and living in a temperate climate, and to provide a safety margin for each vitamin over the minimal level that will normally maintain health (See Table 11–1, Chapter 11.)

With every innovation enthusiasm usually runs high, and in the vitamin era virtually all ailments have been blamed at some time on a shortage of vitamins. Under these circumstances it is not surprising that the vitamins should become imbued in the minds of many lay and professional people with far-reaching therapeutic qualities which they do not possess. However, it is important that sight should not be lost of the nature of these substances and their highly specific role in human nutrition.

Vitamins taken in excess of the finite amount utilized in the metabolic processes are valueless, since they will have no substrate upon which to act. Excessive water-soluble vitamins are excreted, mainly in the urine, and an excessive intake of fat-soluble vitamins will result in increased storage, having little or no beneficial effect, but rather, taken to extreme, producing actual toxicity.

VITAMIN SUPPLEMENTATION There is no reliable evidence that vitamin supplementation increases immunity in the otherwise well-nourished individual, nor will there be that extra surge of energy so confidently expected by some on taking a multivitamin capsule. While certain vitamin requirements may be increased by prolonged muscular

[1]McCollum, E. V.: A History of Nutrition. Boston, Houghton Mifflin Co., 1957.

[2]Food: The Yearbook of Agriculture, 1959. Washington, D.C., U.S. Dept. of Agriculture, pp. 1–23.

[3]Essays on the History of Nutrition and Dietetics. Chicago, American Dietetics Association, 1967.

[4]Lowenberg, M. E., et al.: Food and Man. New York, John Wiley & Sons, Inc., 1968.

TABLE 9–1   NOMENCLATURE OF THE VITAMINS*

ORIGINAL NAME	CURRENT NAME
Vitamin A (anti-infective)	Vitamin A (retinol)
Vitamin B₁ (antiberiberi, antineuritic)	Thiamin (vitamin B₁)
Vitamin G (B₂)	Riboflavin
Pellagra preventative factor	Niacin (nicotinic acid, niacinamide)
Vitamin B-complex	Vitamin B₆ (pyridoxine)
	Vitamin B₁₂ (cyanocobalamin)
Vitamin M	Folacin (folic acid, pteroylglutamic acid)
	Pantothenic acid
	Biotin
Vitamin C	Ascorbic acid
Vitamin D	Vitamin D (calciferol)
Vitamin E	Vitamin E (α-tocopherol)
Vitamin K	Vitamin K (menaquinone and phylloquinones)

*Only those vitamins proved to be essential to human nutrition are listed here.

exertion, the extra vitamins will be automatically provided if the exertion is counterbalanced calorically by the consumption of a reasonably mixed diet. The routine vitamin supplementation of the diet, as a prophylactic measure, is not justified.

A vast amount of money is expended annually on vitamin concentrates that might better be used for providing health-building foods. Healthy persons who eat well-balanced meals rarely require vitamins as medication. Vitamin deficiencies are uncommon in this country except in alcoholics, or in persons with gastrointestinal or mental diseases. It has been stated that vitamin concentrates have a limited but definite use in clinical medicine. However, the enthusiasm for vitamin therapy must not be allowed to run away with itself. It has been estimated that over 500 million dollars are spent annually on vitamin products in the United States. (See Food Fads, Fallacies and Quackery in Chapter 1.)

STANDARDIZATION   The early method of determining the vitamin potency of a food was of necessity based upon the direct measurement of its biological activity in preventing or curing certain specific pathological conditions in a predetermined experimental animal. This is known as the *bioassay* method and expresses measurement in terms of units. At present, only two vitamins are still thought of in terms of "units," namely, A and D. The unitage of these will be discussed subsequently. The other vitamins are discussed in terms of actual weight of material as determined by chemical or microbiological assay.

STABILITY   In general, the fat-soluble vitamins are fairly stable to ordinary cooking methods and are not lost in the cooking water. On the other hand, the water-soluble vitamins may be destroyed by overcooking and are easily dissolved in cooking water. A good rule to follow is to avoid long cooking at high temperature in the presence of air, under alkaline conditions, and to use as little water as is feasible. Washing, dicing and failure to store under refrigeration are among other factors that cause loss of vitamins.

Storage reduces the potency of vitamins in ratio to length of time they are stored.

TERMINOLOGY   Avitaminosis means "without vitamins" and is a term applied to severe vitamin deficiency. For example, in cases of severe or complete deficiency of B-complex, we speak of "avitaminosis B." Less severe grades of deficiency would be "deficiency of B-complex." On the other hand, it is now known that excessive intake of certain vitamins can cause clinical abnormalities, characteristic of "hypervitaminosis." Vitamin deficiencies will be discussed in Chapter 34, Nutritional Deficiency Diseases.

FAT-SOLUBLE VITAMINS

These vitamins are absorbed along with dietary fats, and conditions not favorable to normal fat uptake will also interfere with their absorption. They can be stored in the body to some extent and are not normally excreted in the urine. Mineral oil interferes with absorption, and if used it should be taken on rising or long enough after a meal to prevent interference with the utilization of the fat-soluble vitamins. Antibiotics and certain other drugs and various disease states such as malabsorption syndromes decrease the absorption of vitamins, especially fat-soluble vitamins, from the intestinal tract.

VITAMIN A
(Retinol)

HISTORY   Vitamin A was the first fat-soluble vitamin to be recognized. Two groups of research workers, McCollum and Davis at Wisconsin, and Osborne and Mendel at Yale, made the discovery almost simultaneously in 1913. They found that young animals be-

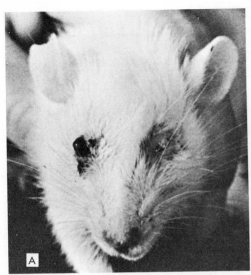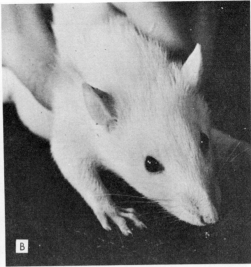

Figure 9–1   A, Typical eye condition produced by lack of vitamin A in the diet. B, Eyes restored to normal by feeding vitamin A. Three U.S.P. units (about 0.001 mg.) of vitamin A daily will cause resumption of growth and cure symptoms of vitamin deficiency in the white rat. (Courtesy of E. R. Squibb and Sons.)

came unhealthy and failed to grow on diets lacking natural fats. They also observed that, following a lack of growth, the eyes became inflamed and infected (see Fig. 9–1, A) but could be quickly relieved by the addition to the diet of a natural fat, such as butter fat or cod liver oil (see Fig. 9–1, B). In 1924, Bloch, working in Denmark, demonstrated that xerophthalmia in children could be prevented by feeding them butterfat or cod liver oil.

Vegetable foods also had vitamin A activity which was found to be related to their content of carotenes, yellow pigments frequently found in association with chlorophyll and largely responsible for the color of red and yellow vegetables. By 1932 it was found that the carotenes were precursors of vitamin A. Beta carotene was the most active, one molecule yielding two molecules of vitamin A; alpha and gamma carotenes yielded only one molecule of vitamin A, the other half of the carotene molecule being inactive. Carotene is referred to as a provitamin. Animals cannot synthesize it but can convert it to vitamin A. The human dietary includes not only the provitamin but the vitamin itself *preformed,* from animal foods and fish oils.

CHEMISTRY AND UTILIZATION   Vitamin A has been isolated in pure form as pale yellow crystals which are fat-soluble and has been synthesized chemically. The condensed formula, $C_{20}H_{29}OH$ indicates that it is an alcohol. It has been named retinol because it has a specific function in the retina of the eye. Natural vitamin A usually is found esterified with a fatty acid (usually palmitic acid).

Metabolically active forms of the vitamin include the corresponding aldehyde and acid.

The dietary vitamin A esters are hydrolyzed in the lumen of the small intestine to form retinol. Retinol passes across the mucosal cell wall where it is again esterified and is carried as retinyl ester to the liver where it is stored. Carotenoids are partially absorbed as such from the intestine and contribute to the yellow color of the blood serum. Most of the carotene is converted in the intestinal mucosa to retinal (vitamin A aldehyde). Both liver and intestinal mucosa have enzymes which catalyze reduction of the aldehyde to the alcohol.

Vitamin A and the carotenoids are fat-soluble. Therefore the factors which affect the absorption of the fat (bile salts, lipases, etc.) affect their absorption. In the blood stream vitamin A is transported with the lipids in the form of chylomicrons and lipoproteins. Mobilization of retinol from the liver depends on adequate dietary protein.

Inadequate vitamin A and protein are probably the two most common causes of malnutrition in the world today and the two deficiencies frequently occur together. It has been shown that protein deficient children afflicted with kwashiorkor have a vitamin A deficiency[5] also (Fig. 9–2).

STABILITY   Vitamin A is rather stable to light and heat, but prolonged heating in contact with air destroys it. It is easily destroyed

[5]Arroyave, G., et al.: Alterations in serum concentration of vitamin A associated with the hypoproteinemia of severe protein malnutrition. J. Pediatrics, 62:920, 1963.

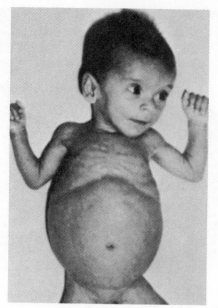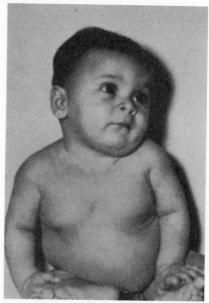

Figure 9–2   Malnutrition led to refractive errors in the eyes of this child from Bealback, Lebanon. Normal eye function returned when he was properly fed. Courtesy of Nutrition Today, March, 1968, p. 5.

by oxidation and ultraviolet light. A cool atmosphere and refrigeration tend to preserve it. Vitamin E may be used with vitamin A to prevent oxidation.

MEASUREMENT   The international unit (IU) of vitamin A activity was originally defined as the amount required per day to promote growth in a white rat receiving an otherwise vitamin A-free diet. This may now be expressed in chemical terms as 0.300 μg. of cyrstalline vitamin A alcohol. The unit for B-carotene is 0.6 μg. Thus dietary carotene has only about one-half the activity of vitamin A. This may be due to poor absorption from the intestinal tract or inefficient conversion of carotene to vitamin A.

RECOMMENDED DIETARY ALLOWANCE
The requirement appears to be proportional to body weight. Levels of intake which provide 20 I.U. (6 mcg.) of preformed vitamin A per kg. of body weight, or 40 I.U. (24 mcg.) of beta carotene, have been demonstrated to meet minimal requirements. The average adult recommended allowance is 5000 I.U. daily. This is about twice that required to meet the minimal needs. During pregnancy 6000 I.U. are recommended, and during lactation 8000 I.U. Children need 1500 to 5000 I.U. daily, the amount increasing with age from infancy to 13 years.

In the United States, according to the Food and Nutrition Board,[6] "the usual foods avail-

able are estimated to provide about 7500 I.U. of vitamin A per day; about 3500 I.U. derived from vegetables and fruits; 2000 I.U. from fats, oils and dairy products; and 2000 I.U. from meat, fish and eggs." Approximately 50 per cent of the vitamin A intake is in the form of the provitamin (carotene). Preliminary data on vitamin A status from the U.S. National Survey[7] shows that 13 per cent of the population sample studied had serum vitamin A levels below 20 μg. per 100 ml., which is considered to be the minimum acceptable level. The greatest percentage, 33 per cent, was in children under 6 years of age. Serum levels of vitamin A for healthy adults are about 30 to 65 μg. per 100 ml. (100 to 200 I.U. per 100 ml.); serum carotenoid levels range from 80 μg. to 225 μg. per 100 ml.

FUNCTION   Vitamin A is essential to the integrity of night vision, being a constituent of the visual purple of the retina, which is necessary for normal dim light vision. The elucidation of the biochemical role of vitamin A in the visual system is a result largely of the investigations of Wald and his co-workers. Retinal is a prosthetic group of photosensitive pigment of both the rods (rhodopsin) and cones (iodopsin), the difference between the two visual pigments being a result of the nature of the protein bound to retinol. The reaction involves the oxidation-reduction   systems   of   retinol-

---

[6]Food and Nutrition Board: Recommended Dietary Allowances. 7th ed. Washington, D.C., National Research Council, National Academy of Sciences, Pub. No. 1694, 1968, p. 22.

[7]Nutrition and Human Needs (III). The National Nutrition Survey. Hearings Before the Senate Committee on Nutrition and Human Needs of the United States Senate, Jan. 22, 23, 27 and 28, 1969.

retinal and stereochemical changes of the vitamin A molecule. When there is a deficiency of vitamin A the rods and cones cannot adjust to light changes, resulting in night blindness. An injection of vitamin A corrects this condition within a matter of minutes. Color blindness and other defects of vision cannot be cured by vitamin A. Vitamin A is necessary for growth and development of skeletal and soft tissues through its effect upon protein synthesis.

Vitamin A also plays a role in the maintenance of normal epithelial structures. A deficiency of this vitamin is accompanied by keratinization of the mucous membranes which line the respiratory tract, the alimentary canal and the urinary tract, and by keratinization of the body skin and epithelium of the eye, which lowers the protective barrier role played by these membranes in protection of the body against infection. Thus, a ready entry for infections is provided. It is from this function that vitamin A has become known as the anti-infective vitamin. Actually, vitamin A has nothing to do with an already present infection, but its lack sets up conditions whereby infection can more easily occur. The keratinization related to the eye is known as *xerophthalmia*. If treatment is initiated early and is adequate (25,000 I.U. vitamin A daily) the pathological changes of xerophthalmia may be remedied. Otherwise, partial or complete blindness may result. Xerophthalmia is a major cause of blindness in underdeveloped countries. A normal intake of vitamin A also helps to provide for normal bone development[8] and profoundly influences normal tooth formation.

The formation of mucus-secreting cells which synthesize glycoproteins and contain mucopolysaccharides depends upon the presence of vitamin A. A role of vitamin A in mucoprotein synthesis is suggested.

The role of vitamin A in normal human metabolism continues to challenge clinicians and biochemists. It must be involved in some fundamental function in most tissues but the nature of this function still is not known. It is probably unrelated to the retinal-retinol interconversion of the visual pigments, since in some, but not all, tissues retinoic acid (which cannot be reduced to retinal) is active.

Animal studies have shown that vitamin A intake must be increased above that required for good growth in order to assure normal reproduction and lactation.

Vitamin A deficiency is one of the most widespread forms of malnutrition in the world.

If the diet is inadequate in vitamin A, a primary deficiency may occur. "Secondary" or "conditioned" deficiencies occur when (1) a bodily dysfunction interferes with the absorption or storage of vitamin A (as in ulcerative colitis, cirrhosis of the liver, obstructions of the bile ducts); (2) a disorder interferes with the conversion of carotene to vitamin A (as in diabetes mellitus, hypothyroidism); (3) any rapid bodily loss of vitamin A takes place (pneumonia, hyperthyroidism, scarlet fever and some respiratory infections in children); and (4) enamel-forming epithelial cells are deprived of vitamin A. See Chap. 34 for Vitamin A Deficiency Disorders.

STORAGE   The liver is considered the storage site of vitamin A, with small amounts in the fat depots, lungs, and kidneys. Through the years the liver accumulates a reserve supply which reaches its peak in adult life. Approximately 90 per cent of the vitamin A in the body is stored in the liver. This savings account of vitamin A in the system may be drawn upon if in any emergency the vitamin is wanting in the diet.

DIETARY SOURCES   The dietary sources of preformed vitamin A are chiefly liver, kidney, butter and fortified margarine, egg yolk, whole milk and cream, and cheese made with whole milk or cream. The carotene forms are found in dark green, leafy and yellow vegetables, (collards, turnip greens, carrots, sweet potatoes, squash) and yellow fruit (apricots, peaches, cantaloupe). The deeper the green or the yellow of a vegetable, the more carotene (provitamin A) it contains. Cod and halibut fish oils are usually sources for therapeutic doses of vitamin A.

TOXICITY   In normal doses no toxic effects are observed. Toxicity from overdose (excess of 50,000 U.S.P. units daily) has been observed in adults and children. It has been noted to stunt growth or has left one leg two to three inches shorter than the other. The difference in leg length usually develops because the child tends to favor whichever leg becomes more painful. Bone fragility, thickening of long bones and deep bone pain, loss of appetite, coarsening and loss of hair, scaly skin eruptions, enlargement of the liver and spleen, irritability, double vision and skin rashes are among the symptoms of prolonged, excessive intake. If vitamin A toxicity is detected and stopped in time, the symptoms disappear in a few days after the vitamin is withdrawn.

VITAMIN D (Calciferol)

HISTORY   The isolation of vitamin D was delayed because of its confusion for a time with vitamin A. Both of these vitamins are fat-soluble; hence, they occur together in nature.

---

[8]Fell, H. B.: Brit. M. Bull., *12*:35, 1956.

Since the Middle Ages cod liver oil has been used as a remedy for rickets, but not until the period of World War I was the cause of rickets and the scientific basis for its cure established. Mellanby produced bone development characteristic of rickets in dogs, and demonstrated that it was related to the anticalcifying effect of some cereals. It was next found that this abnormal development could be counteracted by a fat-soluble factor which McCollum separated from vitamin A in 1922. In 1924 Steenbock and Hess independently and simultaneously discovered that ultraviolet irradiation gave antirachitic properties to certain foods. In 1930 vitamin D was isolated in crystalline form and named *calciferol*. In 1936 Windaus demonstrated that the natural prehormone found in the skin which becomes calciferol on ultraviolet irradiation was 7-dehydrocholesterol.

SOURCES   Vitamin D can be acquired either as preformed vitamin D by ingestion or by exposure to sunlight. It is found in only small and highly variable amounts in butter, cream, egg yolk and liver. The best food sources are the fish liver oils. In recent years approximately 85 per cent of all fluid milk[9] has been fortified with vitamin D, usually 400 I.U. per quart. Most dried whole milk and evaporated milk are fortified as well as some margarines, butter, certain cereals and infant formula products. Vitamin D_3 is formed in the body by the action of sunlight (ultraviolet rays) on 7-dehydrocholesterol in the skin. Since the provitamin can be synthesized in the body and needs only sunlight as an activator, classification of the active compound as a vitamin is not strictly accurate.

STABILITY   Vitamin D is remarkably stable, and preparations or foods containing it can be warmed or kept for long periods without its deterioration.

CHEMICAL AND PHYSICAL PROPERTIES
There are at least 11 sterols with vitamin D activity but only those called D_2 and D_3 are of practical importance. Ergosterol, a plant sterol closely related to cholesterol in structure is provitamin D_2 and 7-dehydrocholesterol is provitamin D_3. They are converted to the active form by irradiation with ultraviolet light. Ergocalciferol (D_2) is prepared commercially for use as a vitamin supplement. Cholecalciferol (D_3) is the form synthesized in animal tissues. It is the chief form in the fish oils.

MEASUREMENT   The International Unit of vitamin D is the equivalent of 0.025 μg. of pure calciferol (D_2), produced by irradia-

tion of ergosterol, and is based on certain biological activities in the rat. For all practical purposes, the U.S.P. unit and I.U. are identical.

ABSORPTION AND STORAGE   Ingested vitamin D is absorbed with the fats from the intestine with the aid of bile. Vitamin D from the skin is absorbed into the blood stream. It is stored in the liver, skin, brains, bones, and probably other tissues. Its exact fate has not yet been fully determined, and its mechanism of action is not completely elucidated, but its importance and function are known.

FUNCTION   Vitamin D is essential for normal growth and development and is important for the formation of normal bones and teeth. Vitamin D is directly related to increasing the rate of calcium and phosphorus accretion and resorption in bone. Vitamin D, along with parathormone and thyrocalcitonin, has an important role in the maintenance of the rather narrow range of serum calcium and phosphorus levels, in the growth and mineralization of the bones of children, and in the maintenance of mineralization of bones of the adult. Tracer studies indicate that vitamin D_3 is converted in the liver to the most biologically active metabolite, 25-hydroxycholecalciferol (25-HCC). It is believed to be transported to the intestinal wall where it acts with nucleoprotein to produce a protein which binds calcium and facilitates its active transport across the brush border of the intestine. This metabolite is thought to act similarly in mobilizing calcium from the bone.[10] To accomplish this, normally functioning kidneys and intestines and the ingestion of adequate amounts of calcium and phosphorus are required. Vitamin D is needed to prevent and to cure *rickets*, a disease formerly prevalent in infants and children, associated with malformation of bones due to deficient deposition of calcium phosphate. In rickets the bones are not strong and rigid and cannot stand the ordinary stresses and strains expected of them, so that knock-knees, bowlegs, pigeon breast, and frontal bossing of the skull appear. When a deficiency of vitamin D occurs, and calcium is not well absorbed, the renal threshold for phosphate excretion is lowered and more phosphate than normal is excreted in order to maintain a balance between calcium and phosphorus in the blood. In the adult, the equivalent disease is *osteomalacia*, in which, however, there is a decalcification of the bone shafts and the tendency is for fractures rather than bending to occur. Vitamin D participates in the absorption and utilization of calcium and phosphorus and the blood level of alkaline phosphatase.

---

[9]Dairy Council Digest: Recent Developments in Vitamin D. Chicago, National Dairy Council, 41: No. 4, July-August, 1970.

[10]*Ibid.*

With the discovery of the need for and function of vitamin D, the incidence of rickets and osteomalacia from vitamin D deficiency has dropped remarkably in the past generation. Renal rickets, caused by a certain type of kidney disease and altered calcium metabolism, has no connection with vitamin D. (See Chapter 34 for Vitamin D Deficiency Disorders.)

TOXICITY   It is known that hypervitaminosis D can occur and cause pathological changes in the body when vitamin D is taken in excess. These changes consist of an exaggeration of the normal changes produced by the vitamin, namely excessive calcification of bone, and metastatic calcification (calcification elsewhere in the body). It encourages the formation of kidney stones. Headache, nausea and diarrhea may be the subjective findings. Infants given excessive amounts of vitamin D may suffer gastrointestinal upsets, calcification of soft tissues (kidney and lungs), bone fragility and retarded growth. However, these difficulties appear only with enormous doses given over an extended period of time, and the usual doses available in vitamin preparations are not likely to be harmful.

Hypercalcemia   Excessive quantities of vitamin D (1000 to 3000 I.U. per kg. per day for children and adults) and hypersensitivity to vitamin D may lead to hypercalcemia (excess calcium in the blood). It can be cured if recognized in time, by medication and omitting vitamin D from the diet. A few infants who receive excessive amounts in association with a liberal calcium intake suffer this syndrome.

RECOMMENDED DIETARY ALLOWANCE
The normal adult is presumed to obtain sufficient vitamin D from exposure to sunlight and from the incidental ingestion of small amounts with food, such as fish and vitamin D fortified milk. The need for supplemental vitamin D by vigorous adults is believed unnecessary unless they are shielded from sunlight, as in the case of persons living in smoggy sunless areas; wearing clothes which cover the body; working at night and staying indoors as elderly persons may do. In these special cases a small daily supplement of vitamin D is believed desirable. The Food and Nutrition Board, National Research Council, sets the daily allowance of vitamin D at 400 international units as sufficient to meet the requirements of practically all healthy individuals who have no exposure to ultraviolet light. When the milk intake is sufficient, 400 international units allowance for infants is provided. Because of more access to sunlight and various food sources of vitamin D, the requirement is more difficult to determine beyond infancy. For women during pregnancy and lactation, adequate vitamin D is needed to promote efficient use of the increased calcium and phosphorus in the diet. The optimum amount of vitamin D is not known, but on the basis of available evidence 400 units is recommended.

It must be emphasized that no good will come from the provision of adequate vitamin D unless the calcium and phosphorus requirements are met also. In cases of vitamin D deficiency, "therapeutic dosages" are needed, namely, 1500 to 2500 I.U. daily for several months.

VITAMIN E (Tocopherol)

HISTORY   Vitamin E was first discovered by Evans and Bishop in 1922 when they found that rats reared on a basic diet failed to reproduce. In 1924 Sure gave it the name of vitamin E or antisterility vitamin. Evans, Emerson and Emerson isolated it from the unsaponifiable fraction of wheat germ oil in 1936, and it was chemically identified in 1938 and named tocopherol [tokos (Gr) = offspring].

CHEMISTRY   Four different tocopherols have been identified (alpha, beta, gamma, delta). They are oily yellow liquids, insoluble in water but soluble in fat solvents. They are stable to heat. Their most important chemical characteristic is their antioxidant property. Of the four tocopherols, alpha is the most active biologically. This may be related to better absorption from the intestine. Delta tocopherol is the most potent antioxidant.

FUNCTION   The function of vitamin E at the molecular level in the biological processes of the body is not fully determined. There is evidence that it acts as a co-factor in the electron transfer system in conjunction with the cytochromes. That it acts *in vivo* as a lipid antioxidant is well documented. It serves to prevent the formation of peroxides from polyunsaturated fatty acids, thus preventing the oxidation of the unsaturated fats.[11] Vitamin E also helps to enhance the activity of vitamin A by preventing its oxidation and loss of activity in the intestinal tract. Vitamin C in foods is similarly protected when vitamin E is present. Vitamin E deficiency is associated with the aging process as manifested in the increased destruction by lipid peroxidation.[12] When insufficient vitamin E is present, the amount of unsaturated fats in the cells decreases. This causes abnormal structure and function of the mitochondria and the lyso-

---

[11]Roels, O. A.: Present knowledge of vitamin E. In: Present Knowledge of Nutrition. 3rd ed. New York, The Nutrition Foundation, Inc., 1967, p. 87.

[12]Tappel, A. L.: Where old age begins. Nutrition Today, 2:2, 1967.

somes.[13, 14] It was reported in 1949 by György and Rose that in *in vitro* experiments normal resistance of red blood cells to rupture by oxidizing agents is reduced in vitamin E deficiency. Increased hemolysis and megaloblastic anemia and creatinuria are found in some children with kwashiorkor and in vitamin E-deficient monkeys. The addition of vitamin E induced a reticulocyte response and urinary excretion of creatine decreased.[15] Newborn infants have low tissue concentrations of vitamin E because of little transfer across the placenta. The amount of vitamin E in human milk is apparently sufficient to meet the infant's requirement. Cow's milk is relatively low in vitamin E content.

Whether or not vitamin E is essential in human nutrition has been a controversial issue. It is generally present in adequate amount in the diet and may be stored for long periods of time so that severe deficiency is rare.

It is well known that a deficiency of vitamin E causes a variety of symptoms in many species of animals. Some symptoms in animals attributed to vitamin E deficiency are listed.[16]

— in the female rat, the fetus dies and is resorbed, and in the male rat the testes atrophy resulting usually in sterility.
— in poultry, low hatchability and embryonic abnormalities and mortalities occur.
— in the dog, guinea pig, rabbit, chick, lamb and monkey, muscular dystrophy, anemia and various hematological symptoms are observed in deficient animals.
— in herbivorous animals, myocardial degeneration is found.
— in pigs, degeneration of skeletal and cardiac muscle and liver develops.
— in chicks, encephalomalacia with its neurological symptoms is manifested.
— in rats, a necrosis of the liver develops. The effect of vitamin E in prevention of this condition is augmented by small amounts of selenium.

The above brief mention of research reported in the literature suggests the possibilities of the role of tocopherols in human nutrition. However, the many previous enthusiastic claims for vitamin E in relieving or preventing rheumatic fever, muscular dystrophy, menstrual disorders, toxemias of pregnancy, spontaneous abortion, fibrositis, and sterility have not been substantiated for the human being, and the reader is cautioned against acceptance of claims for usefulness of this material (and for so many other vitamins and drugs) until long term, controlled, and carefully studied results are forthcoming.

STORAGE Vitamin E is thought to be absorbed in the same way as the other fat-soluble vitamins in the presence of bile salts and fat. Vitamin E is stored primarily in the fatty tissues and not in the liver, unlike the other fat-soluble vitamins. The pituitary and adrenal glands have high concentrations of vitamin E.

STABILITY Vitamin E is fairly stable to heat and acids and unstable to alkalies, ultraviolet light, and oxygen. It is also destroyed when in contact with rancid fats, lead, and iron. Since it is insoluble in water, there is no loss by extraction in cooking. Storage including deep freeze food processing and deepfat frying destroy most of the tocopherol present. Esters of tocopherol such as tocopherol acetate are not appreciably destroyed. As in the intestine, the tocopherols protect vitamin A and carotene in foods from oxidative destruction. Exposure to oxygen, however, and development of rancidity result in the destruction of the tocopherols.

MEASUREMENT One milligram of alpha tocopherol acetate is proposed as the international unit.

RECOMMENDED DIETARY ALLOWANCE Calculation for the recommended allowances provided in the values shown in Table 11-1 is $1.25 \times$ body wt. in kg. 0.75. The allowance for infants is 3 to 6 I.U. of vitamin E; for children and adolescents the range is 10 to 25 I.U.; for the adult male and female 30 I.U. and 25 I.U. respectively; in pregnancy and lactation 30 I.U. The requirement of vitamin E increases as the intake of fat and linoleic acid content in the diet are increased. The vitamin E content of foods in the customary dietary is estimated to range from about 2 to 66 I.U. daily.[17]

No toxic effect of alpha tocopherol is known. Conditions interfering with fat absorption reduce the amount of vitamin E absorbed.

SOURCES Vitamin E is the most widely available of any of the vitamins in common foodstuffs. Wheat germ oil is the richest source of the vitamin, but other cereal germs, green plants, egg yolk, milk fat, butter, meat (especially liver), nuts, and vegetable oils (soybean, corn, cottonseed) also contain it. In the customary United States diet about 64 per cent of the vitamin E intake is supplied by salad oils, margarine and shortening; about 11 per cent by fruits and vegetables and about 7 per cent by grains and grain products.[18] It is produced synthetically, also.

[13]Tappel, A. L.: Where old age begins. Nutrition Today, 2:2, 1967.
[14]Guyton, A. C.: Textbook of Medical Physiology. 4th ed. Philadelphia, W. B. Saunders Company, 1971, p. 1858.
[15]Food and Nutrition Board, *op. cit.*, p. 27.
[16]Roels, O. A., *op. cit.*, p. 87.

[17]Food and Nutrition Board, *op. cit.*, p. 29.
[18]*Ibid.*

VITAMIN K

HISTORY   In 1935 Dam in Copenhagen discovered a severe hemorrhagic disease in newly hatched chickens on a ration adequate in all known vitamins and dietary essentials. By giving hog liver fat or alfalfa, normal clotting time was restored. It was suggested that the hemorrhage in chicks was due to a fall in prothrombin, a compound required for normal clotting of blood. Dam named the antihemorrhage factor vitamin K, or "Koagulationsvitamin." In 1939 vitamin K was isolated and only a few months later it was synthesized.

CHEMICAL AND PHYSICAL PROPERTIES There are at least three forms of vitamin K all belonging to a group of chemical compounds known as quinones. The naturally occurring vitamins are K_1 (phylloquinone), which occurs in green plants, and K_2 (menaquinone), which is formed as the result of bacterial action in the intestinal tract. Vitamin K_1 was isolated from alfalfa and K_2 from putrefied fish meal. Water-soluble forms of K_1 and K_2 are available for use by individuals unable to absorb the fat-soluble form. The fat-soluble synthetic compound, menadione (K_3), is about twice as potent biologically as the naturally occurring vitamins K_1 and K_2 on a weight basis because it lacks the long side chain of the natural vitamin. The body must add the side chain to the menadione before it can function as vitamin K. None of the forms of vitamin K are stored in appreciable amounts.

STABILITY   Vitamin K is fairly resistant to heat, but sunlight destroys the K_1. There is no destruction in ordinary cooking methods and, being fat-soluble, there is no loss in cooking water. All vitamin K compounds tend to be unstable to alkali.

MEASUREMENT   At present no specific unitage of vitamin K has been agreed upon. One of the most commonly used systems, however, states that 1 mg. of pure vitamin K_1 contains 1000 Thayer-Doisy units.

FUNCTION   Vitamin K is absorbed (with the aid of bile) in the upper intestinal tract and transported to the liver where it is essential for synthesis of prothrombin and several related proteins involved in the clotting of blood. The clotting mechanism, of which the final step is the conversion of fibrinogen, which is soluble, to fibrin, which is insoluble, and forms the clot is complex. It involves at least 12 factors (of which prothrombin is factor VII) along with calcium ion. The peptides which become the various glycoproteins of the prothrombin complex cannot be synthesized on the appropriate RNA molecules unless the liver contains vitamin K.[19] A deficiency occurs when the dietary lacks green vegetables and the growth of intestinal microorganisms is inhibited simultaneously by the administration of antibiotics or when the absorption of lipid is impaired.

Deficiencies of vitamin K usually occur from inadequate absorption from the intestinal tract or inability to utilize it in the liver. The latter occurs frequently in severe liver disease and is an instance in which large therapeutic doses of vitamin K are indicated.

Newborn infants are prone to have prothrombin deficiency during the first few days of life and are therefore susceptible to development of *"hemorrhagic disease of the newborn,"* a disease manifested by abnormal bleeding. Therefore, it is necessary at times to administer vitamin K to mothers just before delivery of a child or to the child upon delivery as a preventive measure against this disease. Furthermore, in the use of anticoagulants such as Dicumarol, bleeding occasionally occurs and this can be mitigated by the use of vitamin K. Frequently, it is given to patients before surgery to prevent abnormal bleeding. Excessive use of aspirin can prevent normal clotting of blood by interfering with platelet aggregation.[20]

TOXICITY   Excessive doses of synthetic vitamin K have produced hemolytic anemia in the rat and kernicterus in the infant.[21] Because the toxicity of menadione causes an increase in breakdown of red blood cells and inhibits bilirubin glucuronide formation, menadione in over-the-counter supplements for pregnancy has been prohibited.

RECOMMENDED DIETARY ALLOWANCE No quantitative estimate of vitamin K requirement has been made for human beings, but it is known that materials containing vitamin K activity in doses of 1 to 2 mg. will correct vitamin K deficiency in most cases. The Food and Nutrition Board, National Research Council, suggests that a single dose of 1 mg. of vitamin K_1 immediately after birth is adequate to prevent hemorrhagic disease. Infants born to mothers receiving anticoagulant therapy should be given vitamin K_1 immediately after birth.

Vitamin K occurs in abundant quantities in the average diet, and is synthesized by intestinal bacteria, so that, with the exception of the newborn infant, there should be no dietary deficiency of it in the healthy person.

[19]McGilvery, R. W.: Biochemistry: A Functional Approach. Philadelphia, W. B. Saunders Company, 1970, p. 650

[20]*Ibid.*, p. 653.

[21]Crosse, V. M., et al.: Kernicterus and prematurity. Arch Dis. Child., 30:501, 1955.

Few malnourished individuals have shown a dietary lack of vitamin K.

SOURCES   Vitamin K is found in green leafy vegetables, especially cabbage, spinach, kale and lettuce, cauliflower, tomatoes, wheat bran, soybean and in oil, cheese, egg yolk and liver. It can be synthesized chemically. Vitamin K_2 has been shown to be formed by bacterial action of the flora of the human lower intestinal tract, so that an important supply of this vitamin may be available to the body even if it is not supplied in the diet. However, this source is only partially available for absorption.

WATER-SOLUBLE VITAMINS

These vitamins are not normally stored in the body in appreciable amounts; thus, a daily supply is desirable to avoid depletion and interruption of normal physiologic functions. Most of them are components of essential enzyme systems and are normally excreted in small quantities in the urine.

VITAMIN B-COMPLEX

HISTORY   Originally vitamin B was recognized as the preventive factor in the disease beriberi. Today more than a dozen separate B vitamins have been identified and found to play important roles in nutrition.

In 1897 Eijkman, a Dutch physician in Java, observed that chickens in the prison yard showed symptoms similar to those of his beriberi patients. The chickens ate the polished-rice table scraps discarded from the prisoners' meals, developed the malady and died. Eijkman found that addition of rice bran to the rice cured and prevented the beriberi in fowls. Although the findings were wrongly interpreted and shelved for years, the work of Eijkman laid the foundation for the conduct of future experiments. It was not until about 1911 that Funk and others described vitamin B.

Since later work showed that the original vitamin B actually consisted of several necessary accessory food factors, the anti-beriberi portion was christened B_1 or thiamin, and the other parts labeled B_2 and so forth as they were discovered. Today the members of the B-complex group are commonly referred to by their chemical names. Thiamin is B_1 riboflavin is B_2, pyridoxine is B_6, and we also have niacin (nicotinic acid), pantothenic acid, folacin, biotin, para-aminobenzoic acid, inositol, choline and cyanocobalamin (B_{12}).

The grouping of all these water-soluble compounds under the term "B-complex" is based upon their common source distribution, their close relationship in vegetable and animal tissues, and their intimate functional *interrelations*.

FUNCTION   One should think of the symptoms arising from avitaminosis B as a result of an attempt by the tissue cells to produce the energy needed for normal function in the absence of enough of the members of the B-complex group to accomplish the oxidation of food at the required rate. The B group, in general, plays an essential role in the metabolic processes of all living cells by serving as co-factors in the various enzyme systems involved in the oxidation of food and production of energy. They function as coenzymes or as a prosthetic group bound to an apoenzyme, an enzyme protein. Coenzymes and prosthetic groups function similarly, since both contain one of the active sites of the enzyme complex to which the substrate molecule is attached. The active site for most enzyme systems is a portion of the vitamin molecule. There exists such a close *interrelation* among the B vitamins that a inadequate intake of one may impair the utilization of others. Therefore, single discrete deficiencies of the B group are seldom seen clinically although the signs and symptoms of deficiency of a particular member of the group may predominate. Furthermore, the use of a single member of the group therapeutically may create a vitamin imbalance and precipitate deficiency of other members of the group. Thus, therapy with vitamin B should generally consist of therapy with all vitamin B-complex members rather than with any single substance of the group. Dry yeast is the richest natural source of the B-complex group.

Thiamin (Vitamin B_1)

HISTORY   Thiamin has been known as the antineuritic vitamin because it is needed for normal functioning of the nervous system. Deficiency of it in animals causes hindquarter paralysis. The symptom recognized by Eijkman in chickens and pigeons, and the beriberi described by workers in the Orient, was found to be concerned with the B_1 or thiamin fraction of the original B vitamin. In 1926 Jansen and Donath isolated thiamin in crystalline form, and in 1936 R. R. Williams accomplished the synthesis and determined the chemical formula. The vitamin was named thiamin to designate the presence of sulfur and an amino group in the complex molecule. For more of the history see Beriberi in Chapter 34.

SOURCE   Thiamin is found in a large variety of animal and vegetable materials but in abundance in only a few foods. Lean pork, fresh and cured, and wheat germ are outstanding sources. Liver and all organ meats, liver sausage, lean meats, poultry, egg yolk, fish, dry beans and peas, soybeans, peanuts and whole grains are excellent sources. The whole grain and enriched grain products are the best daily sources of thiamin. The basic foods in the recommended amounts for an adult provide approximately 1 mg. of thiamin per day. Milk and milk products, fruit and vegetables are not good sources but when consumed in sufficient quantities they contribute materially to the day's total intake of thiamin.

CHEMICAL CHARACTERISTICS AND STABILITY Pure thiamin hydrochloride has been isolated and is a crystalline yellowish white powder with a salty, nutlike taste, and is water soluble. The dry vitamin is fairly stable, but solutions of it are unstable in the presence of heat or alkali. It is heat stable in acid solution. Loss of the vitamin in cooking is extremely variable, depending on the pH of the food, time, temperature, quantity of water used and discarded, and the use of sodium bicarbonate to enhance the green color of vegetables. Freezing has little or no effect on the thiamin content of foods.

ABSORPTION, SYNTHESIS AND STORAGE Thiamin is absorbed readily in the acid medium of the proximal duodenum and to some extent, in the lower duodenum and is carried to the liver by the portal circulation. It is not stored in any great quantity in the body and must, therefore, be supplied daily. The vitamin can be synthesized by microorganisms in the intestinal tract of animals and man, but the amount available to the human body to supplement the dietary supply seems to be small. Thiamin is excreted in the urine in amounts that reflect the intake and the amount stored. Fat and protein spare thiamin and a high intake of carbohydrate increases the need for thiamin. Thiaminase present in uncooked clams and fish destroys approximately 50 per cent of the thiamin.

FUNCTION Thiamin is necessary throughout life for tissue respiration. Thiamin combines with phosphorus to form the coenzyme thiamin pyrophosphate (TPP), which functions as cocarboxylase. TPP is required for the oxidative decarboxylation of pyruvate to form active acetate and thence to acetyl Coenzyme A, the central compound of the Krebs metabolic pathway. TPP is required for the oxidative decarboxylation of other alpha-keto acid, alpha-ketoglutaric acid and the 2-ketocarboxylates derived from amino acids methionine, threonine, leucine, isoleucine and valine. TPP is also the coenzyme for the transketolase reaction which functions in the pentose phosphate shunt, an alternate pathway for glucose oxidation.

Thiamin is needed for the metabolism of carbohydrates, fats and proteins. However, all the evidence from the effects of thiamin deficiency link it with disturbance of carbohydrate metabolism, especially in the brain. The thiamin requirement is linked to carbohydrate intake. This indicates that the decarboxylation of pyruvate, which is concerned only with carbohydrate metabolism, is the one which suffers loss of thiamin first. A total blood thiamin below 3.0 μg. per 100 ml. in the absence of anemia is indicative of a state of thiamin deficiency.[22]

THIAMIN DEFICIENCY As previously stated, severe thiamin deficiency of long duration causes beriberi, a disease formerly quite common in the Orient. (See Chap. 34 for Thiamin Deficiency Disorders.) Animals and humans with mild deficiencies may show fatigue, emotional instability, depression, irritability, retarded normal growth, loss of appetite, loss of interest in daily tasks, and general lethargy. (See Fig. 9–3.)

Effect of Thiamin Deficiency on the Nervous System Without thiamin the function of the central nervous system, which depends solely upon glucose for its energy, is greatly impaired. The neuronal cells show chromatolysis and swelling resulting in diminished reflex response. During thiamin deficiency, degeneration of myelin sheaths of nerve fibers in the central nervous system and the peripheral nerves occurs. This causes the nerves to become irritable which produces pain in the pathway of the peripheral nerves. Progressive degeneration may cause paralysis and muscle atrophy.[23]

Effect of Thiamin Deficiency on the Cardiovascular System The heart muscle is weakened in thiamin deficiency and it may cause cardiac failure resulting in peripheral edema and ascites in the extremities. A metabolic deficiency in smooth muscle of the vascular system causes peripheral vasodilatation.[24]

Effect of Thiamin Deficiency in the Gastrointestinal Tract Gastrointestinal symptoms of thiamin deficiency are indigestion, severe constipation, anorexia, gastric atony and decreased hydrochloric acid secretion. This probably results from insufficient energy from carbohydrate metabolism for the smooth muscles and glands of the intestinal tract.[25]

Other Effects of Thiamin Deficiency Alcoholic polyneuropathy and amblyopia are largely due to a thiamin deficiency. When treated early the symptoms of the Wernicke-Korsakoff syndrome respond to thiamin.[26]

[22]Latham, M. C.: Present knowledge of thiamin. In: Present Knowledge of Nutrition. 3rd ed. New York, The Nutrition Foundation, Inc., 1967, p. 56.

[23]Guyton, A. C.: Textbook of Medical Physiology. 4th ed. Philadelphia, W. B. Saunders Company, 1971, p. 853.

[24]Ibid.

[25]Ibid.

[26]Latham, M. C., op. cit., p. 59.

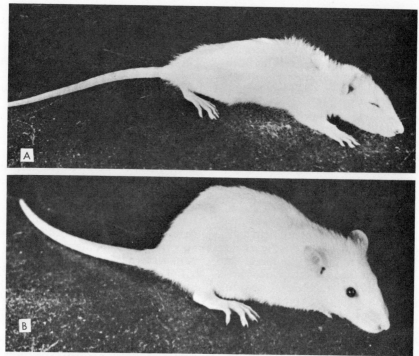

Figure 9–3   A, Prolonged deficiency of vitamin B₁ checks growth in young animals, causes loss of appetite, and results in degenerative changes in the nervous system. B, Animal cured by administration of vitamin B₁ (thiamin chloride). Two to three International Units (0.006 to 0.009 mg.) of thiamin chloride daily will cure symptoms of vitamin B₁ deficiency in these animals. (Courtesy of E. R. Squibb and Sons.)

Individuals whose intake of calories is markedly restricted are prone to development of thiamin deficiency symptoms. Exercise, fever, hyperthyroidism, major surgical operations and other stresses increase cellular energy requirements which increase the thiamin needs. Deficiency may be remedied by giving therapeutic doses of B-complex and thiamin plus an adequate diet.

TOXICITY   There are no known toxic effects from thiamin.

RECOMMENDED DIETARY ALLOWANCE Many factors influence the thiamin needs of an individual. Among these are body weight, calorie intake, and the small amount synthesized in the intestinal tract. The amount of thiamin required is related to calorie needs, specifically to those obtained from carbohydrate. Liberal amounts of fat and protein in the diet exert a thiamin-sparing effect and will require less thiamin than will a high carbohydrate diet of the same caloric value. The Food and Nutrition Board[27] recommends 0.5 mg. per 1000 kcalories for all ages. This allows for a margin of safety. A thiamin intake of 1.0 mg. per day is recommended for older adults even though they consume less than 2000 kcalories daily because it is believed

that older persons use thiamin less efficiently. An additional allowance for pregnancy of 0.2 mg. per day and for lactation 0.5 mg. per day is recommended. (See Table 11–1, Chapter 11.)

Based on the 1968 Food and Nutrition Board allowance for thiamin, dietary surveys in 1965[28] indicate that 17 per cent of the families studied received less than two-thirds of the recommended thiamin intake.

Riboflavin (Vitamin B₂)

HISTORY   The existence of a yellow-green fluorescent pigment in milk whey was recognized in 1879. The biological significance of this pigment was not understood until 1932 when a group of German workers isolated "Warburg's yellow enzyme" from yeast and demonstrated that the material was necessary for activity of an intracellular respiratory enzyme. Almost simultaneously other investigators were studying a food factor that aided growth of laboratory animals. In 1933 Kuhn and his co-workers isolated the

[27] Food and Nutrition Board, op. cit., p. 42.

[28] Davis, T. R. A., Gershoff, S. N., and Gamble, D.: Review of studies of vitamin and mineral nutrition in the United States (1950–1958). J. Nutr. Ed., Vol. 1., No. 2, Supplement 1, Fall, 1969, p. 48.

pigment from milk. They noted, however, that it did not have all the activities ascribed to vitamin B_2. The compound was synthesized in 1935 by Kuhn and his co-workers and given the name *riboflavin*. Later investigations differentiated it from the pellagra-preventive factor with which it had first been confused.

CHEMICAL CHARACTERISTICS AND STABILITY Riboflavin belongs to a group of yellow fluorescent pigments called flavins. The flavin ring is attached to an alcohol related to ribose. It has been synthesized and in pure state appears as yellow crystals. It is stable to heat, oxidation, and acid; it is sparingly soluble in water but disintegrates in the presence of alkali or light, especially ultraviolet. Due to its heat stability and limited water solubility, very little is lost in the cooking and processing of foods. It has been demonstrated that bottled milk left outside the door in sunlight will lose a significant amount of riboflavin. Milk in paper containers is protected against such losses.

FUNCTION Riboflavin combines in the tissues with phosphoric acid to become part of the structure of two flavin coenzymes, flavin mononucleotide (FMN) and flavin adenine dinucleotide (FAD). These coenzymes are the prosthetic group of the flavoprotein enzymes which catalyze oxidation-reduction reaction in the cells as hydrogen carriers in the mitochondrial electron transport system. They are coenzymes of the dehydrogenases which catalyze the first step in oxidation of several intermediates in glucose metabolism and of fatty acids. They are also active in oxidative deamination of amino acids.

Riboflavin is essential for growth. (See Fig. 9-4.) Deficiency of riboflavin leads to cheilosis (cracking at the corners of the lips), glossitis (swollen and reddened tongue), seborrheic type of dermatitis, and ocular disorders such as itching, burning, lacrimation, sensitivity to light, and vascularization of the cornea. Other members of the B group are usually concurrently deficient, and appropriate signs and symptoms of such deficiencies also appear. (See Chapter 34 for Riboflavin Deficiency Disorders.)

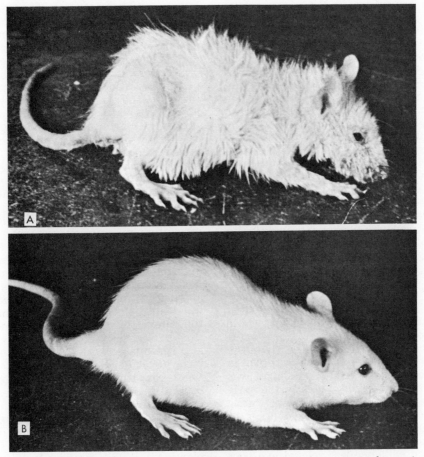

Figure 9-4   *A*, Deficiency of vitamin B_2 (riboflavin) affects growth and also induces certain changes in skin. *B*, Riboflavin deficiency symptoms cured. About 0.012 and 0.015 mg. daily is required. (Courtesy of E. R. Squibb and Sons.)

ABSORPTION AND STORAGE Riboflavin is easily absorbed through the walls of the small intestine where it must be phosphorylated before entering the blood stream. It is carried by the blood to the tissue of the body and excreted in the urine. The amount excreted depends upon the intake and relative need of the tissues. Loss of riboflavin accompanies a loss of protein from the body. Although small amounts of riboflavin are found in the liver and kidney, it is not stored to any great degree in the body and must therefore be supplied in the diet regularly.

TOXICITY There is no known toxicity to riboflavin.

RECOMMENDED DIETARY ALLOWANCE The riboflavin requirements of the human, according to the 1968 revision of the Food and Nutrition Board, are related to body size, metabolic rate and rate of growth. These factors are related to protein and calorie intake of the individual. The recommended amount for the reference adult male and female respectively is 1.7 and 1.5 mg. daily. During pregnancy an increase of 0.3 mg. per day and for lactation an additional daily intake of 0.5 mg. are recommended. The value recommended for infants is 0.1 mg. per kilogram. See Table 11–1 for the amounts of riboflavin needed for children. The FAO/WHO Expert Group recommends 0.55 mg. per 1000 kcalories for all age groups.

SOURCES Riboflavin is widely distributed in foods but in small amounts. The best daily sources in average servings are milk (fresh, canned or dried), cheddar cheese and cottage cheese. Although some of the riboflavin of cheese and cottage cheese is lost to the whey, they are good sources of riboflavin. Variety meats (liver, heart, kidney, liverwurst) contain appreciable amounts of riboflavin and other lean meats, eggs and green leafy vegetables are important sources in the amounts usually consumed. Breads and cereals enriched with riboflavin provide lesser amounts of riboflavin but contribute appreciably to the total daily intake.

Niacin (Nicotinic Acid)

HISTORY It has been known for several centuries that pellagra occurred mainly where people used corn as a staple of the diet. It was described by Casál of Spain early in the 18th century and the disease was common in Italy at about the same time. Pellagra was described first in United States in the early 1900's. The United States Bureau of Public Health selected Dr. Joseph Goldberger to investigate the problem of pellagra that was rampant in the southern states. The condition based on evidence was related to a poor diet (high in cornmeal) as the cause. A diet of good quality protein foods prevented pellagra. Following the discovery in 1937 by Elvehjem that the disease blacktongue in dogs is due to a niacin deficiency, human pellagra was recognized by Spies and others as a niacin deficiency condition. In 1945 Krehl and his associates, in treating pellagra at the University of Wisconsin, found that tryptophan and niacin produce similar results. Since then it has been established that tryptophan is a precursor of niacin. However, recent findings indicate that pellagra is a mixed deficiency and that thiamin and riboflavin are also lacking. In addition, the role of corn in the production of this disease has been recognized. This may be due to lack of tryptophan in corn or to a toxic substance in corn. Pellagra is further discussed in Chapter 34.

SOURCE Both niacin and its precursor, tryptophan, are included in determining the niacin in foods. Lean meats, poultry, fish and peanuts are rich daily sources of both. Organ meats, brewers' yeast, peanuts and peanut butter are the richest sources of niacin. Vegetables and fruits are poor sources. Milk and eggs contain small amounts of niacin but are excellent sources of tryptophan. To a lesser extent, beans, peas, other legumes, most nuts, and whole grains or enriched cereals also contain them. Of particular importance to the South is the niacin enrichment of corn products. Most foods rich in animal protein are also rich in tryptophan. A dietary intake of 60 gm. predominantly complete protein, provides 0.6 gm. (600 mg.) tryptophan. One niacin equivalent (1 mg.) is defined as 60 mg. of dietary tryptophan. A 60-gm. protein dietary would contribute 10 mg. of niacin. Approximately 500 to 1000 mg. of tryptophan (8 to 17 mg. niacin) is provided in a diet containing good quality protein.

CHEMICAL CHARACTERISTICS AND STABILITY Niacin, nicotinic acid, is a whitish crystalline material, stable when dry. It is easily converted to the active form nicotinamide. It is much more stable than thiamin and riboflavin, and is remarkably resistant to heat, light, air, acids and alkalies, although small amounts may be lost in discarded cooking water. It is frequently administered in the amide form, namely nicotinamide for therapeutic doses, since nicotinic acid acts as a vasodilator.

ABSORPTION AND STORAGE Absorption takes place in the intestine. Little storage occurs in the body, and any excess is eliminated through the urine.

FUNCTION Nicotinic acid functions in the body as a component of the coenzymes nicotinamide adenine dinucleotide (NAD) and nicotinamide adenine dinucleotide phosphate

(NADP), known as the pyridine nucleotides. They were formerly known as coenzymes I and II and then DPN and TPN (diphosphopyridine nucleotide and triphosphopyridine nucleotide.) These coenzymes are concerned with glycolysis, tissue respiration and fat synthesis. They serve as hydrogen acceptors capable of accepting and releasing hydrogen atoms as they are removed from food substrates by the many different types of dihydrogenases that are essential in the oxidation-reduction reactions in the release of energy from carbohydrates, fats and proteins. These coenzymes in their reduced forms (NADH and NADPH) deal with reduction of riboflavin-containing coenzymes and enzymes. Hydrogen is passed along from the reduced pyridine nucleotides to the riboflavin-containing coenzymes and then through mediation of the cytochromes finally to oxygen and the formation of metabolic water. Some niacin may be synthesized by the bacteria in the intestinal flora and some may be synthesized from tryptophan. Tryptophan is known as a precursor of niacin and as having a sparing action on the amount of niacin needed in the diet. Experiments with humans indicate that approximately 60 mg. tryptophan are equivalent to 1 mg. of niacin.

The symptoms of niacin deficiency are many. In the early stages muscular weakness, anorexia, indigestion and skin eruptions occur. Severe deficiency of niacin leads to pellagra which is characterized by dermatitis, dementia, diarrhea (the "3 D's" of pellagra) tremors, and sore tongue ("beef tongue"). The skin develops a cracked pigmented scaly dermatitis in the parts exposed to sun irradiations. Lesions appear in many parts of the central nervous system resulting in confusion, disorientation and neuritis. Many digestive abnormalities develop in niacin deficiency causing irritation and inflammation of the mucous membranes of the mouth and the gastrointestinal tract. Clinical symptoms of severe riboflavin deficiency appear. In fact many of the niacin deficiencies are similar, owing to the close interrelationships of riboflavin and niacin in cell metabolism. (See Chap. 34 for further discussion of pellagra.)

TOXICITY   No real *toxic* effects are known, but large doses cause transient side effects such as tingling sensations, flushing of the skin and throbbing in the head due to its vasodilating action.

RECOMMENDED DIETARY ALLOWANCE The 1968 Food and Nutrition Board recommended allowances for niacin are expressed as niacin equivalents, and it is assumed that 60 mg. of tryptophan may be converted to 1 mg. of niacin. Requirement is based on caloric intake and the recommended allowance ex-

pressed in niacin equivalents is 6.6 mg. per 1000 kcalories and not less than 13 equivalents at caloric intakes of less than 2000 kcalories. If the caloric intake falls below 2000 kcalories, the minimum need in adults is 9 mg. per day to prevent pellagra. Daily requirement for niacin is influenced by the amount of tryptophan and thus by the amount and kind of protein available in the dietary. Most diets consumed in the United States average 500 to 1000 mg. or more of tryptophan daily and 8 to 17 mg. of preformed niacin, for total niacin equivalents of 16 to 33 mg. Thus, the daily allowance falls between 13 to 14 mg. for women and 14 to 18 mg. for men, varying with the energy requirement. For pregnancy, the recommended allowance provides an increase of 2 equivalents per day based on the recommended increase in calorie intake. During lactation an additional daily allowance of 7 niacin equivalents is recommended, based on the additional allowance of 1000 kcalories.[29] See Table 11–1 for the niacin mg. equivalents, which includes dietary sources of niacin plus 1 mg. equivalent for each 60 mg. of dietary tryptophan.

Vitamin B$_6$ (Pyridoxine, Pyridoxal and Pyridoxamine)

HISTORY   In 1938 pyridoxine was identified as another fraction of the vitamin B-complex, and synthesized in 1939. Later it was found that two derivatives of pyridoxine, namely *pyridoxamine* and *pyridoxal*, were also active. Therefore, vitamin B$_6$ is a complex of these three closely related chemical compounds of naturally occurring pyridines that are metabolically and functionally interrelated. Pyridoxine or B$_6$ is the term used to designate this group of vitamins.

CHEMICAL PROPERTIES   Pyridoxine, a white, crystalline, odorless compound, is soluble in water and alcohol. It is stable to heat in an acid medium and relatively unstable in alkaline solutions, but very unstable to light. It is absorbed in the upper small intestine and excreted from the body primarily as pyridoxic acid.

FUNCTION   This vitamin plays an essential role in many of the complex biochemical processes by which foods are metabolized in the body. Pyridoxine is found in cells in the active form, pyridoxal phosphate (PLP) a coenzyme that functions in protein, fat and carbohydrate metabolism. Its primary function as a coenzyme for many chemical reactions, however, is related to protein metabolism. Pyridoxal phosphate functions in the

---

[29] Food and Nutrition Board, *op. cit.*, p. 38.

reactions involved in the nonoxidative degradation of amino acids, namely:

— transamination, the transfer of the amino group (NH_2) from one amino acid to form a different amino acid and the keto-analogue of the original amino acid. Transaminase activity in tissues is low in pyridoxine deficiency.

— deamination, the removal of amino groups from some amino acids not needed for growth thus rendering the carbon residues available for energy.

— desulfuration, transfer of sulfhydryl group (HS) from one amino acid (methionine) to another (serine) to form cysteine.

— decarboxylation, the removal of the carboxyl group (COOH) from certain amino acids to form another compound. This decarboxylation is required for the synthesis of serotonin, norepinephrine and histamine from tryptophan, tyrosine and histidine respectively. In addition, pyridoxal phosphate is necessary for the formation of a precursor of porphyrin compounds which are an essential part of the hemoglobin molecule. It is essential for the formation and metabolism of tryptophan and for the conversion of tryptophan to nicotinic acid (niacin). In this reaction pyridoxal phosphate plays a role in niacin supply. An individual with pyridoxine deficiency when given the tryptophan load test will accumulate xanthurenic acid (an intermediary product in the conversion of tryptophan to niacin). The amount can be measured in the urine and is used as an indication of the extent of available pyridoxine.

Pyridoxine as a part of the enzyme phosphorylase facilitates the release of glycogen from the liver and muscle as glucose-1-phosphate. It is also involved in the conversion of the essential unsaturated fatty acid, linoleic acid, to the biologically important arachidonic acid.

DEFICIENCY   Rats deficient in pyridoxine (B_6) develop a dermatitis, decreased rate of growth, fatty liver, anemia, weakness and evidence of mental retardation. (See Figure 9–5.) The skin disturbance cannot be cured with niacin. Hamsters and monkeys given diets deficient in B_6 show an increase in dental caries.[30] Monkeys on a pyridoxine-deficient diet develop arteriosclerotic changes, indicating a possible role for pyridoxine in cholesterol metabolism.

Adults who were given a B_6 antagonist (deoxypyridoxine) developed depression, nausea, vomiting, seborrheic dermatitis,

mucous membrane lesions and peripheral neuritis.[31]

Isoniazid (INH; isonicotinic acid hyrazide), used as a chemotherapeutic agent for tubercular patients, is a potent antagonist of B_6. Patients develop peripheral neuritis and many of the symptoms of pyridoxine deficiency. The enzyme involved in decarboxylation of amino acids apparently is inactivated when isoniazid combines with pyridoxal phosphate. Urinary excretion of vitamin B_6 is greatly increased. The same is true with the medication penicillamine. Several patients with microcytic hypochromic anemia have responded to the administration of vitamin B_6 even though the diets contained the usual amount of the vitamin. The tryptophan load test manifested the deficiency.

Spies found that certain symptoms in some pellagra and beriberi patients which were not relieved by niacin, thiamin or riboflavin responded to pyridoxine.

Vitamin B_6 deficiency has been shown to increase urinary oxalate excretion and has been implicated in renal calculi formation. This has been attributed to inability to convert glyoxalate to glycine and reflects the importance of this vitamin in metabolism of glycine and serine (decrease in transaminase activity). Antibody production appears to be low in pyridoxine deficiency. The synthesis of nucleic acid required for cells which form antibodies is reduced.[32]

Pregnant women on "normal" diets have manifested pyridoxine deficiency when given the tryptophan load test and the abnormality was corrected by the administration of the vitamin. The placenta actively transports pyridoxine to attain a five-fold increase in fetal blood as compared with the mother.[33] The vitamin has been used in the treatment of nausea and vomiting of pregnancy and following radiation treatment with apparently good results. However, its efficiency in this use has not been proved.

Central nervous system abnormalities appear in extreme pyridoxine deficiency. Infants fed a liquid milk formula in which much of the vitamin was unknowingly destroyed in processing (autoclaving, high temperatures) developed irritability and convulsions (see p. 257). Urinary excretion of B_6 decreased and the tryptophan load test was positive with an increase in xanthurenic aciduria. Other infants fed a synthetic formula devoid of vitamin B_6 developed anemia and convul-

[30]Williams, M. A.: Present knowledge of vitamin B_6. In: Present Knowledge in Nutrition. 3rd ed. The Nutrition Foundation, Inc., 1967, pp. 67, 70.

[31]Vitler, R. W., et al.: The effect of vitamin B_6 deficiency induced by desoxypyridoxine in human beings. J. Lab. Clin. Med., 42:335, 1953.
[32]Vitler, R. W., et al., *op. cit.*
[33]Food and Nutrition Board, *op. cit.*, p. 47.

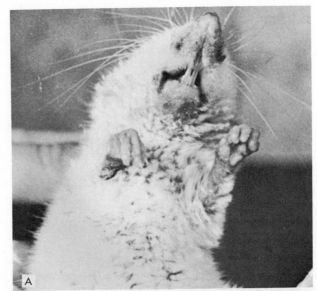

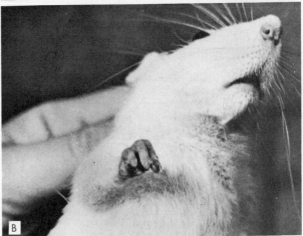

Figure 9-5   A, Typical dermatitis about the nose and paws due to lack of vitamin B₆. B, Animal cured of vitamin B₆ deficiency. A daily dose of 0.01 mg. of vitamin B₆ suffices to erase the symptoms of deficiency. (Courtesy of E. R. Squibb and sons.)

sions.[34] Infants recovered rapidly after an injection of the vitamin. It is apparent that enzyme systems of the central nervous system have a low order of binding capacity with coenzyme pyridoxal phosphate, making them susceptible to deficiency with resultant derangement of cellular metabolism and clinical abnormalities.

A deficiency syndrome has been identified in mentally retarded children with uncontrollable convulsions from birth due to inborn error of B_6 metabolism. Correction of the convulsions requires daily ingestion of large amounts of the vitamin and must be started in the neonatal period in order to prevent the development of irreversible mental retardation. Another form in children with crypto-genic epilepsy which occurs at several years of age requires large doses of pyridoxine in order to correct the tryptophan load test and improve the EEC and seizure manifestations.

SOURCE   The best sources of pyridoxine are yeast, wheat germ, pork, glandular meats (especially liver), whole grain cereals, legumes, potatoes, bananas, and oatmeal. Milk, eggs, vegetables and fruit contain small amounts. It is in most common foodstuffs and probably some can be synthesized by the intestinal flora.

TOXICITY   Side effects, such as sleepiness, may follow injection of large doses (100 mg.).

RECOMMENDED DIETARY ALLOWANCE
Results from a study by Baker et al.[35] with

---

[34]Snyderman, S. E., Carreterro, R., and Holt, L. E., Jr.: Pyridoxine deficiency in the human being. Fed. Proc., 9:371, 1950.

[35]Baker, E. M., et al.: Vitamin B₆ requirement for adult men. Am. J. Clin. Nutr., 15:59, 1964.

young adult male subjects indicate that the requirement is directly related to the protein intake. They conclude that the optimal daily vitamin B_6 requirement (as pyridoxine hydrochloride) for subjects on a high protein intake (100 gm.) appears to be 1.75 to 2.0 mg. per day; on a low protein intake (30 gm.) the requirement appears to be 1.25 to 1.5 mg. per day. In the 1968 revision, the Food and Nutrition Board provides for a margin of safety in recommending for adults a level of 2.0 mg. per day when daily intakes of protein are 100 gm. or more. (See Table 11–1.) The need increases in pregnancy and lactation and possibly with aging and in special situations such as radiation exposure, cardiac failure and in isoniazid therapy.

Pantothenic Acid

HISTORY   The synthesis of pantothenic acid was completed in 1940. It is a part of coenzyme A, which mediates acetylation and many other acylation reactions.

SOURCE   Pantothenic acid is present in all plant and animal tissue, hence its name meaning "widespread." Egg, kidney, liver, salmon, and yeast are the best sources. Cauliflower, broccoli, beef (lean), potatoes (white and sweet), tomatoes, and molasses are good sources. It is also synthesized by the intestinal flora. Approximately 33 per cent is lost in cooking meat and about 50 per cent is lost in the milling of flour.

CHEMICAL CHARACTERISTICS AND STABILITY   Pantothenic acid is a white, crystalline compound (calcium pantothenate), bitter to the taste, more stable in solution than in dry form and easily decomposed by acid, alkali and dry heat. It is water-soluble and stable in moist heat in neutral solution.

FUNCTION   Pantothenic acid is known to be essential in the intermediary metabolism carbohydrate, fat and protein. As part of Coenzyme A it has many metabolic roles in the cells. Because pantothenic acid is incorporated into CoA on which acetylation and other acylation reactions depend, it is involved in the release of energy from carbohydrate and in the degradation and metabolism of fatty acids. Besides functioning in the transfer of acetate groups to the Krebs cycle, CoA is involved as an acceptor acetate groups for amino acids, vitamins and sulfonamides. It is involved in the synthesis of cholesterol, steroid hormones, porphyrin for hemoglobin and phospholipids. It is known to be essential in the metabolism of man, chicks, dogs and rats, and prevents graying of the hair in certain animals.

It is so widely distributed in foods that a deficiency disease due to lack of the vitamin has not been observed in man on an adequate diet. Deficiency induced by administering an antagonist to volunteer subjects produced numerous physical and biochemical disturbances. Some of the subjects experienced pain and sensations in the arms and legs; others noted loss of appetite, nausea, and indigestion. Most became quarrelsome, sullen and depressed. Fainting attacks were common; the pulse tended to be rapid. An increase in susceptibility to infection seemed to follow. Pantothenic acid deficiency in both animals and man results in loss of antibody production. Pantothenic Acid has been reported to improve the stress reactions of well-nourished subjects and to relieve the burning feet syndrome.

TOXICITY   No toxic effects of this substance are known.

RECOMMENDED DIETARY ALLOWANCE According to the Food and Nutrition Board's, 1968 revision, the daily intake of 5 to 10 mg. is probably adequate for children and adults and there is no evidence for or against a greater requirement during pregnancy and lactation. Usual intake of pantothenic acid in the American dietary is about 10 to 15 mg. with a range of 6 to 20 mg. A deficiency is not likely.

Biotin

HISTORY   Biotin was first isolated in 1936 and synthesized in 1943. Previously the factor causing the syndrome manifested by eczema and characteristic alopecia around the eyes observed in rats and chicks fed large amounts of raw egg whites had been named vitamin H. A potent growth factor for yeast was called coenzyme R. These factors proved to be the same and the corrective factor found in egg yolk was called biotin.

CHEMISTRY AND STABILITY   Biotin is a monocarboxylic acid, stable to heat, soluble in water and alcohol, and susceptible to oxidation, to alkali and to strong acids.

SOURCE   Biotin is found in a great many foods, and a considerable amount is synthesized by intestinal bacteria. It is known to occur in liver, milk, meat, egg yolk, most vegetables, mushrooms, a number of fruits (bananas, grapefruit, watermelon, strawberries), peanuts, and yeast in moderate abundance.

FUNCTION   Biotin is essential for the activity of many enzyme systems. It functions as the coenzyme for the process of carbon dioxide fixation (enzymatic reactions involving the addition or removal of carbon dioxide to or from active compounds). The synthesis and oxidation of fatty acids and the oxidation of carbohydrate require biotin as a coenzyme. Biotin has a role in deamination as a coenzyme in the removal of NH_2 from certain amino acids (notably aspartic acid, threonine and serine). It is closely related metabolically to folic acid, pantothenic acid and vitamin B_{12}.

In animals its deficiency is associated with the characteristic dermatitis and can be produced only by adding egg white to a biotin-deficient diet. Thus, it has been known in animal research as the "egg-white-injury" factor. Avidin, a carbohydrate-containing protein material in raw egg white, combines with biotin in the intestine, making it unavailable to the body. Biotin deficiency symptoms have also been induced in human beings by feeding raw egg whites, and the symptoms have been alleviated by giving a biotin concentrate. The experimental diet for man of 200 mg. dried egg white daily[36] induced the deficiency. This amount or its equivalent in raw egg white ingested daily in the American diet is unusual. The occasional raw egg whites would not precipitate a deficiency state. Avidin in raw egg whites is denatured upon cooking.

Biotin is frequently added to multiple vitamin preparations even though its need has not been definitely established.

TOXICITY   There are no known toxic effects from this substance.

RECOMMENDED DIETARY ALLOWANCE In 1968, the Food and Nutrition Board, National Research Council, stated that 150 to 300 mcg. of biotin per day will provide daily needs although the minimum requirement has not been established. This amount is available in the average American diet, plus that furnished by bacterial synthesis in the intestinal tract. An additional amount is needed during pregnancy and lactation. Cow's milk contains approximately 150 mcg. per liter and human milk contains from 1 to 8 mcg. with an average of 4 mcg. biotin per liter.

Folacin (Folic Acid or Pteroylglutamic Acid)

Folacin has been known under several names in the study of unidentified growth factors in bacteria and experimental animals and in the study and treatment of anemias. It was synthesized in 1946 and established as a dietary essential for man, many animals and microorganisms.

CHEMICAL AND PHYSICAL PROPERTIES Folacin is a water-soluble, yellow, crystalline compound which belongs to a group of compounds known as "pterins," (Greek, "wing"; they were found in pigment of butterfly wings) and is also known chemically as pteroylglutamic acid, folic acid and *Lactobacillus casei* factor. Pteroylglutamic acid (PGA) is formed by the linkage of three compounds: pterin and para-aminobenzoic acid (PABA) conjugated with two or six molecules of glutamic acid. Some of the glutamic acid molecules are split off to form an unconjugated folacin molecule with the aid of specific enzymes and vitamin B_{12}. Folic acid in the presence of ascorbic acid and NAD (niacin-containing coenzyme) is reduced to tetrahydrofolic acid (THFA). Folic acid is an indispensable component of tissues, without which there is serious interference with cellular metabolism as shown by the use of folic acid antagonists or blocking agents that cause acute folic acid deficiency (for example, aminopterin). This antagonist, chemically related to folic acid, blocks the action of folacin by interrupting its conversion to tetrahydrobolic acid. Folacin is readily absorbed by the gastrointestinal tract by active transport and diffusion and is stored primarily in the liver. Folate compounds are synthesized by intestinal microorganisms. The utilization of folacin by the body is not fully understood.

SOURCE   It occurs widely in foods, and an adequate supply is easily obtained. The best sources are liver, kidney beans, lima beans, fresh dark green leafy vegetables, especially spinach, asparagus and broccoli. Good sources are lean beef, potatoes, whole wheat bread and dried beans. Poor sources include most meats, milk, eggs, most fruits and root vegetables. Folacin is a potent substance, with 1 mg. causing certain physiological responses which will be discussed subsequently.

STABILITY   Folacin is unstable to heat in acid media, and stable to sunlight when in solution. There is considerable loss of folic acid in vegetables during storage at room temperature. Loss occurs in processing food at high temperatures. In dried milk, for example, folic acid activity is destroyed.

FUNCTION   Five coenzyme forms of folacin are known and their major role is the transfer of one-carbon units to appropriate metabolites in the synthesis of DNA, RNA, methionine and serine.[37] The enzymes which utilize folacin coenzymes are known as pteroproteins.

Tetrahydrofolic acid is carrier for the single carbon groups (formyl, hydroxymethyl, or

[36]Sydenstricker, V. P., et al.: "Egg-White Inquiry" in man and its cure with a biotin concentrate. J.A.M.A., *118*:1199, 1942.

[37]Vitale, J. J.: Present knowledge of folacin. In: Present Knowledge of Nutrition. 3rd ed. New York, The Nutrition Foundation, Inc., 1967, p. 105.

methyl groups) from one substance to another. It plays an important role in the synthesis of the purines guanine and adenine and of the pyrimidine thymine, compounds which are utilized for the formation of nucleoproteins DNA (deoxyribonucleic acid) and RNA (ribonucleic acid) which are essential to cell division and the transmission of inherited traits.

Tetrahydrofolic acid participates in the interconversion of serine and glycine, the oxidation of glycine, methylation of homocysteine, to methionine with B_{12} as co-factor, and the methylation of the precursor ethanolamine to the vitamin choline. The conversion of nicotinamide to N-methyl nicotinamide by addition of a single carbon (methyl group) and the oxidation of phenylalanine to tyrosine require folacin.

Folacin is required for one step in the conversion of histidine to glutamic acid. An impaired metabolism of histidine results in piling up of the intermediary product, formiminoglutamic acid, (F I G L U) which is excreted in the urine.

Folacin is essential for the formation of both red and white blood cells in the bone marrow and for their maturation. It serves as a single carbon carrier in the formation of heme.

Deficiency of folacin results in poor growth, megaloblastic anemia, and other blood disorders, glossitis, and gastrointestinal tract disturbances arising from inadequate dietary intake, impaired absorption, excessive demands by tissues of the body and metabolic derangements.[38] In pernicious anemia, folic acid will produce marked alleviation of the anemia, but the gastrointestinal symptoms and neurologic lesions progress. On the other hand, liver extract and vitamin B_{12} control all the aspects of pernicious anemia, namely, blood cell regeneration and the neurological condition. It does control the macrocytic anemias of pregnancy and sprue and the megaloblastic anemia of infancy. Many patients with malabsorption syndrome have impaired absorption of folacin. Protein malnutrition may impair the utilization and function of folacin and conditions in which the demands for folacin are unusually great such as in hemolytic anemia, leukemia, Hodgkin's disease, certain drugs and carcinomatosis cause a deficiency.[39] (See Ch. 31 for discussion of folacin and anemia.)

RECOMMENDED DIETARY ALLOWANCE
A well-balanced American diet according to the 1968 recommendation of the Food and Nutrition Board contains up to 0.6 mg. by

L. *casei* assay of total folacin activity. Intestinal bacteria which synthesize folacin provide some folacin. The daily recommendations are: 0.4 mg. for adults; 0.8 mg. in pregnancy and 0.5 mg. in lactation. Other stressful situations including disease states and the consumption of alcohol increase the requirement for folacin.[40]

Vitamin preparations without prescription containing more than 0.1 mg. of folacin in a daily dose is prohibited by law. More than 0.1 mg. per day may prevent anemia but not cure the neurological conditions of patients with pernicious anemia.

Para-aminobenzoic Acid (PABA)

This is a derivative of benzoic acid and has been a recognized chemical compound for many years and is known as a growth factor for bacteria but is not considered a vitamin. It is a yellow, crystalline, slightly water-soluble substance. PABA has been isolated from vitamin B-complex sources such as liver, yeast, wheat germ and molasses. It occurs in conjugated form as a part of folic acid.

It has no known metabolic function in man but seems to be of value in the treatment of rickettsial diseases (in man) by inhibiting the growth of the causative organisms. It is used in the therapy of Rocky Mountain Spotted Fever. In animals its deficiency has been associated with growth and premature graying of the hair.

Vitamin B_{12} (Cobalamin)

In 1948 this compound was isolated from liver extract and shown to have high antipernicious anemia potency. It contains the heavy metal cobalt, chelated in a large tetrapyrrole ring very similar to the porphyrin ring of heme. The form of the vitamin originally isolated contained cyanide, which we ordinarily consider to be very toxic. Cobalamin is the generic name of vitamin B_{12} because of the presence of cobalt. Several of the different cobalamin compounds exhibit vitamin B_{12} activity. Of these compounds cyanocobalamin and hydroxycobalamin are the most active forms. The functional forms of the vitamin are called cobamide coenzymes.

Vitamin B_{12} is the extrinsic factor of food so necessary for treatment and prevention of pernicious anemia. It is considered to be identical with the antipernicious anemia factor and the erythrocyte maturation factor of Castle, as well as with the so-called animal protein factor.

---

[38] Food and Nutrition Board, *op. cit.*, p. 36.
[39] *Ibid.*

[40] *Ibid.*

ABSORPTION   It is poorly absorbed from the intestinal tract unless the intrinsic factor (a mucoprotein enzyme called Castle's intrinsic factor) in the gastric secretion is present. The presence of hydrochloric acid is necessary to split vitamin B_{12} from its peptide bonds. The intrinsic factor combines with vitamin B_{12} in the food and in the bound form becomes adsorbed to a receptor in the membranes of the ileum through which it is transported into the cells in pinocytic vesicles. Calcium is necessary for the transfer.

After absorption, it is transported in the blood stream again bound to serum protein (globulins) and circulates to the various tissues. The tissues of normal persons contain vitamin B_{12} in varying amounts, with the highest concentration found in the liver and to some extent in the kidney. It is released as needed to the bone marrow and other tissues of the body. The body store of the vitamin (approximately 2000 μg.) is substantial. It may take five or six years for deficiency symptoms to appear after the body's supply from the natural sources has been restricted. An excess intake of the vitamin is excreted in the urine.

Absorption of B_{12} appears to decrease with aging and with iron and B_6 deficiency and increases during pregnancy. Infant levels are approximately twice that of the mother.[41]

FUNCTION   Cobalamin has various physiological roles at the cellular level. It is essential for normal function in the metabolism of all cells, especially for those of the gastrointestinal tract, bone marrow, and nervous tissue, and for growth. It participates with folic acid, choline and methionine in the transfer of methyl groups in the synthesis of nucleic acids, purines and pyrimidine intermediates. Cobalamin coenzymes are necessary for reducing ribonucleotides to deoxyribonucleotides which function in the promotion of growth and the red blood cell maturation. Vitamin B_{12} affects myelin formation. It is involved in protein, fat and carbohydrate metabolism and associated with folic acid absorption and metabolism.

Failure to absorb vitamin B_{12} because of the absence of intrinsic factor in the gastric secretion results in a deficiency state of the vitamin. Surgical resection of the intrinsic-factor-secreting portions of the stomach (fundus and cardia) or the absorbing surfaces of the ileum may result in a deficiency of vitamin B_{12}. The anemia may not become apparent for several years after the gastrectomy because of storage of the vitamin. Small bowel diverticula, intestinal infestations, sprue and other malabsorption syndromes may induce a vitamin B_{12} deficiency state. These conditions are complicated by deficiencies of folic acid as well as other essential nutrients.[42] Vitamin B_{12} deficiency causes demyelination of the large nerve fibers of the spinal cord.

Vegetarians (persons living exclusively on vegetables) have a low dietary intake of vitamin B_{12}. They usually have low serum levels of this vitamin.[43]

CHEMICAL CHARACTERISTICS AND STABILITY   Vitamin B_{12} is slowly destroyed by dilute acid, alkali, light and oxidizing or reducing agents. It is water-soluble and forms red crystals. Red color is due to the presence of cobalt in the molecule. Its potency has been found to be amazingly high. One microgram of crystalline B_{12} equals 1 U.S.P. unit of purified liver extract. Approximately 70 per cent of the vitamin activity is retained during cooking.

SOURCE   Vitamin B_{12} is present in animal protein foods. Liver and kidney are richest sources; fresh milk, eggs, fish, cheese and muscle meats are good sources. Pasteurized and evaporated milk have lost 40 to 90 per cent of the vitamin.

TOXICITY   No toxic effects are known.

RECOMMENDED DIETARY ALLOWANCE Human requirements for this factor are minute but essential. One to 2 μg., injected parenterally, have relieved pernicious anemia, and large doses have relieved or prevented progression of the neurologic complications of pernicious anemia. It seems to act by allowing maturation of the red blood cells. B_{12} also relieves nutritional anemia (sprue, pregnancy) in many cases. Oral administration is ineffective unless administered in huge doses. Excesses are not absorbed. Limited bacterial synthesis in man occurs in the colon but too far into colon to be absorbed. Therefore, humans apparently do not derive sufficient vitamin B_{12} from endogenous bacterial synthesis and must rely on a supply of the preformed vitamin in the food intake. The usual American diet, adequate in proteins, provides minimum requirements. The 1968 revision of the Recommended Dietary Allowances suggests 5 μg. daily for adults, 6 μg. daily after 55 years of age, and during pregnancy and lactation, 8 and 6 μg., respectively. A diet containing 15 μg. daily will gradually replenish depleted stores.

ASCORBIC ACID (VITAMIN C)

HISTORY   Vitamin C is the antiscorbutic vitamin, the preventive of and cure for scurvy.

[41]Food and Nutrition Board, *op. cit.*, p. 48.

[42]Weser, E.: Intestinal adaptation to small bowel resection. Am. J. Clin. Nutr., 24:133, 1971.

[43]Hines, J. D.: Megaloblastic anemia in adult vegan. Am. J. Clin. Nutr., 19:260, 1966.

Many dramatic stories are in the scientific literature relating the use of citrus fruits for the cure of scurvy, the dreaded disease of explorers and voyagers. This disease was first described during the Crusades, and remained common among soldiers and sailors until the preventive value of lemon juice was discovered. The history of the relation between vitamin C and scurvy is further discussed in Chapter 34.

Although vitamin C was isolated in 1928 by Szent-Györgyi, who found it in adrenal tissue and in orange and cabbage and identified it as hexuronic acid, it was not until 1932 that C. Glenn King at the University of Pittsburgh re-isolated the compound from lemons and identified it as vitamin C, having the properties of preventing and curing scurvy in guinea pigs. Shortly thereafter its correct structural formula was established and synthesis was accomplished. It is known as L-ascorbic acid in the reduced form and as L-dehydroascorbic acid in the oxidized form. Ascorbic acid is the accepted name of the vitamin.

SOURCE   Ascorbic acid is widely found in citrus fruits, raw leafy vegetables, and tomatoes. Canned or frozen citrus fruit, and tomatoes are good and inexpensive sources of ascorbic acid where fresh fruits are not abundant or not obtainable. Strawberries, cantaloupe, cabbage and green peppers are good sources. Potatoes are considered a good source when properly prepared because of the quantity eaten. An average serving of citrus fruit juices ($\frac{1}{2}$ cup) contains 45 to 60 mg. of ascorbic acid, cantaloupe ($\frac{1}{4}$) 30 mg., strawberries (1 cup) 88 mg., sweet green pepper (1 raw) 94 mg. tomato (1 raw) 42 mg. and boiled potato (1 med.) 20 mg. The acerola tree, or Puerto Rican cherry, has an unusually high vitamin C concentration. Values obtained have averaged to 2000 mg. of ascorbic acid per 100 gm. of juice or fruit. A six-ounce glass of the juice contains as much as 8650 mg. of vitamin C — more than 85 times as much as an equal glass of orange juice. Other less common foods rich in ascorbic acid are black currants, and edible hips of the wild rose. Tropical foods high in the vitamin include the sapodilla, ceriman cherry, papaya, soursop, star apple, and guava. Turnip greens, broccoli, cabbage, spinach, Brussels sprouts, berries, and pineapples are good sources. Apples, peaches, pears and bananas are good sources when eaten in large amounts. Milk, eggs, meat and poultry contain little or no ascorbic acid.

CHEMICAL CHARACTERISTICS AND STABILITY   Chemically, ascorbic acid is a white, water-soluble crystalline material that is stable in dry form. In solution it is easily oxidized, especially on exposure to heat. Oxidation can be accelerated by the presence of copper and by alkaline pH. Consequently, much ascorbic acid is lost in cooking or thrown out in the cooking water. Bruising, cutting, and allowing fruit and vegetables to be kept exposed to the air cause much loss of ascorbic acid. Less destruction and more retention of the vitamin occurs when the food is cooked quickly in small amounts of boiling water, and covered tightly. Quick freezing of foods preserves the vitamins. Refrigeration aids retention. Use of sodium bicarbonate in cooking vegetables to preserve and improve the color is very destructive of the vitamin. The ascorbic acid content of fruits and vegetables varies with the conditions under which they are grown, degree of ripeness when harvested, and conditions under which they are stored, and cooked.

Ascorbic acid is a hexose derivative and classified as a carbohydrate closely related to the monosaccharides. The reduced ($C_6H_8O_6$) form is the most active form and is readily oxidized to form dehydroascorbic acid ($C_6H_6O_6$). It may be reduced back to the original form (reversible oxidation-reduction). Both forms are antiscorbutic. Further oxidation of dehydroascorbic acid produces diketogulonic acid with no antiascorbic acid properties and cannot be reduced to form dehydroascorbic acid again. In plants several simple sugars are converted to ascorbic acid but in animals glucose and to some extent galactose are the precursors for the vitamin.

ABSORPTION AND STORAGE   Ascorbic acid is easily absorbed from the small intestine probably by diffusion and carried to the tissues by the blood. It readily passes into tissues of the adrenals, kidney, liver and spleen, most of which appear to be in equilibrium with serum level. It is stored in these tissues to some extent (1 to 5 gm.) through tissue saturation but should be supplied daily. Excess amounts ingested over the saturation level of various tissues are excreted in the urine as oxalic, threonic and dehydroascorbic acids and some is oxidized and exhaled as carbon dioxide. A very small amount is lost in the feces.

FUNCTION   Ascorbic acid has multiple functions in the body, either as a coenzyme or co-factor. Its function at the cellular level has not been resolved. It appears to be present and essential to the normal functioning of all cellular units including subcellular structures such as ribosomes and mitochondria. The ability of ascorbic acid to lose and take on hydrogen gives it an essential role in metabolism.

Ascorbic acid is required for production and

maintenance of collagen, a protein substance found in all fibrous tissue (connective tissue, cartilage, bone matrix, tooth dentin, skin and tendon). The integrity of cellular structure depends on it. Ascorbic acid is involved in the hydroxylation of proline to form hydroxyproline in the synthesis of collagen. Ascorbic acid maintains this intercellular cement substance with preservation of capillary integrity; promotes healing of wounds, fractures, bruises, pinpoint hemorrhages and bleeding gums; and reduces liability to infections. A high level of ascorbic acid is present during healing and in scar tissue.

It is essential for the oxidation of phenylalanine and tyrosine; for the conversion of folacin to folinic acid (the citrovorum factor); for the reduction of ferric iron to ferrous iron in the intestinal tract to facilitate absorption; and for the transfer of iron from plasma transferrin to liver for the conversion of tryptophan to 5-hydroxytryptophan. Hydroxylation reactions appear specific for ascorbic acid. It also participates in the hydroxylation of certain steroids synthesized in adrenal tissue. Under stress, when adrenal cortical hormone activity is high, ascorbic acid concentration in the tissue is decreased. Injection of ACTH causes considerable loss of ascorbic acid from the adrenal cortex.

Fevers and infections require additional amounts of ascorbic acid to maintain tissue levels. Adequate tissue concentration of ascorbic acid helps the body to maintain resistance to infection. The value of large amounts of ascorbic acid to prevent and cure the common cold has been reported.

In the experimental animal large amounts of ascorbic acid change the intestinal flora, resulting in the synthesis of available quantities of the B-complex vitamins.[44]

The earliest signs of ascorbic deficiency may begin during the first month of deprivation, depending on the rate of catabolism. Deficiency appears after the serum level has fallen below 0.2 mg. per 100 ml. Severe deficiency of ascorbic acid causes scurvy. It is characterized by decreased urinary excretion, plasma concentration, tissue and leukocyte concentration. Other symptoms include weakness, poor appetite and growth, anemia, tenderness to touch, swollen and inflamed gums, loosened teeth, swollen wrist and ankle joints, shortness of breath, petechial hemorrhages from the venules, beading or fracture of ribs at costochondral junctions, fracture of

---

[44]King, C. G.: Present knowledge of ascorbic acid. In: Present Knowledge in Nutrition. 3rd ed. New York, The Nutrition Foundation, Inc., 1967.

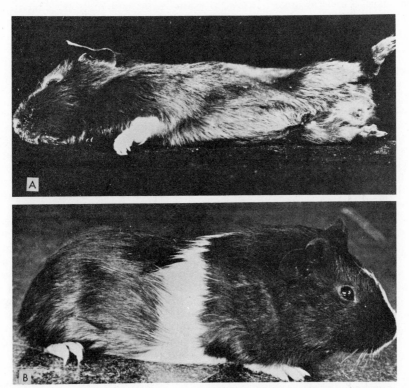

Figure 9–6   *A,* The guinea pig is very susceptible to deficiency of vitamin C and rapidly develops scurvy, one evidence of which is seen in the enlarged joints. If completely deprived of vitamin C, the animals generally die in about 3 weeks. Untreated scurvy is also fatal in man. *B,* Guinea pig cured of scurvy by treatment with crystalline vitamin C (ascorbic acid). (Courtesy of E. R. Squibb and Sons.)

epiphysis, multiple subcutaneous and sub-periosteal hemorrhages with pain on motion of the body.[45] Secondary infections develop easily in the bleeding areas. All these characteristics can be attributed primarily to collagen defects.

Neurotic disturbances consisting of hypochondriasis, hysteria and depression followed by decreased psychomotor performance have been reported in ascorbic acid deficiency.[46] The symptoms of scurvy clear rapidly with therapeutic doses of ascorbic acid. (See Fig. 9–6 A and B.) Although scurvy is rare today, dietary surveys indicate that many Americans receive insufficient amounts of this vitamin for optimum health.

Apparently cigarette smoking adversely affects the body's ability to utilize ascorbic acid. Less ascorbic acid is available in smokers for utilization and storage, indicating the lower amount absorbed. Smokers appear to oxidize more ascorbic acid to dehydroascorbic acid which isomerizes to diketogulonic acid in the gastrointestinal tract due to the secretion of an oxidative enzyme, ceruloplasmin, involved in the oxidation of serotonin. Serotonin is known to be released by nicotine. The average smoker probably needs twice as much ascorbic acid as the non-smoker to have a comparable blood level.[47]

Excess ascorbic acid excreted in the urine gives a false positive test for sugar. It could cause formation of urate, cystine or oxalate stones.[48]

RECOMMENDED DIETARY ALLOWANCE According to the Food and Nutrition Board National Research Council the minimal daily intake of ascorbic acid needed to prevent scurvy is approximately 10 mg. The revised recommended allowances (1968) are 55 mg. daily for a 58 kg. female and 60 mg. daily for a 70 kg. male. Infants need 35 mg. daily the first year. Infants during the first few weeks who receive formulas with two or three times the protein content of milk may need up to 50 mg. daily. A daily allowance of 60 mg. is recommended in pregnancy and lactation. (See Table 11–1, Chapter 11.)

OTHER VITAMIN-LIKE FACTORS

This chapter might be summarized by stating that, to date, the metabolic function in man of the following vitamins has been

clearly demonstrated: vitamins A, D, E, K, ascorbic acid, thiamin, riboflavin, niacin, folic acid, B_{12}, B_6, pantothenic acid and biotin.

Exact minimal quantitative requirements for vitamins are difficult to state. The standards set by the Food and Nutrition Board of the National Research Council are aimed toward generous and safe margins of intake in the light of present knowledge and continued revisions of these figures in the future are to be expected.

There are many other food factors, some of which have no known specific functions, and others which have functions known for certain animal species. A brief presentation of a few with vitamin-like properties follows.

CHOLINE

Choline has been known for over a century as an essential component of animal tissues but only in recent years has it been classified as having vitamin-like activity in experimental animals. Choline is widely distributed in animal and plant tissues, and in an average diet no inadequacy of it will occur. The body can synthesize choline from the amino acid, serine, providing methionine is present to supply methyl groups and with vitamin B_{12} and folacin to act as coenzymes. However, the rate at which it is synthesized is insufficient to meet the need of most higher animals. For this reason choline is considered an essential nutrient. Chemically, it is a colorless, bitter-tasting basic compound, water-soluble, fairly stable to heat and storage but unstable in strong alkali. Choline is a source in the body for labile methyl groups. These are used for various synthetic processes and for detoxification of many toxic compounds. Choline is an integral part of phospholipids, lecithin and sphingomyelin. Lecithin is important in the metabolism of fat in the liver and sphingomyelin is found in brain and nerve tissue. Choline serves also as a precursor of acetylcholine.

FUNCTION Its function in man is in the metabolism of and in the transport of fat from the liver, preventing the development of fatty liver. As a component of several phospholipids, it functions in triglyceride transport. Choline forms lecithin in the liver. In the action fatty acids are removed from the glycerides of the liver, resulting in the decrease of triglyceride content of the liver. As a constituent of acetylcholine, it plays a role in the transmission of nerve impulses. As a dietary source of labile methyl groups it is essential for synthesis of methionine. Betaine, methionine and choline function as donors of methyl groups. Each serves to partially make up for a shortage of one of the others. This

[45] *Ibid.*

[46] Kinsman, R. A., and Hood, J.: Some behavioral effects of ascorbic acid deficiency. Am. J. Clin. Nutr., 24:455, 1971.

[47] Pelletier, O.: Cigarette smoking and vitamin C. Nutrition Today, 5:12, Autumn, 1970.

[48] Lamden, M.: Dangers of massive vitamin C intake. New Eng. J. Med., 284:336, 1971.

process is known as a transmethylation. The action of these substances serves to prevent the development of fatty liver.

Deficiency is associated with fatty deposition in the liver and choline is currently being used in the treatment of fatty liver, in which case it has been shown to increase phospholipid and fat turnover in the fatty liver. Fatty infiltration of the liver is observed in chronic alcoholics and in kwashiorkor.

Choline deficiency in animals leads to many abnormal findings, including hemorrhagic lesions in the kidney and fatty liver.

SOURCE   The richest known dietary source is egg yolk. Other food sources are liver, brain, kidney, heart, lean meat, yeast, soy beans, peanuts, beans, peas and wheat germ. Fruit, fruit juices, milk and vegetables generally are not sources of choline. Neutral fats are essentially devoid of choline.

RECOMMENDED DIETARY ALLOWANCE Daily requirements are not known and no toxic effects have been observed. The average diet has been estimated to contain 500 to 900 mg. per day of choline, including its natural precursor betaine, according to the 1968 revision of the Recommended Dietary Allowances.

INOSITOL

Inositol has long been known as a chemical compound, but only since 1940 has it been considered a vitamin. It is found in fruits, grains, vegetables, nuts, legumes, and organ meats (liver, heart). It occurs abundantly in the average diet. Chemically, inositol is a colorless, water-soluble crystalline material. It is a cyclic 6-carbon compound with 6-hydroxyl groups and so is related to glucose. Myoinositol, known as "muscle sugar," occurs in animal tissues as a component of phospholipids. In plants it is found as phytic acid (hexaphosphate ester of inositol). Phytic acid interferes with the absorption of calcium and iron. It binds both to form an insoluble complex. Inositol is concentrated in the brain and occurs in skeletal and heart muscles and other tissues.

Inositol's physiological role is related to its presence in phosphoinositols and thus to the function of phospholipids. It is considered to have lipotrophic activity. The requirement for man is unknown. Synthesis of inositol occurs within the cell. Small amounts are excreted in the urine normally. Diabetic patients excrete much more.

LIPOIC ACID

Lipoic acid, a fat-soluble, sulfur-containing fatty acid, is not a true vitamin, since it can be synthesized in the body. It functions as a coenzyme and is essential together with the thiamin-containing enzyme, pyrophosphatase (TPP), for reactions in carbohydrate metabolism which convert pyruvic acid to acetyl-coenzyme A. Lipoic acid with two sulfur bonds combines with the TPP to reduce pyruvate to active acetate. It joins the intermediary products of protein and fat metabolism in the Krebs cycle in the reactions involved in producing energy from these nutrients. A metal ion (magnesium or calcium) is involved in this oxidative decarboxylation along with vitamins, thiamin, pantothenic acid, niacin, riboflavin and lipoic acid.

No dietary requirements for lipoic acid for humans is known. The amounts needed to participate in the reactions in the tissues may be synthesized in the body. It is found in liver and yeast.

UBIQUINONE (COENZYME Q)

A lipid-like substance similar to vitamin K, ubiquinone belongs to a group of compounds known as ubiquinones. Ubiquinones are a group of coenzymes. Attached to the basic quinone ring structure are 30 or more carbon atoms in a side chain. Coenzyme Q is present in all cell nuclei and microsomes. It is concentrated in the mitochondria and functions in the respiratory chain in which energy is released from the energy-yielding nutrients as ATP. The ubiquinones appear to be synthesized in the body and cannot be classified as vitamins.

ANTIVITAMINS
(Vitamin Antagonists or Antimetabolites)

There are a growing number of instances of antivitamin activity of special interest in nutrition. An antivitamin or antagonist may be defined as a substance or condition that interferes with the synthesis or metabolism of vitamins. Many vitamin antagonists are compounds similar in structure to the active vitamin molecule. They can prevent incorporation of the vitamin units in the coenzyme structure by attaching themselves to the enzyme. They block the action of the coenzyme, which results in a true vitamin deficiency. Experimental vitamin deficiencies have been produced by using vitamin antagonists. An established example of another type of antivitamin is avidin, found in raw egg white, which combines with biotin and forms a compound which cannot be absorbed from the intestinal tract. A biotin deficiency can be produced in experimental animals and humans who are fed extremely large quanti-

TABLE 9–2   SUMMARY OF INFORMATION ON VITAMINS

FAT-SOLUBLE VITAMINS

Name	Daily Recommended Allowances for Adults	Rich Food Sources	Pharmaceutical Sources	Stability	Biological Role
Vitamin A (retinol; provitamin A; α, β, γ carotene)	5000 I.U.	Liver, kidney, milk fat, fortified margarine, egg yolk, yellow and dark green leafy vegetables, apricots, cantaloupe, peaches.	Fish liver oils.	Stable to light, heat and usual cooking methods. Destroyed by oxidation, drying, very high temperature, ultraviolet light.	Essential for normal growth, development and maintenance of epithelial tissue. Essential to the integrity of night vision. Essential for health of the eyes. Helps provide for normal bone development and influences normal tooth formation. Toxic in large quantities.
Vitamin D (calciferol)	Sunlight and normal diet are adequate. (400 I.U. in children, pregnancy and lactation.)	Vitamin D milk, irradiated foods, some in milk fat, liver, egg yolk, salmon, tuna fish, sardines.	Fish liver oils, concentrates.	Stable to heat and oxidation.	Essential for normal growth and development; important for formation of normal bones and teeth. Influences absorption and metabolism of phosphorus and calcium. Prevents and cures rickets and osteomalacia.
Vitamin E (tocopherols)	25 to 30 mg.	Wheat germ, vegetable oils, green leafy vegetables, milk fat, egg yolk, nuts. (Synthesized in intestinal tract.)	Wheat germ oil, synthetic.	Stable to heat and acids. Destroyed by rancid fats, alkali, oxygen, lead, and iron salts, and ultraviolet irradiation.	Is a strong antioxidant. As such may help prevent oxidation of unsaturated fatty acids and vitamin A in intestinal tract and body tissues. Protects red blood cells from hemolysis. Reproduction (in animals).
Vitamin K (menadione)	Not established. Oral dose of 1–2 mg. considered adequate for prophylaxis. Normal diet adequate for healthy persons.	Liver, soybean oil, other vegetable oils, green leafy vegetables, tomatoes, cauliflower, wheat bran. (Synthesized in intestinal tract.)	Synthetic.	Resistant to heat, oxygen, and moisture. Destroyed by alkali and ultraviolet light.	Aids in production of prothrombin, a compound required for normal clotting of blood. Toxic in large amounts.

WATER-SOLUBLE VITAMINS

Name	Daily Recommended Allowances for Adults	Rich Food Sources	Pharmaceutical Sources	Stability	Biological Role
Thiamin (vitamin B_1)	0.4 mg. per 1000 kcalories; older person 1.0 mg. per day.	Pork, liver, organs, meats, legumes, whole grain and enriched cereals and breads, wheat germ, potatoes. (Synthesized in intestinal tract.)	Yeast, wheat germ, synthetic.	Unstable in presence of heat or alkali or oxygen. Heat stable in acid solution.	Prevents beriberi. As part of cocarboxylase, aids in removal of CO_2 from alpha-keto acids during oxidation of carbohydrates. Essential for growth, normal appetite, digestion and healthy nerves.
Riboflavin (vitamin B_2)	0.6 mg. per 1000 kcalories.	Milk and dairy foods, organ meats, green leafy veg., enriched cereals and breads, eggs.	Yeast, liver concentrates, synthetic.	Stable to heat, oxygen, and acid. Unstable to light (especially ultraviolet) or alkali.	Essential for growth. Essential for health of the eyes. Plays enzymatic role in tissue reproduction, and acts as a transporter of hydrogen ions. Coenzyme forms FMN and FAD. Prevents fissures at corners of mouth, around nose and ears, eye irritation, photophobia.
Niacin (nicotinic acid)	13–18 mg. niacin equivalent or 6.6 mg. per 1000 kcalories.	Fish, liver, meat, poultry, many grains, eggs, peanuts, milk, legumes, enriched grains.	Yeast, liver concentrates, synthetic.	Stable to heat, light, oxidation, acid and alkali.	As part of enzyme system, aids in transfer of hydrogen, acts in metabolism of carbohydrates and amino acids. Prevents pellagra, nervous depression, neuritis.

Table continued on opposite page.

TABLE 9–2 SUMMARY OF INFORMATION ON VITAMINS *(continued)*

WATER-SOLUBLE VITAMINS

Name	Daily Recommended Allowances for Adults	Rich Food Sources	Pharmaceutical Sources	Stability	Biological Role
Vitamin B$_6$ (pyridoxine, pyridoxal and pyridoxamine)	2.0 mg.	Pork, glandular meats, cereal bran and germ, milk, egg yolk and oatmeal, legumes.	Yeast, wheat germ, liver concentrates.	Stable to heat, light and oxidation.	As a coenzyme, aids in the synthesis and breakdown of amino acids and in the synthesis of unsaturated fatty acids from essential fatty acids. Essential for conversion of tryptophan to niacin. Prevents hypochromic anemia, seborrheic dermatitis, mucous membrane lesions and peripheral neuritis. Essential for normal growth.
Pantothenic acid	Level not yet determined but believe 10 mg. adequate. Supplied in normal diet.	Present in all plant and animal foods. Eggs, kidney, liver, salmon and yeast are best sources.	Yeast, wheat germ, liver concentrates.	Unstable to acid, alkali, heat and certain salts.	As part of coenzyme A, functions in the synthesis and breakdown of many vital body compounds. Essential in the intermediary metabolism of carbohydrate, fat, and protein.
Biotin	Not known but 150 to 300 mcg. will provide daily needs.	Liver, mushrooms, peanuts, yeast, milk, meat, egg yolk, most vegetables, banana, grapefruit, tomato, watermelon, and strawberries. (Synthesized in intestinal tract.)	Yeast, liver concentrates.	Stable.	Probably an essential component of a coenzyme. Appears to be involved in synthesis and breakdown of fatty acids and amino acids through aiding the addition and removal of CO$_2$ to or from active compounds, and the removal of NH$_3$ from amino acids. It is closely related metabolically to folic acid and pantothenic acid.
Folacin (folic acid)	Not yet determined but probably 0.1 to 0.2 mg. is adequate.	Green leafy vegetables, organ meats (liver), lean beef, wheat, eggs, fish, dry beans, lentils, cowpeas, asparagus, broccoli, collards, yeast. (Synthetized in intestines.)	Yeast, concentrates.	Stable to sunlight when in solution; unstable to heat in acid media.	Appears essential for biosynthesis of nucleic acids and probably for normal fat metabolism. Appears essential for normal maturation of red blood cells. Functions as a coenzyme: tetrahydrofolic acid.
Vitamin B$_{12}$ (cyanocobalamin)	5 μg.	Liver, kidney, milk and dairy foods, meat, eggs.	Concentrates, synthetic.	Slowly destroyed by acid, alkali, light and oxidation.	Involved in the metabolism of single-carbon fragments. Essential for biosynthesis of nucleic acids and nucleoproteins, and thereby in normal red blood cell formation; role in metabolism of nervous tissue; probably essential for normal fat metabolism. Related to certain anemias, especially pernicious anemia. Related to growth.
Ascorbic acid (vitamin C)	70 mg.	Puerto Rican cherry, citrus fruits, tomatoes, melons, peppers, greens, raw cabbage, guava, strawberries, pineapple, potatoes.	Synthetic.	Unstable to heat, alkali, and oxidation, except in acids. Destroyed by storage.	Essential for growth. Possibly functions as coenzymes in the metabolism of amino acids, particularly phenylalanine and tyrosine; facilitates conversion of folic acid to folinic acid and is essential for many hydroxylation reactions. Role in tooth and bone formation. Maintains intracellular cement substance with preservation of capillary integrity. Promotes healing of wounds and fractures; and reduces liability to infections. Enhances absorption of iron. Essential for production of collagen, the basic substance of connective tissue. Related in some way to biosynthesis of steroid hormones. Prevents scurvy.

ties of raw egg white. Antibiotics used in medical and surgical treatment may destroy the bacteria in the intestinal tract which are necessary to synthesize certain vitamins (K and several members of the B-complex group). Isonicotinic acid hydrozide (INH), which is used as a chemotherapeutic agent in the treatment of tuberculosis, is an antagonist for pyridoxine. Aminopterin, an antagonist of folacin, has reduced the number of leukocytes in leukemia. Dicumarol, which is an anticoagulant, acts as an antagonist to vitamin K.

PROBLEMS AND SUGGESTED TOPICS FOR DISCUSSION

1. Evaluate your dietary pattern for the foods high in vitamins A, D, thiamin, riboflavin, niacin, and ascorbic acid. Make suggestions for improvement.
2. Select references from the suggested reading list pertaining to vitamins and vision, thiamin and mentality, folic acid and anemia, vitamin B_6 deficiency, and the relationship of enzymes and vitamins, for either an oral or written report.
3. What are the functions of vitamins A, D, and K?
4. List the fractions of the vitamin B-complex that are recognized as necessary for humans. What is the function of each?
5. What effects may handling, storage, and cooking of foods have on vitamins A, B-complex fractions, D, and ascorbic acid?
6. Does the normal healthy person on an adequate well-rounded diet need vitamin supplements? Explain.
7. Search the literature, and make a list of examples of antivitamin activity that are of special interest in nutrition.
8. List the vitamins that should be supplied daily. List the vitamins stored in the body. List the vitamins that are known to be synthesized in the body.

SUGGESTED ADDITIONAL READING REFERENCES

Abt, A. F., et al.: Vitamin C requirements of man re-examined. Am. J. Clin. Nutr., 12:21, 1963.

Ames, S. R.: Factors affecting absorption transport and storage of vitamin A. Am. J. Clin. Nutr., 22:934, 1969.

Armstrong, B. K.: Absorption of vitamin B_{12} from human colon. Am. J. Clin. Nutr., 21:298, 1968.

Baker, E. M.: Vitamin C requirements in stress. Am. J. Clin. Nutr., 20:583, 1967.

Baker, E. M., et al.: Vitamin B_6 requirement for adult men. Am. J. Clin. Nutr., 15:59, 1964.

Bergen, S. S., Jr., and Roels, O. A.: Hypervitaminosis A, report of a case. Am. J. Clin. Nutr., 16:265, 1965.

Brin, M.: Erythrocyte as a biopsy tissue for functional evaluation of thiamine adequacy. J.A.M.A., 187:762, 1964.

Burton, B. T. (ed.): Heinz Handbook of Nutrition. 2nd ed. New York, McGraw-Hill Book Company, Inc., 1965, Chapters 10 and 11.

Campbell, J. A., and Morrison, A. B.: Some factors affecting the absorption of vitamins. Am. J. Clin. Nutr., 12:162, 1963.

Chopa, J. G., and Kevany, J.: Hypovitaminosis A in the Americas. Am. J. Clin. Nutr., 23:231, 1970.

Council on Foods and Nutrition. Importance of vitamin D in milk, J.A.M.A., 159:1018, 1955.

Coursin, D. B.: Present status of vitamin B_6 metabolism. Am. J. Clin. Nutr., 9:306, 1961.

Coursin, D. B.: Vitamin B_6 requirements. J.A.M.A., 189:27, 1964.

Davis, T. R. A., et al.: Review of studies of vitamin and mineral nutrition in the United States (1950–1958). J. Nutr. Ed., Vol. 1, No. 2, Supplement 1, Fall, 1969.

DeLuca, H. F.: Recent advances on the metabolism and function of vitamin D. Fed. Proc., 28:1678, 1969.

Dicks-Bushnell, M. W., and Davis, K. C.: Vitamin E content of infant formulas and cereals. Am. J. Clin. Nutr., 20:262, 1967.

Drapanas, T., et al.: Role of the ileum in the absorption of vitamin B_{12} and intrinsic factor (NF) J.A.M.A., 184:337, 1963.

Duncan, G. G.: Diseases of Metabolism. 5th ed. Philadelphia, W. B. Saunders Company, 1964, Chapter 7.

Elliott, R. A., and Dryer, R. L.: Hypervitaminosis A. J.A.M.A. 161:1157, 1956.

Food: The Yearbook of Agriculture, 1959. Washington, D.C., United States Department of Agriculture, pp. 130–161.

Food and Nutrition Board: Dietary Recommended Allowances. 7th ed. Washington, D.C., National Research Council, National Academy of Sciences Pub. No. 1694, 1968.

Guyton, A. C.: Textbook of Medical Physiology. 4th ed. Philadelphia, W. B. Saunders Company, 1971.

Herbert, V.: Nutritional requirements for vitamin B_{12} and folid acid. Am. J. Clin. Nutr., 21:743, 1968.

Herting, D. C.: Perspective on vitamin E. Am. J. Clin. Nutr., 19:210, 1966.

Horwitt, M. K.: Vitamin E and lipid metabolism in man. Am. J. Clin. Nutr., 8:451, 1961.

Horwitt, M. K., et al.: Polyunsaturated lipids and tocopherol requirements. J. Am. Dietet. A., 38:231, 1961.

Hsu, J. M.: Effect of deficiencies of certain B vitamins and ascorbic acid on absorption of vitamin B_{12}. Am. J. Clin. Nutr., 12:170, 1963.

Jacobs, F. A.: Role of Vitamin B_6 in intestinal absorption of amino acids in situ. J.A.M.A., 179:523, 1962.

Jeghers, H., and Marraro, H.: Hypervitaminosis A: Its broadening spectrum. Am. J. Clin. Nutr., 6:335, 1958.

Johnson, B. C.: Dietary factors and vitamin K. Nutr. Rev., 22:225, 1964.

Jolliffe, N.: Clinical Nutrition. 2nd ed. New York, Harper & Brothers, 1962, Chapters 13 through 22.

Mangay Chung, A. S., et al.: Folic acid, vitamin B_6 pantothenic acid and vitamin B_{12} in human dietaries. Am. J. Clin. Nutr., 9:573, 1961.

McGilvery, R. W.: Biochemistry: A Functional Approach. Philadelphia, W. B. Saunders Company, 1970.

Nutrition and Human Needs (III). The National Nutrition Survey. Hearings Before the Senate Committee on Nutrition and Human Needs of the United States Senate. January 22, 23, 27, and 28, 1969.

Orr, M. L.: Pantothenic acid, vitamin B_6 and vitamin B_{12} in foods. Home Economics Research Report No. 36, Washington, D.C., Agricultural Research Service, U.S. Department of Agriculture, 1969.

Oski, F. A., and Barnes, L. A.: Vitamin E deficiency: a previously unrecognized cause of hemolytic anemia in the premature infant. J. Pediat., 70:211, 1967.

Pearson, W. N.: Biochemical appraisal of the vitamin nutritional status in man. J.A.M.A., 180:49, 1962.

Pearson, W. N.: Flavonoids in human nutrition and medicine. J.A.M.A., 164:1675, 1957.

Pereira, S. M., et al.: Vitamin A therapy in children with kwashiorkor. Am. J. Clin. Nutr., 20:297, 1967.

Polansky, M. M., and Murphy, E. W.: Vitamin B_6 in fruits and nuts. J. Am. Dietet. A., 48:109, 1966.

Present Knowledge of Nutrition. 3rd ed. New York, The Nutrition Foundation, Inc., 1967.

Report. Vitamin B_{12}–Microbiological assay methods and distribution in selected foods. Home Econ. Res. Report No. 13, Washington, D.C., Department of Agriculture, Agriculture Research Service, 1962.

Review, Interrelationships between vitamins A and E. Nutr. Rev., 23:82, 1965.

Review. The metabolic role of vitamin E. Nutr. Rev., 23:90, 1965.

Review. Toxic reactions of vitamin A. Nutr. Rev., 22:109, 1964.

Review. Vitamin B₆ components in various foods. Nutr. Rev., 23:78, 1965.

Revin, R. S.: Riboflavin metabolism. New Eng. J. Med., 13:626, 1970.

Santini, R., et al.: The distribution of folic acid active compounds in individual foods. Am. J. Clin. Nutr., 14:205, 1964.

Sauberlich, H. E.: Biochemical alterations in thiamine deficiency—their interpretation. Am. J. Clin. Nutr., 20:528, 1967.

Schwartz, F. W.: Ascorbic acid in wound healing—a review. J. Am. Dietet. A., 56:497, 1970.

Shaffer, C. F.: Ascorbic acid and atherosclerosis. Am. J. Clin. Nutr., 23:27, 1970.

Sherlock, P., and Rothchild, E. O.: Zen diets and scurvy. J.A.M.A., 199:794, 1967.

Strieff, R. R., and Little, A. B.: Folic acid deficiency in pregnancy. New Eng. J. Med., 276:776, 1967.

The Nutrition Foundation, Inc.: Further studies of pantothenic acid deficiency in man. Nutr. Rev., 17:200, 1959.

Toepfer, E. W., and Polansky, M. M., Richardson, L. R., and Wilkes, S.: Comparison of vitamin B₆ values of selected food samples by bioassay and microbiological assay. Agricultural and Food Chemistry, 11:523, 1963.

Udall, J. A.: Human sources and absorption of vitamin K in relation to anticoagulation stability. J.A.M.A., 194:127, 1965.

Vietti, T. J., Stephens, J. C., and Bennett, K. R.: Vitamin K₁ prophylaxis in the newborn. J.A.M.A., 176:791, 1961.

Williams, J. N., Jr.: Some metabolic interrelationships of folic acid, vitamin B₁₂, and ascorbic acid. Am. J. Clin. Nutr., 2:20, 1954.

Wilson, T. H.: Intrinsic factor and B₁₂ absorption—a problem in cell physiology. Nutr. Rev., 23:33, 1965.

Wirtschafter, Z. T., and Walsh, J. R.: Hepatocellular lipoid changes in pantothenic acid deficiency. Am. J. Clin. Nutr., 10:525, 1962.

Wolf, G.: Some thoughts on the metabolic role of vitamin A. Nutr. Rev., 20:161, 1962.

Wohl, M. G., and Goodhart, R. S. (ed.): Modern Nutrition in Health and Disease. 4th ed. Philadelphia, Lea & Febiger, 1968, Chapter 11, The Vitamins.

Chapter 10
WATER
AND
ELECTROLYTES

DISTRIBUTION OF WATER WITHIN THE BODY

Water constitutes about two-thirds of the total body weight and is the body's principal component from the anatomical as well as the physiological point of view. Next to oxygen, it is the most important constituent for maintenance of life. A person can live for several weeks without food but only a few days without water. Dehydration (water loss) will kill far quicker than starvation.

A man can lose most of his fat and glycogen and half his protein (40 per cent loss of body weight) and survive, but a 20 per cent loss of body water may cause death, and a loss of only 10 per cent of water causes severe disorders.

Life goes on in a milieu of water. Water is an essential component of all protoplasm and plays a major role in cellular metabolism. Structurally 70 per cent of the mass of fat-free body weight consists of water. It is classified as intracellular and extracellular water. Intracellular water is within the cells of the body. Extracellular water includes the water in the blood, lymph, spinal fluid and secretions, and the intercellular or interstitial water that is found between and around the cells. (Fig. 10-1)

The water in the blood constitutes about 5 per cent and the interstitial water about 15 per cent of body weight. The intracellular water will approximate 50 per cent of the body weight. The distribution of body water is not fixed but can vary under differing circumstances, but the total amount in the body remains relatively constant.

FUNCTIONS OF WATER IN THE BODY

Water is the solvent in which all of the metabolic changes take place. It is not only a solvent but acts catolytically as well.

Water functions in digestion, absorption, circulation and excretion. It leaves the body through the skin, lungs, kidneys and feces. Water helps to maintain the electrolytic balance of the body. Only so long as the osmotic pressure exerted by solutes remains in equilibrium is it possible to have good health.

Water plays a role in the maintenance of

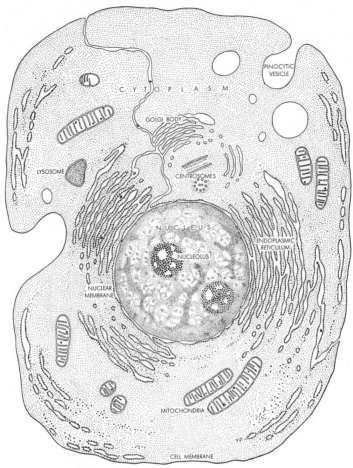

Figure 10–1   Diagram of a typical cell based on what is seen in electron micrographs. (From the living cell by J. Brachet. Copyright 1961 by Scientific American. All rights reserved.)

body temperature. Perspiration during warm weather and in fevers keeps the skin moist; by evaporation of perspiration the body is cooled.

Water acts as a transporting medium for nutrients and all body substances.

Metabolic waste products generated in the cells of the body are transported in the water solution via the blood to the kidneys where the wastes are excreted in urine.

Water substances in the body act as lubricants. Special water-soluble substances are in saliva to make foodstuffs slippery and around bones to lubricate the joints.

Water serves as a building material for growth and repair of the body. It is a part of all body tissues and fluids.

Water as a bulk in the intestinal tract aids elimination.

WATER BALANCE

Because the water content of the fat-free body weight remains fairly constant, it is evident that balance must exist. That is, the amount of water taken in daily is approximately equivalent to the amount of water lost.

WATER INTAKE   Water intake is controlled largely by thirst sensations. The thirst control center located in the hypothalamus is apparently activated when osmotic pressure of the body fluids increases. The sensation of thirst occurs and serves as a signal to seek fluids.

Water is ingested as such and as part of ingested food. Most adults in the United States consume 1.5 to 2.0 liters of fluids daily. Almost all foods contain some water. They may be composed of from 4 to 98 per cent water. Table 10–1 shows the percentage of water in some common foods.

In addition to the water contained in ingested foods, the oxidation of these foods in the body also produces water as an end-product. The oxidation of 100 gm. of fat, carbohydrate or protein yields 107, 55 and 41 gm. of water, respectively. Such water is known as "metabolic water" and must be

TABLE 10-1 PERCENTAGES OF WATER IN SOME COMMON FOODS

Lettuce (iceberg)	96
Snapbeans, radishes, celery	94
Watermelon	93
Cabbage (raw)	92
Broccoli, carrots, beets, collards	91
Orange	88
Milk	87
Cereals (cooked)	87
Apples	85
Potatoes (boiled)	80
Bananas	76
Eggs	74
Corn	74
Chicken (boiled)	71
Fish (baked)	68
Prunes (cooked)	66
Beef (lean)	60
Cheese	40
Bread	36
Cake (sponge)	32
Butter	16
Nuts	5
Soda crackers, dry cereals	4
Sugar (white)	trace
Oils	0

From Nutritive Value of Foods, U.S. Department of Agriculture. Home Garden Bull. No. 72, revised 1964. Appendix Table 1.

considered in the calculations of water balance. The amount of water as a result of the oxidation of food is 10 to 14 grams per 100 kcalories.

In addition to water taken into the digestive tract by mouth, a large amount of extracellular fluid is transferred daily into the stomach and intestines. Gamble[1] estimates that this may amount to 8200 ml. daily. The sources of this fluid are shown in Table 10-2. These fluids function in digestion and absorption (Chapter 2) and then pass on into the ileum and colon. Here the water is almost entirely reabsorbed except for a small amount excreted in the feces. Because this volume of fluid is twice that of the blood plasma (3500 ml.) the loss of large amounts from the gastrointestinal tract (diarrhea) may be of serious consequence to the individual.

[1]Gamble, J. L.: Chemical Anatomy, Physiology and Pathology of Extracellular Fluids. Cambridge, Harvard University Press, 1954.

TABLE 10-2 SOURCES OF WATER IN THE DIGESTIVE JUICES*

Saliva	1500 ml.
Gastric secretions	2500 ml.
Bile	500 ml.
Pancreatic secretions	700 ml.
Intestinal mucosa secretions	3000 ml.
Total	8200

*Gamble, J. L.: Chemical Anatomy, Physiology and Pathology of Extracellular Fluids. Cambridge, Harvard University Press, 1954.

When water cannot be taken orally, it may be given intravenously, subcutaneously or rectally in the form of salt solutions which resemble closely the fluids of the body. Water also may be given intravenously as glucose solutions or as blood, plasma or protein hydrolysate mixtures.

Water is absorbed rapidly from the digestive tract into blood and lymph because it moves freely by diffusion through membranes. The movement of water is controlled mostly by osmotic forces generated by the inorganic ions found in solution in the body.

WATER ELIMINATION Water is lost from the body through the kidneys as urine, through the bowel in feces, through the lungs with expired air, and through the skin as perspiration.

Insensible water loss is that which goes on constantly and usually unconsciously, namely through the skin and lungs. Sensible water loss is that excreted through the bowel and kidneys.

Lung water goes out of the body as tiny droplets in the expired air. Water lost through the kidneys, perspiration and feces carries out waste products and minerals with it, thus accounting for the need to replace minerals daily by the diet, as discussed in Chapter 8.

Abnormal losses of water occur through vomiting, diarrhea, hemorrhages, draining fistulas and exuding of burns. When water intake is insufficient or water loss occurs, the kidney attempts to compensate by conserving water and thereby excretes a more concentrated urine. This action of the kidney is controlled by the pituitary antidiuretic hormone (ADH), which stimulates the renal tubules to increase the reabsorption of water. When water is lost, changes in electrolyte balance occur. When the water losses are excessive (dehydration), the extracellular fluid becomes concentrated and osmotic pressure drains water from the cells into the extracellular fluid to compensate. Usually the individual becomes extremely thirsty and nauseated. According to Snively[2] there are many recognized specific imbalances of body fluids.

WATER BALANCE Water balance is directly related to the homeostatic functioning of the internal environment: hydrogen ion concentration, water and electrolyte concentration, osmotic pressure, temperature, and other balances of the interstitial fluids.

For a person to be in metabolic equilibrium, water intake must equal water output. The

[2]Snively, W. D.: Sea Within. Philadelphia, J. B. Lippincott Company, 1960, p. 55.

TABLE 10–3   WATER BALANCE

WATER INTAKE	
Fluids	1250 ml.
Water in food	900 ml.
Water from oxidation of food in the body	350 ml.
Total	2500 ml.

WATER OUTPUT	
Urine	1400 ml.
Water in feces	100 ml.
Skin (perspiration)	700 ml.
Lungs (expired air)	300 ml.
Total	2500 ml.

typical daily water intake and output is shown in Table 10–3.

This table could be changed markedly by varying environmental conditions. For example, in cold weather, less water would be lost through the skin and more would then be passed as urine. In very hot weather, both skin and lung water output would be much greater, urine output would be less, and intake of drinking water would be greater.

The body has no place to store water. Water held in the bladder is of no metabolic use. Therefore, the amount lost every 24 hours must be replaced to maintain health and efficiency.

WATER IN FOODS

Vegetables and fruits contain approximately 90 per cent water (Table 10–1). Milk is 87 per cent water, meat 60 to 75 per cent water. Even dried foods such as figs and raisins contain about 20 per cent water. Only truly dried foods, the commercially dehydrated foods, do not contain water. In addition to the actual water present in foods is the water that becomes available as an end product of food metabolism, as previously stated.

RECOMMENDED ALLOWANCE OF WATER The water requirement depends upon the losses through the various routes – sensible and insensible. The Food and Nutrition Board in 1968 states that under the most favorable conditions (low solute diet), minimal physical activity and absence of sweating, the total water supplied from food, beverages and metabolic water should be at least 1.5 liters per day.[3] A reasonable allowance based on recommended caloric intake is suggested to be 1 ml./kcal. for adults and 1.5 ml./kcal. for infants. A suitable daily allowance for adults

in most instances is 2½ liters or approximately 2½ to 3 quarts. A large percentage of this is contained in prepared foods.

Thirst is usually an adequate guide for water intake except for infants and the sick. In cases of extreme heat or excessive sweating thirst may not keep pace with the actual water requirement. Special attention to water needs should be given to infants on high protein formulas; to comatose patients; to those individuals with fever, excessive urine loss or diarrhea or who are consuming high protein diets; and to all persons in hot environments.[4]

WATER AND ELECTROLYTES

WATER AND ELECTROLYTES When a salt, acid or base is dissolved in water it dissociates into its constituent ions. Because these charged particles can conduct an electric current they are known as electrolytes. Glucose, alcohols, urea, protein and many other substances involved in metabolism which do not separate into charged particles are called nonelectrolytes because these molecules do not ionize.

There are some major differences in the electrolyte composition of extracellular and intracellular fluids. The composition of the extracellular fluid is well known because blood, the main extracellular fluid, is readily accessible for study. Obtaining representative samples of intracellular fluids for analysis is no easy task. Thus the data on their composition is less reliable than that of extracellular fluids. The substances present in the fluid between the cells (interstitial fluid) closely resemble those found in blood plasma except that the concentration of proteins is lower.

Electrolytes are of importance in relation to their concentration (number of particles per unit volume) and because of their number of charges. Electrolyte concentrations are conventionally expressed in terms of milliequivalents (mEq.). When the concentrations of each ionic constituent of extracellular or intracellular fluids are expressed in terms of milliequivalents per liter, the sum of all the positively charged ions (cations) exactly equals the sum of all the negatively charged ions (anions). Thus, every positively charged ion is exactly balanced by a negatively charged ion. This concept will be evident from perusal of the values in Table 10–4. The average sum of the concentration of all the cations in serum is about 150 mEq. per liter. This is balanced by 150 mEq. per liter of anions.

[3]Food and Nutrition Board: Recommended Daily Allowances. 7th ed. Washington, D.C., National Research Council, National Academy of Sciences. Pub. No. 1694, 1968, p. 65.

[4]Food and Nutrition Board, *op. cit.,* p. 67.

TABLE 10–4   NORMAL ELECTROLYTE
CONCENTRATIONS OF THE EXTRACELLULAR
AND INTRACELLULAR FLUIDS
(in mEq/liter)

	IN EXTRACELLULAR FLUID	IN INTRACELLULAR FLUID
Cations		
Sodium	135 to 147	10
Potassium	3.5 to 5.5	150
Calcium	4.5 to 5.5	1 to 2
Magnesium	1.5 to 3.0	40
Anions		
Chloride	98 to 106	4
Bicarbonate	26 to 30	10
Phosphate	2 to 5	140
Sulfate	2 to 5	10
Organic Acids (lactic, pyruvic)	3 to 6	
Proteins	15 to 19	40

Adapted from Gamble, J. L.: Chemical Anatomy, Physiology and Pathology of Extracellular Fluids. Cambridge, Harvard University Press, 1954.

OSMOTIC PRESSURE   The body seeks to equalize the total salt concentrations (in milliequivalents) of the intracellular and extracellular fluids. Reference is being made to cation and anion concentrations and not the concentrations of individual ions because it has already been noted that sodium and potassium, for example, are normally distributed in quite a different manner between intracellular and extracellular fluid.

In an effort to maintain these equal concentrations, small shifts of water may take place. These shifts are due to a force called osmotic pressure which is directly proportional to the number of particles in solution. If the salt content of the tissues (intracellular fluid) gets too high, water passes from the surrounding fluid (extracellular fluid) which tends to reduce the salt concentration in the tissues and also increases somewhat the concentration of salt in the extracellular fluid. If, on the other hand, the salt concentration in the intracellular fluid is too low, water passes out of the tissues into the extracellular fluid. It is convenient (although not entirely accurate) to consider that the osmotic pressure of the intracellular fluid is largely a function of its content of potassium because this cation predominates, whereas the osmotic pressure of the extracellular fluid may be conveniently considered to relate to its content of sodium—this being the major cation present. Shifts in the distribution of these ions are the principal cause of shifts of water between the various fluid compartments.

Proteins, non-diffusible because of their size, also play an important part in maintaining osmotic equilibrium. Their presence in the plasma exerts a colloidal osmotic pressure which helps to retain water and thereby prevents the leakage of water from the plasma into the interstitial fluid. In some disease states, when the protein content of plasma is exceptionally low, water does leak into the interstitial fluids, resulting in edema.

ELECTROLYTE CONTROL OF BODY HYDRATION   An important difference in the distribution of sodium and potassium has been noted (i.e., sodium is largely confined to extracellular fluids, whereas potassium occurs largely within the cells). Also it has been noted that phosphate anions predominate within cells and chloride anions predominate in the extracellular fluids.

Sodium and potassium concentrations are of major influence in directing the movement of water from one body compartment to another (i.e., from extracellular fluid into cells and vice versa). These two cations are in control of total hydration of the body (i.e., control over the amount of water to be retained in any given compartment). The shifts in water from one compartment to another are due to changes occurring in the extracellular concentrations of electrolytes. When water loss exceeds electrolyte loss, the extracellular fluid becomes hypertonic to the intracellular fluid (i.e., the osmotic pressure of the extracellular fluid is higher than the osmotic pressure of the intracellular fluid) and water shifts from the cells to the extracellular space to compensate. When water enters the extracellular fluid with the electrolytes in amounts insufficient to maintain normal density of the solutions, the extracellular fluid becomes hypotonic to the intracellular fluid (i.e., the osmotic pressure of the extracellular fluid is lower than the osmotic pressure of the intracellular fluid) and water shifts from the extracellular space to the cell. The reduction of the extracellular fluid continues until osmotic equilibrium between intracellular and extracellular fluids is reestablished. When the body is unable to maintain osmotic equilibrium, dehydration or edema may result. Causes of dehydration or edema are discussed later in the text.

ACID-BASE REGULATION

ACID-BASE BALANCE   The reaction of the body fluids is slightly basic (pH 7.35 to 7.4). The body normally maintains this narrow range of pH with remarkable precision even though large amounts of acid are produced during metabolism and various amounts of acids are ingested in foodstuffs. The reason that pH is maintained in the face of these threats is that the food and metabolic acids are rapidly neutralized by buffers present in the blood. The main buffers operating in this regulatory system are the bicarbonate-carbonic acid system, the phosphate system and the protein systems.

When acids are ingested or formed in metabolism the hydrogen ion combines with bicarbonate ion in the blood plasma to form carbonic acid which is only slightly ionized and traps the hydrogen ion in non-ionized form. In the lungs the carbonic acid is decomposed to form carbon dioxide and water. The carbon dioxide is excreted. The organic anion is excreted in the urine along with a cation (usually sodium). This process, if allowed to continue, would deplete the amount of sodium ion in the body. There are two main mechanisms in the kidney for saving cation. The urine is usually more acid than blood, with a pH of 6.0 to 7.0 and may be as low as 4.7. This is accomplished through the phosphate buffer system. In the plasma most of the phosphate is present as Na_2HPO_4, with smaller amounts of NaH_2PO_4. In the urine the ratio may be reversed. Hydrogen ion is exchanged for sodium ion in the kidney, and the sodium returned to the plasma. Also ammonium ion (NH_4^+) may be formed in the kidney chiefly by hydrolysis of the amino acid glutamine. The ammonium ion is excreted and a sodium ion saved.

ACIDS AND BASES An acid is defined as a substance (ion, molecule) that yields hydrogen ion (protons) in solution. Conversely, a base is anything that combines with hydrogen ions. Accordingly, when the common acids dissociate into their respective cations and anions, the anionic component may be considered to be a base. Bases are weak or strong depending on their affinity for the hydrogen ion. HCO_3^-, $HPO_4^=$, $H_2PO_4^-$, and protein are relatively strong because they have a strong affinity for hydrogen ion. On the other hand, HCl is almost completely ionized, thus Cl^- is an extremely poor base because it has little ability to bind hydrogen ions. Clinically the term base is frequently applied to the cations (Na^+, K^+, Mg^{++}, Ca^{++}) of the body fluids and the term acid is commonly applied to the anions (Cl^-, HCO_3^-, $SO_4^=$, $HPO_4^=$). The term

"total base" is frequently used in reference to the sum of the cations.

The term alkali reserve is frequently used by clinicians to refer to plasma bicarbonate concentration. This anion is available to neutralize acids that might enter the plasma. The term alkali reserve should really refer to all the relatively strong buffer bases of the body fluids, i.e., HCO_3^-, $H_2PO_4^-$, $HPO_4^=$, protein, etc., but under ordinary conditions the bicarbonate levels will reflect the condition of the entire buffer complex. It must be remembered that carbon dioxide is constantly being formed in metabolism and though carbonic acid is a much weaker acid (HCO_3^- a much stronger base) than those we have been discussing and serves as a buffer for them, the amount formed would cause an appreciable change in the pH of the blood if it were not buffered. Hemoglobin is in large measure responsible for the buffering of the metabolic CO_2. Conditions in which respiration is depressed (pneumonia, emphysema, etc.) cause retention of carbon dioxide and a condition referred to as respiratory acidosis.

POTENTIAL ACID-BASE REACTION OF FOODS Foodstuffs, when burned in the body, yield mineral residues which are acidic or basic in reaction. If approximately equal quantities of cations and anions are left in the residue, then the residue will be essentially neutral and the body will not have to make any particular adjustment in the pH of its fluids. If, on the other hand, there is an excess of cations (Na^+, K^+, Ca^{++}, Mg^{++}), the body must draw on its anion reserve to restore pH of blood. The cations will be excreted in the urine largely as dicationic phosphate (Na_2HPO_4, K_2HPO_4) and the urine will be more alkaline in reaction. If there is an excess of anions ($SO_4^=$, $PO_4^=$), the urine will be acid, as described in the previous section, and ammonium ion may be formed.

In general, meats and cereal produce acidic residues such as phosphates and sulfates which result in an acid urine. Conversely, vegetables and fruits produce basic residues

TABLE 10–5 POTENTIAL ACID-BASE REACTION OF CERTAIN FOODS

ACID ASH FOODS	BASIC ASH FOODS	NEUTRAL ASH FOODS
Breads and crackers	Fruits (except prunes,	Butter and margarine
Cakes and cookies, plain	plums, cranberries)	Cooking fat and oils
Cereals and cereal products	Jams, jellies, honey	Cream
(macaroni, spaghetti, noodles)	Milk	Starch
Cheese	Nuts (Cocoanut)	Sugars and sirups
Eggs	(Almond)	
Fish	(Chestnut)	
Meats	Vegetables (except corn	
Peanuts, walnuts	and lentils)	
Poultry		
Prunes		
Plums		
Cranberries		
Corn		
Lentils, dried		

which tend to produce alkaline urine. It would seem a curious anomaly that the consumption of citrus fruits and tomatoes results in an alkaline urine. This is because the cations in fruits (chiefly Na^+, K^+) are associated with weak organic anions such as malate or citrate which can be oxidized in the body leaving a cationic residue. A typical mixed diet contains a reasonable balance of acidic and basic substances. Thus the body often does not have to draw strenuously upon its buffering systems to take care of these ingested compounds. The principal threat to the buffer systems of the body are the many acidic products of metabolism. Fortunately, its buffer defenses are quite biased toward the excretion of excess acid and the usual pH of the body fluids is maintained. For this reason, the usual pH of urine is on the acid side of neutral.

Occasionally, foods that will produce acid, basic or neutral ashes are used to produce acidic or basic urine for various therapeutic purposes. Table 10–5 contains a list of foods and indicates their potential acid-base reaction.

FUNCTIONS OF ELECTROLYTES OF BODY FLUIDS   The most important cations and anions of body fluids have been listed in Table 10–4 and other mineral elements essential for many vital processes in human metabolism are listed in Table 8–3, page 111. They are delivered to the body in the food ingested daily.

The functions of sodium, potassium and chloride, the electrolytes which are the major constituents in extracellular and intracellular fluids, along with the other mineral elements essential in nutrition are presented in Chapter 8, The Minerals.

PROBLEMS AND SUGGESTED TOPICS FOR DISCUSSION

1. Keep a record of your water and fluid intake for a period of 24 hours. Evaluate.

2. Select references from the suggested list pertaining to water and salt relationship for either an oral or written report.
3. What are the routes of water elimination from the body?
4. What is insensible water loss?
5. List the functions of water in the body.
6. List the conditions that affect water balance in the body.
7. What is the relationship between water and electrolytes in the body?
8. What is meant by the acid-base regulation of the body? Evaluate your food intake as to whether it is predominately acid or alkaline.

SUGGESTED ADDITIONAL READING REFERENCES

Baker, E. M., Plough, I. C., and Allen, T. H.: Water requirement of men as related to the salt intake. Am. J. Clin. Nutr., 12:394, 1963.
Bland, J. H.: Clinical Metabolism of Body Water and Electrolytes. Philadelphia. W. B. Saunders Company, 1963.
Brooke, C. E.: Oral fluid and electrolytes. J.A.M.A., 179:792, 1962.
Burton, B. T. (ed.): Heinz Handbook of Nutrition. 2nd ed. New York, McGraw-Hill Book Company, Inc., 1965. Chapter 3, Fluid Electrolyte and Acid-Base Balance.
Camien, M. N., et al.: A critical reappraisal of acid-base balance. Am. J. Clin. Nutr., 22:786, 1969.
Chow, B. F., et al.: Diet and urinary output of water. Am. J. Clin. Nutr., 12:333, 1963.
Duncan, G. G. (ed.): Diseases of Metabolism. 5th ed. Philadelphia, W. B. Saunders Company, 1964. Chapter 6, Water Balance in Health and Disease.
Gamble, J. L.: Chemical Anatomy, Physiology and Pathology of Extracellular Fluid. 6th ed. Cambridge, Harvard University Press, 1954.
Goldberger, E.: A Primer of Water Electrolyte and Acid-Base Syndromes. 2nd ed. Philadelphia, Lea and Febiger, 1962.
Jolliffe, N. (ed.): Clinical Nutrition. 2nd ed. New York, Harper & Bros., 1962. Chapter 12, Sodium, Potassium and Chloride Malnutrition, including Water Balance and Shock.
Snively, W. D.: Sea Within. Philadelphia, J. B. Lippincott Company, 1960.
Statland, H.: Fluids and Electrolytes in Practice, 3rd ed. Philadelphia, J. B. Lippincott Company, 1970.
Weisberg, H. E.: Water Electrolytes and Acid-Base Balance, Normal and Pathological. Baltimore, Williams & Wilkins, 1962.
Wohl, M. G., and Goodhart, R. S. (eds.): Modern Nutrition in Health and Disease. 4th ed. Philadelphia, Lea & Febiger, 1968. Chapter 12, Fluid and Electrolyte Balance.

UNIT THREE
APPLIED NUTRITION: RECOMMENDED DIETARY ALLOWANCES, FOOD SELECTION, MEAL PLANNING AND FOOD ECONOMICS

Chapter 11
AN
ADEQUATE
DIET

INTERPRETATION OF AN ADEQUATE DIET

An adequate diet is composed of the various nutrients which the body needs for maintenance, repair, the living processes and growth or development. It is a diet which meets in full all the nutritional needs of the person. There is no *ideal* diet, since such a diet is a matter of individual requirement. It is the purpose of the daily meals to supply the essential elements. Regional availability of foods, socioeconomic conditions, taste preferences, food habits, age of the family members, storage and preparation facilities, and cooking skills are factors to consider when nutritious meals are planned.

In the preceding chapters the various nutrients needed by the body have been discussed. In this chapter, application of the information gained will be made by translating the nutrients into a daily diet. This chapter is important in that it is the translation of principles of nutrition into the selection of an adequate diet and the foundation of therapeutic nutrition.

DIETARY INTERRELATIONSHIPS

All studies of the interaction of nutrients indicate the need for a balanced diet. Clinical reports show that often when an individual is found deficient in one nutrient, such as a vitamin, deficiencies in others are also found. For example, a deficiency of vitamin A may result also in symptoms and damage associated with deficiency of ascorbic acid. Scurvy has been produced in animals by depriving them of vitamin A. Today it is an established fact that the presence or absence of one essential nutrient may affect the availability, absorption, metabolism, or dietary need for others.

Interrelationships exist not only among the vitamins but among the minerals, between vitamins and minerals, between vitamins and proteins, between vitamins and carbohydrates, and between vitamins and fats. Multiple relationships also exist. Numerous experiments have extended understanding of the broad nutritional import of interrelationships or "balance" among nutrients. While certain interrelationships have long been known, the recognition of the large number of them re-emphasizes the basic soundness of the principle of maintaining variety in foods in order to provide the most complete diet. Much current research is being devoted to dietary interrelationships.

PROGRESS IN DETERMINING HUMAN DIETARY NEEDS

The history of the development of the science of nutrition and dietary standards is outlined in Chapter 1. The dietary standards set up by the Food and Nutrition Board of the National Academy of Sciences–National Research Council (Table 11–1) are universally accepted as the guide or yardstick for planning and evaluating diets and food supplies for population groups and individuals in the United States. These standards represent years of research by many workers on both animals and human beings. The standards, revised in 1968 (seventh revision; original edition published in 1943), represent the latest interpretation of human nutritional needs by a large number of nutrition authorities.

RECOMMENDED DAILY DIETARY ALLOWANCES (RDA)

The purposes and the applicability of the recommended dietary allowances can best be explained by quoting from the 1968 revised publication.[1]

"The allowances are intended to serve as goals for planning food supplies and as guides for the interpretation of food consumption records of groups of people. The actual nutritional status of groups of healthy people or individuals must be judged on the basis of physical, biochemical, and clinical observations combined with observations of food or nutrient intakes. If the RDA are used as reference standards for interpreting records of food consumption, it should not be assumed that malnutrition will occur whenever the recommendations are not completely met. . . .

Except for calories, the allowances are designed to afford a margin sufficiently above average physiological requirements to cover variations among practically all individuals in the general population. The allowances provide a buffer against increased needs during common stresses and permit full realization of growth and productive potential, but they are not necessarily adequate to meet the additional requirements of persons depleted by disease, traumatic stresses, or dietary inadequacies. However, the allowances are generous with respect to temporary emergency feeding of large groups under conditions of limited food supply and physical disaster.

The margin above normal physiological requirements varies for each nutrient because of differences in body storage capacity, in individual requirements, in the pre-

[1] Food and Nutrition Board: Recommended Dietary Allowances. Revised 7th ed. Washington, D.C., National Academy of Sciences–National Research Council, 1968.

cision of assessing requirements, and in the possible hazard of excessive intake of certain nutrients.

With the exception of iron, patterns of food consumption and food supplies in the United States permit ready adaptation to and compliance with the RDA. The primary objective of the RDA is to permit and encourage the development of food practices by the population of the United States that will allow for greatest dividends in health and in disease prevention."

The RDA have been used as guides in planning nutritionally adequate diets for groups. They are used in the interpretation of the adequacy of nutrient intakes of individuals in dietary surveys. They are to be used as a reference. Any deviations of the individual intakes from the recommended nutrient allowances should be regarded as significant only in terms of the individual's total health status. The nutritional status is the sum total of the food consumption present and past nutrient intake; clinical signs and symptoms; growth and development; biochemical data and excretory levels of nutrients.

Individuals whose diets do not meet the RDA standards are not necessarily inadequate nor does it indicate that the individual is suffering from malnutrition. The RDA allow for a margin of safety for individual variations. The recommended allowances are designed for the population of the United States and are revised about every five years in order to include new research findings. Nutritional surveys are needed periodically to determine the nature, causes and location of malnutrition in the United States.

In the 1968 revision recommended allowances have been added for vitamins E, B_6, B_{12} and folacin and for minerals iodine, magnesium and phosphorus. The age and sex groupings include three periods of infancy up to one year, six age groupings for children and seven age groups of males and females from 10 years to 75 years of age and beyond. The "reference" man, 22 years of age (wt: 150 lbs. or 70 kg., ht: 69 in. or 175 cm.) and "reference" woman, 22 years of age (wt: 128 lbs. or 58 kg., ht: 64 in. or 160 cm.) with three age groups are used. They are presumed to live in an environment with a mean temperature of 20°C. (70°F.). Their physical activity is considered "light" (neither sedentary nor heavy physical activity).

Some of the changes in the 1968 revision are as follows:

Calories: Calorie recommendations for infants to one year of age have been added for the convenience of those preparing infant foods. Because of the concern over the fact that a considerable segment of the American population is overweight, and the belief that the average adult exerts much less energy than was allowed in the 1958 and 1964 reference man and woman, the 1968 calorie allow-

TABLE 11–1   RECOMMENDED DAILY DIETARY ALLOWANCES,[1] REVISED 1968

Designed for the Maintenance of Good Nutrition of Practically All Healthy Persons in the U.S.A.
(Allowances are intended for persons normally active in a temperate climate)
Food and Nutrition Board, National Academy of Sciences—National Research Council

Age[b] From-Up to	Weight kg (lb)	Height cm (in)	Kilocalories	Protein gm	Fat-Soluble Vitamins A activity IU	D IU	E activity IU	Water-Soluble Vitamins Ascorbic acid mg	Folacin mg	Niacin mg equiv[d]	Riboflavin mg	Thiamine mg	Vitamin B₆ mg	Vitamin B₁₂ mcg	Minerals Calcium gm	Phosphorus gm	Iodine µg	Iron mg	Magnesium mg
Infants																			
Birth–1/6	4 (9)	55 (22)	kg.×120[c]	kg.×2.2	1,500	400	5	35	0.05	5	0.4	0.2	0.2	1.0	0.4	0.2	25	6	40
1/6–1/2	7 (15)	63 (25)	kg.×110[c]	kg.×2.0	1,500	400	5	35	0.05	7	0.5	0.4	0.3	1.5	0.5	0.4	40	10	60
1/2–1	9 (20)	72 (28)	kg.×100[c]	kg.×1.8	1,500	400	5	35	0.1	8	0.6	0.5	0.4	2.0	0.6	0.5	45	15	70
Children																			
1 – 2	12 (26)	81 (32)	1,100	25	2,000	400	10	40	0.1	8	0.6	0.6	0.5	2.0	0.7	0.7	55	15	100
2 – 3	14 (31)	91 (36)	1,250	25	2,000	400	10	40	0.2	8	0.7	0.6	0.6	2.5	0.8	0.8	60	15	150
3 – 4	16 (35)	100 (39)	1,400	30	2,500	400	10	40	0.2	9	0.8	0.7	0.7	3	0.8	0.8	70	10	200
4 – 6	19 (42)	110 (43)	1,600	30	2,500	400	10	40	0.2	11	0.9	0.8	0.9	4	0.8	0.8	80	10	200
6 – 8	23 (51)	121 (48)	2,000	35	3,500	400	15	40	0.2	13	1.1	1.0	1.0	4	0.9	0.9	100	10	250
8 – 10	28 (62)	131 (52)	2,200	40	3,500	400	15	40	0.3	15	1.2	1.1	1.2	5	1.0	1.0	110	10	250
Males																			
10 – 12	35 (77)	140 (55)	2,500	45	4,500	400	20	40	0.4	17	1.3	1.3	1.4	5	1.2	1.2	125	10	300
12 – 14	43 (95)	151 (59)	2,700	50	5,000	400	20	45	0.4	18	1.4	1.4	1.6	5	1.4	1.4	135	18	350
14 – 18	59 (130)	170 (67)	3,000	60	5,000	400	25	55	0.4	20	1.5	1.5	1.8	5	1.4	1.4	150	18	400
18 – 22	67 (147)	175 (69)	2,800	60	5,000	—	30	60	0.4	18	1.6	1.4	2.0	5	0.8	0.8	140	10	400
22 – 35	70 (154)	175 (69)	2,800	65	5,000	—	30	60	0.4	18	1.7	1.4	2.0	5	0.8	0.8	140	10	350
35 – 55	70 (154)	173 (68)	2,600	65	5,000	—	30	60	0.4	17	1.7	1.3	2.0	5	0.8	0.8	125	10	350
55 – 75+	70 (154)	171 (67)	2,400	65	5,000	—	30	60	0.4	14	1.7	1.2	2.0	6	0.8	0.8	110	10	350
Females																			
10 – 12	35 (77)	142 (56)	2,250	50	4,500	400	20	40	0.4	15	1.3	1.1	1.4	5	1.2	1.2	110	18	300
12 – 14	44 (97)	154 (61)	2,300	50	5,000	400	20	45	0.4	15	1.4	1.2	1.6	5	1.3	1.3	115	18	350
14 – 16	52 (114)	157 (62)	2,400	55	5,000	400	25	50	0.4	16	1.4	1.2	1.8	5	1.3	1.3	120	18	350
16 – 18	54 (119)	160 (63)	2,300	55	5,000	400	25	50	0.4	15	1.5	1.2	2.0	5	1.3	1.3	115	18	350
18 – 22	58 (128)	163 (64)	2,000	55	5,000	400	25	55	0.4	13	1.5	1.0	2.0	5	0.8	0.8	100	18	350
22 – 35	58 (128)	163 (64)	2,000	55	5,000	—	25	55	0.4	13	1.5	1.0	2.0	5	0.8	0.8	100	18	350
35 – 55	58 (128)	160 (63)	1,850	55	5,000	—	25	55	0.4	13	1.5	1.0	2.0	5	0.8	0.8	90	18	300
55 – 75+	58 (128)	157 (62)	1,700	55	5,000	—	25	55	0.4	13	1.5	1.0	2.0	6	0.8	0.8	80	10	300
Pregnancy			+200	65	6,000	400	30	60	0.8	15	1.8	+0.1	2.5	8	+0.4	+0.4	125	18	450
Lactation			+1,000	75	8,000	400	30	60	0.5	20	2.0	+0.5	2.5	6	+0.5	+0.5	150	18	450

[a] The allowance levels are intended to cover individual variations among most normal persons as they live in the United States under usual environmental stresses. The recommended allowances can be attained with a variety of common foods providing other nutrients for which human requirements have been less well defined.

[b] Entries on lines for age range 22-35 years represent the reference man and woman at age 22. All other entries represent allowances for the midpoint of the specified age range.

[c] Assumes protein equivalent to human milk. For proteins not 100% utilized, factors should be increased proportionately.

[d] Niacin equivalents include dietary sources of the vitamin itself plus 1 mg equivalent for each 60 mg of dietary tryptophan.

[e] The folacin allowances refer to dietary sources as determined by *Lactobacillus casei* assay. Pure forms of folacin may be effective in doses less than 1/4 of the RDA.

ances were again reduced. The 1968 RDA for men and women are 2800 and 2000, respectively. It is estimated on a per capita basis, that Americans consume 76 kcalories of alcohol per day, making this product an important factor in the consideration of kcaloric intake. Since this calculation includes children and non-users, the actual intake of the remaining population is significantly higher.

Protein: Protein allowances for adults have been decreased from 1.0 gm. to 0.9 gm. per kilogram per day (65 gm. per day for the reference man and 58 gm. for the reference woman). An additional 10 gm. per day is recommended during pregnancy and 20 gm. per day during lactation.

Vitamin E: The RDA is 30 I.U. and 25 I.U. per day for the reference man and woman.

Ascorbic Acid: The RDA is reduced from 70 mg. per day to 60 mg. per day for the reference man and woman.

Folacin: The RDA is 0.4 mg. per day from dietary sources based on *Lactobacillus casei* assay.

Niacin: The RDA is 6.6 mg. per 1000 kcal. (18 mg. per day for men and 13 mg. per day for women).

Riboflavin: The RDA is 1.7 mg. per day and 1.5 mg. per day for men and women, respectively.

Vitamin B_6: The RDA for adults is 2.0 mg. per day.

Vitamin B_{12}: The RDA is 5 μg. per day.

Calcium and Phosphorus: The RDA is based on 1:1 ratio except for infants which is 2:1. The adult RDA remains 0.8 gm. per day.

Iodine: The RDA is 5 μg. per 100 kcal. (140 μg. per day for men and 100 μg. per day for women).

Iron: Because of the wide individual variability in its absorption and availability from from various foods, iron is the most problematic nutrient. Absorbability is assumed to be about 10 per cent of the food intake of iron. For males the 10 mg. per day recommended may be attained readily from the average American diet but the RDA of 18 mg. per day for females on 2000 kcal. per day may be difficult to obtain from the dietary sources. Fortification of foods is indicated.

Magnesium: The RDA is approximately 150 mg. per 1000 kcal. (350 mg. per day for men and 300 mg. per day for women).

Nutrients without well-defined requirements: Vitamin K, Vitamin D, essential fatty acids, choline, chromium, cobalt, manganese, molybdenum, selenium and brotin.

The RDA for a 70-kg. man is summarized in Figure 11–1. Differences in single nutrients due to age and sex are insignificant.

About 10 gm. of nitrogen is present in the 65 gm. of protein required. Leucine and tryptophan are shown in the figures to represent the extremes of essential amino acid need. The amounts are calculated from the provisional amino acid pattern of the Food and Agricultural Organization of the United Nations. Values for vitamins A and E are based on retinol and *dl-α*-tocopherol acetate, respectively.

Dietary standards have been formulated for other countries, which differ in philosophy and purpose from those of the American standards, and thus specific recommendations differ. The allowances proposed in the Canadian standard[2] approach minimal requirements but are considered to be adequate for the maintenance of health among the majority of people (Table 11–2); values recommended in the British standard are for maintenance of good nutrition in the average person; allowances recommended in the United States standards are for the maintenance of good nutrition in substantially all normal persons. Comparative dietary standards of selected countries and UN agencies may be found in the Appendix of the DRA, published by the National Research Council.

Although the recommended daily dietary allowances are designed for *groups* of people, with proper interpretation and use, they can serve as a helpful criterion to judge, evaluate and plan the nutritional status of an *individual* and are referred to repeatedly throughout this text. When new research findings alter the previous recommendations new standards are issued.

The scientific bases for the Recommended Dietary Allowances are described in full in the publication, and for proper and intelligent use of this table, it is strongly recommended that the report be read in its entirety.

ESSENTIALS OF AN ADEQUATE DIET

The task of planning nutritious meals centers on the inclusion of the essential nutrients and adequate calories. In the underdeveloped countries where food is scarce and there is much ignorance concerning adequate nutrition, the United Nations World Health Organization (WHO) is working constantly to

---

[2]"Dietary Standard for Canada," Canadian Bulletin on Nutrition, Vol. 6, No. 1, 1964, from the Dept. of Public Printing and Stationery, Ottawa, Canada.

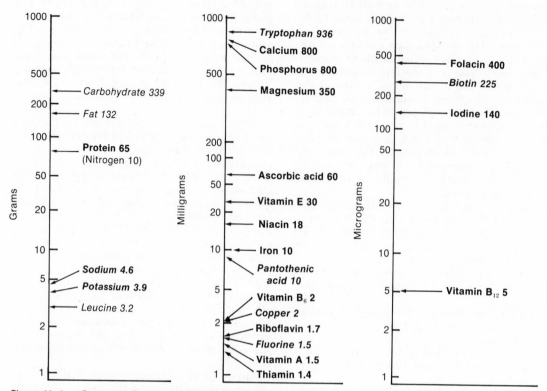

Figure 11–1   Summary of recommended dietary allowances for reference man (70 kg.). Tabulated values are in Roman type: Bold-face italics are best estimates and italics indicate calculated values. (Adapted from Klevay, L. M.: Teaching the Recommended Daily Allowances. Am. J. Clin. Nutr. 23:1639, 1970.)

TABLE 11–2   SUMMARY OF RECOMMENDED DAILY NUTRIENT INTAKES FOR CANADIANS

SEX	AGE	WEIGHT	ACTIVITY CATEGORY	CALORIES	PROTEIN*	CALCIUM	IRON	VITAMIN A	VITAMIN D	ASCORBIC ACID	THIAMIN	RIBOFLAVIN	NIACIN
	yr.	*lb.*			*gm.*	*gm.*	*mg.*	*I.U.†*	*I.U.*	*mg.*	*mg.*	*mg.*	*mg.*
Both	0– 1	7–20	usual	360–900	7–13	0.5	5	1,000	400	20	0.3	0.5	3
Both	1– 2	20–26	usual	900–1,200	12–16	0.7	5	1,000	400	20	0.4	0.6	4
Both	2– 3	31	usual	1,400	17	0.7	5	1,000	400	20	0.4	0.7	4
Both	4– 6	40	usual	1,700	20	0.7	5	1,000	400	20	0.5	0.9	5
Both	7– 9	57	usual	2,100	24	1.0	5	1,500	400	30	0.7	1.1	7
Both	10–12	77	usual	2,500	30	1.2	12	2,000	400	30	0.8	1.3	8
Boy	13–15	108	usual	3,100	40	1.2	12	2,700	400	30	0.9	1.6	9
Girl	13–15	108	usual	2,600	39	1.2	12	2,700	400	30	0.8	1.3	8
Boy	16–17	136	B‡	3,700	45	1.2	12	3,200	400	30	1.1	1.9	11
Girl	16–17	120	A#	2,400	41	1.2	12	3,200	400	30	0.7	1.2	7
Boy	18–19	144	B‡	3,800	47	0.9	6	3,200	400	30	1.1	1.9	11
Girl	18–19	124	A#	2,450	41	0.9	10	3,200	400	30	0.7	1.2	7
Male	adult	154	B	3,582	47	0.5	6	3,700	–	30	1.1	1.8	11
Female	adult	124	A	2,390	40	0.5	10	3,700	–	30	0.7	1.2	7

*Protein recommendation is based on normal mixed Canadian diet. Vegetarian diets may require a higher protein content.
†Vitamin A is based on the mixed Canadian diet supplying both vitamin A and carotene. As preformed vitamin A, the suggested intake would be about 2/3 of the indicated.
‡Expenditure assessed as being 113% of that of a man of same weight and engaged in same degree of activity.
#Expenditure assessed as being 104% of that of a woman of the same weight and engaged in the same degree of activity.
From Sabry, Z. I.: The Canadian dietary standard. J. Am. Dietet. A., 56:198, 1970.

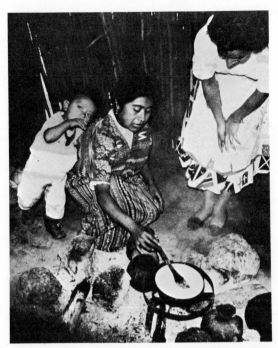

Figure 11–2   Guatemalan mother learns to prepare nourishing meals for her family with help of INCAP nutritionist. (Courtesy of UNICEF. Photo by Bernard Cole.)

teach the population how to prepare nourishing meals (Fig. 11–2). Proteins, carbohydrates, fats, vitamins, minerals, cellulose and water need to be provided through the daily meals in sufficient quantity to meet the needs of the body.

Animal proteins are furnished through meats (muscle and organs), fish, fowl, eggs, milk and products made from milk, such as cheese. Vegetable proteins are furnished through nuts, legumes, grains, and some of the vegetables and fruits. A blend of the two types of proteins is needed to provide the essential amino acids.

Carbohydrates are supplied through grains, fruits, vegetables, starches and sugars.

Fats are furnished through the "invisible" fat content of meats, eggs, cheese, and nuts, and the "visible" fats, such as butter, fortified margarine, oil, cream, and products made from cream.

Vitamins and minerals are supplied through meats, fish, fowl, eggs, milk and products made from milk, and through nuts, legumes, grains, and some of the fruits and vegetables. Some foods have higher vitamin and mineral content than others. It is important to know the best sources in relation to the availability in the region and the socioeconomic status. The tables of food values are used as guides. (See Appendix Tables 1 and 2.)

Cellulose is furnished through the skins,

peelings and pulp of fruits and vegetables, and the hulls of grains.

Water is supplied as such, and through the water content of foods and liquids.

APPLICATION OF DIETARY ALLOWANCES

In the previous discussion and chapters the physiological necessities for specific nutrients have been presented. These nutrition facts can be arranged now into a basic pattern to assist in the planning of meals. This pattern is essentially the same as the four food groups outlined by the Institute of Home Economics (see Fig. 2–1).

The various quantities of nutrients recommended as allowances may generally be obtained from usual portions of commonly available foods in the United States. As previously pointed out, variety in foods is of considerable advantage in the selection of an adequate diet, since it offers the potential of affording many essential nutrients in natural proportions. Some foods are unique because of their important contributions to the diet. For example, milk is an important source of calcium, protein, and riboflavin; citrus fruits and tomatoes provide relatively large amounts of ascorbic acid. Table 11–3 offers a guide to the foods that should be included daily in meals.

This basic pattern forms a *foundation* for a good diet providing the essential nutrients. It will supply the adult with approximately one half the caloric allowance, all the protein, vitamin A and riboflavin, ascorbic acid and calcium. Almost all the thiamin and niacin allowances are provided but the iron supply is about half that needed by the female adult. Other foods are added, as necessary, to meet the caloric requirement and to add palatability. These may be more of the same foods listed above, or others. Since butter, margarine, other fats, oils, sugars, and refined cereal foods are usually combined with other specified foods, they are not included in the food plan. See Table 11–4 for an evaluation of the foundation of an adequate diet for an adult.

The Milk Group is counted on to provide most of the calcium requirement. In addition, it provides riboflavin, high quality protein, other vitamins and minerals, carbohydrates, and fat. The milk allowance is used in the form of fluid whole or skim milk, buttermilk, evaporated milk, dry milk, and cheese. A portion may be used in cooking. Approximate equivalents of 1 cup of fluid milk, according to calcium content, are outlined in Chapter 38, Milk.

TABLE 11–3   DAILY FOOD GUIDE

FOOD GROUP	DAILY AMOUNTS	MAIN CONTRIBUTION
I. Milk and cheese or equivalents*	Children under 9: 2 to 3 cups Children 9 to 12: 3 or more cups Teenagers: 4 or more cups Adults: 2 or more cups Pregnancy: 3 or more cups Lactation: 4 or more cups	Calcium Protein Riboflavin Vitamin D
II. Meat: Beef, veal, pork, lamb, poultry, fish, eggs Alternates: Dry beans, dry peas, lentils, nuts, peanut butter	2 or more servings Serving size: 2–3 ounces lean, boneless cooked meat, poultry, fish 2 eggs 1 cup cooked dry beans, dry peas or lentils 4 tablespoons peanut butter	Protein Thiamin Iron Niacin Riboflavin
III. Breads and cereals (whole-grain or enriched)	4 or more servings Serving size: 1 slice bread 1/2 to 3/4 cup cooked cereal, macaroni, spaghetti, hominy grits, kasha, rice, noodles, bulgur 1 ounce (1 cup) ready-to-eat cereal 5 saltines or 2 Graham crackers	Thiamin Riboflavin Niacin Iron Protein
IV. Vegetables and fruits	4 or more servings Serving size: 1/2 cup dark green or deep yellow every other day 1/2 cup or 1 medium citrus fruit (or any raw fruit or vegetable rich in ascorbic acid) Other vegetables and fruit including potato (1 medium)	Vitamin A Ascorbic Acid Other vitamins and minerals
Water	6 to 8 glasses	

*Milk equivalents: 1 cup whole or skimmed milk, 1 cup buttermilk, 1/2 cup evaporated milk, 1/4 cup non-fat milk powder, 1 ounce cheddar cheese, 2 cups ice cream, 1-1/2 cups cottage cheese. (The amount given is figured on the basis of calcium content.)

The Meat Group provide generous amounts of protein of high quality. In addition, iron, thiamin, riboflavin and niacin are supplied. At least once a week, liver, kidney and salt water fish such as salmon, oysters and mackerel are included in the animal protein allowance. See Chapter 39.

The Bread and Cereal Group furnish thiamin, protein, iron, and niacin at a relatively low cost. The enrichment of breads and cereals with iron, thiamin, riboflavin, and niacin substantially contributes additional amounts of these nutrients to the diet. See Chapter 41, Bread-Cereal Group.

The Vegetable and Fruit Group are important suppliers of vitamins and minerals, particularly vitamins A and C. Dark green and deep yellow vegetables are especially valuable for vitamin A, and citrus fruits for vitamin C. See Chapter 40.

The above foods in adequate amounts along with fat and oil taken into the body, vitamin E, vitamin K, vitamin B_6, vitamin B_{12}, pantothenic acid, biotin, folic acid and minerals (trace), will also be provided for the normal healthy adult.

Salt pork, fatback and bacon are considered fat, not meat. Molasses, syrups, honey, jellies, jams, sugars, and candies are considered sweets.

If perspiration is excessive, the water allowance is increased to make up for any dehydration.

FAMILY MEAL PLANNING AND SAMPLE MENUS

Contrary to beliefs that different age members of the family require specific foods, the suggested basic pattern for meals applies to the entire family group. Deviations may be made from it to meet the requirements of children or the aging members, and for activity. For example, some of the custard filling of a pie may be baked separately and

TABLE 11-4   EVALUATION OF THE FOUNDATION OF AN ADEQUATE DIET FOR AN ADULT

| FOOD | AVERAGE SERVING | | KILO-CALORIES | PRO-TEIN GM. | FAT GM. | CARBO-HYDRATE GM. | MINERALS | | VITAMINS | | | | |
	Household Measure	Weight Gm.					Calcium Mg.	Iron Mg.	A. (I.U.)	Ascorbic Acid Mg.	Thiamin Mg.	Riboflavin Mg.	Niacin Mg.
Milk, whole (or equivalent)	1 pt.	488	320	18.0	18	24	576	.2	700	4	.16	.84	.2
Meat group													
Eggs	1	50	80	6.0	6	tr.	27	1.1	590	—	.05	.15	tr.
Meat, poultry, fish[1]	3 oz. (cooked)	85	237	23.0	15	0	10	2.4	10	—	.09	.21	4.7
Vegetable–fruit group													
Vegetables:													
Deep green or yellow[2]	1 salad or cooked	50 raw or 75 cooked	27	1.4	tr.	6	36.7	.6	3016	20.5	.046	.08	.4
Other, cooked[3]	1/2 cup	80	41	2.5	tr.	7.7	15	.93	225	11	.12	.06	1.5
Potato, peeled, boiled	1 medium	122	80	2.0	tr.	18	7	.6	tr.	20	.11	.04	1.4
Fruits:													
Citrus[4]	1 serving	125	57	.8	tr.	14	28	.35	302	58	.09	.03	.36
Other (fresh and canned)[5]	1 serving	150	92	.5	tr.	24	8	.5	164	5	.03	.04	.4
Bread–cereal group													
Cereal (whole grain and enriched)[6]	1/2 cup cooked	28 (dry)	88	2.2	1	17.7	7.7	.6	—	—	.11	.02	.3
Bread (whole grain and enriched)	3 slices	69	180	6.0	3	36	57	1.8	tr.	tr.	.18	.15	1.8
Totals[7]			1202 (5000 k.J.)	62.4	43	147.4	772.4	9.1[8]	5007[8]	118.5[9]	.986[9]	1.62	11.6[10]
Recommended Daily Dietary Allowances*													
Man (age, 35–55; wt, 70 kg, ht, 173 cm.)			2600	65			800	10	5000	60	1.3	1.7	17[11]
Woman (Age, 35–55; wt, 58 kg, ht, 160 cm.)			1900	55			800	18	5000	55	1.0	1.5	13[11]

Evaluation based on Table 91 in the Appendix.
[1] Evaluation based on figures for cooked (lean and fat) beef, lamb, and veal.
[2] Evaluation based on lettuce, cooked carrots, green beans, winter squash and broccoli.
[3] Evaluation based on average for cooked peas and beets.
[4] Evaluation based on Florida orange and white and pink grapefruit; whole and juice.
[5] Evaluation based on canned peaches, applesauce, raw pears, apples and bananas.
[6] Evaluation based on oatmeal and cornflakes.
[7] With the addition of more of the same foods, or other foods, to meet calorie requirement, the totals will be increased.

[8] With the use of liver this figure will be markedly increased.
[9] With the use of pork, legumes and liver this figure will be markedly increased.
[10] The average diet in the United States, which contains a generous amount of protein, provides enough tryptophan to increase the niacin value by about a third.
[11] These figures are expressed as niacin equivalents, which include dietary sources of the preformed vitamin and the precursor, tryptophan.
*Recommended Dietary Allowances. Washington, D.C., National Research Council, Publication 1694, 1968.

served to the children and grandparents while the custard pie is served to the adults.

If the working members of the family and schoolchildren carry lunch, then some of the vegetable and meat allowances may be chopped into a sandwich filling. There are also dessert types of sandwiches which have fillings of chopped raisins and peanuts, sliced banana and peanut butter, orange marmalade or jam with cottage cheese, and chopped prunes and peanut butter.

The art of planning nutritious meals incorporates the knowledge of nutrition facts, the regional availability of foods, and cookery skills. Thought should be given to texture and color for "eye appeal," which is important for both the well and the sick. If meals are planned in advance there is less chance of guesswork or the omission of essential nutrients. A shopping list is made from the menus, checking the supplies needed against those which are on hand. However, the shopping list should be sufficiently flexible to take advantage of economical, abundant foods in the market.

There are many choices of food around the world which will provide adequate meals for the day. From the nutrition point of view, a meal should contain a complete protein (single food or mutual supplement combination), sufficient calories for energy needs and satisfying qualities. An adequate diet pattern for the daily meals for a family is suggested below.

BREAKFAST

Fruit or fruit juice
Egg and/or ham, sausage, bacon, or fish
Whole grain or enriched toast; griddle cakes; or rolls; or cereal with milk and sugar
Butter or fortified margarine
Milk or milk drink for children
Coffee or tea for adults

DINNER

Main dish of meat, fish, fowl, cheese, eggs or other protein-rich food combination
Potato or other starch food (rice, grits, spaghetti, macaroni, noodles)
Cooked green or yellow vegetable
Raw vegetable salad
Whole grain or enriched bread, biscuits or roll and butter or fortified margarine
Dessert
Milk or milk drink for children
Coffee or tea for adults

SUPPER OR LUNCH

Casserole, stew or soup
Sandwich with filling of meat or peanut butter or cheese and chopped vegetable, tuna or egg salad
Cooked or raw fruit
Milk, milk shake

SNACK

(during day or evening)
Milk for children and teenagers
Cereal, graham cracker, roll, cookies, pizza or hamburger.

OMITTING A MEAL   It is important to stress again that meals should be served regularly at approximately the same time each day. If any meal is omitted or neglected, there is too much nutritional load put on the remaining meals in the day's meal plan. For example, if breakfast is omitted, the intake of nutrients for the day is inadequate or one's food intake is concentrated later in the day instead of divided throughout the twenty-four hours. Many times poor snacks, which are mainly "empty" calorie foods and drinks, comprise the entire day's food intake for teenagers.

The neglect of breakfast is more common in cities than in rural areas and does not seem to be related to income. Eating breakfast has been found essential for maximum efficiency —both physical and mental—during the morning hours. Skipping or slighting breakfast results in decreased output and decreased mental alertness. Four separate studies conducted at the University of Iowa Medical School showed the basic or medium breakfast, providing 25 per cent of the day's calories, permits, in most cases, a greater work output than a breakfast supplying 40 per cent of the day's calories. Unfortunately, one may not recognize the damage being done to the body through poor food habits until too late.

SAMPLE MENUS   Sometimes five or six small meals are preferable to the usual three meals, in which case the milk and/or fruit allowance could be taken between meals. Some authors report this increases efficiency. It is important to prepare the foods tastily, and serve them attractively to favorably influence the appetite. Contrast in textures and color are other influential factors.

When planning meals, some nutritionists classify foods into (1) the essential protective foods and (2) the energy foods. The essential protective foods form the framework of the meal plans and the calorie requirements are completed by the energy foods. A sample menu using the adequate diet pattern follows:

BREAKFAST

Large glass of orange juice
Cereal with milk or cream
Poached egg on toasted enriched bread with fortified margarine or butter
Milk for children   Tea or coffee for adults

DINNER

Roast chicken
Baked sweet potato   Cooked green beans
Tomato, lettuce salad
Whole wheat rolls   Butter or fortified margarine
Ice cream with fruit sauce
Cookies
Milk for children   Tea or coffee for adults

SUPPER OR LUNCH

Cheese souffle
Bran muffins   Butter or fortified margarine
Fruit salad
Milk

The same meal pattern may be adjusted to any socioeconomic status. For example, here is a sample menu suggested for a minimum cost adequate diet.

BREAKFAST

Stewed prunes
Cooked oatmeal with milk
Toasted whole wheat or enriched bread
Fortified margarine
Milk* for children   Tea or coffee for adults

DINNER

Meat or fish or fowl stew with
potatoes, carrots, and onions
Cole slaw
Enriched bread   Fortified margarine
Apple cobbler
Milk* for children   Tea or coffee for adults

SUPPER OR LUNCH

Cream of corn soup*
Sandwiches with fillings of:
(1) baked beans,
(2) chopped hard cooked egg
mixed with chopped greens, and
(3) peanut butter and jam
Tomato juice

COST COMPARISON   To determine the economy of a choice of food, it is helpful to make a cost comparison. For example, to decide the form of milk which is most economical for the family food budget, the following cost analysis could be made:

Whole milk: 7 quarts at. . . cents a quart would cost. . .

Evaporated milk: 7 tall (14½ oz.) cans at . . . cents a can would cost. . .

Skim milk: 7 quarts at. . . cents a quart would cost. . .

Dry whole milk: 23 ounces at. . . cents an ounce would cost. . .

Dry skim milk: 23 ounces at. . . cents an ounce would cost. . .

For food values, Tables 1 and 2 in the Appendix should be consulted.

The same procedure may be followed to determine the most economical source of the other foods and nutrients, as for example, vitamin C, to fit the family food budget: orange juice, canned or frozen grapefruit juice, canned tomatoes, fresh strawberries, raw cabbage, raw turnips or rutabagas. The Daily Food Guide (Table 11–3) and the Food Selection Score Card (Table 2–1) have been devised to assist with meal planning in order to include all the nutrients in the daily diet.

*Reconstructed powdered milk.

NUTRITION IN THE MIDDLE-AGE PERIOD

Nutrition to prevent precocious aging and declining resistance to disease should start early in life.

Increased attention is being given to geriatrics, largely devoted to the prevention of chronic disease and unnecessary disability. Geriatric nutrition will be discussed in Chapter 18.

The middle-age period, from 45 to 60, also needs careful attention. These are the years just prior to senescence. Leaders in the field of nutrition point to these years as the most promising period for discovery and prevention of advancing and preventable illness and disability. It can be called the last chance for effective prevention of unnecessary aging. The middle-age period is frequently referred to as the active, productive period of life. Wise eating habits can play a profound role in prolonging these years and in maintaining vitality and general well-being. It is during these years that the body is most generally neglected and abused, that stress and nervous strain of business and work are greatest; this can only be combated by a body in top physical condition. Hurried meals, frequently skipped meals, irregular eating times and improper selection of foods take their toll.

Overweight and underweight are also problems, but the former is much more common and serious from the standpoint of longevity. It is during middle age that metabolism and activity are slowing down, and adequate modifications in food intake should be taken to extend the productive years of life. Obese individuals are prone to develop the common chronic diseases, such as diabetes, hypertension, osteoarthritis, and the degenerative cardiovascular diseases. (See Chapter 29, Overweight and Underweight.)

RECOMMENDED DAILY DIETARY ALLOWANCES   The Food and Nutrition Board lists the recommended daily dietary allowances for ages 35 to 55 (see Table 11–1), which can be attained with a great variety of common foods, as previously described in this chapter.

ADEQUATE NUTRITION FOR ASTRONAUTS IN SPACE

Space nutrition is a whole new concept and is only touched on here. Adequate nutrition for man in space offers many problems. The astronaut is a particularly healthy man by virtue of selection. He requires all the nutritional factors required by earth man. Individual requirement demands calorie intake that will not increase body mass or lose body weight. Lack of knowledge concerning the influence of the space conditions on man— weightlessness—makes it difficult to predict the energy required for activity. The main tasks in flight are classified as largely sedentary. The precise estimation of energy requirements are critical and based on the need for oxygen. Calloway[3] estimates a 2800 calorie diet as a safe allowance for routine space missions. Consideration of calorie density suggests that 50 per cent of the diet, or approximately 150 gm. should be derived from fat. On the basis of present knowledge, 0.9 gm. protein/kg. of body weight, or approxi-

mately 75 gm./day is allowed. Therefore, a total of approximately 285 gm. of carbohydrate is needed to make up the balance of calories. The minerals calcium, sodium, potassium and magnesium are provided in amounts 10 per cent above normal requirements to meet needs of anticipated stress. All other minerals are supplied by a mixed diet of processed foods. Animal research indicates that increased levels of ascorbic acid, vitamin E, and possibly thiamin are beneficial at high altitude. Liberal allowances of all vitamins are recommended, particularly ascorbic acid and vitamin E.

FOODS   Foods must be compact, conveniently prepared and easily eaten in space.

[3]Calloway, D. H.: Nutritional aspects of gastronautics. J. Am. Dietet. A., 44:347, 1964.

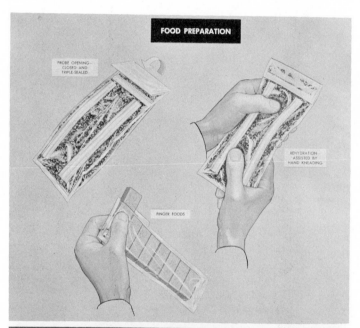

Figure 11–3   Food package which will serve as storage vessel, food preparation utensil, and eating device. (Courtesy of Beatrice Finkelstein and J. Am. Dietet. A.)

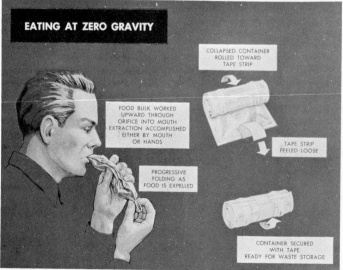

Figure 11–4   Eating at zero gravity by expelling food from food package. (Courtesy of Beatrice Finkelstein and J. Am. Dietet. A.)

(See Figs. 11–3 and 11–4). Conditions dictate the predominant use of precooked, dehydrated, spray- or drum-dried foods. Some can be obtained from commercial sources and some will need to be custom produced. It is emphasized that "gas-producing" foods must be avoided in space diets on the basis that the gases produced are noxious and flammable. In addition, at reduced atmospheric pressure, expansion of gas volume can cause incapacitating pain due to distention.

Food preparation in the first missions consisted of the addition of water (hot or cold) in specified amounts. Food packaging and eating devices were designed and developed by the Food and Container Division of the U.S. Army Natick Laboratories, Natick, Massachusetts[4] working with the National Aeronautics and Space Administration (NASA) (See Fig. 11–5). Twenty-three bite-size foods and 37 dehydrated foods were included in the early missions. An average of 45 ounces (1330 ml.) water was required to reconstitute one day's menu. Approximately 2500 ml. water (5.5 lb.) was required per man per day for drinking and for the reconstitution of foods and beverages. A feeding system for one man per day contained 1.5 lb. of food which when packaged weighed approximately 1.67 lb. and occupied 225 cu. in. of space.[5]

In the voyage to the moon the astronauts Armstrong, Aldrin and Collins enjoyed a variety of food, enough to satisfy their hunger and to enable them to maintain performance. The first meal on the moon consisted of a light meal of fortified candy sticks, intermediate-moisture fruit, ham salad sandwich and rehydratable beverage. The food consumption on this mission (Apollo XI) was estimated to average 1800 to 2000 kcal. a day. In this mission the food supply came closer to meeting all the engineering, physiological and psychological requirements than in any previous flight. The problem of acceptability of foods in space is present. Eating habits are not easily changed or ignored. The food presented to man in the manner to which he is accustomed provides good nutrition. Astronauts now help plan the menus. The reader will recall the comments made when Borman, Lovell and Anders opened a surprise food package on Christmas Day and found natural chunks of turkey and brown gravy, bright red cranberry applesauce and an honest-to-goodness spoon. That meal proved it was possible to have familiar and tasty

[4]Klicka, M. V.: Development of space foods. J. Am. Dietet. A., 44:358, 1964.

[5]Finkelstein, B., and Symons, J.: Feeding concepts for manned space stations. J. Am. Dietet. A., 44:353, 1964.

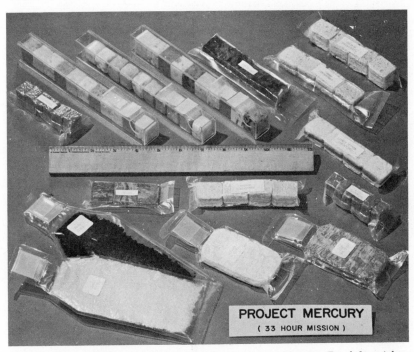

Figure 11–5   Bite-size foods available for astronauts' selection in Project Mercury. Top, left to right: cornflake cubes; three dispensers containing nine varieties of bite-size dessert-type cubes; fruit cake; beef sandwiches, and chicken sandwiches. At the end of the ruler; peanut butter sandwiches. Below the ruler; orange juice, grape juice, bacon squares, cheese sandwiches, chicken and gravy; and rice-cornflake cubes. (U.S. Army photo.)

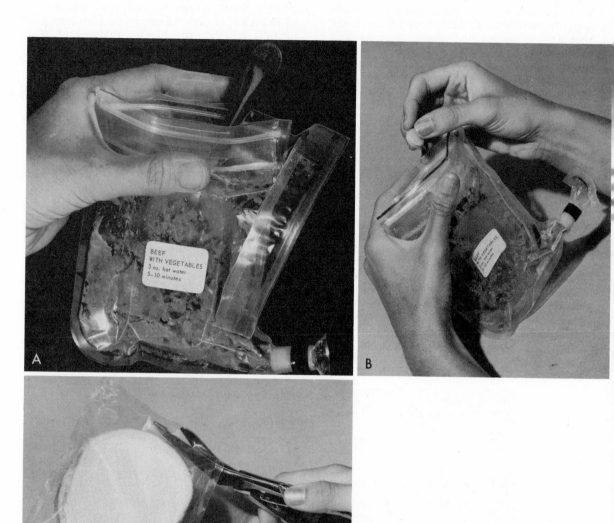

BEEF
WITH VEGETABLES
3 oz. hot water
5–10 minutes

Figure 11–6 Familiar and tasty foods and using utensils in space missions. (Courtesy of NASA.)

foods and be able to eat them with utensils, too (Fig. 11–6). The moon flight recorded considerable information about energy requirements. Every food program is influenced by the health of the people for which it is planned and the astronauts are no exception. Engineers, biologists, physicians and nutritionists have a challenge to design a feeding program for the space food system that will stimulate the appetite, allay hunger, be easy to prepare, be familiar in texture and flavor, provide pleasure and impart a sense of security.[6]

PROBLEMS AND SUGGESTED TOPICS FOR DISCUSSION

1. List your food intake for a week and compare with the basic food pattern on page 18. List any necessary adjustments for improvement.
2. Compare the daily nutritional allowances suggested for each member of the following family as determined from Table 11–1: Mother, age 35, overweight 30 pounds, who does own housework; father, age 40, who works as a mason and carries his lunch; girls, ages 3 and 6; active boy, age 12, 10 pounds underweight, who goes to school and comes home for lunch.
3. Compare costs of different available sources of milk to meet the daily calcium allowance. Follow the same procedure to compare costs of foods containing ascorbic acid; iron.
4. Why should a student nurse start the habit of eating adequate nutritious meals?

SUGGESTED ADDITIONAL READING REFERENCES

Bulletin. Conserving the Nutritive Values in Foods. Washington, D. C., U.S. Department of Agriculture, Home and Garden Bulletin Number 90, 1963.
Bulletin. Facts About Nutrition. Washington, D.C., U.S.

[6]Smith, M., and Berry, C. A.: Dinner on the moon. Nutrition Today, 4:37, 1970.

Army Department of Health, Education, and Welfare, Public Health Service Pub. No. 917, 1963.
Bulletin. Family Fare: A Guide to Good Nutrition. Washington, D.C., U.S. Department of Agriculture. Home and Garden Bulletin Number 1, Revised, 1970.
Bulletin. Food for the Young Couple. Washington, D. C., U.S. Department of Agriculture, Home and Garden Bulletin No. 85, 1967.
Bulletin. Food for Fitness—A Daily Food Guide. Washington, D.C., U.S. Department of Agriculture, Leaflet 424.
Burton, B. T. (ed.): Heinz Handbook of Nutrition. 2nd ed. New York, McGraw-Hill Book Company, 1965, Chapter 15, The Normal Adult Diet.
Church, C. F., and Church, H. N.: Food Values of Portions Commonly Used. 11th ed. Philadelphia, J. B. Lippincott Company, 1970.
Dairy Council Digest: Recommended Dietary Allowances Reviewed, 1968. Chicago, National Dairy Council, 39: Nov.-Dec., 1968.
Hayes, J. (ed.): Food for Us All. Yearbook of Agriculture, 1969. U.S. Government Printing Office, Washington, D.C.
Leverton, R. M.: Basic nutrition concepts. J. Home Econ., 59:346, 1967.
Maynard, L. A.: An adequate diet. J.A.M.A., 170:457, 1959.
McLean, B. B.: Planning Meals for the Family. Food: The Yearbook of Agriculture, 1959. Washington, D.C., U.S. Department of Agriculture, pp. 510–518.
Ohlson, M. A., and Hart, B. P.: Influence of breakfast on total day's food intake. J. Am. Dietet. A., 47:282, 1965.
Recommended Dietary Allowances. 7th revised ed. Washington, D.C., Food and Nutrition Board, National Academy of Sciences—National Research No. 1694, 1968.
Sabry, Z. I.: The Canadian dietary standard. J. Ann. Diet. A., 56:195, 1970.
Smith, M., and Berry, C. A.: Dinner on the Moon, Nutrition Today, 4:37, 1969.
Turner, D.: Handbook of Diet Therapy. 5th ed. Chicago, University of Chicago Press, 1970, Chapters 1 and 2.
Tuttle, W. W., Daum, K., Meyers, L., and Martin, C.: Effect of omitting breakfast on the physiologic response of men. J. Am. Dietet. A., 26:332, 1950.
Walker, A. R. P.: Optimal intake of nutrients. Nutr. Rev. 23:231, 1965.
Wilson, E. D., et al.: Principles of Nutrition. 2nd ed. New York, John Wiley & Sons, 1965. Importance of breakfast, p. 438.
Williams, R. J.: We abnormal normals. Nutrition Today, 2:19, 1967.
Wohl, M. G., and Goodhart, R. S. (ed.): Modern Nutrition in Health and Disease. 4th ed. Philadelphia, Lea & Febiger, 1968.

Chapter 12
FOOD ECONOMICS

Economics may be defined as the science dealing with the production, distribution, exchange and consumption of wealth. This chapter will deal with economics as it relates to food, with special emphasis on food economy. During the past half century the science of food economics has made tremendous progress. The growing, processing, and packaging of food so that it can be transported for thousands of miles and remain in good condition for months or even years are among the wonders of modern living.

The food plans, menu planning suggestions and examples, market order, economy hints for planning, marketing and cooking provided in this chapter are basic guidelines primarily. They are the information and tools helpful to those counseling individuals and families. The counselor using the principles of teaching-learning (see Chap. 2) assists homemakers in improving their dietary patterns, in changing improper habits and in providing adequate nutrition. The problem solving begins with the amount of money the homemaker or individual has to spend for food and the kind of food she purchases. From this data, the counselor and the homemaker would plan the appropriate steps toward the goals desired.

THE COST OF AN ADEQUATE DIET

BUDGET ALLOWANCE FOR FOOD   Food takes the greatest share of the family budget at a low or moderate income level. This is particularly true of the large family when as much as half or even more of income may be allotted to food. As a rule, when the income is high, the food allowance is proportionally small. It costs more to feed a large family, but the average cost per person is less, as the small family generally cannot buy and prepare the meals as economically as the large one.

In the United States more than 100 billion dollars a year is spent for food. This represents a little more than 17 per cent on the average of the take-home pay (about 5 per cent less than that spent for food in 1950). A recent study indicated that the percentage of income spent for food varied from about 30 per cent for families with incomes below 3000 dollars to approximately 12 per cent for those earning 15,000 dollars or more. A larger share of food preparation is done outside the home than it was two decades ago. The highest income group spent approximately a third of the money spent for food for meals and snacks eaten away from home.[1]

Food prices tend to follow the general economic trend in the nation. They represent costs and profits earned by farmers, processors and retail operators. One way in which the U.S. Department of Agriculture measures trends in prices of food that originate on farms in the United States is by changes in the cost of a "market basket." The quantities and qualities of foods in this market basket are kept constant. The market basket is based upon the average quantities of food purchased per year by the families of the urban wage earner and clerical worker and by single workers living alone. The cost is estimated using retail prices that are published by the Bureau of Labor Statistics. During the past decade the retail cost of the market basket has increased about 14 per cent. Rising marketing costs have been the main cause for higher prices; approximately two-thirds of the increase in retail cost is due to marketing costs. Currently the populace tends to purchase expensive and higher quality foods than it did a decade ago.[2]

The average family will spend approximately one-half its food budget for milk, meat and eggs and about one-fifth for vegetables and fruits. The rest is almost equally divided between grain products, oils, sugars and miscellaneous. Nearly one-fifth of the money spent in supermarkets is not for food. It is for something to wear, read, clean with, listen to, smoke, as well as alcoholic beverages and drugs.

THE FOOD PLAN   To assure adequate nutrition for each member of the family, it is wise to use a plan. The Recommended Daily Dietary Allowances of the Food and Nutrition Board are used as the yardstick for planning the adequate diet as described in Chapter 11, An Adequate Diet, and can also serve as the basis for determining the cost of an adequate diet as shown in Tables 12-1, 12-2, and 12-3. These three food plans—a low cost, a moderate cost, and a liberal plan, based on the latest information on food consumption and nutritional recommendations—were worked out and published in booklet form by the Consumer and Food Economics Research Division, Agriculture Research Service, U.S.D.A.[3] Each plan can be used as a guide for weekly budgeting, marketing and individual or family food planning, as it shows the approximate amount of food needed by each member of a family. Table 12-4 shows the estimated cost of each of three low, moderate and liberal food plans for one week's and one month's food supplies for four family groups as well as for sex-age groups, and pregnant and lactating women, estimated on the basis that all meals are served at home or from the home food supply. Meals away from home cost about twice as much as when prepared in the home. In the food survey of United States diets for men, women and children for one day in spring (1965) some 62 per cent of the farm families spent on the

[1]Heimstron, S. J.: Telescoping 20 years of change in the food we eat. Food For Us All, 1969 Yearbook of Agriculture, U.S. Department of Agriculture.

[2]Durham, D. F., and Frye, R. E.: Shedding light on the prices we pay for our food. Food For Us All, 1969 Yearbook of Agriculture, U.S. Department of Agriculture.

[3]Family Food Plans and Food Costs, Home Economics Research Report No. 20, Agricultural Research Service, U.S.D.A., revised 1964.

TABLE 12–1   FOOD PLAN AT LOW COST: SUGGESTED WEEKLY QUANTITIES OF FOOD[1]

(As Purchased) for 17 Sex-Age Groups, Pregnant and Lactating Women

SEX-AGE GROUP[2]	MILK, CHEESE, ICE CREAM[3]	MEAT, POULTRY, FISH[4]		EGGS	DRY BEANS, PEAS, NUTS		FLOUR, CEREALS, BAKED GOODS[5]		CITRUS FRUIT, TOMATOES		DARK GREEN AND DEEP YELLOW VEGETABLES		POTATOES		OTHER VEGETABLES AND FRUITS		FATS, OILS		SUGARS, SWEETS	
	Qt.	Lb.	Oz.	No.	Lb.	Oz.	Lb.	Oz.	Lb.	Oz.	Lb.	Oz.	Lb.	Oz.	Lb.	Oz.	Lb.	Oz.	Lb.	Oz.
Children:																				
7 months to 1 year	4	1	4	5	0	0	1	0	1	8	0	4	0	8	1	0	0	1	0	2
1 to 3 years	4	1	12	5	0	1	1	8	1	8	0	4	0	12	2	4	0	4	0	4
3 to 6 years	4	2	0	5	0	2	2	0	1	12	0	4	1	4	3	4	0	6	0	6
6 to 9 years	4	2	4	6	0	4	2	12	2	0	0	8	2	4	4	4	0	8	0	10
Girls:																				
9 to 12 years	5½	2	8	7	0	6	2	8	2	4	0	12	2	4	5	0	0	8	0	10
12 to 15 years	7	2	8	7	0	6	2	12	2	4	1	0	2	8	5	0	0	8	0	12
15 to 20 years	7	2	12	7	0	6	2	8	2	4	1	4	2	4	4	12	0	6	0	10
Boys:																				
9 to 12 years	5½	2	8	6	0	6	3	0	2	0	0	12	2	8	5	0	0	8	0	12
12 to 15 years	7	2	8	6	0	6	4	4	2	0	0	12	3	4	5	4	0	12	0	12
15 to 20 years	7	3	8	6	0	6	4	12	2	0	0	12	4	4	5	8	0	14	0	14
Women:																				
20 to 35 years	3½	3	4	7	0	6	2	8	1	12	1	8	2	0	5	0	0	6	0	10
35 to 55 years	3½	3	4	7	0	6	2	4	1	12	1	8	1	8	4	8	0	4	0	10
55 to 75 years	3½	2	8	5	0	4	2	0	2	0	1	0	1	4	3	12	0	4	0	6
75 years and over	3½	2	4	5	0	4	1	8	2	0	1	0	1	4	3	0	0	4	0	6
Pregnant[6]	5½	3	12	7	0	6	2	12	3	4	2	0	1	8	5	8	0	6	0	10
Lactating[6]	8	3	12	7	0	6	3	12	3	4	1	8	3	4	5	8	0	10	0	10
Men:																				
20 to 35 years	3½	3	8	6	0	6	4	4	1	12	0	12	3	4	5	8	0	12	1	0
35 to 55 years	3½	3	4	6	0	6	3	12	1	12	0	12	3	0	5	0	0	10	0	12
55 to 75 years	3½	3	0	6	0	4	2	12	1	12	0	12	2	4	4	8	0	10	0	10
75 years and over	3½	2	12	6	0	4	2	8	1	8	0	12	2	0	4	4	0	8	0	8

[1]Food as purchased or brought into the kitchen from garden or farm.

[2]Age groups include the persons of the first age listed up to but not including those of the second age listed.

[3]Fluid whole milk, or its calcium equivalent in cheese, evaporated milk, dry milk or ice cream. (See Ch. 38 for factors to convert milk products to calcium equivalents of whole fluid milk.)

[4]Bacon and salt pork should not exceed 1/3 pound for each 5 pounds of meat group.

[5]Weight in terms of flour and cereal. Count 1 1/2 pounds bread as 1 pound flour.

[6]Three additional quarts of milk are suggested for pregnant and lactating teenagers.

From Family Economics Review, Consumer and Food Economics Research Division, Agricultural Research Service, U.S. Department of Agriculture, October, 1964.

TABLE 12–2   FOOD PLAN AT MODERATE COST: SUGGESTED WEEKLY QUANTITIES OF FOOD[1] (AS PURCHASED) FOR 17 SEX-AGE GROUPS, PREGNANT AND LACTATING WOMEN

SEX-AGE GROUP[2]	MILK, CHEESE, ICE CREAM[3]	MEAT, POULTRY, FISH[4]		EGGS	DRY BEANS, PEAS, NUTS		FLOUR, CEREALS, BAKED GOODS[5]		CITRUS FRUIT, TOMATOES		DARK GREEN AND DEEP YELLOW VEGETABLES		POTATOES		OTHER VEGETABLES AND FRUITS		FATS, OILS		SUGARS, SWEETS	
	Qt.	Lb.	Oz.	No.	Lb.	Oz.	Lb.	Oz.	Lb.	Oz.	Lb.	Oz.	Lb.	Oz.	Lb.	Oz.	Lb.	Oz.	Lb.	Oz.
Children:																				
7 months to 1 year	5	1	8	6	0	0	0	14	1	8	0	4	0	8	1	8	0	1	0	2
1 to 3 years	5	2	4	6	0	1	1	4	1	8	0	4	0	12	2	12	0	4	0	4
3 to 6 years	5	2	12	6	0	1	1	12	2	0	0	4	1	0	4	0	0	6	0	8
6 to 9 years	5	3	4	7	0	2	2	8	2	4	0	8	1	12	4	12	0	10	0	14
Girls:																				
9 to 12 years	5½	4	4	7	0	4	2	8	2	8	0	12	2	0	5	8	0	8	0	12
12 to 15 years	7	4	8	7	0	4	2	8	2	8	1	0	2	4	5	12	0	12	0	14
15 to 20 years	7	4	8	7	0	4	2	4	2	8	1	4	2	0	5	8	0	8	0	12
Boys:																				
9 to 12 years	5½	4	4	7	0	4	2	12	2	4	0	12	2	4	5	8	0	10	0	14
12 to 15 years	7	4	12	7	0	4	4	0	2	4	0	12	3	0	6	0	0	14	1	0
15 to 20 years	7	5	4	7	0	6	2	8	2	8	0	12	4	0	6	8	1	2	1	2
Women:																				
20 to 35 years	3½	4	12	8	0	4	2	4	2	4	1	8	1	8	5	12	0	8	0	14
35 to 55 years	3½	4	12	8	0	4	2	4	2	4	1	8	1	4	5	0	0	6	0	8
55 to 75 years	3½	4	4	6	0	2	1	8	2	4	0	12	1	4	4	4	0	6	0	8
75 years and over	3½	3	8	6	0	2	1	4	2	4	0	12	1	0	3	12	0	4	0	8
Pregnant[6]	5½	5	8	8	0	4	2	12	3	4	2	0	1	8	5	12	0	6	0	8
Lactating[6]	8	5	8	8	0	4	3	12	3	8	1	8	2	12	6	4	0	12	0	12
Men:																				
20 to 35 years	3½	5	0	7	0	4	4	0	2	4	0	12	3	0	6	8	1	0	1	4
35 to 55 years	3½	4	12	7	0	4	3	8	2	4	0	12	2	8	5	12	0	14	1	0
55 to 75 years	3½	4	8	7	0	2	2	8	2	4	0	12	2	4	5	8	0	12	0	14
75 years and over	3½	4	8	7	0	2	2	4	2	4	0	12	2	0	5	4	0	8	0	12

[1]Food as purchased or brought into the kitchen from garden or farm.
[2]Age groups include the persons of the first age listed up to but not including those of the second age listed.
[3]Fluid whole milk, or its calcium equivalent in cheese, evaporated milk, dry milk or ice cream. (See Ch. 38 for factors to convert milk products to calcium equivalents of whole fluid milk.)
[4]Bacon and salt pork should not exceed 1/3 pound for each 5 pounds of meat group.
[5]Weight in terms of flour and cereal. Count 1 1/2 pounds bread as 1 pound flour.
[6]Three additional quarts of milk are suggested for pregnant and lactating teenagers.
From Family Economics Review, Consumer and Food Economics Research Division, Agricultural Research Service, U.S. Department of Agriculture, October, 1964.

TABLE 12–3   FOOD PLAN AT LIBERAL COST: SUGGESTED WEEKLY QUANTITIES OF FOOD (AS PURCHASED) FOR 17 SEX-AGE GROUPS, PREGNANT AND LACTATING WOMEN

SEX-AGE GROUP[1]	MILK, CHEESE, ICE CREAM[2]	MEAT, POULTRY, FISH[3]		EGGS	DRY BEANS, PEAS, NUTS		FLOUR, CEREALS, BAKED GOODS[4]		CITRUS FRUIT, TOMATOES		DARK GREEN AND DEEP YELLOW VEGETABLES		POTATOES		OTHER VEGETABLES AND FRUITS		FATS, OILS		SUGARS, SWEETS	
	Qt.	Lb.	Oz.	No.	Lb.	Oz.	Lb.	Oz.	Lb.	Oz.	Lb.	Oz.	Lb.	Oz.	Lb.	Oz.	Lb.	Oz.	Lb.	Oz.
Children:																				
7 months to 1 year	6	1	4	7	0	0	0	12	1	12	0	2	0	8	1	8	0	2	0	2
1 to 3 years	6	2	4	7	0	1	1	0	1	12	0	4	0	12	2	12	0	4	0	4
4 to 6 years	6	3	0	7	0	1	1	8	2	4	0	8	0	12	4	8	0	8	0	12
7 to 9 years	6	3	12	7	0	2	1	12	2	12	0	8	1	8	5	4	0	10	1	0
10 to 12 years	6½	4	12	7	0	4	2	12	3	0	0	12	2	4	6	0	0	10	1	0
Girls:																				
13 to 15 years	7	5	8	7	0	2	2	8	3	0	0	12	2	4	6	0	0	12	1	2
16 to 19 years	7	5	4	7	0	2	2	4	3	0	0	12	1	12	5	12	0	10	1	0
Boys:																				
13 to 15 years	7	5	8	7	0	4	4	0	3	4	0	12	3	0	6	8	0	14	1	4
16 to 19 years	7	6	4	7	0	6	5	0	3	8	0	12	4	4	7	4	1	4	1	2
Women:																				
20 to 34 years	4	4	12	6	0	1	2	0	3	0	0	12	1	4	6	4	0	8	1	2
35 to 54 years	4	4	12	6	0	1	1	12	3	0	0	12	1	0	6	0	0	8	1	0
55 to 74 years	4	4	12	6	0	1	1	8	3	0	0	12	1	0	4	8	0	6	0	12
75 years and over	4	4	4	6	0	1	1	8	3	0	0	12	0	12	4	0	0	6	0	10
Pregnant	7	4	12	7	0	1	2	0	4	8	1	8	1	4	6	4	0	8	1	0
Lactating	10	5	12	7	0	2	2	12	5	8	1	8	2	8	6	4	0	12	1	2
Men:																				
20 to 34 years	4	6	0	7	0	4	3	12	3	0	0	12	2	12	7	12	1	0	1	8
35 to 54 years	4	5	8	7	0	4	3	8	3	0	0	12	2	4	6	8	0	14	1	4
55 to 74 years	4	5	4	7	0	2	3	4	3	0	0	12	2	0	6	0	0	12	1	2
75 years and over	4	5	4	7	0	2	2	12	2	12	0	12	1	12	5	12	0	10	1	0

[1]Quantities of food suggested here are based on growth needs and activity levels suitable for people in the U.S.A.

[2]Fluid whole milk, or its equivalent in cheese, evaporated milk, dry milk, or ice cream. See Ch. 38 for factors to convert milk products to calcium equivalent of whole fluid milk.

[3]Includes bacon and salt pork not to exceed ⅓ pound for each 5 pounds of meat group.

[4]Weight in terms of flour and cereal. Count 1 pound bread or baked goods as 0.6 pound flour or cereal.

From Family Food Plans and Food Costs. Home Economics Research Report No. 20, Agricultural Research Service, USDA, 1962, and Family Food Budgeting for Good Meals and Good Nutrition. Home and Garden Bull. No. 94, U.S. Department of Agriculture, 1964.

TABLE 12–4 COST OF FOOD AT HOME

Cost of food at home estimated for food plans at three cost levels, March 1971, U.S. average[1]

SEX-AGE GROUPS[2]	COST FOR ONE WEEK (in dollars)			COST FOR ONE MONTH (in dollars)		
	Low-cost plan	Moderate-cost plan	Liberal plan	Low-cost plan	Moderate-cost plan	Liberal plan
FAMILIES						
Family of 2:						
20 to 35 years[3]	18.50	23.50	28.90	80.20	102.10	125.50
55 to 75 years[3]	15.10	19.70	23.60	65.70	85.10	102.40
Family of 4:						
Preschool children[4]	26.80	34.20	41.60	116.30	148.20	180.40
School children[5]	31.10	39.80	48.90	135.10	182.80	212.10
INDIVIDUALS[6]						
Children:						
Under 1 year	3.60	4.50	5.10	15.50	19.60	21.90
1 to 3 years	4.60	5.80	6.90	19.80	25.00	29.90
3 to 6 years	5.40	7.00	8.40	23.60	30.40	36.40
6 to 9 years	6.60	8.50	10.60	28.70	36.90	46.00
Girls:						
9 to 12 years	7.50	9.70	11.40	32.60	42.20	49.40
12 to 15 years	8.30	10.80	13.10	36.00	46.80	56.60
15 to 20 years	8.50	10.70	12.80	36.80	46.50	55.30
Boys:						
9 to 12 years	7.70	9.90	12.00	33.50	43.10	52.00
12 to 15 years	9.10	11.90	14.20	39.30	51.60	61.50
15 to 20 years	10.40	13.30	16.00	45.30	57.50	69.50
Women:						
20 to 35 years	7.80	9.90	12.00	33.80	43.00	51.90
35 to 55 years	7.50	9.60	11.50	32.40	41.50	49.90
55 to 75 years	6.30	8.20	9.80	27.50	35.60	42.50
75 years and over	5.80	7.30	9.00	25.00	31.70	38.80
Pregnant	9.30	11.60	13.70	40.20	51.20	59.40
Nursing	10.80	13.40	15.70	46.70	58.00	68.00
Men:						
20 to 35 years	9.00	11.50	14.30	39.10	49.80	62.20
35 to 55 years	8.40	10.70	13.10	36.30	46.30	56.60
55 to 75 years	7.40	9.70	11.70	32.20	41.80	50.60
75 years and over	7.00	9.30	11.20	30.10	40.20	48.60

[1] Estimates computed from quantities in food plans published in Family Economics Review, October, 1964. Costs of the plans were first estimated by using average price per pound of each food group paid by urban survey families at three income levels in 1965. These prices were adjusted to current levels by use of Retail Food Prices by Cities, released by the Bureau of Labor Statistics.

[2] Persons of the first age listed up to but not including the second age.

[3] 10 per cent added for family size adjustment.

[4] Man and woman, 20 to 35 years; children 1 to 3 and 3 to 6 years.

[5] Man and woman, 20 to 35 years; child 6 to 9; and boy 9 to 12 years.

[6] Costs given for persons in families of 4. For other size families, adjust thus: 1-person, add 20 per cent; 2-person, add 10 per cent; 3-person, add 5 per cent; 5-person, subtract 5 per cent; 6-or-more-person, subtract 10 per cent.

Data received from U.S. Department of Agriculture, Agricultural Research Service, Consumer and Food Economics Research Division, June, 1971.

TABLE 12-5   FOOD PLANS ATTAINABLE BY URBAN FAMILIES OF DIFFERENT SIZE
AND INCOME WHEN THEY SPEND AVERAGE PROPORTIONS OF INCOME FOR FOOD

AFTER-TAX FAMILY INCOME (in dollars)	SIZE OF FAMILY				
	2 Persons	3 Persons	4 Persons	5 Persons	6 Persons
2,000 to 4,000	Low-cost	Economy* or low-cost	Economy*	Economy*	Economy*
4,000 to 6,000	Moderate-cost	Low-cost	Low-cost	Economy*	Economy*
6,000 to 8,000	Liberal	Moderate-cost	Low-cost or moderate-cost	Low-cost	Economy* or low-cost
8,000 to 10,000	Liberal	Moderate-cost or liberal	Moderate-cost	Low-cost or moderate-cost	Low-cost
10,000 to 15,000	Liberal	Liberal	Liberal	Moderate-cost or liberal	Low- or moderate-cost
15,000 and over	Liberal	Liberal	Liberal	Liberal	Moderate-cost or liberal

*For families on very limited food budgets. The economy plan (not included in the regular table published quarterly) costs about 20 per cent less than the low-cost plan. All meals are eaten at home or carried from home.

From Budgeting for the Family's Groceries. J. Am. Dietet. A., 57:218, 1970. Taken from Family Economics Review, Agricultural Research Service, U.S. Department of Agriculture, June, 1970.

average per week $6.16 for either meals or snacks away from home. Some 72 per cent of the urban families spent on the average $9.42 per family. Total expenditure for between-meal food and drinks for farm and urban families was approximately the same—25 per cent farm and 22 per cent urban.[4] Table 12-5 recommends the applicable budget level according to family size and income. For further study refer to Family Food Plans and Food Costs, U.S.D.A. Report No. 20. An additional bulletin is available, designed for the consumer[5] using this information and would be especially helpful for the public health or welfare nurse working with population groups.

CHARACTERISTICS OF DIETS AT DIFFERENT LEVELS OF COST   The *basic low-cost* plan (Table 12-1) provides for a diet typical of food patterns in the United States. It is the plan usually used by social welfare and public health agencies for calculating allotments and planning family food budgets. An Economy Food Plan (Table 12-6) includes larger amounts of flour for home baking, more rice and corn products, and some fats. The economy plan is designed for use when funds are limited. The quantities of food provide an adequate diet for 20 per cent less than the

low-cost plan and are suitable for food habits of many groups. (See Table 12-4.) The low-cost and especially the economy plans require skill in buying, storing and preserving food to ensure that the family is well fed nutritionally. The *moderate-cost* plan (Table 12-2) is suitable for the average American family. It includes larger quantities of milk, eggs, meats, fruits and vegetables than the low-cost plans. It also has more variety and less home preparation. The *liberal* plan (Table 12-3) allows for more variety, more animal products, and more fruits and vegetables.

In general, the quantity of milk and milk products, leafy, green, and yellow vegetables, and tomatoes and citrus fruits should not be changed very much, regardless of the amount to be spent for food. The greatest reduction in the cost of food can be made by reducing somewhat the quantities of meat, fish, poultry, and the group described as "other vegetables and fruits," and by increasing the intake of potatoes, cereals, and dry beans and peas. Within any food group there are both expensive and less expensive sources of the essential nutrients. For example, evaporated or powdered milk can be used in place of fresh bottled milk; cereals cooked at home cost less than the ready-to-eat varieties; lower grades and cheaper cuts of meat can be used on the lower cost levels. Additional adjustments are listed in this chapter under "Economy Hints." The housewife who knows how to bake and cook can lower the cost of meals. Ready-to-serve or partially prepared foods are proportionally expensive.

[4]Clark, F.: A scorecard on how we Americans are eating. Food For Us All, 1969 Yearbook of Agriculture, U.S. Department of Agriculture.

[5]Family Food Budgeting for Good Meals and Good Nutrition. U.S. Department of Agriculture, Home and Garden Bulletin No. 94, 1964. Washington, D.C., 20402, Superintendent of Documents. U.S. Govt. Printing Office, 10 cents.

TABLE 12-6 ECONOMY FOOD PLAN—AMOUNTS OF FOOD[1] AND COST FOR A WEEK

SEX-AGE GROUP	MILK, CHEESE, ICE CREAM[2] (Qt.)	MEAT, POULTRY, FISH[3] (Lb. Oz.)	EGGS (No.)	DRY BEANS, PEAS, NUTS[4] (Lb. Oz.)	FLOUR, CEREALS, BAKED GOODS[5] (Lb. Oz.)	CITRUS FRUIT, TOMATOES (Lb. Oz.)	DARK GREEN AND DEEP YELLOW VEGETABLES (Lb. Oz.)	POTATOES (Lb. Oz.)	OTHER VEGETABLES AND FRUITS (Lb. Oz.)	FATS, OILS (Lb. Oz.)	SUGARS, SWEETS (Lb. Oz.)	ESTIMATED COST, U.S. AVERAGE JUNE 1969[6] (dollars)
Children:												
7 months to 1 year	4	1 0	4	0 0	1 0	1 0	0 4	0 12	1 0	0 2	0 2	2.70
1 to 2 years	4	1 4	4	0 1	1 12	1 0	0 4	1 0	2 0	0 0	0 4	3.50
3 to 5 years	3½	1 8	4	0 4	2 4	1 4	0 4	1 8	2 8	0 6	0 6	4.10
6 to 8 years	3½	1 12	5	0 6	3 0	1 8	0 8	2 8	3 0	0 10	0 10	5.00
Girls:												
9 to 11 years	5	1 12	5	0 10	2 12	1 12	0 12	2 8	3 4	0 8	0 10	5.70
12 to 14 years	6	2 0	6	0 6	3 0	1 12	1 0	3 0	3 8	0 10	0 10	6.30
15 to 19 years	6	2 0	6	0 8	2 12	1 12	1 4	2 8	3 4	0 8	0 10	6.40
Boys:												
9 to 11 years	5	2 0	5	0 8	3 4	1 8	0 12	2 12	3 4	0 10	0 12	5.90
12 to 14 years	6	2 0	5	0 10	4 4	1 12	0 12	3 8	3 8	0 14	0 12	6.80
15 to 19 years	6	2 8	5	0 10	5 0	1 12	0 12	4 12	3 8	1 0	0 14	7.90
Women:												
20 to 34 years	3	1 12	6	0 10	2 12	1 8	1 8	2 12	3 0	0 8	0 12	5.90
35 to 54 years	3	1 12	6	0 10	2 8	1 8	1 8	2 8	2 12	0 6	0 8	5.70
55 to 74 years	3	1 8	4	0 6	2 0	1 12	1 0	2 8	2 12	0 6	0 6	4.80
75 years and over	3	1 4	4	0 6	1 12	1 12	1 0	2 0	2 4	0 4	0 6	4.40
Pregnant[7]	5½	2 0	7	0 10	3 0	3 0	2 0	2 8	4 8	0 6	0 6	7.00
Nursing[7]	8	2 0	6	0 10	4 0	3 0	1 8	3 0	4 8	0 12	0 12	8.10
Men:												
20 to 34 years	3	2 0	5	0 8	4 8	1 8	1 12	4 4	3 8	0 14	1 2	6.80
35 to 54 years	3	1 12	5	0 8	4 4	1 8	0 12	3 8	3 4	0 12	0 14	6.30
55 to 74 years	3	1 8	5	0 6	3 4	1 8	0 12	2 12	3 0	0 12	0 10	5.60
75 years and over	3	1 8	5	0 6	3 0	1 8	0 12	2 8	2 12	0 10	0 6	5.30
Total for Family												

[1] Amounts are for food as purchased or brought into the kitchen from garden or farm.

[2] Fluid milk and beverage made from dry or evaporated milk. Cheese and ice cream may replace some milk. Count as equivalent to a quart of fluid whole milk: Natural or processed Cheddar-type cheese, 6 ounces; cottage cheese 2½ pounds; ice cream 1½ quarts.

[3] Bacon and salt pork should not exceed ⅓ pound for each 5 pounds of meat group.

[4] Weight in terms of dry beans and peas, shelled nuts, and peanut butter.

[5] Weight in terms of flour and cereal. Count 1½ pounds of bread and bakery products as 1 pound flour.

[6] Cost estimates are for families who buy all of their food, and eat all meals and snacks at home or carried from home. They are based on selections within food groups and prices paid by survey families with low incomes. Costs given are for individuals in 4-person families. For individuals in other size families, the following adjustments are suggested: 1 person—add 20 per cent; 2 persons—add 10 per cent; 3 persons—add 5 per cent; 5 persons—subtract 5 per cent; 6 or more persons—subtract 10 per cent.

[7] 3 additional quarts of milk a week are suggested for pregnant and nursing women less than 20 years of age.

Taken from Hearings before the Select Committee on Nutrition and Human Needs of the United States Senate, 92nd Congress, First Session, Part 1: Review of the Results of the White House Conference on Food, Nutrition and Health, Washington, D.C., February 23, 24; March 2, 1971.

COST VERSUS ADEQUACY   Studies have shown that there is some relationship between income and an adequate diet. Education, or its lack, is as important as income in determining eating habits. In low-income groups, some diets were found good, while in high-income groups some diets were poor. Education as to the foods which make up an adequate diet is essential. Studies of the food buying practices of urban low-income consumers indicate that they demonstrate considerable grocery shopping sophistication. The majority of these consumers purchase groceries at supermarket stores. They tend to stretch the food bill by buying canned and dried milk, canned fruits and vegetables, breads, potatoes, rice and other cereals in part for meat, fresh milk, fruit and frozen foods.[6]

EMERGENCY FOOD PROGRAM

U.S.D.A. FOOD STAMP PLAN   Through the Food Stamp Plan, eligible low-income households exchange an amount of money for an allotment of food stamps. Stamps are used to purchase any food except alcohol and certain imported items from retail stores at prevailing prices. The purpose is to assist low-income households to increase their food purchasing power to improve their diets. The program is conducted under the auspices of U.S.D.A. in many counties in the United States. The New Food Stamp Amendment (January, 1971) allows older persons eligible for food stamps to use them for food prepared and delivered by a private non-profit organization such as the "meals-on-wheels" program.

U.S.D.A. COMMODITY DISTRIBUTION PROGRAM   Some counties utilize U.S.D.A.'s Commodity Distribution Program for improving diets of low-income households. Food items are distributed free of charge.

Information about the programs may be obtained through the consumer Food Program District Offices of the Consumer and Marketing Service, U.S.D.A.

MEAL PLANNING

Menus are usually planned several days in advance to be certain the essential nutrients and calories are included. These menus should be flexible, however, to make use of leftovers and to take advantage of special food buys.

There are many sources of help for planning attractive, appetizing and economical meals. Food editors of newspapers, maga-zines, radio and television programs regularly discuss plentiful foods and newer, more appetizing ways of serving them. Many food companies distribute leaflets and booklets containing tested recipes and other cooking information helpful to the housewife and for teaching. Many official bulletins related to food and nutrition, meal planning, food preparation, budgets, buying, preservation and production are available from government agencies in most states, as well as from the United States Department of Agriculture, at a small cost or are free of charge. Family Fare, Food Management and Recipes, Home and Garden Bulletin Number 1, United States Department of Agriculture, is complete and easily understood. It can be used as a helpful guide for weekly shopping and family meal planning. The suggested food allowances are grouped to assure good nutrition for all members of the family. The same material is available with the recipes omitted.[7] Additional Nutrition Up to Date Up to You. Additional planning guides are listed at the end of this chapter.

Although wise planning of menus is the first step, the second step emphasizes careful selection of quality foods, and the third step is focused on cookery standards and attractive service.

Following are menus for one week, planned to furnish a family adequate meals at low cost.

Low-Cost Menus for One Week[8]

SUNDAY

Orange juice
Pancakes   Syrup
Butter or margarine
Bacon

Fried chicken[9]
Browned potatoes   Snap beans
Lettuce salad — cottage cheese dressing
Ready-to-serve rolls   Butter or margarine
Apple brown betty[9]

Baked beans with cheese
Toasted rolls
Celery, carrot strips
Plums

●

MONDAY

Orange juice
Oatmeal   Sugar   Milk
Toast   Butter or margarine

Split-pea soup
Deviled egg sandwiches
Raw relishes

[6]Coltrin, D. M., and Bradfield, R. B.: Food buying practices of urban low-income consumers — a review. J. Nutr. Ed., *1*:16, No. 3, 1970.

[7]Nutrition Up to Date Up to You, U.S. Department of Agriculture.

[8]Family Economics Review. Consumer and Food Economics Research Division, Agricultural Research Service, U.S. Department of Agriculture, 1964.

Meat loaf[9]
Scalloped potatoes[9]   Carrots
Green Salad
Cronbread[9]   Butter or margarine
Peach upside-down cake[9]

TUESDAY

Bananas
Ready-to-eat cereal   Sugar   Milk
Toast   Butter or margarine

Tomato juice
Peanut butter and lettuce sandwiches
Apples

Frankfurters and boiled potatoes
Coleslaw and shredded carrots
Bread   Butter or margarine
Peach upside-down cake (left from Monday)

WEDNESDAY

Farina
Sugar   Milk
Toast   Butter or margarine

Meat loaf sandwiches
(meat loaf left from Monday)
Apple-celery-raisin salad

Chili con carne with beans[10]
Crackers
Rice   Raw carrot strips
Oranges

THURSDAY

Grapefruit and orange juice
Omelet
Toast   Butter or margarine

Corn chowder[9]   Crackers
Spiced beet salad
Oatmeal cookies[9]

Braised steak and onions[9]
Boiled potatoes
Green salad
Bread   Butter or margarine
Vanilla pudding

FRIDAY

Grapefruit juice
Fried mush (farina left from Wednesday)
Syrup
Toast   Butter or margarine

Vegetable soup   Crackers
Coleslaw
Oatmeal cookies

Broiled fish[9]
Potatoes   Spinach
Bread   Butter or margarine
Pineapple and cottage cheese salad

SATURDAY

Tomato juice
French toast   Syrup
Butter or margarine
Bacon

Cheese rarebit on toast
Green peas
Cookies

Ragout of beef[9]
Noodles   Chopped broccoli   Celery sticks[11]
Biscuits   Butter or margarine
Cherry crisp

Following is the market order of food to supply the menus on page 177 and this page for the family outlined in Table 12–7.

Food for the Week's Menu[8]

Milk, Cheese, Ice Cream

14 quarts fluid whole milk
1/2 to 3/4 pound Cheddar cheese
1 12-ounce carton cottage cheese

Meat, Poultry, Fish
4 pounds frying chicken
1 pound round steak
2 1/2 pounds ground beef
1 to 1 1/2 pounds stew beef
1 pound fish fillets
1/2 pound bacon
1/2 pound pork sausage
1 pound frankfurters

Eggs
2 dozen eggs

Dry Beans, Peas, Nuts
1/3 pound dried navy beans
1/3 pound dried or 1 No. 303 can red kidney beans
4 ounce package dried split-pea soup
1/3 pound peanut butter

Flour, Cereals, Baked Goods
5 loaves enriched white bread
1 loaf whole-wheat bread
1 loaf cracked-wheat bread
12 ready-to-serve rolls
1 pound crackers
2 pounds all-purpose flour
2/3 pound pancake mix
1/2 pound ready-to-eat cereal
1/2 pound rolled oats
3/4 pound farina
1/2 pound rice
1/3 pound cornmeal
1/3 pound noodles

---

[9]Recipes from "Family Fare," Home and Garden Bulletin No. 1.
[10]Recipe from "Dry Beans, Peas, Lentils . . . Modern Cookery," Leaflet No. 326.

---

[11]Replace with tomato-cucumber salad when vegetables are in season.

Note: There will be milk to drink at each meal for the children, and at one meal a day for parents. Also coffee or tea as desired.

Citrus Fruit, Tomatoes

1½ to 2 pounds oranges
   1 46-ounce can orange juice
   2 No. 2 cans tomato juice
   1 No. 2½ can tomatoes
   1 No. 2 can grapefruit juice
   1 pound tomatoes (when in season)

Dark-green, Deep-yellow Vegetables

1¼ pounds carrots
   ⅔ pound salad greens in season
   1 to 1½ pounds spinach
   1 10-ounce package frozen chopped broccoli

Potatoes

10 pounds white potatoes

Other Vegetables and Fruits

   1 pound green beans
1½ to 2 pounds cabbage
   1 bunch celery
   1 cucumber (in season)
   1 head lettuce
   1 pound onions
   1 No. 303 can beets
   1 No. 303 can corn
   1 10-ounce package frozen green peas
   3 pounds apples
   3 bananas
   1 No. 2 can cherries
   1 No. 303 can sliced peaches
   1 No. 1 flat can pineapple slices
   1 No. 303 can plums
   4 ounces raisins

Fats and Oils

   1 pound butter or margarine
   ½ pound shortening
   ½ pint salad dressing
   ⅛ pint salad oil

Sugars, Sweets

   1 pound granulated sugar
   ½ pound brown sugar
   1 pint syrup
   1 4½-ounce package vanilla pudding

Note: There is a money allowance for coffee, tea, and accessories such as vinegar, baking powder, and spices in the estimated cost of each food plan. Sufficient money is allowed in the estimated cost of food for the low-cost plan to buy about ⅓ pound coffee and 4 tea bags per adult as well as the necessary accessories.

How to select *quality* foods is of major importance. Availability of foods varies according to regions and seasons. The economic status also influences the choice of foods, although nutritious foods may be procured to meet any of the levels. Following the basic rules of nutrition plus the consultation of food value charts is good strategy when diet programs are planned for either the well or the sick.

MARKETING LIST MADE FROM MENUS

After the menus are planned for the week, the foods included in the meals are listed. The list is checked against the foods on hand, which determines the items to keep on the marketing list. To facilitate shopping, foods are classified into 11 groups (see Tables 12–1, 12–2 and 12–3). The group totals should approximate the quantities suggested in the family food plan (Table 12–7) required for the menus. Some adjustments may be needed at first to get the correct proportion of foods from each group into menus. With a little practice, however, these plans will prove easy to follow.

Regardless of the economic status of the family, these steps are followed in the procedure of making a marketing list from the planned menus. The amount of the food budget determines only the selection of foods within the groups. Some types are less expensive than others. On page 177 is a sample set of low-cost menus for one week, and on page 178 the accompanying market order of food to supply these menus for the family listed in Table 12–7. The quantities of food needed in one week in each of the 11 food groups to provide three meals at home are taken from Table 12–1, which is based on the daily food pattern for an adequate diet (page

TABLE 12–7   SAMPLE WORKSHEET (LOW-COST FOOD PLAN)

FAMILY MEMBERS (sex and age)	MILK, CHEESE, ICE CREAM		MEAT, POULTRY, FISH	EGGS	DRY BEANS, PEAS, NUTS		FLOUR, CEREALS, BAKED GOODS		CITRUS FRUIT, TOMATOES		DARK-GREEN AND DEEP-YELLOW VEGETABLES		POTATOES		OTHER VEGETABLES AND FRUITS		FATS, OILS		SUGARS, SWEETS	
	Qt.	Lb.	Oz.	No.	Lb.	Oz.	Lb.	Oz.	Lb.	Oz.	Lb.	Oz.	Lb.	Oz.	Lb.	Oz.	Lb.	Oz.	Lb.	Oz.
1. Father, 33 years	3½	3	8	6	0	6	4	4	1	12	0	12	3	4	5	8	0	12	1	0
2. Mother, 33 years	3½	3	4	7	0	6	2	8	1	12	1	8	2	0	5	0	0	6	0	10
3. John, 11 years	5½	2	8	6	0	6	3	0	2	0	0	12	2	8	5	0	0	8	0	12
4. Mary, 8 years	4	2	4	6	0	4	2	12	2	0	0	8	2	4	4	4	0	8	0	10
Total	16½	11	8	25	1	6	12	8	7	8	3	8	10	0	19	12	2	2	3	0
Range	16 to 18	11 to 12 lb.		2 to 2½ doz.	1¼ to 1½ lb.		12 to 14 lb.		8 to 9 lb.		3 to 4 lb.		10 lb.		20 to 22 lb.		2 to 2½ lb.		2½ to 3½ lb.	

From Consumer and Food Economics Research Division, Agricultural Research Service, U.S. Department of Agriculture, 1964.

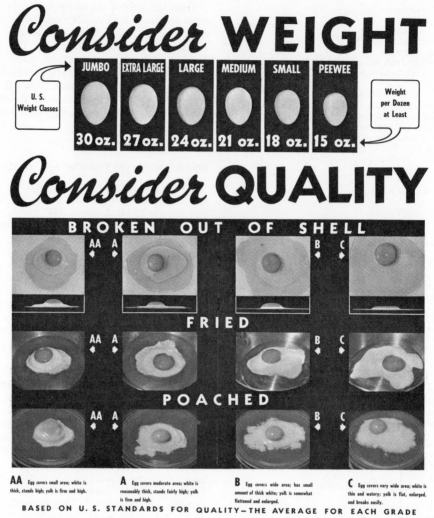

Figure 12–1 Standards for judging the quality of eggs. (U.S. Department of Agriculture, Poultry Division.)

162 to fulfill the nutritional requirements as outlined in Table 11-1.

The U.S. Department of Agriculture issues bulletins giving buying hints for all classes of foods. An example is Shopper's Guide to U.S. Grades for Food, Home and Garden Bulletin No. 58; Tips on Selecting Fruits and Vegetables, Marketing Bulletin No. 13, is another. Charts are also available, such as Figure 12-1 on eggs. Additional buying information is printed on the back.

ECONOMY HINTS

A limited food budget does not necessarily mean an inadequate diet. The budget can be stretched without sacrificing either variety or essential foods in the menu. The following hints for menu planning, marketing, storage and cooking are suggested when it is necessary to reduce costs. (See Figs. 12-2 and 12-3.)

ECONOMY HINTS FOR MENU PLANNING

1. Follow the papers for weekly market specials and seasonal, plentiful foods that are economical.
2. Plan menus a week in advance, with flexibility for leftovers and good buys.
3. In season, use foods that are plentiful and locally produced.
4. Use economical cuts and lower grades of meat. The food value is essentially the same as that of the higher priced. For example, beef liver is much less expensive than calves' liver and is equal in nutritive value.
5. Use nutritious low-cost foods, such as dried peas and beans, frequently.
6. Use leftovers in appetizing combinations.
7. Use canned or frozen fruits and vegetables when fresh products are too expensive or out of season.
8. Poultry is usually an expensive source of protein, while fish is generally cheaper.
9. Bread is less expensive than rolls.

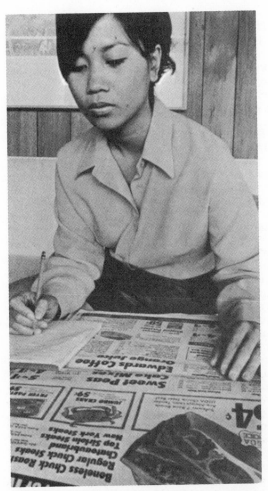

Figure 12–2 A listing of needed items, a week's menu, and newspaper ads are useful in planning a shopping list. At grocery store, adjust plans to take advantage of specials. (Courtesy of Ullrich, H. D.: Food Planning for Families at 3 Different Cost Levels. Yearbook of Agriculture 1969, Food For Us All, U.S. Department of Agriculture, Washington, D.C.)

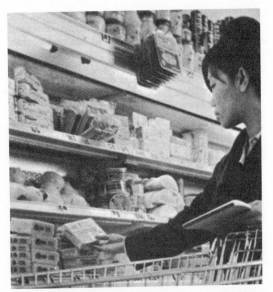

Figure 12–3 Choose package size that best suits family needs. Read labels for information on nutritive value, weight, and price. Compare prices per serving. (Courtesy of Ullrich, H. D.: Food Planning for Families at 3 Different Cost Levels. Yearbook of Agriculture 1969, Food For Us All, U.S. Department of Agriculture, Washington, D.C.)

ECONOMY HINTS FOR MARKETING

Armed with a carefully planned market list, you may save money in the following ways:

1. Shop in person and choose the most economical method, such as in the cash-and-carry chain stores or supermarkets. Shop at several stores if bargains are available.
2. Take advantage of sales and specials.
3. Buy foods in season, and buy those that are plentiful.
4. Buy foods in bulk if sold under sanitary conditions.
5. Buy foods in quantity if storage space is adequate and if they will be used before becoming stale.
6. Be familiar with brands and grades of foods. The less expensive standard brands are essentially the same in nutritive value as the more expensive, fancy grades and brands. Study the labels to become familiar with quality, size and weight.
7. Compare relative cost of different forms and packs of food (bulk, packaged, fresh, canned, frozen and dried).
8. Consider edible value of purchases. For example, a cheaper cut of meat with a high proportion of bone and fat may have so much waste it would be false economy. Wilted or decayed fruits or vegetables are usually a waste in both edible portion and nutritive value of vitamins.
9. When buying flour, get the "enriched," "restored," or whole grain for extra B vitamins and minerals. The cost is no more.
10. Buy the less expensive forms of food whenever possible. For example, evaporated, skim, or dried skim milk is cheaper than fresh milk, satisfactory for cooking, and has some use as a beverage. Fortified margarine can be used in place of butter.
11. In choosing eggs, remember the color of the shell does not affect the food value or taste. Grade B eggs are usually cheaper than grade A and are just as nutritious.
12. Home processing of foods (freezing and canning) is good economy when the foods are home-produced or purchased at the time the supply is plentiful.

ECONOMY HINTS FOR STORING FOODS

No matter how good a buy, foods must be properly stored after their purchase to avoid loss of vitamin values and to prevent spoilage, or the result will be false economy.

1. Be sure there is adequate storage *space* for food.
2. All perishable foods need refrigeration, namely meat, eggs, fresh milk, cheese, butter, margarine, and certain fruits and vegetables, such as salad greens and tomatoes.
3. Bread should be stored in a bread box with a few holes for circulation of air. If there is room in the refrigerator or freezer, it will stay fresh longer.
4. Store dried fruits in sealed containers in a cool place.
5. Store potatoes, root vegetables, and cabbage in a dark, cool, dry place with good ventilation.
6. Keep frozen foods frozen until ready to use. Never refreeze after food has thawed.
7. Keep dry milk and cereals in covered containers in a cool, dry place.

ECONOMY HINTS FOR COOKING FOODS

Much food value can be lost by improper cooking. Economy does not end with menu planning, buying, and storage; the "proof of the pudding" is in the eating.

1. Use raw or cooked fruits and vegetables with the skin, or peel very thinly. Much of the mineral and vitamin content is in the skin.
2. Save fat and meat drippings to use in other cooking.
3. Use leftover vegetable water in soups and sauces.
4. To retain the vitamins use as little liquid in cooking as possible, and do not overcook.
5. Use accurate measurements and tested recipes to eliminate failure.
6. In cooking, substitute fortified margarine for butter; inexpensive forms of milk for fresh milk; dried eggs for fresh.
7. Foods prepared in the home are usually less expensive than the ready-to-eat. Cereals, breads and rolls are examples.
8. Prepared foods, bought in the delicatessen, are an expensive practice.
9. Use bits of food in soups or in combination with other foods in casseroles and salads.
10. Use oven to best advantage by baking several foods at one time.

FOOD TECHNOLOGY

During the past fifty years, there has been tremendous progress in food technology. The ever-growing food industry markets food fresh, frozen, dried and canned, especially processed for convenience to meet the public demands. The improved methods of food preservation through canning, freezing, and irradiation, plus the growth of transportation systems have made seasonal variation in food consumption less important. Trains, trucks, planes, and barges are making longer but quicker trips from the farm and production centers to the cities. The increased use of certain fruits and vegetables in the dietary is due largely to these improvements. The improvements in the *production of food* have grown out of the improvement of agricultural methods. Insecticides, selective seeds, and soil chemistry are some of the contributions from scientific agriculture. Better livestock, better quality of produce, and better production are some of the contributions of genetics.

The number of easy-to-cook foods found in markets today were not in the stores five years ago and more are expected. It is predicted that the use of these "convenience" foods will increase. New names appear on lists of ingredients on packages. New items have different combinations of foods and some are synthesized to represent natural foods. Many contain preservatives of various kinds, to ensure better keeping qualities, and stabilizers and emulsifiers, to provide the desired texture and flavors. New equipment, methods for processing, preservatives, packages and methods of getting foods to the stores have been developed. Technology has given us new varieties of foods which are now grown on farms and can be harvested more readily by machines. Breeds of cattle and special rations have been selected which will give meat the desired qualities demanded by consumers. Farmers raise a breed of hogs with less fat and young broilers come to the market cleaned and ready to cook. One farmer with a more mechanized farm now feeds about twice the number he did a decade ago.

New methods are used in processing foods. To keep foods from spoiling or ripening too fast the temperature and moisture and the oxygen or carbon dioxide of the air are controlled. More ready-to-serve canned products ranging from soup to desserts are now available. One of the new kinds of dairy products available is aseptically canned pudding (container and contents are sterilized separately). New combinations of frozen foods are available: vegetables in cream sauce, entrées for one person or for family size, frozen egg noodles, canapés. In fact, almost every food prepared at home can be bought frozen. Soon frozen lettuce and salad mixes and other hard-to-freeze items using new freezing techniques will be on the market. More dehydrated foods such as dry whole milk will soon be available. The freeze-drying method of preservation will add more items that will keep without refrigeration and can be quickly reconstituted. The newest items are imitation foods such as meatless meats, filled milk, imitation ice cream and imitation milk, whipped toppings, non-dairy coffee whiteners. These can be kept a long time without refrigeration. Packaging materials have been developed that will lengthen the shelf-life of the product considerably. Marketing new products relies on advertising through mass media. The cost of these new foods in comparison to their made-at-home counterparts varies. Most cost more, some cost less. The shopper has to decide. The choice the shopper makes will depend upon the value put on time necessary for preparation of an item. The development of new varieties of foods on the farm, new processes by the manufacturers and new ways to get the products to the market and finally to the family table and eating places outside the home are insights into what technology will be in the future. The demand for better food and marketing services is an ongoing endeavor.[7]

The *distribution of food* is the effort to provide foods to meet the pressures and demands of population. When the population is concentrated in metropolitan areas, foods must be transported from various areas to provide canned goods, dairy products, fish,

---

[7]Harp, H. H.: Thousands of new foods give you a wide choice. Food For Us All, 1969 Yearbook of Agriculture, U.S. Department of Agriculture.

frozen foods, ingredients for bread and baked goods, meat, perishable fruits and vegetables, poultry products, and staple supplies. Food production centers are usually located convenient to the site of available foods.

Food service includes the preparation and service of food. Home cooking is influenced by the type of utensils, facilities and standards of the person responsible for the preparation and service of food. In institutional cooking the habits of the cook or chef may reveal different standards from those of the consumer. Large quantity cookery takes place in hospitals, school cafeterias, industrial cafeterias, in dormitories and clubs, hotels, restaurants and other public eating places.

Food handling laws enforce food hygiene. (See Chapter 14.)

THE PRODUCTION OF FOODS

The scientific advancements made in agriculture, animal husbandry, dairying, and poultry raising have produced improvements in quality. Hog cholera, tick fever of cattle, and hookworm are some of the animal diseases brought under control. In bacteria control, milk pasteurization has been promoted along with the improvements in the manufacture of butter and cheese. To bring about control in plant diseases, insecticides were introduced and the chemistry of the soil promulgated.

SCIENTIFIC AGRICULTURE Agricultural science is a blend of many different areas. It includes a search for improvement in technical skills, better breeds of livestock, high-yielding, disease-resistant pasture, animal nutrition, control of pests, knowledge of marketing, storage and transportation, organization of the farm, farm machinery, and careful management of expenditure. At first, tests are made in the laboratory, then enlarged to pilot tests in the field before farmers are encouraged to try the improved techniques. Results from different regions are classified, correlated and the facts redistributed. State Experimental Stations cooperate with the U.S. Department of Agriculture to put across the research findings on a practical scale. Grains, fruits, berries, vegetables, and legumes are yielding more quality produce per acre than during former years.

SCIENTIFIC ANIMAL HUSBANDRY AND POULTRY RAISING To bring about genetic improvement, the breeder selects the animals carefully, then inbreeds and crossbreeds. The results are evident in the production of better milk and better meats.

Parasites infest animals. For instance, arthropods live on the skins of animals, and worms and protozoa occur inside the body of the animal. Control plans, which include sanitation, vaccination and treatment with drugs, have been the tools used by veterinarians and farmers to fight an aggressive battle against animal plagues. Animal nutrition has introduced new ideas in feeding to produce better quality livestock. Artificial breeding has been one of the greatest advancements in scientific animal husbandry during the past decade.

To meet consumer demands, poultry breeds have been changed to furnish more white meat on breasts, and turkeys that are smaller for the family of fewer members. In some areas brown shells on eggs are preferred while in other regions the white shell egg draws a premium price. Since both furnish equally good nutrition, the poultry raiser feeds his flocks according to the newer theories.

SCIENTIFIC DAIRYING The improved dairy starts with a better breed of cows. Because the greatest money value of whole milk is in the butterfat, the emphasis is placed on the fat content of milk. Thus we see surplus whole milk converted into products such as butter, whole-milk cheese, evaporated and sweetened condensed milk, and dried whole milk. From the production of butter, cheese, cream, and ice cream, there are by-products of skim milk, buttermilk, and whey. Some of the skim milk is converted into cottage cheese, flavored milk drinks and cultured buttermilk, and some, in concentrated form, is used in ice cream, bread, and food products.

THE MARKETING AND DISTRIBUTION OF FOODS

The increased cost of food has been due to the increased cost of marketing. About 7 to 10 per cent of the retail cost of food goes into packaging. For some items the cost is slight, but for others the cost may equal the cost of the food itself. The public demands convenient packages for handling and storage plus built-in maid service, such as premixed foods and heat-and-serve dinners, all of which increase food cost.

Milk is marketed in various forms. *Certified* milk is high quality, raw milk, with no more than 10,000 bacteria per cubic centimeter of milk, and not older than 36 hours when delivered. Grade A raw milk should have an average bacterial count not exceeding 50,000 bacteria per cubic centimeter at the time of delivery. *Pasteurized* milk has been subjected to "a temperature not lower than 145° F. for not less than thirty minutes." (See Fig. 12–4.) Milk *fortified* with vitamin D has 400 I.U. of the vitamin per quart. *Ho-*

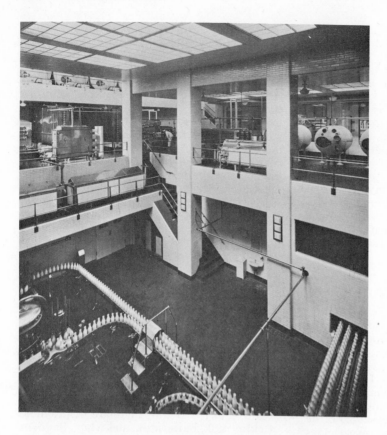

Figure 12–4   A modern plant for pasteurization of milk. (Courtesy of the National Dairy Council.)

mogenized milk has the fat content emulsified to prevent cream separation. *Evaporated* milk has some of the water content removed, and *condensed* milk has some of the water removed but sugar added. *Fermented* milk, *buttermilk*, and *acidophilus* milk have specific desirable bacteria added to act upon the milk. *Dried* milk has most of the water content removed, and *dried skim* milk has the water content removed to reduce the product to a white powder. Milk is discussed further in Chapter 38. *Filled* milk is any milk (skimmed, evaporated, powdered etc.) or cream in which the butterfat has been removed and replaced with a vegetable fat. Filled milks usually have skimmed milk as their base. They cannot be shipped in interstate commerce. Imitation milk resembles milk but contains no milk ingredients. A typical imitation milk contains sodium caseinate or some vegetable protein, vegetable fat and corn syrup solids. Additives such as artificial flavoring and coloring, emulsifiers and stabilizers are used. They can be shipped in interstate commerce because they are not covered by the Federal Milk Act (1923) as is filled milk.

Cream contains 20 to 40 per cent fat, and the remaining milk with the lessened fat content is known as *skim* milk.

Cheese is made from the casein and fat of milk, and coagulation takes place because of the action of the rennin on the casein. The variations in cheese flavor and texture are brought about by the bacteria, the type of milk, the ripening process, and the temperature.

Ice cream is made from cream or milk fat, sugar, flavoring, and a binder (gelatin is frequently used). Ice milk is made of whole milk.

Butter, according to Federal food laws, is "the clean sound product, made by gathering in any manner the fat of fresh or ripened milk or cream into a mass, which also contains a small portion of other milk constituents, with or without salt, and contains not less than 80 per cent of milk fat."

Eggs are sold fresh by the dozen according to size, and are graded for quality through a candling process. Frozen and dried eggs are used for cooking and baking.

Meat, according to Federal food laws, is "the properly dressed flesh derived from cattle, from swine, from sheep, or from goats," and flesh is defined as "any clean, sound, edible part of the striated muscle of an animal." Meat is sold fresh, frozen, canned, dried, smoked, and it is marketed in packages, ground, sliced into chops, steaks, cutlets, or cut into roasts. Certain parts of the edible animal are preferred, and the choice cuts bring premium prices.

Fish is obtained from local lakes, streams, and coastal waters. Fish from salt water and shellfish are rich in iodine. Fish are sold fresh, frozen, dried, smoked, and canned.

Poultry is sold fresh, frozen or canned. Current marketing practices have encouraged the sale of parts of chickens rather than the whole, which is convenient for the family that prefers white meat or other particular parts. Turkeys are sold whole, halved or quartered. Ducks and geese are popular fare in some regions.

Fats and *oils* are sold as margarine, hydrogenated shortening, lard, olive oil, corn oil, soy bean oil, and cottonseed oil. Modern processing is designed to provide some degree of polyunsaturation. This is in keeping with the current concepts of the prevention of atherosclerosis and heart disease.

Cereals are produced from the edible portions of grains, and grain is defined by the Federal food laws as "the fully matured, clean, sound, air-dry seed of wheat, maize, rice, oats, rye, buckwheat, barley, sorghum, millet or spelt." Wheat is the most popular grain consumed in the United States and it is eaten in breads and other bakery products, cereal products, such as spaghetti and macaroni, and breakfast cereals.

Sugar is derived from the sugar cane and the sugar beet, and molasses is the liquor remaining after the removal of part of the cane sugar from the boiled juice. Sugar is made into granular form, tablets or small loaves, powdered or confectioners', and varying degrees of brown sugar.

Other sweetenings include syrups from the maple sap and cornstarch, honey, and sorghum.

The popular varieties of *vegetables* number in the twenties and most of them are produced commercially in California, New York, Texas, and Wisconsin. Vegetables are sold fresh, canned, frozen, or dried. Within recent years the quick-freezing of vegetables has become a popular form of marketing.

Fruits are grown in commercial areas and sold fresh, canned, frozen, or dried. Fruit juices are the most recent popular form of marketing fruits, and the juices are sold either in cartons or cans or in frozen concentrated form.

ENRICHED, RESTORED AND FORTIFIED FOODS   The words enriched, restored and fortified are frequently confused. *Enriched* applies to flour, bread, degerminated corn meal and corn grits, and standards have been established as to how much of the food values can be added. Iron, niacin, and thiamin are returned in about the same amounts as are lost in milling white flour from the whole grain, while riboflavin is added in larger amounts than found in whole wheat, and calcium and vitamin D may be added.

In *restored* foods the manufacturer puts back the nutrients lost in the processing. It is a voluntary move and not compulsory.

In *fortified* foods, the manufacturer adds nutrients that were not present in the food originally. For example, margarine is fortified with vitamin A and milk may be fortified with vitamin D.

The 1953 joint report of the Food and Nutrition Board and the American Medical Association Council on Food and Nutrition approved the enrichment of flour, bread, degerminated corn meal, and corn grits with thiamin, riboflavin and niacin.[12,13] It also approved the nutritive improvement of whole grain corn meal and white rice; the retention or restoration of thiamin, niacin and iron in processed food cereals; and the addition of vitamin D to milk (400 I.U. per quart), vitamin A to margarine (15,000 I.U. per pound) to bring it up to the average vitamin A content of butter, and iodine to table salt (1 part sodium or potassium iodide to 5000 parts salt).

Definite limits had to be set to the addition of nutrients to food products in order to protect the public from combinations that are irrational or even harmful. Most states have based their laws on the recommendations of the Food and Nutrition Board and the Council on Food and Nutrition. There is good evidence that the policies recommended have benefited the public and have encouraged sound nutritional practices.

Although the report endorses, in principle, the addition of specific nutrients to certain staple foods, it stresses the desirability of meeting the nutritional needs of the people by the use of natural foods insofar as possible. See Chapter 4, Carbohydrates, and Chapter 41, Bread-Cereal Group, for additional information on enriched, restored and fortified bread, flour, and cereals.

WORLD FOOD SUPPLY

Sixty per cent of the world population lives in underdeveloped countries where there is great need of more and better food. Food problems of many countries will continue to be critical for some time in spite of large

---

[12] The Addition of Specific Nutrients to Foods. Public Health Report 69, March, 1954, p. 275.

[13] A Statement of General Policy Concerning the Addition of Specific Nutrients to Foods. Report of the Council on Foods and Nutrition. J.A.M.A., *154*:145, 1954.

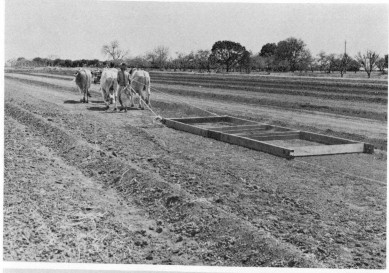

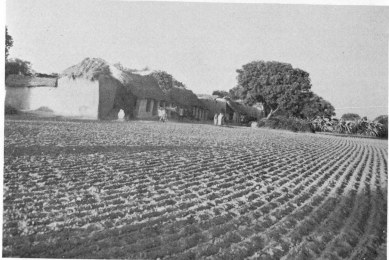

Figure 12–5 (Top).   Using wooden floats to smooth the land in Central India. (Courtesy of A.I.D., India.)
Figure 12–6 (Bottom).   Graded contour furrows for efficient irrigation and drainage in Etawon area, India. (Courtesy of A.I.D., India.)

surpluses in countries such as the United States. It is not practical or advisable for the regions of abundance and efficient production to supply the countries of need and low production indefinitely. They must be educated to produce their own food supply. The World Health Organization of the United Nations is taking measures to increase the food supply in these countries through scientific agriculture. Cultivation projects, such as irrigation and flood control works, drainage projects, and leveling of land for rice fields, require time and an abundance of manual labor. In Asia, for example, where rice is the chief crop, mechanized agriculture on a large scale is impractical because of the topography of the countries. In countries such as India, China, and Pakistan, which contain about 40 per cent of the world's population, erosion is a serious problem. (See

Figures 12–5 and 12–6.) However, production of adequate food supply in the needy areas depends chiefly on the adoption of more scientific agricultural practices. In a scientifically ignorant, tradition-bound population the progress is necessarily slow. Death rates are declining in these areas despite widespread malnutrition and, consequently, the population is growing, but the supply of food is not keeping pace. The recent World Food Survey made by the United Nations Food and Agriculture Organization shows that amounts of animal protein ranged from 8 gm. per person per day in the Far East and 14 gm. in the Near East to 62 gm. in Oceania and 66 gm. in North America.[14]

---

[14]Clark, F.: A score card of how we Americans are eating. Food For Us All, 1969 Yearbook of Agriculture, U.S. Department of Agriculture.

PROBLEMS AND SUGGESTED TOPICS FOR DISCUSSION

1. a. Using the family in Problem 2, page 169 (Chapter 11), list the family members and their ages. By referring to Table 12–1, copy the amount of food in each food group according to age and sex. (See sample worksheet, Table 12–7). Add the amounts in each of the groups. These will provide 21 meals for the family (3 meals a day for 1 week).

b. Plan low-cost meals for 1 week for the above family.

c. Prepare the marketing list for the above family. Check to make sure the market list and food allowances from the 11 food groups are approximately the same.

d. Calculate the cost of the market list using current prices in your locality from either:
 (1) A supermarket
 (2) A regular delivery store.

2. If possible, visit a local dairy plant, a large supermarket, a meat packing plant, bakery and other food manufacturing and distribution centers.

3. Give reports on the advancements made in scientific farming and production of high quality foods.

ADDITIONAL PLANNING GUIDES

Better Health Care for People with Low Incomes. U.S. Department of Health, Education and Welfare, Bureau of Family Services, Washington, D.C., 1966.

Family Fare: A Guide to Good Nutrition. Home and Garden Bulletin No. 1, Consumer and Food Economics Research Division, Agricultural Research Service, U.S. Department of Agriculture, 1970.

Family Food Buying. A Guide for Calculating Amounts to Buy: Comparing Costs. Home Economics Research Report No. 37, Agricultural Research Service, U.S. Department of Agriculture, 1969.

Family Food Plans, Revised 1964. Consumer and Food Economics Research Division Agricultural Research Service, U.S. Department of Agriculture, Hyattsville, Maryland.

Food for Families with School Children. Home and Garden Bulletin No. 13, Revised, 1963.

Food for the Family with Young Children. Home and Garden Bulletin No. 5, Revised, 1963.

Food for the Young Couple. Home and Garden Bulletin No. 85, 1967.

Food Guide for Older Folks. Home and Garden Bulletin No. 17, 1963.

Shopper's Guide to U.S. Grades of Food. Home and Garden Bulletin No. 58, U.S. Department of Agriculture.

Your Money's Worth in Foods. Home and Garden Bulletin No. 183, U.S. Department of Agriculture, 1971.

SUGGESTED ADDITIONAL READING REFERENCES

Adelson, S. F.: Changes in diets of households 1955–1965 —implications for nutrition education. Nutrition Program News, U.S. Department of Agriculture, Washington, D.C., May–June, 1968.

Agriculture, Volume III. Science, Technology, and Development. U.S. papers prepared for the UN Conference on the Application of Science and Technology for the Benefit of the Less Developed Areas. Washington, D.C., U.S. Govt. Printing Office, 1962, 75 cents.

Family Economics Review, Consumer and Food Economics Research Division. U.S. Department of Agriculture, Hyattsville, Maryland (Quarterly).

Hames, P. J., and Robertson, E. C.: Nutritive value of low-income families' diets, J. Am. Dietet. A., 30:766, 1954.

Hayes, J. (ed.): Food For Us All, Yearbook of Agriculture, 1969. U.S. Government Printing Office, Washington, D.C.

Irelan, L. M.: Low-income life styles. U.S. Welfare Administration, Pub. No. 14, 1966.

Larrick, G. P.: The nutritive adequacy of our food supply. J. Am. Dietet. A., 39:117, 1961.

Monge, B., and Throssell, D.: Good nutrition on a low income. Am. J. Nursing, 60:1290, 1960.

Moore, M. L.: When families must eat more for less. Nurs. Outlook, 14:66, 1966.

Stefferud, A. (ed.): Food: The Yearbook of Agriculture, 1959. Washington, D.C. United States Department of Agriculture. Food Costs: Pp. 557–566, Waugh, F. V., and Ogren, K. E.: What your food money buys; pp. 567–575, Page, L., and Cofer, E.: Your money's worth; pp. 576–588, Cofer, E., and Clark, F.: Food plans at different costs.

Thompson, W. S.: World population and food supply. J.A.M.A., 172:1647, 1960.

Chapter 13
*GEOGRAPHIC
AND
CULTURAL
DIETARY
VARIATIONS*

UNIT FOUR
DIETARY
VARIATIONS:
NUTRITION AND
COMMUNITY
HEALTH

FOOD PATTERNS

Food patterns of a country are molded by agricultural resources, technical progress, buying power and cultural patterns. Some factors influencing food habits of individuals are nationality, race, and regional locality. When people come to the United States to make their homes, they bring along food tastes of their native lands. An example is in the many varieties of breads, which vary with national heritage. (See Figure 13–1). The firmly rooted habits of social groups are not readily relinquished, nor are the reasons for an unwillingness to taste a new food to be ignored. The new food may have a kindred association with a similar food which was either barred or honored at an ancient festival. The regional availability of food plays another strong influence in food selection. Sometimes the familiar foods are not available and the adjustment to different tastes is not made willingly. (See Food Habits, page 11.) Many food customs of the foreign born are excellent, both nutritionally and economically, and contribute to our pattern of living in the United States. Familiarity with the food patterns of the various nationality groups may help us to better understand and appreciate our neighbors abroad, as well as those living in the United States.

Since World War II, many people from European and Asiatic countries have migrated to Canada. Most large Canadian cities contain a variety of ethnic groups. The Toronto Nutrition Committee compiled a food customs guide to assist nutrition workers in Canada in evaluating traditional eating habits in terms of Canada's Food Rules, and in establishing good eating habits among the new Canadians.[1]

Social and cultural influences on food patterns are not well understood. The habit of eating is culturally based. Some cultures such as the middle class urban American generally have the largest meal of the day in the early evening and consider it a social occasion. It is served on a table on plates with utensils and napkins and with a minimum amount of eating sounds. In some cultures, people eat on the floor, use their fingers and smack their lips to show appreciation of what they are eating. Food patterns are interwoven with the culture of a people. These must be considered and utilized by all members of the health team. Whenever changes are desired in the nutritional behavior they must be accomplished with a minimum of disruption in the lives of individuals.

Food patterns are based on the type of food production and presentation in a culture. Distinct differences in the diet are reflected in areas where almost all food (plant and animal) consumed is self produced or gathered contrasted with those areas where the food is supplied from large-scale commercial agriculture (domestic and foreign). The ability of a people to preserve food is shown in the food pattern. Some cultures preserve food for future needs or for periods of scarcity. Other cultures do not preserve food and thereby experience a feast or famine way of life. *The distribution* of food (transportation, storage,

---

[1]Food Customs of New Canadians. Revised 1967. Available from Toronto Nutrition Committee, Box 744, Terminal A, Toronto 1, Ontario.

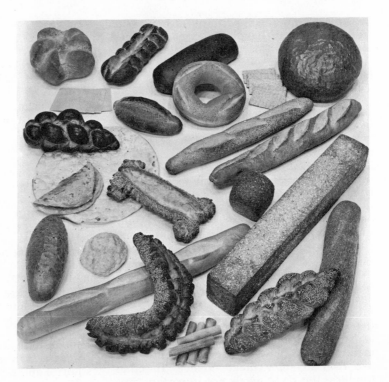

Figure 13–1   Bread varies with the national heritage of the baker. Included are the big, round corn rye popular in Jewish neighborhoods; the long, square, dark pumpernickel of German shops; seed topped Italian white loaves in different shapes; slim, smooth French breads; a ring of Greek kouloura, and braided coils of the Jewish challah; lavash, the wide and flat Armenian bread, and wafers of Swedish and Norwegian flatbreads; the small golden puff of the East, puri, and the brittle bread sticks of Italy. (New York Times Magazine, August 30, 1953.)

marketing facilities) affects the food pattern. People who travel extensively are able to find familiar foods in the large cities as a rule because the food is imported. Different methods of *food preparation* influence food patterns as well as the nutritive value of foods. One-pot dishes are used by some cultures and to other cultures baking and roasting in ovens are unfamiliar ways of preparing food. Scarcity of fuel also affects the method of cooking. (See Figure 13–2.)

Food patterns are based on edible materials one's culture considers to be food. Many foods may not be considered food by some cultures but others eat them. In almost every culture, man eats only a portion of the food supply

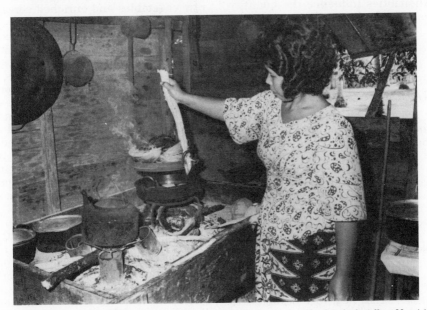

Figure 13–2   Food preparation in Malay kitchen. (Taken from Wilson, C. S.: "Food Beliefs Affect Nutritional Status of Malay Fisherfolk." Journal of Nutrition Education, Winter, 1971, p. 97.)

available to him. Food patterns, although not fully understood, have categories identified and applicable to various cultures.[2]

FOOD AND BEHAVIOR

Investigators realize the close relations between food habits and social and religious beliefs. They define the study of food habits as "the study of the way in which individuals or groups of individuals, in response to social and cultural pressures, select, consume and utilize portions of the available food supply." One school of thought may condemn the practice which another praises. To understand the behavior of individuals within social groupings, their reactions to environment and their survival at different levels of efficiency and reproduction requires the integration of various sciences: anthropology, biochemistry, soil chemistry, economics, genetics, physiology and sociology.

Food has varying values to the members of the different social groupings. To some, food is used to discipline children or to exhibit maternal affection, while adolescents may use food to show independence. In other families, the daily meals are important as a get-together, and lavish expenditures may be made on food to compensate for deprivations in other areas. Individuals may eat food for pleasure or from a sense of duty and the nourishment derived. The amount of food consumed, the number of meals per day, and the distribution of meals through the day have nationality heritage. The afternoon tea of the English, the early and late breakfasts of other nationalities influence the quantity of food consumed. Review Food Habits, page 11.

REGIONAL DIETARY VARIATIONS IN THE UNITED STATES

THE SOUTH Traditionally, hot breads have been one of the characteristic features of the Southern diet. This may be attributed to the climate, because the heat seems to influence the keeping qualities of ingredients. Vegetable greens of all kinds are used. Vegetables are usually cooked a long time and often with fat pork. Much of the vitamin content is destroyed in the long cooking; however, a saving factor is the general use of the pot-liquor. Sweet potatoes seem preferable to the white potato. Southern fried

---

[2]Wenkaw, N. S.: Cultural determinants of nutritional behavior. Nutrition Program News, U.S. Department of Agriculture, July-August, 1969.

chicken is a favorite of the South, as are hominy grits and corn pone. Fish is used abundantly along the coast—fried shrimp being especially popular. Nuts are abundant. Fresh milk is limited, so buttermilk, canned evaporated milk, and/or dried milk are used.

The elegance of entertaining still prevails in Southern homes. In New Orleans and the neighboring country the early influence of French cookery is still prevalent. New Orleans is considered one of the cities in the nation where gourmets may relish the French cuisine.

Negroes in the South are apt to use cornmeal, hominy, hominy grits, rice, cornbread, hoe cakes and hot biscuits extensively. Mustard, collard and turnip greens are favorites. Salt pork, fat back, ham hocks or bacon ends are cooked with the greens and other vegetables such as kale and cabbage. This gives the flavor desired. Black-eyed peas, marrow fat and kidney beans are popular. Sweet potatoes and yams are more often used than white potatoes. All fresh fruits, especially melons, are favored. Pork in all forms, chicken, fish and, when available, rabbit, squirrel and raccoon are used.

Economy is important to the Negroes. A typical main meal is a boiled dinner: fresh or smoked pork, fish or chicken, greens, sweet potatoes and cornbread. Butter, margarine and drippings from pork are used. Sorghum or molasses is used on the hot bread frequently. They need to use more whole-grain cereals and milk products. Because they prefer vegetables "well done" (overcooked) and the refined cereals, they need to include more raw vegetables and enriched cereals in their diet.

With the new emphasis on the black people's contribution to the American culture "soul food" has received prominence. Food discarded or disfavored by masters of slaves during pre-Civil War years was prepared in slave kitchens. These were pork snout and tail, bacon ends, ribs, chitlins and chicken wings. Animals from the field, such as opossum, squirrel and rabbit, and fish and turtles from the waters along with local vegetables were used. Much originality and feeling or "soul" went into the preparation of these foods. Currently they are served on special occasions. (See Figure 13-3.)

THE SOUTHWEST In the Southwestern states and along the Pacific coast the infiltrations of several cultures are noticeable, namely the early nomadic tribes of Indians, the Spanish and Mexicans from Central and South America, the Chinese, Japanese, Filipinos, and Hawaiians from across the Pacific ocean. The vegetarian habits of the

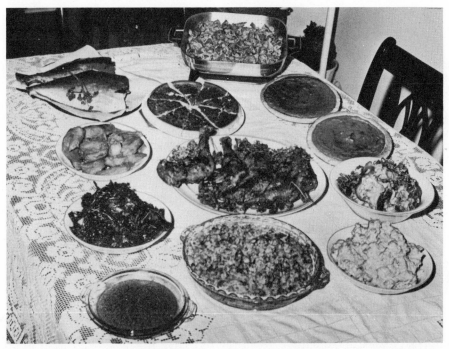

Figure 13-3   These dishes are considered to be the pièce de résistance of soul food cookery. From top, clockwise: chitlins or wrinkled steak, sweet potato pie, pigs' feet, potato salad, hopping johns, pot likker, collard greens, candied yams, porgies, and (center) cornbread and fried chicken. (Courtesy of the Evening and Sunday Bulletin, Philadelphia.)

Chinese, Japanese, Filipinos, and Hawaiians have been brought along, and the habits are reflected in their garden produce. Most vegetables are cooked too long. Foods which have been used for generations and, therefore, are considered typical are tortillas, tamales, pinto beans, chili, and certain forms of corn. The Spanish and Mexican influence is strong in Texas and Southern California. More recently, Oriental and Hawaiian dishes have become more popular in California. Some of the old recipes brought to Nevada from England by Cornishmen who came to work in the mines are saffron buns and Cornish pasties. Big, gregarious cookouts, with the menu ranging anywhere from poultry, such as turkey, to a whole steer which may be barbecued over an open fire, date back to the early days of ranching and cattle raising. Along the varied coastline and terrain can be found native products such as sand dabs, Gulf shrimp, Dungeness crab, avocados, almonds, and ripe olives, which are used in ingenious ways and distinctive dishes. The custom of serving the salad as a first course originated in California, which is especially famous for Caesar salad.

The hot spiced foods from Spain are reflected in the seasoning of foods, and the slow preparation and cooking processes of enchiladas and chilis may be associated with the temperament of the people and their limited cooking facilities.

THE MIDDLE WEST   Into the fertile, widespreading valley of the Mississippi and its tributaries, and along the shores of the Great Lakes, the Scandinavians, Swiss, Germans, English and other enterprising nationalities have migrated. First generation families maintain many of their native eating habits, while the second and third generations, who are born in this country, adjust to the social grouping and their diet becomes a blend of Americana and traditional native food. The third generation homemakers prepare some of the characteristic native dishes, and on the festival days the menus are replicas of former eating customs. Ingenuity has assisted in the creation of tasty dishes from the regional choice of ingredients. Fish from the Great Lakes and rivers are favorites, along with the game hunted in marshes, plains and forests. The well kept farms produce vegetables and fruits and raise dairy cattle. Butter, cheese and ice cream are made from the milk fat. Wisconsin has become famous as a dairy state and ranks along with California, New York and Texas in the production of vegetables. Iowa agriculture is the epitome of high-protein production. This is the heart of the great American corn belt, and here, more than in any other area in the world, man concentrates on the conversion of feed grains and forage crops into meat, milk and eggs. The homemakers of the Middle Western states take pride in their cookery skills, and their hospitality is reflected by the bountiful table.

The Middle Western states are now regarded as industrial states, and agriculture is no longer the chief occupation. The migration of workers has brought industrial feeding problems.

THE EASTERN SEABOARD   Historical events are reflected in the summation of food characteristics of the people who reside in New England and other states along the Eastern seaboard. Every schoolchild knows the story of the Pilgrims and the education they received from the Indians in the use of available fowl, fish, corn, and other products. Baked beans, fish or clam chowder, fish cakes, lobster, and turkey for holidays or special occasions are some of the old New England customs. The molasses and spices shipped in from the West Indies, the retention of some of the food habits from the countries in Europe, plus the acquisition of new food tastes, characterize the meals of easterners, with the exception of the metropolitan areas, New York, Philadelphia, and Washington. Philadelphia is known for "sticky buns" and scrapple.

In the large seaboard cities, emigrants arrive and stay with relatives until they are familiar with the ways of their new home. Gradually an adjustment is made to dress and living conditions, while eating habits become a blend of the traditional along with the current trends. For example, New York has areas which have food shops (see Fig. 13–1) and restaurants catering to the food tastes of the Jews, Italians, Spanish, Puerto Ricans, French, Germans, Irish, Armenians, and many others. In these sections, the sophisticates take their international gourmet tours.

DIETARY PATTERNS OF NATIONALITY GROUPS

Current food habits of individuals are related to their social strata in a contemporary culture. The evolvement may be traced to the early establishment of social groupings. In the pre-Biblical period, the occupations of fishing, pastoral tending of sheep, farming of grain and fruits, and taking care of vineyards dominated the business of living for the roving nomadic tribes. The learned occupied the priestly positions. The East Mediterranean Sea area was the birthplace of three great religions, the Christian, the Hebrew, and the Mohammedan. The festivals attained religious significance, and to the Hebrews dietary laws were given. In contemporary society in all sections of the world, the Jews continue to observe their religious festivals with the same choice of ceremonial foods. (See page 205.)

NATIONAL RECIPES   There are a number of regional and national recipe books available for those who wish to prepare and eat dishes of other peoples.

FOOD PLANS   Following are dietary patterns of a number of countries to assist the student in a better understanding of various foreign-born individuals and families needing aid in meal planning, food budgeting and dietary instruction. It is a very large undertaking to provide food and dietary information for persons who emigrate to the United States under stress conditions. The rapid influx of the Cubans to Florida, for example, led to crowded conditions, linguistic problems and unfamiliar foods.

Rapid change is taking place in all countries, and it should be kept in mind that, while the dietary patterns listed here consist of the typical native foods and customs, all nations are being benefited by the United Nations educational programs on food and agricultural practices. Thus, what is typical today may not be true in a few years or so.

THE BELGIAN FOOD PLAN

THE SELECTION OF FOODS	PREPARATION
Meats: Beef, mutton, pork, and veal.	Meats are stewed or cooked into soups. All parts of animal used; sausage liked.
Fish: Salt water fish (fresh, dried and smoked), and shellfish.	Fish is stewed or boiled.
Other proteins: Eggs, split peas, and navy beans.	Eggs are used in cooking and in casserole dishes. Dried legumes are boiled or cooked into soups.
Vegetables: Beets, Brussels sprouts, cabbage, carrots, green beans, mushrooms, onions, potatoes, spinach, turnips, chicory, endive, lettuce, tomatoes, and some citrus fruits.	Potatoes served daily either boiled, mashed, or fried, or cooked with other vegetables and meats. Leafy vegetables served raw in salads, and tomatoes are used in cooking. Other vegetables are boiled in soups and stews, or served in cream sauce.

Fruits: Apples, berries, cherries, dried fruits, melons, pears and plums.

Fresh fruits in season are served raw, and stewed or used in baking; some are preserved for winter. Dried fruits are used in baking.

Cereals and breads: Oats and wheat.

Oatmeal is cooked into porridge, and wheat is used in white bread, rusks, rolls, and baked goods.

Milk: Cows' milk.

Fresh milk is the beverage for children, and used by adults in coffee and chocolate and in cooking.

Cheese: Soft and mild cheese.

Fats: Butter and lard.

Butter is spread on bread and used in baking; lard is used in baking.

Seasonings: Celery leaves and seeds, chervil, cinnamon, chocolate, honey, nuts, mustard, parsley, and thyme.

Beverages: Coffee, cocoa, wine, and beer.

Coffee is usually served as café au lait.

THE FOOD PLAN OF THE BRITISH ISLES

THE SELECTION OF FOODS

PREPARATION

Meats: Bacon, beef, lamb, mutton, and glandular organs.

Bacon is broiled. Beef, lamb and mutton are boiled, roasted, or cooked in a pie with vegetables. Steak and kidney pie is a favorite.

Fish: Locally available, such as cod, haddock, and herring.

Fish is boiled or fried in bacon drippings.

Other proteins: Eggs, game.

Eggs are cooked medium to hard consistency, and served in the shell. Available game is stewed with vegetables.

Vegetables: Brussels sprouts, cabbage, potatoes, and turnips.

Vegetables are boiled. Cabbage is cooked with bacon drippings. Potatoes are boiled and eaten abundantly.

Fruits: Apricots, berries, cherries, peaches, plums, rose hips, Seville oranges.

Berries and small fruits are stewed and served as fruit sauce. Rose hips are cooked into jam. Seville oranges are cooked into marmalade.

Cereals and breads: Oatmeal for cereal; oaten cake, rye, whole wheat, and white bread.

Oatmeal is cooked and served as breakfast porridge; it is also served frequently at evening meal. Bread is served with afternoon tea. Scones or biscuits and some bread are baked at home. Yorkshire pudding is served traditionally with roast beef.

Milk: Buttermilk, milk, very little cream, unless clotted into Devonshire cream.

Hot milk is served with cereal and also with tea.

Cheese: Cheddar type, Stilton, and soft cheeses.

Cheese is served with bread or biscuits at evening meal.

Fats: Bacon drippings; butter is imported.

Bacon drippings used in cooking; butter is spread on bread.

Seasonings: Herbs, salts, spices.

Herbs and spices used in cooking; salt flavor is enjoyed.

Beverages: Tea, alcoholic beverages.

Tea is served at the three daily meals and as a refreshing beverage between meals. Ale, stout, wine, and whisky are the alcoholic beverages.

THE BULGARIAN FOOD PLAN

THE SELECTION OF FOODS

PREPARATION

Meats: Beef, goat, lamb, mutton, pork, veal and poultry.

Meats are stewed with vegetables (mandja). Ground meat is used and organ meats are liked; the brains and kidneys are cooked in soups.

Fish: Some salt water fish.

Other proteins: Eggs; navy, dark, white, horse beans; and lentils.

Eggs are fried, hard boiled or scrambled. Beans are boiled or stewed.

Vegetables: Beets, green beans, cabbage, carrots, celery, cucumbers, eggplant, onions, potatoes, peppers, pumpkin, spinach, squash, vine leaves, and tomatoes.

Vegetables are stewed, baked into a pie (banitsa), or stuffed. Slices of pumpkin are baked and served with cheese.

Fruits: Apples, berries, cherries, dried fruits, grapes, melons, peaches, pears, and plums.

Fresh fruits in season are eaten raw, sun-dried for winter use and preserved. Apples are used in pastry, and prunes are baked with lamb.

Cereals and bread: Maize, rice, rye, and wheat.

Maize is used as cornmeal in polenta, rice is used to stuff vegetables, and rye (rural) and wheat (urban) are used in breads.

Milk: Cows' and sheeps' milk; yogurt, and sour cream.

Cold boiled milk is beverage for children, and adults like hot sugared milk. Sour milk is served with vegetables, and sour cream is put in soups.

Cheese: Soft and mild, and hard and dry.

Cheese is served at breakfast and with vegetables (to fill banitsa).

Fats: Butter, black olives, lard, olive oil, poultry fat, sunflower seed oil.

Oils are used in cooking, and butter is preferred for baking.

Seasonings: Caraway, poppy and sesame seeds, herbs, honey, garlic, paprika, parsley, vinegar, and walnuts.

Foods are highly seasoned. Nuts and honey are used in pastry.

Beverages: Coffee and tea (or other leaves).

Tea is served at breakfast, and Turkish style coffee at dinner.

THE CHINESE FOOD PLAN

THE SELECTION OF FOODS

PREPARATION

Meats: Pork (favorite), lamb, goat and poultry. Entire animal is eaten, including organs, brain, spinal cord, skin and coagulated blood.

Quantity is small and usually cut into small thin slices about 2 inches long and cooked in sesame or peanut oil with soy bean sauce, spices, and a little water; and served mixed with vegetables. Many methods for preserving and drying. Sweet and pungent pork or duck is a favorite (meat cubes rolled in batter and fried in oil, then simmered in sauce made of pineapple, green peppers, molasses, brown sugar, vinegar and seasonings.)

Fish: Fish and shellfish liked.

Frequently baked with native spices or prepared as sweet-sour dishes. Many dried.

Other proteins: Eggs: hen, duck and pigeon in abundance when afforded; soybean products; legumes.

Eggs are preserved and dried; also combined with chicken, mushrooms, bean sprouts, and served with soy sauce (looks like vegetable omelet), termed *egg foo yung.* Egg roll served at beginning of meal is made of shrimp or meat and chopped vegetables rolled in thin dough, and fried in deep fat. Soybeans used as sauce, as milk for infants in China, and many products. Legumes as substitute for meat.

Vegetables: Many plants and weeds such as carrots, onions, leeks, peas, cabbage, white turnips, corn, cucumbers, green and yellow beans, squash, shepherd's purse, radish leaves, sprouts (bean, bamboo, etc.), some white but more sweet potatoes.

Cut into uniform pieces and simmered or steamed with eggs or meat, or added to meat and widely used in soups.

Fruits: Kumquat is favorite.

Preserved dessert.

Cereal and bread: Rice used freely. Some wheat, barley, corn and millet seed. Noodles are popular. Rice is main dish; others are side dishes.

Rice is used as main dish, plain or fried. Millet seed is made into cakes or used as a gruel. Noodles are small and fried. Steamed bread is eaten at breakfast.

Milk: Very little, and generally not used. Given to children and invalids.

Cheese: Little used.

Fats: Chief oil is peanut oil. Some soy oil, rice oil, sesame oil or lard. Practically no butter or cream used.

Used in cooking.

Seasonings: Sesame seed, salt, ginger, garlic, fresh herbs, red pepper.

Beverage: Tea is national beverage.

Beverage at all meals, when afforded.

THE CUBAN FOOD PLAN
(PRE-CASTRO REGIME)

THE SELECTION OF FOODS	PREPARATION
Meats: Beef, pork, lamb, veal, poultry, sausages.	Pork is either roasted or fried. Beef and chicken are used in soups, stewed, roasted, broiled or barbecued. The sausages are used with beans.
Fish: All varieties of fish (fresh, salted, smoked and canned).	Fried, boiled, marinated, roasted or grilled.
Other proteins: Beans (black, red, kidney, navy, yellow, lima, green); split peas; eggs.	Black beans with rice and roast pork is a favorite dish and is eaten on Christmas day. Eggs are eaten daily: fried, scrambled or in dessert.
Vegetables: Native tubers such as yuca, ñame, malanga (white and yellow), boniato (white yams), chayote, berenjena, plantain, potatoes, lettuce, tomatoes, carrots.	The tubers are boiled and served with *mojo* (made with sour orange, crushed garlic, sliced onions, and hot oil), or mashed with butter and milk. Fried ripe or green plantains are a favorite side dish.
Fruits: Anón, mamey, guanábana, chirimoya, papaya, banana, zapote, marañón, mangoes, grapefruit, oranges (sweet and sour), cocoanuts, caimito.	Eaten fresh, in juice, or in desserts such as pastes, jellies, puddings.
Cereals: Rice, cornmeal, cornstarch, imported breakfast cereals such as oatmeal, corn flakes.	The favorite is white (long grain) steamed rice; sometimes bijol is added to make it yellow as in *arrez con pollo* (yellow rice with chicken). White rice is eaten daily for dinner and supper.
Milk: Fresh cows' milk (whole, skimmed), condensed, evaporated, dry; sour cream; goats' milk for the sick, usually.	Adults use it in coffee; children use as beverage. Also used in cream sauces, gravies, desserts, etc.
Cheese: Gouda, cream, *queso de mano*.	The native cheese is *queso de mano* (hard cheese) made from milk, lactate of calcium and salt, which looks like compressed cottage cheese; is usually eaten with guava paste.
Fats: Pork lard, olive oil, peanut oil, soy oil, butter, margarine and shortening.	Pork lard is most popular. Oil is used in salads and beans.
Desserts: Fruits, ice cream, cakes, pies, custards, puddings; guava, prune and mango pastes; guava shelves, morón cookies, terrejas, boniatillo, buñuelos, cafiroleta.	Eaten after each meal and also as snacks. *Raspadura* is very sweet and the most typical native dessert.
Seasonings: Oil, vinegar, cumin, oregano, bijol, salt, pepper, garlic, onion, green peppers.	
Beverages: Coffee, beer, wines, tea, carbonated beverages.	Dark strong coffee served demitasse, with or without sugar.

THE CZECHOSLOVAKIAN FOOD PLAN

THE SELECTION OF FOODS	PREPARATION
Meats: Beef, pork (fresh and smoked), veal, poultry, and game.	Smoked ham, fresh pork, organ meats, and sausage are preferred.
Fish: Fresh water fish.	
Other proteins: Eggs, lentils, yellow peas, kidney and white beans.	Eggs are used in cooking and baking. Legumes are boiled, cooked in soups or stews, or served as a relish.
Vegetables: Beets, cabbage, carrots, cauliflower, celeriac, kale, leeks, mushrooms, parsnips, potatoes, spinach, turnips, and tomatoes.	Potatoes and vegetables are boiled and served with cream. Cabbage is made into sauerkraut.
Fruits: Apples, apricots, berries, cherries, pears, plums, and some imported bananas, pineapple, dried fruits, citrus fruits.	Fresh fruits in season are eaten raw, or preserved. Dried fruits are used in baking.
Milk: Cows' milk, fermented milk and buttermilk.	Fresh milk is the beverage for children. Buttermilk and clabber milk are preferred by adults.
Cheese: Soft and mild cheese from sheep's milk.	Soft and hard cheese are used in baking and dumplings.

Fats: Butter, lard, poultry fat.

Poultry fat spread on bread. Lard is used in cooking and butter is preferred for baking.

Cereals and breads: Maize, rye, and wheat.

Maize cooked into mush. Sour rye bread with caraway seeds is liked. White flour used in pastries and dumplings.

Seasonings: Caraway, poppy and sesame seeds, garlic, honey, dried mushrooms, nuts, and spices.

Beverages: Coffee, cocoa, beer, and wine.

Coffee consumed during entire day. Czechs enjoy beer, and Slovaks like wine.

THE DANISH FOOD PLAN

THE SELECTION OF FOODS

PREPARATION

Meats: Beef, mutton, pork, veal, and poultry.

Meats are roasted, stewed, braised with or without vegetables; organ meats are liked; sausages are liked, too.

Fish: Salt water fish and shellfish (fresh, smoked or canned).

Fish is boiled or broiled, and used in puddings. Smoked fish roe is liked.

Other proteins: Eggs and yellow peas.

Eggs used in cooking, and yellow peas are cooked in soup.

Vegetables: Beets, Brussels sprouts, cabbage, carrots, cauliflower, celery, celeriac, cucumbers, dandelion and sorrel greens, leeks, onions, peas, potatoes, radishes, lettuce, tomatoes.

Potatoes are popular, and are boiled, mashed, fried, in soups, and casserole dishes. Vegetables are served in cream sauce. Tomatoes, cucumbers and lettuce used in salads.

Fruits: Apples, bananas, berries (all varieties), cherries currants, pears, plums, raisins, rhubarb, some oranges and lemons, and rose hips.

Fresh fruits in season and those preserved for winter use are served as stewed fruits, fruit soups, and in pastry fillings.

Cereals and breads: Barley, oats, rye, and wheat.

Barley is cooked in soup; oats are cooked into porridge; rye and wheat are made into breads, rolls and cakes.

Milk: Cows' and goats' milk, cream.

Fresh milk is popular beverage for children and adults, and used in cooking to make sauces and desserts.

Cheese: Soft and mild, hard and dry varieties.

Fats: Butter, margarine (made of vegetable, whale or other fish oils), lard, and salt pork.

Butter or margarine is used on bread, in cooking and baking. Butter is considered "cash crop."

Seasonings: Cinnamon, cloves, dill, mace, pepper, and thyme.

Beverages: Coffee, tea, and beer.

Coffee served with cream or as café au lait.

THE FRENCH FOOD PLAN

THE SELECTION OF FOODS

PREPARATION

Meats: Beef, mutton, pork (fresh and cured), veal and poultry.

Meats are boiled, stewed, broiled, roasted, fried, or cooked into soups. Sausage is either eaten separately or cooked with other foods. All parts of the animal are used. Poultry is stewed, sautéed or cooked into soup.

Fish: Fresh water and salt water fish, and shellfish.

Fish is boiled, broiled, fried, baked or cooked into soup.

Other proteins: Eggs, lentils, dried peas, and kidney beans.

Eggs are prepared in many different ways. Lentils and legumes are boiled or cooked into soups and stews.

Vegetables: Asparagus, artichokes, beets, broccoli, Brussels sprouts, cabbage, carrots, celery, endive, green beans and peas, leeks, mushrooms, onions, peppers, potatoes, salsify, turnips, tomatoes, salad greens.

Potatoes are boiled, fried or cooked into soups and stews. Regional differences are noticed in cooking of vegetables. Salad greens are dressed with oil and vinegar.

Fruits: Apples, apricots, berries, cherries, dates (imported), figs (South), grapes, melons, pears, peaches, plums, and some citrus fruits.

Fresh fruits in season are served raw or stewed. Grapes are pressed into wine, and apples and pears are pressed into cider.

Cereals and breads: Barley, maize, rice, and wheat.

Barley and rice are cooked in soups; wheat is used in breads, rolls and baked goods.

Milk: Cows' milk.

Boiled milk is served to children, and adults use boiled milk in coffee and chocolate.

Cheese: Various types made from cows' and goats' milk.

Cheese is used in cooking and also served for snacks or dessert.

Fats: Butter, poultry fats, lard, olives, seed oils, and salt pork.

Butter is used in cooking but little is spread on bread; olive oil used in salads and in the South used for cooking, too.

Seasonings: Allspice, bayleaves, chervil, chives, cloves, cinnamon, capers, garlic, parsley, saffron, tarragon, truffles, and vinegar.

Beverages: Beer, cider, cocoa, coffee, and wine.

In the North cider is popular and all ages drink wine. Coffee is mixed with chicory and served as café au lait. Chocolate has hot milk added. Much wine is used in food preparation.

THE GREEK FOOD PLAN

THE SELECTION OF FOODS

PREPARATION

Meats: Lamb is main meat. Some beef, goat, mutton, pork products; poultry is popular.

Meat is either cut into small pieces or ground. Poultry is cooked into broth. Lamb is cooked on skewers or cut up and browned in oil or fat with rice or flour and vegetables.

Fish: Salt water fish (fresh, smoked or salted), shellfish, smoked roe, squid, and octopus.

Fish is fried or steamed with vegetables. Used frequently.

Other proteins: Eggs, white beans and legumes.

Legumes are boiled, mashed, stewed, and eaten either hot or cold. Soup made of dried beans, onions, celery and carrots is a national dish. Eggs are popular.

Vegetables: Cabbage, cauliflower, cucumbers, eggplant, greens, okra, onions, peppers, some potatoes, vine leaves, zucchini, tomatoes, salad greens, oranges, and lemons.

Vegetables boiled or fried in a small amount of olive oil and served hot or cold. Many vegetables are stuffed. Potatoes or vegetables are cooked with meat or fish. Lemon juice is used to dress salads and cold foods.

Fruits: Apricots, cherries, dates, figs, grapes, melons, nuts, plums, peaches, pears, quinces, and raisins.

Fruits in season are eaten raw, grapes are pressed into wine or dried as raisins. Fruit for dessert.

Cereals and breads: Maize, rice and wheat.

Maize is used in polenta; rice is an ingredient for pilawi and stuffing for vegetables; and wheat is made into bread. Bread is used abundantly and white preferred.

Milk: Cows', goats' and sheep's milk.

Milk is boiled for children. Fermented milk or yaourti is eaten as dessert or with pastry.

Cheese: Soft and mild, and hard and dry cheese.

Cheese is popular.

Fats: Olive oil, seed oils, salted black olives, and little butter.

Olive oil is used to dress salads and hot or cold vegetables, and in cooking.

Seasonings: Caraway and pumpkin seeds, herbs, honey, nuts (hazel, pignolia, and pistachio), and sesame.

Seeds are eaten between meals, and nuts are served as dessert.

Beverages: Coffee and wine.

Coffee (American) is the beverage served in the mornings. At other meals it is made and served Turkish style. Wine is served at meals.

THE GERMAN AND HUNGARIAN FOOD PLAN

THE SELECTION OF FOODS

PREPARATION

Meats: Beef (muscle and organs), pork, veal, bacon, sausage, poultry (especially goose), and game.

Stews served with dumplings or noodles. These combinations are frequent: chicken and anchovies, beef and noodle soup, beans with pork, veal and peas, and crawfish and tomatoes.

Fish: Fresh water fish and shrimp.

Other proteins: Eggs.

Used in noodles, as thickening agent or garnish.

Vegetables: Cabbage (red and white), carrots, cauliflower, cucumbers, beets, beans, broccoli, kale, kohlrabi, onions, potatoes, sauerkraut, tomatoes, and lettuce.

Lettuce served with bacon and hot vinegar, red cabbage with bacon sauce, and potato salad with herring. Vegetables eaten rarely as separate dish.

Fruits: Apples, apricots, bananas, cherries, berries, grapes, melons, oranges, quinces, pears, peaches, and prunes.

Served for dessert.

Cereals: Barley, farina, mehl (Hungarian flour), and rye.

Breads: Noodles, spaetzel (dumplings), and strudel (sweet bread).

Milk: Buttermilk, milk, sour milk, and sour cream.

Milk and cream used in cooking rather than as beverage.

Cheese: Cottage, cream, and brick cheese.

Cottage cheese used in strudels, cheese cake and noodle dishes.

Fats: Butter and meat fats.

Butter used in cooking and sparingly on breads; jam is preferred on breads.

Desserts: Fruits, cheese cakes, and strudels.

Seasonings: Caraway seed, horseradish, garlic, onions, paprika, peppers, pickles, poppy seed, parsley, and vinegar.

Beverages: Tea, coffee, beer, Tokay wine, schnapps, and Hungarian whisky.

THE ITALIAN FOOD PLAN

THE SELECTION OF FOODS

PREPARATION

Meats: Beef, lamb, veal, pork, fowl; and sausages, bologna and salami.

Small quantity of meat slow simmered, served with sauce such as tomato sauce prepared with garlic, onion, green peppers, tomato; or fried. Usually cut up and stewed, fried or ground and cooked with pasta. Some favorite dishes are chicken *cacciatora*, veal (cutlet) *scallopine*, meat balls with tomato or clam sauce on spaghetti.

Fish: All fish, and clams, mussels, octopus, fresh sardines, squid, and snails.

Other proteins: Eggs; dried beans, lentils and peas.

Eggs fried plain or with spinach, onions and peppers; used as thickening agent; and omelet with cheese. Dried beans, lentils, and peas cooked in thick soups such as *minestrone* and *pastafasiole*.

Vegetables: Artichokes, string beans, broccoli, cauliflower, celery, chicory, Savoy cabbage, dandelion greens, endive, eggplant, fennel, garlic, mushrooms, peas, few potatoes, peppers, radishes, romaine, scallions, spinach, Italian squash, and tomatoes.

Greens are served raw and flavored with oil and wine vinegar; other vegetables are parboiled and fried in oil, or served with olive oil or olive oil and vinegar; tomatoes are cooked into sauce, soups, or cooked with meat or fish.

Fruits: Fresh, glazed and dried fruits, grapes, pears, plums, melons, quinces, cherries, peaches, figs, dates, apricots, apples, oranges, persimmons, and raisins.

Served for dessert.

Nuts: Almonds, chestnuts, hazelnuts, pistachios, and walnuts.

Cereals: Chestnut flour, cornmeal (polenta), farina, macaroni and spaghetti.

Cooked pasta (spaghetti, noodles, macaroni) served with sauces and cheese.

Breads: Crusty Italian white bread, pizza and facaccia (whole wheat bread).

Breads served with each meal. Also used for stuffings. Fried bread dough (pietsa) served with sugar.

Milk: Very little used, no cream. Goat's milk preferred.

Beverage for children.

Cheese: Casicavallo, locatelli, Parmesan, provolone, Roman mozzarella, and ricotta (Italian cottage cheese).

Italian cheeses (*mozzarella* and *ricotta* for cooking; *parmesan* and *romano* for grating; *gorgonzola*) are well liked and used in liberal amounts. Grated parmesan cheese served on spaghetti and vegetables; soft cheese used as fillings in sandwiches.

Fats: Olive oil, cotton seed oil, lard, salt pork, very little butter.

Olive oil used to cook meats and in vegetables; to season salads; in sauces.

Desserts: Fruit, fancy cakes, chestnuts, gelati (brick ice cream), marzapane (almond cakes), spumone ice cream, and tortoni.

Desserts served on feast days and special occasions.

Seasonings: Aniseed, cloves, garlic, onions, parsley, pepper, salt, thyme, and vinegar.

Foods are highly seasoned.

Beverages: Coffee, dry wines and liquors.

Coffee with hot milk and sugar. Wine in cooking and as beverage for adults.

THE JAPANESE FOOD PLAN

THE SELECTION OF FOODS

PREPARATION

Meats: The Buddhist tradition of not eating meat conforms with the physical necessities of agriculture. The Japanese masses consume very little meat, except beef. Since the war, however, protein intake has increased; from 1950 to 1960 the protein intake increased 10 per cent and animal protein almost doubled.

Quantity is small and usually cut into small pieces and served mixed with vegetables and cereal products. (See Fig. 13-4).

Fish: Liked and one of staple foods.

Prefer fish, shellfish, and other marine life to meats of all types. Certain kinds of raw fish are considered great delicacies. Others cooked or dried.

Other proteins: Soybean preparations used freely. Eggs used when available.

Variety soybean preparations.

Vegetables: Prefer plants and weeds such as seaweed, bamboo shoots. Onions, large radishes, dried mushrooms (shiitake) and beans. Potatoes and others when available.

Pickled is favorite. Others cooked with meat or fish.

Figure 13-4   A Japanese meal. Sukiyaki, made with beef and vegetables, may be served with tea, rice and a small marinated salad. (New York Times Magazine, April 24, 1955.)

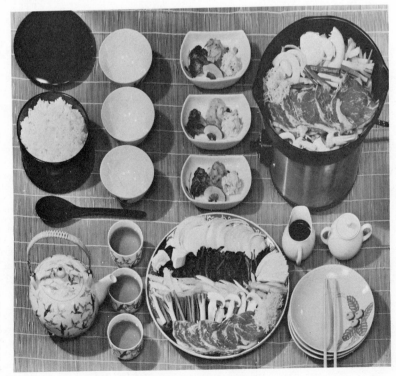

This is an example of a meal, Japanese in inspiration, American by adaptation. The ingredients of sukiyaki are beef suet, paper-thin sliced tender beef, sliced onions, sliced celery, steamed spinach, scallions, sliced mushrooms, sliced bamboo shoots, cubes of soybean curd, vermicelli, sugar, soy sauce and sake. A very hot skillet is rubbed with the suet, and meat is seared on both sides. The heat is turned low, and the remainder of ingredients are added. The entire contents of the skillet are then simmered five to seven minutes longer. Vegetables should be crisp when eaten. In preparing sukiyaki, Japanese often use dried mushrooms (shiitake) of very intense flavor and fragrance. These are soaked a couple of hours before they are added to the dish. They are available in Japanese groceries.

"Suki" means plow and "yaki" means roasted. According to a story, probably apocryphal, this dish originated in Japan a century or more ago at a time when Buddhism forbade the eating of beef. A farmer slaughtered a steer in secret on a lonely mountain and then cooked it, using part of his plow as a grill over the fire. Hence, the term "plow-roasted" – sukiyaki.

Fruits: Principal fruit is nasi (tastes somewhat like pear, shaped like an apple; yellow, rough skin). Some persimmons and mulberries. Tangerines in mountain regions. Postwar increase in variety.

Dessert.

Cereal and bread: Rice is main food. Some barley, oats and rye.

Rice is main dish of food. Rice is mixed with barley by farmers and the poorer classes. Wheat bread, especially in urban communities.

Milk: Enjoy when available; mainly import evaporated or dry milk powder.

For children mainly.

Cheese: Very little.

Fats: Soy oil, rice oil. Suet when available. Practically no butter and cream.

Used in cooking.

Seasonings: Salt, sake (liquor distilled from rice).

Beverages: Tea, sake.

Tea freely used when afforded.

THE JEWISH FOOD PLAN

THE SELECTION OF FOODS

PREPARATION

Meats: Koshered forequarters only and organs of beef, lamb and veal; smoked, salted and spiced beef and tongues; poultry. Pork prohibited.

Meats are boiled or cooked with vegetables and in meat soups. Meat and dairy products are not prepared at the same time. Poultry is usually eaten on Sabbath eve (Friday).

Fish: Carp, cod, flounder, haddock, herring (smoked and salted fish). Fish without scales or fins prohibited.

Fish is boiled in sweet and sour sauce, fried, pickled and stuffed (gefülte).

Other proteins: Eggs, lentils, dried peas and beans.

Eggs are cooked and served or used in soups, particularly to make small dumplings or noodles.

Vegetables: Root vegetables (beets, onions, potatoes, turnips), corn, cabbage, sauerkraut, legumes, tomatoes, cucumbers, lettuce, and sorrel.

Cooked with meats into soups (borscht), served rarely as a separate dish; eaten raw with sour cream; pickled and salted vegetables liked.

Fruits: Apples, dried fruits, grapes, oranges, pears, and plums.

Eaten raw or stewed and served in compote.

Cereals: Barley, buckwheat, oatmeal, rye, rice, and wheat.

Barley and kasha cooked in soups.

Breads: Matzoth, noodles, pumpernickel bread, rye bread, white seed rolls, and challah (rich white bread).

Matzoth are served during Passover. Noodles are cooked in soup.

Milk: Cows' milk and sour cream.

Dairy products are never combined with meat dishes.

Cheese: Cream, cottage, Swiss, and Muenster.

Fats: Sweet butter, beef fat and chicken fat, sour cream, vegetable oil and shortening.

Butter is not used in meat dishes.

Desserts: Pancakes (blintzes); rich pastries filled with fruits and nuts: fruit compote; cheese cake and sponge cake; macaroons.

Seasonings: All of the spices and many relishes used (garlic, horseradish, lemon, mustard, onion, pepper, salt, vinegar); conserves and preserves.

Beverages: Coffee, tea, wine.

Wine is served as part of ceremonial rites on Sabbath, feast days, and holidays.

(See p. 205 for Jewish Food Customs and Dietary Laws.)

THE FOOD PLAN OF THE NETHERLANDS

THE SELECTION OF FOODS

PREPARATION

Meats: Beef and pork most popular. Some veal and poultry.

Meats are stewed and braised; broths and gravies are popular; smoked beef is liked.

Fish: Salt water fish; herring (fresh, smoked or pickled); and shellfish.

Fish is boiled or broiled in stews and soups, and the salted, smoked or pickled varieties are eaten as snacks. Fish at least once a week.

Other proteins: Eggs, yellow split peas, kidney and navy beans.

Eggs are used in cooking and served many ways when available. Split pea soup is served with sausages.

Vegetables: Beets, broccoli, Brussels sprouts, green beans, cabbage, carrots, cauliflower, cucumbers, kohlrabi, onions, potatoes, turnips, lettuce and few tomatoes.

Potatoes are usually boiled or mashed and served daily; other vegetables are served boiled or in cream sauce. Tomatoes, cucumbers and lettuce served raw. Hutspot is a combination of boiled carrots and potatoes. Combinations are popular.

Fruits: Apples, cherries, citron, currants, pears, plums, raisins, strawberries, and some citrus fruits.

Fresh fruits in season are served raw, also preserved into jams and jellies, and dried fruits are used in baking.

Cereals and breads: Barley, cornstarch, oats, rice, rye, and wheat.

Barley and rice cooked in soups; cornstarch is an ingredient in baked goods and puddings; barley, rice and oats cooked into porridge; rye and wheat are made into bread. Oatmeal cereal popular for breakfast.

Milk: Cows' milk.

Fresh milk is the beverage for children, and used in cooking, coffee and chocolate. Buttermilk is liked.

Cheese: All varieties of cheese, especially Edam and Gouda.

Fats: Butter, margarine (made of vegetable oils and butter), and lard.

Butter is used in baking and on bread when available (a luxury), margarine is used for most purposes, and lard is used extensively in baking.

Seasonings: Allspice, capers, chocolate, cinnamon, cloves, curry, dill, ginger, honey, mace, nuts, and peppercorns.

THE NORWEGIAN FOOD PLAN

THE SELECTION OF FOODS

PREPARATION

Meats: Beef, mutton, pork, veal, game, and poultry.

Braised, boiled, stewed, roasted, alone or with vegetables; smoked and salted meats; cooked in broths and soups.

Fish: Fresh and salt water fish (fresh, salted, smoked, and canned).

Boiled, broiled, used in puddings, fish balls, soups, and served several times during week. Evening meal consists of smoked or salted fish or meat and bread.

Other proteins: Eggs; navy and kidney beans; yellow split peas.

Eggs used in cooking; dried peas and beans cooked in soups.

Vegetables: Beets, string beans, cabbage, carrots, celeries, cucumbers, dandelion greens, leeks, parsley, peas, potatoes, rutabagas, mushrooms, turnips, tomatoes, lettuce.

Potatoes served daily, boiled, mashed, fried, in salads, and cooked with meats or fish; other vegetables served boiled, steamed, cooked with meat, creamed. Tomatoes and cucumbers served raw.

Fruits: Apples, berries, cherries, cloudberries, currants, dried fruits, lingon berries, rose hips, and rhubarb.

In season, used in fruit, soups, sauces and puddings; stored in water in crocks, in preserves and jams, or as juice.

Cereals and breads: Barley, oats, rice, rye, sago, and wheat.

Barley cooked in soups; rice or sago used in fruit soups and puddings; oats cooked into porridge; rye is made into bread; whole wheat is used in leavened bread; and white flour is used in pastry, cake and rolls.

Milk: Cows' and goats' milk.

Milk is beverage for children, and used by adults in coffee; used in cooking porridge, cream sauces and gravies.

Fats: Butter, margarine (from fish oils), lard, cod livers, poultry fat, and salt pork.

Butter is spread on bread, to flavor vegetables, in baking; salt pork and lard used in cooking; in winter, fish oil is supplemented to cod livers.

Cheese: Mild and soft cheese, and gjetøst from goats' milk.

Seasonings: Bay leaves, caraway and cardamon seeds, chives, citron, dill, honey, black pepper, and thyme.

Beverages: Coffee, tea, cocoa, beer.

Coffeepot is on stove all day; chocolate is a popular afternoon beverage.

THE POLISH FOOD PLAN

THE SELECTION OF FOODS	PREPARATION
Meats: Beef, pork (ham), veal (lungs, tongue, tripe, brain, liver, kidneys), fowl, geese, rabbit, and salami.	Stews are preferred. Meat is smoked with fumes of juniper wood, seldom fried.
Fish: All varieties of fish.	Fresh fish eaten in summer, pickled fish is selected in winter.
Other proteins: Eggs.	Eggs used in soups and dumplings.
Vegetables: Butter beans, cabbage, carrots, cucumbers, kale, lettuce, mushrooms, onions, parsnips, potatoes, sauerkraut, sorrel, radishes, leeks, turnips, beets, and split peas.	Potatoes served at most of the meals. Vegetables cooked with meat (pig's knuckles) and noodles. Frequent combinations are cabbage and split peas, stuffed cabbage, potato pancakes, and borscht (beet soup). Cabbage (sauerkraut) and root vegetables main ones used.
Fruits: Apples, apricots, cherries, grapes, pears, plums, prunes, and strawberries.	Cooked into fruit soups, and eaten dried and raw.
Cereals and breads: Barley, buckwheat, cornmeal, kasha (mixture of barley, buckwheat, oats, and millet), oats, rice, rye, and whole wheat.	Oatmeal and cornflakes eaten in United States. Rice cooked with meats and vegetables. Barley and kasha are cooked in soups. Dark rye bread served with each meal.
Milk: Cows' and goats' milk; sour cream.	Cream used in soups. Milk and sour cream popular. Sour cream served on vegetables, salad, and used in cooking meats.
Cheese: Cottage, cream and brick cheese.	Cottage cheese used in dumplings and kuchens.
Fats: Butter, flaxseed oil, pork fat, and sesame oil.	Small amounts of butter used in cooking and on bread. Luxury.
Desserts: Fruits, cookies, small cakes, and pancakes with preserves.	
Seasonings: Almonds, chili sauce, dried mushrooms, horseradish, mace, onions, pickles, poppy seeds, peppers, and saffron.	
Beverages: Tea and coffee are popular; Polish beer.	

THE PUERTO RICAN FOOD PLAN

THE SELECTION OF FOODS	PREPARATION
Meats: Pork and chicken are favorite meats. Also use ham butts, sausages, beef.	A little goes a long way in flavoring stew and vegetables. Beef and pork, cut in small pieces, cooked with potatoes, and served with refrito. (Refrito is a mixture of seasonings.) Chicken cooked with rice well liked and called *arroz con pollo;* and eaten with red kidney beans.
Fish: Fresh fish along coast; dried and salted fish inland. Dried codfish a favorite.	Salad of salt cod, hard cooked eggs, and raw onions, served with oil and vinegar; well liked. *Viandas* (starchy vegetable) with codfish plus avocado in season, and eggs when income permits, is called *serenata* and is a staple dish; onion for flavor.
Other proteins: Legumes: Lima, navy, pinto, and red beans; chick peas. Eggs when available.	Legumes are basic food. Stew is common method of preparing beans and rice with lard or olive oil added for flavor. Annato is added to fat for color. Rice and beans form main meal several times a week. Refrito often cooked with beans and/or rice. Variety is obtained by using various kinds of legumes. Dried beans sometimes cooked with tomatoes, onions and seasonings. Eggs also hard cooked and used in salad.
Vegetables: Chayote (eggplant), ñame, cassava, malangas, yams, and yautias; onions, green peppers, beets, tomatoes, green beans, carrots, and okra.	Use in stew; salad of cooked tubers and onions, served with oil and vinegar.
Fruits: Plantain and banana are favorites. Also oranges, acerola, mango, guava, papaya, cashew nut fruit and pineapple.	Plantain is mashed and mixed with chopped onion. Green banana and plantain used as a vegetable with fish or meat in place of potato. Other fruit eaten raw or cooked in syrup.

Cereals: Rice, wheat, oatmeal and cornmeal.	Rice is a staple food as described above. When rice is not available, use cornmeal. Also spaghetti and noodles widely used. Oatmeal for breakfast.
Breads: White chiefly.	
Milk: Fresh cows' milk when available and consumer can afford it. Milk always boiled.	Used as beverage for children; in coffee (4–5 ounces per cup) for adults. Also, used in very sweet cocoa and chocolate drink.
Cheese: Native white (*queso blanco*) when available and consumer can afford it.	Use *queso blanco* with pastas.
Fats: Lard, ham fat, olive oil, very little butter.	Lard, ham fat and olive oil used in cooking. Olive oil also on salads.
Desserts: Fruits (see above); and pastas.	
Seasonings: Garlic, onion and vinegar favorites.	
Beverages: Coffee, chocolate and cocoa.	Strong coffee served with half milk at each meal (Café con leche).

THE RUMANIAN FOOD PLAN

THE SELECTION OF FOODS	PREPARATION
Meats: Beef, lamb, mutton, pork (fresh and smoked), veal, poultry, and game.	All parts of the animal used; cooked in soups or stews, or grilled. Lamb, mutton and pork are everyday meats, while beef, veal, and poultry are served on holidays.
Fish: Fresh water fish (fresh and smoked); and shellfish.	Fish is boiled, steamed, grilled, or marinated.
Other proteins: Few eggs; white and other beans.	Eggs are used in baking for holiday foods; beans are cooked in soup or boiled and served with oil.
Vegetables: Beets, green beans, cabbage, carrots, cucumbers, eggplant, leeks, mushrooms, okra, peppers, potatoes, pumpkin, radishes, turnips, and tomatoes.	Potatoes and other vegetables are cooked in soups or stews, stuffed and then steamed. Fermented or pickled vegetables are liked.
Fruits: Apples, berries, cherries, dried fruit, grapes, melons, peaches, pears, plums, and some lemons.	Fruits in season are eaten raw and preserved. Grapes are pressed into wine.
Cereals and breads: Barley, maize, rice, rye, and wheat.	Barley is cooked in soups; rice is cooked in soups, with meats, or in stuffings. Yellow maize meal is boiled (mamaliga), and wheat is used in bread dumplings and paste.
Milk: Cows', goats' and sheep's milk, fermented milk, sweet and sour cream.	Boiled milk is served to children. Sweet or sour cream is served with soup.
Cheese: Soft and mild, or dry and hard.	Cheese is eaten with bread or served with cooked vegetables.
Fats: Butter, black olives, lard, olive oil, poultry fat, and seed oils.	Oil is used to dress vegetables, and lard and seed oils are used in cooking.
Seasonings: Garlic herbs, horseradish, nuts, paprika, seeds, spices, and vinegar.	Foods are highly seasoned.
Beverages: Coffee and wine.	Coffee is made Turkish style.

THE SWEDISH FOOD PLAN

THE SELECTION OF FOODS	PREPARATION
Meats: Beef, pork (ham and bacon), veal, kidneys, sausages, reindeer meat, and wild birds.	Assorted fish and meat served at smorgasbord; jellied meats; and meats in cream gravies.
Fish: Anchovies, caviar, crayfish, herring, smoked salmon, shrimp, and Lutfisk.	Herring is served most mornings.
Other proteins: Eggs.	Eggs are cooked and stuffed or used in omelets.
Vegetables: Asparagus, cabbage, mushrooms, onions, peas, and potatoes.	Potatoes are cooked in skins and then fried.

Fruits: Apples, cherries, cranberries (Lingon conserve), currants, and prunes.

Served with meats or as dessert.

Cereals and breads: Oatmeal, rye bread, white bread, and Limpa (Swedish bread).

Milk: Cows' milk, goats' milk, cream, and whipped cream.

Children receive milk at meals.

Cheese: Cream and cottage cheese.

Fats: Butter and cream.

Used generously on bread and in cooking.

Desserts: Almond wafers, cookies, glacé, ginger cakes, and ginger snaps.

Cookies and ginger cake served at breakfast.

Seasonings: Almond, cloves, cinnamon, dill, ginger, molasses, mustard, onion, peppercorns, and vinegar.

Beverages: Coffee, beer and wines.

Large quantities of coffee consumed, enjoyed with bread and cheese.

THE SYRIAN FOOD PLAN

THE SELECTION OF FOODS

PREPARATION

Meats and fish: Lamb is the choice.

Lamb is prepared barbecued style on hickory skewer, or in Keib (a national dish of lamb and ground wheat).

Other proteins: Lentils, nuts, dried peas and beans.

Vegetables: Artichokes, cabbage, cucumbers, eggplant, garlic, grape leaves, okra, onions, peppers, olives, squash, and tomatoes.

Vegetables are fried in olive oil or meat fat, then boiled in meat stock. Many are stuffed with wheat, rice, meat, nuts or beans, then cooked in oil (called pilaf).

Fruits: Dates, dried apricots, figs, grapes, oranges, and raisins.

Fruit compotes for dessert.

Cereals and breads: Barley, rice, whole or cracked wheat, and white and dark breads.

Cereals are combined with meat for main dish, or with fruits for dessert.

Milk: Goats' milk or camels' milk, Liben-cured milk, and clotted cream.

Fermented and soured milk called yoghurt and matzoon.

Cheese: Hard, Kasher, and Greek cheese.

Fats: Olive oil, sheep's butter, and meat fats.

Nuts: Chestnuts, hazelnuts, peanuts, and pistachios.

Nuts used in place of meats with cracked wheat and rice.

Desserts: Fruit compotes; bread, honey and cream; apricot candy; and Turkish paste.

Seasonings: Cloves and other spices, honey, hickory embers for broiling, molasses from grapes, and rose water.

Beverages: Milk for children; Turkish coffee (Giaour).

THE YUGOSLAVIAN FOOD PLAN

THE SELECTION OF FOODS

PREPARATION

Meats: Beef, mutton, pork (fresh and smoked), veal, poultry, and game.

Meats are stewed, roasted or grilled or cooked into soups. Poultry is served on holidays.

Fish: Fresh water and salt water fish (fresh, salted and smoked).

Fish is either grilled or cooked in pilaf.

Other proteins: Eggs and all types of beans.

Beans are boiled, and served hot or cold.

Vegetables: Beets, green beans, cabbage, carrots, cucumbers, eggplant, greens, onions, peppers, potatoes, turnips, salad greens, and tomatoes.

Vegetables are cooked, in soups or stuffed. Sauerkraut is liked. Cabbage slaw and green salads with chives; garlic and onion are liked.

Fruits: Apples, apricots, cherries, dates, dried fruits, figs, grapes, melons, peaches, pears, plums, strawberries, and some citrus fruits.

Fresh fruits in season are eaten raw, and apples, pears and plums are dried for winer use. Fruit fillings are put into strudels and dumplings.

Milk: Cows', goats' and sheep's milk, yoghurt and sour cream.

Boiled milk is served to children and adolescents. Adults drink fresh, fermented milk and buttermilk.

Cheese: Soft and hard, sharp cheese from sheep's milk.

Cheese is eaten with bread or used in cooking, baking and in pancakes.

Fats: Butter, lard, olive oil, and poultry fat.

Fats used in cooking, some butter spread on breads.

Seasonings: Caraway, poppy and sesame seeds, garlic, paprika, and spices.

Beverages: Coffee, beer, and wine.

Coffee is served Turkish style. Wine is served on holidays.

SOUTHEAST ASIA AND SOUTH VIETNAM   Rice is the principal food and is eaten at least once a day. Fish and vegetables (manioc, maize and sweet potatoes) are ingested with or in place of rice. Nuoc mam, a fish sauce made by a salt pickling process, is served with most foods. Soybeans, coconuts, peanuts and sugar cane are important foods. Cane juice is used to sweeten food and the sugar cane is eaten raw. Cabbage, spinach, squash, watercress are plentiful and reasonable in price. Poultry and pork back are served two or three times a week, but beef is very expensive and seldom eaten. Little fresh milk is used. Tea is the beverage served at meals by all classes. Chinese influence in the choice of foods and methods of preparation prevails. French cooking has been acquired to some extent but the rice and fish sauce is included in the meal. In the city the noon meal is the largest but in rural areas during periods of intense work the morning and evening meals are heavy meals with only a bowl of rice at noon. Food is eaten with chopsticks usually and the family may sit on mats on the floor or a wooden platform or at a table.

DIETARY RESTRICTIONS AND PATTERNS OF RACIAL AND RELIGIOUS GROUPS

JEWISH FOOD CUSTOMS AND DIETARY LAWS[3]

The Jewish dietary laws are Biblical ordinances codified and interpreted into rules regarding food. The rules pertain chiefly to the selection, slaughter, and preparation of meat. Animals allowed for food are the quadrupeds with a cloven hoof that chew a cud, specifically cattle, sheep, goats and deer; they are considered "clean." Permissible fowls are chicken, turkey, goose, pheasant and duck. All animals and fowl must be inspected for disease and slaughtered by a ritual slaughterer according to specific rules. Only the forequarter of the quadruped may be used. Only if the hip sinew of the thigh vein can be removed is the hindquarter allowed.

Blood is forbidden as food, since blood is synonymous with life. Thus, the traditional process of "koshering" the meat and poultry gets rid of all blood before it is cooked. This is a process of soaking the meat in water, salting it thoroughly, allowing it to drain and then washing it three times to remove the salt.

Meat and milk cannot be combined in the same meal. Milk or milk foods may be eaten immediately before the meal, but not with it. After meat has been eaten, 6 hours must elapse before milk products may be used. Because of this rule, traditional orthodox Jewish homes must keep two completely separate sets of dishes, silver, and cooking equipment, one for meat meals and one for dairy meals.

Fish allowed are only those with fins and scales. This bars all shellfish and eels. Fish may be eaten with either dairy or meat meals.

Eggs, too, may be used with either meat or milk. However, any egg yolk containing a drop of blood may not be used, since the blood is considered an embryo chick or a sign of a new life.

Fruits, vegetables, cereal products and all of the other foods that make up a normal adequate diet may be used without restrictions.

Bakery products and prepared food mixtures must be produced under acceptable kosher standards to satisfy the orthodox Jew.

HOLIDAY OBSERVANCE   The most important of the holy days is the Sabbath, or day of rest, observed on Saturday. The meal on Friday night is the choicest of the week and usually includes both fish and chicken. No food is allowed to be cooked or heated on Saturday, so all food eaten on the Sabbath is cooked the previous day and either kept warm in the oven or eaten cold.

The festival holidays are Rosh Hashanah, the New Year in September; Succoth, the Fall harvest holiday; Chanukah, the feast of lights in midwinter; and Purim, a gay holiday in spring, and each has associated delicacies.

Yom Kippur, or the Day of Atonement, occurs 10 days after Rosh Hashanah and is a day of fasting, with abstinence from all food and drink, including water, from sundown on the eve of the holiday to sundown on the holiday. Pregnant women and those who are ill are urged to refrain from fasting.

Passover, a spring commemorative festival lasting 8 days, requires special dietary consideration. During this period, leavened bread or cake is prohibited. Matzoth, an unleavened bread, is eaten and all cake and baked products are made from flour of ground up matzoth or potato starch, leavened only with beaten egg whites. No salt is allowed in the traditional Passover matzoth. Variations of fried matzoth or matzoth meal pancakes are prepared with generous amounts of fat. See page 200 for the Jewish Food Plan.

MOHAMMEDAN RELIGIOUS DIETARY CODE

The following dietary restrictions are followed by the Mohammedan:
1. Pork is prohibited.
2. Alcoholic beverages are prohibited.
3. All meat used for food must be slaughtered according to ritual letting of blood.

ROMAN CATHOLIC DIETARY LAWS[4]

On Abstinence

1. Everyone, after the 7th birthday, is bound to observe the law of abstinence.
2. On days of complete abstinence, meat and soup or gravy made from meat may not be used at all. At the present time, these days are Ash Wednesday and the Fridays during Lent.

---

[3]Based on Kaufman, M.: Adapting therapeutic diets to Jewish food customs. Am. J. Clin. Nutrition, 5:676, 1957.

[4]The dietary restrictions on abstinence and on fast have been liberalized. Customs vary in different localities and with individuals.

On Fast

1. Everyone, from the 21st birthday to the 59th birthday inclusive, is also bound to observe the law of fast except pregnant women and nursing mothers.
2. The days of fast vary because church laws have been changed in recent years.
3. On days of fast, only one full meal is allowed. Two other *light meatless* meals, sufficient to maintain strength, may be taken according to each one's needs. Meat may be taken at the principal meal on a day of fast, except on Ash Wednesday.
4. When health or ability to work would be seriously affected, the law does not oblige.

VEGETARIANS

Cultural philosophies of the so-called pure vegetarians are based mainly on Eastern religions and they have many similarities, yet they are distinctly different.[5] Some regimens are nutritionally adequate and others are not.

Lacto-ovo-vegetarian dietary consists of vegetables supplemented with milk, cheese and eggs. Many legumes and nuts are included and used in a variety of ways. Meat of all kinds, fish and poultry are prohibited. The Seventh Day Adventists follow this program. Lacto-vegetarians eat all vegetables supplemented with milk and cheese only. No other animal protein is permitted. Pure vegetarians ingest vegetables only and prohibit the use of animal foods, dairy products and eggs. The fruitarian diet consists of raw or dried fruits, nuts, honey and olive oil.

The pure vegetable and fruit diets are nutritionally inadequate in all respects, especially protein, iron, calcium, vitamin B_{12}, vitamin D and possibly vitamin A. Mutual protein supplementation, a mixture of vegetables which supplies essential amino acids and the proper vitamin and mineral supplements, should be included in these regimens. See Chapters 6, 8 and 9.

The Zen Buddhist believes that one's health and happiness depends on a proper balance between the "yin and yang" foods. This way of eating is known by some American groups as the Zen Macrobiotic diet. The dietary pattern progresses through ten steps ranging from the lowest level diet, which includes 30 per cent vegetables, 30 per cent animal products, 15 per cent salad and fruits, 10 per cent soups, 10 per cent cereals and 5 per cent desserts, to the highest level, which contains 100 per cent cereals. Erhard[7] explains how the philosophy of eating can be used in a nutrition program to improve their dietary pattern.

SOUL FOODS

Soul foods in present-day meals do not refer to any particular food or group of foods. They can be chicken wings, plantain, apple pie, a famous jelly layer cake, yams, shrimp or any food into which the one who cooks the food puts a great deal of feeling and pride during its preparation and serving. It is a "natural" feeling and if one's attitude is natural, imaginative and creative, soul food will be served at the table, regardless of nationality, race or creed.

PROBLEMS AND SUGGESTED TOPICS FOR DISCUSSION

1. What changes in food patterns have taken place in the United States? What caused these changes?
2. Interview the patients with different ethnic origin who are in the wards of the hospital and find out about their native food habits and social customs.
3. Evaluate one of the above dietary patterns to make sure it contains the basic foods.
4. Plan field trips to restaurants and food shops offering foods of various nationalities.
5. From the suggested reading list, select references and report on topics pertaining to the regional food habits in the United States.
6. Select a family representing the most prevalent nationality in your neighborhood. Interview the homemaker of this family to determine the quality of the menus served for one week. How do they rate? What improvements in them are needed? How does the homemaker perceive the changes?

SUGGESTED ADDITIONAL READING REFERENCES

Adolph, W. H.: Nutrition in the Near East. J. Am. Dietet. A., *30*:753, 1101, 1954.

Bulletin. The Toronto Nutrition Committee, 1959. Food Habits of New Canadians, published by the Bakery Foods Foundation of Canada, Ontario, Canada.

Cantoni, M.: Adapting therapeutic diets to the eating patterns of Italian-Americans. Am. J. Clin. Nutr., 6:548, 1958.

Cassel, J.: Social and cultural implications of food and food habits. Am. J. Pub. Health, 47:732, 1957.

Community Nutrition Section. The American Dietetic Association: Selected List of References of National Food Patterns and Recipes, 1954.

Cornely, P. B., et al.: Nutritional beliefs among a low-income urban population. J. Am. Dietet. A., 42:131, 1963.

Council of Foods and Nutrition: Zen macrobiotic diets. J.A.M.A., *218*:No. 3, 1971.

Drummond, J. C.: The Englishman's Food: A History of Five Centuries of English Diet. London, J. Cape, 1939.

Ellis, F. R., and Montegriffo, V. M. E.: Veganism, clinical findings and investigations. Am. J. Clin. Nutr., 23:249, 1970.

Erhard, D.: Nutrition education for the "now" generation. J. Nutr. Ed., 2:135, 1971.

Hacker, D. B., and Miller, E. D.: Food patterns of the Southwest. Am J. Clin. Nutrition, 7:224, 1959.

Hardinge, M. G., et al.: Nutritional studies of vegetarians. J. Am. Dietet., A., 43:550, 1963, and 48:25, 1966.

Harris, R. S., Wang, F. K. C., Ying, H. W., Tsao, C. H. S., and Loe, L. Y. S.: The composition of Chinese foods. J. Am. Dietet. A., 25:28, 1949.

Hawks, J. E.: Preparation and composition of foods served

---

[5] Erhard, D.: Nutrition education for the "now" generation. J. Nutr. Ed. 2:135–136, 1971.

[6] Council of Foods and Nutrition: Zen macrobiotic diets. J.A.M.A., *218*:No. 3, 1971.

[7] Erhard, *op. cit.*

in Chinese homes. J. Am. Dietet. A., 12:136, 1936.

Hegsted, D. M.: World wide opportunities. J. Am. Dietet. A., 31:236, 1955.

Joseph, S., et al.: Composition of Israeli mixed dishes. J. Am. Dietet, A., 40:125, 1962.

Judd, J. E.: Century-old dietary taboos in 20th century Japan. Am. J. Dietet. A., 33:489, 1957.

Koroff, S. I.: The Jewish dietary code. Food Technology, 20:76, 1966.

Lee, D.: Cultural factors in dietary choice. Am. J. Clin. Nutrition, 5:166, 1957.

Lowenberg, M. E., et al.: Food and Man. New York, John Wiley & Sons, Inc., 1968.

Marsh, A. G., et al.: Metabolic response of adolescent girls to lacto-ovo-vegetarian diet. J. Am. Dietet. A., 51:441, 1968.

Mayer, J.: The nutritional status of American Negroes, Nutr. Rev. 23:161, 1965.

McCann, M. B., and Trulson, M. F.: Our changing diet. J. Am. Dietet. A., 33:358, 1957.

Mead, M.: Food habits research: Problems of the 1960's. National Academy of Sciences, National Research Council, Pub. No., 1225, 1964.

Mitchell, H. S., and Joffe, N. F.: Food Patterns of some European countries: Background for study programs and guidance of relief workers. J. Am. Dietet. A., 20:676, 1944.

New, P. K–M., and Priest, R. P.: Food and thought: A sociologic study of the food cultist. J. Am. Dietet. A., 51:13, 1967.

Pongborn, R. M., and Bruhn, C. M.: Concepts of food habits of other ethnic groups. J. Nutr. Ed., 2:106, 1971.

Queen, G. S.: Culture, economics, and food habits. J. Am. Dietet. A., 33:1044, 1957.

Report of the Committee on Food Habits. Manual for the Study of Food Habits. National Academy of Sciences, National Research Council, Bull. No. 111, 1943. Reprinted 1964.

Review. Some nutrition studies in Mexico. Nutr. Rev., 7: 12, 1949.

Roberts, L. J.: Basic food pattern for Puerto Rico. J. Am. Dietet. A. 30:1097, 1954.

Stitt, K. R.: Nutritive value of diets today and fifty years ago. Nutr. Rev., 21:257, 1963.

Torres, R. M.: Dietary patterns of the Puerto Rican people. Am. J. Clin. Nutr., 7:349, 1959.

White, H. S., et al.: Dietary surveys in Peru. J. Am. Dietet. A, 30:856, 1954.

Chapter 14

COMMUNITY NUTRITION AND FOOD SANITATION

The nurse functions in a patient-care centered capacity in the hospital and extended health care facilities which are an integral part of the community. The division between the two facilities is becoming more difficult to distinguish because the "bedside" is no longer confined to the hospital structure. Nursing in the community involves working with the physicians, nurses, social workers, nutritionist and other related health personnel. Nurses are involved in coordinated planning for the provision and continuity of patient care not only with the person who is ill but with each member of the household. The nurse is concerned with the goals of community health in (1) the prevention of disease, (2) the development of healthy bodies and minds and (3) rehabilitation and longevity. Nurses function as care-givers, health teachers and counselors and are available to persons of any income within the community.

Other matters that concern the health of the community and require cooperative effort are food inspection and sanitation, control of epidemics and the water supply. This chapter is devoted to community health as it is related to nutrition status and food sanitation.

Many organizations, groups, and individuals have a part in protecting and advancing health—local, state, national, international, both official and voluntary; universities and medical schools; hospitals and research institutions. Approximately one out of every 30 employed persons in the United States now works in the "health" service industries according to the Health Information Foundation. This is a total of two and a half million people, and about three-fifths of these persons are connected with hospitals or related institutions. Effort is directed toward prevention and treatment of dietary imbalances.

NUTRITION EDUCATION IN COMMUNITY HEALTH PROGRAMS The health department has always been charged with the responsibility for food sanitation and safety. In addition, in more recent years it has been made responsible for nutrition and nutrition education. In the beginning, improved nutrition was directed almost exclusively to the health and welfare of infants, growing children and women during pregnancy and lactation. However, the physical examination of the men inducted in the Armed Forces revealed the great need for extending the educational program to all of the adult population so that everyone contributing to the war effort would be able to maintain a high level of health efficiency. It is said that the science of nutrition was born during World War I and came of age during World War II. Current interest and effort embraces the senior citizen, schoolchild and teenagers. Geriatric nutrition is discussed in Chapter 18; maternal and child health nutrition are detailed in Part Two. An important function of the nutrition service is to conduct surveys for the purpose of establishing nutritional programs related to such problems as child development and stress conditions. Included in the latter category are chronic illness, pregnancy, obesity, and old age. See Chapter 2, Teaching Nutrition, for discussion of community nutrition education programs.

All nurses and nutritionists, along with their co-workers, whether they work at the bedside, in the clinic or in the home, have a challenging, inspiring and rewarding role in counseling families regarding food practices. A booklet entitled *Nutrition Handbook for Family Food Counseling* was written by the National Dairy Council to aid community health and family life education leaders in interpreting nutrition to families and individuals. Finding ways in which people become motivated to improve food practices is one of the significant challenges to health workers. The improvement of human nutrition on a national scale usually requires greater production and more efficient conservation of food as well as better dietary habits. Conservation of food includes the use of chemicals and/or fertilizers in the field, improved storage conditions, and better consumer distribution. Of potential value to underdeveloped areas are the various new means of preserving food such as freeze-drying. Ionizing radiation (p. 232) is being used to extend the life of foods. Enrichment of foods (p. 52) is recognized as making foods more effective in human nutrition.

Another booklet, *Facts About Nutrition,* is a brochure prepared by the National Institute of Arthritis and Metabolic Diseases of the National Institutes of Health and is designed to answer a variety of questions on nutrition directed to the U.S. Public Health Service. It discusses nutritive needs, food habits and common sources of important nutrients. Overweight, nutrition in pregnancy and lactation, infant nutrition and nutrition in old age are stressed.

FOOD SURVEYS

FOOD SURVEY 1948 TO 1955 A summary of food consumption surveys made by the United States Department of Agriculture[1] covering a period of 47 years, Table 14–1 is shown listing the nutritive value of diets per person in the United States from 1909 to 1955. The figures are based upon total available food and not on actual consumption and thus are difficult to interpret accurately. However, they do give some insight into trends. A marked decrease in carbohydrate intake, particularly from grain products and potatoes, occurred during this period. Sugar and syrup consumption increased sharply until 1930, fell during World War II when rationed and remained fairly stable during the rest of this period. Fat consumption increased in spite of the decrease in total calories, with a concurrent increase in the use of hydrogenated fats. Increased consumption of meat, poultry, fish and dairy products resulted in more animal protein in the diet to compensate for the vegetable protein lost with decreased grain consumption. Fruits and vegetables increased steadily until about 1948 and then decreased, resulting in the lowering of ascorbic acid levels of intake. The drop in calories was reflected in the sharp curtailment in the consumption of cereals, breads and potatoes. A noticeable change in the selection of a greater variety of food was noted. Enrichment and fortification of staple products resulted in a marked rise in essential nutrients—thiamin, riboflavin, niacin and iron.

Figure 14–1 shows the comparison of dietary adequacy in 1948 and 1955. In 1955 approximately the same proportion of urban households had diets furnishing recommended amounts of calcium, vitamin A, thiamin and riboflavin as in 1948. There was some increase in the percentage of households meeting the recommended dietary level of protein, iron and niacin, but the percentage meeting the allowance for ascorbic acid was lower. A greater consumption of meat, poultry and fish accounted chiefly for the improvement in protein, iron and niacin levels. A shift in the pattern of consumption of fruits and vegetables accounted chiefly for the lowering of ascorbic acid. The amounts of milk, fats and oils consumed were about the same in the two periods, while grain products continued their downward trend.

On the basis of the percentage of family diets which did not meet the recommended

[1]Consumption of Foods in the United States 1909–1952. Supplements for 1956 Agricultural Handbook No. 62, Washington, D.C., U.S. Department of Agriculture, Agricultural Marketing Service, 1957.

TABLE 14–1   NUTRITIVE VALUE OF DIETS PER PERSON IN THE UNITED STATES*

YEAR	CALORIES	PROTEIN (gm.)	FAT (gm.)	CARBO-HYDRATE (gm.)	CALCIUM (gm.)	IRON (mg.)	VIT. A (i.u.)	THIAMIN (mg.)	RIBO-FLAVIN (mg.)	NIACIN (mg.)	ASCORBIC ACID (mg.)	CALORIES FROM FAT (per cent)	CALORIES FROM CARBO-HYDRATE (per cent)	CALORIES FROM PROTEIN[2] (per cent)
1910	3,500	101	123	498	.84	15.3	7,000	1.63	1.86	17.8	107	32	57	11.5
1920	3,280	93	122	460	.88	14.9	7,400	1.53	1.86	16.2	107	33	56	11.3
1930	3,450	92	134	477	.90	14.3	7,800	1.55	1.89	15.9	108	35	55	10.6
1940	3,340	92	142	432	.96	14.8	8,200	1.55	1.95	16.5	122	38	52	11.0
1950	3,250	95	144	401	1.03	17.1	8,200	1.90	2.31	19.4	112	40	49	11.7
1955	3,220	96	148	386	1.04	16.4	7,400	1.85	2.34	19.7	108	43	48	11.9
1955[1]	3,200	103	155	350	1.15	17.6	8,540	1.56	2.70	18.7	106	44	44	12.8

*Trulson, M. F.: The American Diet—Past and Present. Am. J. Clin. Nutrition, 7:93, 1959. Compiled from "Supplement for 1956, Consumption of Food in the United States, 1904–1952," Agriculture Handbook No. 62.

[1]Taken from "Dietary Levels of Households in the United States," Agricultural Marketing Service and Agricultural Research Service Report No. 6.
[2]The factors 9, 4, 4, respectively, were used to figure calories from fat, protein, and carbohydrate for the calculation of the percentages.

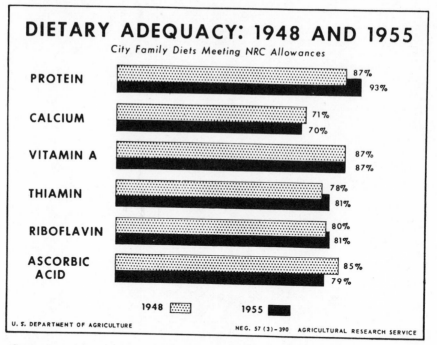

Figure 14–1   Comparison of dietary adequacy in 1948 and 1955 as measured by percentage of city family diets meeting Recommended Dietary Allowances. (Courtesy of Faith Clark, Director, Household Economics Research Division, Institute of Home Economics, Agricultural Research Service, U.S. Department of Agriculture, Washington, D.C., and J. Am. Dietet. A., *34*:379, 1958.)

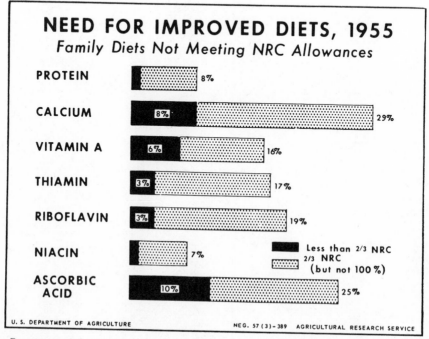

Figure 14–2   Percentage of family diets in 1955 not meeting the Recommended Dietary Standards. (Courtesy of Faith Clark, Director, Household Economics Research Division, Institute of Home Economics, Agricultural Research Service, U.S. Department of Agriculture, Washington, D.C., and J. Am. Dietet. A., *34*:378, 1958.)

TABLE 14–2 AVERAGE AMOUNTS OF FOOD EATEN IN ONE DAY

Food (as served)	Unit	Men	Women
Milk and milk products:			
Milk, milk drinks	cups	1¼	¾
Cream, ice cream	cups	¼	¼
Cheese	ounces	⅓	⅓
Eggs	each	1	½
Meat, poultry, fish:			
Beef	ounces	4	2¼
Pork	ounces	3½	2
Other meat	ounces	¼	¼
Poultry	ounces	1¼	¾
Fish, shellfish	ounces	½	¼
Mixtures	ounces	2¾	1¾
Legumes, nuts:			
Legumes, mixtures	tablespoons	2	1¼
Nuts, nut butter	tablespoons	½	¼
Grain products:			
Bread, rolls, biscuits	slices	5¼	3
Other baked goods	ounces	2¾	1¾
Cereals, pastes	ounces	1½	1¼
Mixtures	ounces	1½	1½
Tomatoes, citrus fruits:			
Tomatoes	cups	¼	¼
Citrus fruit	cups	¼	¼
Dark green and deep yellow vegetables	tablespoons	1¼	1¼
Potatoes	cups	½	¼
Other vegetables and fruit:			
Other vegetables	cups	½	½
Other fruit	cups	½	¼
Sugars, sweets:			
Sugar	teaspoons	4¼	3¼
Sirup, honey, molasses	teaspoons	1	½
Jelly, jam, gelatin desserts	teaspoons	2¾	2¼
Candy	ounces	¼	¼
Fats, oils:			
Table fats	tablespoons	1¼	¾
Other fats, oils	tablespoons	1¾	¾
Beverages other than milk, juices, and alcoholic drinks:			
Tea	6-ounce cups	¾	¾
Coffee	6-ounce cups	2¼	2¼
Soft drinks	12-ounce bottle	½	½

Average amounts of food eaten in one day (Spring 1965) by men and women 20 to 34 years of age. Taken from Food for Us All, 1969 Yearbook of Agriculture, U.S.D.A.

daily dietary allowances in 1955, it was found, as in 1948, that calcium and ascorbic acid were the nutrients in which diets are most in need of improvement. (See Figure 14–2.)

In general, relatively little improvement in dietary levels of city families took place in the period from 1948 to 1955. Farm diets furnished larger amounts of all nutrients except vitamin A and ascorbic acid.[2]

FOOD SURVEY 1965[3] In the spring of 1965, over a period of 13 weeks, a survey of the food intake and nutritive value of diets of men, women and children in the United States was made. Information was obtained on the food intake for one day of individual members of the households interviewed. This represents the first time an estimate of the food eaten by individuals has been obtained on a nation-wide basis. Approximately 15,000 reports of food eaten at home and away from home by men, women and children living in housekeeping households were collected.

The 1965 survey showed that men and boys eat larger quantities of most types of foods than women of the same age. It is especially true for cereals, bread and other baked goods; meat, fish and poultry; fats and oils; and sweets and sugars. For vegetables and fruits, namely, tomatoes and citrus fruit, dark green and deep yellow vegetables and fruit, average quantities eaten by women and girls equaled or exceeded quantities eaten by men and boys at the same ages. Average amounts of all foods used by men and women 20 to 34 years of age are shown in Table 14–2.

The 12 food groups tabulated in kinds and amounts as shown in Table 14–2 were milk and milk products; eggs; meat, poultry, fish, legumes and nuts; grain products; tomatoes and citrus fruits; dark green and deep yellow vegetables; potatoes; other vegetables and fruits; sugars and sweets; fats and oils; and beverages other than milk and juices.

The highest level of consumption of milk and milk products (butter not included) was by children under 1 year and the next highest

---

[2]Dietary levels of households in the United States. Household Food Consumption Survey, Report No. 6, U.S. Department of Agriculture, 1955.

[3]Fincher, L. J., and Rauschert, M. E.: Diets of Men, Women and Children in the United States. Nutrition Program News, U.S. Department of Agriculture, September-October, 1969.

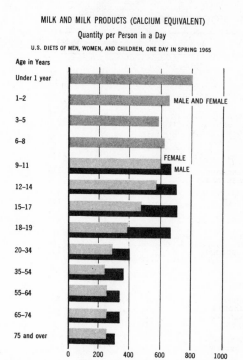

MILK AND MILK PRODUCTS (CALCIUM EQUIVALENT)

Quantity per Person in a Day

U.S. DIETS OF MEN, WOMEN, AND CHILDREN, ONE DAY IN SPRING 1965

Figure 14–3   U.S. diets of men, women and children one day in Spring, 1965. (From Food For Us All, 1969 Yearbook of Agriculture, U.S. Department of Agriculture, p. 269.)

by boys of ages 9 through 19. Boys and men used more milk products than girls and women at all ages past 9 years. As noted in Figure 14–3, the milk consumption of females decreased from age 12 years on and was lowest in the 35 to 54 age group, when the average milk or the calcium equivalent of milk products used was less than 1 cup per day. Males showed a sharp decrease in consumption of milk and milk products between the ages 18 to 19 and 20 to 34 to about 1 cup.

There was a steady increase in the consumption of meat, poultry and fish until the 20 to 34 age group and thereafter the consumption declined. The amounts of meat, poultry and fish eaten by males were considerably higher than those by females. (See Figure 14–4.) On the day of the survey, over 85 per cent reporting (except very youngest children) used one or more of these foods.

The peak years for consumption of grain products by boys were ages 15 through 19. Their average consumption of grain products was the equivalent of 6 slices of bread plus 7 ounces of other grain cereals. Bread products (including rolls and biscuits) were preferred by more persons in larger quantities than other items in this group of foods. Larger quantities of grain products were used by

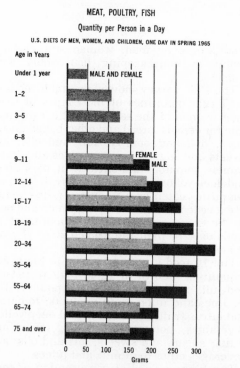

MEAT, POULTRY, FISH

Quantity per Person in a Day

U.S. DIETS OF MEN, WOMEN, AND CHILDREN, ONE DAY IN SPRING 1965

Figure 14–4   U.S. Diets of men, women and children one day in Spring, 1965. (From Food For Us All, 1969 Yearbook of Agriculture, U.S. Department of Agriculture, p. 268.)

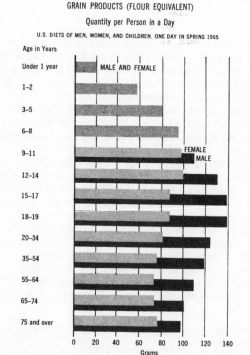

GRAIN PRODUCTS (FLOUR EQUIVALENT)

Quantity per Person in a Day

U.S. DIETS OF MEN, WOMEN, AND CHILDREN, ONE DAY IN SPRING 1965

Figure 14–5   U.S. diets of men, women and children one day in Spring, 1965. (From Food For Us All, 1969 Yearbook of Agriculture, U.S. Department of Agriculture, p. 268.)

VEGETABLES AND FRUITS

Quantity per Person in a Day

U.S. DIETS OF MEN, WOMEN, AND CHILDREN, ONE DAY IN SPRING 1965

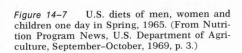

Figure 14–6   U.S. diets of men, women and children one day in Spring, 1965. (From Food For Us All, 1969 Yearbook of Agriculture, U.S. Department of Agriculture, p. 269.)

boys and men than girls and women in all age groups above 9 years (Fig. 14–5).

The consumption of citrus fruits ranged from 19 per cent by infants under 1 year to 50 per cent by men and women in the 20 to 34 age group. More tomatoes and citrus fruits were consumed by women than men. Men generally ate more of all food groups than did women in the 55 through 74 age group. Use of dark green and deep yellow

vegetables was low. Only 10 to 20 per cent of all persons in the various age groups ate any of these vegetables on the day of the survey. The highest users were males aged 65 through 74. Males consumed almost twice as much potatoes. More than half the persons in most of the sex-age groups used potatoes. Over half the vegetables and fruits eaten were other vegetables and fruits. On the day of the survey more than 75 per cent of most groups used one or more foods from other vegetable and fruit groups. The total quantity of vegetables and fruits used on this day is shown in Figure 14–6.

Beverages other than milk and fruit juices included coffee, tea, soft drinks and alcoholic beverages. (See Figure 14–7.) The highest consumption was by men and women in the 35 through 54 age group. The increase in coffee consumption occurred between the 18 to 19 and 20 to 34 age groups. Almost one third of the children and one half of the adolescents reported using soft drinks on the day of the survey. The average quantities of milk and milk products generally ingested by persons in different age groups varied inversely with the average quantities of other beverages used.

When the average nutritive content of the food and beverages consumed by the different sex and age groups in the 1965 survey was compared with the 1968 Recommended Dietary Allowances the results showed the following:

Average diets approached (90 to 100 per cent) or were above the recommended allowances for calories and five of the seven nutrients studied: protein, vitamin A, thiamin, riboflavin and ascorbic acid. Calcium and iron were the nutrients below the recommended allowances. (See Figure 14–8.)

Calcium and iron (Figs. 14–9 and 14–10) in

Figure 14–7   U.S. diets of men, women and children one day in Spring, 1965. (From Nutrition Program News, U.S. Department of Agriculture, September–October, 1969, p. 3.)

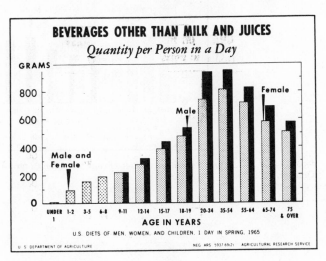

NUTRIENT INTAKE BELOW RECOMMENDED ALLOWANCE

Average Intake of Group Below Recommended Dietary Allowance, NAS–NCR, 1968

U.S. DIETS OF MEN, WOMEN, AND CHILDREN, ONE DAY IN SPRING 1965

Sex-Age Group	Protein	Calcium	Iron	Vitamin A value	Thiamine	Riboflavin	Ascorbic acid	
MALE AND FEMALE:								
Under 1 year			• • • •					
1– 2 years			• • • •					
3– 5 years			• •					
6– 8 years								
MALE:								
9–11 years		•						
12–14 years		• •	• • •		•			
15–17 years		•	•					
18–19 years								
20–34 years								
35–54 years		•						
55–64 years		• •						
65–74 years		• •						
75 years and over		• • •		•		• •	•	
FEMALE:								
9–11 years		• • •	• • • •		•			
12–14 years		• • •	• • • •	•	•			
15–17 years		• • • •	• • • •		• •			
18–19 years		• • •	• • • •	•	•			
20–34 years		• • •	• • • •		•	•		
35–54 years		• • • •	• • • •		•	• •		
55–64 years		• • •			•	•		
65–74 years		• • • •	•		• •	• •		
75 years and over		• • • •	•	• •	• •	• • •		

BELOW BY:
1–10% •
11–20% • •
21–29% • • •
30% OR MORE • • • •

Figure 14–8.   Average intake of nutrients below Recommended Dietary Allowance. U.S. diets of men, women and children one day in Spring, 1965. (From Food For Us All, 1969 Yearbook of Agriculture, U.S. Department of Agriculture, p. 270.)

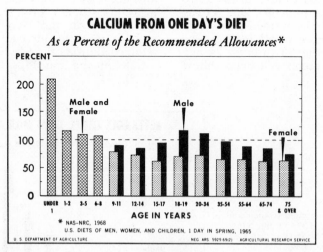

Figure 14–9   Calcium from one day's diet. (From Nutrition Program News, U.S. Department of Agriculture, September-October, 1969.)

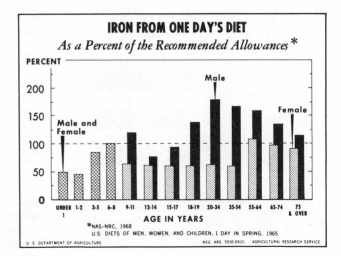

Figure 14–10   Iron from one day's diet. (From Nutrition Program News, U.S. Department of Agriculture, September–October, 1969.)

the day's food were more than 30 per cent below the recommended dietary allowances for girls and women especially. The average diets of girls (15 to 17 years) and of women (from 35 years on) were about 35 per cent below recommended dietary allowances for calcium. Diets of girls and women 9 through 54 years were on the average approximately 40 per cent below the amounts suggested for iron. The iron in diets of children under 3 years was about 50 per cent below recommended amounts but the average amounts of calcium for this age group were above recommendations. The Food and Nutrition Board indicates that the recommended allowances for iron for some age groups cannot be met with ordinary food products by all sex-age groups.[4] Ordinary diets provide about 6 mg. of iron per 1000 calories of food. That level was not reached in the diets of children under six years of age and boys 12 to 14 years and females under 55 years.

Males consumed approximately the same calories as recommended by the Food and Nutrition Board and the females about 10 per cent below the recommendations.

The fat in the diets ranged from an average of 39 per cent to 45 per cent of the calories for infants and men 20 to 64 years of age respectively. The average intake of protein for all age groups in the study was over 100 per cent of the recommended amounts. The average intakes of vitamin A, thiamin and riboflavin in the diets of several groups of females were 5 to 15 per cent below the recommended allowances. The amounts of these vitamins in the diets of men were well above the

recommended amounts. Men 75 years and over had diets below the recommended allowance for ascorbic acid.

Nutritive content of vitamin supplements were not recorded and were not taken into account in the calculation of the nutritive value of the diets. Approximately 55 per cent of the infants under 1 year of age and 43 per cent of children 1 through 2 years had vitamin or mineral supplements. Persons over 3 years of age ranged from about 12 per cent for girls 15 to 17 years and boys and men 15 to 34 years to about 34 per cent for men and women 75 years of age and over.

On the basis of this survey (Figs. 14–2 to 14–8) the groups which need dietary improvement to meet recommended allowances are infants and children under 3 years; adolescent girls and women, ages 9 through 64; and older women, 65 years and over; and men 75 years and over. Infants and children under 3 years: Iron in the diets of this age group averaged about 50 per cent below the recommended allowance. Other nutrients including calories were found to be in excess of recommended amounts. Adolescent girls and women, ages 9 through 64: Calcium and iron intake was under the recommended allowances 20 and 30 per cent, respectively. The exception for iron was the women in the 55 to 64 age group. All these groups had slightly below recommended amounts for thiamin. Older women and men: Women 65 years and over were below recommended allowances for calcium (30 per cent), thiamin, riboflavin, vitamin A value and iron. The diets of men 75 years and over were below allowances for calcium (24 per cent), vitamin A, riboflavin and ascorbic acid.

The quality of the diet and income are closely related[5] (See Figure 14–11). In the 1965 household survey about one third of the

[4]Food and Nutrition Board: Recommended Dietary Allowances. 7th ed. Washington, D.C., National Academy of Sciences, National Research Council, No. 1694, 1968.

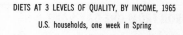

DIETS AT 3 LEVELS OF QUALITY, BY INCOME, 1965

U.S. households, one week in Spring

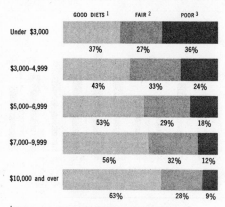

¹ Met recommended dietary allowances (1963) for 7 nutrients.
² Met at least ⅔ RDA for 7 nutrients but less than RDA for 1 to 7.
³ Met less than ⅔ RDA for 1 to 7 nutrients; is not synonymous with serious hunger and malnutrition.

Figure 14–11   Diets in U.S. households for one week in Spring, 1965, showing three levels of quality by income. (From Food For Us All, 1969 Yearbook of Agriculture, U.S. Department of Agriculture, p. 271.)

families with incomes under 3,000 dollars and about one tenth (a sizable proportion) of the families with incomes over 10,000 dollars had poor diets. Ignorance of or indifference to the selection of a good diet was observed at almost all income levels.

Improvements in processing, transportation and storage have made it possible to have consumptions of the same foods in the four regions (Northeast, North Central, South and West). Differences in regional food patterns are smaller than they were formerly. However, the South still has important differences.

Households in the South had the lowest average consumption of milk and milk products, used the smallest amount of bread but the most flour, sugar, fat and eggs and were doing more home baking than in the other regions. Although the South used about the same amount of meat, poultry and fish as the other regions, Southern families used more pork, poultry and fish and smaller amounts of beef and lunch meats.

Farm families now produce about one third of their food (10 years ago it was 40 per cent). In 1965, farm households used more than twice as much flour and cereals as urban families. They also use more fats and sugars than urban families and purchase smaller amounts of baking products, soups, mixes

and all types of beverages. In 1965, approximately 62 per cent of the farm families and 72 per cent of urban families ate meals or snacks away from home.

The implications of the 1965 survey indicate the need to develop and intensify nutrition education programs. The survey indicates that there are individuals in many families at all income levels who need guidance in meeting their nutritional needs. The age groups which need special emphasis are teenage girls, women and older men. They need assistance in selecting foods which will provide increased amounts of calcium, iron, thiamin, riboflavin and vitamin A. Some low-income families need assistance in extending their purchasing power through food assistance and education programs that help them make better use of their money spent for food. Many higher-income families also need help in meeting their nutritional needs. Nutrition education programs need to be adapted to

 – Needs of different age groups
 – Different income groups
 – Selection of foods within framework of food habits and preferences of the various age groups
 – Wise selection of foods at different cost levels
 – Mass media and other means to reach people

Emphasis must be placed on

 – Nutrients most often found to be below the daily recommended allowance in the age group
 – Low-income families which need to extend their purchasing power through food assistance programs
 – Higher-income families which need guidance in meeting their nutritional needs from the abundance of foods available
 – Wide selection of foods to provide the nutrients found to be below recommended allowance

NATIONAL NUTRITION SURVEY 1968[6] According to preliminary reports of the National Nutrition Survey, Department of Health, Education and Welfare, findings of surveys conducted in 10 states in the United States indicate that many people in low-income areas are seriously malnourished. The survey was done according to the Manual for Nutrition Surveys (published by the Interdepartmental Committee on Nutrition for National Defense, National Institutes of Health) and was part of an undertaking to

[5]Clark, F.: A scorecard on how we Americans are eating. Food For Us All, 1969 Yearbook of Agriculture, U.S. Department of Agriculture, p. 266.

[6]Schaefer, A. E., and Johnson, O. C.: Are we well fed? The search for the answer. Nutrition Today, 4:No. 1, 1969, p. 3.

assess the nutritional status of the population of the United States. The trends in this preliminary survey suggest that the economic status may be an important underlying factor in the families' nutritional patterns along with lack of concern, lack of knowledge of what foods to buy or the right foods to eat and ignorance of health care. The clinical findings of the prevalence of anemia and reduced levels of serum albumin, vitamin A and ascorbic acid, urinary thiamin and riboflavin clearly indicate the seriousness and magnitude of the problem. Another concern of the investigators in this study of the nutritional status of low-income families related to the food fortification programs in existence. The programs are voluntary and most people do not know the difference. Anyone can sell bread that is not enriched, milk that contains no vitamin D and milk from which vitamin A is removed and salt that is not iodized. Evidence of inadequate intake of calories, protein, minerals and vitamins of boys 5 years of age and under in the 1968 preliminary nutrition survey concerning the relationship between height and age is shown in Figure 14–12.

Copies of hearings before the Select Committee on Nutrition and Human Needs of the United States Senate; Reports on the White House Conferences on Food, Nutrition and Health; and the White House Conferences on Children and Youth and Aging are available from U.S. Government Printing Office, Wash-

ington, D.C. Implications for more effective nutrition education in community health programs are indicated.

FOOD POISONING

Food poisoning may be caused by different agents: bacteria, poisonous chemicals, and foods which are intrinsically poisonous, such as certain mushrooms and mussels. Most food poisoning is caused by bacteria. The general public often speaks of any food poisoning as synonymous with *ptomaine poisoning*. True ptomaines are formed in the latter stages of food decomposition, and the foods are so obviously decayed that people would not eat them. Hence, such food poisoning is extremely rare.

BACTERIAL FOOD POISONING

The distinctive feature of an outbreak of food poisoning is the sudden illness of several individuals following ingestion of a common meal. Usually a particular item of food served at the meal is the source of the poisoning. The victim suffers any one or all of the following symptoms: diarrhea, cramps, nausea, vomiting and fever. The symptoms may or may not be severe enough to require treatment. In the absence of specific diagnosis, the conditions may be grouped under the general heading of *gastroenteritis*.

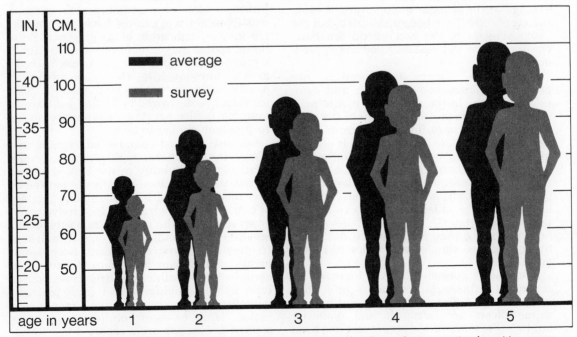

Figure 14–12   Height and age relationship for boys five years of age and under: preliminary national nutrition survey, 1968, of low income groups. (From Nutrition Today, 4:No. 1, 1969, p. 10.)

DIET THERAPY   Small amounts of cracked ice, barley water, and tea are taken as soon as the stomach has settled down. Later, custards, gelatin, eggs, toast, milk, broth, or cream soups are added if they can be retained. Solid foods usually are resumed on the second or third day.

STAPHYLOCOCCAL AND SALMONELLA FOOD POISONING   Physicians now distinguish two main subgroups. One is *enterotoxic,* usually induced by a poison secreted by *staphylococci.* The other is *infectious,* induced by invasions of *salmonella, shigella, streptococci* and other organisms.

It is estimated that at least three-fourths of the gastroenteritis outbreaks reported are caused by staphylococcal enterotoxins. Salmonella infections appear to be the next most common cause, and shigella infections seem to follow in order.

The human carrier is the most common vector of both the staphylococci and salmonella. Approximately 25 out of every 10,000 people are Salmonella carriers. It is estimated that the nation may suffer as many as 1,000,000 enterotoxic cases a year, without counting the vast number of mild subclinical, undiagnosed, and, therefore, unreported cases.

Staphylococcal Poisoning   Staphylococcal food poisoning is caused by a toxin formed in the food before ingestion. The enterotoxin is relatively heat-stable. The staphylococcus multiplies rapidly in certain foods at room temperature. These organisms hibernate when refrigerated and are revitalized when exposed again at room temperature. A wide variety of foods have been implicated, but the usual vehicles of the enterotoxin are ham, poultry, cream and custard-filled baked products.

Prevention   Since staphylococci are present in abundance in nature and commonly present in the secretions of the nose and throat and in purulent lesions of the skin, it is impossible to exclude them from foods exposed to air. There is no perceptible change in flavor to warn one eating the offending food. The best control is cleanliness, elimination of flies, adequate refrigeration of all perischable foods, and education. Staphylococcus can be killed by heating to boiling temperature, but if toxins had developed before heating *they may not* be destroyed by boiling. See simple basic rules to follow on page 219.

Salmonella Poisoning   An increase in reports of salmonella food-borne infections has been noted. The major sources of human salmonellosis are livestock and domestic animals. Presence of the organisms has been demonstrated in animal feeds, in food processing places, among people who prepare and handle food, and in other situations where their presence invites the spread of disease. The natural habitat of salmonella is the gastrointestinal tract of animal and human hosts. Salmonellosis is thus primarily an excremental disease transmitted by the fecal-oral route. The cycle of infection usually involves the transfer (direct or indirect) of viable salmonellae from one host to another and finally to man, with food and water the most often implicated agents. Although salmonellosis may occur at any age, the highest incidence and most severe forms are observed in infants under 1 year of age and in aging persons. The foods most often implicated appear to be poultry, prepared meats, desiccated coconut, cake mixes, custard-filled bakery products which are lightly cooked and subject to much handling, milk and milk products, and eggs.

Prevention   Heat and refrigeration are the main tools to combat germ growth. The dangerous temperatures for food at which germs thrive are between 40 and 120° F. To ensure destruction of salmonella in food, the temperature must be raised throughout the food to an appropriately high degree for a sufficiently long time, such as 140° F. for 20 minutes or 149° F. for 3 minutes. Refrigeration does not kill the bacteria but will prevent multiplication. See simple basic rules on page 219.

BOTULISM   *Botulism* is the most serious form of food poisoning; the mortality average is about 68 per cent. The *Clostridium botulinum,* which may sometimes be present, usually in nonacid canned foods, may or may not give an indication of its presence. Botulinum spores may remain resistant to 212° F. temperature despite several hours of processing. Subsequently, they can produce a deadly toxin in the canned product. This toxin can be destroyed by boiling for 10 to 15 minutes before serving—a wise precaution for the homemaker to take.

Because of good commercial canning and preserving practices, botulism now occurs relatively infrequently in the United States. Outbreaks of botulism usually are caused by the consumption of home-canned vegetables or other foods which are inadequately cooked or preserved. In the past, the majority of outbreaks were found due to type A, and less frequently, to type B botulism. Recent outbreaks of botulism have caused grave concern. In 1963 fatalities occurred from canned tuna fish in Michigan, and from prepared whitefish originating in the Great Lakes region. Three cases of botulism from home-canned gefilte fish were reported in 1969. It was prepared from Great Lakes whitefish cooked and stored in a sealed jar in a refrigerator for seven weeks before it was opened. It was eaten cold. All outbreaks appeared to have been due to the type E toxin, which had not previously been common in this country. This form of toxin has been associated primarily with marine products. The exact manner of contamination of the tuna and whitefish has not been found. No defect in the technique of canning was detected in relation to the canned tuna; the whitefish was prepared by a method in use commercially for many years without previous difficulties. Type A and B outbreaks are usually due to contaminated vegetables and meats and type E to fish. Botulism organisms occur in garden and farm soil, in vegetables, in silt and in aquatic life. It appears that new and more stringent public health regulations relating to commercial processing are indicated.

Prevention   Some simple basic rules to follow are:

1. Wash the hands before preparing a meal.

2. Never touch food with infected hands. Pimples, boils, paronychia, felons, and infected scratches teem with bacteria, especially staphylococci. These microorganisms multiply rapidly in certain foods such as custards, potato salad, and cream-filled pastries when exposed to room temperature. If there is a lesion on a finger, it should be kept well covered or gloves worn while preparing meals or handling food.

3. Infections in the nose and throat increase the chances of contamination unless a mask is worn while handling food.

4. Keep perishables in the refrigerator until ready for use. This is essential for chopped and processed meats, custards, pastries, cream, butter, and similar products.

5. Wash uncooked fruits and vegetables thoroughly.

6. Cook meats thoroughly.

7. Inspect all leftovers and discard if signs of spoilage exist, such as changes in color and foul odor.

8. Inspect prepared foods for insect and rodent contamination.

9. Never eat partly spoiled foods.

10. Destroy cans that bulge. The same applies when the contents bubble out when the can is opened. Botulism may be present even though there are no changes in taste and smell.

11. Leftovers or food cooked for later use should be refrigerated immediately and not held until food reaches room temperature.

FOOD- AND WATER-BORNE DISEASES AND THEIR PREVENTION

Milk and water have long been known as carriers of disease, and we now know that other foods and food utensils are also carriers. Food, water and utensils can be contaminated with bacteria, parasites or poisons. Food-borne diseases are brucellosis, tuberculosis, typhoid fever, paratyphoid, scarlet fever, diphtheria, tularemia, salmonellosis, septic sore throat, and a variety of other disorders. Trichinae, tapeworms, and other parasites, and botulin, staphylococcal enterotoxin, and other toxins, too, can contaminate the food supply. The possibilities of utensil-borne disease are suggested by the fact that the bacterial count on spoons, glasses, and cups in many restaurants is relatively high. (See

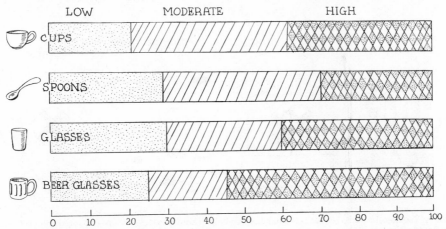

BACTERIAL COUNTS OF FOOD UTENSILS

Figure 14–13   The possibilities of utensil-borne diseases are suggested by the relatively high bacteria count on cups, spoons, glasses, and beer glasses in many restaurants. (Adapted from Publication No. 84, U.S. Public Health Service.)

Fig. 14–13.) Health workers aim to install sanitation programs in all food handling and food processing establishments where there may be a hazard to community health. Despite the progress which has been achieved, however, food-borne illness continues to be a major public health problem. To reduce the incidence of such illness, the basic principles of food protection must be applied. The "Food Service Sanitation Manual," issued in 1962 with recommendations of the Public Health Service, U.S. Department of Health, Education, and Welfare, was developed for the improvement of food protection programs throughout the United States.

TRICHINOSIS Uncooked or partially cooked meat is a serious cause of infection and disease such as *trichinosis*. It is suggested that up to 6 per cent of the hogs fed uncooked garbage in the country are infested with trichinous worm cysts. Trichinae are microscopic worms whose larvae burrow their way from the intestine into the muscles and mesenteric organs of swine and humans. The parasites are carried only if the host has eaten uncooked flesh of an infested animal. When man eats infected pork, he in turn becomes host to trichinae.

Prevention To prevent infection, pork should be *thoroughly cooked;* that is, cook large, thick cuts at least 30 minutes to the pound or until the internal meat is white. Thorough cooking is necessary for fresh, cured, or smoked pork and for pork products, such as sausages and frankfurters, and also for hamburgers if they contain pork. As gauged by a meat thermometer, tenderized picnic shoulders should be heated to an internal temperature of 170° F., cured hams to 160° F., and fresh pork to 185° F. Freezing pork for 20 days at a temperature of minus 5° F., or at minus 0.4° F. for 24 hours, is another way of killing trichinae. Tenderized hams with the stamp "Federally Inspected

and Passed" have been processed to kill parasites and can be safely eaten with less cooking. From the standpoint of public health trichinosis can be practically eliminated if garbage is cooked before it is fed to hogs. (See Fig. 14–14.) It is reported that 40 per cent of infected swine get the disease from eating commerical raw garbage. Many cities dispose of their garbage by selling or giving it away for hog feed. However, cooking garbage intended for feed is now required by law in most states.

The most recent method for making contaminated meat safe for human consumption utilizes *radioactive cobalt.* Neither the meat nor taste is harmed. The rays sterilize the female parasites, and if infested meat is ingested the parasites, though still present, cannot multiply. (See Radiation Preservation, p. 232.)

TULAREMIA Although tick bites are considered much more of a factor than rabbit meat in transmitting tularemia, the latter is a factor.

Prevention Rabbits should never be handled with the bare hands, and the flesh must be *thoroughly cooked.*

TAPEWORMS In certain lake regions fish are hosts to tapeworm, which is transmitted to man. As a rule, infections occur when housewives taste chopped fish as they season it for cooking.

Prevention Infected fish are not safe to eat unless they have been frozen or thoroughly cooked. If infected they produce in the host a blood condition resembling pernicious anemia.

SHELLFISH In 1924 an outbreak of typhoid fever was reported and traced to oysters taken from contaminated waters off Long Island, New York. In 1964 and 1969 outbreaks of infectious hepatitis were associated with eating raw clams. As a result the Public Health Service has developed a pro-

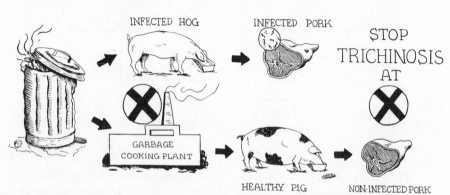

Figure 14–14 Cooking the garbage that is fed to hogs will help to eliminate trichinosis. (Adapted from Publication No. 84, U.S. Public Health Service, 1951.)

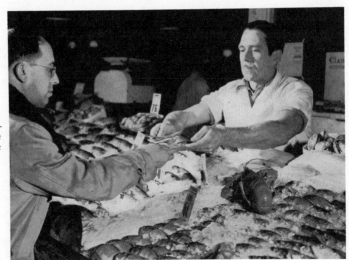

Figure 14–15 From shucker to consumer, the handling of shellfish must be sanitary. (Publication No. 84, U.S. Public Health Service, 1951.)

gram to strengthen sanitary regulations. Contaminated waters are restricted, and plants are inspected periodically.

Recently, shellfish sanitation experts have become concerned with the apparent ability of shellfish to concentrate radioactive material, insecticides, or other chemicals from the environment. Steps have been taken to meet this problem. The entire shellfish control program is one of interlocking and joint cooperation by industry, the states, and the Public Health Service, to assure that only safe shellfish are sold in the market. (See Fig. 14–15.)

TUBERCULOSIS Through inspection of animals and the pasteurization of milk, the Public Health Service and state legislation have almost completely eliminated bovine tuberculosis.

FOOD POISONS OF NATURAL ORIGIN

Some of the most potent poisons to man are of natural origin, coming from plants, seeds, roots and animals. Certain varieties of mushrooms containing alkaloids are poisonous and extremely common in all parts of the United States. Dermatitis from handling pascal green summer celery has been reported among farm workers. Rhubarb leaves contain considerable oxalic acid, cause illness and should not be used. The green part of sprouting white potatoes contains sufficient solanine (a narcotic alkaloid) to produce illness or even death. Ingestion of the fava bean or the inhalation of pollen causes a severe form of hemolytic anemia in susceptible individuals. Many wild plants are poisonous. Clams and mussels found in the Pacific along the coast from California to Alaska may contain a poisonous alkaloid similar to strychnine. During the summer they feed on plankton, a marine organism, which infects the fish. Poisoning incurred by eating fresh, unspoiled fish of species not ordinarily poisonous was reported in 1957[7] in the South Pacific, Philippines, Hawaii and the West Indies. Food poisoning caused by carbophenothion resulted after eating tortillas made from flour contaminated with Carbophenothion, an organo-phosphate insecticide which acts by inhibiting cholinesterase. Swordfish has been reported in 1970 to contain a sufficient amount of mercury to be toxic. In the spring and summer of 1954 there were four outbreaks in Florida, all caused by eating barracuda. Victims of the poisoning observed that the fish tasted better than any they had ever eaten. Only one fish, the puffer, is regarded as inherently poisonous. Puffer fish have a gland containing neurotoxin tetraodontoxin. Death ensues from the poison soon after ingestion. Yet, to list a few examples, herring is toxic in Cuba and Tahiti from May to October; many species of the fish native to New Hebrides waters are most toxic from April to July; some of these are poisonous at all times at one location, and harmless 20 miles away. This is a real public health problem, since with the increased use of freezing to preserve foods and in transporting of frozen foods, fish poisoning may appear in parts of the world where it has hitherto been unknown.

PESTICIDES

Pesticides have played a major role in agriculture's phenomenal success and are

[7]Editorial. Poisonous Fish. J.A.M.A., *162*:118, 1957.

expected to continue as the chief deterrent against pests which menace production. A disadvantage in their use is the poisonous nature which gives rise to harmful residues. The effects of pesticides on other organisms in the environment and varying amounts of residues on agricultural produce have been the subject of much debate and controversy. The current system for regulating residues on food is based on the "tolerance principle" which assumes that all pesticide chemicals can be poisonous at high levels while there are low levels at which injury does not occur. There is evidence that, in general, adherence to tolerances is good.

The Food and Drug Administration (FDA) made determinations in market basket samples[8] for residues of 20 chlorinated hydrocarbons, including DDT, and for organic phosphate-type insecticides. Most of the samples were reported to contain no residues or mere traces of chlorinated hydrocarbons; a few contained amounts measurable by extremely sensitive techniques; only a few traces of organic phosphate residues were found. These findings were interpreted to mean that the protection program provided by the Pesticides Amendment of the Federal Food, Drug and Cosmetics Act (p. 233) is adequate. The FDA's third annual "total diet" study (1967) showed that pesticide residues found in food remained well below acceptable daily intake levels established by the World Health Organization and the Food and Agricultural Organization of the United Nations.

A weakness in the current system of regulating residues is that the FDA regulations apply only to the products in interstate commerce. Individual state programs are needed to fill the gap left in the federal regulations. The search for compounds of lower mammalian toxicity is meeting with encouraging results and similar progress is expected in finding substitutes for broad spectrum insecticides. The system currently employed in regulating the agricultural use of pesticides is directed chiefly to the problems of residues on agricultural products.

It is well recognized that traces of pesticides, retained on fruits, vegetables, and forage material, may be ingested either directly by man or by edible animals that are in turn consumed by man. The chlorinated hydrocarbon pesticides are more likely than others to be biologically magnified in a food chain because of their relative stability and their solubility and persistence in animal fat.

The question of the danger of spraying DDT on surfaces, and thus contaminating and endangering food, is still open. Studies have been made on the most popular items consumed at breakfast, lunch and dinner in restaurants and institutions. Chemical analysis disclosed minute traces of DDT in every food. Fatty dishes and foods cooked in fat contained more of the insecticide because DDT is soluble in oil, grease and fat. When fed to animals and humans, it is stored in their fatty tissues. The more absorbed the more stored, until the saturation point is reached, but nothing adverse happens. Evidence shows that DDT is changed into another chemical, which leaves the body via the kidneys.

Persons sensitive to DDT may develop dermatitis, bleeding tendencies or destruction of blood cells. Acute, uncomplicated DDT poisoning is a recognized condition, but so far no one has been reported to have died from this cause. Fatalities have been reported after swallowing the compound with other products, but in each instance one of the other products has proved to be responsible. In one suicide, in which DDT powder was used, possible involvement of other poisons in the compound was not excluded.

To investigate the nature and extent of the storage of chlorinated pesticides in human fat, Hoffman et al.[9] analyzed fat specimens obtained at autopsy from 282 persons who had died of various diseases. The data obtained confirmed earlier conclusions that for any chronic intake level of DDT, equilibrium between intake of DDT and excretion of the sum of its metabolic derivatives is eventually achieved, after which the concentration of total DDT in the fat tends to remain constant. The most significant finding of the analysis is that the results indicate that there has been no progression of storage of DDT in the general population since 1951 when the first studies were made. Also, the intake of lindane, dieldrin, and other pesticides is so low and/or the rate of excretion is so rapid, that apparently the fat levels of these pesticides are either insignificant when measurable, or not even measurable by the most sensitive methods now available. We need to intensify our national effort to understand and weigh the long-term effects of using pesticides on health and total environment. It is very important that anyone who uses a pesticide understand its purpose and properties.

RADIOACTIVITY IN FOODS

Atomic energy has assumed an important role in our civilization and the relationship of

[8]J.A.M.A., *182*:27, 1962.

[9]Hoffman, W. S., et al.: J.A.M.A., *188*:819, 1964.

foods to fallout contamination has been questioned frequently. Comar[10] reported that it could be concluded that there is no indication for a change in our dietary habits or food technology as a result of fallout contamination. This has been confirmed. However, broad-scale research on the problem of radioactivity in foods and its implications is continuing for future public welfare.

Strontium-90, the dangerous element of radioactive fallout, is absorbed like calcium, and if a significant amount were to find its way into the food supply, a serious health problem would result. Like calcium it concentrates in bone, and radiation of bone tissue may cause cancer or leukemia. Calcium appears to reduce the amount of radioactive strontium-90 that may be deposited in the body. The relation of the amount of strontium-90 to the amount of calcium is referred to as the strontium-to-calcium ratio. Plants take up the strontium-90 along with their necessary calcium. Animals eat the plants, and human beings eat both plants and animal products such as milk, meat, and eggs.

In a survey made by the U.S. Public Health Service,[11] a slight increase in the average daily dietary intake of strontium-90 during 1962 was observed at 21 boarding schools and institutions throughout the country. The strontium-90 intake ranged from 9 to 46 picocuries (pc) per day; the average was 25 pc per day. The 1961 average was 19 pc per day. These averages are well below those which the Federal Radiation Council's radiation guide lists as acceptable health risks. Two-hundred picocuries per day is listed as compatible with the orderly development of nuclear industry in the United States. The guidelines are not intended to be limits of safe radiation levels but are meant to indicate when there is need for detailed evaluation of possible exposure risks and when there is need to consider whether any protective action should be taken. A warning system is in operation in the United States so that should radiation levels exceed the guidelines and standards which have been established, the public will be informed.

FOOD FOR SURVIVAL

In the instance of an atomic or hydrogen bomb attack, it would be necessary for many survivors to rely on their own food and water reserves for approximately 2 weeks. The United States Department of Agriculture in cooperation with the Office of Civil and Defense Mobilization, has prepared a publication[12] suggesting a food and water stockpile plan to use so as to prevent overexposure to fallout radiation. Services such as gas, electricity, and water may be disrupted and, therefore, the stockpile must supply all items necessary for survival until the local health authorities declare it safe and possible to get other foods and water. The basic foods should be in cans, jars or tightly sealed paper containers; foods that will keep without refrigeration and that can be eaten with little or no cooking. The kinds and quantities of food suitable to store for use in such an emergency are listed in Table 14-3. The amounts suggested will supply adequate calories for an adult for 2 weeks. If there are four adults in the family, four times the amount listed should be stored. Teen-agers are likely to need more than listed; younger children need less.

By including, each day, foods from each of the eight groups outlined in Table 14-3, a reasonably nutritious diet can be obtained. Special kinds of milk and strained, chopped, or other specially prepared foods required for infants, toddlers, elderly persons and other limited diets can be included. Jars and cans in sizes suitable for the family's needs for only one meal are preferable to prevent deterioration and spoilage of food. This is especially important for meat, poultry, fish, vegetables and evaporated milk. If a food freezer is available in the shelter area, these foods are safe to use. Food spoilage in a well-filled freezer does not begin until about 72 hours after the power goes off.

Sample meal plans using (a) no cooking facilities and (b) limited cooking facilities are outlined in Table 14-4, and use the foods suggested in Table 14-3.

COOKING AND SERVING EQUIPMENT The equipment recommended for cooking and serving includes a small, compact, cooking unit, such as the type used by campers; one or two cooking pans; disposable knives, forks, and spoons; paper plates, towels, cups and napkins; can and bottle openers; nursing bottles and nipples if there is a baby in the family; measuring cup; medicine dropper for measuring water purifier if this becomes necessary; matches; and a pocketknife. Plastic dishes, cups, forks, knives, and spoons may be used instead of disposable tableware if preferred. They will take less storage space, but water for washing them may not be available after an attack.

WATER One-half gallon of water per person per day (7 gallons per person for a 2-week period) is suggested for drinking and food preparation. Some of this can be in the

[10]Comar, C. L.: Radioactivity in Foods, J.A.M.A., *171*: 1221, 1959.

[11]J.A.M.A., *182*:27, 1962.

[12]Family Food Stockpile for Survival. Home and Garden Bulletin No. 77, U.S. Department of Agriculture, 1961.

TABLE 14–3   GUIDE FOR EMERGENCY RESERVE FOOD SUPPLY*

KIND OF FOOD	AMOUNT PER PERSON FOR–		REMARKS
	1 Day	*2 Weeks*	
1. Milk	Equivalent of 2 glasses (fluid)	Equivalent of 7 quarts (fluid)	Each of the following is the equivalent of 1 quart of fluid milk: Evaporated milk: three 6-ounce cans; one 14½-ounce can. Nonfat dry milk or whole dry milk: three to 3½ ounces
2. Commercially canned meat, poultry, fish, cooked dry beans, and peas	2 servings	28 servings (8 to 9 pounds)	Amounts suggested for one serving of each food are as follows: Canned meat, poultry: 2 to 3 ounces. Canned fish: 2 to 3 ounces. Canned mixtures of meat, poultry, or fish with vegetables, rice, macaroni, spaghetti, noodles, or cooked dry beans: 8 ounces. Condensed soups containing meat, poultry, fish, or dry beans or dry peas: one-half of a 10½-ounce can.
3. Fruits and vegetables†	3 to 4 servings	42 to 56 servings (about 21 pounds, canned)	Amounts suggested for one serving of each food are as follows: Canned juices: 4 to 6 ounces, single strength. Canned fruit and vegetables: 4 ounces. Dried fruit: 1½ ounces.
4. Cereals and baked goods	3 to 4 servings	42 to 56 servings (5 to 7 pounds)	Amounts suggested for one serving of each food are as follows (selection depends on extent of cooking possible): Cereal: Ready-to-eat puffed: ½ ounce. Ready-to-eat flaked: ¾ ounce. Other ready-to-eat cereal: 1 ounce. Uncooked (quick-cooking): 1 ounce. Crackers: 1 ounce. Cookies: 1 ounce. Canned bread, steamed puddings, and cake: 1 to 2 ounces. Flour mixes: 1 ounce. Flour: 1 ounce. Macaroni, spaghetti, noodles: Dry: ¾ ounce. Cooked, canned: 6 ounces.
5. Spreads for bread and crackers	According to family practices		Examples: Cheese spreads. Peanut and other nut butters. Jam, jelly, marmalade, preserves. Syrup, honey. Apple and other fruit butters. Relish, catsup, mustard.
6. Fats and vegetable oil		Up to 1 pound or 1 pint	Amount depends on extent of cooking possible. Kinds that do not require refrigeration.
7. Sugars, sweets, and nuts		1 to 2 pounds	Sugar, hard candy, gum, nuts, instant puddings.
8. Miscellaneous	According to family practices and extent of cooking possible		Examples: Coffee, tea, cocoa (instant). Dry cream product (instant). Bouillon products. Flavored beverage powders. Salt and pepper. Flavoring extracts, vinegar. Soda, baking powder.

Home and Garden Bulletin No. 77, U.S. Department of Agriculture.
†If nonacid vegetables are included, those commercially canned are recommended.

TABLE 14–4   SAMPLE MEAL PLANS: NO COOKING FACILITIES*

FIRST DAY	SECOND DAY	THIRD DAY
Morning		
Citrus fruit juice.[1]	Fruit juice.[1]	Grapefruit segments.[1]
Ready-to-eat cereal.	Corned beef hash.[1]	Ready-to-eat cereal.
Milk, cold coffee,[2] or tea.[2]	Crackers.	Vienna sausage.[1]
Crackers.	Spread.	Milk, cold coffee,[2] or tea.[2]
Peanut butter or other spread.	Milk, cold coffee,[2] or tea.[2]	
Noon		
Spaghetti with meat sauce.[1]	Baked beans.[1]	Chile con carne with beans.[1]
Green beans.[1]	Brown bread.[1]	Crackers.
Crackers.	Tomatoes.[1]	Fruit.[1]
Spread.	Fruit.[1]	Cookies.
Milk, cold coffee,[2] or tea.[2]	Milk, cold coffee,[2] or tea.[2]	Milk, cold coffee,[2] or tea.[2]
Between Meals		
Fruit-flavored drink or fruit drink.	Milk.	Tomato juice.
Night		
Lunch meat.[1]	Pork and gravy.[1]	Sliced beef.[1]
Sweet potatoes.[1]	Corn.[1]	Macaroni and cheese.[1]
Applesauce.[1]	Potatoes.[1]	Peas and carrots.[1]
Milk, cold coffee,[2] or tea.[2]	Instant pudding.	Crackers.
Candy bar.	Fruit juice.[1]	Milk, cold coffee,[2] or tea.[2]

[1] Canned.
[2] Instant.
*Home and Garden Bulletin No. 77, U.S. Department of Agriculture.

TABLE 14–4   SAMPLE MEAL PLANS: LIMITED COOKING FACILITIES* *(Continued)*

FIRST DAY	SECOND DAY	THIRD DAY
Morning		
Citrus fruit juice.[1]	Citrus fruit juice.[1]	Prunes.[1]
Ready-to-eat cereal.	Hot cereal (quick-cooking).	Ready-to-eat cereal.
Milk.	Milk.	Milk.
Hot coffee,[2] tea,[2] or cocoa.[2]	Hot coffee,[2] tea,[2] or cocoa.[2]	Crackers.
		Cheese.
		Hot coffee,[2] tea,[2] or cocoa.[2]
Noon		
Vegetable soup.[1]	Beef-and-vegetable stew.[1]	Chile con carne with beans.[1]
Potato salad.[1]	Green beans.[1]	Tomatoes.[1]
Crackers.	Crackers.	Crackers.
Ham spread.[1]	Peanut butter.	Hot coffee,[2] tea,[2] or cocoa.[2]
Milk.	Milk.	
Candy bar.		
Between Meals		
Fruit-flavored drink or fruit drink.	Tomato juice.[1]	Fruit-flavored drink or fruit drink.
Night		
Beef and gravy.[1]	Tuna fish,[1] cream of celery soup,[1] mixed sweet pickles[1] — combined in one dish.	Lunch meat.[1]
Noodles.[1]	Fruit.[1]	Hominy.[1]
Peas and carrots.[1]	Cookies.	Applesauce.[1]
Instant pudding.	Hot coffee,[2] tea,[2] or cocoa.[2]	Cookies.
Hot coffee,[2] tea,[2] or cocoa.[2]		Peanuts.
		Hot coffee,[2] tea,[2] or cocoa.[2]

[1] Canned.
[2] Instant.
*Home and Garden Bulletin No. 77, U.S. Department of Agriculture.

form of fruit juice and soft drinks. In an emergency, the water in home hot-water tanks and toilet tanks can be used. Water to be stored for emergency use should be put in thoroughly washed, clean containers, preferably of heavy plastic with tight-fitting caps. Water from open sources, such as uncovered cisterns, streams, and ponds that have been exposed to radioactive fallout may be unsafe to drink after an attack. Water from wells and springs is safe if protected from surface contamination. Melted ice cubes from the refrigerator are safe, if available.

Foods in the stockpile should be rotated, or the regular food supply can be increased so that there will always be a 2-week supply on hand. As the food is used it should be replaced. Thus, the stockpile is always fresh.

CARE OF FOOD EXPOSED TO RADIATION FALLOUT   In the event of radiation fallout, all foods such as fruits and vegetables should be carefully washed before cooking or eating. Cooking does *not* remove radioactive contamination but the ordinary radioactive dust can, at least in part, be washed off. Experiments of the FDA have shown that processing fruit and vegetables in commercial plants reduces the strontium-90 content from 20 to 60 per cent, depending on the type of food. These amounts, though, are extremely small and the particles microscopic. Because the current amounts are so tiny, the FDA does not advocate peeling, coring or scraping every fruit and vegetable. These practices may remove essential food ingredients and actually cause greater dietary harm than would, at present, be caused by residual radiation contamination.

Although there is a high content of strontium-90 in milk compared to other foods, milk is also high in calcium content. Since both strontium-90 and calcium concentrate in bone tissue, if there is a reduction of calcium in the diet by lowering milk intake, the bones may take up more strontium from other sources, such as vegetables. Experiments under the joint auspices of the Public Health Service, the Department of Agriculture and the Atomic Energy Commission have shown that strontium-90 can be removed from milk. Other ways being studied to reduce radioactive material in food are agricultural practices to lessen fodder and crop contamination and different cattle feeding practices. At present, cows in the United States do not take in enough strontium-90 to make milk dangerous.

Foods which are in cans, jars, and tightly sealed paper containers are safe for use following a nuclear attack. However, the container should be washed before opening or breaking the seal to remove the radio-active substance. Foods in a closed refrigerator or freezer are safe to use.

FOOD SANITATION

Sanitation in the home and in restaurants, soda fountains, bars and similar places is essential to prevent spread of food-borne diseases. The Public Health Service plays a large part in establishing sanitation programs for all public food handling and food processing establishments.

Following is a summary of the Public Health Service activities, as related to food-borne diseases.[13]

"The Public Health Service engages in the following activities to protect the nation from food-borne, including milk-borne, disease:

1. Develops and revises standards.
2. Promotes State and local programs based upon uniform standards and operations.
3. Advises and consults with State and industry officials on technical and administrative problems relating to sanitation of milk, shellfish, and other foods.
4. Encourages the training of food handlers and food sanitarians.
5. Certifies State ratings of milk and shellfish shipped interstate.
6. Prepares educational materials to train sanitarians and food handlers.
7. Evaluates State and local programs, upon request of State and local officials.
8. Consults with industry representatives on design and construction of food handling equipment and participates in joint industry-government development of equipment standards.
9. Inspects food handling facilities and practices in Federal prisons, National parks, in Indian Service installations, and on interstate carriers serving food to the public.
10. Conducts and advises on food sanitation and related research.
11. Compiles and publishes annual summaries of outbreaks of disease traced to food.
12. Serves on national and international bodies concerned with food sanitation.

"Food has both a positive and negative effect on health. On the positive side, there are the complex and imperfectly understood effects of food on long life, vigor, mental alertness, and resistance to disease. On the negative side, there are hazards from swallowing food-borne organisms or poisons. Hazards may result from individual idio-

---

[13]Public Health Service Publication No. 84.

syncrasies of the food or the person fed, but many are peculiarly a product of the environment: of polluted water, of careless handling, of contamination by insect vectors, and of improper processing. To the extent that it is possible to do so, the Public Health Service seeks to provide assistance in eliminating these hazards."

FOOD SPOILAGE

The spoilage of foods is a fairly common phenomenon. The souring of milk, the molding of bread, and the putrefaction of foods of animal origin are examples. The primary causes of this spoilage are microorganisms known as yeasts, molds and bacteria. They grow and flourish on foods by virtue of the fact that they use the food for their nutrition and thus support their life cycles. As a result of this growth, the natural characteristics of the foods are changed either chemically or physically, or both, to produce the condition known as *spoilage*. Alterations of odor, texture and flavor are manifest.

FOOD PRESERVATION

The increasing complexity of present-day civilization makes the growing use of preserved foods a necessity in order that they can be safely carried long distances. The nutritive value now receives careful consideration, and should be improved whenever possible and desirable from the point of view of health safety.

Like all living organisms, yeasts, molds and bacteria cannot survive and flourish unless the environmental conditions are favorable. Unfavorable conditions are extreme heat or cold, deprivation of water and sometimes oxygen, excess acidity in the medium in which they are suspended, and the presence of certain chemicals. Treatment of food in one or more of these ways is the basis of food preservation. The method used to preserve a food product will vary with the type of food.

HEAT

Heat is a valuable defense against the growth of bacteria, but its effectiveness will depend upon the length of time it is used and the temperature maintained.

BOILING Boiling (212° F.) will kill bacteria if the heat is maintained for a sufficient length of time to completely penetrate the food, but spores of the bacteria such as those of the botulinus or of molds may not be destroyed.

PRESSURE COOKER The pressure cooker, which permits a temperature above boiling (240° F.), will kill the very resistant bacteria and molds. The pressure cooker is a popular and safe method for preserving food in the home. Recipes and directions, which accompany a pressure cooker, give the recommended pressure and length of time for cooking specific foods.

BAKING AND ROASTING These are methods that permit temperatures up to 500° F. Standard cookbooks give the recommended time and temperature for cooking meats, fish, poultry and all baked foods, and should be followed accurately.

CANNING Commercially canned foods are considered safe from botulinus toxin. The canning methods generally recommended for home canning or processing are the *boiling water bath* for fruits and tomatoes, and the *steam-pressure* cooker for meats and all vegetables (low acid foods) except tomatoes. In the boiling water bath a temperature of no higher than 212° F. is reached. This is considered adequate for canning fruits and tomatoes, but not for other vegetables and meats because these require the higher temperatures of the pressure cooker to kill spores of bacteria.

For the maximum nutritional value of all methods of canning, only the freshest and best food should be used. But freshness and safety are not synonymous. Safe canning means first that foods must be made free of bacteria which might cause ferments. If such bacteria are not destroyed, the result of their work is obvious, for the molds, color changes, acids and gases they cause are easily seen, tasted or smelled; such products should, of course, be discarded at once.

Other methods of canning sometimes used by homemakers include the so-called *open-kettle* method and *oven* canning. These are not recommended. In the open-kettle method, cooking of the food probably destroys the organism that causes spoilage of fruits and tomatoes, but yeasts, molds, and bacteria may come in contact with food while it is being transferred from the kettle to the jar. In addition, there may not be enough heat present to give a tight seal. If this method is used in canning fruits and tomatoes, the precaution to process the product for 10 minutes before serving should definitely be taken. The open-kettle method is not satisfactory for other vegetables and meats.

Oven canning is influenced by so many variables that it cannot be recommended as a safe method of food preservation for any product. One main reason is that when jars seal during processing in the oven, steam builds up inside the jars and can cause an explosion. Oven canning has resulted in some serious accidents.

Details of canning are not listed here. Those interested in further information on the subject are referred to the excellent national and state government bulletins, as well as state college and university extension service bulletins.

NUTRITIVE VALUE   Some loss of nutritive value occurs in the process of canning, but losses are not so great as at one time supposed. Vitamin A, vitamin D, riboflavin and niacin appear to be little affected in most foods. There is some loss of ascorbic acid and thiamin. Meat, particularly, has been shown to lose considerable thiamin content. Because of better controlled conditions, commercial canning will show less loss than home methods.

COLD

Modern refrigeration is particularly effective in preventing the growth of dangerous numbers of bacteria. Most outbreaks of food poisoning have been caused by serving perishable foods which have been allowed to stand at room temperature after contamination.

COLD STORAGE   Nearly every home has some form of cold storage, such as the refrigerator, for storing perishable foods and thus limiting the growth of organisms and food decay. (See Chapter 12 for economy hints for storage of foods.) Commercial firms preserve foods, such as meat, eggs, fruit and vegetables, for long periods of time in cold rooms.

FREEZING   Commercially frozen foods have been on the market for many years. However, only comparatively recently have foods been successfully frozen in the home. Freezing takes from one-third to one-half the time and labor needed for canning. Busy homemakers find frozen foods a real time saver. Besides fruits, vegetables, and meats, a quantity of baked goods, such as cookies, cakes, pies, bread and rolls, may be prepared and stored in the freezer. Single-frozen food items are now available, which is of practical value to the housewife. Each individual vegetable, for example, is separate instead of the package contents being frozen in a solid block; thus, it is possible to remove and use only the desired amount. The development of frozen foods and concentrates has greatly influenced the eating habits and nutrition of man today. Per capita annual consumption has risen from 6 to 30 pounds since World War II.

For those interested in further information on freezing foods, the national and state government bulletins, as well as the state college and university extension service publications, are suggested.

NUTRITIVE VALUE   The family freezer in the home, the locker in a community plant, or a combination of both makes possible a varied and satisfying diet. The frozen foods compare favorably in vitamin content with fresh foods. The only loss is in the blanching process, when approximately 10 per cent of the water-soluble vitamins are lost. In good commercial practice, crops are harvested at prime maturity and are frozen within 3 to 4 hours after harvesting. Fruits are packed under a sugar syrup with added ascorbic acid to retard oxidation and loss of color. Poultry is killed, bled, dressed, and chilled, then frozen before any spoilage due to microbial action can occur. Not all the microorganisms are killed in freezing, and it is recommended that thorough cooking or reheating of frozen foods always be practiced.

DRYING OR DEHYDRATION

The oldest method of food preservation is removal of water from foods, or *drying*. This method has been greatly improved during the last 20 years, and is used for meats, fish, fruits, legumes, potatoes, cereals, soups, beverages and numerous cake, bread and dessert mixes. Microorganisms cannot grow in the absence of water. However, ascorbic acid is almost completely destroyed in the process, and there is a great loss of carotene, the precursor of vitamin A. If sulfur dioxide is used in the process, the ascorbic acid is protected, but the thiamin suffers. Eggs and milk, especially skim milk, are successful dried products. Foods which contain fat become rancid by oxidation if kept too long. Dehydrated foods were used extensively during the world wars, since they take a minimum of space for shipping and storing. Today, homemakers use the popular package mixes of cakes, cookies, quick breads and puddings almost exclusively. Potatoes are dried and packaged to prepare in various ways, such as mashed, scalloped, baked, and fried. They save time in preparation, and require fewer ingredients from the pantry shelf. Instant coffee, instant fruit juices, instant sauces and instant soups are also widely used. Substitutes for cream in coffee, which contain vegetable fat rather than butter fat, are available and quite economical.

FREEZE-DEHYDRATION   One of the newer processes in food preservation is freezing a food and then placing it in a special drying chamber. Freeze-dehydration products retain their shape. For example, a lamb chop looks like a lamb chop in the dry state and after reconstitution. Also, they retain good color, a fresh taste, texture, and appearance, require no refrigeration until reconstituted, and can be made ready to eat in a few seconds or minutes. Among products available are shrimp, crab meat, chicken, and several of the red meats, eggs, and vegetables.

DEHYDROFREEZING   Dehydrofreezing is another new process which is just the opposite of freeze-dehydration. Here the food is first partially dehydrated and *then* frozen. Not all the moisture is removed and the products must be kept in frozen storage until reconstituted. Mashed potatoes processed by this method result in an excellent product and hold well on the steam table.

NUTRITIVE VALUE   The nutrient content of a dehydrated food[14] reflects the effect of the specific preparatory treatment and process used by the manufacturer, growth conditions, and harvesting methods. The products, in general, compare favorably with canned foods, and in the case of very low temperature dried foods, with frozen and fresh foods.

CHEMICAL PRESERVATIVES

The public is often concerned by the word "chemical" not realizing that all food is chemical in nature. The practice of adding chemicals to food for preservation is a very old one which probably began when man first learned to preserve his meat by putting salt on it. Sugar, salt, vinegar and spices are common preservatives used in the home. For centuries jellies, jams, preserves, pickles, sauerkraut, smoked hams and bacon have been made both commercially and in the home. Government regulations limit the amount and kind of chemicals used. For example, benzoic acid or sodium benzoate may be used up to a concentration of 0.2 per cent if the labels so specify. Some additives have been banned because of questionable safety or unethical use. An extensive listing of additives and the level of their use in foods may be found in "Food Values of Portions Commonly Used" by Bowes and Church, 7th edition.

FOOD ADDITIVES

Food additives come from natural sources or from chemicals made in the laboratory. Lecithin is an example of an additive from a natural source. It comes from soybeans and corn. It is used primarily as an antioxidant and an emulsifier. Additives synthesized in the laboratory are often the same as those found in food. For example, vitamins and minerals added to foods are identical to the vitamins and minerals found naturally in food.

Various chemicals are added during the production, processing and storage of almost everything we eat. By definition, a chemical additive is "A chemical or a mixture of chemicals of known or reproducible composition used in addition to the basic foodstuff in the production, processing, or storage of a food, and present in the food as purchased. A chemical additive may be either nutritive or non-nutritive and its presence in the food may be either intentional or incidental.[15] They improve the nutritional value, appearance, texture and flavor of food. Some additives retard rancidity and spoilage. Without additives in food, it would be nearly impossible to provide urban communities in America with sufficient untainted food daily. Additives help to overcome soil deficiencies and to protect growing crops against insects and plant disease.

An intentional additive is a chemical added by the processor to carry out a number of functions. In contrast, an incidental or non-intentional additive such as pesticide residue or detergent or substances from the packages get into food accidentally during its production, processing or storage. More than 2000 substances are used as direct additives. The essential purpose of any intentional additive in food must be (a) to improve the nutritive value; (b) to increase acceptability of the food item to the consumer through better physical appearance, flavor, color and texture; (c) to facilitate production and the keeping qualities; and (d) to lower cost. The functions of additives are numerous. A few of the commonly used additives, their use and some of the foods in which they are used are shown in Table 14–5. Without additives Rice Provence, Whip'n'Chill and Awake would not be possible. Sara Lee's Cherry Cream Cheesecake, because of limited shelf-life might not be commercially feasible. New food products such as the convenience foods require more additives than conventionally cooked food largely because of the conditions under which they are processed. They require additives to make up for partial loss of flavor, color and texture. Because these foods are not eaten immediately after they are prepared they need special preservatives, antioxidants and other additives to maintain their freshness and desired physical properties over long periods of time. The public is becoming more

---

[14]Nutr. Rev. 20:257, 1962.

[15]Food Protection Committee, Principles and Procedures for Evaluating the Safety of Intentional Chemical Additives in Foods, National Research Council, 1954 (Reprinted 1957).

TABLE 14–5   COMMON FOOD ADDITIVES' FUNCTION AND USE IN FOODS

FUNCTIONS	ADDITIVES USED	EXAMPLES OF FOOD IN WHICH ADDITIVES ARE USED
To improve nutrition value of certain foods.	Thiamin, riboflavin, niacin, iron, vitamin A, vitamin D, ascorbic acid, potassium iodide.	Wheat, flour, bread, rolls, biscuits, breakfast cereals, macaroni and noodle products, cornmeal, margarine, milk, iodized salt.
To maintain appearance, palatability and wholesomeness in certain foods (delaying undesirable changes in food caused by oxidation or microbial growth; preventing food spoilage caused by molds, bacteria, yeast).	Propionic acid, calcium and sodium salts of propionic acid, ascorbic acid, butylated hydroxyanisole, butylated hydroxytoluene (BHT or BHA), propylene glycol.	Bread, pie filling, cake mixes, potato chips, crackers, cheese, syrup, fruit juices, frozen and dried fruits, margarine, shortenings, lard.
To enhance flavor of certain foods.	Spices (cloves, ginger, cinnamon, etc.), citrus oils, amyl acetate, carvone, benzaldehyde, monosodium glutamate, vanilla.	Spice cake, gingerbread, ice cream, candy, carbonated beverages, fruit-flavored gelatins, toppings, sausage.
To give characteristic color to certain foods.	Annotto, carotene, cochineal chlorophyll, Citrus Red No. 2.	Baking goods, candy, carbonated beverages, cheese, ice cream, jams, jellies, oranges.
To maintain desired consistency in certain foods (emulsifiers and stabilizers).	Lecithin, mono- and diglycerides, gum arabic, carboxymethyl cellulose, carrageenan.	Bakery products, cake mixes, salad dressings, frozen desserts, ice cream, chocolate milk, candy, beer.
To control acidity or alkalinity in certain foods (leavening and neutralizing agents).	Potassium acid tartrate, tartaric acid, sodium bicarbonate, lactic acid, citric acid, adipic acid, fumaric acid.	Cakes, cookies, biscuits, crackers, waffles, muffins, butter, process cheese, cheese spreads, chocolates, carbonated beverages, confectionery.
To serve as maturing and bleaching agents.	Chlorine dioxide, chlorine, potassium bromate and iodate.	Wheat flour to make it white, certain cheeses.
To help retain moisture (humectants) or prevent caking or act as curing agents.	Glycerin, magnesium carbonate, sodium nitrate, saccharin, calcium phosphate.	Coconut, marshmallows, table salt, garlic and onion powder, frankfurters, sausages, dietetic foods.

Adapted from Food Additives—Every Day Facts. Manufacturing Chemists Association, 1825 Connecticut Ave. N. W., Washington, D.C., 20009.

interested in more sophisticated, flavorful, exotic and ethnic foods. Foods are shipped greater distances and stored for greater lengths of time. These foods require additives to prevent or retard food deterioration.

Much progress has been made in the removal of non-intentional additives from food by FDA inspectors (Fig. 14–16).

There has been considerable public concern with respect to safety of foods in relation to the number and kind of chemicals that enter the food supply. The big problem which concerns chemists is the long-term effect on the body as a result of exposure to these chemicals. Several years of feeding tests on different kinds of animals are required to appraise these chronic after effects (Fig. 14–17). In 1950, this led to an investigation by the Delaney committee, appointed by the U.S. House of Representatives, of the use of chemicals in foods. This committee reported that about 200 substances used as food additives were judged by experts to be generally recognized as safe (GRAS) under the conditions of the current practice. Twenty years later the list has grown to approximately 600 items. About half of these are natural flavorings and spices. Another large group is the vitamins and minerals and other dietary supplements. Other agents such as preservatives, buffers, emulsifiers, stabilizers and antioxidants are included in the GRAS list. Out of consideration of the public concern, and because of the postwar release of a large number of new materials used in some way in crop production or food processing, the Food and Nutrition Board, National Research Council established the Food Protection Committee in the summer of 1950. This committee serves as a fact-finding and advisory body for government and industry in respect to the use of chemicals in food. All of the committee's work is in the interest of public welfare. (See Additives Legislation, page 233.)

ANTIBIOTICS FOR FOOD PRESERVATION

Preservation of foods by antibiotics has been under study for a considerable time.[16] However, reports on research were prematurely publicized, and additional tests did not

[16]Vaughn, R. H., and Stewart, G. F.: Antibiotics as food preservatives. J.A.M.A., *174*:1308, 1960.

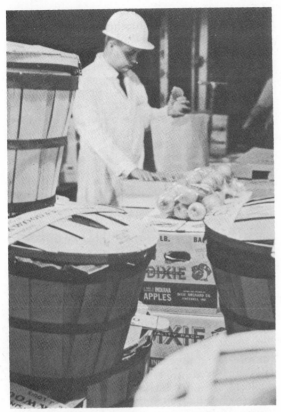

Figure 14–16   Samples of fresh foods are collected from the 800 carloads passing daily through Chicago's South Water Market. Inspector selects apples to be analyzed for pesticide residues. (From FDA Papers, July–August, 1970, p. 12.)

justify all the early enthusiasm. In spite of the setbacks, work has gone forward.

One of the big problems[17] in using antibiotics for food preservation is the question of toxicity, and much work still is being carried out to make sure requirements of the Food and Drug Administration are met for protection of consumers' health. A small per cent (approximately 10 per cent) of the population react unfavorably to contact with antibiotics, manifested by allergic symptoms. On the other hand, repeated human consumption of the chemical may produce an immunity in other persons so that they do not respond to therapeutic doses administered in the treatment of disease.

Antibiotics have recently been introduced into commercial food preservation. Two antibiotics, chlortetracycline (November, 1955) and oxytetracycline (1956), have been approved for use as antiseptic washes on eviscerated poultry. Any residues of the antibiotics are destroyed by heat when the poultry is cooked. The tolerance level in raw poultry for both antibiotics was established at 7 parts per million in any part of the bird. In August, 1959, a tolerance level of 5 parts per million was established for chlortetracycline in preserving certain kinds of fish and shellfish. When used under controlled conditions these antibiotics prevent the spoilage of fresh

---

[17]Welch, H.: Problems of antibiotics in foods. J.A.M.A., *170*:2093, 1959.

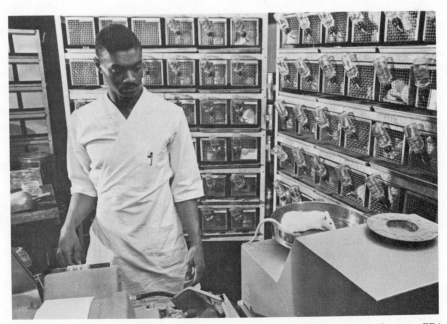

Figure 14–17   Technician records growth rate in long-term food additive toxicity test. (Courtesy FDA photo.)

poultry and fish during processing, transport and storage. They extend the shelf-life from almost a week to 10 days by inhibiting spoilage organisms.

Numerous investigations of the usefulness of antibiotics in the preservation of meats, vegetables, milk, and baked goods have also been explored. However, conclusive evidence has not been presented that such use is not detrimental to health and, therefore, approval has not been granted to date. Antibiotics are used in feed for animals to stimulate growth and prevent disease. Proper use of antibiotics is essential and additional research is needed.

ANTIBIOTICS IN MILK   Indirect means of contaminating foods with antibiotics poses a problem.[18] Penicillin in milk supplied from cows treated for mastitis is an example. The U.S. Department of Agriculture has attempted to control this through education of the farmer. Milk from penicillin-treated cows is supposed to be withheld from human consumption for at least 72 hours after the last treatment. However, this is not always adhered to, and it has created a public health problem by exposure of consumers who are allergic, or who may become sensitized to penicillin by the milk supply. Other antibiotics in milk, arising from similar use, do not appear to constitute a similar hazard. Legislative action may have to be resorted to, to combat the problem.

RADIATION PRESERVATION

Another method in the research stage for the preservation of foods is that of *ionizing radiation or irradiation.*[19] It is reported to destroy food spoilage bacteria, but in many foods studied there are changes in color, flavor and texture. Extensive tests, since 1950, point to the safety of this method of food preservation, but no irradiation process can be used until the U.S. Food and Drug Administration, and possibly other government agencies, approve it. Such approval is unlikely until present research, involving animal-feeding studies, rules out harmful effects. Radiation affects vitamins, especially thiamin and vitamin E, but these losses are comparable to those in other preservation methods and are not considered highly important. No heat is developed in the process. Raw meat, for example, remains raw. Considerable evidence is available to show that the irradiation at low dosages of prepackaged

meat extends storage life in the refrigerator five to twenty times. Further research on this process should be followed. By regulating the *amount* of radiation applied, it is possible to stop the sprouting of onions, potatoes, and carrots; kill insect eggs deposited on fruit, vegetables, and grain; prevent the transmission of trichinosis through pork; prevent insect life in dry foods; stop molding on baked goods; extend the refrigerated shelf life of meats, fruits and vegetables; and produce a sterile product that can be stored at room temperature. However, the method is still expensive.

CITY, STATE AND FEDERAL CONTROL OF FOOD QUALITY

Most cities have food handling laws which apply to workers in the kitchens of institutions, hotels, clubs, hospitals, restaurants, and food manufacturing plants. The workers are inspected by a doctor for the presence of any communicable disease or other illnesses which may contaminate foods.

States vary in the laws pertaining to food handlers and processors. It is when foods are sold or distributed into another state that Federal laws are enforced because this constitutes interstate commerce.

The Wiley Act or "Pure Food and Drug Law" of 1906 was the first effective food law: "An Act for preventing the manufacture, sale, or transportation of adulterated or misbranded or poisonous or deleterious foods, drugs, medicines and liquors, and for regulating the traffic therein, and for other purposes."

Several amendments were made, and three were retained although the Wiley Act was repealed when the 1938 Federal Food, Drug and Cosmetic Act was enacted by the 75th Congress. The "Weight and Measure Amendment" of 1913 clarified the rules about stating the quantity of the contents of packaged foods, and the Kenyon amendment of 1919 extended the rules to cover packaged meats. In 1923 "the Butter Standard Amendment" was passed and it established the minimum milk fat content of butter as 80 per cent.

The McNary-Napes Amendment passed in 1930 authorized the Secretary of Agriculture to establish minimum standards of quality, condition and fill of containers, which were required to be met by all canned foods except meat products and milk. Products which did not comply with the standards were required to be labeled to show that they were "Below U.S. Standard." While such food was entirely wholesome, this required statement served to identify the quality of the product for the prospective consumer.

[18]Council on Drugs; Penicillin and other antibiotics in milk. J.A.M.A., *170*:49, 1959.

[19]Robinson, H. E., and Urbain, W. M.: Radiation preservation of foods. J.A.M.A., *174*:1310, 1960.

The Sea Food Inspection Amendment, passed in 1935, authorized "the Secretary of Agriculture to provide government inspection of the packing of any sea food which might enter into interstate commerce for those packers desiring such inspection service."

The Meat Inspection Act of 1907 requires that "all meat and meat food products in interstate commerce be prepared under the supervision of the U.S. Department of Agriculture."

In 1957 a law was passed requiring inspection of dressed poultry and poultry products, similar to the Meat Inspection Act. The Production and Marketing Administration of the U.S. Department of Agriculture also offers a grading service to determine the quality of canned fruits and vegetables. Labeling of food products, food adulteration and food poisoning are also regulated by the 1938 Food, Drug and Cosmetic Act.

PESTICIDE LEGISLATION   In 1954, the Miller Pesticide Chemicals Amendment to the Federal Food, Drug and Cosmetic Act was passed to establish tolerances for pesticide chemical residues on raw agricultural commodities (fruit and vegetables). Under this amendment, the applicant must demonstrate "usefulness" to the satisfaction of the U.S. Department of Agriculture and "safety" (tolerance, or exemptions from tolerance) for useful pesticide chemicals to the Food and Drug Administration of the Department of Health, Education, and Welfare. The regulations cover 26 pesticides, ranging from those which are virtually harmless to some which are among the most potent poisons known to man. Each pesticide is listed with the amount of tolerance (based upon results of animal tests which the pesticide manufacturer is required to submit) and the food crops to which each applies.

The Food and Drug Administration, an agency of the Department of Health, Education, and Welfare, has the responsibility of enforcing the Food, Drug and Cosmetic Act and thereby carrying out the purpose of Congress to insure that foods are safe, pure, and wholesome, and made under sanitary conditions; and that all of these products are honestly labeled and packaged. It carries on research and public education. Food standard regulations governing definition and standard of identity, standards of quality, standards of filling container and labeling are established to promote honesty and fair dealing in the interest of the consumer. Standards of identity have been established for a number of common foods such as jellies, jams, mayonnaise, salad dressing, catsup, cheese, macaroni and noodles. The list of ingredients is not listed if they are prepared

by a fixed standard. Standards of these foods may be obtained from the FDA without charge. Minimum standards of quality have been established concerning certain properties such as tenderness, color and freedom from defects. Standards of fill ensure that no air, water or space is sold as food and that the container fits the food. Standards for enrichment of foods are set. The product labeled "enriched" or "fortified" must contain the exact specified amount of added nutrients.

ADDITIVES LEGISLATION   In September, 1958, a bill was signed into law requiring that the safety of chemicals used in processing food must be proved by industry before they can be sold for use in foods. It became fully effective for all new chemicals on March 5, 1959. Up to this time, it was necessary for the government to prove a chemical unsafe after a food item was already on the market and then to bring court action to remove it from the market.

Under the Delaney clause of the 1958 Food Additive Amendment, a food additive must be tested for safety on animals by the manufacturer or promoter, and the results submitted to the Food and Drug Administration (FDA). If the food additive is found to produce cancer when ingested in any amounts by test animals of any species its use is prohibited. The statutes led to the ban of cyclamates in 1969. The safety of the additive applies equally to substances added directly to foods including animal feeds, and to substances likely to contaminate food as a result of some incidental use in food processing. If the FDA is satisfied that no harm will result from use of the proposed additive, it will issue a regulation specifying the amount which may be used and any other necessary conditions of use.

The use of any additive that tends to deceive the customer or otherwise result in adulteration or in misbranding within the meaning of the Federal Food, Drug and Cosmetic Act is forbidden by law.

In 1960 the Color Additive Amendment was passed which requires that manufacturers prove that their color additives are safe, and authorizes FDA to establish and enforce tolerances for the use of color additives in foods, drugs, and cosmetics. It was estimated that 18,000 firms use color additives in their products.

In 1966, the "truth in packaging" law was enacted, and it took effect in July, 1967. It requires fuller and more prominent information on the labels of packaged foods. Four basic regulations have been specified:[20]

---

[20]Fredelson, I.: Fair packaging: synopsis of food packaging and labeling regulation. FDA Papers, *1*:21, 1967.

1. A statement of the food's identity must appear on the principal display panel in bold type.
2. The name and address of the manufacturer, packer and distributor must be conspicuously stated.
3. A statement of the net contents must appear in concise standard measure. No qualifying terms such as "giant quart" or "jumbo pound" may appear.
4. A statement listing ingredients, when required, must appear in type of legible size, on a single panel of the label. The common names of the ingredients must appear in decreasing order of predominance.

The new regulations include proposals for special diet foods with particular reference to vitamin and mineral supplementation and low calorie foods. Guidelines for nutritional qualities of foods such as main dishes, snack foods, staples important in the diets of ethnic groups known to be malnourished, new foods such as meat analogues, dairy products and fruits are under study by the National Research Council Food and Nutrition Board. In order for the consumer to gain a clearer understanding of the nutritional value of foods, a review of a new form and policy of labeling is forthcoming.[21] In June, 1971, the Food and Drug Administration announced the regulatory proposal requiring food manufacturers to list on the labels the name and source of all fat ingredients and on some foods the kinds of fatty acids present in the food. On special dietary products the label will show the fat content and quality of fat. "The purpose of the proposed fat labeling regulations is to help consumers identify the amount, source and type of fat in the foods they buy."[22]

A survey of the substances generally recognized as safe was conducted in 1970 by the Food Protection Committee, National Academy of Sciences, to establish the nucleus of a new GRAS list or its equivalent. The effects of monosodium glutamate, saccharin, mercury and further studies on the cyclamates and pesticides are under way. Extrapolating findings from animal experimentation to man is a problem.

DRUGS AND ADDITIVES IN LIVESTOCK FEEDS   Most commercial feeds currently contain some type of medication added to control animal diseases, increase yield of meat per pound of feed, shorten the period of feeding prior to marketing, or improve the texture and tenderness of meat.

Drugs that leave any residue in meat, milk, eggs, or other human food products must be proved safe before they can be marketed, just as are animal feed and human food additives (Fig. 14–18). Also, the Federal agencies responsible for inspection of meat and poultry products prevent the slaughter and processing of food animals that have been improperly fed with medicated foods. State and local officials cooperate with FDA inspectors in enforcing the feed additives safety rules.

GENERAL POLICY ON FOOD ADDITIVES   In 1953 the Food and Nutrition Board of the National Academy of Sciences and the Council on Foods and Nutrition of the American Medical Association published jointly a policy entitled "Statement of General Policy in regard to the Addition of Specific Nutrients to Foods." In May, 1961, a revised statement of policy was published, which follows in abbreviated form:

1. The principle of the addition of specific nutrients to certain foods is endorsed, with defined limitations, for the purpose of maintaining good nutrition in all segments of the population at all economic levels.
2. The desirability of meeting nutritional needs by the use of an adequate variety of foods as far as practicable is emphasized strongly.
3. Foods suitable as vehicles for the distribution of additional nutrients are those which have a diminished nutritive content as a result of loss in refining or other processing or those which are widely and regularly consumed.
4. Scientific evaluation of the desirability of restoring an essential nutrient or nutrients to the diet is necessary whenever technological or economic changes lead to a nutritionally significant reduction in the intake of a nutrient or nutrients.
5. The endorsement of the following is affirmed: the enrichment of flour, bread, degerminated corn meal, corn grits, whole grain corn meal, and white rice; the retention or restoration of thiamin, riboflavin, niacin, and iron in processed food cereals; the addition of vitamin D to milk, fluid skim milk, and nonfat dry milk; the addition of vitamin A to margarine, fluid skim milk, and nonfat dry milk; and the addition of iodine to table salt. The protective action of fluoride against dental caries is recognized and the standardized addition of fluoride to water is endorsed in areas where the water supply is low in fluoride.
6. The above statements and endorsements apply to conditions existing in the United States.

[21]Annual Report of U.S. Department of Health, Education and Welfare, 1970, p. 241.

[22]News Release, U.S. Department of Health, Education and Welfare. Public Health Times. Rockville, Maryland, Food and Drug Administration, June 14, 1971.

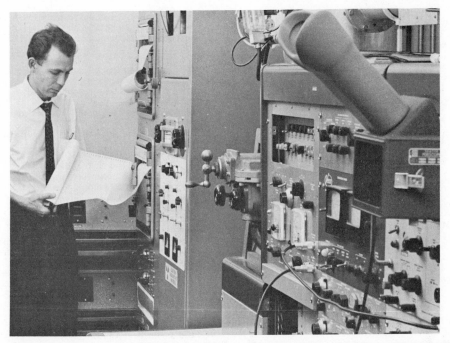

Figure 14–18   Advanced instrumentation detects and measures minute amounts of additives. (Courtesy FDA photo.)

PROBLEMS AND SUGGESTED TOPICS FOR DISCUSSION

1. Explain food poisoning. How can it be prevented?
2. What are the main types of bacterial food poisoning, and how can they be prevented?
3. List four food poisons of natural origin.
4. List the food-borne diseases, and explain how each can be controlled.
5. Describe four methods of preventing food spoilage.
6. What are the possible dangers of the use of pesticides on fruits and vegetables?
7. What methods of food preservation retain the most nutritive value? List the advantages and disadvantages for (a) canned foods, (b) frozen foods, (c) dehydrated foods, (d) freeze-dehydrated foods, (e) dehydrofrozen foods.
8. Report on the Nutrition Community Health program in your community.
9. Discuss the purpose of and legislation on food additives. List seven classes of food additives and give an example of each. Read the labels on ten canned or packaged foods and list the additives in each. What purpose does each of the additives listed serve?
10. What is the role of the nurse in the health of society?
11. Discuss the public health hazards of antibiotics in the milk supply. To what purpose are antibiotics used in food preservation? To what purpose is radiation preservation used?
12. What precautions should be taken with food exposed to radioactive fallout? Outline the foods needed for survival for the family in Problem 2, Chapter 11, in the event of a nuclear attack. Plan menus for 2 weeks using the foods listed.

SUGGESTED ADDITIONAL READING REFERENCES

Agar, E. A., and Dolman, C. E.: Type E botulism. J.A.M.A. *187*:538, 1964.

Anderson, L., and Browe, J. H.: Nutrition and Family Health Service, Philadelphia, W. B. Saunders Company, 1960.

Beacham, L. M.: Food standards. FDA Papers, *1*:4, 1967.

Bond, R. G., and Stauffer, L. D.: Food sanitation and/or the infectious process. J. Am. Dietet. A., *31*:993, 1955.

Brooke, M. M.: Epidemiology of amebiasis in the U.S. J.A.M.A., *188*:519, 1964.

Burgess, A.: A nutrition education in Public Health Programs—What we have learned. Am. J. Pub. Health, *51*:1715, 1961.

Burr, H. K., and Elliott, R. P.: Quality and safety in frozen foods. J.A.M.A., *174*:1178, 1960.

Burton, B. R. (ed.): Heinz Handbook of Nutrition. 2nd ed. New York, McGraw-Hill Book Company, Inc., 1965. Chapter 42, Nutrition in relation to community health.

Cannon, P. R.: Why we have a safe and wholesome food supply, Am. J. Pub. Health, *53*:626, 1963.

Coon, J. M.: Protecting our internal environment. Nutrition Today, 5:14, 1970.

Darby, W. J.: Food additives in animal production. National Live Stock and Meat Board, Food and Nutrition News, *33*(No. 1), 1961.

Duggan, R. E., and Dawson, K.: Pesticides: a report on residues in food. FDA Papers, *1*:4, 1967.

Dunning, G. M.: Radioactivity in the diet. J. Am. Dietet. A., *42*:17, 1963.

Eadie, G. A., et al.: Type E botulism. J.A.M.A., *187*:496, 1964.

Ebbs, J. C.: New horizons for food, J. Am. Dietet. A., *39*: 101, 1961.

Editorial. Salmonella control. J.A.M.A., *189*:691, 1964.

Editorial. The most deadly poison. J.A.M.A., *187*:530, 1964.

Food for Us All, 1969 Yearbook of Agriculture, U.S. Department of Agriculture, Washington, D.C.

Food Protection Committee, Food and Nutrition Board, National Research Council, Washington, D.C. Chemicals used in food processing, Pub. No. 1274, 1965; An evaluation of public health hazards from microbiological contamination of foods, Pub. No. 1195, 1964.

Friedelson, I.: Fair packaging: synopsis of food packaging and labeling regulations. FDA Papers, *1*:21, 1967.

Friedman, L.: Safety of food additives, FDA Papers, *4*:4, 1970.

Hoffman, W. S., et al.: Pesticide storage in human fat tissue. J.A.M.A., *188*:819, 1964.

Hussemann, D. L.: Food-borne disease – A continuing problem. J. Am. Dietet. A., *31*:253, 1955.

Ireland, L. M.: Low-Income Life Styles, U.S. Department of Health, Education and Welfare, 1967.

Irmiter, T. F.: New trends in foods. J. Am. Dietet. A., *43*: 15, 1963.

Kupchik, G. L.: Environmental health in the ghetto. Am. J. Pub. Health, *59*:220, 1969.

Larrick, G. P.: The role of the Food and Drug Administration in Nutrition, Am. J. Clin. Nutr., *8*:377, 1960.

Lindsay, D. R.: Food Safety. FDA Papers, *4*:4, 1970.

Lowenberg, M. E., et al.: Food and Man. New York, John Wiley & Sons, Inc., 1968.

Most, H.: Trichinellosis in the United States. J.A.M.A., *193*:871, 1965.

Patterson, M. L., and Marble, B.: Dietetic foods, Am. J. Clin. Nutr., *16*:440, 1965.

Piper, G. M.: Nutrition in coordinated home care programs. J. Am. Dietet. A., *39*:198, 1961.

Protecting Our Food: 1966 Yearbook of Agriculture, U.S. Department of Agriculture, Washington, D.C.

Queries and Minor Notes. Trichinosis. J.A.M.A., *160*:341, 1956.

Report: Analysis of pesticide residues. FDA Papers, *1*:17, 1967.

Report. Council on Foods and Nutrition: General policy on addition of specific nutrients to foods. J.A.M.A., *178*:1024, 1961.

Report. Council on Foods and Nutrition: Safe use of chemicals in foods. J.A.M.A., *178*:749, 1961.

Report. Food Protection Committee: The Use of Chemical Additives in Food Processing. National Research Council Pub. No. 398, 1956.

Review. Freezer storage and vitamin stability in beef. Nutr. Rev., 23:18, 1965.

Review. Radionuclides in American diets. Nutr. Rev., *21*:105, 1963.

Robinson, H. E., and Urbain, W. M.: Radiation preservation of foods, J.A.M.A., *174*:1310, 1960.

Rountree, J. I.: The place of nutrition in the health education program. Am. J. Pub. Health, *42*:293, March, 1952.

Sanders, H. J.: Food additives. Chemical and Engineering News, October 10, 1966, p. 100.

Select Committee on Nutrition and Human Needs of the U.S. Senate 90th Congress. Part B: The National Nutrition Survey, U.S. Government Printing Office, Washington, D.C.

Sipple, H. L.: Opportunities in nutrition education. J. Am. Dietet. A., 42:140, 1963.

Smillie, W. G., and Kilborne, E. D.: Preventive Medicine and Public Health. 3rd ed. New York, The Macmillan Company, 1963.

Smith, E. H.: Problems in the safe and effective use of pesticides in agriculture. Nutr. Rev., 22:193, 1964.

Stare, F. J., Myers, M.L., and McCann, M. B.: Nutrition education via the public press. J. Am. Dietet. A., *39*:124, 1961.

Stoll, N., and Miyauchi, D.: Acceptability of irradiated fish and shellfish. J. Am. Dietet. A., *46*:111, 1965.

Vaughn, R. H., and Stewart, G. F.: Antibotics as food preservatives. J.A.M.A., *174*:162, 1960.

Walsh, H. E.: The changing nature of public health. J. Am. Dietet. A., *46*:93, 1965.

Welch, H.: Problem of antibiotics in foods. J.A.M.A., *170*:2093, 1959.

Werrin, M., and Krondich, D.: Salmonella control in hospitals. Am. J. Nurs., *66*:528, 1966.

WHO Report. The Public Health Aspects of the Use of Antibiotics in Food and Feedstuffs.

Wohl, M. G., and Goodhart, R. S. (ed.): Modern Nutrition in Health and Disease. 3rd ed. Philadelphia, Lea & Febiger, 1964, Chapter 16A, Chapter 16B, and Chapter 40.

Chapter 15
NUTRITION FOR PREGNANCY AND LACTATION

PREGNANCY

Many studies have shown that the nutritional state of the mother previous to and during pregnancy plays an important role in her health and in that of the fetus. Nutrition surveys in pregnancy,[1] controlled animal investigations,[2] and observations in Holland of the effect of war starvation on pregnancy[3] affirm this fact. The body requirements for food differ from those of a normal non-pregnant woman. Immediately following fertilization, the maternal organism begins a readjustment to provide the environment it needs to support life and the normal growth of the fetus. The metabolic and physiologic changes involving all organs and systems of the mother's body take place during pregnancy. For the child, 9 months old at birth, the intrauterine months represent the period of most rapid growth and development of the entire life cycle. All dietary essentials are increased proportionately to supply the additional demands of the mother and the growing fetus.

Although the adage that the pregnant woman must "eat for two" is not accurate quantitatively, it does denote the increased nutritional demands of the woman during pregnancy. Although the fetus is parasitic on the mother to a degree which depends on her nutritional state and her diet during pregnancy, research data has consistently shown that if the mother is sufficiently depleted nutritionally, the fetus may suffer to spare the mother. A statistically significant relationship has been found[4] between the diet of the mother during pregnancy and the condition of her infant at birth and within the first 2 weeks of life, the better diet producing babies in better physical condition. Stillborn, premature, and congenitally defective infants are more frequently born to mothers who have had an inadequate diet prior to and during pregnancy. It appears the mother also benefits from being in a good nutritional condition during pregnancy. Burke et al.[5] found a greater incidence of complications, due largely to a higher percentage of toxemia, among women whose diets were given a rating of poor. Most authorities agree that the nutritional status of the mother prior to conception is important. Baird concluded that the nutritional status of the mother, the result of her lifetime dietary habits, had a greater influence on the outcome of pregnancy than the diet during pregnancy.[6] Foundations are laid down during prenatal life and early childhood. Many other factors—genetic, biological, socioeconomic and psychological—are involved. An understanding of the role of nutrition in reproduction is based on the concept that pregnancy is a normal state and not a pathological one.

[1]Ebbs, J. H., Tisdall, F. F., and Scott, W. J.: J. Nutrition, 22:515, 1941; Woodhill, J. M., et al.: Am. J. Obstet. Gynec., 70:987, 1955; Burke, B. S.: J. Am. Dietet. A., 20:735, 1944.

[2]Hogan, A. G.: Ann. Rev. Biochem., 22:299, 1953.

[3]Smith, C. A.: Am. J. Obstet. Gynec., 53:599, 1947.

[4]Burke, B. S., et al.: Am. J. Obstet. Gynec., 46:38, 1943; Burke, B. S., et al.: J. Nutrition, 38:453, 1949.

[5]Burke, B. S., et al.: Am. J. Obstet. Gynec., 46:38, 1943.

[6]Baird, D.: Variations in fertility associated with changes in health status. J. Chron. Dis., 18:1109, 1965.

PHYSICAL AND BIOCHEMICAL CHANGES[7]
Many physical and biochemical changes occur in normal pregnancy that are found in pathological conditions. (Special diets or therapeutic supplements are not indicated.) As the blood volume increases, concentrations of hemoglobin are reduced. Plasma albumin falls. Amino acids may be excreted in urine. Edema is sometimes present. Changes occur in cardiac and pulmonary functions. Serum alkaline phosphatase may rise markedly and other enzymes increase in amounts. Most plasma lipid fractions rise during pregnancy. Thyroid glands often enlarge due to loss of inorganic iodine in the urine. A renal loss of folate in some individuals occurs. During late pregnancy, the ability to excrete a water load is below normal and the water may pool in the lower limbs. The stomach shows signs of depressed function (histamine is depressed and pepsin production is reduced). A reduced secretion of hydrochloric acid could have a depressing effect on calcium and iron absorption. Reduced motility of the gastrointestinal tract has been noted, resulting in constipation. A relaxed cardiac sphincter may produce regurgitation into the esophagus and "heartburn." Appetite and thirst increases during the first trimester. Once the early morning nausea subsides the ravenous appetite often returns. Cravings for or aversions to certain foods are common. Pica develops in a few pregnant women. Digestion and assimilation of foods is generally efficient. The following is a quote from the Committee of the World Health Organization (WHO): "From the standpoint of physiological function, pregnancy cannot be regarded as a process of foetal growth superimposed on the ordinary metabolism of the mother. Foetal development is accompanied by extensive changes in maternal body composition and metabolism . . . . Many of the adjustments begin in early pregnancy before foetal growth is appreciable and therefore cannot be interpreted as reaction to stress. Undoubtedly many of them are under hormonal control, although the precise mechanisms are poorly understood . . . . It is clear that clinical standards considered 'normal' for the non-pregnant woman cannot be used as standards for pregnant women."[8]

Weight gain reflects the physiological effects of pregnancy. The average weight gain in the United States is 24 pounds. Weight gain, however, varies considerably. Young women tend to gain more weight than older women, primigravidas more than multigravidas and thin women more than fat women. The difference is slight, however.[9]

The height of women appears to be an important factor in the course and outcome of pregnancy. In 1952 Baird showed that the incidence of stillbirths and difficult labor was common among short women. Macy and Hunscher (1951) and Burke et al. (1959) presented evidence that growth and ultimate height are related to childhood nutrition. It seems to follow that women who in their childhood had a high standard of living tend to grow to the full height permitted by their genetic development and those on poor standards may be stunted in growth.

The incidence of low birth weight infants and closely related neonatal mortality rates appears to be affected by the socioeconomic status of the mother. Other factors such as biological immaturity (under 17 years of age), low pre-pregnancy weight for height, low gain in weight during pregnancy, short stature, poor nutritional status, smoking, infectious agents, chronic disease, history of unsuccessful pregnancies and complications of pregnancy are affected by the socioeconomic status of the mother. The most vulnerable individuals are those born and brought up in poor homes and in large families. Access to food, education and medical care are inadequate. However, women who have had sufficient income may also arrive at childbearing age with poor nutritional status and poor health habits.

Investigations into the psychological factors associated with fetal and infant mortality and morbidity have not come to firm conclusions. Anxiety has been shown to be a predictor of poor outcome of pregnancy when it occurs late in pregnancy. In addition, anxiety usually affects an adequate intake of the protective foods and thus leads to poor nutrition. The pregnant woman may overeat or may suffer deprivation.

THE FETUS AND THE PLACENTA[10]   The placenta's role in feeding the fetus is as yet poorly understood in terms of controlling factors. The placenta is responsible from early gestation for the transfer of sufficient amounts of all substances needed for growth and development to the fetus and for the return of nutrient excesses and waste products to the maternal circulation. Transfer of the nutrient

[7]Hytten, F. E., and Thomson, A. M.: Maternal physiological adjustments. Maternal Nutrition and the Course of Pregnancy, National Research Council, National Academy of Sciences, Washington, D.C., 1970, Chapter 3.

[8]World Health Organization. Technical Report, Series 302, 1965.

[9]Siegel, E., and Morris, N.: The epidemiology of human reproductive casualties with emphasis on the role of nutrition. Maternal Nutrition and the Course of Pregnancy, National Academy of Sciences, Chapter 2, 1970.

[10]Working Group: Coursin, D. B. (Chairman): Relation of nutrition to fetal growth and development. Maternal Nutrition and the Course of Pregnancy, National Academy of Sciences, 1970, p. 125.

takes place in several stages. Diffusion may be at one stage and active transport at another. Conversions and syntheses probably go on in the substances as they pass through.

Most of the nitrogen reaches the fetus as amino acids. Concentration of amino acids, calcium and phosphorus are higher in fetal than in maternal blood. Active transport apparently takes place at the stage of their passage through the placenta. Glucose is transported to the fetus. From glucose the fetus receives energy and makes its own glycogen and fat. Essential fatty acids are transferred. Other fats are synthesized from glucose. The level of blood glucose apparently influences the rate of fetal growth. If the blood sugar is low near term, the fetus fails to store glycogen in its liver.

Sufficient amounts of iron, ascorbic acid, pyridoxine, folacin and cobalamin are transported to meet the demands of the fetus even at the expense of maternal reserves. The fetus and maternal tissue compete for riboflavin, thiamin and vitamin D. More vitamins A and E are present in maternal circulation than in the fetus.

The DNA increases linearly to about 35 weeks gestation and then diminishes. Protein and RNA increase linearly to term. In infants with intrauterine growth retardation, placentas have a reduced DNA, a markedly elevated RNA-DNA ratio and a decrease in total cell number. The high RNA-DNA ratio in the placenta may be a useful tool for study of malnutrition in the fetus. At present, no substantial proof exists that placental failure per se limits the supply of nutrients to the fetus when the placenta is intact and when the supply is sufficient on the maternal side. Other factors such as circulatory factors and biochemical defects may be more important determinants in causing abnormal development or growth retardation of the fetus. It is suspected that some circulatory changes brought about by smoking may interfere with normal transport of nutrients to the placenta. More research is needed to determine the maternal factors that influence the supply line to the fetus.

ADOLESCENCE[11]   Currently, marriage and childbearing occur at a relatively earlier stage of life than in previous generations. If the prospective mother is an adolescent (under 17 years of age) her diet requires individual attention to include the needs for her growth as well as that of the developing fetus. Many of these girls enter into pregnancy with inadequate nutritional stores and are poorly equipped to meet the demands of motherhood. (See Chapter 17, Nutrition in Childhood and Adolescence.) Girls who become pregnant before they are 17 years of age are at great risk both biologically and psychologically. The infant mortality rates are high among infants born to very young mothers. Girls 17 to 20 years are comparable biologically to women 20 to 24 years of age. Growth is usually complete at age 17 and the nutritional requirements for them are similar to those of adult women. The psychological aspects of adolescence superimposed on those inherent in pregnancy add to the emotional burden carried by the adolescent.

The increase in the nutritional requirements for the adolescent and the woman in the second half of pregnancy in relation to those of the normally active and healthy nonpregnant woman are shown in the recommendations of the Food and Nutrition Board of the National Research Council. They are given in Table 15–3 (from Table 11–1, Chapter 11). The increased allowances are only guides and must be carefully adjusted to the need of the individual; they will vary with the age, the weight and the activity of the mother. The increased amounts recommended for the second half of pregnancy assume that the woman is in sound nutritional condition at conception and continues to eat a good diet during the early months of gestation.

NUTRITION IN PREGNANCY

CALORIES   During the course of pregnancy the new tissues that form account for nearly 50,000 kcal. of heat stored (Table 15–1). There are approximately 35,000 kcalories in the maternal fat reserves (9 pounds). The total energy cost of storage plus maintenance (additional work of the maternal heart and uterus and the steady rise in basal metabolism) amounts to approximately 80,000 kcal. Decreased activity of the mother during pregnancy amounts to about 40,000 kcalories. This leaves 40,000 kcalories as the energy cost of pregnancy or about 200 kcalories a day. The components of the maternal weight gain are shown in Table 15–2. The weight of the blood volume and the enlargment of the reproductive organs are fairly constant. If the weight gain is less than the weight of the maternal components in pregnancy the growth of the fetus calls on the reserves of the mother. Weight gain varies. General agreement is found in the literature that the normal curve of weight gain is sigmoid in shape. During the first trimester there is a small gain, a more rapid gain the second

[11]Working Group: McGanity, W. J. (Chairman): Relating nutrition to pregnancy in adolescence. Maternal Nutrition and the Course of Pregnancy. National Academy of Sciences, Chapter 6, 1970.

TABLE 15–1 COMPONENTS OF WEIGHT GAIN AND THE HEAT EQUIVALENT OF EACH (ACCUMULATIVE TOTALS)*

STAGE OF PREGNANCY (Weeks)	PROTEIN (Gm.)	FAT (Gm.)	HEAT OF COMBUSTION (kcal.)
10	35	367	3,700
20	210	1930	19,500
30	535	3614	37,300
40	910	4464	47,500

*Taken from Maternal Nutrition and the Course of Pregnancy, National Academy of Sciences, Chapter 3, p. 67, 1970.

TABLE 15–2   MATERNAL WEIGHT GAIN

TISSUE	WEIGHT (Pounds)
Fetus	7.5
Uterus	2.0
Placenta	1.5
Amniotic fluid	2.0
Blood volume	3.0
Extracellular fluid accretion	2.0
Breast tissue	1.0
Fat	9.0
Total	28.0

trimester and a slower rate of gain in weight during the third trimester (Fig. 15–1).

The committee on Maternal Nutrition and the Course of Pregnancy recommended an average gain in weight during pregnancy of 24 pounds (range 20 to 25 lbs.). This amount the committee believes is commensurate with a better than average course and outcome of pregnancy. The shape of curve would be that shown in Figure 15–1. A gain of 1.5 to 3.0 lbs. during the first trimester and a gain of 0.8 lb. per week during the remainder of pregnancy is a guideline. The pattern of weight gain is more important than the total amount gained. A sudden gain in weight after the 20th week of pregnancy may indicate water retention and the possible onset of pre-eclampsia. The energy stored as fat in the maternal tissue (Table 15–2) is found in fat deposits primarily, with a small deposit in the mammary glands.

Fat serves as energy reserve and prevents catabolism of the mother's tissues. After delivery of the baby the added fat is lost in a short time.

Approximately 1800 to 2000 kcalories of foods carefully selected for their nutritive value (protein, minerals, vitamins) are necessary to meet essential requirements. Any regimen below this would be inadequate in nutrients. Severe calorie restriction limits the nutrients essential for the growth and development of the fetus and those essential to the mother. Weight control should be based on an adequate dietary program and not on the restriction of water and salt. An overweight woman should not correct her weight problem during pregnancy unless under supervision of the physician. It is better to increase exercise when possible than to restrict food. An adolescent under 17 years

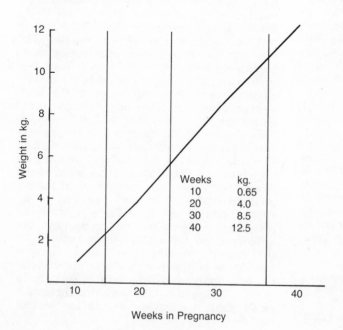

Weeks	kg.
10	0.65
20	4.0
30	8.5
40	12.5

Figure 15–1   The pattern of weight gain in normal pregnancy. Adapted from Maternal Nutrition and the Course of Pregnancy. National Academy of Sciences, Chapter 3, p. 63. Based on documentation found in Hytten, F. E., and Leitch, I.: The Physiology of Human Pregnancy. Oxford, Blackwell 1964.

TABLE 15–3   MATERNAL DAILY DIETARY ALLOWANCES

	RECOMMENDED DAILY ALLOWANCES FOR NONPREGNANT WOMEN					RECOMMENDED DAILY ALLOWANCES ADDED FOR PREGNANCY	DAILY ALLOWANCES ADDED FOR LACTATION
	12 to 14[a] years old	14 to 16[b] years old	16 to 18[c] years old	18 to 22[d] years old	22 to 35[d] years old		
Calories (kcal.)	2300	2400	2300	2000	2000	200	1000
Protein (gm.)	50	55	55	55	55	10	20
Vitamin A (I.U.)	5000	5000	5000	5000	5000	1000	3000
Vitamin D (I.U.)	400	400	400	400	–	0	0
Vitamin E (I.U.)	20	25	25	25	25	5	5
Ascorbic acid (mg.)	45	50	50	55	55	10	5
Folacin (mg.)	0.4	0.4	0.4	0.4	0.4	0.4[e]	0.1
Niacin (mg. equiv.)	15	16	15	13	13	2	7
Riboflavin (mg.)	1.4	1.4	1.5	1.5	1.5	0.3	0.5
Thiamin (mg.)	1.2	1.2	1.2	1.0	1.0	0.1	0.5
Vitamin B_6 (mg.)	1.6	1.8	2.0	2.0	2.0	0.5	0.5
Vitamin B_{12} (μg.)	5	5	5	5	5	3	1
Calcium (gm.)	1.3	1.3	1.3	0.8	0.8	0.4	0.5
Phosphorus (gm.)	1.3	1.3	1.3	0.8	0.8	0.4	0.5
Iodine (μg.)	115	120	115	100	100	25	50
Iron (mg.)	18	18	18	18	18	f	f
Magnesium (mg.)	350	350	350	350	300	150	150

From Appendix C, Maternal Nutrition and the Course of Pregnancy—Summary Report, Public Health Service Pub. No. 2114, 1970.
[a]Body size, 44 kg.; height, 154 cm.
[b]Body size, 52 kg.; height, 157 cm.
[c]Body size, 54 kg.; height, 160 cm.
[d]Body size, 58 kg.; height, 163 cm.
[e]The diet may be supplemented with 0.2 to 0.4 mg. of folacin daily.
[f]It is recommended that the diet be supplemented with 30 to 60 mg. of iron per day.

should not be restricted in calories below energy needs for her own growth and the fetus. If obese, the young adolescent should be expected to gain weight. The standardized diets used in most prenatal clinics are unsuited to the nutritional needs of the adolescent. It is expedient to plan with the individual the dietary program that can be adopted. The expectant mother should not be concerned particularly about increasing the quantity of food consumed until the second half of pregnancy.

PROTEIN   The Food and Nutrition Board of the National Research Council suggests adding 10 gm. of protein daily for the second half of gestation in addition to the usual 0.9 gm. per kg. body weight. The additional protein provides for the increase in maternal tissue and for the growth of the fetus. Two thirds of the proteins should be of animal origin of the highest biologic values (meat, milk, eggs, cheese, poultry and fish) since they furnish all the essential amino acids.

If protein needs are met, all other nutrients except ascorbic acid, vitamin A and vitamin D will probably be provided because of their association with protein in food. If protein is inadequate in the pregnant woman's diet, calcium, phosphorus, iron and B vitamins will usually also be inadequate.

Inadequacies in the protein content of the diet of the pregnant woman may lead to nutritional edema. Some research workers believe that a diet low in proteins may be a cause of toxemia of pregnancy. Other disorders of pregnancy which may result from a low protein intake are anemia, poor muscle tone of the uterus, abortion, lowered resistance to infection, and insufficient lactation. The studies of Burke and co-workers[12] carried on at the Harvard School of Medicine show that the weight, length and general condition of the infant at birth are in a direct ratio to the

[12]Burke, B. S., et al.: J. Pediat., 23:506, 1943.

grams of protein consumed by the mother. As a result of this study, the investigators suggest that "less than 75 gm. of protein daily during the latter part of pregnancy result in an infant who will tend to be short, light in weight, and most likely receive a low pediatric rating in other respects." More recent observations, however, have not completely corroborated these studies.

An extensive study by Dieckmann et al.[13] revealed that women who consumed increased protein diets throughout pregnancy had less anemia, no miscarriages and healthier babies, as compared with women who did not receive extra protein foods. No correlation was found, however, between the weight and length of the infants and the protein intake of the mother. According to McGanity,[14] "There is satisfactory evidence that one cannot materially influence the birth weight or birth length of her infant by the caloric or protein intake of the mother during her pregnancy. There is, however, a direct relationship between the prepartum weight of the mother and the delivery weight of her child."

Of special interest is the research work of McCane, Widdowson and Lehman[15] which shows the interrelation of the high protein diet and calcium absorption during pregnancy. They report that in the presence of a high protein intake 15 per cent of the calcium was absorbed, while in the low protein diet only 5 per cent of the calcium was absorbed. The report suggests that probably the amino acids facilitate calcium absorption. The findings of this study are significant in cases in which the calcium intake is low and absorption is poor. A high protein diet may convert a calcium deficiency into sufficiency.

In Iowa, studies by Stearns[16] indicate that many women receive insufficient protein and calcium during pregnancy. These poorly nourished mothers have more premature babies and/or babies who are too weak to live or who have deformities. A low intake of protein is associated with a decrease in the number of cells in the tissues of the fetus at birth. This would affect brain development.

CALCIUM, PHOSPHORUS AND VITAMIN D
Calcium is one of the most important elements of the diet for the pregnant woman. Since phosphorus and vitamin D are linked so closely with calcium metabolism, their values are considered at the same time. An adequate supply of vitamin D is essential for the utilization of the calcium and phosphorus necessary for the calcification of the fetal bones and teeth, as well as for the gravid patient's own needs. If the diet of the pregnant woman is inadequate in calcium she will have to sacrifice the calcium of her bones in the interests of the developing fetus. It has been shown that the calcium and phosphorus retained in the fetus during the last two lunar months are 65 and 64 per cent, respectively, of the total body content of the full term fetus. Despite the fact that there is evidence that calcium absorption is increased during pregnancy and lactation, the daily intake of calcium must be increased from the standard nonpregnant adult daily allowance of 0.8 gm. to 1.2 gm. to satisfy these additional needs. The calcium recommendations for the non-pregnant young adolescent is 1.3 gm. and during pregnancy 1.7 gm. Approximately 30 gm. of calcium is deposited in the infant at birth. Phosphorus is less likely to be inadequate in the average diet. The phosphorus intake should be at least equal to that of calcium during the latter part of pregnancy. If the protein and calcium requirements are observed, the need for phosphorus will likely be met. The daily vitamin D requirement during pregnancy is estimated at 400 I.U. (See Table 15–3.)

IRON   During pregnancy there is a noticeable increase in the need for iron to supply the growing fetus. Iron is stored in the liver of the fetus for use during the first three to six months of life. The World Health Organization's Expert Committee on Nutrition in Pregnancy and Lactation[17] has calculated the iron balance during pregnancy, shown in Table 15–4. The mother transfers to the fetus and placenta 200 to 300 mg. of iron during the second half of pregnancy. This amounts to nearly 6 mg. of iron daily. The 1.5 to 1.0 mg. iron lost through the intestine, urinary tract

[13]Dieckmann, W. J., et al.: J. Am. Dietet. A., 27:1046, 1951.

[14]McGanity, W. J.: J.A.M.A. (Medical News), 186:39, 1963.

[15]McCane, R. A., Widdowson, E. M., and Lehman, H.: J. Biochem.,36:686, 1942.

[16]Stearns, G.: National Live Stock and Meat Board, Food and Nutrition News, 25:3, 1953; J.A.M.A., 168:1655, 1958.

[17]World Health Organization Technical Report, Series 302.

TABLE 15–4   IRON BALANCE DURING PREGNANCY*

Extra iron in:	mg.
Product of conception	370
Maternal blood	290
Total	660
Minus iron "saved" by cessation of menstruation	120
Total	540

*Hytten, F. E., and Thomson, A. M.: Maternal physiological adjustments. Maternal Nutrition and the Course of Pregnancy, National Academy of Sciences, Chapter 3, p. 68, 1970.

and the integument must be added. The sources of iron needed during pregnancy come from the maternal stores, her diet and supplementary iron (ferrous). Iron stores are very often insufficient to meet the requirements of pregnancy. Young healthy American women average about 300 mg. of storage iron. Women in the United States usually ingest 9 to 12 mg. of iron daily or 1.5 to 1.8 mg. of absorbable iron, an amount below the daily recommended allowance of 18 mg. It is believed that the rate of absorption of iron is increased in pregnancy. The Food and Nutrition Board in the 1968 revision of Daily Dietary Allowances did not increase the amount suggested for the non-pregnant woman to meet the demands for pregnancy (see Table 15-3). Because an otherwise adequate diet contains approximately 6 mg. of iron per 1000 kcalories and women enter pregnancy with suboptimal stores and low hemoglobin values, a supplement of 30 to 60 mg. of iron in the form of ferrous salt daily during the second and third trimesters is recommended. WHO committee "feels that the indiscriminate issue of [iron] preparations to all pregnant women in situations where there is no obvious indication for them is to be deplored." An adequate diet prior to and continuing through pregnancy is recommended. Hemoglobin production requires an adequate supply of protein to furnish essential amino acids, sufficient calories to protect the protein from catabolic degradation, iron and other minerals such as copper, zinc, folic acid, vitamin B_{12} and other co-factors involved in the synthesis of heme and globin. If the additional demands for iron are not met, varying grades of hypochromic anemia may result. (See Anemia, p. 246, and Chapter 31, Diseases of the Blood and Blood-forming Organs.)

IODINE   This mineral is of special importance in pregnancy to meet the added demands placed upon the metabolism by the thyroid gland, to meet the needs for fetal development and to provide for the deficiency of iodine due to urinary loss during pregnancy. An inadequate intake of iodine may result in goiter in the mother, especially the adolescent. The child may have a goiter also or, in the case of severe iodine deficiency, the child may develop cretinism. The regular use of iodized salt is recommended. Provisions for iodine supplementation are indicated when salt in the diet is severely restricted.

OTHER MINERALS   Routine sodium restriction in pregnancy is now questioned. Evidence of increased need of sodium in pregnancy has been demonstrated and a severe restriction is hazardous. Undesirable changes in the fetus have been associated with very low or excessive levels of intake of zinc, magnesium and manganese.

VITAMINS   The Food and Nutrition Board, National Research Council in the 1968 revision suggests a small increase in most of the vitamins (see Table 15-3). The 1967 report of a Joint FAO/WHO Expert Committee reviewed the evidence of need for vitamin A, thiamin, riboflavin and niacin. This committee found no need for increasing vitamin A during pregnancy. The needs for thiamin, riboflavin and niacin would be met when the intake would be increased proportionately to the increase of calories. Adequate provision for all the vitamins, other than vitamin D, usually can be realized by including in the dietary sufficient protective foods without relying on special products. In most climates supplementary amounts of vitamin D should be given. Vitamin D fortified milk is now available and 1 quart contains the 400 I.U. required daily for maximum calcium retention. On the other hand, there is evidence that excessive vitamin D intake during pregnancy may cause abnormal calcium deposition in the fetus, producing increased density of the bones, especially the base of the skull, and chalky deposits in the aorta.

Considerable experimental research has been carried on to show the relation between vitamin E and reproduction. No conclusive results have been demonstrated. Experimental and clinical data suggest that vitamin E is necessary for the normal development of the fetus and the completion of pregnancy.

Vegetable oils that supply the essential polyunsaturated fatty acid also supply vitamin E. A deficiency may occur when the diet contains excessive amounts of polyunsaturated fatty acids.

In animals, Warkany demonstrated congenital malformations during early stages of gestation and poor reproductive performance when deficient in vitamin A.

For a margin of safety the B vitamins (thiamin, riboflavin, niacin, pyridoxine) are increased. They are not stored and are important as co-factors in a number of metabolic activities which are increased in pregnancy. Folacin is essential for normal fetal growth and the prevention of megaloblastic anemia. A supplement is recommended when a deficiency or poor absorption of the vitamin is apparent. A large amount of B_{12} (cobalamin) absorbed in pregnancy provides fetal needs.

When the vitamin K status of the mother has been unsatisfactory or is unknown at the time of labor, it is advisable to give the mother 0.5 to 1.0 mg. parenterally or 1.0 to 2.0 mg. orally before the birth of the baby to stabilize the prothrombin level of the infant until food is taken. If this has not been done,

1 to 2 mg. can be given to the infant. It is recommended that infants born to mothers receiving anticoagulant therapy should be given 2 to 4 mg. immediately after birth.

ASCORBIC ACID A 10 per cent increase of ascorbic acid is recommended daily (60 mg.) for pregnancy. Ascorbic acid is essential in the formation of intercellular cement substance in connective tissue and vascular systems of the fetus.

FOOD ALLOWANCES FOR THE NORMAL PREGNANT WOMAN

The selection of food for the pregnant woman is important. All the essential nutrients in the amounts recommended must be included in the daily dietary. To be certain this is accomplished, the adequate diet pattern (Chapter 11) is used plus a few important changes and additions.

One way of providing the additional kcalories, protein, calcium, phosphorus and vitamins recommended is shown below.

	Amount	Protein (gm.)	Kcalories
Skim milk	1 cup	8	80
Bread	1 slice	2	68
Citrus fruit	1 serving	–	60
Total		10	208

A number of choices for milk are available: whole milk, skim milk, fluid and non-fat powdered, buttermilk, evaporated milk, yogurt and cheese. Those patients who find drinking milk disagreeable may utilize the required amount in soups, custards, puddings, ice cream, or flavored beverages. Also, milk products, such as evaporated, homogenized or the powdered variety, may be incorporated into the meal plan. The use of non-fat skim powder is an inconspicuous and acceptable way to add milk to the diet. Approximately 1½ ounces (5 tablespoons) of dried skim milk will equal 1 pint of fluid milk. Dried non-fat milk may be used as a dry ingredient in the preparation of meatloaf, soups, mashed and scalloped potatoes, sandwich spreads, cooked cereals, hot breads, cookies, pastries, or puddings with little difficulty. A palatable drink may be prepared by adding approximately 2½ tablespoons of dried skim milk and flavoring (vanilla, cocoa) if desired to 1 glass (8 ounces) of fluid milk. Sugar, molasses or honey can be added to make it more palatable, if the calorie allowance permits. The non-fat milk powder may be added also as a dry ingredient to cottage cheese, scrambled eggs, macaroni or spaghetti, and cake.

With the exception of lactose, American Cheddar cheese contains the nutrients of milk. If milk or milk products are not tolerated, commercial calcium preparations may have to be prescribed, although they are not always efficient because they may be unabsorbed in their passage through the intestinal tract.

The daily consumption of whole-grain or enriched bread and cereals, leafy green and yellow vegetables, fresh and dried fruits should be encouraged to provide additional minerals and vitamins. Careful attention to the selection of foods that are good sources of iron within the food groups is stressed to provide as much dietary iron as possible. Liver should be included in the diet at least once a week. The daily egg in the diet regimen is very important because of its protein and iron content.

Three to 4 cups of milk fortified with vitamin D provides 300 to 400 I.U. of the

---

TABLE 15–5   DAILY FOOD PATTERN TO ENSURE OPTIMAL NUTRITION DURING PREGNANCY

FOOD	AMOUNT	PROTEIN (gm.)
Milk, whole	3 or 4–8 oz. glasses.	24 to 32
Meat (lean), poultry, fish, liver is desirable at least once each week, cheese	2 servings/day, in all at least 4 oz. or equivalent in grams of protein.	28
Egg	One	7
Fruit	At least 2 servings. Two servings of citrus fruit or equivalent should be eaten. (1 serving equals 4 oz. of orange juice, 1 med. orange, 8 oz. of tomato juice, or ½ med. grapefruit.)	2
Potato	1 med. (150 gm.), preferably cooked in skin.	3
Other vegetables cooked and/or raw	2 or more servings (1 serving equals ½ cup). Dark green leafy or deep yellow vegetables often.	
Bread and cereal	3 to 4 servings. (1 serving equals 1 slice of bread or ½ cup of cereal.) Whole grain or enriched.	4
Vegetable oil or special margarine, butter or fortified margarine	1 tablespoon	6 to 8
Vitamin D	An amount to supply 400 I.U. such as vitamin D fortified milk (1 qt.)	0
Total		74 to 84

TABLE 15–6 SAMPLE MENU FOR THE SECOND HALF OF PREGNANCY

Breakfast
Orange juice, 4 oz.
Oatmeal, ½ cup
Soft cooked egg
Whole grain or enriched toast, 1 slice
Butter or fortified margarine, 1 pat
Coffee or tea

Mid-Morning
Orange juice, 4 oz.
Wheaties, ¾ cup
Milk, 4 to 8 oz.

Lunch
Meat or cheese sandwich with rye or whole wheat bread and
1 pat butter
Lettuce and tomato salad
Grapefruit, half
Milk, 8 oz.

Midafternoon
Milk, 8 oz.

Dinner
Broiled beef liver, 4 oz.
Baked potato with 1 pat butter or fortified margarine
Peas and carrots
Crisp celery
Baked custard

Bedtime
Hot or cold milk, or cocoa, 8 oz.

Kcalories are adjusted for desired weight. If the gravid individual is an adolescent, additional milk, fresh fruits or vegetables, whole-grain bread and butter or margarine are suggested.

vitamin. If milk is used in limited amounts, fish liver oil is recommended.

See Table 15–5, Food Pattern To Ensure Optimal Nutrition during Pregnancy; and Table 15–6, Sample Menu for the Second Half of Pregnancy.

TOTAL FLUIDS The drinking of 6 to 8 glasses (2 liters) of water daily is encouraged. Intestinal stasis is often encountered as a result of the necessary restrictions of activities and the pressure of the enlarging uterus. However, for most individuals the bulky content of the protective diet plus the suggested amount of water will counteract any difficulty. Mineral oil is discouraged, since it interferes with the absorption of the fat-soluble vitamins.

NUTRITION EDUCATION

Usually the prospective mother is anxious for a normal, healthy baby, and seeks obstetric care early. Nutrition advice, well presented at this time, is more apt to be accepted than at any other stage or period in life. Unless such advice is based on previous food habits, customs and food budget, it may not be followed. Any improvement in food pattern depends upon how the person perceives the task of change. With few exceptions, a woman whose diet is poor in pregnancy can be considered as having been on a poor diet previous to conception. The average gravid adolescent girl especially requires individualized counseling on the basis of her specific needs. A printed diet list is of little or no value. Full discussion on individual needs with involvement of the person in planning for the necessary changes is the only effective approach. (Review Food Habits, Chapter 1; Diet Instruction, Chapter 2.)

To gain cooperation for diet improvement from the prospective mother, a discussion on the dietary habits of the prospective father and any other members of the family is also necessary. A prospective father, convinced that it is an essential part of his duties as a father, will join his wife in improving their food pattern and food habits. The counselor utilizes this interest and helps them to move in the direction of changes needed to provide an adequate diet. If each parent tends to guard the other's diet, both will improve their food habits. Thus, if both parents adopt an adequate diet, another family is started in good nutritional habits. Good nutritional habits of parents and family increase the number of well-born infants.

COMPLICATIONS OF PREGNANCY IN WHICH DIET IS A FACTOR

OBESITY

An obese woman at conception and one who gains an excessive amount of weight during pregnancy is in jeopardy. Complications develop that affect the course and outcome of pregnancy. Quite apart from the dangers to both mother and child of overweight in pregnancy, another hazard of excessive antepartum weight gain is the development of permanent obesity and the resultant complications, some of which may not appear until later in life. While many patients who gain excessive weight during pregnancy lose it again spontaneously after delivery, too many women do not return to normal weight unless they make positive attempts to do so, either alone or with help. An adequate diet with sufficient calories to provide the energy required for the fetus and activity of the woman is an essential approach to weight control in the preventive concept of medicine. The present day expectant mother usually relies upon modern work-saving devices and therefore needs very few (200) additional kcalories over the non-pregnant state.

The obese pregnant woman can control her rate of gain in weight without compromising the basic dietary requirements simply by decreasing the total calorie content through restriction of fats and carbohydrates. Skim milk (350 kcalories per quart) may be substituted for whole milk (670 kcalories per quart). Sugar and "empty" calorie foods can be restricted or omitted. Protein intake is maintained at the prescribed level, and the diet is adequate in minerals and vitamins unless total calories are below 1500, in which case specific nutritional supplements may be required.

Jacobson, Burke, Smith and Reid[18] studied 89 obese pregnant women placed on a 1500 kcalorie, 95 gm. protein, diet supplemented with iron and thiamin. They found that those who followed the diet (as indicated by weight loss) had fewer complications of pregnancy, and there was no demonstrable adverse effect on the condition of the infant at birth. From this study it would appear safe and beneficial during pregnancy to restrict calories in an otherwise adequate diet if the individual is overweight or gaining weight too rapidly.

The diet in pregnancy should not, as a rule, be less than 1500 kcalories and preferably 1800 to assure nutritional adequacy. McGanity[19] believes it is dangerous to reduce an individual more than 5 to 10 per cent during the 40 weeks of gestation. (See Chapter 29, Overweight and Underweight.)

Allen et al.[20] report the birth of a normal infant whose mother was maintained on a 900 kcalorie nutritionally adequate formula throughout pregnancy. The patient experienced an average weight loss of 3.7 pounds (1.7 kg.) per week. The average nitrogen retention during pregnancy was 1.2 gm./day, with a maximum negative nitrogen balance of 2.93 gm./day during the 11th week, and a maximum positive nitrogen balance of 3.31 gm./day during the 25th week. This carefully controlled instance is insufficient evidence for widespread practice of such a severe reduction in calories.

In a study of 12,847 cases of teen-age gestation, excess weight gain was the most frequent complication, occurring in over 30 per cent of the patients.[21] The incidence of pre-eclampsia and eclampsia are correlated with increasing weight gain, and perinatal mortality increases with the severity of the disease. As pointed out, it is the rate of gain during pregnancy that is important. Any sharp or sudden gain is indicative of possible onset of complications.

ANEMIA

During pregnancy there is a high incidence of various types and degrees of anemia. In the second and third trimesters, physiologic hemodilution lowers the red blood cell count, hematocrit and hemoglobin readings, so that normochronic normocytic anemia (hydremia) must be distinguished from *true* anemia.

True anemias of mild degree are managed with appropriate medications. Hydrochromic anemia, the most common variety, is treated with iron and cobalt preparations. Megaloblastic anemia is relatively uncommon in pregnancy. Pernicious anemia is treated with liver extract and vitamin B_{12}. Other macrocytic anemias (megaloblastic) respond to folic acid.

True anemia is most commonly the result of iron deficiency or impaired utilization of iron or acute loss of blood, or low storage of iron. In pregnancy, the maternal and fetal hemoglobin synthesis requires considerable iron. Maternal iron is lost to the fetus during the gestation period, and maternal blood is lost in association with delivery. A diet inadequate in animal protein of high biologic value is another significant cause of anemia.

Iron stored in the body in sufficient amount prior to pregnancy, plus an adequate diet for pregnancy, will usually provide the necessary iron during pregnancy. The amount required for pregnancy is more than most women have stored. If the diet or absorption has been faulty and the iron stores are insufficient, iron must be provided through the food intake or through medication if iron deficiency anemia is to be avoided. It is well known that once anemia becomes established, it is impossible to raise the iron level by diet, regardless of the amount made available. In such cases, it is necessary to provide supplemental iron.

Some obstetricians believe it is advantageous to provide the mother with iron therapy as a prophylaxis against iron deficiency anemia, especially those with a history of anemia or frequent pregnancies. Others maintain that an adequate diet for pregnancy is sufficient. Inorganic ferrous preparations are the most effective and least irritating forms of medical iron to administer.

Angulo and Spies[22] have shown that the diets of patients having macrocytic anemia of pregnancy are low in folic acid content. Although megaloblastic anemia due to maternal folate deficiency is relatively uncommon, it does occur. Folate deficiency may be present in the absence of iron deficiency

[18] Jacobson, H. N., et al.: Am. J. Obstet. Gynec., *83*:1609, 1962.

[19] McGanity, W. J.: J.A.M.A., *186*:39, 1963.

[20] Allen, C. E., et al.: J.A.M.A., *188*:392, 1964.

[21] Semmens, J. P.: Implications of teen-age pregnancy. Obstet. Gynec., 26:77, 1965.

[22] Angulo, J. J., and Spies, T. D.: The determination of the folic acid content of foods usually consumed by patients with tropical sprue. Am. J. Trop. Med., 27:317, 1947.

anemia. The deficiency may be common in late pregnancy and multiple fetuses. Administration of folic acid produces a prompt hematologic response.[23] (See Anemias, Chapter 28.)

CARDIAC DISEASE

Cardiac diseases during pregnancy are treated in much the same fashion as in the nonpregnant state. Dietary regulation in pregnant cardiac patients is concerned mainly with obesity and vascular congestion as contributory causes of failure (Chapter 30). Overweight must be avoided to minimize the work of the heart and adequate rest is essential.

SODIUM AND FLUIDS   The relation of vascular congestion to fluid balance is discussed in Chapter 30, Cardiovascular Diseases. Since sodium and fluids are frequently restricted to certain cardiac diseases, the diet of the pregnant woman requires careful, supervised planning.

Current medical concepts regarding dietary control of fluid balance emphasize the restriction of sodium, and there is an increasing trend not to limit the fluid intake. In pregnancy, however, because of the tendency to retention of sodium and of water, it is difficult to achieve satisfactory regulation of fluid balance without restricting both sodium and liquids. This has specific implications in the management of heart disease (and of toxemia), in which, in most subjects, it is advisable to limit the daily fluid intake to 1500 ml. or less, depending upon the individual problem.

Because milk is usually considered a fluid and is relatively high in sodium chloride content, the daily three-fourths to one quart of milk necessary for calcium requirements may have to be restricted. If it is necessary to reduce the amount of milk to less than three-fourths of a quart a day, it may be advisable to use a low sodium milk (Chapter 30) or to supply part of the needed calcium by medication.

IODINE   The iodine content of the diet needs special evaluation when iodized salt cannot be used because of sodium restriction. Iodine may have to be prescribed if the iodine content of the diet and of the local drinking water is inadequate, as in the goiter belt (see Chapter 34).

CHOLESTEROL   With the current emphasis on the influence of cholesterol as a cause of vascular sclerosis, it seems appropriate to mention that serum cholesterol

values may rise as high as 350 to 400 mg. during the last trimester of *normal* pregnancy. (The normal serum of cholesterol range is approximately 150 to 250 mg. per 100 ml., with an average of 180, in the nonpregnant state.)

DIABETES

The diet of the pregnant diabetic woman must be adequate to meet the maternal and fetal nutritional needs. Statistics reveal that pregnancy may aggravate uncontrolled cases or may initiate imbalance in controlled ones. The instance of toxemia is high, and fetal mortality is significantly greater than in normal pregnancy. Successful pregnancy depends upon adequate dietary and insulin management to meet the growth needs of the fetus and to prevent depletion of the mother's nutritional stores. Needs for increased diet go hand in hand with needs for increased insulin. The nutritional fetal demands of pregnancy may impose an initial need for insulin in a diabetic gravid woman otherwise adequately controlled solely by diet in the nonpregnant state.

There is no fixed rule about the amount of insulin administration during pregnancy. The insulin requirements usually increase, but only temporarily. The increase occurs rather abruptly during the fifth month and may last through the ninth month. Frequent changes in the diet and insulin dosage may be necessary.

Infants born to diabetics are, as a rule, larger than those of nondiabetics. At least 25 per cent of the infants weigh more than 10 pounds at birth. The hazards of labor are increased and, in many cases, cesarean section is advised. It must be emphasized that unfavorable effects are in proportion to the care the mother receives; when the diabetes is under control, complications are rare. Early prenatal care is an important factor.

TOXEMIA

For many years nutrition has been related to the occurrence of toxemias of pregnancy. Prevention and treatment have been largely empirical. The Committee on Maternal Nutrition, Food and Nutrition Board, National Research Council in a report of their review of the literature considered toxemia under two classifications: pre-eclampsia and eclampsia. Pre-eclampsia was defined as acute hypertension with proteinuria or edema or both appearing after the twentieth week of pregnancy and accompanied by edema of the tissues. Eclampsia was defined as the oc-

---

[23] Prichard J. A.: Anemias complicating pregnancies. Maternal Nutrition and the Course of Pregnancy. National Academy of Sciences, Washington, D.C., 1970.

currence of one or more convulsions with the criteria for the diagnosis of pre-eclampsia.[24]

A dramatic decline in maternal mortality from toxemias has occurred in the United States during the past 25 years. The mortality rates by states has varied widely. The most striking association of the differences is related to per capita income. In those states with low per capita income the incidence of maternal mortality from toxemia is higher than in those states with higher per capita income. Since severe toxemia of pregnancy occurs most frequently among women in the lower socioeconomic strata whose diets are often substandard, the hypothesis has been generally advanced that malnutrition may be a causative factor. Brewer and associates in their studies indicate that impairment of the liver detoxification mechanism may be involved in the toxemia process rather than malnutrition.[25, 26]

Tompkins et al. found that pre-eclampsia tends to be more severe when it develops in markedly underweight women at conception and when they fail to gain weight normally during the neonatal period.[27] Pre-eclampsia is more common among the very young primigravidas and those over age 30, diabetics, multiple pregnancies and those with a hypertensive disorder. The Committee reported that little scientific evidence was found to indicate calorie restriction and the restriction of accumulation of fat as means for preventing toxemia. Since the work of Strauss, protein deficiency resulting in hypoproteinemia and water retention is considered by many to be a primary factor in the cause of toxemia.[28] In the United States the decreased incidence of toxemia may be attributed to improvement in diet especially in the protein intake. The proportion of calories from protein has remained at 11 to 13 per cent over the past half century. Two thirds of the protein now comes from animal sources compared with one half in the 1904 to 1913 period. In order to avoid protein depletion, appropriate dietary regulation is required. It may be necessary to increase the protein to as much as 120 gm. or more. However, when nitrogen retention is present, as in certain renal dis-

eases, the protein intake must be individualized and this may even necessitate less than normal requirement. (See Chapter 32, Nutrition in Renal Diseases).

The edema of pre-eclampsia is largely extracellular sodium retention. The concentration of sodium in plasma is essentially normal. It has been shown that the pre-eclampsia condition becomes more serious when extra salt is taken, as when women indulge in salty foods. Pike has demonstrated deleterious effects of sodium depletion in experimental studies on pregnant rats.[29] The Committee on Maternal Nutrition believes that the matter of routine salt restriction in pregnancy as a means of preventing pre-eclampsia requires further research and assessment.

Some physicians believe that the restriction of sodium and fluid is desirable for the control of edema in pregnancy. Sodium-restricted diets are outlined in Chapter 30, Cardiovascular Diseases. Protein foods of animal origin contain relatively high amounts of sodium, and most low sodium foods also are low in protein, or their protein is low in biologic value. Sodium deficient milk is, therefore, the most satisfactory source for providing added protein, within the limits of fluid allowance. Special unsalted nuts and legumes or other low sodium products may be used. (See Chapter 30.)

Some workers (Robinson, M.,[30] Mengert, W. F., and Tacchi, D. A.[31]) have questioned the importance of restricting salt in toxemia and report equal or better results when the salt intake was high. Gray et al.[32] studied 28 normal pregnant women in an attempt to define the role of dietary sodium in salt and water retention during normal pregnancy. They report the amount of sodium retained could not be influenced by differences in the average quantity of sodium ingested during this time. Some increase in sodium was observed during the last month of gestation.

In the studies of Klieger and associates, placentas from patients with toxemia contained one third the normal content of B_6 and decreased pyridoxal kinase activity. This would result in insufficient enzymes available to convert pyridoxal to the active enzyme pyridoxal phosphate. The relationship between insufficient B_6 metabolism and toxemia needs further study.[33]

[24]Holly, R. G. (Chairman): Relation of nutrition to the toxemias of pregnancy. Maternal Nutrition and the Course of Pregnancy, National Academy of Sciences, Washington, D.C., 1970.

[25]Brewer, T. H.: Am. J. Obstet. Gynec., 84:1253, 1962.

[26]Brewer, T. H., and Miale, J. B.: Obstet. Gynec., 20:345, 1962.

[27]Tompkins, W. T., et al.: The underweight patient—an increased obstetric hazard. Am. J. Obstet. Gynec. 69:114, 1955.

[28]Strauss, M. B.: Observations on the etiology of the toxemias of pregnancy. The relationship of nutritional deficiency, hypoproteinuria, and elevated venous pressure to water retention in pregnancy. Am. J. Med. Sci., 190:811, 1935.

[29]Pike, P. L.: Sodium intake during pregnancy. J. Am. Dietet. A., 44:176, 1964.

[30]Robinson, M.: Salt in pregnancy. Lancet, 1:178, 1958.

[31]Mengert, W. F., and Tacchi, D. A.: Pregnancy toxemia and sodium chloride. Am. J. Obstet. Gynec., 81:601, 1961.

[32]Gray, M. J., et al.: Regulation of sodium and total body water metabolism in pregnancy. Am. J. Obstet. Gynec., 89:761, 1964.

[33]Klieger, J. A., et al.: Abnormal pyridoxine metabolism in toxemia of pregnancy. Am. J. Obstet. Gynec., 94:316, 1966.

NAUSEA AND VOMITING IN PREGNANCY

Morning sickness or nausea is not uncommon during the early months of pregnancy, and the condition usually disappears just as spontaneously as it appears. However, when early pregnancy is characterized by excessive vomiting, an acute protein deficit and loss of minerals, vitamins and electrolytes may be produced, which will require a return to an adequate diet as soon as possible.

In cases of *pernicious vomiting*, fats are a fairly common offender. Many obstetricians achieve benefits for the patient by advising the withholding of fluids from 1 to 2 hours before and following meals, plus the prescription of a dry diet. Milk may be skimmed if the fat in the whole milk is not well tolerated.

Frequent small meals consisting of such foods as thickly cooked cereal, Melba toast with jelly, saltines, and baked potato served at 2 hour intervals, usually are well tolerated initially. If the food is retained, fluids may be tried 1 hour before and after the serving of food. A dry, soft diet may be given as soon as all fluids and foods are retained. Fats and fluids, as tolerated, are gradually added to the meals.

DRY DIET

Foods Allowed

Meats: Lean meat, fish, chicken, and crisp bacon (prepared by broiling or roasting methods).

Eggs: Hard cooked.

Cheese: American Cheddar and Swiss cheese.

Breads: Toasted enriched white bread and saltines.

Cereals: Thick cooked cereals and the dry ready-to-eat variety.

Potatoes: Baked, boiled, or mashed.

Fats: Butter or fortified margarine and peanut butter in limited amounts.

Desserts: Arrowroot cookies, sponge cake, pound cake, angel food cake, baked custard, vanilla ice cream (if tolerated).

Sugar: Sugar, jelly, jam, and honey.

Liquids: At the beginning of the diet regimen, all liquids are served between meals; later on, if liquids are tolerated, liquids may be allowed with the meals.

Meal Plan

8:00 A.M. Cereal with sugar, fortified margarine or butter
Toasted enriched white bread with jelly
Crisp bacon or hard cooked egg

10:00 A.M. Orange juice

11:00 A.M. Milk

12:00 NOON Lean meat, small serving
Baked potato
Toasted enriched white bread, lightly buttered
Jelly
Dessert

2:00 P.M. Milk

4:00 P.M. Fruit juice

6:00 P.M. Meat or cheese, small serving
Potato or dessert
Crackers or toast
Jelly, jam, or peanut butter

8:00 P.M. Milk

DIET FOR PATIENTS IN LABOR

Patients who are in early labor frequently make the mistake of eating a hearty meal before entering the hospital. They believe erroneously that large amounts of food are required to give strength for parturition.

It has been demonstrated that during labor the stomach does not readily empty itself. It is not uncommon for patients at delivery to vomit food which was ingested 24 to 48 hours previously.

The pregnant patient should be warned against ingestion of solid foods or liquids once labor has commenced. Food particles may remain in the stomach and later on be vomited and aspirated during general anesthesia, thereby causing serious obstructive reactions of the respiratory tract. Suffocation and massive atelectasis may result.

Unfortunately, it is common hospital practice to urge water, tea and fruit juice throughout the first stage of labor. Mendelson[34, 35] has reported that such practice is fraught with danger because during labor the gastric emptying time of liquids is also prolonged. He has described a syndrome due to the aspiration of liquid gastric contents during anesthesia. Gastric hydrochloric acid is responsible for the changes described. Mendelson advocates omitting all oral feedings during labor. If the patient has ingested solid or liquid food recently, he suggests the alkalinization and emptying of the stomach contents prior to the administration of a general anesthesia for delivery. Should fluid and calorie balance be disturbed in the event of prolonged labor, parenteral feedings may be given.

[34] Mendelson, C. L.: The aspiration of stomach contents into the lung during obstetric anesthesia. Am. J. Obstet. Gynec., 52:191, 1946.

[35] Haussman, W., and Lunt, R. L.: The problems of the treatment of peptic aspiration pneumonia following obstetric anesthesia. "Mendelson's Syndrome." J. Obstet. Gynaec. Brit. Emp., 62:509, 1955.

DIET DURING LACTATION

The preparation for assuring an adequate supply of good quality breast milk must begin with the onset of pregnancy. Most of the dietary essentials are increased over and above the requirements during pregnancy to meet the demands of milk production for an infant who doubles the birth weight in five months. These increased requirements are expressed by the allowances recommended by the Food and Nutrition Board of the National Research Council in Table 15–3.

CALORIES The actual mechanism involved in the production of milk by the maternal organism does not demand a great expenditure of energy. The additional food necessary for the maternal organism to produce and secrete milk is not appreciable when an adequate diet has been consumed during pregnancy. The chief concern during lactation is the loss of the food material in the milk and the storage of a certain amount of food which cannot be accounted for entirely by the chemical composition of the milk. It is known that the conversion is not complete. Also, extra calories may be needed for additional activity necessitated by the care of the infant.

The extra calories required for lactation depend on the amount of milk produced. The food requirements are not uniform during the entire period of lactation but depend on the demands of the infant. It is generally suggested that the extra food calories should be approximately 120 kcalories for each 100 ml. of milk produced. The National Research Council recommends an increase of 1000 kcalories of protective foods a day during the lactation period above the normal requirement of a healthy nonpregnant woman, for an average production of 850 ml. (30 ounces) of milk. Approximately 400 kcalories are required for the synthesis and secretion of milk and 600 kcalories for the energy content of milk. (One ounce of human milk contains 20 kcalories and 30 ounces contain 600 kcalories.) (See Table 15–3.)

PROTEIN An adequate intake of protein of high biologic value during pregnancy is essential in the preparation for lactation. Lactation makes large demands on the human nitrogen stores. The food intake of a nursing mother must contain sufficient protein to supply both the maternal needs and the essential amino acids to be transferred through her breast milk to the growth of the baby. Human milk contains 1.2 gm. of protein per ml. The amount of protein in 850 ml. is 10 gm. If the amount of protein in the mother's diet is inadequate to meet the body maintenance needs and the protein of the milk secreted, a loss of maternal body tissue will result. An increase of 20 gm. of protein daily in addition to the usual 0.9 gm. per kg. body weight requirement of the nonlactating woman is the amount recommended by the Food and Nutrition Board of the National Research Council (Table 15–3). The diet properly provides this only if it is otherwise well balanced in mineral and vitamin content and adequate in calories.

FAT The kind of fat in breast milk is reflected in the composition of fat in the maternal diet. Medium chain fatty acids predominate in human milk. The polyunsaturated fatty acids in the mother's diet contribute about 6 to 9 per cent of the calories in human milk as linoleic acids.

CALCIUM AND VITAMIN D In order to prevent depletion of calcium, the mother needs approximately 500 mg. above the normal amount of 800 mg. during lactation. (Approximately 5 cups of milk.) The intake of 400 I.U. of vitamin D for the utilization of calcium and phosphorus in bone formation is recommended.

IRON Some lactating women tend to become anemic unless the iron allowance in the diet is maintained at the same level as during pregnancy. During lactation there is loss of iron which, if considered on an annual basis, is probably similar in quantity to that lost in the menstrual flow.

VITAMINS There is an increased demand for vitamin A, riboflavin, thiamin, niacin and ascorbic acid during lactation above the requirements of pregnancy. The additional amount of vitamin A (3000 I.U.) is readily supplied by the dark green and deep yellow vegetables and fruit. The B-complex vitamins are increased as caloric intake increases. Ascorbic acid need is easily obtained from a serving of citrus fruit or fruits and vegetables of comparable value. The increases are expressed in the table established by the Food and Nutrition Board of the National Research Council (Table 15–3).

FOOD ALLOWANCES FOR THE NORMAL LACTATING WOMAN

The selection of foods to provide the increased calories over and above the requirements of a normal diet includes all the nutrients, especially protein, calcium, vitamin A, thiamin, riboflavin, niacin and ascorbic acid. These are supplied by an additional serving of meat, dark green and deep yellow vegetables or fruit, whole-grain breads or cereal, a citrus fruit and 2 cups of fortified milk or equivalent. Five or six small meals daily is recommended. See pattern suggested in Table 15–6. The volume of milk produced is reduced when the maternal diet is inadequate in quantity. However, the milk remains balanced because the underfed mother draws on her own tissues. Smoking may reduce the volume of milk. Nicotine, a highly toxic drug, is fat soluble and is transmitted through milk to the infant. The kinds and amounts of drugs, pesticides and toxicants a baby can be exposed to and their effect on the composition of maternal milk are not well known.[36]

FLUIDS   The total daily intake of fluids should be at least 2 quarts, because fluids tend to increase the volume of milk.

PROBLEMS AND SUGGESTED TOPICS FOR DISCUSSION

1. What are the special nutritional needs during pregnancy? What kinds and amounts of food supply these needs?
2. Why are diet and good nutrition important during the prenatal period? During lactation?
3. Visit a patient in the prenatal clinic and obtain an average dietary intake for a day. Check diet for nutritional adequacy. How does it need to be nutritionally improved?
4. Visit a patient in the postnatal clinic and obtain an average dietary intake for a day. Check diet for nutritional adequacy. Is her weight normal? Help her with the necessary corrections.
5. Visit a patient in your hospital who has toxemia complications along with her pregnancy. Obtain a typical dietary intake. Calculate it to determine adequacy of proteins. Plan a correct diet with mild sodium restriction for this patient which is adequate in all nutrients. Follow the progress of the patient.
6. Make a survey in your hospital noting if fluids and food are served to patients who are in labor.
7. Survey the complications of pregnancy in your hospital. What part does diet play in each?
8. How does the diet during lactation differ from that of a non-lactating woman? Take a diet history of a lactating woman and assist her with the changes she needs to make in her dietary pattern.

SUGGESTED ADDITIONAL READING REFERENCES

Allen, C. E., et al.: Vigorous weight reduction during pregnancy—Nitrogen balance before and during normal gestation. J.A.M.A., 188:392, 1964.
Arena, J. M.: Contamination of the ideal food. Nutrition Today, 5:2, 1970.
Benjamin, F., et al.: Serum levels of folic acid, B_{12} and iron in anemia of pregnancy. Am. J. Obstet. Gynec., 96:310, 1966.
Burke, B. S.: Nutrition during pregnancy: A review. J. Am. Dietet. A., 20:735, 1944.
Burke, B. S.: Diet and nutrition during pregnancy. Am. J. Nursing, 52:1378, 1952.
Burke, B. S.: Diet during pregnancy. Am. J. Clin. Nutr., 2:425, 1954.
Burke, B. S., et al.: Nutrition studies during pregnancy. Am. J. Obstet. Gynec., 46:38, 1943.
Cellier, K. M., and Hankin, M. E.: Studies of nutrition in pregnancy. I. Some considerations in collecting dietary information. Am. J. Clin. Nutr., 13:55, 1963.
Committee on Maternal Nutrition: Maternal Nutrition and the Course of Pregnancy. Food and Nutrition Board. National Academy of Sciences, Washington, D.C., 1970.
Everson, G. J.: Basis for concern about teenagers' diets. J. Am. Dietet. A., 36:1, 1960.

Gold, E. M.: Interconceptional nutrition. J. Am. Dietet. A., 55:27, 1969.
Gray, M. J., et al.: Regulation of sodium and total body water metabolism in pregnancy. Am. J. Obstet. Gynec., 89:761, 1964.
Holly, R. G.: Dynamics of iron metabolism in pregnancy. Amer. J. Obstet. Gynec., 93:370, 1965.
Hytten, F. E.: Is breast feeding best? Am. J. Clin. Nutr., 7:259, 1959.
Jacobson, H. N., Burke, B. S., Smith, C. A., and Reid, D. E.: Effect of weight reduction in obese pregnant women in pregnancy, labor and delivery, and on the condition of the infant at birth. Am. J. Obstet. Gynec., 83:1609, 1962.
Larson, R. H.: Effect of prenatal nutrition on oral structures. J. Am. Dietet. A., 44:368, 1964.
Luhby, A. L., et al.: Survey of folic acid deficiency in pregnancy. Am. J. Clin. Nutr., 12:332, 1963.
Macy, I. G.: Metabolic and biochemical changes in normal pregnancy. J.A.M.A., 168:2265, 1958.
Macy, I. G., and Hunscher, H. A.: Calories—A limiting factor in the growth of children. J. Nutr., 15:189, 1951.
Macy, I. G., et al.: The composition of milks. Washington, D.C., National Research Council, Pub. No. 254, 1953.
McGanity, W. J.: Obesity, and the obstetrician. J.A.M.A., 186:39, 1963.
McGanity, W. J., et al.: The Vanderbilt Cooperative Study of Maternal and Infant Nutrition. VIII. Some nutritional implications. J. Am. Dietet. A., 31:582, 1955.
McGanity, W. J., et al.: The Vanderbilt Cooperative Study of Maternal and Infant Nutrition. XII. Effect of reproductive cycle on nutritional status and requirements. J.A.M.A., 168:2138, 1958.
Mengert, W. F., and Tacchi, D. A.: Pregnancy, toxemia and sodium chloride. Am. J. Obstet. Gynec., 81:601, 1961.
Metz, J., et al.: Effect of folic acid and vitamin B_{12} supplementation on tests of folate and vitamin B_{12} nutrition in pregnancy. Am. J. Clin. Nutr., 16:472, 1965.
Mullick, S., et al.: Serum lipid studies in pregnancy. Am. J. Obstet. Gynec., 89:766, 1964.
Mullins, A.: Weight gain in pregnancy with special reference to diet. Nutrition, 16:150, 1962.
Nutrition in pregnancy and lactation. Report of the Joint FAO/NRC Expert Committee, Technical Report, Series 302, 1965.
Payton, E., et al.: Dietary habits of 571 pregnant Southern Negro women. J. Am. Dietet. A., 37:129, 1960.
Pike, R. L.: Sodium intake during pregnancy. J. Am. Dietet. A., 144:176, 1964.
Pike, R. L., and Gursky, D. S.: Further evidence of deleterious effects produced by sodium restriction during pregnancy. Am. J. Clin. Nutr., 23:883, 1970.
Prenatal Care. Washington, D.C., U.S. Department of Health, Education, and Welfare, Children's Bureau Publication No. 4, 1962.
Report: Sodium intake in pregnancy: two views. J.A.M.A., 200:42, 1967.
Semmens, J. P.: Implications of teen-age pregnancy. Obstet. Gynec., 26:77, 1965.
Seifrit, E.: Changes in belief and food practice in pregnancy. J. Am. Dietet. A., 39:455, 1961.
Shank, R. E.: A chink in our armor. Nutrition Today, 5:2, 1970.
Spies, T. D.: Observations on the macrocytic anemia associated with pregnancy. Surg. Gynec. Obstet., 89:76, 1949.
Stearns, G.: Nutritional state of the mother prior to conception. J.A.M.A., 168:1655, 1958.
Thomson, A. M., et al.: The energy cost of human lactation. Brit. J. Nutr., 24:565, 1970.
Warkany, J.: Production of congenital malformations by dietary measures (experiments in mammals). J.A.M.A., 168:2020, 1958.
White, H. S.: Iron deficiency in young women. Am. J. Pub. Health, 60:659, 1970.
Wohl, M. G., and Goodhart, R. S. (ed.): Modern Nutrition in Health and Disease. 4th ed. Philadelphia, Lea & Febiger, 1968. Chapter 36, Nutrition in pregnancy.

[36]Arena, J. M.: Contamination of the ideal food. Nutrition Today, 5:2, 1970.

Chapter 16
NUTRITION
IN
INFANCY

The infant continues to grow and develop rapidly after birth. Postnatal life is a continuum in human development. Normal growth and development depend largely upon the nutritional status of the infant. Nutritional status is related directly to the nutrition of the mother, to the inherited characteristics and to a dietary intake of the essential nutrients. The infant born with a poor nutritional rating is handicapped from the beginning of life. Stunted growth and depressed brain and neurological development may result from dietary inadequacies or restrictions at the early stage of physical development. In many underdeveloped countries where infant mortality is high the nutritional status is poor largely because of an inadequate intake of dietary essentials at the appropriate stage of development. Infant mortality in the United States has declined but ranks thirteenth among the nations of the world.

NUTRITIONAL ALLOWANCES FOR THE INFANT

The nutritional requirements of the normal full-term infant at birth are considered fulfilled. During the first few days of life, the infant usually loses a few ounces, which is of no serious consequence. A daily intake of the dietary essentials, without feeding problems, will result in a gain in weight within a week or 10 days.

CALORIES During infancy the body grows faster than at any other time of life, and the caloric requirements per unit of body weight are high. While the calorie allowance *per kg.* decreases progressively from birth, the needs of the infant increase from month to month. At birth a baby requires about 350 to 500 kcalories, and at one year from 800 to 1200 kcalories. Milk provides all the calories at birth. At six months, it supplies about 70 per cent of the calories. Cereal, vegetables, fruit, meat and egg introduced provide the remaining energy needs. The variation in the caloric requirements is due chiefly to differences in activity of individual infants. A placid infant requires fewer calories than one who cries frequently. The Food and Nutrition Board of the National Academy of Sciences – National Research Council recommends that during the first year of life calorie allowances be reduced in suitable steps from a level of 120 kcalories per kg. (2.2 pounds) of body weight at birth and for the first two months to 100 kcalories per kg. by the end of one year. (See Table 16–1.) There are wide individual variations in physical activity and individual adjustments, of course, must be made.

WEIGHT AS A DIETARY INDICATOR The infant requires approximately 2½ to 3 ounces of breast milk per day per pound of body weight. To determine whether the infant is getting an adequate amount of milk, it is advisable to weigh the baby before and after each feeding during a 24-hour period about once a week. The differences in weight at each feeding are totaled, which gives an accurate, quantitative figure for the amount of breast milk consumed within the 24-hour period. Insufficient intake is also indicated by the infant's reactions after completion of the feeding. If he is restless, cries, and fails to fall asleep after nursing, the feeding may be inadequate and may require supplementary bottle feedings or food. Between the fourth and fifth month the weight of the baby should double, and at the end of the year the birth weight of the baby is usually trebled. Because the poundage is dependent upon the baby's weight at birth, no definite standards or guides

TABLE 16–1   DAILY DIETARY ALLOWANCES FOR INFANTS* AND NUTRIENT CONTENT OF HUMAN AND COW'S MILK†

| NUTRIENT | AGE (MONTHS) | | | HUMAN MILK | COW'S MILK |
	0–2	2–6	6–12	(per 100 ml. of milk)	
kilocalories	kg. × 120	kg. × 110	kg. × 100	77.0	65.0
Protein (gm.)	kg. × 2.2	kg. × 2.0	kg. × 1.8	1.1	3.5
Vitamin A (I.U.)	1500	1500	1500	240.0 (45)[a]	140.0 (63)[a]
Vitamin D (I.U.)	400	400	400	42.0	41.0
Vitamin E (I.U.)	5.0	5.0	5.0	0.56	0.13
Ascorbic acid (mg.)	35.0	35.0	35.0	5.0	1.0
Folacin (mg.)	0.05	0.05	0.1	0.018	0.006
Niacin (mg. equiv.)[b]	5.0	7.0	8.0	0.2 (mg.)[b]	0.92
Riboflavin (mg.)	0.4	0.5	0.6	0.04	0.17
Thiamin (mg.)	0.2	0.4	0.5	0.01	0.03
Vitamin B_6 (mg.)	0.2	0.3	0.4	0.011	0.04
Vitamin B_{12} (µg.)	1.0	1.5	2.0	–	0.4
Calcium (gm.)	0.4	0.5	0.6	0.033	0.118
Phosphorus (gm.)	0.2	0.4	0.5	0.014	0.093
Iodine (µg.)	25.0	40.0	45.0	–	35.0
Iron (mg.)	6.0	10.0	15.0	0.1	0.057
Potassium (mg.)				51.0	144.0
Magnesium (mg.)	40.0	60.0	70.0	4.0	13.0
Sodium (mg.)				16.0	50.0
Fat (gm.)				4.0	3.5
Lactose (gm.)				7.0	4.9
Casein (gm.)				0.4	2.8
Lactalbumin (gm.)				0.8[b]–0.3	0.4

*From the Food and Nutrition Board, National Research Council, National Academy of Sciences. Revised, 1968. (See Table 11–1, Chapter 11).
†Composition of Foods, Agriculture Handbook No. 8, United States Department of Agriculture, Revised, 1963, and Dairy Council Digest, National Dairy Council, 42:January–February, 1971.
[a]Carotene I.U.
[b]Niacin equivalent is the composite of the niacin already in food and that which may be formed from tryptophan (1 mg. equivalent for each 60 mg. of dietary tryptophan). Milk is a good source of tryptophan.

are provided stating that all babies must weigh a specific number of pounds at one year.

Since a newborn baby's stomach holds about two tablespoons of food, the feedings must be small and frequent. The number of feedings given within a period of 24 hours depends on the size and age of the infant. The average number of feedings ranges between five and eight. (See feeding schedule, p. 263.)

An excessive weight gain is undesirable and a large overweight baby is not considered in the best state of health. An overweight baby during the first year of life is more likely to grow up to be an obese adolescent or adult than is one weighing within the normal range.[1] Early feeding of solids may lead to ingestion of excessive calories.[2] Hirsch and Kittle in their work with rats and young children have found that overfeeding in early life produces excess and large fat cells which are needed for the storage of fat. These cells are permanent. The regulation of weight is made more difficult because these cells remain filled with fat.[3]

PROTEIN Protein requirements during infancy, when there is rapid growth, are relatively higher than those of the adult or older child; nitrogen must be provided for the formation of new tissue, the maturation of tissue, and the maintenance of tissues. In

[1]Mac Keith, R. C.: Is a big baby healthy? Proc. Sci., 22:128, 1963.

[2]Bakwin, H.: Feeding programs for infants. Fed. Proc., 23:66, 1964.
[3]Hirsch, J., and Kittle, J. L.: The cellularity of obese and non-obese human adipose tissue. Fed. Proc., 29:1516, 1970.

early infancy, some form of milk comprises the only protein food. Since the protein of milk contains all the amino acids essential for growth, the protein needs of the infant are believed to be met automatically through human milk or formulas designed to simulate human milk. The utilization efficiency of mother's milk by the infant is assumed to be 100 per cent. Based on the composition of human milk (see Table 16–1), the recommended daily allowance for infants during the first year of life is 1.8 gm. per 100 kcal. The allowance on the basis of body weight (kg.) for the first two months is 2.2 gm., from two to six months 2.0 gm. and from six months to one year 1.8 gm. When proteins of lower biological value than those of human milk are fed, the intake of protein should be higher. If the dietary protein is more than 8 per cent of calories as provided by human milk, the protein requirement is usually met. Below 8 per cent it is impossible to feed the infant enough food to meet protein requirements. Higher than 10 per cent of the calories from protein of high biological value makes no difference in nitrogen retention. Any protein not needed for growth and maintenance undergoes deamination in the liver and the non-nitrogenous residue can be oxidized to provide energy or converted to fat and stored as energy reserve. The nitrogenous end-products must be excreted. This requires a sufficient quantity of water. Sensitivity to the high protein content of cow's milk has been reported. Human milk is reported to have antibodies desirable for the prevention of children's diseases. Infants fed cow's milk have a higher rate of infection than infants on human milk. The mechanisms concerned with formation of antibodies are believed to be used to combat foreign milk protein. Histidine, an essential amino acid for the infant, is needed in addition to the eight required by the adult. The minimum requirement is 34 mg. per kg. per day[4] and is amply supplied by human and cow's milk as well as the standard formulas.

FAT   A small amount of essential fatty acid, linoleic, has been found to be necessary for growth and dermal integrity in human infants. Both human milk and cow's milk contain it but human milk normally contains about three times as much linoleate as cow's milk. Human milk contains 6 to 9 per cent of calories as linoleate. Linoleic acid in the range of 3 per cent of total calories is reported to meet the infant requirement. For most full-term babies, milk containing not

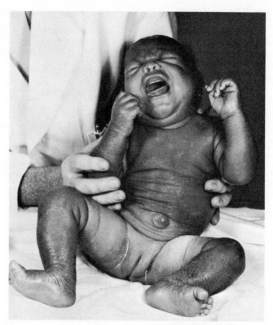

Figure 16–1   Thickening and dryness of the skin, oozing in the body folds and eruption in the diaper region in infant on low fat intake due to linoleic acid deficiency. (Courtesy Dr. Arild E. Hansen, and The National Live Stock and Meat Board Food and Nutrition News, 29, No. 5, 1958.)

more than 3.5 to 4 per cent fat causes no difficulty. Infants and children probably have a greater need for fats than do adults. During the first 3 months of life, infants store large amounts in the skin and internal organs. Tests show that fat is added until age 1, when the situation changes; during the next 4 years, there is a steady loss of this tissue. From the fifth to the eighth year, there is neither loss nor gain. Thereafter, fat is added gradually until adult life. The only exception is the year or two before the adolescent growth spurt. Young infants lacking fat in their diet have been reported to develop certain types of eczema (p. 57, Fig. 5–1). Hansen[5] reported thickening and dryness of the skin, oozing in the body folds and eruption in the diaper region (Fig. 16–1) in infants on low fat intake and has established[6] the abnormalities as a manifestation of linoleic acid deficiency, and not the total fat content. The percentage of linoleic acid and the principal sources of fat in human milk and the standard formulas are shown in Table 16–2.

CARBOHYDRATE   As a rule, approximately half of an infant's calorie allowance is supplied as carbohydrate. The disaccharide lactose, which is found only in milk, appears

[4]Holt, L. E., and Snyderman, S. E.: Report to the Council: The amino acid requirements of infants. J.A.M.A., *175*:100, 1961.

[5]Hansen, A. E.: National Live Stock and Meat Board Food and Nutrition News, 29:No. 5, 1958.
[6]Hansen, A. E., et al.: Role of linoleic acid in infant nutrition. Pediatrics, *31*:171, 1963.

TABLE 16-2   APPROXIMATE ANALYSES OF COMMONLY USED INFANT FORMULAS AND HUMAN MILK

STANDARD FORMULA	NORMAL DILUTION	Kcal/(oz.)	PERCENTAGES				APPROXIMATE VITAMIN AND MINERAL CONTENT PER QUART												
			FAT	LINOLEIC ACID	PROTEIN	CHO*	A UNITS	D UNITS	E UNITS	ASCORBIC ACID (mg.)	NIACIN (mg. equiv.)	THIAMIN (mg.)	RIBOFLAVIN (mg.)	B₆ (mg.)	Na (mEq.)	K (mEq.)	Ca (mEq.)	P (mEq.)	Fe (mg.)
Standard Formulas																			
Baker's Infant	1:1	20	3.3	16[i]	2.2	7.0	2500	400	5.0	50	5.0	0.6	1.0	0.4	16	22	40	35	7.5
Bremil	1:1	20	3.5	27[h]	1.5	7.0	2500	400	5.0	50	6.0	0.4	1.0	0.4	12	21	33	17	trace(8)
Carnalac	1:1	20	2.7	2[a]	2.4	8.2	1035	400	1.0	80	6.4	0.4	1.1	0.2	17	24	40	35	trace
Cow's milk (undiluted)	–	20	4.1	2[a]	3.5	5.0	946	38	0.5	17	8.0	0.4	1.6	0.5	24	34	58	50	1.4(8)
Enfamil	1:1	20	3.7	24[d]	1.5	7.0	1500	400	5.0	50	6.6	0.4	1.0	0.3	10	17	30	30	trace
Evaporated 1:2	1:2	15	2.7	2[a]	2.4	3.4	800	265	–	–	5.0	0.3	1.1	–	17	24	40	35	trace(8)
Formil	1:1	20	3.5	15[g]	1.65	7.0	2500	400	–	50	7.0	0.5	0.9	0.3	12	17	29	26	trace
Lactum	1:1	20	2.8	3[a]	2.7	7.8	400	400	–	2	–	0.3	–	–	16	26	47	45	trace
Modilac	1:1	20	2.7	53[b]	2.15	7.7	1500	400	5.0	45	6.0	0.7	1.0	0.7	15	25	39	33	10
Optimil	1:1	20	3.8	18[f]	1.47	7.2	2500	400	8.5	80	8.7	0.7	1.0	0.4	8	14	18	15	8
Purevap	1:2	20	2.6	3[a]	2.3	8.0	800	400	–	–	5.0	0.3	1.1	–	17	24	42	38	trace
Similac	1:1	20	3.4	30[c]	1.7	6.6	2500	400	5.0	50	5.7	0.7	1.0	0.4	10	22	32	28	trace(12)
SMA S-26	1:1	20	3.6	22[e]	1.5	7.2	2500	400	7.0	50	9.5	0.7	1.0	0.4	7	13	20	20	7.5
Soy Formulas																			
Isomil	1:1	20	3.6	30[c]	2.0	6.8	1419	378	4.7	47	5.7	0.4	0.6	0.4	12	17	33	26	11.4
Mull-Soy	1:1	20	3.6	53[k]	3.1	5.2	2000	400	10.0	40	9.0	0.5	0.8	0.4	15	39	57	44	5
Neo-Mull-Soy	1:1	20	3.5	53[k]	1.8	6.4	2000	400	10.0	50	7.0	0.5	1.0	0.4	16	24	40	23	8
Pro Sobee	1:1	20	3.4	37[k]	2.5	6.8	1500	400	5.0	50	11.3	0.5	1.0	0.4	23	26	44	40	8
Sobee	1:1	20	2.6	45[l]	3.2	7.7	1500	400	5.0	50	12.1	0.5	1.0	0.4	21	31	47	30	8
Soyalac	1:1	20	4.0	53[k]	2.1	5.9	1500	400	5.0	50	6.0	0.4	0.6	0.4	13	22	20	20	10
Human Milk	1:1	20	3.8	8[j]	1.25	7.0	1419	95	5.3	41	5.0	0.2	0.4	0.1	7	13	16	9	trace

[a] Butterfat
[b] Corn oil
[c] Corn, coconut oil
[d] Coconut, corn, oleo
[e] Corn, coconut, soy, oleo
[f] Corn, coconut, olive oil
[g] Coconut, corn, butterfat
[h] Coconut, corn, peanut oil
[i] Coconut, corn, soy oil
[j] Human milk fat
[k] Soy oil
[l] Coconut, soy oil

Adapted from Handbook of Infant Formulas, J. B. Roerig, Division Chas. Pfizer & Co., Inc., New York, 1967.

*Lactose in standard formulas and sucrose in soy formulas predominately.

( )Indicates formula with iron added.

TABLE 16–3   COMPOSITION OF COMMON CARBOHYDRATES USED IN INFANT FORMULAS

CARBOHYDRATE USED	KARO	DEXTRI-MALTOSE	DEXIN	BETA LACTOSE	SUGAR CANE
Dextrose (%)	8	—	—	—	—
Maltose (%)	22	56	25	—	—
Dextrins (%)	37	44	75	—	—
Lactose (%)	—	—	—	100	—
Sucrose (%)	7	—	—	—	100
Kcal./tablespoon	60	30	20	40	60

to be the carbohydrate of choice in infant feeding. A mixture of carbohydrates has been found to provide a slower rate of digestion and absorption and a lower incidence of excessive fermentation. Dextrose, maltose, dextrins, sucrose and lactose are used in formulas. In Table 16–3 lactose is the dominant carbohydrate in the standard formulas and sucrose in the soy formulas. Maltose, dextrose and dextrins are also used in some formulas. Table 16–3 shows the composition of the commonly used carbohydrates in infant formulas. Maltose is usually used with dextrose and dextrins.

MINERALS   Breast milk supplies about 60 mg. of calcium per kilogram. The infant retains about two thirds of this amount. An infant fed a standard type of formula receives about 170 mg. of calcium per kilogram but retains only 35 to 50 per cent of it. Although the calcium available to the breast-fed infant is less, it is assumed that the calcium needs are met fully. The recommended daily allowances of 400 to 600 mg. per day for the first year of life apply only to the bottle-fed infant (Table 16–1). A ratio of approximately 1.2:1.0 calcium to phosphorus occurs in cow's milk compared to the ratio of 2:1 in human milk. It is recommended that the calcium to phosphorus ratio in an infant's diet be maintained at a 1.5:1.0 ratio. Later the amount of phosphorus can be raised to a ratio similar to cow's milk. If the mother's diet is adequate during pregnancy, the baby has adequate stores of iron at birth to permit maintenance of a normal hemoglobin level for about 3 months. At about 3 months when iron reserves are depleted as manifested by a drop in the hemoglobin level, approximately 10 mg. of iron per day is recommended. Enriched cereals, meat and egg yolk provide the iron needed. The low birth weight infant (under 2500 gm.), the premature and the infant of a multiple birth with significant reduction in total hemoglobin levels require 2 mg. per day beginning soon after birth.

Fluoride is considered to be an essential nutrient in the structure of teeth and is necessary for resistance to tooth decay. It has a protective role during the period of calcification of dental tissues. A lactating mother drinking fluoridated water or formulas using fluoridated water will protect the infant. See Table 16–1 for mineral allowances recommended.

WATER   Special attention to water needs of bottle-fed infants must be given. The recommendation for infants is 1.5 ml./kcal. The infant's surface area per unit of body weight and the basal metabolic rate are each twice that of an adult. Therefore there are greater heat and water losses and more metabolic wastes with the infant than the adult. A high protein formula, excess sodium and potassium intake and high environmental temperature require more water to eliminate body metabolic wastes and replace water loss.

VITAMINS   If the diet of a nursing mother is nutritionally adequate, the vitamins necessary for the infant will be contained in the milk with the exception of vitamin D and possibly vitamin C. The same is true for cow's milk except that vitamin C is rarely adequate. Therefore, it seems desirable to administer tomato or orange juice very early in life regardless of whether the baby is breast-fed or formula-fed. Vitamin D should be given to all infants either as a supplement or in the formula or fortified milk.

The vitamin A requirement of human infants has not been determined. The amount stored in the infant's liver at birth depends largely on the vitamin A intake of the mother. The infant consuming 850 ml. of human milk receives about 1500 I.U. of vitamin A and this is taken as the recommended daily allowance for the first year of life.

The recommended allowances (RDA) for vitamin D in infancy are well established. An intake of 100 I.U. per day will prevent rickets and 300 I.U. per day will cure rickets. With a sufficient calcium intake, the ingestion of 400 I.U. per day promotes calcium absorption and metabolism, provides for skeletal growth and prevents rickets in normal full-term and premature infants. Excessive intake of vitamin D (1000 to 3000 I.U. per kg. per day) may be toxic and may lead to hypercalcemia.

Very little placental transfer of vitamin E occurs and infants have low tissue concentration of the vitamin. The content in human milk ranges from 2 to 5 I.U. per liter. This amount meets the infant's requirement (RDA). Cow's milk contains about one tenth to one half the amount in human milk. A supplement to cow's milk formula of 5 I.U. is needed during the first year of life. The requirement increases for infants receiving formulas high in polyunsaturated fatty acid content.[7]

The recommended allowance (RDA) of 35 mg. of ascorbic acid is supplied daily in 850 ml. of human milk. Infants fed formulas with two or three times the protein in human milk may need 50 mg. of ascorbic acid daily. Infants fed cow's milk need a daily dietary supplement.

Thiamin content of human milk is usually adequate if the dietary intake is adequate. Human milk contains an average of 0.015 mg. of thiamin per 100 ml. as compared with 0.04 mg. per ml. in cow's milk. The minimum thiamin requirement for the human infant based on intake from mother's milk or formula and urinary excretion studies seems to be approximately 0.2 mg. per 1000 kcal. and the recommended daily allowance (RDA) is 0.5 mg. per 1000 kcal. Enriched cereals are good sources of thiamin in the infant's diet.

The riboflavin requirement for tissue saturation has not been determined. The recommended allowance (RDA) for infants to 2 months of age is 0.4 mg.; for 2 to 6 months, 0.5 mg.; and for 6 to 12 months, 0.6 mg. Human milk contains 0.042 mg. per 100 ml. and cow's milk 0.157 mg. per 100 ml. An average of 0.17 mg. of niacin and 22 mg. of tryptophan or a niacin equivalent of 0.50 per 100 ml. is contained in human milk. The recommended daily allowance (RDA) for infants is 5 to 8 niacin equivalents.

The infant's storage of pyridoxine (B_6) at birth protects him against a diet containing very little of the vitamin. The recommended allowances (RDA) are 0.2 mg. to 2 months of age, 0.3 mg. from 2 to 6 months and 0.4 mg. from 6 months to one year. The amount of B_6 in human milk gradually increases from 0.01 to 0.02 mg. per liter during the first month of lactation to 0.10 mg. per liter from then on. If the mother is undernourished and the B_6 content of breast milk falls below 0.06 to 0.08 mg. per liter, chemical and biochemical abnormalities may occur. Cow's milk contains 0.35 to 0.60 mg. of vitamin B_6 per liter. The higher content of vitamin B_6 correlates with the higher protein found in cow's milk as compared to human milk. Though there is considerable variation in the amount of B_6 present in the commercially prepared formulas,[8] they contain more than adequate amounts of pyridoxine in relation to protein provided by them. Meats in general are a good source of B_6, fish is a fair to good source and dairy products are a poor to good source. Pyridoxine is destroyed during sterilization of formulas in ratio to the degree of temperature and the length of time of the heat. The infant develops a vitamin deficiency which is manifested by convulsive seizures.

Folacin requirement for infants according to the Food and Nutrition Board is approximately 0.005 to 0.020 mg. per day. The recommended daily allowance (RDA) is 0.05 mg. for the infant 2 months to 6 months and 0.10 mg. for 6 to 12 months.

The infant serum levels of cobalamin (vitamin B_{12}) are approximately twice that of the mother. Human milk supplies the infant between 0.15 and 0.25 μg. of vitamin B_{12} daily. The recommended daily allowance (RDA) for infants during the first year of life ranges from 1.0 to 2.0 μg. (See Table 16–1 for Daily Dietary Allowances for Infants and Nutrient Content of Human and Cow's Milk.)

BREAST FEEDING VERSUS FORMULA FEEDING

Although advancement in the planned formula nutrition of newborn infants has been made in recent years, many pediatricians still hold a preference for breast feeding. Holt and Snyderman[9] report the results of ideal artificial feeding as comparable to breast feeding; there is no longer any important nutritional advantage to human milk, but advantages to breast feeding may remain. The chief advantages are freedom from bacterial contamination; it is economical, requires no elaborate preparation, improves the parent-child relationship and is less likely to be associated with infant allergic manifestations. Breast feeding also has the advantage of immunizing the baby against certain infectious diseases through the action of the antibodies received in his mother's milk. The healthy woman with firm, healthy nipples who prefers to nurse her baby should be encouraged to do so. On the other hand, the mother with small

---

[7]Hassan, H., et al.: Syndrome in premature infants associated with low plasma vitamin C levels and high polyunsaturated fatty acid diets. Am. J. Clin. Nutr., 19:147, 1966.

[8]Polansky, M. M., and Toepfer, E. W.: Vitamin B_6 components in some meats, fish, dairy products and commercial infant formulas. Agricultural and Food Chemistry, 17:1394, 1969.

[9]Holt, L. E., Jr., and Snyderman, S. E.: In Wohl, M. G., and Goodhart, R. S. (ed.): Modern Nutrition in Health and Disease. 3rd ed. Philadelphia, Lea & Febiger. 1964, Chapter 37.

delicate or inverted nipples should be discouraged from nursing. Regardless of the mother's physical condition, a patient who harbors psychological reasons for an aversion to nursing should not be threatened about the future welfare of her baby if she does not breast feed. If the mother has a chronic illness or wishes to use contraceptives, it is not wise for her to breast feed the baby. Contraceptives may produce estrogenic effects in the infant. All drugs ingested by the lactating mother are found in breast milk to some degree. Little is known about the kind and amount of drugs and toxicants an infant can safely tolerate. Heavy cigarette smoking may reduce the volume of milk excreted. Nicotine is highly toxic, is fat soluble and is transmitted through breast milk to the infant.[10] In other cases, nursing may interfere with the mother's well-being, especially if labor has been complicated by severe hemorrhages or a blood stream infection.

In a study[11] to determine whether behavior problems of children were related to breast feeding, the length of the nursing period (breast or bottle, or both), and the family attitude during the nursing period, none of the variables was found to be significantly related to breast feeding. Also, the study gave no evidence that breast feeding is more positively related to favorable growth or general health of the child than bottle feeding.

TECHNIQUE OF BREAST FEEDING AND BOTTLE FEEDING   Details on the techniques of breast and bottle feeding will be acquired in the pediatric lectures and experience and therefore will not be duplicated in this text. Babies instinctively know how to suck but may need some help in getting started. The infant is laid close to the mother with his cheek against her breast. The mother can help by holding the breast so that the baby can easily get the nipple into his mouth. The bottle baby should be held as though he is being breast fed in order to establish security and companionship. It is not safe to reheat any formula that is not taken.

Should the reader be interested in further information on the subject, the following booklet is recommended: Infant Care. U.S. Department of Health, Education, and Welfare, Children's Bureau Publication No. 8, 1963.

Complemental Feeding   When the mother's milk supply is inadequate to meet the entire nutritional needs of the infant, the baby is given one or more supplementary bottle feedings. This is known as complemental or mixed feeding.

A comparison between cow's milk and human milk is shown in Table 16–1.

Cow's milk is higher in proteins and calcium (the calf matures within a few months while a human needs years to reach maturity). Human milk is higher in carbohydrates (lactose) and iron. Williams[12] reports striking differences in the pattern of minerals, fatty acids, vitamins, and several amino acids in the two milks. It is suggested that some of these differences may be significant in the utilization of milk by the human infant. For example, there is reported to be an association between a high intake of phosphorus, such as that provided by cow's milk, and the occurrence of hypocalcemic tetany of the newborn.[13] Because of the distinctive curd formed in the stomach, cow's milk is more difficult to digest than human milk unless treated with heat (such as takes place during terminal sterilization of formulas), which coagulates the lactalbumin into fine particles. The heat treatment (depending on how high and how long) may, however, destroy or render unutilizable certain nutritive properties of milk — ascorbic acid (especially), vitamin B_6, thiamin, certain amino acids (notably lysine) — which may need to be replaced. As previously noted, ascorbic acid in some form should always be given to artificially fed infants as a supplement.

PROPRIETARY MILKS   Usually either whole cow's milk, canned evaporated milk or dried milk is used as the basis for the infant's formula feeding. The infant may tolerate evaporated milk or dried milk more easily than whole cow's milk because the curd formed in digestion is very fine. Additional advantages of canned evaporated milk and dried milk are economy, consistency of the product, convenience and availability. Canned evaporated milk, which has no additional sugar, should not be confused with sweetened condensed milk!

There are also available specially prepared formulas designed to meet the needs of the infant. Some are fortified with ascorbic acid and/or iron. These prepared formulas save time and labor but are more expensive.

SPECIAL MILK PREPARATIONS   In cases of digestive disturbances, diarrhea or an allergy, special milk preparations are

[10] Arena, J. M.: Contamination of the ideal food. Nutrition Today, 5:7, 1970.

[11] Heinstein, M. I.: Influence of breast feeding on children's behavior. Children, 10:93, 1963.

[12] Williams, H. H.: Differences between cow's and human milk. J.A.M.A., 175:104, 1961.

[13] Gardner, L. I., et al.: Etiologic factors in tetany of newly born infants. Pediatrics, 5:228, 1950; Tetany and parathyroid hyperplasia in the newborn infant: influence of dietary phosphate load. 9:534, 1952.

prescribed. Since babies with diarrhea experience more difficulty digesting fats than proteins, boiled skim milk is often used in the basic formula. Many commercially prepared formulas derive better tolerance by replacing cow's milk fat with vegetable oils. (See Table 16-2.) Acid milk is sometimes used in cases of digestive disturbances, particularly if the intestinal tract is involved. The acid milk produces a very fine curd which is readily digested in the stomach. Scraped raw apple or its equivalent in canned apple powder is sometimes prescribed for diarrhea.

Protein milk formulas are often prescribed in cases of severe diarrhea. This kind of milk can be prepared in the laboratory or at home, or in a preparation purchased in a dried or liquid form.

In cases of allergy in infants, the protein of milk is usually the offending ingredient. Goat's milk is sometimes tolerated by infants who have an allergy to cow's milk. Goat's milk has a fine curd, and the fat particles are so small they will not separate. There are several commercial preparations especially formulated for this condition, such as the meat base formula which consists of strained meat with suitable additives. It approximates cow's milk (in content of complete proteins, fats, carbohydrates and minerals), or predigested casein with certain additives. In some cases, it may be necessary to exclude all animal protein, and use vegetable base milk.[14] This contains no milk, and the chief protein ingredient is soy bean or other suitable plant protein. See Table 16-2, Approximate Analyses of Commonly Used Infant Formulas and Human Milk.

VEGETABLE PROTEIN IN INFANT FEEDING Soy bean protein is unique among vegetable proteins by virtue of its high biologic value. While soy protein is biologically inferior to milk protein, growth rates and general development are satisfactory in the majority of cases. One hope for improved nutrition of innumerable children in the newly developed countries, and overpopulated countries such as Japan,[15] lies in the judicious use of *available* vegetable protein sources.[16] Incaparina (p. 71), named after the Institute of Nutrition of Central America and Panama, is a vegetable protein mixture on the market in a number of Central American countries, where it is saving countless lives of needy infants and children.

INFANT FORMULAS

A feeding formula is individualized for the baby and it is determined in specific amounts by considering the requirements for protein, vitamins, minerals and calories. Whole cow's milk, evaporated milk or dried milk is usually selected as the basis for the formula. The nutrient value of human and cow's milk is summarized in Table 16-1 to compare with the Recommended Dietary Allowances.

MILK AND FLUID ALLOWANCE The amount of milk should be sufficient to meet the infant's individual needs and satisfy his hunger. A 20 kcal. per fluid ounce formula consisting of $2\frac{1}{2}$ to 3 fluid ounces per pound of body weight will supply a caloric intake of 50 to 60 kcalories per pound (110 to 130 kcal. per kg.). The amount of milk allowed in the formula varies from 1.5 to 2 ounces per pound of body weight. Boiled water is added to meet a satisfactory volume intake for the day. The fluid requirement (water) in addition to milk is approximately 150 ml. (5 ounces) per kg. of body weight per 24-hour period, or 1.5 ml. per kcal. In tropical or subtropical climates the amount may have to be increased. This is included in the formula, or given (boiled) between feedings.

SUGAR ADDED TO FORMULA The carbohydrate content of cow's milk is increased to meet the energy requirements. Five to 6 per cent of the total formula volume is the quantity of sugar added. The forms of sugar used are white corn syrup, milk sugar, malt sugar (Dextri-Maltose), lactose, granulated sugar, brown sugar and thick cereal preparations.

Several commercially prepared formulations are available. Some consist of powder or concentrated liquid to which only water is added. Other preparations come ready-to-use. (Refer to Table 16-3 for the approximate composition of carbohydrates commonly used in infant formulas.) Ready-to-eat preparations may be purchased in 8-oz. and 32-oz. cans. Ready-to-use preparations in the bottle cost more than the completely home-mixed formulas. Economy in infant feeding is especially important to families on limited incomes. In low income groups, the lowest cost combination of foods and supplements consistent with safety and facilities for home preparation is desirable especially if other members in the family are deprived of adequate food.[17]

TECHNIQUE OF FORMULA PREPARATION

The amount of formula needed for a 24-hour period is prepared at one time and

[14]Vegetable protein in infant feeding. Nutr. Rev., 21:173, 1963.

[15]Muto, S., et al.: Soybean products as protein sources for weaning infants. J. Am. Dietet. A., 43:451, 1963.

[16]Nutritional value of leaf proteins—Human studies. Nutr. Rev., 21:231 and 232, 1963.

[17]Heseltine, M. M., and Pitts, J. L.: Economy in nutrition and feeding of infants. Am. J. Pub. Health, 56:1756, 1966.

divided into the number of bottles which will be used for feedings. The bottles are stoppered and kept in the refrigerator until feeding time. When needed, the nursing bottle containing its portion of formula is placed in warm water until body temperature is reached. The formula and bottles are sterilized, either during preparation of the formula or at some other time before the infant is fed.

FORMULA MAKING EQUIPMENT[18]

The nurse is frequently responsible for making the formula, and teaching the new mother how to do so before she leaves the hospital. Following is a standard set of utensils for use in the hospital or home. Keeping a set of equipment to use only for preparing the formula will make the sterilizing and formula preparation go more easily.

Kettle for sterilizing. Such a kettle has a tight-fitting cover and a rack inside to hold the bottles.

A wire rack, or a pie tin punched with holes (upside down) that fits the bottom of the kettle, for holding the bottles.

A bottle brush with a long handle and with stout bristles to scrub the inside of the bottles. It should be one that is bent at the tip, so that the bristles clean the bottom of the bottle and not just the sides.

A measuring tablespoon.

A measuring cup, marked in ounces, with a pouring lip.

A 2-quart saucepan or jar with a pouring lip to mix the formula in.

A small saucepan with a lid, in which to boil and keep the nipples (if you use the standard clean technique, p. 261).

A funnel makes it easier to pour the formula into the bottles. If you get a plastic funnel, make sure it is the kind that can be boiled.

A long-handled spoon.

A can opener that punches holes (if you use canned milk).

A small wide-mouthed jar with a cover, for used nipples.

Bottles to hold a 24-hour supply of formula.

Nipples and nipple caps.

A pair of tongs is convenient to handle hot bottles and other sterile equipment.

Nursing bottles. The standard-sized nursing bottle holds 8 ounces. Ounces are marked, so there need be no guesswork when you pour the formula. Wide-mouth bottles are easiest to clean.

Bottles of heat-resistant glass or of boil-able plastic cost more but will probably be cheaper in the long run.

Have as many bottles as are needed in a 24-hour period, plus extras for possible breakage. Two to three 4-ounce bottles will be needed for water and orange juice.

Bottles are easier to clean if rinsed after each feeding and filled with cold water.

Nipples. Have one nipple for each feeding, and one for each drink of water or orange juice.

The holes in the nipples may have to be made larger. Try out the nipple by putting it on a bottle with water in it, and turning it upside down. Watch to see if there is a steady drip. Remember that water will come through faster than milk because it is thinner. If the holes seem too small, heat the point of a fine needle in the flame of a match. While the point is red hot, poke it through one or more holes in the nipple.

After each feeding, wash the nipple and squeeze water through the holes. Dry it, and keep it in a covered jar until ready to sterilize the day's supply.

Nipple covers. Nipple caps or covers are made of glass, plastic, aluminum, or paper. Paper caps are inexpensive but can be used only once.

METHODS OF FORMULA PREPARATION

In general there are 2 methods of preparing the formula to make it safe, namely, terminal heating and standard clean technique. The first method is to mix the formula, pour it unboiled into bottles that have been washed but not sterilized, put on the nipple and, last, sterilize the filled bottles. This method eliminates possibility of contamination and is simple to carry out. It is suitable for all types of formulas except those that would be affected by the heat of sterilization, such as lactic acid milk.

The second or standard clean technique method is to sterilize the equipment, bottles, nipple collars, nipple covers or disc seals and measuring equipment and then pour the boiled or sterile formula into the sterilized bottles. Any water added must first be boiled. It is suitable for all types of formulas, including acid milk formulas. When acidified milk is used in the formula, the milk is boiled and then cooled. When the milk is cold, the acid is added slowly, drop by drop, and stirred continuously.

Following is a detailed description of the technique of each method.

TERMINAL HEATING METHOD (See Fig. 16-2, p. 262.)

1. Wash thoroughly with hot water and detergent all the articles to be used. Scrub the insides of the bottles and nipple covers and the insides and outsides of the nipples

---

[18] Adapted from Infant Care. U.S. Dept. of Health, Education, and Welfare, Children's Bureau, Publication No. 8, 1963.

with the bottle brush.

2. Rinse all articles well. Drain. Squeeze clean water through nipple holes.

3. Measure the milk, water, and sugar (or syrup) into the large saucepan. If granulated sugar is used, level off the measuring spoon with back of table knife. If syrup is used, pour from the bottle into the measuring spoon. If the milk used is not homogenized, shake the bottle well to mix the cream before measuring. If evaporated milk is used, wash the top of the can with soap and water, and rinse it off well before opening. If dried milk is used, mix powder with water according to amounts prescribed, and beat with an egg beater to blend.

4. Divide the milk mixture among the number of bottles needed in 24 hours.

5. Put nipples and nipple covers on the bottles. Do not push or screw nipple covers down tight, because during sterilization the hot air may blow the caps off.

6. Put the bottles of formula on the rack in the kettle. Put one or two bottles of drinking water, covered with nipple and cap, in at the same time. Pour water into the kettle until it comes about half way up on the bottles. Cover the kettle.

7. Bring the water in the kettle to a boil. *Boil actively for 25 minutes* by the clock. As soon as the bottles are cool enough to handle, take them out of the kettle. Tighten nipple caps.

8. After the bottles cool, put them in the refrigerator at once. In an ice refrigerator, place the bottles near the ice. A rack to hold the bottles upright is very convenient. (See Fig. 16-2.)

STANDARD CLEAN TECHNIQUE METHOD: Sterilizing the equipment

1. Wash the bottles, nipple covers, funnel and nipples thoroughly in hot water with a detergent. With the bottle brush scrub the insides of the nursing bottles and nipple covers, disc seals and collars, and the insides and outsides of the nipples.

2. Rinse all these articles well. Squeeze clean water through the nipple holes.

3. If the sterilizing kettle has a rack to hold the bottles, set each bottle in it, upside down. Fit nipple covers, funnel, tongs, can opener, measuring cup and spoons between the bottles. If the kettle has no rack, lay the bottles on their sides in the kettle, with the other equipment on top.

4. If the kettle has a rack and a tight-fitting cover, pour in about 5 inches of water and put on the cover. When the water boils actively, steam will form and will sterilize the equipment. Keep the water boiling for at least 5 *minutes* by the clock. If the kettle does not have a tight-fitting lid, put in enough

water to completely cover the bottles and all the other things to be sterilized. Boil for at least 5 minutes after the water has come to a boil.

5. Drain off some of the water. Leave the things in the covered kettle until ready to use them, or remove with tongs, and place bottles on clean towel or rack.

6. Drop the nipples into boiling water in a small pan, cover, and let boil for 5 minutes. Then pour the water off, let the steam escape and leave the nipples in the covered pan until needed.

Boiling nipples too long, or letting them stand in water, wears them out.

7. Boil water for formula (and drinking water) for five minutes and measure required amount.

8. Add evaporated milk* and carbohydrate or a commercially processed formula to the boiled water. Wash top of container with soap and water and rinse.

9. Pour into bottle. If funnel is used remove it from the sterilizer without touching its rim or stem and set it in one of the bottles. Attach nipples and cover. For disc seals invert nipples in bottle, apply disc and screw collar down tight. Do not touch any part of the nipple that goes into baby's mouth. Use tongs. (Follow directions that come with the kind of nipple and bottle used.)

10. Store in refrigerator.

Previously sterilized bottles, nipples and nipple covers are required for use in the commercially prepared formulas such as concentrated liquid and powder formulations and the ready-to-use preparations. These preparations are sterile in the cans and bottles. Tops should be washed and rinsed before opening the can. When opened, canned or bottled formulas should be refrigerated and used within 48 hours. Follow instructions given on the bottle or cans for best procedure.

WARMING THE PREPARED FEEDING

Formulas are generally warmed before each feeding but several investigators believe that this practice may be unnecessary. Ice-cold formulas apparently are well tolerated by 50 per cent of very young infants and 75 per cent of older infants. Studies indicate that feedings given directly from the refrigerator tend to lower gastric temperature to decrease proteolytic enzyme activity and to delay digestion. For heating the bottle before feeding, the following directions should be followed: Remove the formula-filled nursing bottle from the refrigerator and set it upright in a small deep saucepan with 3 to 4 inches of

---

*Bottled milk or other unsterilized milk is boiled with the water. Stir constantly while it is boiling.

a good way to make the baby's formula is

HEATING AFTER BOTTLING

① Wash your hands with soap and water.

② Wash a 1½ to 2-quart jar, jar top, baby bottles, bottle caps or nipple covers, tablespoons, nipples and can opener with soap and hot water.

③ Wash the top of the evaporated milk can.

④ Rinse all with clean water.

⑤ Put the needed amount of water, evaporated milk, syrup or sugar into the jar.

⑥ Stir with the clean spoon.

STEP 1   STEP 2   STEP 3

⑦ Pour the amount of formula for one feeding into each of the clean bottles. Usually this is 4, 6, or 8 ounces.

⑧ Put the nipples and bottle caps or nipple covers on the bottles.

⑨ Put a wire rack, or a clean cloth in the bottom of a large pot and add about 3 or 4 inches of water.

⑩ Put bottles filled with the formula into the pot. Be sure the bottle caps are loose.

⑪ Cover the pot. After the water starts to boil, boil for 25 minutes.

⑫ Remove the pot from the fire. Leave cover on. Let cool slowly so that milk won't clog the nipples. When you can hold your hands against the sides of the pot remove the bottles. Tighten the caps and place the bottles in the refrigerator or icebox.

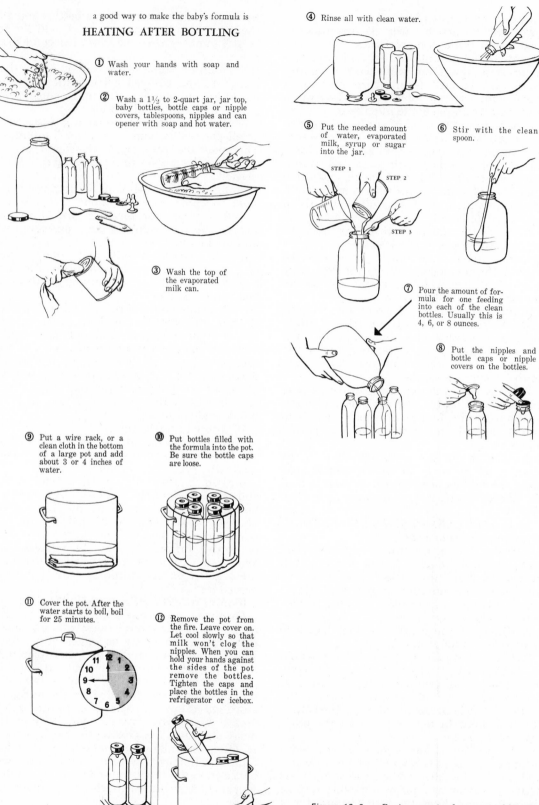

Figure 16–2   Basic steps in the terminal heating method of making a baby's formula. (From U.S. Department of Health, Education and Welfare, Children's Bureau.)

warm water. Place the pan over high heat and leave until the water is ready to boil. Shake bottle several times so that milk is warmed through.

Remove nipple cover, being careful not to contaminate the nipple.

Test the temperature of the milk by letting a few drops trickle onto the inner side of the wrist. It should feel warm but not hot.

Two typical infant feeding formulas are presented:

Formula I

Whole cow's milk	1½ oz./lb. body weight
Sucrose	1 oz./each 10 oz. milk used
Water	added to *total* 2½ oz. formula/lb. body weight

Formula II

Evaporated milk	1½ oz./lb. body weight *after* reconstitution with an equal amount of water
Cane sugar or corn syrup	1 oz./each 10 oz. reconstituted milk used
Water	added to *total* 2½ oz. formula/lb. body weight

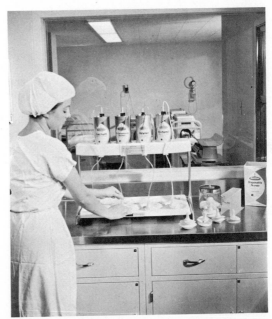

Figure 16–4   Sterile nursers (Beniflex) are filled with ready-to-use formulas via a "closed" system to simplify infant feeding and provide added safeguards against bacteria. (Courtesy of Mead Johnson Laboratories.)

DISPOSABLE BOTTLES   Recently, a number of disposable plastic bottles of various shapes and sizes have been designed to simplify infant feeding and provide safeguards against bacteria. Ready-to-use formulas supplied in quart cans, requiring no rewarming, are drained into the bottle through a plastic tube inserted by needle into the nipple (Beniflex[18])—a process requiring only 15 seconds. (See Figs. 16–3 and 16–4.) As the infant nurses, the plastic dispenser contracts (the bottom of the bottle draws into the hollow of the top), thus avoiding intake by the infant of excess air. These have been tried out and are currently being used in several hospitals with satisfactory results. The cost is generally greater in the home, however, than if the mother made and sterilized the formula, reusing the same bottles from day to day.

FEEDING SCHEDULE

The following feeding schedules for infants are typical and are dependent upon the number of required daily feedings.

Five feedings per day:
  6 and 10 A.M.; 2, 6 and 10 P.M.
Six feedings per day:
  2, 6 and 10 A.M.; 2, 6 and 10 P.M.
Seven feedings per day:
  3, 6, 9 and 12 P.M.; 6, 9 and 12 A.M.
Eight feedings per day:
  3, 6, 9 and 12 P.M.; 3, 6, 9 and 12 A.M.

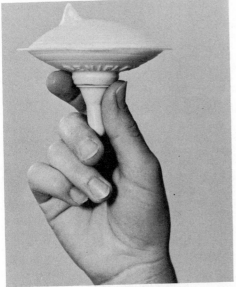

Figure 16–3   A sterile plastic disposable nursing bottle for infant feeding. (Courtesy of Mead Johnson Laboratories and called Beniflex Disposable Nurser System.)

[18]Mead Johnson Laboratories.

Babies thrive better when fed regularly. However, this does not mean rigidly set intervals of 3 to 4 hours, regardless of how much sooner or later they get hungry. Some years ago it was widespread practice for babies to be fed "by the clock." Today the baby is allowed to develop a feeding schedule of his own, known as "self-regulation," or "self-demand feeding." A baby's hunger is considered the best clock to go by. During the first few weeks, a baby may wake up and appear to need food a dozen times in 24 hours. By the end of the first month, there may be 3 hours between feedings. By the time the baby is 2 months old, he frequently sleeps through the night after the late feeding (10 P.M.), and is established on the 5-feeding schedule (see p. 263). When they are between 2 and 3 months old, the majority of babies are on a 4-hour feeding schedule.

SUPPLEMENTARY FOODS

Infants have supplementary foods added to the formula or breast feeding during the first year of life to provide the essentials that milk does not supply in adequate amounts, especially iron and vitamin C. These supplements are added gradually, guided by the age, developmental growth, and condition of the infant. The age at which solid foods are given varies widely, reflecting divergent opinions on the ability of the infant's gastrointestinal tract to properly process the foods. The Academy of Pediatrics Committee on Nutrition states that a normal full-term infant can thrive on human milk or formula for the first 2½ to 3 months of life when diet is appropriately supplemented with vitamins (ascorbic acid and vitamin D). Smith[19] reports on a case which demonstrates that milk is occasionally fed to infants (or children) in such excessive amounts that other essential foods, notably foods containing iron, may be excluded, causing one or more deficiencies. Although milk is an excellent food for all ages, especially infants and children, it should not be given to the exclusion of other equally necessary foods.

Bakwin[20] suggests that the time to introduce solid foods is determined by changes in the behavior of the oral musculature. At about 3 months of age when the spoon is inserted between the lips, the lips part, the tongue depresses and food placed at the tip forms into a ball. It is then thrown to the back of the pharynx and swallowed. Earlier, when the spoon is placed between the lips, the baby purses his lips, raises his tongue and pushes against the spoon. Few infants are ready for anything but liquid food until 10 to 12 weeks of age. Salivary enzymes are necessary for the digestion of complex starches. Salivary amylase in the saliva is present between 2 and 3 months of age. When the infant is fed milk only the disaccharide (lactose) does not require the salivary enzymes. Forcing solid foods may be frustrating to the infant. It may result in an unpleasant experience for both mother and infant and a beginning of food problems. Biting movements begin also at about 3 months. This appears the best time to begin feeding solids. When chewing movements begin (about 7 to 9 months) foods requiring chewing should be introduced. It is considered a good rule to limit the daily intake of milk to a maximum of one quart. When an infant seems hungry after taking 26 ounces of formula in 24 hours it is generally time to introduce a semi-solid food.

The sequence given below is the usual order in which the formula supplements are added. There may be considerable variations, depending upon the physical and physiological development of the infant. No set guideline is feasible. The eating process is a learning experience and each child develops at his particular rate. There would be restrictions if the child were known to have an allergic background. Such foods as orange juice, eggs, and foods containing cow's milk may be introduced in small quantities and increased gradually as tolerated.

FOOD	AVERAGE AGE WHEN ADDED
Cod liver oil or equivalents	2 weeks
Orange juice	2 weeks
Cereal (whole grain or enriched)	2 to 3 months
Vegetable purée, meat purée	4 to 5 months
Fruit purée	5 to 6 months
Potatoes, boiled or baked, may sometimes be used in place of cereal	6 months
Zwieback or dried bread	8 months
Egg yolk	7 to 8 months (or 2 to 4 months)
Meat	6 to 10 months

Orange juice and cod liver oil or equivalents are introduced into the baby's dietary in the early days of life. One fourth to one third of a cup of orange juice supplies approximately 35 mg. of ascorbic acid. If either orange or tomato juice is not tolerated, a supplement containing 35 mg. ascorbic acid should be given daily. Because tomato juice is only half as rich in ascorbic acid as orange juice, it is necessary to give twice as much tomato juice as the amount of orange juice.

The need for vitamin D is believed to exist from birth. Fish liver oils can be given without difficulty to the average infant beginning

[19]Smith, C. A.: Overuse of milk in the diets of infants and children. J.A.M.A., 172:567, 1960.

[20]Bakwin, H.: Current feeding practices of infants. Nutrition News, National Dairy Council, 28:3:10, 1965.

within 2 weeks following birth. Milk fortified with vitamin D is a good source if the intake of milk provides 400 units daily of vitamin D. Commercial preparations are fortified with vitamin D and ascorbic acid.

CEREALS Cooked cereal is the customary first supplementary food added to the infant's diet. Because the infant's storage of iron is depleted after the first 3 or 4 months of life, one of the reasons for introducing solid foods is to replenish iron. Fortified (enriched with B vitamins and iron) cereals are used. The approximate compositions of commonly used cereals are recorded in Tables 16–4 and 16–5. It is best to begin with finely divided enriched refined cereal. Regular cereals must be cooked thoroughly in the top of a double boiler or in a pressure cooker, then strained while hot. However, there are quick-cooking cereals available that are timesaving and satisfactory. The ready-prepared dry cereals and commercially canned strained cereals, prepared especially for infants, are of great convenience to the mother. The ready-prepared baby cereals need only to be mixed with a little warm formula, warm boiled milk, or warm boiled water. Anderson and Fomon[21] found that mothers generally fed infants less than one-third ounce of dry cereal to approximately two ounces of cereal-milk or cereal-formula mixture (one part dry cereal, six parts milk).

Labels list the nutrient content on the basis of one serving (one ounce) of dry cereal. The mixed cereals are made from wheat, oats and corn primarily. High protein cereals are made with soy, wheat and oat flours. The cost of the cereals is approximately the same. In situations in which cost per unit of protein is important, one would choose the high protein cereals. (See Table 16–4.) The per cent of recommended dietary allowances (RDA) for vitamins and minerals for an infant 6

to 12 months of age supplied by 100 gm. of cereal-milk and cereal-water mixture is shown in Table 16–5.

EGGS Only the egg yolk in very small amounts of one-fourth teaspoon is offered to the young baby. Because some infants are sensitive to the protein of egg yolk, it is advisable to increase gradually the amount of whole yolk served daily. The raw yolk may be given alone, or may be added to the milk, cooked with milk into a custard, added to vegetables or cereals; or the yolk may be coddled, poached, or cooked. Egg yolk simmered for about 10 minutes and put through a sieve is an easy method of preparation. The sieved yolk can be mixed with a small amount of milk or added to the cereal. An idiosyncrasy to egg white seems to be more prevalent than to the egg yolk. Until about the end of the first year, care should be exercised in separating the egg yolk from the egg white.

VEGETABLES AND FRUITS Opinions differ as to which should be introduced first — fruits or vegetables. Some believe that if fruit (especially sweetened) is introduced first, the vegetables are poorly accepted. The fruits and vegetables served to the baby may be either canned or freshly cooked and strained. Use green or deep yellow vegetables, such as carrots, squash, spinach, green beans, or turnip greens. Mashed raw banana is acceptable. In the beginning only a teaspoonful is given; the amount is increased gradually until the year old baby receives 3 to 4 tablespoons of fruits and vegetables. To familiarize the child with different flavors, a variety of fruits (such as applesauce, peaches, apricots, pears and cooked prunes) and vegetables should be offered. By 6 months boiled or baked potatoes may sometimes take the place of cereal. Before the end of the first year more coarsely mashed or chopped vegetables should be substituted for the strained varieties. Near the end of the year, butter or fortified margarine can be added to vegetables for flavor.

---

[21] Anderson, T. A., and Fomon, S. J.: Commercially prepared infant cereals. J. Pediat., 78:789, 1971.

TABLE 16–4 AVERAGE CALORIE AND PROTEIN CONTENT OF CEREAL-MILK AND CEREAL-WATER MIXTURE*

CEREALS	DRY CEREAL MIXED WITH (in kilocalories per 100 gm.)		DRY CEREAL MIXED WITH (in per cent protein)	
	Milk†	Water	Milk†	Water
Barley, mixed Oatmeal, Wheat	109	53	5.2	2.2
High Protein	107	52	8.1	5.1
Rice	108	52	3.9	0.9

*One part cereal, six parts milk or water by weight. Averages of Gerber, Beech-Nut and Heinz nutritional data.
†Values of 100 gm. of whole milk used—67 kcalories and 3.5 protein. Taken from Anderson and Fomon, J. Pediat., *18*:790, 1971.

TABLE 16-5 PROXIMATE AVERAGE COMPOSITION OF GERBER, BEECH-NUT AND HEINZ INFANT CEREALS (VITAMINS AND MINERALS)

CEREAL BRAND	NIACIN (mg./100 gm.)			RIBOFLAVIN (mg./100 gm.)			THIAMIN (mg./100 gm.)			CALCIUM (mg./100 gm.)		PHOSPHORUS (mg./100 gm.)		IRON (mg./100 gm.)	
	Dry Cereal	Cereal and Milk*†	Cereal and Water*	Dry Cereal	Cereal and Milk	Cereal and Water	Dry Cereal	Cereal and Milk	Cereal and Water	Cereal and Milk*†	Cereal and Water*	Cereal and Milk	Cereal and Water	Cereal and Milk	Cereal and Water
GERBER Barley, high-protein, mixed, oatmeal, rice	14.1	2.1 (26)‡	2.0 (25)	2.1	0.4 (67)	0.3 (50)	2.8	0.4 (80)	0.4 (80)	191 (32)‡	89 (15)	179 (36)	99 (20)	14 (93)	14 (93)
BEECH-NUT High protein, mixed, oatmeal, wheat	3.5	0.6 (8)	0.5 (6)	1.6	0.4 (67)	0.2 (33)	1.6	0.2 (40)	0.2 (40)	215 (36)	114 (19)	191 (33)	111 (22)	7 (47)	7 (47)
Rice	17.7	2.6 (33)	2.5 (31)	3.2	0.6 (100)	0.5 (83)	2.8	0.4 (80)	0.4 (80)						
HEINZ Barley, high-protein, mixed, oatmeal	52.6	7.6 (95)	7.5 (94)	0.34	0.20 (33)	0.05 (8)	5.2	0.8 (160)	0.7 (140)	242 (40)	141 (24)	196 (39)	117 (23)	10 (67)	10 (67)
Rice	47.2	6.8 (85)	6.7 (84)	0.18	0.18 (30)	0.03 (5)	4.4	0.7 (140)	0.6 (120)						

Adapted from: Anderson, T. A., and Fomon, S. J.: Commercially Prepared Infant Cereals, J. Pediat., 78:788, 1971.
*Mixed one part (by weight) cereal and 6 parts milk or water (diluent).
†Whole milk: niacin 0.09 mg., riboflavin 0.18 mg., thiamin 0.04 mg., calcium 118 mg., phosphorus 39 mg., iron trace per 100 gm.
‡Numbers in parentheses refer to percentage of Recommended Daily Allowance for an infant 6 to 12 months of age supplied by 100 gm. of cereal-diluent mixture.

MEAT AND FISH   Scraped lean meat or liver cooked in little or no fat can be added before the baby has teeth. Leverton et al.,[22] conducted a study in which they included strained meat in the diet as early as 6 weeks with favorable results. They report that the infants who received a dietary supplement of strained meat showed higher hemoglobin values as a result. However, meat is usually added to the diet between the fourth and sixth month. When the secretion of the proleolytic enzymes in the intestinal juice increases, the infant is able to digest most proteins. Canned puréed and chopped varieties, as well as meat soups, prepared for babies and ready to use, save time and effort. See Chapter 39 for directions on how to prepare a scraped meat patty.

Toward the end of the first year, white-fleshed fish, such as cod or haddock (baked, steamed or broiled; see Chapter 39), can be served in place of meat once or twice a week. Canned salmon or tuna, with fat removed, can also be used. Start with a teaspoon and gradually increase; when teeth and chewing movements appear, the baby may have thinly sliced liver, chicken or other fowl, beef, veal or well-cooked, lean pork.

BREAD   Bread, dried in the oven, or zwieback can be added when the baby's first teeth have come in. He can have it after meals, or for midmorning or midafternoon lunches. The main purpose of the dried bread is to exercise his jaws.

OTHER FACTORS   The renal solutes (nitrogenous substances and electrolytes) must be excreted from the kidney. Infants fed strained meats, egg yolk and high meat dinners have comparatively high renal solute excretion (loads). Those infants fed fruit juices, fruit puddings and desserts have low renal solute loads and the other infant foods are intermediate renal solute loads. The choice of infant foods is important at various times when volume of food is low, when extrarenal losses of fluid are abnormal and when renal concentration is low. Kidney function generally becomes efficient by 6 to 8 weeks, after which protein foods can be handled.[23]

Sodium and monosodium glutamate are used in commercially strained and junior foods. These appear to be added to these foods primarily to satisfy the tastes of the mothers. Study was conducted by Fomon et al.[24] to compare the consumption of salted and unsalted strained foods by 4-month-old and 7-month-old infants. On the basis of an average daily food intake infants appeared to accept the unsalted foods as well as the salted foods. The unsalted foods usually fed to infants contain sufficient sodium to meet the infant's need. From a nutritional point of view there is no justification for adding salt to strained foods for infants. Animal studies have suggested that the large amount of sodium chloride present in commercially strained and junior foods may predispose susceptible infants to development of hypertension later in life. Studies on the salt intake of infants in the first year of life varied widely but were rather high. About 60 per cent of the total sodium in the diet of the infant is contributed by processed vegetables, meats and eggs. An infant eating these foods to which salt has been added commercially or by the mother at four months of age may be receiving three times the sodium recommended. The safety of the added sodium chloride and monosodium glutamate in infant food is not resolved. In 1970 the National Academy of Sciences recommended to the Food and Drug Administration that the level of salt added to strained and junior foods not exceed 0.25 per cent.

MEAL PLAN

At the age of 12 months, the infant should be consuming a varied diet and eating from the family table. The transition from strained to coarser textured foods begins around 6 months of age. The following list shows the foods infants who are 9 to 12 months old usually eat. The amount and type of foods served are adjusted to the child's age.

Foods
    Milk: Homogenized.
    Eggs: Poached, scrambled, or soft cooked.
    Meats, fish or poultry: Beef juice; ground beef, lamb, veal, liver, well-cooked, lean pork, or chicken; chopped bacon, flaked fish.
    Cheese: Cottage cheese.
    Breads: Fine whole grain or enriched white bread; toast; crackers; zwieback.
    Cereals: Fine-grained, cooked cereal, or fortified ready-to-eat (without sugar).
    Cereal products: Plain cooked spaghetti, macaroni, noodles, rice or grits (enriched).
    Fats: Butter and fortified margarine.
    Vegetables: Mashed vegetables, vegetable purée, or cooked vegetables of low fiber.
    Fruits: Cooked fruit purée; cooked fruit without skins or seeds; mashed ripe banana; and fruit juices.
    Soups: Vegetable and cream soups.

[22]Leverton, R. M., et al.: Further studies of the use of meat in the diet of infants and young children. J. Pediat., 40:761, 1952.

[23]Anderson, T. A., and Fomon, S. J.: Commercially prepared strained and junior foods for infants. J. Am. Dietet. A., 58:520, 1971.

[24]Fomon, S. J., et al.: Acceptance of unsalted strained foods by normal infants. J. Pediat., 76:242, 1970.

Desserts: Custard, rennet pudding, blanc-mange; gelatin, bread, cream, rice, and tapioca puddings; and plain ice cream.

The meal plan may look something like this:

Breakfast: Cereal, egg, milk (orange juice).
Midmorning: Orange juice if not given at breakfast and/or crusty bread.
Noon meal: Vegetables, meat, milk.
Midafternoon: Milk, crusty bread or crackers.
Evening meal: Cereal, fruit, milk.

WEANING

In the milk consumption pattern survey of over 2000 infants from New York City and San Francisco, Riveria[25] reported that canned formulas were the most common sources of milk used during the first three months of life. Among middle income families about 25 per cent were breast fed during the first month. Among low income families less than 5 per cent of mothers breast fed their infants. After six months the majority of the infants drank fresh cow's milk. Infants under 6 months of age from lower income families used evaporated milk more often than did infants from higher income families.

The breast-fed baby is weaned by the sixth month. Many mothers wean their babies earlier. Since supplements are advised during the early months, preparation for the weaning begins when supplementary foods are served to the baby. The addition of solid foods to the dietary teaches the baby to rely less on the breast as a food source. Besides, cow's milk, fresh or evaporated, is added to the cooked cereal and vegetables which supplement one breast feeding when indicated. Cow's milk from a bottle or cup replaces all the breast feedings. The mother's mammary glands respond to the decreased demand and secrete smaller amounts until the flow is finally exhausted. Through a gradual weaning, the mother's discomfort is minimized and the infant rarely experiences any indigestion.

The bottle-fed baby is weaned to milk in a cup when he is ready and usually before the end of the first year. It is wiser to diminish gradually the number of bottle feedings, although the morning and bedtime feedings may be continued for some time. The addition of solid foods to the baby's diet decreases the need for bottle feedings, and ultimately the bottle feedings are abandoned for whole milk and solid foods.

FEEDING OF THE PREMATURE INFANT

An infant who weighs less than 5½ pounds at birth is considered premature. The feeding of the premature infant requires special attention. He usually has difficulty in sucking and in swallowing. Although the need for calories is high, the infant has a limited capacity to digest a quantity of nutritious food.

In former years, human milk was preferred for the premature infant. It was considered the only suitable milk, and if the mother was unable to nurse her baby, human milk was secured either from some nursing woman or a human milk station. However, further research indicates that heated cow's milk mixtures are preferred in the routine feeding of young premature infants. Gordon, Levine and McNamara's studies[26] showed that many of these infants have difficulty in digesting and absorbing fat. Thus, dietary calories should be derived chiefly from proteins and carbohydrates. They fed three different types of milk: processed human milk, a diluted evaporated milk-carbohydrate mixture, and a mixture of powdered, partially skimmed cow's milk with added carbohydrate and water. Infants fed cow's milk mixtures gained more weight than those fed human milk. Disadvantages of cow's milk are increased requirement for vitamin C and postulated disorders of water balance resulting from renal disability in excreting added solutes. Water and electrolyte balance is very important. The rapidly growing body of the premature infant demands higher protein and calcium. (Consult Table 16–1, comparing values of human milk with cow's milk.) There is evidence that the premature infant can retain larger amounts of nitrogen from a high-protein diet. Providing these infants with a relatively high-protein modified cow's milk formula is usually recommended.[27] Gordon[28] recommends liberal protein intake in properly constituted cow's milk mixtures in which protein supplies 16 to 20 per cent of the daily calories—4 to 6 gm. protein, 100 to 120 kcalories per kg. body weight.

The average daily kcalorie requirement of the premature infant is 120 to 125 kcalories per kg., which is only slightly higher than the requirements of the normal full-term infant. If human milk is fed in amounts to comply with the higher requirements for

[25]Riveria, J.: The frequency of use of various kinds of milk during infancy in middle and lower income families. Am. J. Pub. Health, 61:277, 1971.

[26]Gordon, H. H., Levine, S. Z., and McNamara, H.: Feeding of premature infants; A comparison of human and cow's milk. Am. J. Dis. Child., 73:442, 1947.

[27]Waisman, H. A., and Kerr, G. R.: Amino acid and protein metabolism in the developing fetus and the newborn infant. Pediat. Clin. N. Amer., 12:569, 1965.

[28]Gordon, H. H.: Protein allowances for premature infants. J.A.M.A., 175:107, 1961.

maintenance and growth, it furnishes 180 ml. of fluid per kg. of body weight (2.7 ounces per pound), 2.2 gm. of proteins (1 gm. per pound), 6.7 gm. of fats (3 gm. per pound), and 13 gm. of carbohydrates (6 gm. per pound). The fluid intake and amount of fats are excessive for the tolerance of the very small infant who weighs 1500 gm. (3 pounds and 6 ounces) or less.

On the other hand, cow's milk mixtures may be prepared to provide less total fluid and fat, higher amounts of protein, and the equivalent or larger amounts of carbohydrates, totaling the desired calories per kilogram.

In Table 16–6 are examples of such mixtures reported by Gordon[28] and Levine[29].

Premature infants, who are heavier in weight, older, and tolerate fats and high fluid intake, do equally well on human milk. When the infant reaches normal growth rates, the protein intake of the cow's milk mixture can be reduced correspondingly to the recommended daily level of 3 to 4 gm. per kg. of body weight.

Barness, et al.[30] report satisfactory results with a low protein-low ash formula. The formula used is based on cow's milk. About one-half of the protein content is from skim milk, the rest from electrodialyzed whey (chiefly lactalbumin and lactoglobulin). The resultant formula has the same fat, carbohydrate, sodium, potassium, magnesium, and chloride as human milk. Calcium content is only about 50 per cent higher, and phosphorus content twice that of human milk. Total protein content is 1.5 per cent, compared to 1.2 per cent for breast milk.

Since premature infants are often unable to suck, other methods of administering the nourishment must be employed. For such cases there are special nipples available, but some pediatricians prefer tube feeding. In any case, the feeding must be administered slowly to lessen the tendency to regurgitate and aspirate. The number of feedings given depends on the size and age of the infant; the hours intervening between feedings vary between 2 to 4. No feedings are given until 12 to 36 hours after birth, depending on the size and condition of the infant. However, saline solution with or without glucose should be given every 2 to 3 hours.

Ascorbic acid is administered in the amount of 100 mg. daily during the early weeks. Ascorbic acid is continued until the baby is able to take adequate quantities of orange juice. Vitamins A and D are required in larger amounts than for full-term infants. Vitamin D is started when the baby is approximately 2 weeks old. Large quantities of vitamin D are given since premature infants are more susceptible to rickets than full-term infants and the rapid bone growth of the premature infant requires ample vitamin D. Iron storage usually is incomplete, and iron is administered in the form of ferrous sulfate when the baby is about 1 month old to prevent the development of an iron deficiency anemia. Schulman[31] recommends a total daily intake of about 2 mg. per kg. body weight by the third month, gradually decreasing to about 1 mg. per kg. by the end of the first year. Some physicians prescribe vitamin B-complex for the premature infant.

EATING HABITS AND THE PSYCHOLOGY OF INFANT AND CHILD FEEDING

Eating patterns begin with the first introduction to food and they follow a sequence when an infant is old enough emotionally and physically, and the culture in which he is raised influences this pattern of eating habits.

[29]Levine, S. Z.: Protein nutrition in pediatrics. *In* Protein Nutrition in Health and Diseases. Chicago, The American Medical Association, 1945. This material is available in a Manual for Physicians, by Gordon, H. H., in Dunham, E. C.: Premature Infants, New York, Paul B. Hoeber, Inc.

[30]Barness, L. A., et al.: Progress of premature infants fed a formula containing demineralized whey. Pediatrics, 32:52, 1963.

[31]Schulman, I.: Iron requirements in infancy. J.A.M.A., *175*:118, 1961.

TABLE 16–6   FORMULAS FOR FEEDING PREMATURE INFANTS
(per Kilogram of Body Weight and in Percentages of Dietary Calories)

MILK Type	AMOUNT (cc.)	SUGAR (grams)	WATER (cc.)	PROTEIN (grams)	(%)	FAT (grams)	(%)	CARBO-HYDRATES (grams)	(%)	KCAL-ORIES
Human	180		0	2.2	7	6.7	50	12.9	43	120
Cow's										
Whole	100	13	50	3.5	13	3.5	27	17.8	60	120
Lactic acid	140	6	—	4.8	16	5.5	41	12.9	43	120
Evaporated	70	6	80	4.8	16	5.5	41	12.9	43	120
Powdered half Skimmed (Alacta)	18	11	150	6.0	20	2.2	16	19.4	64	120

Anorexia is one of the most common complaints about child feeding. Frequently, the origin of the indifferent appetite displayed by a child is traced to the food habits started in infancy. The feeding formula prescribed by the physician may be the initial cause. The conscientious parent may overlook the variation in appetite, being too zealous in fulfilling the prescribed time schedule and amount of feedings. Rebellion against food can begin because of a rigid instead of a flexible feeding schedule.

Feeding problems often not recognized until age 2 when a child's growth rate slows, his appetite lessens and his burgeoning sense of independence leads him to balk at many requests and expectations for the sheer assertive joy of refusal to secure attention. Because appetite can be strongly influenced by emotions and attitudes, as well as physical hunger, the first aim is to keep eating enjoyable. The feeling of being loved and feeding are closely intertwined. One does not give the child food alone; attitudes are also being fed. An unloved child may lose his appetite, and nutritional deficiency may cause retarded growth.[32] Too much excitement or distraction at mealtime, particularly in the early stages of learning, may cause a child to neglect eating. The nurse's approach is important in the formation of good eating habits. (See Fig. 16–5.) She, as well as the child's parents, needs to understand the child and his feelings about food. It is important to see food as a

child sees it and to maintain respect for the child. Focus attention on the learner as well as what is to be learned.

LEARNING TO EAT

In the weaning stage an infant has to learn many things: not to suck food, to want solid food, to learn not to be held during eating, and to learn how to eat—new manipulative skills which include chewing and swallowing solid food.

Babies are individualists! Baby John's gluttonous appetite is no criterion for judging baby Mary's diminutive appetite. Some babies have an idiosyncrasy of gulping down a large feeding to satiate their appetites, while other babies enjoy frequent small feedings.

Pushing a fist full of food into his mouth is the cue a baby usually gives when he wants to feed himself. If the doting parent misses the cue, a feeding problem can easily develop. Very young children should be encouraged to feed themselves. They will spill and scatter the food at first but should be encouraged to keep on trying (See Fig. 16–6.) Too much help and attention from the mother or nurse will slow down the child's efforts, because he dislikes being interfered with, and will build up his resistance to eating. Eating will cease to be fun.

At the beginning of a meal the child is hungry and should be allowed to feed himself; when he becomes tired, he can be quietly helped. Emphasis on table manners and the fine points of eating should be left

[32]Witten, C. F.: T.L.C. and the Hungry Child. Nutrition Today, 7:10, 1972.

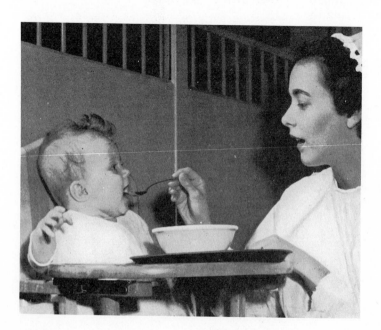

Figure 16–5   The nurse's approach is important in the formation of good eating habits. (Sellew and Pepper: The Nursing of Children, 7th edition.)

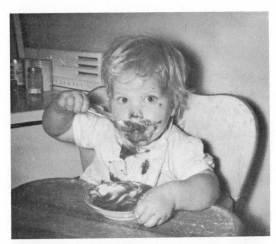

Figure 16-6   Very young children should be encouraged to feed themselves. They will spill and scatter the food at first but should be encouraged to keep on trying. This youngster is learning to eat with a spoon. She is making a mess but will gradually make a go of it.

until later when he has matured and developed to be ready for it. If he wants to eat with his fingers instead of the spoon—let him! (See Fig. 16-7.) But, if he plays with the food, just squeezing it or daubing it on himself and furniture, it should be put out of reach. He has probably had enough.

The food should be in a form that is easy to handle and eat. Meat should be cut into bite sizes, potatoes and vegetables mashed so a spoon can be used easily. Raw fruits and vegetables should be in sizes that can be picked up in the hands. In addition, the dishes and silver should be small and easy to handle. The cup should be easy to hold and other dishes so designed that they do

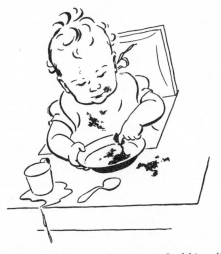

Figure 16-7   This baby is learning to feed himself. He prefers to use his fingers instead of the spoon. All right! (Infant Care. U.S. Department of Health, Education, and Welfare, Children's Bureau.)

not tip over easily. (See Fig. 16-8.) Child psychologists agree that the food habit pattern is established, for better or worse, when the first bottle is fed to the newborn infant. It is important to establish good food habits during infancy because they form the basis of the individual's food habits carried throughout life.

SIZE OF SERVINGS   The size of servings offered a child is very important. A baby's stomach at birth holds about two tablespoons of food, and at one year the stomach holds about a cupful of food. The stomach enlarges gradually until in adult life it holds approximately two quarts of food. A child cannot be expected to eat as much as an adult. A large serving of food will often discourage the dainty, fastidious eater. At 1 year, the baby will eat one third to one half, at 3 years, one half or a little more, and at 6 years he will eat about two thirds the amount an adult consumes. A little child should not be served a large plate full of food; the size of the plate and amount should be kept in proportion to his age. A tablespoonful (not heaping!) of each food offered for each year of age is a good guide to follow. Serving him less than you think or hope he will eat helps a child to eat successfully and happily. He will ask for more food if his appetite is not satisfied.

TYPE OF FOOD   Because the baby's stomach is so small, it should not be considered a reservoir for food. There is no room in the stomach for foods which do not serve a purpose. Pastry, candy, sweet drinks and highly sweetened foods take the place of nourishing foods. Bulky foods are avoided. Instead, strained fruits and vegetables, chopped meats, eggs and milk are served. At the age of 6 months the baby may be fed chopped or mashed vegetables so he will become accustomed to the coarser foods early in life and start the mechanism of chewing along with swallowing. Children, in general, prefer simple, uncomplicated foods. Lowenberg[33] found that a stew in which vegetables and meat were ground and cooked together was considerably more popular with young children than one with separate pieces of vegetables and meat. It was found that children of ages 2 to 6 years often prefer raw to cooked vegetables and fruits. Food from the meal planned for adult members of the family may be adapted to the child in child size portions. Highly seasoned sauces are omitted from the child's plate, and the filling of pies is served as pudding. Children

[33]Lowenberg, M. E. F.: National Food Conference, Washington, D.C., Feb. 24, 1958; and Lowenberg, M. E. F.: For the young child—success promotes success in eating. Food and Nutrition News, 40:No. 6, 1969.

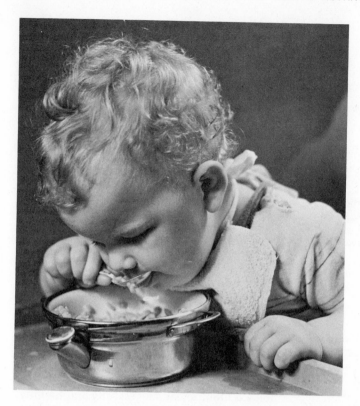

Figure 16-8   The child's spoon is easy to handle and the dish will not easily tip over. (Harold M. Lambert Studios.)

under 6 usually prefer very mild-flavored foods, even those which an adult would consider too bland. Because the child's stomach is small, he may require a supplement between meals of milk, milk and crackers or sandwich, or fruit.

VARIETY OF FOODS   It is especially desirable that the baby should receive foods varied both in texture and flavor. The infant who is accustomed to many kinds of food is less likely to grow up with definite food dislikes. To add variety to the infant's diet, one of the two cereal feedings during the day may be supplemented with different sieved vegetables and fruits.

Food attitudes do not change markedly during childhood. Many factors influence preferences. It is important to offer a variety of dishes and not allow the youngster to continue on a diet consisting of one or two favorite foods.

NEW FOODS   Introduction of new foods may be a problem with some children. The old advice was to encourage the child to "try just a taste." At Merrill-Palmer Institute, Detroit, the researchers found the children did exactly that—nibbled one leaf of a Brussels sprout or took a "lick" of a beet and called it quits. More successful is an approach that intrigues a child's curiosity in a new food: the look, the smell, the feel of it—even before

it is cooked—perhaps at the marketing stage. Give only a small portion of an unfamiliar food the first time. If rejected, do not force, but wait a few days and give it another trial. If he himself asks for a bite of it when it is served the next time he is farther along to learning to like it, according to Lowenberg, than if he is forced to eat even a bite of it. The less said the better. A child will find it much easier to learn to like beets, for example, if he does not have to live up to the reputation of being a beet hater. Any new food should be given along with a familiar food the infant likes, at a time when he is hungry, happy and not tired.

Many studies on food attitudes have been made. Breckenridge[34] made a survey of the preferences of 51 grammar school pupils. They were questioned first about 25 specific food items. Fat meat was the one food disliked by more than half the children. All but one liked meat when prepared alone (not in a stew) and ice cream. Fish was the second least popular; cheese and meat mixtures were not far behind. Potatoes, bread, crackers, milk, raw fruits and cereal were high on the list of favorites. Candy and sweets were liked by 86 per cent of the children. Raw vegetables were

[34] Breckenridge, M. E.: Food attitudes of five- to twelve-year-old children. J. Am. Dietet. A., 35:704, 1959.

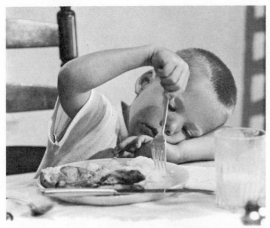

Figure 16–9   "Really tired or just dawdling?" (From Good Housekeeping, Feb., 1960. Courtesy of Suzanne Szasz.)

more popular than cooked, and raw fruits and juices were preferred to the canned or cooked products.

The largest number of specific dislikes was among the cooked vegetables, carrots and cabbage heading the list. Eggs were next, especially soft cooked. Grapefruit juice was not too popular. Antipathies to fish were common, but some admitted that what they objected to was "fish with bones."

FORCED FEEDING   A child should not be forced to eat; instead the cause for the unwillingness to eat should be determined. He may have a very good reason. A normal healthy child will eat without coaxing. Sometimes refusal of food is due to a child's being too inactive to make him hungry, or too active and overtired (Fig. 16–9). Overfatigue can be avoided by planning a short rest before meals or quiet enjoyment of a picture book (Fig. 16–10). An over-anxious parent can affect the appetite of the infant or child. Emotions can retard the flow of gastric juice and inhibit digestion.

If the child refuses to eat, the reason may be too much attention. Children enjoy the attention of their parents and soon learn that refusal to eat is one way to obtain it. Seeking of attention is necessary to satisfy the need for affection, a feeling of belonging. Food and eating contribute to cultural and emotional life as well as to physiological needs. Through food, the infant and child form a basic concept of the world in which they live, the people in it and their relationship to them.

If a child refuses to eat, the meal should be completed without comment and the child's plate removed. When mealtime again appears, he will be hungry enough to enjoy meat, vegetables, and milk. Such denial and discipline is usually harder on the parent than

on the child! However, the parent can display affection toward the child to prevent a feeling of not belonging.

WHERE THE CHILD SHOULD EAT   The subject of where the child should eat his meals is controversial. Some contend the child should eat his meals at the family table; others believe the child should sit in a small chair at a small table. Modern psychologists contend that it seems unfair to set the child apart from the family group. The child has an opportunity to learn table manners while enjoying meals with a happy, well-established family group. Sharing the family fare strengthens ties and makes mealtime a pleasure period. However, if the adult meal is delayed or there are adult guests, the child should receive his meal at the usual time. If the child has young visitors, he may wish to entertain them at his own little table at the usual meal hour. Regular meal hours are followed.

If a child does eat with the family, everyone must be careful not to make unfavorable comments about any food. Children are great imitators of someone they admire, so if father turns up his nose at squash, for example, they are likely to do the same. Parents sometimes have to learn to eat what they want their infant to like!

So much has been written about feeding both the problem and the well child that the nursery school bulletins and government sponsored pamphlets should be consulted.

FAMILY FOCUS IN FEEDING   From the nutritional standpoint the infant and/or child

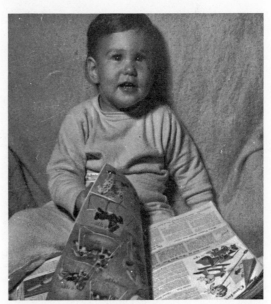

Figure 16–10   Overfatigue at meals can be avoided by planning a short rest before meals or quiet enjoyment of a picture book.

is not an isolated member of the family. While guiding parents in feeding the young, the nurse indirectly improves the entire family's diet, for the present and the future. By choosing and adapting suitable family foods for the baby and growing children, the whole family benefits by being well fed. Simple, wholesome foods, so good for the young members, can prove economical and adaptable when part of an over-all food plan, especially when the budget is restricted.

Most normal healthy children do best when their feeding is integrated with the total family food plan. This is sound child care as well as sound family economics. Each age and stage in life has its special nutritional requirements; and a family well fed has all its members on the road to good health. Infant feeding should be aimed toward life-long healthful living. In choosing the baby's diet, selection should be based on whole family foods.

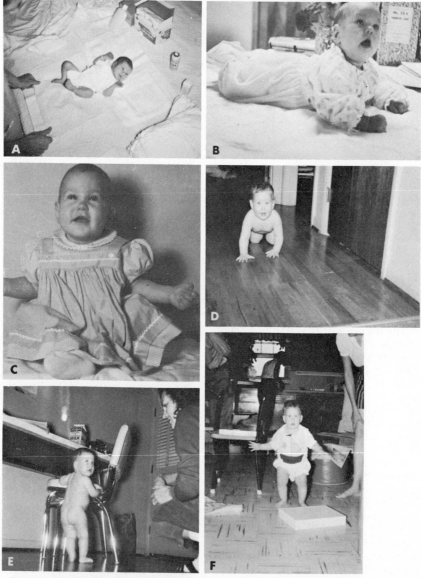

Figure 16–11   Stages in developmental growth of an infant during the first year. *A*, A newborn infant stays in the position in which he is placed. *B*, Lifting his chin and finally his head when lying on his stomach, a baby shows early signs of beginning muscle control, usually around 3 to 5 months. *C*, Sitting up unaided is the next big achievement, reached commonly between 6 and 8 months. *D*, Crawling starts between 7 and 9 months. *E*, He pulls himself up to standing at about 9 to 10 months. *F*, Standing alone and then walking alone may appear anywhere from 9 to 15 months.

DEVELOPMENTAL GROWTH

As the infant grows in size, height and weight, he is also making progress in what he does with his body and mind. He gains in understanding and body coordination. This is developmental growth. No two babies develop at the same rate, but each sets his own pace. Each is influenced by his environment, to which he reacts according to his own capacities. However, all babies follow the same general pattern. Figure 16–11 illustrates the usual order of a few of the significant physical achievements of a healthy well nourished infant during the first year. All stages are influenced by the diet and are subject to setbacks and deformities, both physical and mental, if the child is not properly nourished. (See Chapter 34, Nutritional Deficiency Diseases, and Chapter 36, Diet Therapy in Diseases of Infancy and Childhood.)

Infants should be encouraged to develop their natural desire to explore by being given surroundings and care that allow freedom for using their abilities. Let a baby finger and explore the food as much as he wishes. It is part of his development to find out the feel of scrambled eggs and oatmeal as well as their taste and smell. Food texture is important in forming likes and dislikes. The crispness of lettuce and carrots makes chewing fun; it is possible that infants consider whether this or that food is worth chewing by feel and appearance in much the same way as we look upon taste as a criterion in judging a meal.

PROBLEMS AND SUGGESTED TOPICS FOR DISCUSSION

1. Make a survey of the feeding formulas ordered for babies in your hospital. List the contents of the various formulas. What type of milk is used most frequently for the basis of the formula?
2. Observe for one week the feeding habits of a newborn baby who is bottle fed. How often is the infant fed and how much food is taken at each feeding? Observe and record the feeding habits of a breast-fed baby. Compare.
3. Are there any benefits in breast feeding over bottle feeding? Explain. When should formula feeding take precedence over breast feeding?
4. Make a study of the following proprietary foods: dried milk, acidified milk, vegetable-protein formulas, liquid whole milk, and meat base formula. Compare cost and food values. What are the major factors which determine the feeding used?
5. What procedure is used in your hospital for calculating infant formulas for the well baby? Calculate a feeding formula for a newborn baby in your hospital, using whole cow's milk as the basis for the formula.
6. When are supplementary foods usually added to the infant's diet? List the order in which the various foods may be introduced and reason for giving.
7. How much food is an infant in your hospital eating who is 1 year old? Check the diet for nutritional adequacy.
8. How do a premature baby's needs differ from those of a full-term baby?
9. How can you help the children in your family or friend's family form good food habits?
10. What special techniques and precautions need to be observed in the preparation of infant formulas? What method of formula preparation and sterilization is used in your hospital? Why? What is used in the out patient well baby clinic?
11. At what age are feeding problems likely to occur? What effect do emotions and attitudes have on an infant's eating habits?
12. What is meant by developmental growth? Do all infants develop at the same rate? Explain.

SUGGESTED ADDITIONAL READING REFERENCES

Adams, S. F.: Use of vegetables in infant feeding through the ages. J. Am. Dietet. A., 35:692, 1959.

Anderson, T. A., and Fomon, S. J.: Commercially prepared infants' cereals: Nutritional considerations. J. Pediat., 78:788, 1971.

Anderson, T. A., and Fomon, S. J.: Commercially prepared strained and junior foods for infants: Nutritional consideration. J. Am. Dietet. A. 58:520, 1971.

Arena, J. M.: Contamination of the ideal food. Nutrition Today, 5:2, 1970.

Beal, V. A.: An acceptance of solid foods and other food patterns of infants and children. Pediatrics, 20:448, 1957.

Beal, V. A.: Breast and formula feeding of infants. J. Am. Dietet. A., 55:31, 1969.

Bernstein, N.: Rehabilitating a child with a severe feeding problem. J. Am. Dietet. A., 36:131, 1960.

Farquhar, J. D.: Iron supplementation during first year of life. Am. J. Dis. Child, 106:201, 1963.

Fomon, S. J.: Infant Nutrition. Philadelphia, W. B. Saunders Company, 1967.

Fomon, S. J., Thomas, L. N., and Filer, L. J.: Acceptance of unsalted strained foods by normal infants. J. Pediat., 76:242, 1970.

Fries, J. H.: Milk allergy—Diagnostic aspects and the role of milk substitutes. J.A.M.A., 165:1542, 1957.

Gordon, H. H.: Protein allowances for premature infants. J.A.M.A., 175:107, 1961.

Guthrie, H. A.: Infant feeding practices—a predisposing factor in hypertension? Am. J. Clin. Nutr., 21:863, 1968.

Guthrie, H. A.: Nutritional intake of infants. J. Am. Dietet. A., 43:120, 1963.

Guthrie, H. A.: Evaluation of infant diets—Daily versus weekly collection; Physician versus nutritionist requests. Am. J. Clin. Nutr., 14:202, 1964.

Hansen, A. E., et al.: Role of linoleic acid in infant nutrition. Pediatrics, 31:171, 1963.

Hauck, H. M., and Tabrah, F. L.: Infant feeding and growth in Awo Omamma, Nigeria, J. Am. Dietet. A., 43:327, 1963.

Heinstein, M. I.: Influence of breast feeding on children's behavior. Children, 10:93, 1963.

Heseltine, M. M., and Pitts, J. L.: Economy in nutrition and feeding of infants. Am. J. Pub. Health, 56:1756, 1966.

Hirsch, J., and Knittle, J. L.: Cellularity of obese and nonobese human adipose tissue. Fed. Proc., 29:1516, 1970.

Holt, E. J., Jr., et al.: A study of premature infants fed a cold formula. J. Pediat., 61:556, 1962.

Holt, L. E., and Snyderman, S. E.: The effect of high caloric feeding on premature infants. J. Pediat. 58:237, 1961.

Holt, L. E., and Snyderman, S. E.: Protein and amino acid requirements of infant and children. Nutr. Abstr. Rev., 35:1, 1965.

Infant Care. U.S. Department of Health, Education, and Welfare, Welfare Administration, Children's Bureau, Publication No. 8, 1963.

Joint FAO/WHO Expert Committee on Protein Requirement. Nutr. Meet Report, Series No. 37, WHO Technical Report Series No. 301 (Rome), 1965.

Lahey, M. E.: Iron and copper in infant nutrition. Am. J. Clin. Nutr. 5:516, 1957.

Lowenberg, M. E.: Philosophy of nutrition and application in maternal health services. Am. J. Clin. Nutr., 16:370. 1965.

Lubchenko, L. O.: Formulas and nutrition. Am. J. Nursing, 61:73, 1961.

Matoth, Y., et al.: Studies on folic acid in infancy. III. Folates in breast fed infants and their mothers. Am. J. Clin. Nutr., 16:356, 1965.

Meyer, H. F.: Breast feeding in the United States. Clin. Pediat., 7:708, 1968.

Muto, S., et al.: Soybean products as protein sources for weaning infants. J. Am. Dietet. A., 43:451, 1963.

Owen, J. M.: Modification of cow's milk for infant formulas. Current practices. Am. J. Clin. Nutr., 22:1150, 1969.

Polansky, M. M., and Toepfer, E. W.: Vitamin B_6 components in some meats, fish, dairy products and commercial infant formulas. Agricultural and Food Chemistry, 17:1394, 1969.

Potgieter, M., and Morse, E. H.: Food habits of children. J. Am. Dietet. A., 31:794, 1955.

Pratt, E. L.: Dietary prescription of water, sodium, potassium, calcium and phosphorus for infants and children. Am. J. Clin. Nutr., 5:555, 1957.

Review. Cow's milk versus human milk protein in infant feeding. Nutr. Rev., 20:67, 1962.

Review. Diet and growth in infancy. Nutr. Rev., 21:327, 1963.

Review. Feeding premature infants. Nutr. Rev., 21:227, 1963; 22:108, 1964.

Review. Growth failure associated with maternal deprivation. Nutr. Rev., 21:229, 1963.

Review. Histidine requirement in infancy. Nutr. Rev., 22: 114, 1964.

Review. Linoleic acid in infant nutrition. Nutr. Rev., 22: 45, 1964.

Review. Nutrition functions of maternal and child health programs in technically underdeveloped areas. Nutr. Rev., 20:33, 1962.

Review. Tocopherol requirements in infancy. Nutr. Rev., 22:132, 1964.

Review. Vegetable protein in infant feeding. Nutr. Rev., 21:173, 1963.

Riveria, J.: The frequency of use of various kinds of milk during infancy in middle and lower-income families. Am. J. Pub. Health, 61:277, 1971.

Schulman, I.: Iron requirements in infancy. J.A.M.A., 175:118, 1961.

Stearns, G.: Food, The Yearbook of Agriculture, 1959. Washington, D.C., U. S. Department of Agriculture, pp. 283-295, Infants and Toddlers.

Stitt, G., and Heseltine, M. M.: Some practical consideration of economy and efficiency in infant feeding. Am. J. Pub. Health, 52:125, 1962.

Vaughan, V. C., III, et al.: A study of techniques of preparation of formulas for infant feeding. J. Pediat., 61: 547, 1962.

Williams, H. H.: Differences between cow's and human milk. J.A.M.A., 175:104, 1961.

Wohl, M. G., and Goodhart, R. S. (ed.): Modern Nutrition in Health and Disease. 4th ed. Philadelphia, Lea & Febiger, 1968.

Wood, A. L.: The history of artificial feeding of infants. J. Am. Dietet. A., 31:474, 1955.

Chapter 17
NUTRITION IN CHILDHOOD AND ADOLESCENCE

HEALTHY GROWTH AND DEVELOPMENT

Heredity and environment determine the way a child grows and the size and shape that he becomes. His genetic inheritance specifies how much his bones will grow and what kind of a physique he will have. His environment during the period of growth when cells multiply and increase in size may encourage or inhibit genetic possibilities. Growth of the young reflects individual health. Adequate nutrition and freedom from disease play important roles in determining whether an individual attains his potential. A harmful environment such as malnutrition and dis-

ease disrupts normal growth patterns. Development, that is, the changes in growth of an individual, is a continuous orderly process. It is progressive and leads eventually to maturity. The rate (or age) at which growth and development takes place varies with each individual. The danger of accepting any "standard measurement" of growth and development is the tendency to hold too rigidly to exact figures. An individual must be assessed according to many factors attributing to his growth and development. The nutritional requirements vary with chronological age, growth rate, maturational stage, physical activity, efficiency of absorption and utilization of the nutrients.

Healthy growth and development depend more upon good nutrition than any other factor. Oettinger[1] states that "From the beginnings of growth in the prenatal period to the time when the child attains his full size as an adult, the food that he eats and his ability to convert that food into energy and new body tissues will influence the state of his health not only as a child but throughout life."

For convenience in classification, the following age grouping is used in this text to designate the various *stages of growth and development* of the child:

Infant—Birth to 1 year.
Preschool child—1 year to 6 years.
School child—6 years to 12 years.
Adolescent—13 years to 19 years.
Adult—20 years and on.

RATES OF GROWTH   There are four phases of growth (height and weight): a period of very rapid growth during infancy; a period of slower but fairly uniform gain throughout early and middle childhood; a period of marked acceleration during adolescence; and a period of gradual decline of growth until its cessation.

NUTRITIONAL ALLOWANCES

It is very important that the diet be nutritionally adequate throughout childhood. (See Table 11–1, Chapter 11.) The recommended dietary allowances (RDA) represent the level of intake of the nutrients children in each age group require for optimal health. They are designed to provide a margin above physiological requirements of individuals in the general population. The recommendations applied to an individual child may be misleading. One cannot assume that a child is inadequately nourished if his intake falls below the recommended allowances. Another child's intake of the nutrients may come close to the recommended allowances and yet the child may be overweight. The requirements of children vary widely even within the same age group, the short versus the tall, the small frame versus the large frame, the boy versus the girl. Throughout infancy and early middle childhood, boys are usually taller and heavier than girls. However, during early or preadolescence the reverse is true. When girls are 11 to 12 years old, they grow very rapidly and, during this period, they are actually larger than boys of the same age. They require almost the same amount of food es-

sentials as boys, and often more than their mothers. Their growth impulse reaches its maximum at approximately 13 years and starts to slacken about the period that the boys start their accelerated growth. Boys grow rapidly when they are about 15 years old, and soon regain their superiority in size.

During the period of adolescence, the nutritional requirements are increased to such an extent that it is sometimes difficult to meet them. To provide for this accelerated growth, the diet must include adequate amounts of all food essentials.

There are three functions of the diet for the child: The food must (1) provide fuel for muscular activity, (2) supply the necessary chemical elements and compounds the child's body requires for building new tissues (growth) and the repair of worn-out tissues, and (3) give pleasure and satisfaction to the child.

Because growing children are building bones, teeth, muscles and blood, they need more nutritious food in proportion to their weight than adults. If children are to grow strong and be normal and healthy, they must eat, digest and absorb enough proteins, fats, carbohydrates, minerals and vitamins to meet the body needs. All the body organs do not develop at the same rate of speed. After infancy, height assumes greater importance than weight. Although heredity determines stature, diet and disease exert a marked influence. The progressive increase in height of children over the years is believed to be due, in part, to improved economic conditions, better diets, and advances in medical care and health services.

CALORIES   The energy or calorie requirement of the child is determined by his basal metabolism, age and activity. To simplify the process of calculation, consult Table 19–2, p. 309, which gives the recommended calorie allowances for energy requirements for all age groups. Of the total calorie intake, a suggested proportion is 50 to 60 per cent in carbohydrates, 25 to 35 per cent in fats, and the remaining amount (10 to 15 per cent) in protein. (See also Table 19–3, p. 313.) Because of the wide individual variation in physical activity in children, it is difficult to determine a standardized amount of food. However, checking on the child's weight, growth, and general state of well-being will help to serve as a guide.

The Recommended Dietary Allowances for different age groups issued by the Food and Nutrition Board, National Academy of Sciences—National Research Council, serves as an excellent guide for the calorie needs of children for the heights and weights given in the table. However, variations for the

[1]Oettinger, K. B.: Nutrition and healthy Growth. Children's Bureau Pub. No. 352, 1955, U.S. Dept. of Health, Education, and Welfare, Social Security Administration, p. ii.

individual child must be considered. (See Table 11–1, Chapter 11.)

FLUIDS   The total daily fluid requirement for a normal healthy child is 4 to 6 glasses, 1 to 1½ quarts, or 1000 to 1500 ml.

PROTEIN   The child's protein requirements are relatively higher in relation to body weight than those of an adult. While exact protein requirements have not been established for children, there is considerable evidence that low levels of protein intake are harmful. (See Protein Deficiency, Ch. 34.) The recommended daily allowances indicate that the protein need per kg. of body weight decreases from 2.5 to 3 gm. in early childhood to 1.5 to 2 gm. in late childhood and adolescence. (See Table 11–1, Chapter 11.) The Food and Nutrition Board protein calculations indicate that the proportion of dietary protein requirement for growth is large in the early years of life only. The total need for unit body weight falls continuously to the adult level, and the increased rate of growth during puberty does not greatly increase the need.

There is considerable variation in the time of growth phases among individuals, but all phases follow the same general pattern. An adequate protein intake for the child is one which contains sufficient amounts of all the known essential amino acids in palatable and digestible form to cover maintenance needs besides providing an extra amount for protein deposition compatible with normal growth. Therefore, the protein should be of high biologic value. The Food and Nutrition Board protein allowances recommended for children after infancy provide approximately 10 to 15 per cent of the child's total calorie intake as protein, of which one half to two thirds of the protein is derived from animal or other sources of high quality. These allowances are estimated to provide approximately twice the minimal need for the average child and allow a reasonable margin for the rapidly growing child.

Research studies with rats have revealed that when any one of the essential amino acids of proteins is omitted from the diet, normal growth does not follow (Fig. 6–1). It can be interpreted that some of the amino acids assume an important role, similar to the important role of the vitamins, to maintain normal nutrition and promote healthy life processes.

Milk is one of the important foods needed to meet the protein requirements. Children under 9 years should have two to three cups daily, and those from 9 to 12 years of age, three or more cups; teen-agers need one quart or more. The child of 2, 3 or even 4 years prefers his milk room temperature or lukewarm, and not icy cold. It has been observed that the amount a child takes is related to the temperature. Meats and eggs are equally important foods to provide protein in the diet. The remainder of the protein requirements can be met by including breads, cereals, potatoes, fruits, vegetables and desserts.

MINERALS AND VITAMINS   Minerals and vitamins are necessary for normal growth and development. Insufficient vitamin and mineral intake can cause many varied deficiency diseases which are described in Chapter 34, Nutritional Deficiency Diseases, and Chapter 36, Diet Therapy in Diseases of Infancy and Childhood. Adequate milk intake will cover many of the mineral and vitamin requirements. Three cups of milk contain approximately 0.8 gm. of calcium and enough phosphorus to ensure proper bone and tooth formation. For good measure, it adds a rich supply of vitamin A, riboflavin, vitamin D and vitamin B_{12}, and some thiamin and niacin.

The iron requirement will be met by an adequate intake of the protective foods but calls for careful attention to the selection of foods that are good sources of iron and foods that are fortified with iron. The Food and Nutrition Board daily iron allowances recommended were 15 mg. for the age period 1 to 3 years; 10 mg. for the age period 3 to 10 years and 18 mg. for ages 12 to 18 for both girls and boys. After 18 years of age 10 mg. is believed to be sufficient for males. The allowance remains at 18 mg. for females for adequate storage of iron against the hazard of drain on reserves of iron during the menses or pregnancy and lactation. The need for iodine is increased during puberty and should be given consideration.

Some source of vitamin D (400 I.U. daily) is needed throughout the growth period, and continued use of fish liver oil or fortified milk is recommended through the school years and adolescence. The Recommended Dietary Allowances for different age groups, set up by the Food and Nutrition Board, National Academy of Sciences–National Research Council, list the various mineral and vitamin requirements. (See Table 11–1, Chapter 11.) In a study[2] concerning nutritive value of food fed to 40 infants ranging in age from 9 months to 2 years, ascorbic acid, thiamin and iron were the nutrients most frequently found to be below the recommended allowances. In young children calcium, iron, ascorbic acid and vitamin A are the most common deficiencies. These deficiencies are found in older children as well.

[2]Guthrie, H. A.: Nutritional intake of infants. J. Am. Dietet. A., 43:120, 1963.

THE ADEQUATE DIET

The nucleus of an adequate diet for the child is presented. Such a pattern is the basis for all normal and therapeutic diets for children. If these foods are included in the daily diet, the protein, mineral and vitamin requirements will be met. Additional foods are added to this nucleus to meet the individual energy requirements. (See p. 162.)

THE NUCLEUS OF AN ADEQUATE DIET PATTERN FOR A CHILD

FOOD	AMOUNT PER DAY
Milk, vitamin D fortified	Children 1 pt. to 1 qt. depending on age Adolescents 1 qt. or more
Butter or fortified margarine and vegetable oil	At least 4 teaspoons
Eggs	1
Meat, fish, poultry or equivalent	1 or 2 servings
Whole grain or enriched cereals and breads	4 or more servings
Vegetables	2 servings besides potatoes, 1 dark green, leafy or deep yellow
Fruits	2 servings, 1 of them a citrus fruit

TABLE 17–1   FOODS INCLUDED IN A GOOD DAILY DIET
(AVERAGE AMOUNTS FOR EACH AGE)

FOOD	PRE-SCHOOL 3–5 YEARS OLD	EARLY ELEMENTARY 6–9 YEARS OLD	LATER ELEMENTARY 10–12 YEARS OLD	EARLY TEENS 13–15 YEARS OLD
Milk	2 cups	2–3 cups	3 cups or more	3–4 cups or more
Eggs	1 whole egg	1 whole egg	1 whole egg	1 or more whole eggs
Meat, poultry, fish	2 ounces ($1/4$ cup) (1 small serving)	2–3 ounces (1 small serving)	3–4 ounces (1 serving)	4 ounces or more (1 serving)
Dried beans, peas (Also an occasional replacement for meat, poultry or fish)	3–4 tablespoons	4–5 tablespoons	5–6 tablespoons	$1/2$ cup or more
Potatoes (May occasionally be replaced by equal amount enriched macaroni, spaghetti or rice)	3–4 tablespoons	4–5 tablespoons	$1/2$ cup or more	$3/4$ cup or more
Other cooked vegetables (Often a green leafy or deep yellow vegetable)	3–4 tablespoons at one or more meals	4–5 tablespoons at one or more meals	$1/3$ cup or more at one or more meals	$1/2$ cup or more at one or more meals
Raw vegetables (Lettuce, carrots, celery, etc.)	2 or more small pieces	$1/4$ cup	$1/3$ cup	$1/2$ cup or more
Vitamin C food (Citrus fruits, tomatoes, etc.)	1 medium-size orange or equivalent	1 medium-size orange or equivalent	1 medium-size orange or equivalent	1 large orange or equivalent
Other fruits	$1/3$ cup at one or more meals	$1/2$ cup or more at one or more meals	$1/2$ cup or more at one or more meals	2 servings
Cereal, whole grain restored or enriched	$1/2$ cup or more	$3/4$ cup or more	1 cup or more	1 cup or more
Bread, whole grain or enriched	2 or more slices	2 or more slices	2 or more slices	2 or more slices
Butter or fortified margarine	1 tablespoon	1 tablespoon	1 tablespoon or more	1 tablespoon or more
Sweets	$1/3$ cup simple dessert at 1 or 2 meals	$1/2$ cup simple dessert at 1 or 2 meals	$1/2$ cup or more simple dessert at 1 or 2 meals	$1/2$ cup or more at 1 or 2 meals
Vitamin D source	Enough to provide 400 U.S.P. units of vitamin D daily			
Recommended allowances	1600 kcal. 40 grams protein	2100 kcal. 52 grams protein	Girls: 2200 kcal. 55 grams protein Boys: 2400 kcal. 60 grams protein	Girls: 2500 kcal. 62 grams protein Boys: 3000 kcal. 75 grams protein

From Foods for Growing Boys and Girls. Department of Home Economics Services, Battle Creek, Mich., The Kellogg Company, 1964. (Personal Communication)

THE PRESCHOOL CHILD
(AGE 1 TO 6 YEARS)

By the time the baby is 1 year old, good feeding habits should be established. The baby's meals have been increased to include milk, cereals, eggs, breadstuffs, butter or fortified margarine, meats, soups, vegetables, crisp bacon, fruits, and puddings. (See Chapter 16, Nutrition in Infancy.) Because the baby's teeth have developed, the selection of food should include those which will encourage chewing. Although the baby's size and individual requirements govern the amount of foods, the choice for daily meals is selected from whole grain or enriched breads and cereals, milk, egg, meat, fish or poultry, butter or fortified margarine, vegetables, fruits, fruit juices, cheese, and ice cream or milk puddings. If good eating habits are to be established early in the child's life, many bothersome complaints can be avoided. Solid protein foods containing iron (meat, eggs) should be fed along with milk. Unlimited milk consumption which leads to neglect of other necessary foods should be discouraged. A wide variety of foods is the best plan to assure an adequate diet at all ages. (See Table 17–1.)

As the child passes the fast-growing period of infancy, and into the 1 to 3 year age, he becomes more selective and more independent about food. This period is sometimes difficult because the appetite wanes, the rate of growth is slow and irregular, weight often drops, and the child is beginning to find wider horizons of activity offering greater interests. Desire for food becomes erratic and reaches a noticeable drop in consumption of food between the second and third years, and the child may go for weeks or even months without gaining an ounce. The "won't eat" era is a normal phase of development, and is much harder on the parents than the child. Table 17–2 shows the mother's concern about the eating behavior of preschool children of various ages. It is during this period that the nurse and parents must be careful not to foster poor eating habits by overanxious urging or bribing the child to eat. Appetite usually tends to improve as the child approaches school age, and an increase in growth and weight is bound to follow.

Protein-calorie malnutrition—as pointed out (Chapter 34)—is prevalent in preschool children around the world. The preschool child belongs to the most vulnerable age group with respect to certain physical and social needs. Unfortunately, this is the age group being reached least effectively. Younger children in the home place priority demands on the mother and are most difficult to reach with services from outside the home. If the child attains school age he has a reasonably good chance of matriculating where special aids to health and social development are available. (See Figs. 17–1 and 17–2.) The World Food Program (WFP), UNICEF, FAO, WHO, and government projects have organ-

TABLE 17–2   MOTHER'S CONCERN OF EATING BEHAVIOR OF PRESCHOOL CHILDREN

CONCERNS	0 TO 3 MOS. (%)	3 TO 6 MOS. (%)	6 TO 9 MOS. (%)	9 TO 1 YR. (%)	1 TO 1½ YR. (%)	1½ TO 2 YR. (%)	2 TO 3 YR. (%)	3 TO 4 YR. (%)	4 TO 5 YR. (%)	5 TO 6 YR. (%)	TOTAL (%)
Chooses limited variety	2.6	8.7	12.0	24.6	34.1	37.6	40.3	41.2	44.8	34.2	35.8
Dawdles with food	10.3	3.1	15.5	14.6	34.1	25.7	36.8	43.8	39.7	33.3	33.5
Eats too little fruits and vegetables	0.0	2.4	12.9	14.5	15.8	29.4	27.2	27.5	27.9	27.1	23.9
Eats too many sweets	0.0	0.0	0.0	1.4	4.7	7.8	26.3	28.9	27.9	26.4	20.7
Eats too little meat	0.9	4.7	7.2	22.5	22.6	30.3	22.3	21.6	24.0	17.7	20.5
Eats too little food	8.5	2.4	8.2	10.1	14.7	13.8	21.6	28.3	21.1	22.8	19.9
Drinks too little milk	0.0	3.9	4.8	10.9	10.8	16.5	20.1	18.6	18.7	18.5	16.3
Drinks too much milk	9.4	7.9	7.1	5.1	10.0	13.8	10.0	7.1	7.1	5.9	8.0
Eats too much food	7.7	4.7	8.2	8.7	5.1	3.7	2.7	3.1	5.4	6.4	4.9
Eats too much meat	0.0	0.0	0.0	0.0	1.4	5.0	3.5	4.4	4.3	5.9	3.7
Number	117	127	84	138	279	218	551	610	691	628	3444

From Eppright, E. S., et al.: Eating behavior of preschool children. J. Nutr. Ed., 1:16, 1969. (This paper is published as Journal Paper No. J-5983 of the Iowa Agriculture and Home Economics Experiment Station, Ames, Iowa. Project No. 1532 contributing to North Central Regional Project No. 75.)

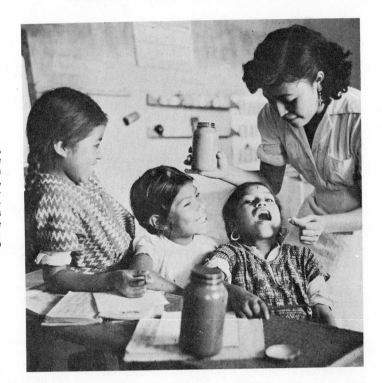

Figure 17–1   Babies, young children, expectant and nursing mothers are the first victims of the shortage of certain key foods. Under the direction of INCAP, field workers carry out surveys and initiate measures to combat deficiency diseases. In an Indian village, a nurse gives prophylactic vitamin B_{12} tablets to the schoolchildren. (Courtesy of Pan-American Sanitary Bureau, Regional WHO Office.)

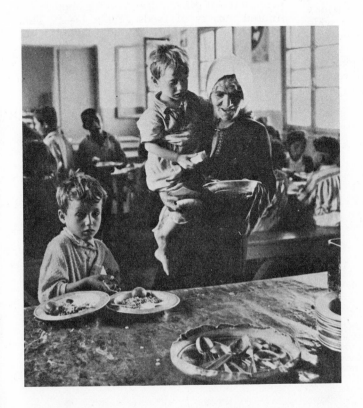

Figure 17–2   Refugee children are seen eating a supplementary meal at the Jebel Hassein Camp near Amman, Jordan. To protect vulnerable groups—pregnant and nursing mothers, children, TB outpatients—supplementary feeding centers provide meals in each camp. (Courtesy of FAO of United Nations.)

ized a program[3] to establish permanent distribution channels (mainly commercial) which provide special food mixtures for preschool children. These mixtures are cereal-based, precooked foods designed for children and are similar to those available in supermarkets of developed countries. The projects are planned to provide a vehicle for use of new protein-rich foods.

Two-, 3- and 4-year-olds want to identify food. They seem to prefer simple foods rather than mixed dishes. Finger foods are enjoyed. Gravies and cream sauces are not popular. Food jags are common with the 4- and 5-year-old. The 5- and 6-year-old youngsters are imitators. Lewin determined how children perceive food—as conflict, praise or scold food, according to the authority in the home. Food aversions, based on those foods actually tasted and rejected, develop for many reasons. Emotional experiences at the table, unpleasant associations aroused by food, fear of the new and strange foods are some of the attitudes toward food that are learned in childhood. They need to be recognized and prevented early in life.

Colorful, attractive and easy to handle and eat foods are appealing. The environment and utensils which are conducive to enjoyment and ease of handling foods encourage curiosity and successful eating patterns.

An adequate meal contains sufficient calories for energy needs and a complete protein (one protein food or a combination of foods which supply all essential amino acids). A good meal may be obtained from a wide selection of foods to provide the necessary nutrients.

The following is a suggested meal plan[4] for a preschool child which would require very little, if any, adjustments in the pattern to use for the whole family.

BREAKFAST

Fruit or juice
Cereal with milk or meat, eggs, fish
Toast or roll
Butter or margarine
Milk

LUNCH OR SUPPER

Main dish—mainly meat, eggs, fish, poultry,
   dried beans or peas, cheese, peanut butter
Vegetable or salad
Bread
Butter or margarine
Dessert or fruit
Milk

DINNER

Meat, poultry, or fish
Vegetable
Potato or substitute
Raw vegetable
Bread
Butter or margarine
Fruit or pudding
Milk

Midmorning and midafternoon snacks usually continue for this age group, unless they interfere with the appetite at mealtime. Good snacks, which are part of the whole day's plan and will make a real contribution to his nourishment, might include (see Fig. 17–3):[4]

Dry cereal, with milk or out of the box
Simple cookie or Graham cracker
Raw vegetables
Canned, fresh, or dried fruit
Toast, plain or cinnamon
Cheese wedge
Fruit sherbet or ice cream
Fruit juice
Milk
Fruit drinks made with milk and juice

A survey[5] of the eating behavior of over 3000 preschool children ranging in age from birth to 6 years representing 2000 households of moderate to marginal income living in the North Central Region of the United States revealed that mothers have many concerns about eating habits of their preschool children. The major concern for the greatest percentage of the children was the choice of a limited variety of foods (Table 17–2). The concern about dawdling and playing with food and eating too little food reached the highest peak in the 3- to 4-year-olds. An appreciable concern for eating too many sweets

---

[5]Eppright, E. J., et al.: Eating behavior of preschool children. J. Nutr. Ed., 1:16, 1969.

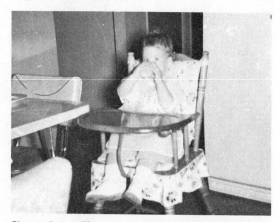

Figure 17–3   This 14-month-old child is enjoying a between-meal glass of milk but also eats meals of good variety.

---

[3]Teply, L. J.: Nutritional needs of the pre-school child. Nutr. Rev., 22:65, 1964.
[4]From: Your Child from One to Six. U.S. Department of Health, Education, and Welfare, Children's Bureau Publication No. 30, 1962.

appeared in mothers of children 2 years of age and remained through the sixth year in over 25 per cent of the group surveyed. Consumption of milk for children less than 1 year of age averaged 3 or more cups daily. From one year of age on, the mean daily milk intakes approximated 2½ cups. The peak of the consumption of milk reported in this survey and others[6] appeared around 6 months of age and decreased toward the end of the first year or early in the second year. Boys averaged greater intake of milk than did girls. The vegetables most frequently disliked are spinach, carrots, green beans and peas (in the order listed). Dislikes of vegetables are closely associated with those of older siblings. The tendency for the foods disliked by the children was associated more with the dislikes of the fathers and older brothers than with mothers and older sisters. Preschool children, beginning in the 2- to 3-year-old group, in this survey made food selection decisions more often at breakfast and snack periods than at other times. However, the study indicated that almost half the children enter school with little experience in making decisions about food selection.

Beal observed that a smooth curve representing nutrient requirements by age tends to correspond to weight and height curves. Early in infancy the curve rises rapidly but with decreasing acceleration. Appetite, food intake and weight gain are usually erratic in the preschool years. These have been associated with changes in growth rate. Much more investigation of the eating behavior of children needs to be done. A lack of understanding of the physiological and psychological changes taking place in children as they pass through the toddler phase into the early preschool years may cause problems. The resolution of the problems and concerns of mothers has implications for nutrition education.

THE SCHOOL CHILD (AGE 6 TO 12 YEARS)

During the early school years growth in height and weight is slow but steady. A child may add 10 or 12 inches to his height and 30 to 35 pounds to his weight. There is a relatively constant increase in food intake.

Going to school brings new problems. The meal schedule must be spaced in relation to the school routine, rather than to the child's needs or desires. He has to decide whether he wants to eat lunch in the school cafeteria or carry it from home. The decision often rests on the practices of his peers. However, the excitement of school, new contacts and

routine when approached as a new challenge helps to continue or promote good eating habits and regular meals. There should be sufficient time for eating all meals, including an adequate breakfast. Calm, unhurried meals contribute to good digestion and appetite.

The school child, 6 to 12 years of age, requires the same basic foods as when he was younger, but the quantities are increased to take care of his greater needs. His energy needs gradually increase and approach the same as adults during this period. His eating habits and attitudes toward food vacillate. Teachers and scout leaders as well as peers influence the selection of food positively and negatively. He seems to prefer meat, potatoes, bread, crackers, milk, ice cream, cereals and raw fruit and dislikes fat meat, fish, cooked vegetables, cheese, mixed meat and egg dishes. His intake of protein, calcium, vitamin A and ascorbic acid is apt to be low. The intake of highly seasoned, poorly fried foods, pastries, tea, coffee, chocolate and sweets should be discouraged. They provide empty calories and usually take away appetite for nutritious foods.

At school, the child should be provided with a hot lunch from the school lunch program, or brought from home, rather than candies, cookies, and sweetened bottled beverages from a snack bar. (Review section on School Lunch Programs in Chapter 2.) Instruction in how to select a good lunch—kinds and amounts of foods needed daily to develop a healthy body—should be started early in the home and continued at school. One way to help the child to want to eat wisely is to convince him that what he eats really does make a difference in the way he grows. Children at this age all desire to grow normally and to be like their peers. They are ready to learn about the relationship of food to a healthy body.

THE ADOLESCENT OR TEENAGER (AGE 12 TO 18 YEARS)

As previously stated, the adolescent years are the second period of rapid rate of growth, but vary greatly for individuals even of the same chronologic age. These years are also about the most active period of life. Because of the double demands of activity and growth, food needs are high and extremely important. (See Table 17–3 for daily dietary requirements for ages 12 to 18 years.)

The adolescent boy usually has a tremendous appetite, and if provided with adequate amounts of protective foods, will have no trouble meeting the dietary needs. Adolescent girls sometimes have finicky appetites, and nutritional counseling is advisable to assist them improve their dietary. Both sexes tend to assert their independence as "almost

[6]Beal, V.: Dietary intake of individuals followed through infancy and childhood. Am. J. Pub. Health, 51:1107, 1961.

TABLE 17–3   RECOMMENDED DAILY DIETARY ALLOWANCES FOR PUBESCENTS AND ADOLESCENTS (12 TO 18 YEARS)

	BOYS		GIRLS		
	12–14 YEARS	14–18 YEARS	12–14 YEARS	14–16 YEARS	16–18 YEARS
WEIGHT	43 KG. (95 POUNDS)	59 KG. (130 POUNDS)	44 KG. (97 POUNDS)	52 KG. (114 POUNDS)	54 KG. (119 POUNDS)
HEIGHT	151 CM. (59 INCHES)	170 CM. (67 INCHES)	154 CM. (61 INCHES)	157 CM. (62 INCHES)	160 CM. (63 INCHES)
K calories	2,700	3,000	2,300	2,400	2,300
Protein	50 gm.	60 gm.	50 gm.	55 mg.	55 gm.
Fat-soluble vitamins					
Vitamin A activity	5,000 I.U.	5,000 I.U.	5,000 I.U.	5,000 I.U.	5,000 I.U.
Vitamin D	400 I.U.	400 I.U.	400 I.U.	400 I.U.	400 I.U.
Vitamin E activity	20 I.U.	25 I.U.	20 I.U.	25 I.U.	25 I.U.
Water-soluble vitamins					
Ascorbic acid	45 mg.	55 mg.	45 mg.	50 mg.	50 mg.
Folacin[a]	0.4 mg.	0.4 mg.	0.4 mg.	0.4 mg.	0.4 mg.
Niacin equivalents[b]	18 mg.	20 mg.	15 mg.	16 mg.	15 mg.
Riboflavin	1.4 mg.	1.5 mg.	1.4 mg.	1.4 mg.	1.5 mg.
Thiamin	1.4 mg.	1.5 mg.	1.2 mg.	1.2 mg.	1.2 mg.
Vitamin B_6	1.6 mg.	1.8 mg.	1.6 mg.	1.8 mg.	2.0 mg.
Vitamin B_{12}	5 μg.	5 μg.	5 μg.	5 μg.	5 μg.
Minerals					
Calcium	1.4 gm.	1.4 gm.	1.3 gm.	1.3 gm.	1.3 gm.
Phosphorus	1.4 gm.	1.4 gm.	1.3 gm.	1.3 gm.	1.3 gm.
Iodine	135 μg.	150 μg.	115 μg.	120 μg.	115 μg.
Iron	18 mg.	18 mg.	18 mg.	18 mg.	18 mg.
Magnesium	350 mg.	400 mg.	350 mg.	350 mg.	350 mg.

[a]The folacin allowances refer to dietary sources as determined by *Lactobacillus casei* assay. Pure forms of folacin may be effective in doses less than ¼ of the RDA.

[b]Niacin equivalents include dietary sources of the vitamin itself plus 1 mg. equivalent for each 60 mg. of dietary tryptophan.

From the Food and Nutrition Board, National Academy of Sciences—National Research Council: Recommended Daily Dietary Allowances (1968).

adults," and as a demonstration of rejecting parental restriction may reject the basic foods in favor of sweets, soft drinks and "snack" foods with empty calories. Of particular concern are the teenage girls who decrease their food intake when their need for nutrients is greatest. Girls, more often than boys, are likely to omit or restrict essential foods, particularly milk, bread and potatoes, in an effort to reduce or to keep thin for the sake of appearance. Skipping breakfast and other meals often results from the teenager's time schedule not coinciding with the family meal schedule. For example, meeting the "gang" or being on time for a date are more important than meals. Teenagers want to be popular with their peers.

Nutritional counseling of teenagers requires a careful approach in order to arouse their interest and motivation to do something about their nutritional status. They welcome challenging problem-solving situations. Efforts to involve them in the problems of obtaining and maintaining good nutritional status are rewarding and usually have a lasting effect. Teenagers respond to your acceptance of what they eat, emphasis on what is good about their diet and eating habits, and involvement in the resolution of their own problems. When given the information needed to improve their own diet, teenagers are apt to convince themselves of the relationship between good nutrition, appearance, energy, growth and development. Appearance is important to adolescents. Girls are interested in their dress size, skin, hair, eyes, body curves; boys are interested in their skin and development of muscles. With an understanding of the relationship of nutrition to appearance and physical prowess these motivating forces play an important role in improving nutritional status. Teenage leaders who exemplify good nutritional appearance are more effective counselors with their peers than are adults. Cooperative efforts on the part of parents, teachers, community leaders, school lunch supervisors, nurses, doctors, nutritionists, extension agents and others are essential in meaningful nutrition education for effective changes in the behavior of teenagers.

UNDERWEIGHT AND OVERWEIGHT

The problems of weight are of considerable concern to the adolescent. A significant number of this group are underweight or overweight. More girls than boys have underweight and overweight problems. Undernutrition implies that the individual has not had a sufficient supply of calories and one or more of the essential nutrients over a long period of time. His nutritional status is poor as the result of several factors. When an individual is 10 per cent or more below the standard appropriate for his height and body frame, he is considered to be underweight. The incidence of tuberculosis is high in adolescence. Evidence suggests that the onset of tuberculosis, speed of recovery and rate of re-infection is related to poor nutritional status, especially in the underweight teenager.

About one third of adolescents studied are overweight. Overnutrition implies that the individual's caloric intake has been in excess of energy needs over a period of time. The problem of teenage obestity is a very real one in the United States and is a subject for considerable physiological and psychological study. Teenagers are "dieting" whether they need to or not. Girls especially have a fear of becoming fat. Many girls who are not overweight as well as overweight girls put themselves on diets and are easy marks for current "reducing fads." The resulting erratic eating habits leads to a poor nutritional status. The fluctuation in weight which many overweight teenagers experience when dieting is physiologically unsound and psychologically frustrating. Inadequate levels of nutrients are unavailable to the body at times when the demand for growth is high and the inability to maintain loss of weight is discouraging. When calories and activity balance, weight is maintained. Activity of the overweight teenager plays a role in the weight control problem. The consideration of both calorie restriction, including all essential nutrients, and suitable activity for the overweight individual are important in any weight reduction program. (See Chapter 29, Overweight and Underweight.)

FOOD HABITS The nutritional problems of teenagers appear to be correlated or related to eating habits. Their dietary intake is cause for much concern for several reasons. During this period of accelerated physical and emotional growth very often the adolescent is under considerable stress and anxiety, which are reflected in physiological, psychological and social behavior. All these interrelated behaviors are manifested in poor eating habits, poor selection of foods, irregular hours of eating and omission of meals. These dietary practices extended for any length of time result in poor nutritional status. Attitudes about and aversions toward food during this period of life may continue indefinitely and may be passed on to future generations. In girls experiencing an excessive amount of excitement and emotional stress negative nitrogen and calcium balances have been noted.

The adolescent who becomes pregnant during this period of growth and development faces many more physiological and psychological conditions than older females. Most of these are due to the fact that her own body growth and development between the ages of 12 and 17 are not completed. (After 17 years of age growth in the majority of girls is generally completed.) When the younger teenager approaches conception, she has difficulty providing for her own physical (and psychological) needs and the demands of the growing fetus, especially if her nutritive intake has been inadequate. Pregnancy at this time presents many risks which are related to nutrition.

Athletes eagerly rely on foods to provide the physical stamina to participate in school sports. Belief that certain foods will enable the athlete to do more and better work, win more medals or gain greater victories has existed for some time. Coaches have been known to promote special regimens and to advocate certain restrictions. Many theories have been advanced such as a high protein diet, and diets including no milk or a considerable amount of milk have been suggested to promote better performance. It is known that a well-balanced diet of normal foods provide all the protein an athlete requires for maximum performance. He may need 3000 to 4000 or more kcalories daily to meet the energy needs. The foods to supply energy may include more protein than the non-active individual requires. Exercise does not lead to a significant increase in the amount of protein metabolized even after glycogen stores have been used. Protein is not a special fuel for working muscle cells but fats and carbohydrates are. Fat is the fuel source during mild exercise and carbohydrate for more vigorous exercise. Glycogen stores are very important for larger and better performance. A program of no milk or considerable milk has shown no difference in athletic performance. Excessive weight reduction or a strenuous dietary regimen is deplored in adolescent athletes. Water and salt intake is important during strenuous exercise.

BREAKFAST An important meal of the day most often skipped or hurried is breakfast. Studies conducted at the University of Iowa show that it is difficult to supply the recommended nutrients for the day without a good morning meal. Foods usually eaten for breakfast provide nutrients such as calcium, riboflavin and ascorbic acid and these may not be obtained at any other time of the day either in meals or as snack foods. Children who did not eat breakfast or had inadequate breakfasts were more fatigued, less attentive and were unable to achieve as much as those who had better breakfasts. Those who ate breakfast worked, played and were sharper in thinking and action during the late morning hours. Breakfasts of equal calorie value but low in protein and high in fat or carbohydrate do not have this effect. Breakfasts with adequate protein elevate the blood glucose level above fasting level for approximately four hours after the meal while meals with less than adequate protein but high in fat and carbohydrate elevate the glucose level for about two and three hours respectively. Within approximately an hour after a carbohydrate breakfast of the same isocaloric value, the blood glucose rises to a peak and by the end of the second hour it falls to the fasting level. One fourth to one third of the day's food allowance at breakfast is recommended. A variety of foods other than the traditional breakfast foods could meet the criteria of an adequate breakfast. Many rationalizations are given for not eating breakfast—lack of time, lack of appetite in the morning, preference for sleeping longer, no one to prepare food.

SNACKS   Snack time is an important social occasion, especially to teenagers, and seems to be here to stay. Choice of foods eaten at snack time is influenced by members of the group. They often may not improve the diet that needs improvement. It has been observed among teenage girls that as calories from snacks in the form of candy and soft drinks increase, calories from breakfast decrease. Choice of food for snacks can be those that supply essential nutrients and need not spoil the appetite for meals. Sandwiches, fruits and milk products are appropriate snack foods. Foods such as candy, carbonated beverages and concentrated sweets supply empty calories and usually take away appetite for other foods. Snacks should be considered as a part of the day's food and should contribute to the total nutrient supply.

In addition to supplying energy for activity and meeting the demands of rapid growth, proper food habits in growing-up years contribute to the individual's good health and well-being as an adult. As parents of tomorrow, these young people will be better able to bear children and teach their own children sound food habits. This is also sound advice for the student nurse.

DIETARY ALLOWANCES   Up to ten years of age the calorie allowance for children of both sexes is about 80 kcalories per kg. of body weight. After 10 years of age, the kcalorie values gradually decline to 50 for adolescent males and 35 for adolescent females (RDA). After nine years of age, three are major differences in growth rates between the sexes and therefore separate recommended allowances are given for boys and girls. (See Table 17–3.) Interpretation of the values requires caution. Physical activity of individuals varies considerably. Inactive individuals may become obese even when calorie intake is below the recommended allowances and extremely active children need larger allowances. Approximately 15 per cent of the total calories should be derived from protein in order to maintain a positive nitrogen balance. Approximately one half to two thirds of the protein should be supplied from complete protein foods—milk, eggs, meat, cheese. Retention of 400 mg. per day of calcium may be needed for adequate mineralization of the rapidly growing skeleton during prepubertal and pubertal growth. Diets supplying the recommended 1400 mg. of calcium permit adequate retention. A quart of milk is needed to supply the calcium. Milk also contains vitamin D (400 I.U. per quart) which is necessary for the absorption of calcium. The amount of iron (18 mg.) probably cannot be

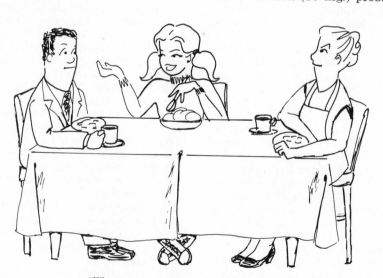

"What's wrong with ice cream for breakfast?"

supplied in the food usually ingested. (See Appendix Table 8 for foods high in iron.) Some of these, such as breads and cereals, are fortified with iron and other foods are under consideration for iron enrichment.

Dietary surveys indicate that many adolescents obtain less than two thirds of the Recommended Dietary Allowances (RDA) for ascorbic acid, vitamin A, calcium and iron.

INDICATIONS OF GOOD OR POOR NUTRITION

Growth, muscular development, and appearance are the hallmarks of good or poor nutrition (Fig. 17-4). Careful observation of the child will reveal many facts about his state of nutrition.

HEIGHT-WEIGHT   There are available numerous height-weight-age tables to consult and note whether the child is within normal limits. (See Appendix Tables 15 and 16.) Obviously not all children have the same body build. Some are large boned and anatomically robust, while other children are small boned and appear more delicate and dainty. This differentiation is important to consider when checking the child's weight and height. A deviation from the average weight for height and age may be perfectly normal for a particular child. All healthy children grow, but each child has his own pathway of development. Thus, height and weight are best evaluated in terms of the child's previous periodic records. Falkner[7] has recently presented "growth" standards for white North American children which are

---

[7] Falkner, F.: The physical development of children. A guide to interpretation of growth—charts and development assessments; and a commentary on contemporary and future problems. Pediatrics, 29:448, 1962.

generally higher than the Iowa and Harvard charts. Growth is subject to many different influences; disease, sex, heredity, hormonal activity, physical condition, seasonal fluctuations and nutrition (food) are some of the factors.

APPEARANCE   Does the child look well? The color and turgor of skin, and musculature condition are revealing factors. The skin should look firm, healthy, smooth, and elastic, and not appear flabby nor fat. A fat child is no longer considered a healthy child! He may be in a poor state of nutrition. A child or adult can be overweight from a diet composed of fats and carbohydrates but lacking in minerals, vitamins and proteins.

A child in a good state of nutrition whose emotional needs are satisfied tends to be happy, active, alert, and playful while a child in a poor state of nutrition will be listless, unhappy and whiney.

POSTURE   The healthy child experiences little difficulty in exhibiting good posture traits (Fig. 17-5); head and chest held high, abdomen in, weight distributed evenly on balls of feet, knees flexed, no curvature of the back and all parts of the skeleton in good alignment (Fig. 17-6). The child in a poor state of nutrition has a difficult task to show good posture. He is listless, pale, weak, chronically tired and slouches (Fig. 17-7). A continuous infection of tonsils and adenoids may add to the poor state of health. Along with the well-balanced, nutritious diet, the child should receive ample rest and sleep, fresh air, sunshine and exercise to stimulate the appetite. (See Fig. 17-8.)

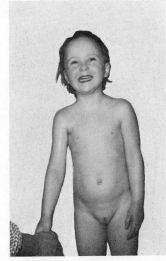

Figure 17-4   Growth, muscular development and general appearance reflect good nutrition in a 5 year old.

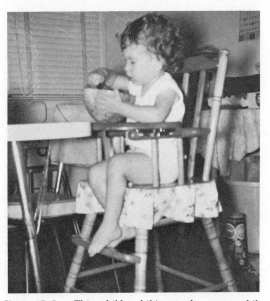

Figure 17-5   This child exhibits good posture while eating.

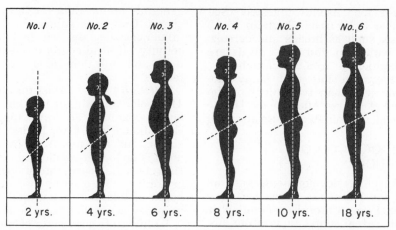

No. 1	No. 2	No. 3	No. 4	No. 5	No. 6
2 yrs.	4 yrs.	6 yrs.	8 yrs.	10 yrs.	18 yrs.

Figure 17–6   Silhouette copies of photographs of children of various ages who were considered to have acceptable posture. These illustrations are not drawn to scale. The apparent kyphosis at ages 6 and 8 is caused by scapular winging, which is commonly seen at these ages. The relative tilt is illustrated. (McMorris, R. O.: Faulty posture. Pediat. Clin. N. Amer., Vol. 8, No. 1, Feb., 1961.)

Figure 17–8   Along with a well-balanced nutritious diet, this 23-month-old child enjoys ample outdoor play – sun, air, water, fun – all contribute toward a healthy body and a good appetite.

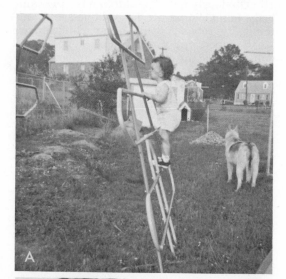

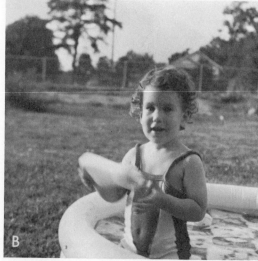

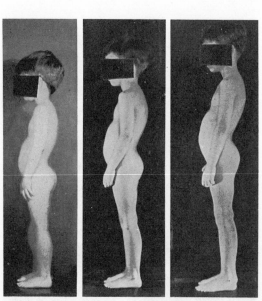

Figure 17–7   Poor postural pattern of a child persisting at different age levels. Note sharp angle of pelvic tilt, prominent abdomen, lordosis, round back, flat chest, forward shoulders and forward head.

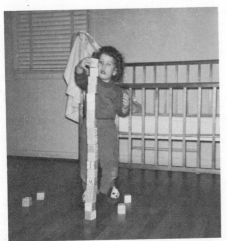

Figure 17–9   Good muscle control and coordination reflects a well-nourished, well-adjusted child. This child is 2½ years old.

MUSCLE CONTROL   Children should have good control of their muscles either at play (Fig. 17–9) or at the table (Fig. 17–10). There will be noticeable posture changes as the baby grows into childhood. The infant of a few months will squirm, kick and wave arms for exercise. At the age of 6 months, the average baby will roll about and attempt to sit up. This is followed by crawling, creeping and attempts to stand (Fig. 16–11). After the first wobbly steps are taken, practice is needed before the muscles are strong enough to permit running and jumping. Children should stand and walk erect. The legs should not be bowed, and the head should be of normal shape and size. Children who suffer from avitaminosis D, the condition described in Chapter 31, Nutritional Deficiency Dis-

eases, have bowed legs, abnormal head and chest development, and in extreme cases the result is rickets. (See Figs. 34–15 and 34–16.)

Also observe these factors:

Does the child sleep well?

Does the child eat well?

Does the child have good daily elimination?

Does the child's hair look glossy and healthy instead of stringy and lifeless?

Are the eyes clear and bright?

Does the child have an alert and happy expression?

The child's teeth and gums are also a good indication of either desirable or poor nutrition. The gums are firm, hugging the teeth, and light pink in color, with no bleeding tendencies. The approximate number of teeth expected for his age are listed:

6 teeth at 1 year of age

12 teeth at 1½ years of age

16 teeth at 2 years of age

20 teeth at 2½ years of age

24 teeth at 6 years, 4 of which are permanent molars

PROBLEMS AND SUGGESTED TOPICS FOR DISCUSSION

1. Check the children in your Children's Ward against the height-weight-age table. Account for variations.
2. What and how much is a child who is 1 year old, a child who is 2 years old, a child who is 6 years old, and an adolescent who is 14 years old eating? Check the food record for nutritional adequacy.
3. Obtain an average day's intake of food from a boy in the clinic who is 15 years old. How does he rate his diet? How may it be improved?
4. Follow the same procedure suggested in problem 3 for a child who is 10 years old.
5. Follow the same procedure suggested in problem 3 for an adolescent girl who is 14 years old.
6. How does nutrition affect healthy growth and development? What are the visible signs? How do a girl's growth and development differ from those of a boy? Give the general growth and development pattern of a child from age 1 to 18.
7. What changes in eating habits take place from ages 1 to 18? Account for the changes.
8. Milk is an excellent food for children, but under what circumstances may it need to be limited?
9. Why is malnutrition prevalent in the preschool children? What is being done about it?
10. What are the food needs of teenagers? What nutrients have been found to be inadequate or low in the diets of adolescent girls? Adolescent boys? Give reasons for the poor diets of teen-agers.
11. How can you help a teenage girl to improve her nutrition and health habits?
12. Why are adequate breakfasts and lunches of importance to the school child? Or what does a good breakfast consist? What is a good lunch?
13. What are the implications for teaching mothers concerned about the eating behavior of their preschool children?

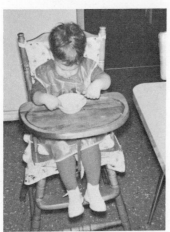

Figure 17–10   This 19-month-old child shows good muscle control in feeding herself. She can use either hand and do a good job!

SUGGESTED ADDITIONAL READING REFERENCES

Astrand, P.: Something old and something very new—very new. Nutrition Today, 3:9, 1968.

Beal, V. A.: Dietary intake of individuals followed through infancy and childhood. Am. J. Pub. Health, *51*:1107, 1961.

Breckenridge, M. E.: Food attitudes of five-to-twelve-year-old children. J. Am. Dietet. A., 35:704, 1959.

Bryan, M. S., and Lowenberg, M. E.: The father's influence on young children's food preferences. J. Am. Dietet. A., 34:30, 1958.

Burke, B. S., et al.: A longitudinal study of animal protein intake of children from one to eighteen years of age. Am. J. Clin. Nutr., 9:616, 1961.

Burke, B. S., et al.: A longitudinal study of the calcium intake of children from one to eighteen years of age. Am. J. Clin. Nutr., 10:79, 1962.

Burke, B. S., et al.: Relationship between animal protein, total protein, and total caloric intakes in the diets of children one to eighteen years of age. Am. J. Clin. Nutr., 9:136, 1961.

Committee on Nutrition, American Academy of Pediatrics: Factors affecting food intake. Pediatrics, 33:135, 1964.

Dierks, E. C., and Morse, L. M.: Food habits and nutrient intakes of preschool children. J. Am. Dietet. A., 47:292, 1965.

Eppright, E. S., and Swanson, P. P.: Distribution of calories in diets of Iowa school children. J. Am. Dietet. A., 31:144, 1955; II. Distribution of nutrients among meals and snacks of Iowa school children. 31:256, 1955.

Eppright, E. S., et al.: Eating behavior of preschool children. J. Nutr. Ed., 1:16, 1969.

Everson, G. J.: Bases for concern about teenagers' diets. J. Am. Dietet. A., 36:17, 1960.

Food for the Family with Young Children. U.S. Department of Agriculture, Home & Garden Bulletin No. 5, Revised, 1960.

Food for Families with School Children. U.S. Department of Agriculture, Home and Garden Bulletin No. 13, Revised, 1969.

Gyorgy, P.: Concerence Notes (preschool child). Am. J. Clin. Nutr., 14:65, 1964.

Hathaway, M. L.: Heights and Weights of Children and Youth in the United States. Washington, D.C., U.S. Department of Agriculture, Home Economics Research Report No. 2, October, 1957.

Hinton, M. A., et al.: Eating behavior and dietary intake of girls 12 to 14 years old. J. Am. Dietet. A., 43:223, 1963.

Kerry, E., et al.: Nutritional status of preschool children. Dietary and biochemical findings. Am. J. Clin. Nutr., 21:1274, 1968.

Leverton, R. M.: The paradox of teenage nutrition: J. Am. Dietet. A., 53:13, 1968.

Lowenberg, M. E.: Food preferences of young children. J. Am. Dietet. A., 24:430, 1964.

Mitchell, H. S.: Nutrition in relation to stature. J. Am. Dietet. A., 40:521, 1962.

Ohlson, M. A., and Hart, B. P.: Influence of breakfast on total day's food intake. J. Am. Dietet. A., 47:282, 1965.

Owens, G. L., et al.: Nutritional status of preschool children—A pilot study. Am. J. Clin. Nutr., 22:1444, 1969.

Pate, M.: The preschool child protection program (P.P.P.). Am. J. Clin. Nutr., 14:63, 1964.

Peckos, P. S., and Heald, F. P.: Nutrition of adolescents. Children, 11:27, 1964.

Review. Body fat in adolescent boys. Nutr. Rev., 22:72, 1964.

Review. Growth standards for infants and children. Nutr. Rev., 21:141, 1963.

Review. The effects of a balanced lunch program on the growth and nutritional status of school children. Nutr. Rev., 23:35, 1965.

Roth, A.: The teen-age clinic. J. Am. Dietet. A., 36:27, 1960.

Smith, C. A.: Overuse of milk in the diets of infants and children. J.A.M.A., 172:567, 1960.

Spindler, E. B., and Acker, G.: Teen-agers tell us about their nutrition. J. Am. Dietet. A., 43:228, 1963.

Teply, L. J.: Nutritional needs of the pre-school child. Nutr. Rev., 22:65, 1964.

U.S. Department of Agriculture: Food, The Yearbook of Agriculture, 1959. Lowenberg, M. E.: Between infancy and adolescence, pp. 296–302; Storvick, C. A., and Fincke, M. L.: Adolescents and young adults, pp. 303–310.

U.S. Department of Health, Education, and Welfare: Nutrition and Healthy Growth. Children's Bureau Publication No. 352, Reprinted, 1958; The Adolescent In Your Family. Children's Bureau Publication 347, Revised, 1955.

Wohl, M. G., and Goodhart, R. S. (ed.): Modern Nutrition in Health and Disease. 4th ed. Philadelphia, Lea & Febiger, 1968.

Your Child from One to Six. Federal Security Agency, Children's Bureau Publication No. 30, Revised 1962.

Your Child from Six to Twelve. Federal Security Agency, Children's Bureau Publication No. 324, 1966.

Chapter 18
NUTRITION
AND AGING

There are at present 20 million persons in the United States over age 65, constituting about 10 per cent of the total population. Life expectancy in 1900 was approximately 47 years. In 1967, it had increased to 67.8 for males and 75.1 years for females. This was due largely to a marked reduction in infant and early mortality. Between 1900 and 1960 the general population doubled but the number of persons past 65 years of age quadrupled. It is predicted that by 1975 there will be 22 million or 12 per cent of the population over 65 years of age.

THE PROCESS OF AGING

Aging is a normal process. It begins with conception and ends only with death, but may progress at varying rates, depending upon several factors—among them nutrition. Since good nutrition and good health are inseparable, the effects of a faulty diet appear sooner or later. Advancements in medical knowledge, improvements in socioeconomic conditions and research in nutrition have increased life expectancy. Scientific investigations in Gerontology* Centers promise insight into the aging process. The role of nutrition in geriatric* nutrition is to conserve the health and prolong the life of the individual and delay the onset of chronic degenerative diseases, such as chronic heart disease, cancer, atherosclerosis, cerebral hemorrhage, kidney disease, diabetes, arthritis osteomalacia and osteoporosis.

One must begin early in life to prepare for healthy senior citizenship. Shock has suggested that the best preparation for a healthy old age begins in early childhood. The practice of good food habits is a lifetime endeavor. Indeed the woman's eating habits prior to and during pregnancy may influence the subsequent aging process in her offspring. At any rate, the earlier in life a start is made in achieving and maintaining optimum health, the more productive the effort will be. Nutrition is a vital, active process of biochemistry on which every cell of the body depends for nourishment and maintenance throughout life.

Aging occurs at different rates in different individuals. The state of nutrition of the body is determined by the nutrition of the individual cells. From conception and during the period of growth, the anabolic processes exceed the catabolic or degenerative changes. When the body has reached physiologic maturity, the rate of degenerative changes is greater than the growth process. These changes impair the function of any organ to some degree. The decreased efficiency is caused by a loss of cells of organs, leaving the functioning capacity of the organ to the remaining cells. It is believed that in the aging process the cells form defective RNA from the DNA. The defective RNA then designates the synthesis of defective enzymes. Cells are unable to function and they are lost (die). Tissues vary in their loss of functions. The percentages of remaining functions of some tissues are shown in Table 18–1. A decrease in the number of mitochondria with age has been reported. This results in diminished function of a cell to release energy. Structural changes associated with collagen occur. Collagen

*Gerontology is a scientific study of the phenomena of aging and of the problems, including social problems, of the aged.

Geriatrics is a branch of medicine dealing with the problems and diseases of old age and aging people.

TABLE 18–1   PERCENTAGE OF FUNCTIONS OR TISSUES REMAINING IN A 75-YEAR-OLD MALE COMPARED TO A 30-YEAR-OLD MALE

TISSUE	PER CENT REMAINING IN 75-YEAR-OLD MALE
Body water content	82
Number of glomeruli in kidney	56
Number of nerve trunk fibers	63
Brain weight	56
Number of taste buds	36

becomes less elastic and more fibrous as the cell ages. The aging appearance of the skin may be due to the accumulation of collagen in the skin.

The aging process, according to another theory,[1] depends upon the way vitamin E and ascorbic acid are used by the body. Aging seems to be influenced by an intracellular struggle going on between two factors acting on the third: the duration and intensity of radiation, which can penetrate every cell, the polyunsaturated lipids upon which they act and the available vitamin E present to protect the lipids from excessive destruction. When radiant energy strikes a polyunsaturated lipid, the radiation will have little effect if enough vitamin E is present.

If there is an intracellular deficiency of vitamin E, the radiant energy will strike a lipid molecule, release a hydrogen atom and initiate peroxidation of polyunsaturated lipid, which produces free radical intermediates. The latter fly about within the cell and cause considerable damage. Free radicals collide with a lysosome, puncture its membrane and release hydrolytic enzymes which spread through the cell and destroy cellular components. The mitochondria and endoplasmic reticulum are vulnerable to peroxidation. The energy-generating processes of electron transport and phosphorylation cease. The cell dies and only a "clinker" remains. Cell age of a tissue is determined by the ash or "clinker" that remains when the cell has been burned out by peroxidation.

Vitamin E, as noted, is an important antioxidant in the prevention of lipid peroxidation. Ascorbic acid plays a role in the enzyme functions relating to the hydroxylation of proline in collagen biosynthesis. It reacts with glutathione, and through antioxidant synergism ascorbic acid increases its protective role. It has the ability to act as a synergist with vita-

[1]Tappel, A. L.: Where old age begins. Nutrition Today, 2:2, 1967.

min E. Both vitamin E and ascorbic acid appear to be important in retarding the process of cellular aging.

Selenium, present in trace amounts in a wide variety of foods, seems to have an important antioxidant role, although it is not defined in humans. Glutathione, cysteine and sulfhydryl proteins provide a pool of reducing compounds. They function as antioxidants. Further research in these areas is in progress. Although the cause of aging is not fully understood, it is agreed that the changes which occur are irreversible.

NUTRITION NEEDS OF SENIOR CITIZENS

The needs of aging people do not differ significantly from those of young adults. The chief changes observed in dietary surveys and studies are in the speed and completeness of digestion and absorption; glucose tolerance; utilization of protein, fat, calcium and thiamin; and decreased appetite. Lowered metabolism and decreased activity decrease the caloric need.

Poor food habits, common among the aged, tend to speed up these changes. Oversimplification of diet, with excess calorie intake from empty calories such as sugar and fats, and with too little intake of meat, fish, poultry, eggs, milk and cheese, fruits and vegetables, is widely practiced among the elderly population. There is speculation that these food habits may contribute toward the atherosclerotic and degenerative changes so general in the aged.

Review Chapter 11, An Adequate Diet, and see the Food and Nutrition Board, National Academy of Sciences-National Research Council Recommended Daily Dietary Allowances (Table 11–1). The charts in Chapter 14 show the quantities of the nutrients ingested by this age group one day in Spring, 1965.

CALORIES

The hope of prolonging the period in which the characteristics of youth can be maintained is the goal of most dietary research. McCay and co-workers[2] contributed a series of studies on longevity, in which it was shown that restriction of calories was the most important single factor. There is general agreement that McCay's observations – that lean rats live longest – are probably applicable to humans as well. In man, insurance statistics indicate that overweight in adults is associated with shortened life span.

MALNUTRITION Rigidity of eating habits is probably the reason for such universal malnutrition in the aged. Malnutrition, associated with underweight or overweight, is frequently observed in individuals 60 years and over. Poor appetite, impaired digestion and/or absorption, lowered gastric acidity and/or inadequate food intake, as well as poor choice of foods, and low incomes are some factors that may contribute toward underweight. Increasing the caloric intake with concentrated nutritive foods prepared and served to suit the individual taste will usually correct this condition.

OVERWEIGHT More often the tendency is to eat more food than needed, with resultant gain in weight. The tendency toward overweight seen in many older adults is not without basis. There is a normal decline in metabolism by some 10 to 15 per cent (or more) after the age of 50. The body size diminishes in height with advancing years. In addition, there is almost always a slackening of physical activity, which lowers the need for calories still further. Unfortunately, there is not always a decrease in appetite to accompany the decrease in need for calories. With the loss of teeth, and the dulling of taste sensitivity, there is a tendency to eat softer, more bland foods, which often have more calories in relation to their value than do the fruits and vegetables which they tend to replace. When the calorie intake is not decreased to fit the lowered rate of metabolism and reduced activity, weight is gained, which is inadvisable because obesity hastens the degenerative processes. Psychological factors, especially emotions, also play an important role in obesity during old age. Much has been said and written on older people eating as compensation for unmet emotional needs.

RECOMMENDED CALORIE ALLOWANCE FOR AGED The National Research Council (NRC) has indicated in the 1968 revision of Recommended Daily Allowances (RDA) that the approximate decline in rate of resting metabolism is known to be 2 per cent per

TABLE 18–2   AGE ADJUSTMENT: PERCENT OF KCALORIE ALLOWANCE AT AGE 22*

AGE	% ADJUSTMENT	% BASAL ENERGY NEEDS
22–35	100–95	98
35–45	95–92	96
45–55	92–89	94
55–65	89–84	92
65–75	84–79	90
75–85	72	88

[2]McCay, C. M., Maynard, L. A., Sperling, G., and Osgood, H. S.: Nutrition requirements during the latter half of life. J. Nutrition, 21:45, 1941.

*Daily Recommended Allowances. 7th ed. Washington, D.C., National Research Council, National Academy of Sciences, Pub. No. 1694, 1968, p. 5.

decade in adults. It is difficult, however, to estimate the degree of reduction in physical activity of individuals in later years of life. The reduction of physical activity and the decline in basal metabolic needs (loss of cells and tissue mass) varies with individuals. The NRC proposes (Table 18–2) that calorie allowances be reduced by 5 per cent between ages 22 and 35, by 3 per cent per decade between ages 35 and 55, by 5 per cent per decade from ages 55 to 75 and by 7 per cent for 75 and over. The reference man and woman at age 22 need approximately 2800 and 2000 kcal., respectively (RDA). Assuming that they maintain good health, normal activity and about the same weight at age 65, they need approximately 2400 and 1700 kcal. per day, respectively. If the weight is more at age 65 than it was at age 22 there has been a replacement of muscle tissue by fat.

It seems advisable that most of the reduction in calories should come from a reduction in the carbohydrate and fat. Since aged persons require fewer calories, the foods eaten should obviously contain the essential food elements, namely, proteins, minerals and vitamins. When calories are limited to less than 1800, careful planning is required to provide an adequate diet. This was clearly demonstrated by Swanson.[3] Food intakes falling below 1800 calories provided inadequate amounts of protein, calcium, iron and vitamins for nutritional safety. Too often "empty calories" are consumed; e.g., tea with cream and sugar instead of a nutrient-rich food such as milk; or cake instead of a fresh or cooked fruit for dessert.

CARBOHYDRATE AND FAT

CARBOHYDRATE It is suggested that elderly people have a reduced capacity to maintain stable blood sugar levels and, therefore, are more subject to temporary hypo- or hyperglycemia than a younger person. When the blood sugar levels are increased by an undue load of sugar, the rate of return to lower values is significantly slower in an older person than in the young. The use of sugar and sweets may well be restricted to prevent an undue load on the sugar-regulating mechanism of the body. Starchy foods are mobilized and burned more slowly than sugar, and in many instances the starchy foods, such as whole grains or enriched cereals, potatoes, and dried beans, carry B vitamins, iron, and other essential food elements.

[3]Swanson, P., et al.: Iowa Agricultural and Home Economics Experimental Station, Research Bull. 468, 1959; and Swanson, P.: Adequacy in old age. I. Role of nutrition. J. Home Econ., 56:651, 1964.

FAT Because of the current research concerning a possible relationship between serum cholesterol, saturated fatty acids, and atherosclerosis (Ch. 30), and because of the possible parallelism between dietary fat and the level of serum cholesterol, it may prove advisable to decrease the proportion of fat in the diet in the later years of life. However, studies indicate that metabolic cholesterol, rather than dietary cholesterol, is the offender. Food sources of cholesterol are among the protective foods (egg yolk, whole milk), and rigid restriction of these might lead to malnutrition. Until long-term results prove otherwise, it would not seem advisable to rigidly restrict these foods in the daily diet. An excessive or severely restricted intake of fat interferes with the absorption of calcium.

Fats are often a cause of indigestion, which may be due to the reduction of gastric, liver, and pancreatic activity. The fats that are used in the diet for flavor and satiety value should be largely those which are low in saturated fatty acids and those which carry vitamins A and D. The recommended daily intake (RDA) of the essential fatty acids is 2 per cent of the calorie intake. This is supplied by polyunsaturated fats (also a good source of vitamin E).

PROTEIN

Dietary studies of older people frequently show low intakes of the foods which are good sources of protein. Dietary studies show that average intake of protein is approximately 45 gm. daily. A low protein intake usually occurs with a low caloric intake. Meat consumption decreases and the number of eggs eaten increases. The reason may be economic, lack of cooking facilities, poor advice, lack of teeth, or any number of other reasons. Negative nitrogen balances of greater or less degree are often found when balance studies are made, and clinical protein deficiencies are also frequently observed. Such deficiencies contribute to edema, itching of the skin, chronic eczema, fatigue and/or tissue wastage. Wounds heal slowly and body resistance is lowered. It is known that there is reduced gastric hydrochloric acid in older persons. However, the question arises as to whether the protein deficiencies seen are caused solely by low intake or by a combination of low intake with incomplete digestion and assimilation and insufficient calories.

Protein is used in the adult for the maintenance of cells and for the synthesis of enzymes needed for digestion and cellular metabolism. The cell cannot function when enzymes are not produced and it dies. The loss of cells causes a decrease in size of organs and a reduction in function of organs. Protein foods supply essential vitamins and minerals (thiamin, riboflavin and niacin, iron and calcium). A low intake of protein results in a deficiency of these nutrients also.

RECOMMENDED DIETARY PROTEIN ALLOWANCE FOR THE AGED

Since protein is the food element particularly inadequate in the aged, it is important that this inadequacy be corrected either by adequate nutritional intake or by the use of protein supplements (Chap. 43). Ravetz[4] reports that 11 of 22 aged patients who were given a protein supplement for 3 weeks to 3 months, plus the regular diet, had increased mental tone and physical vigor. Two-thirds of the subjects studied had a slight weight gain. Since proteins are not stored in the body, they must be eaten daily. The need for adequate proteins of good quality for older people is essential in spite of the fact that the stomach secretes less acid and pepsin. The Food and Nutrition Board, National Research Council, in 1968 recommended that the protein allowance of 0.9 gm. per kg. per day be maintained for adults at all ages.

MINERALS

Of the minerals, *calcium* and *iron* are probably of greatest importance in the nutrition of the aged. Fragility of bones and capillaries may be attributed to a low intake of calcium-rich foods, such as milk, and ascorbic acid-rich foods, such as the citrus fruits. The interrelations of the minerals and vitamins are obvious from previous discussion. The 1965 U.S.D.A. Nationwide Food Consumption Survey showed that diets of people 65 years and over averaged more than 30 per cent (women) and 24 per cent (men) below the RDA for calcium. The women studied in the survey used the equivalent of less than 1 cup of milk daily. The men used slightly more. Women showed below average amounts for iron. (See Figures 14–9 and 14–10.)

Many of the symptoms attributed to senile weakness may be due to dietary lacks over a period of years. When vitamin and mineral deficiencies manifest themselves at any age they often show some of the characteristics associated with old age. In many older persons nutritional deficiency may even be found in the presence of an adequate diet if there is impaired digestion and absorption, impaired circulation, nutritive loss, or endocrine imbalance, thus increasing the nutritional needs.

OSTEOPOROSIS

This is one of several conditions that develop when more calcium is lost than is taken in and is more common in the later years of life. Although other factors are present in osteoporosis, it has been pointed out that one factor may be inadequate calcium intake over a period of years. Gradual demineralization of the bony tissues takes place. They become thin and fragile. The best protection against osteoporosis in old age is to include daily an adequate amount of calcium in the diet during adulthood. Osteoporosis is discussed in Chapter 34, Nutritional Deficiency Diseases.

OSTEOMALACIA

This is a condition commonly referred to as adult rickets and is believed to be caused by poor utilization of calcium induced by lack of vitamin D. Elderly individuals living alone on an inadequate income or having developed bizarre food habits often ingest a diet extremely low in calcium. Because not enough calcium (and vitamin D) is available for normal bone upkeep, the bones gradually weaken and fractures frequently result. Osteomalacia is further discussed in Chapter 34, Nutritional Deficiency Diseases.

NUTRITIONAL ANEMIA

This is frequently found in older persons and may be due to deficiencies of iron, protein, the B vitamins (especially B_{12} and folacin), ascorbic acid, or, more likely, to a combination of factors, again including reduced gastric acidity. (See Nutritional Anemias in Chapter 31.)

RECOMMENDED DIETARY MINERAL ALLOWANCES FOR THE AGED

The Food and Nutrition Board of the National Research Council recommends 800 mg. daily to promote optimum calcium nutrition in older adults. The allowance of iron for men and women is 10 mg. daily. The daily food should be selected to include foods rich in all minerals.

VITAMINS

In the studies of longevity which Sherman conducted on laboratory animals, he found that it was vitamin A and calcium that made the significant difference between the merely adequate diet and the diet that promoted longer, more vigorous life. A number of studies have shown that increases in vitamin intakes of the aged give general health improvement.

The 1965 U.S.D.A. Nationwide Food Consumption Survey showed that the diets of men and women 65 years and over were below amounts recommended for thiamin, riboflavin, vitamin A and ascorbic acid. The foods most neglected were those in the milk and meat groups. The choice of vegetables and fruits did not include enough of those

---

[4]Ravetz, E.: The effect of a protein supplement in the nutrition of the aged. Geriatrics, *14*:567, 1959.

high in ascorbic acid and vitamin A. The importance of maintaining normal niacin blood levels as prophylaxis against the "psychoses of senility" has been emphasized by Gregory.[5] Some workers have shown that health is improved by giving B vitamins and vitamin C, while others have found that it takes large doses of the water-soluble vitamins to correct deficiencies of long standing in older people. Many of the so-called "normal" or "typical" characteristics of aging, such as slow dark adaption, follicular hyperkeratosis, and certain conjunctival lesions, have been improved by prolonged and increased administration of vitamin A.

Some individuals may need to supplement the diet with vitamin concentrates. However, with the accessibility and widespread use of vitamins, studies have shown that many people take vitamins that are already in their diet in sufficient amounts and not those they need. Guidance is needed to assist those who need a supplementary vitamin to select the right ones. The amount of money spent for vitamins by older people very likely could be spent more profitably on food. Foods containing vitamins provide calories, protein and minerals. Vitamin supplements do not. See Chapter 9, Vitamins.

WATER

The importance of water in the diet of the older person has been emphasized by Keys[6] and others. With diminished kidney function, water becomes increasingly important as a carrier and is reported to ease rather than burden the kidney. Drinking adequate amounts of fluids (5 to 8 glasses daily) also aids digestion and helps in the control of constipation, which so frequently plagues older people.

FOODS IN THE DIET OF THE AGED

Older people, just like people in other age groups, need a well-balanced diet that includes the protective foods. (See Chapter 11.)

The protective protein from *meat, fowl, fish, eggs, milk* and products made from milk are essential along with the provision of vitamins and minerals. *Fruits* and *vegetables* are other important protective foods. Dentures may limit consistency of food to the softened varieties, such as mashed, chopped or strained. *Whole grain bread* and *cereals* are encouraged because they aid in

maintaining normal bowel functions, as well as adding valuable food nutrients. In the aged it is quite likely that under conditions of restricted activity and the associated diminished food intake, the resultant intestinal residue will not stimulate normal bowel movement. Thus, the older adult should be protected from the alluring claims of the food faddist and be reassured that the natural roughage in the fruits, leafy vegetables and whole-grain cereals of a good diet will promote satisfactory intestinal evacuation.

Milk is an important food in the diet of the aged. Yet, too frequently it is omitted, or replaced by tea or coffee. Some older people even resent being encouraged to drink milk, while others dislike it. As has been pointed out, it is the chief source of calcium, plus being a good source of protein, a rich source of riboflavin and, when fortified, an excellent source of vitamin D. The consensus seems to favor the use of at least two glasses (16 ounces) or more daily, which can be served as a beverage as well as being used in cream soups and milk desserts.

Foods which furnish few or no essential nutrients but many calories, such as rich sauces, gravies, pies, frosted cakes, sugar, conserves, candies, oils, fried and fatty foods, are all on the list of products that are better decreased if not actually eliminated. These are the empty calories.

The general principles governing the planning of a diet for the aged are not fundamentally different from those for the mature younger adult. However, modifications may be necessary because of certain characteristics inherent in the process of aging and peculiar to the elderly, such as poor dentures, lack of appetite, diminished sense of taste and smell, physical inability to get around with ease to obtain proper food, difficulties in manipulating eating utensils, in swallowing, or inadequate cooking and refrigeration facilities. Fixed food habits and a low income are barriers in obtaining a variety of foods. False notions about economy too frequently misguide the aging person into a deficient, monotonous diet of tea and toast, or their equivalents. Some aged persons do not know how to choose a good diet. Many eat snacks instead of regular meals. Most older people include a small variety of food in the daily meals. The senior citizen who chooses a wide variety of foods is likely to enjoy his later years more than one whose food habits limit him to a few monotonous foods.

For those with sensitive digestive systems the suggestions are for something hot at each meal, four or five light meals rather than three substantial ones, and eating the dinner meal at noon rather than at night. Concentrated

[5]Gregory, I.: Nicotinic acid therapy in psychoses of senility. Am. J. Psychiat., *108*:888, 1952.

[6]Keys, A.: Nutrition for the later years of life. Pub. Health Rep. 67:484, 1952.

foods in liquid mixtures may be necessary as supplements between meals. If calories need restriction, eliminate those foods which furnish few or no essential nutrients (empty calories).

FOOD PLANS FOR THE AGED

With many elderly persons, the income is a major factor in determining the adequacy of their diets. In 1968 about 30 per cent of the families headed by an aged individual had annual incomes under $3000; 7 per cent had less than $1500. Of the single individuals 42 per cent had less than $1500. Social Security was the major source of income. The estimated cost of food (December, 1970) at home for the low-cost plan calls for $780 a year to provide an adequate diet for a couple 55 to 75 years of age (see Table 18–3). This represents 50 per cent of the total income for some older persons who are unable to buy the food they need. Food stamps, available to supplement incomes, assist in obtaining food to be prepared at home. The Food Stamp Amendment provides for home delivery of meals to homebound elderly.

For the individuals who prepare food at home, the three food plans in Table 18–3 are guides for weekly shopping and meal planning. The amounts listed are for food as purchased. They allow for discarding inedible parts, such as rinds, but not for careless waste. The amounts in each food group, namely, Low-cost Plan, Moderate-cost Plan and Liberal Plan, are for a healthy man and woman about 60 years of age and assume they are somewhat less active than in younger years. The amounts can be adjusted for more or less activity.

Each plan will provide for nutritional requirements. The main difference is: meals will be less varied on the Low-cost Plan. The Moderate-cost and Liberal Plans provide for larger amounts of meat, eggs, fruit and vegetables. In addition, more expensive items within the groups, such as foods out of season and more highly processed foods, can be included. The cost of each food plan, listed at the top of the plan, is based on small-scale buying typical of an elderly couple.

Table 18–4 shows *one* way well-balanced (easy to prepare) meals can be planned from the amounts of food suggested in the Low-cost Plan. They demonstrate the use of planned leftovers. For example, chocolate pudding is made for Sunday noon and the leftover kept in the refrigerator until Monday night; enough stew is prepared for Monday evening and Tuesday noon. If five small meals are preferred to three regular ones, some food can be saved for midmorning and afternoon or evening. An adequate meal contains foods supplying sufficient calories and a complete protein or a combination of foods to provide all the essential amino acids. Wise

TABLE 18–3   THREE FOOD PLANS—LOW-COST, MODERATE-COST, AND LIBERAL*
(Quantities for a couple for one week)

KIND OF FOOD	LOW-COST PLAN $15–$17		MODERATE-COST PLAN $19–$22		LIBERAL PLAN $23–$25	
	Man	*Woman*	*Man*	*Woman*	*Man*	*Woman*
Milk, cheese, ice cream (milk equivalent)	3½ qt.	3½ qt.	3½ qt.	3½ qt.	4 qt.	4 qt.
Meat, poultry, fish	3¼ lb.	2½ lb.	5 lb.	4¼ lb.	5¼ lb.	4¾ lb.
Eggs	6	5	7	6	7	6
Dry beans and peas, nuts	4 oz.	4 oz.	2 oz.	2 oz.	2 oz.	1 oz.
Grain products—whole-grain, enriched, or restored (flour equivalent¹)	3½ lb.	2¼ lb.	3¼ lb.	1¾ lb.	3¼ lb.	1½ lb.
Citrus fruits, tomatoes	2¼ lb.	2 lb.	2¾ lb.	2¼ lb.	3 lb.	3 lb.
Dark-green and deep-yellow vegetables²	¾ lb.	¾ lb.	¾ lb.	¾ lb.	¾ lb.	¾ lb.
Potatoes	2½ lb.	1¼ lb.	2¼ lb.	1¼ lb.	2 lb.	1 lb.
Other vegetables and fruits	4¾ lb.	3½ lb.	5½ lb.	4¼ lb.	6 lb.	4½ lb.
Fats and oils	⅔ lb.	¼ lb.	¾ lb.	⅜ lb.	¾ lb.	⅜ lb.
Sugars, sweets	⅔ lb.	⅜ lb.	⅞ lb.	½ lb.	1⅛ lb.	¾ lb.

*Cost of food at home, December 1970, U.S. average. Estimates computed from quantities in food plans published in Family Economics Review, 1964. Agriculture Research Service, U.S. Department of Agriculture.
¹Count 1½ lb. bread or other baked goods as 1 lb. flour or cereal.
²If choices within the group are such that the amounts specified are not sufficient to provide the suggested number of servings, increase the amounts and use less from the "other vegetables and fruits" group.

TABLE 18-4   LOW-COST SAMPLE MENUS FOR A WEEK*

Butter or margarine would be served with these meals, a glass of milk at least once a day, tea or coffee as desired

SUNDAY	MONDAY	TUESDAY	WEDNESDAY	THURSDAY	FRIDAY	SATURDAY
Orange juice Scrambled egg Toast	Orange juice Oatmeal Milk Toast	Prunes French toast Syrup	Orange slices Soft-cooked egg Toasted rolls	Prunes Ready-to-eat cereal Milk Peanut butter biscuits	Tomato juice Milk toast Jelly	Orange juice Oatmeal Milk Toasted corn muffins
Swiss steak Mashed potatoes Broccoli Bread Chocolate pudding	Frankfurters stuffed with mashed potatoes and cheese Scalloped tomatoes Hot rolls Apple brown betty	Lamb stew Beets Tossed green salad Bread Rice and raisin pudding	Meat loaf Scalloped potatoes Steamed cabbage Peanut butter biscuits Fruit in season	Cream of tomato soup Egg salad–shredded lettuce sandwich Gingerbread	Creamed egg and mushrooms on noodles Cabbage, carrot, raisin salad	Braised liver Potatoes boiled in jackets Green peas Grated carrot salad Bread Orange milk sherbet
Welsh rarebit Crisp bacon strip Apple-raisin salad Ice cream Cookies	Lamb stew with potatoes Snap beans Bread Chocolate pudding	Spaghetti, tomato, chopped meat casserole Broccoli Bread Grapefruit segments	Cheese fondue Snap beans Bread Peaches Gingerbread	Meat loaf– tomato sauce Creamed potatoes Spinach Bread Tapioca pudding	Baked fish Baked potato slices Green peas Corn muffins Tapioca pudding	Vegetable-bean soup Toasted cheese sandwich Fruit in season

*Food Guide for Older Folks. Home and Garden Bulletin No. 17, U.S.D.A. (1963) page 9.

selection of foods for the day provides the minerals and vitamins. A suggested meal pattern for senior citizens is shown in Figure 18–3.

FOOD HABITS AND PROBLEMS OF THE AGED

Assisting older persons to provide an adequate diet for themselves often presents many problems. As a rule, the senescent individual is set in his ways. Radical changes in habits of eating, as well as changes in foods, are not always welcomed. Food habits are firmly established by this age and, if poor, they are difficult to replace with better ones. Superstitions and food fallacies are relinquished reluctantly. The known is familiar; the results of the unknown are mysterious! Food shopping is difficult for some older persons. Some are confused by the variety of items in the stores. The distances from the stores and the inability to carry groceries are handicaps. Transportation to and from the market may be a problem, as well as obtaining food stamps or donated food. Many do not know how to prepare foods and claim that food does not taste good.

Special problems arise when the aged lack variety in the diet or become disinterested in food. According to Davidson,[7] the primary causes for the failure to obtain an adequate diet are social isolation (separation) and re-

[7]Hashim, S.: The difficult patient—how do you feed him? Nutr. Rev., 20:2, 1962.

tirement. Because of the greater amount of leisure time, the senescent person has time to think about his next meal, either relishing the idea of eating or becoming critically despondent over its monotony. This is most likely to happen with persons who live alone or do their own cooking. They find it easier to eat the same thing day after day and, unless watched carefully, may suffer from malnutrition, even though overweight. In general, a more varied diet provides a more nutritious diet. The obese individual can manifest signs of malnutrition as well as the underweight. Eating patterns are very erratic in some older persons. They may overeat one day and nibble on foods the next day. Swanson found one case in which a woman's daily intake varied from 800 to 3700 kcalories. To overcome the fallacy that a fat person is a healthy person is one of the problems in geriatric education. Chronic disease, combined with economic and psychological factors, operates to develop an oversimplified dietary program—one that is too frequently inadequate in protective foods. (See Fig. 18–1.) Studies by Swanson indicate that many older women in Iowa receive insufficient amounts of calcium, protein, ascorbic acid and vitamin A. Cereal products furnish a larger percentage of the total calories than in earlier life; meat, fish and poultry a somewhat smaller proportion.

The nurse should consider all problems before attempting to help an aged person with his diet. The nurse works *with* the food pattern of the person. Together *with* the individual she helps plan a pattern which he can

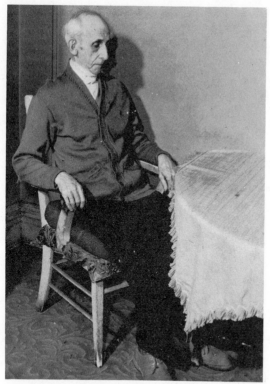

Figure 18–1 The chronically ill, elderly person who fails to eat becomes listless and apathetic, and may spend his days vegetating away. Remarkable changes can be effected by an abundant diet. (S. L. Halpern: Nutrition and Chronic Disease; reprinted from Health News, monthly publication of the New York State Department of Health, September, 1955.)

be expected to adopt. Helpful pamphlets, charts and booklets are available, giving hints and simple information about food for the aged. One such pamphlet is published by the Department of Health, City of New York. (See Figures 18–2 and 18–3.) Others are available from the Bureau of Human Nutrition and Home Economics, Washington, D.C.,[8] and from the American Dietetic Association.[9, 10]

EMOTIONAL, PHYSICAL AND MENTAL HEALTH

Degenerative changes in aging affect digestion, absorption and metabolism of food. Poor mastication of food; decreased saliva; diminished secretion of most digestive enzymes, hydrochloric acid and bile secretions; slower movements of the gastrointestinal tract; impaired liver and kidney function; loss of

[8] Food Guide for Older Folks. Home and Garden Bull. No. 17, U.S.D.A., revised, 1963.
[9] Eating is Fun for Older People, Too.
[10] Forget Birthdays – Enjoy Good Eating.

ability to do extra work and difficulty in excreting excessive waste products are factors affecting the digestion and absorption of food in the aged. Oxidative processes slow down. The capacity of lungs and the amount of blood the heart can pump diminish with age. The rate of blood flowing through the kidney decreases and the number of nephrons in the kidney diminishes. The composition of the blood may be modified, depending upon the functioning of the cells. Loss of elasticity of blood vessels occurs with aging. Changes in the secretion of hormones have a profound effect on the nutrition of cells and the response to stress. Aging proceeds at different rates in different individuals. One of the characteristics of aging is a reduction in reserve capacities. One factor contributing to the loss of reserve capacities with aging is the gradual loss of functioning cells from many organs and tissues of the body.

Closely associated with geriatric nutrition is the mental health status of the individual. The person who refuses to eat may be anxious or depressed and thus have a poor appetite and an inadequate intake. He may be a compulsive nibbler and overeat. He may use food to obtain attention or to escape from reality. Any condition of stress or deprivation may affect attitudes toward food. Food may denote security and comfort. Grief for loved ones, commonly observed, as well as a feeling of insecurity and despondency affect food intakes. The nurse must appraise food practices and identify needs and base her guidance on this foundation.

Signs of senility are noted in lagging memory and chronic degenerative diseases. It is supposed by some scientists that the normal average life span could reach 150 years if the degenerative diseases could be prevented.

The aged must help to minimize the incidence of disease by following the same rules of hygiene that are recommended for younger people. This includes weight control, more sleep, and moderation in exercise and other endeavors. To be well adjusted, the aged person needs some interests and activity – both mental and physical – plus a feeling of usefulness and being wanted.

The nutritional problems of old age are commanding increasing attention in research. The longitudinal study which is in progress at the Gerontology Research Center, National Institutes of Health, should provide insight into the problems and processes of aging. Gerontology is a field of study which has ripened with the increased proportion of the population over 65 and the improvement of nutrition knowledge. The resulting larger number of older persons has focused attention on the health and nutrition needs of this

FOOD TO KEEP FIT
AS THE YEARS GO BY

As the years go by, we want to live as interesting and full lives as ever. It is necessary to keep fit if we are to keep on doing the things we like to do.

Eating good food is part of this job of keeping fit. Eating the same good foods that every person needs, regardless of age, is necessary for health and well being. However, as we grow older we are usually less active and need smaller amounts of high calorie foods.

THE STAR SHOWN BELOW
FORMS THE BASIS OF GOOD MEALS THROUGHOUT LIFE

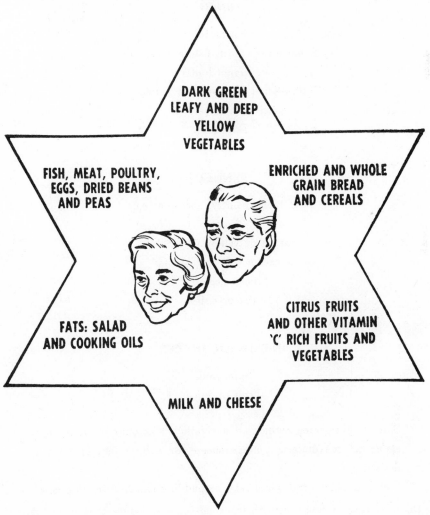

DARK GREEN LEAFY AND DEEP YELLOW VEGETABLES

FISH, MEAT, POULTRY, EGGS, DRIED BEANS AND PEAS

ENRICHED AND WHOLE GRAIN BREAD AND CEREALS

FATS: SALAD AND COOKING OILS

CITRUS FRUITS AND OTHER VITAMIN 'C' RICH FRUITS AND VEGETABLES

MILK AND CHEESE

Figure 18–2   A guide to good meal planning for older people. (Courtesy of Bureau of Nutrition, Department of Health, City of New York.)

SUGGESTED MEAL PATTERN

BREAKFAST

Citrus fruit or juice
Cereal or egg
Toast and spread*
Tea, coffee or cocoa (made
with skim milk)

LUNCH

Soup or juice
Sandwiches (meat, fish, cheese, egg
or peanut butter)
Raw salad or cooked vegetable
Simple dessert**
Skim milk

DINNER

Fish, meat, poultry, cheese or egg
Potato
Green or yellow vegetable
Bread or roll and spread*
Simple dessert**
Tea or coffee

IN-BETWEEN SNACKS

Skim milk
Fruit or juice

* Spread: Margarine containing a significant amount of *liquid vegetable oil,* mayonnaise, cottage cheese, or a little jam or jelly, if desired.
** Simple dessert: Fruit, plain cake, or pudding (made with skim milk)

Figure 18-3   This is a suggested meal pattern for senior citizens, based on the guide to good meal planning in *A.* (Courtesy of Bureau of Nutrition, Department of Health, City of New York.)

age group. In the years ahead more research will be devoted to this field to add life to years, not just years to life. The later years must be active, physically fit and socially interesting if they are to be enjoyed and not merely endured in empty survival.

PROBLEMS AND SUGGESTED TOPICS FOR DISCUSSION

1. List the ways in which the nutritional needs and food intake of a senior citizen may differ from a normal younger mature adult's.
2. What are the main food habits and problems of the aged?
3. Interview an aged man living alone. Identify the problems that he encounters in providing meals. Assist him to plan an adequate diet.
4. Take a diet history from an elderly woman in the hospital or clinic. Assist her with improvements in her dietary, taking into consideration any problems she may have connected with her diet. Check for adequacy.

SUGGESTED ADDITIONAL READING REFERENCES

Beeuwkes, A. M.: Studying the food habits of the elderly. J. A. Dietet. A., 37:215, 1960.

Burton, B. T. (ed.): Heinz Handbook of Nutrition. 2nd ed. New York, McGraw-Hill Book Company, Inc., 1965, Chapter 19, Geriatric nutrition.

Bymers, G. J., and Murray, J.: Food marketing practices of older households. J. Home Econ., 52:172, 1960.

Campbell, V. A., and Dodds, M. L.: Collecting dietary information from groups of older people. J. Am. Dietet. A., 51:29, 1967.

Consumer and Food Economics Research Division, Agricultural Research Service: Food Guide for Older Folks. Home and Garden Bulletin 17. Washington, D.C., U.S. Department of Agriculture, Revised 1963.

Dallas, I., and Nordin, B. E. C.: The relation between calcium intake and roentgenologic osteoporosis. Am. J. Clin. Nutr. 11:263, 1962.

Davidson, C. S., et al.: The nutrition of a group of apparently healthy aging persons. Am. J. Clin. Nutr., 10:181, 1962.

Donahue, W. T.: Psychologic aspects of feeding the aged. J. Am. Dietet. A., 27:461, 1951.

Esposito, S. J., et al.: Nutrition in the aged. Review of the literature. J. Am. Geriat. Soc., 17:790, 1969.

Fry, P. C., et al.: Nutrient intakes of healthy older women. J. Am. Dietet. A., 42:218, 1963.

Goodman, J. I.: The problem of malnutrition in the elderly. J. Am. Geriat. Soc., 5:504, 1957.

Goodman, J. I.: Nutrition, life tenure, and the degenerative diseases. Geriatrics, 13:359, 1958.

Hayes, O. B., Bowser, L. J., and Trulson, M. F.: Relation of dietary intake to bone fragility in the aged. J. Gerontol., 11:154, 1956.

Howell, S. C., and Loeb, M. B.: Nutrition and aging: A monograph for practitioners. St. Louis Gerontological Society, 660 South Euclid, St. Louis, 1969.

Le Bovit, C.: The food of older persons living at home. J. Am. Dietet. A., 46:285, 1965.

Mayer, J.: Nutrition in the aged. Postgrad. Med., 32:394, 1962.

McHenry, E. W.: Nutrition and older people. Canad. J. Pub. Health, 51:101, 1960.

Mitchell, D. L., and Goldfarb, A. I.: Psychological needs of aged patients at home. Am. J. Pub. Health, 56:1716, 1966.

Morgan, A. F.: Programs for the aging: Nutrition. J. Home Econ., 52:817, 1960.

Nutrition and Human Needs. Part 14–Nutrition and the Aged. Hearings before the Select Committee on Nutrition and Human Needs of the United States Senate, Ninetieth Congress (Second Session) and Ninety-first Congress (First Session), Sept. 9, 10, and 11, 1969, Washington, D.C.

Pelcovitz, J.: Nutrition in older Americans. J. Am. Dietet. A., 58:17, 1971.

Portis, S. A., and King, J. C.: The gastrointestinal tract in the aged. J.A.M.A., 148:1073, 1952.

Ravetz, E.: The effect of a protein supplement in the nutrition of the aged. Geriatrics, 14:567, 1959.

Reddout, M. J., and Sister Anne de Paul: Nutrition and the geriatric patient. J. Am. Geriat. Soc., 8:463, 1960.

Shock, N. W.: Physiology of aging. Sci. Am., 206:100, 1962.

Shock, N. W.: Physiologic aspects of aging. J. Am. Dietet. A., 56:491, 1970.

Steinkamp, R. C., Cohen, N. L., and Walsh, H.: Resurvey of an aging population–fourteen year follow-up. J. Am. Dietet. A., 46:103, 1965.

Swanson, P.: Adequacy in old age. Role of nutrition. J. Home Econ., 56:651, 1964.

Swanson, P.: Nutrition in the later years. National Live Stock and Meat Board, Food and Nutrition News, 35(No. 7): April, 1964.

Tappel, A. L.: Where old age begins. Nutrition Today, No. 4, 2:2, 1967.

Tappel, A. L.: Will antioxidant nutrients slow aging processes? Geriatrics, 23:97, 1968.

Watkins, D. M.: The impact of nutrition on the biochemistry of aging in man. World Rev. Nutr. Diet., 6:124, 1966.

Wohl, M. G., and Goodhart, R. S. (ed.): Modern Nutrition in Health and Disease. 4th ed. Philadelphia, Lea & Febiger, 1968, Nutrition for the Aging and the Aged.

Part Two
DIET
THERAPY

This section of the book deals with the role of nutrition in the prevention and treatment of disease. All the therapeutic diets are modifications of the normal adequate diet pattern based on the Recommended Dietary Allowances as suggested by the Food and Nutrition Board of the National Research Council, with amounts of nutrients adjusted to cover the additional requirements created by disease or injury. Space does not permit the inclusion of all diets in use for each disease. Only those diets most generally accepted are outlined here.

DEVELOPMENT OF DIET THERAPY

Nursing and medicine have always been concerned with the feeding of the sick. From the time of the Egyptian medical era, a relationship has been recognized between food and disease and some form of diet therapy has been practiced. Celsus emphasized the role of foods in preventative medicine about 25 B.C. when he wrote ". . . we come to those which nourish, namely food and drink. Now these are of general assistance not only in disease of all kinds but in preserving health as well." In 1671 Nicolai Venette recognized the efficacy of using vegetables and fresh fruits as antiscorbutics; and Bachstrom's writings in 1734 demonstrate that he recognized scurvy as a deficiency disease. As early as 1843, Jonathan Pereira, a member of the Royal College of Physicians in London, published a book in collaboration with Dr. Charles A. Lee of New York based on experimental work in the feeding of "paupers, lunatics, criminals, children and the sick in metropolitan institutions." In 1854, during the Crimean War, Florence Nightingale and her staff, located at Scutari, were as devoted to the problems of feeding the sick and wounded as they were to the other phases of nursing. Florence Nightingale is historically recorded as the founder of dietetics, as well as of nursing. Between 1854 and 1865 there seemed to have been a lull in the study of dietetics until after the Civil War. History appears to repeat itself in that it takes the increased demands of war to further the interest and study of foods and nutrition. In the early 1870's, Dr. F. W. Pacy, Fellow of the Royal College of Physicians, London, began a treatise on food and dietetics. It is recorded that in his lectures he emphasized that the correct feeding of the well and sick should be of deep concern. He stated, "Ill management of food kills off the weak and ruins the middling." Thus, the role of nutrient requirements in disease and the necessity of supplying certain essential nutrients as a preventative to disease were recognized by the earliest physicians.

Others became interested and approached and treated the subject from various angles. Cooking schools were founded in the East (New York, Boston and Philadelphia). In the 1880's, graduates from these various schools began taking positions as instructors in foods and cookery in nurses' training schools, to teach the nurses how to prepare foods for the sick. The next step was a diet kitchen, supervised by a graduate from a cooking school. And so on down to our present-day system of having graduate dietitians in charge of food service in the hospital. It has been a long road, one in which the nurse has played a major role. The nurse continues to function as a very vital and necessary member of the team in feeding the sick. She sees more of the patient than anyone else, and when the tray is served, she should be able to observe, encourage, and intelligently guide the learning process. With the cooperation of all — nurse, doctor, dietitian and patient — effective management of the dietary needs of patients may be obtained.

Chapter 19
THERAPEUTIC
DIETS

UNIT SIX
MODIFICATIONS
OF THE
ADEQUATE
NORMAL DIET

THE CHANGING PICTURE OF NUTRITIONAL DISEASES

The importance of diet in the treatment of disease was emphasized by the ancient Greek and Roman physicians. However, a true conception of the value of good nutrition in the maintenance of health and the prevention and effective treatment of disease has received increasing recognition in more recent years. Currently, some of the most dramatic research in experimental medicine is being done on problems which involve the nutritional factor. The role nutrition is occupying in the routine, educational and investigational programs of the hospital is a vital one. The judicious use of foods or their specific constituents as therapeutic agents is revolutionizing the practice of medicine. The prevention of nutritional disease through the application of this knowledge is bringing benefits to many individuals.

Scientific progress is changing the picture of nutritional disease in America. In the early 1900's frank deficiency diseases — pellagra, beriberi, scurvy and rickets — were endemic. Today fully developed cases are rare or, at least, are uncommon. In fact, in 1955 the United States Public Health Service discontinued reporting the occurrence of pellagra and other deficiency diseases. Today, the majority of current cases of pellagra, beriberi, and xerophthalmia are the result of special conditioning circumstances, e.g., the existence of a primary disease which produces secondary nutritional deficiency disease. Nevertheless, sporadic cases do occur and diagnosis is apt to be overlooked if these diseases are not borne in mind.

Reasons for the changing face of nutritional disease include advance in research, steady improvement of the general economic status, and education of the public. Along with these advancements there has been rapid and wide-reaching technological progress in the food industry itself. However, while certain nutritional diseases are largely disappearing in America, there is a steady increase in recognition of new disorders, most of which fall into one of four categories: (1) lack or imbalance of nutrients (disorders of magnesium deficiency, vitamin E deficiency anemia); (2) inborn errors of metabolism (phenylketonuria); (3) iatrogenic diseases (antibiotics and chemicals affecting the intestinal flora, appetite, absorption and utilization); and (4) overnutrition (obesity, toxicity, imbalances, atherosclerosis). These are only a few of the changes; with continuing study and research more are bound to follow.

During the past decade studies have been reported on the relations between diet and wound healing, stress, burns, gastrointestinal diseases, infectious diseases, diseases of the liver, diseases of the heart and circulatory system, plus the new disorders mentioned above. The latest results of these findings, showing the relation between nutrition and disease, will be described in the subsequent chapters.

STRESS   A person subjected to stress is one upon whom external forces (often severe) are acting. Examples of such forces are war wounds, industrial injury, starvation, surgical operations, burns, extreme heat and extreme cold. There are many variables involved in relation to nutrition, such as the severity of the injury, the previous state of nutrition of the individual, and the nutrients consumed following stress. The problem of maintaining adequate nutrition in times of stress is often a major one. The mechanism of the metabolic changes in stress is not entirely clear. The metabolic response that defends the body against stress is an increased secretion of adrenocorticotropic hormone (ACTH) which stimulates the adrenal cortex to oversecrete the adrenocortical hormones, glucocorticoid and mineralocorticoid hormone. (See Chapter 28, Metabolic Disorders Related to Nutrition.) Under stress, individuals develop hypertension with cardiovascular disease, gastric ulcers, headache or neurosis. Stress superimposed on a nutritional disorder worsens the condition.[1] Some individuals react more to outside forces than do others and often have a sustained rise in blood pressure. These hyper-reactors are considered potential hypertensives and should avoid stimulants such as coffee and tea. They should also be moderate in the use of salt and animal fats (saturated fats), and lose weight if overweight. Psychological factors, emotional states, anxiety, as well as trauma and infection, under severe stress induce loss of nitrogen, carbohydrate, lipids, potassium and increased utilization of ascorbic acid.[2] For this reason the FAO/WHO Expert Group on Protein Requirements included a 10 per cent additional allowance for stress at each recommended level. The well-balanced diet is therapeutic treatment during stress. Excessive amounts of one or more of the nutrients is seldom, if ever, of value unless indicated for specific conditions. More research is needed on the subject.

ADEQUATE NORMAL DIET AS A BASIS FOR THERAPEUTIC DIETS

All the therapeutic diets are modifications of the normal or adequate diet pattern. The hospital house diets are the basis for the therapeutic diets. Regardless of the type prescribed, the aim and purpose of the diet are to supply needed nutrients to the body. Before discussing any therapeutic diets, either general or specific, the adequate normal diet will be reviewed. Also review Chapter 11, An Adequate Diet.

There are many ways to plan a diet that will be nutritious and adequate. To be certain that the dietary allowances are fulfilled the safest procedure is to include certain specified amounts of foods in the daily diet. The Basic Food Groups (p. 18) are recommended as a pattern to follow when planning the basic house diets. Furthermore, it will serve as a guide when planning adequate therapeutic diets, considering the adjustments and changes necessary to meet the abnormal conditions.

For the normal healthy adult the foundation of an adequate diet provides approximately 63 gm. of proteins and 1200 calories. (See Table 11–4.) To provide heat and energy and to produce or maintain normal weight, more of the foods listed or other foods are added. These additional foods will also raise the required nutrients to adequate amounts.

In evaluating the foundation of an adequate diet, the amount of proteins allowed is adequate but not excessive. The fruits and vegetables recommended provide bulk to avoid hunger and residue to prevent constipation. Mineral salts and vitamins are furnished by the foods. Iodized salt is used unless contraindicated. Since every food is needed in the specified amount, any omitted item should be replaced by another food of equal value.

The Recommended Dietary Allowances developed by the Food and Nutrition Board of the National Research Council (Table 11–1) have been used extensively as a guide for good dietary planning in hospitals, institutions, civilian life, and the Armed Forces. The foundation of an adequate diet, which has already been described, is patterned after the recommended allowances. There are many combinations of food which would include the allowances. When normal or therapeutic diets are planned, correct translations should be made of the allowances by using foods which are available in the locality and particularly suited to the nationality and specific income level of the group, with amounts adjusted to cover the needs of illness.

The normal diet is not rigid. It is a flexible diet which supplies the body with all the nutrients needed in the *normal* processes of metabolism. Each nutrient must be supplied in sufficient amount with reasonable relation to each other so the dietary will be both adequate and correctly balanced.

BALANCED DIET   A diet that supplies all the food essentials needed for good health in the right amounts and right relations to each other is what nutritionists call a *balanced diet*. Balance can be attained by eating a large variety of protective foods. These would include the Basic Food Groups (p. 18), or the Foundation of An Adequate Diet, described here and in Chapter 11. Sufficient total calories to supply the requisite energy for work and the desired body weight must be adapted to each of the above.

NORMAL DIET   A *normal diet* is an adequate diet which furnishes the body with all of the nutrients needed for the growth and

[1]Selye, H.: On just being sick. Nutrition Today, 5:2, 1970.

[2]Hodges, R. E.: The effect of stress on ascorbic acid metabolism in man. Nutrition Today, 5:11, 1970.

repair of the tissues and the normal functioning of the organs. The body's needs are very definite. It needs proteins for building and repairing body tissue, carbohydrates and fats for providing heat and energy, and minerals for making bones and teeth, maintaining the proper reaction of the body fluids, and regulating the various body processes. Vitamins play an indispensable role in regulating the body functions. Water is needed in every cell, in the blood and in all of the secretions. For optimum health the body must have foods which supply the nutrients in correct amounts and proportions.

STANDARDIZATION The term *diet standardization* is not readily accepted by people who have been accustomed to the freedom of selection. It sounds perilously like regimentation and it is apt to produce a feeling of physical and spiritual limitation among those whom it affects. Diets should not be standardized even though the basic requirements have been established. The selection from a wide variety of foods permits catering to individual likes and dislikes.

PRINCIPLES OF DIET IN THE TREATMENT AND PREVENTION OF DISEASE

Modifications of the normal diet pattern may be indicated in the case of a number of diseases. In the dietary management for a specific disease some general principles are as follows:

1. The therapeutic diet should vary from the adequate normal diet as little as possible.
2. The diet should meet the body requirements for essential nutrients as generously as the disease condition permits.
3. The diet regimen should take cognizance of the patient's food intake habits, preferences, economic status, religious practices, and any environmental factors that have bearing on the diet, such as where the meals are eaten and who prepares them.

Dietary practices in hospitals have not always kept up with the current advances in the field of therapeutic nutrition. It has been reported[3] that the majority of therapeutic diets outlined in the various hospital manuals do not supply the nutrients necessary to maintain good nutrition during the acute phase of an illness, and insufficient attention is given the extra requirements for the convalescent and rehabilitation phase of medical care. The Daily Dietary Allowances are intended for healthy, active people and would not be adequate for most sick and injured individuals. Diets ordinarily adequate

for the individual may be inadequate under prolonged experience of physical and emotional stress and use of drugs. These conditions may interfere with the utilization of food and bring about a nutritional deficiency. The Committee on Therapeutic Nutrition[3] suggests that "the nutritional requirements for the hospital patient will be determined by:

(a) the previous nutritional state of the individual,
(b) the amount and character of the nutrient which is being lost from the body, and
(c) the anticipated duration of the injury and disease."

THE FOOD PRESCRIPTION

The food prescription in nutrition serves the same purpose as the drug prescription in medicine. It includes the daily caloric requirements based on the individual's desirable weight and activity plus the amounts needed of proteins, fats, carbohydrates, minerals, and vitamins. The food prescription is used for sick or well persons. The Recommended Dietary Allowances for different age groups may be used as a *guide*, since variations or deviations from the average person are not considered. In the food prescription the individual variations are taken into account. The construction of the food prescription will be discussed in detail.

CALORIE ALLOWANCE TO MEET ENERGY REQUIREMENT

Calories are needed to keep the body warm and to furnish energy for muscular work. Therefore, the caloric allowance of the individual is expressed as energy requirement. It is quite possible to estimate roughly the calories required by a normal person or even a person ill with a specific disease. Nature supplies a very good checking device, the appetite, and in most normally active persons it regulates the weight with surprising accuracy. However, the appetite cannot be trusted nor depended upon in disease and in obesity.

The average adult afebrile patient at bed rest with minor injury or illness can be maintained in caloric balance by an intake of about 2000 kcalories per day. Severe injury or illness may increase the needs to 2500 or 4000 kcalories per day. A previously severely depleted individual may require an intake of 3500 kcalories or more. Other situations

[3]Pollack, H., and Halpern, S. L.: Therapeutic Nutrition. Washington, D.C., National Research Council, Publication 234, 1952.

TABLE 19–1   RECOMMENDED CALORIE ALLOWANCES FOR ENERGY REQUIREMENTS

ADULT *Calories per day for varying grades of activity based on desirable weight*		CHILD *Calories per day according to age*
	A Kcals./Kg. per day	B Increase over basal calories	Both sexes

	A Kcals./Kg. per day	B Increase over basal calories	Both sexes
Basal or Standard	25		1–2 years of age: 100–95 Kcal./Kg.
Minimal (bed rest)	27.5	10%	3–5 years of age: 95–80 Kcal./Kg.
Very light (typist)	30–35	20– 40%	6–9 years of age: 80–75 Kcal./Kg.
Light (medical student, teacher, nurse)	35–40	40– 60%	10–13 years of age: 75–60 Kcal./Kg.
			Girls:
Moderate (homemaker, metal worker)	40–45	60– 80%	14–15 years of age: 50–45 Kcal./Kg.
Hard (carpenter, housemaid at hard work)	45–50	80–100%	16–17 years of age: 45–40 Kcal./Kg.
Severe (farmer, laundress at hard work)	50–70	100–180%	18–19 years of age: 40–35 Kcal./Kg.
			Boys:
Very severe (miner, lumberman)	75	200%	14–17 years of age: 60–65 Kcal./Kg.
			18–19 years of age: 55–50 Kcal./Kg.

requiring increased calories will be discussed in the forthcoming chapters. Mention should be made that caloric requirement must be considered in relation to other nutrients. In diseases or injuries in which there is a tendency to lose protein, the administration of 50 to 100 per cent more calories than the calculated requirement has, at times, made it possible to maintain protein equilibrium.

For practical purposes, the energy requirement of an individual may be determined by either (1) calculating the number of calories per kilogram per day; or, (2) calculating the per cent increase over basal demands. To make the determinations, the desirable weight based on sex, age, height, and body build (frame) is used. The desirable weight for an individual is obtained from Appendix Tables 13 to 16. The daily caloric allowances are determined according to the activity of the individual. (See Table 19–1.) Restlessness of a bed patient may increase the requirement 10 to 20 per cent. Fever increases calorie requirements. Desirable weight is used instead of actual weight because the present weight of the individual may be abnormal due to undernutrition or obesity. Synonyms for desirable weight are *ideal, standard, normal, average,* and *expected* weight.

The determination of the energy requirement of an individual is illustrated in the following example.

Example: A 20-year-old nursing student (female) with a height of 162.5 centimeters (5 feet, 5 inches) and medium body build, according to Appendix Table 14 has a desirable weight of 53.6 kg. (118 lbs.). She is classified as doing light activity, which, according to Table 19–1, shows that she requires 35 to 40 kcalories per kilogram per day. Thus, her average calorie allowance would be 53.6 multiplied by 35 to 40, or 1876 to 2144 (average 2010) kcalories per day.

Or the energy requirement could be calculated by determining the percentage increase over the basal calorie requirement. By consulting column B in Table 19–1 one finds that there would be 40 to 60 per cent increase over the student's basal demands. Review Chapter 3, Energy.

RAPID CALORIE REQUIREMENT CALCULATIONS Food specialists in the USDA worked out a formula for rapidly calculating a person's daily energy requirement. The desirable weight in pounds is multiplied by 21 for a man and by 18 for a woman. The result is the approximate number of calories used daily by a moderately active adult. For very active individuals, 25 per cent more calories are required; for a sedentary individual, 25 per cent less.

Example: Using the same subject as above, the calories used daily would be:

118 pounds × 18 or 2124 kcalories

PROTEIN ALLOWANCE

After calculating the daily calorie allowance, the protein fraction of the diet is determined. At least one third of the adult protein fraction should consist of animal or complete protein which contains the essential amino acids. Vegetable proteins are termed incomplete proteins because they do not contain all the essential amino acids.

Protein is essential to life. The recommended daily allowance based on the utilization value of 70 per cent for food proteins is 0.9 gm of protein per kg. of body weight for adults (65 gm. and 55 gm. for the reference man and woman, respectively). The RDA is usually considered adequate for previously well-nourished individuals who are ambulatory patients or require only brief periods of hospitalization. The minimum protein for nitrogen equilibrium ranges from approximately 25 to 40 gm., depending upon the quality of protein ingested. The bed patient who requires more than 10 days' hospitalization, as well as the patient losing formed protein (from burns, exudates, ascites or renal disease), and the patient not forming sufficient protein (hepatic disease) will frequently require an increase. Currently, the trend is to use a liberal protein allowance rather than limit the fraction. Therefore, optimum rather than adequate protein levels are recommended. Review Chapter 6, Proteins.

Severe depletion of body protein can lead to prolonged convalescence, poor wound healing, an increase in complications after surgery, increased susceptibility to infections and anemia, as well as other complications.

The protein foods of high biologic value are usually the more expensive diet items. Thus, there is often a tendency among individuals in the low income groups to consume less animal protein than the recommended amount. If the income is limited, less expensive proteins such as fish, cheese, canned evaporated or powdered milk, beans, and legumes are used, since most animal proteins (meat, eggs, fresh milk, and poultry) are frequently most expensive.

Cultural customs, individual food habits and the supply of foods available are additional factors which influence the protein intake.

The determination of the protein fraction of an individual's diet is illustrated in the following example.

Example: Using the same 20-year-old nursing student previously mentioned, the protein allowance would be:

53.6 × 0.9 equals 48 gm.
of protein per day

FAT AND CARBOHYDRATE ALLOWANCES

Following the calculation of the protein fraction, the remainder of the calories in the diet are determined and they are assigned to fats and carbohydrates. What is the correct or optimum proportion of fat to carbohydrate, particularly meeting the calorie requirements of the body under various conditions? Exact

data on this ratio are scarce. Economic factors dictate the diets of large portions of the population and they select a high percentage of the cheaper carbohydrates. This situation influenced the early diet standards and Voit's diet is an example. It called for 60 to 70 per cent of the total calories in the form of carbohydrates. More recent knowledge of nutrition emphasizes the role of vitamins and minerals, the biologic value of protein, and the possible harm of too much fat. A suggested distribution of proteins, fats and carbohydrates in the diet is shown in Table 19–2. Review Chapter 4, Carbohydrates; and Chapter 5, Lipids.

The average daily food intake of an individual without dietary restrictions amounts to about 60 to 90 gm. of proteins, 90 to 120 gm. of fats, and 300 to 400 gm. of carbohydrates. This proportion may have to be varied to meet the need of certain diseases and will be discussed where indicated.

A rapid, satisfactory clinical method for calculating the constituents of a food prescription consists of dividing the total calorie allowance into approximately 10 to 15 per cent proteins, 25 to 35 per cent fats, and 50 per cent carbohydrates.

Example: Continuing with the same 20-year-old female nursing student used in the examples for calorie and protein allowances, the fat and carbohydrate needs are calculated.

Fat and carbohydrate allowances : to total calories.

Fats average 1 to 2 gm./kg. of desirable body weight or approximately 25 to 35 per cent of total calories.

53.6 × 1.5 equals 80 gm. of fats per day.

Carbohydrates average 4 to 6 gm./kg. of desirable body weight or approximately 50 per cent of total calories.

53.6 × 5 equals
268 gm. of carbohydrates per day.

MINERALS AND VITAMINS

In addition to total calorie, protein, fat and carbohydrate allowances, the diet must satisfy the requirements for the essential minerals

TABLE 19–2   SUGGESTED PROTEIN, FAT AND CARBOHYDRATE ALLOWANCES

AGE	PROTEINS (gm./kg.)	FATS (gm./kg.)	CARBOHYDRATES (gm./kg.)
Under 1 year	2.2	2 to 3	6 to 10
1– 3 years	1.8	2 to 3	6 to 10
3– 6 years	1.8	2 to 3	6 to 10
6– 9 years	1.5	2 to 3	6 to 10
10–20 years	1.3	2 to 3	6 to 10
Adult	0.9	1 to 2	4 to 6
Pregnancy	1 + 10 gm.	1 to 2	4 to 6
Lactation	1 + 20 gm.	1 to 2	4 to 6

and vitamins. All of the foods included in the basic plan were selected particularly because of their essential mineral and vitamin contributions.

MINERALS The requirements for sulfur, phosphorus and potassium, which are laid down with nitrogen in the formation of tissue protoplasm, are increased in certain conditions such as starvation, injury, burns and diabetic acidosis. The efficiency of a high protein diet may be decreased if these minerals are not supplied in sufficient amounts. In acute or relatively acute conditions, sodium and chloride are also of special concern. (See Chapter 8.) The Recommended Dietary Allowances (Table 11–1) are considered adequate for the other minerals in acute or semi-acute situations, but in long-term mineral imbalances, calcium, iron and iodine are of major importance. The amount of iron in normal diet is believed to be about 6 mg. per 1000 kcal. For the adult male 10 mg. daily is recommended. The adult female in the childbearing years needs 18 mg. according to the RDA revised in 1968. A supplement of iron or fortified foods is indicated. In severe sodium restricted diets the iodine content may be below the requirements of approximately 1 μg. per kg. These will be considered in subsequent chapters with the various diseases. Review Chapter 8, The Minerals.

VITAMINS Vitamin requirements under stress situations have never been completely determined. Common practice has been to give up to ten times the normal Recommended Dietary Allowances. However, in many instances, these large intakes are probably not indicated. Since accurate metabolic studies of vitamin requirements during and after disease and injury are lacking, the requirements must be approximated. In arriving at suggested allowances, Pollack and Halpern consider the following factors: (1) requirements for normal individuals, (2) the nature of the disease or injury, (3) the known capacity of the body to store certain vitamins, (4) known losses through the skin, urine or intestinal tract produced by various phenomena, and (5) the interrelations of nutrient requirements. Review Chapter 9, Vitamins.

Thiamin Evidence indicates that thiamin requirement is related to body weight and the caloric content of the diet. (See p. 130.) The requirement is further influenced by the amount of carbohydrate in the diet, since the enzymes containing thiamin are involved in carbohydrate metabolism. A liberal allowance of thiamin is advisable when patients are receiving glucose intravenously. There is no evidence that in minor injuries or illness the thiamin requirements are greatly increased above normal. However, in severely injured

and diseased individuals the thiamin allowance may be increased to about 5 mg. daily. When a definite depletion exists, 10 to 25 mg. of thiamin per day may be indicated for the first week to ten days, to be followed by a maintenance dose of 5 mg. daily until convalescence is well along. Thiamin deficiency is sometimes precipitated during the refeeding of starved persons. The increased calorie and carbohydrate intake sharply increases the body demands for this vitamin. When oral antibiotics are administered, thiamin requirements, as well as those of the other B-complex vitamins, may be increased due to interference with biosynthesis of thiamin.

Example: Continuing with the same 20-year-old female nursing student, the thiamin allowance would be: 0.5 mg./1000 kcalories/day or 1.0 mg./2000 kcalories diet/day.

Riboflavin The allowances recommended by the Food and Nutrition Board, National Research Council, are based on calorie intake and body size, which takes into account body size and metabolic rate but does not consider rate of growth. Riboflavin requirements in disease have not been clearly defined to date. Minor illnesses and injuries should not alter the requirement, providing food consumption is normal. After a severe injury, illness, or burn, requirements may be increased five to ten times normal.

Example: Continuing with the same 20-year-old female nursing student, the riboflavin allowance would be: 0.7 mg./1000 kcalories/day or 1.4 mg./2000 kcalorie diet/day.

Niacin Niacin requirements in health and disease are related to tryptophan-containing protein intake. The amino acid tryptophan can serve as a precursor of niacin. Like thiamin it plays an important role in the intermediary carbohydrate metabolism. The current Food and Nutrition Board recommendations are based on calorie intake and expressed as niacin equivalents, including dietary sources of the preformed vitamin and the precursor tryptophan. (See p. 134.)

Little is known concerning the metabolism and requirement of niacin in stress situations. It has been suggested that following severe injury, infection, and burns, the metabolism of niacin is altered similar to that of other members of the B-complex. During the acute phase of and also in the early period of convalescence, at least 50 to 100 mg. of niacinamide has been recommended. In cases of previous depletion or deficiency, niacinamide is administered up to 500 mg. per day during the first seven to ten days, or longer.

Example: Continuing with the same 20-year-old female nursing student, the niacin allowance would be:

6.6 mg./1000 kcalories/day or 13.2 mg. niacin equivalent/2000 kcalorie diet/day.

Pantothenic Acid and Vitamin B$_6$ (Pyridoxine)   It is generally believed that the amount of pantothenic acid needed is 10 mg. (10 times the thiamin requirement). A 2000 kcal. diet will provide about 10 mg. Authorities recommend that these vitamins be included in the dietary supplements of individuals who have undergone nutritional depletion or who are forced to subsist on processed rations for any length of time.

There has been no evidence produced to indicate that the requirements for these two substances are related to calories. A specific relationship exists between vitamin B$_6$ and the metabolism of tryptophan; the requirement for vitamin B$_6$ increases with the protein in the diet. (See p. 135.) The Food and Nutrition Board, National Research Council, recommended an intake of 2 mg. per day, which they believed would be adequate for the metabolism of 100 gm. of protein.

Folic Acid and Vitamin B$_{12}$ During certain stress situations, the hematopoietic system may be depressed. Both vitamin B$_{12}$ and folic acid have some relation to normal hematopoiesis. Folacin is used in the treatment of nutritional megaloblastic anemia caused by folate deficiency. The amount needed is influenced by body size and metabolic rate. RDA for adults has been set at 0.4 mg.

Many pregnant women manifest a folacin deficiency in the last trimester. Stressful conditions such as hemolytic anemia, leukemia, Hodgkin's disease, carcinomatosis, hyperthyroidism, malabsorption syndromes and consumption of alcohol increase the requirement of folacin.

Folacin does not relieve the neurological symptoms of pernicious anemia. If absorption is normal, a dietary intake of 5 μg. per day of vitamin B$_{12}$ is required to meet the needs of adults. Pernicious anemia patients will respond to as little as 0.1 μg. by intramuscular injection or 5 to 15 μg. taken orally with the intrinsic factor. A diet of 15 μg. will gradually replenish body stores. Strict vegetarians who develop neurological symptoms from a dietary deficiency of vitamin B$_{12}$ do not develop anemia as a rule.

Ascorbic Acid   Ascorbic acid requirements in stress are reported to be abnormally high. This is most likely due to increased utilization, not necessarily to a pre-existing deficiency. However, opinions differ fairly widely regarding normal and therapeutic requirements of vitamin C. The Committee on Therapeutic Nutrition recommends as much as 1 to 2 gm. daily during acute stages of stress, and 300 mg. thereafter. Burns, excessive trauma, and long bone fractures probably necessitate 1 gm. of ascorbic acid daily during the acute phase, and 300 mg. until convalescence is established. Thereafter, 70 to 100 mg. daily is believed adequate. Under moderate stress circumstances about 300 mg. daily is advised. (See p. 142.)

Vitamin A   There is no evidence to date of an *increased* need for fat-soluble vitamin A for short time illnesses *except* in hepatic disease where storage or availability may be less than normal. However, the normal requirement of 5000 I.U. should always be ensured.

Vitamin D   There have been no studies to indicate that acute febrile bacterial diseases, surgical procedures, and burns in any way alter the metabolism of vitamin D in adults. For fracture cases, however, because of the role of vitamin D in calcium and phosphorus metabolism, 400 I.U. of vitamin D should be ensured.

Vitamin E   Therapeutic use of vitamin E has been under considerable study in the treatment of a large number of conditions. Some evidence supports its use among women who have repeated spontaneous abortions. Some types of ulcers have responded to the vitamin E therapy. Claims have been made for its effectiveness in complications of menopause, muscular dystrophy, diabetes, male infertility and heart disease but evidence is lacking to support these claims. Those conditions which interfere with the absorption of fat (biliary tract diseases, pancreatic insufficiency and ingestion of mineral oil) interfere with the absorption of vitamin E. Vitamin E requirement is increased when polyunsaturated fat intake is increased and in severe protein deficiency conditions.

Vitamin K   It is believed that vitamin K requirements are fulfilled by any mixed diet, except in certain stress conditions which may interfere with the absorption or metabolism of the vitamin to result in a deficiency. Oral administration of streptomycin greatly reduces the synthesis of vitamin K by intestinal organisms. There is clinical evidence that other antibiotics and the sulfonamides are capable of inducing certain signs and symptoms which respond to the administration of the B-complex vitamins with folic acid. It is therefore suggested that vitamin K always be given when antibiotics or sulfonamides are given orally. (See p. 129.) Menadione (vitamin K$_3$) is prohibited in prenatal supplements because of its toxicity qualities.

FLUIDS

Water, although not considered a food, is an indispensable nutrient and plays an important

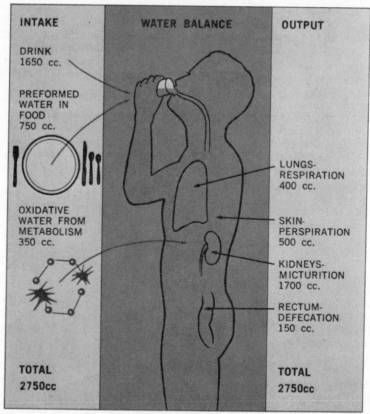

Figure 19–1   Man maintains the osmotic pressure of his body fluids at optimum level by adjusting his water intake and output. Most of his need of water comes from the liquid itself. Some he draws from the moisture in his food and the remainder he manufactures himself. The importance of this "water of oxidation" varies according to species: the kangaroo rat, for example, drinks no water at all. His water need, proportionately the same as man's, is met by the moisture in his diet and that which he manufactures himself. (From Nutrition Today, 5:22, 1970.)

role in the proper functioning of the human body. It is always listed along with foods.

Optimum convalescence demands normal tissue hydration. The Therapeutic Committee estimates that 1800 to 2500 ml. of water is required daily by a normal, not sweating, healthy adult at rest, to provide for urinary secretion, and to replace losses from insensible perspiration. Additional fluids must be added to replace water lost by excessive sweating, vomiting, diarrhea, or other conditions in which there is increased water loss. (See Chapter 10, Water and Electrolytes.) If sufficient water is not obtained through fluid intake and food (Figure 19–1), it must be supplied parenterally.

SUMMARY OF A FOOD PRESCRIPTION

The sample in Table 19–3 shows how a completed food prescription for a normal adult, as described in the preceding pages, is finally assembled.

MODIFICATIONS OF NORMAL DIET

The normal diet may be modified and thereby become a specific therapeutic diet. The substitutions and modifications are made to help compensate for the dysfunction of the affected body part or to meet the specific needs of a disease.

The adjustment in diet may take place in any of the following forms:
1. Change in consistency of foods.
   Examples: Liquid diet; soft diet; low fiber diet; high fiber diet.
2. Increase or decrease in energy value of diet.
   Examples: Reduction diet; high calorie diet.
3. Increase or decrease in type of foods.
   Examples: High acid ash diet; sodium-restricted diet; vitamin deficiency diet.
4. Omission of specific foods.
   Example: Allergy diet.
5. Adjustment in the ratio and balance of

TABLE 19–3   CONSTRUCTION OF DAILY FOOD PRESCRIPTION FOR A NORMAL ADULT

STANDARD ALLOWANCES	TYPICAL APPLICATION
Desirable weight for: (see Tables 13 to 15 in Appendix)	53.6 kg. (118 pounds)
Sex	Female (nursing student)
Age	20 years
Height	162.5 centimeters (5 feet 5 inches)
Protein allowances:	
0.9 gm./kg. desirable body weight or approximately 10 to 20% total calories.	53.6 × 0.9 = 48 gm. proteins per day
Fats and carbohydrate allowances:	
Fats average 1 to 2 gm./kg. desirable body weight or approximately 25 to 35% total calories	53.6 × 1.5 = 80 gm. fats per day
Carbohydrates average 4 to 6 gm./kg. desirable body weight or approximately 50% total calories	53.6 × 5 = 268 gm. carbohydrates per day
Energy or calorie allowance:	
Activity: light	
Calories required per kilogram desirable body weight per day (see Table 19–1): 35 to 40	53.6 × 35 to 40 = 1876 to 2144 (average 2010) calories per day.
Calories from food constituents:	
Protein equals 4 kcalories per gram	48 × 4 = 192 kcalories
Fat equals 9 kcalories per gram	80 × 9 = 720 kcalories
Carbohydrate equals 4 kcalories per gram	268 × 4 = 1072 kcalories
	1984 total kcalories per day
Mineral allowances:	
Calcium: 0.8 gm. per day	Calcium: 0.8 gm. per day
Iron: 18 mg. per day	Iron: 18 mg. per day
Vitamin allowances:	
Vitamin A : 5000 I.U. per day	Vitamin A : 5000 I.U. per day
Thiamin : 0.5 mg./1000 kcalories per day	Thiamin : 1.0 mg. per day
Riboflavin : 0.7 mg./1000 kcalories per day	Riboflavin : 1.5 mg. per day
Niacin equiv. : 6.6 mg./1000 kcalories per day	Niacin equiv. : 13.2 mg. per day
Ascorbic acid : 55 mg. per day	Ascorbic acid : 55 mg. per day
Vitamin D : (?) I.U. per day	Vitamin D : (?) I.U. per day

Food Prescription: Kcalories, 2000; proteins, 48 gm.; fats, 80 gm.; carbohydrates, 265 gm.; calcium, 0.8 gm.; iron, 18 mg.; vitamin A, 5000 I.U.; thiamin, 1.0 mg.; riboflavin, 1.5 mg.; niacin equivalent, 13.2 mg.; ascorbic acid, 55 mg.; and vitamin D, (?) I.U.

food constituents: proteins, fats, and carbohydrates.

Examples: Diabetic diet; ketogenic diet; high protein diet; low fat diet.

6. Rearrangement of the number and frequency of meals.

Example: Gastric ulcer diet.

Some of the modifications may overlap in individual diets. For example: a patient may be on a diabetic diet but because of acute indigestion or poor teeth he may also require a soft diet.

Diets must be flexible to be practical and usable. Therefore, it is quite impossible to draw a final and decisive line to divide diets into separate and distinct categories.

The same standards of recommended dietary allowances for food constituents established for the normal body requirements are considered, with amounts of nutrients adjusted to cover the needs created by disease or injury, when modifications in the diet are indicated.

CLASSIFICATION OF THERAPEUTIC DIETS

Therapeutic diets may be classified as qualitative and quantitative modifications of the normal diet. The qualitative diet is an adjusted adequate diet according to the type of food allowed. The quantitative diet is calculated with an increase or decrease in the amount of the food constituents. To illustrate: the gastrointestinal diets are qualitative while a diabetic diet is quantitative.

THE PRINCIPAL SOURCES OF FOOD CONSTITUENTS

To be familiar with the various foods included in a diet, it is necessary to know their analysis. For that reason Table 19–4 was planned as an aid in learning the contents of various foods. Knowing the nutrients contained in the different foods is essential information for correctly evaluating therapeutic diets.

A set of colorful charts illustrating the various food nutrients (approved by the Council on Foods and Nutrition of the American Medical Association), to serve as an aid in teaching or calculating the nutritional adequacy of a diet, is available from the National Live Stock and Meat Board.[4] Each chart gives a "capsule" story of a key nutrient.

---

[4]36 South Wabash Ave., Chicago, Illinois 60603.

TABLE 19–4   THE PRINCIPAL SOURCES OF THE VARIOUS FOOD CONSTITUENTS*

Stars on the chart below give a rough idea of how servings from groups of familiar foods contribute toward dietary needs—the more stars, the better the food as a source of the nutrient. The percentages given below the chart are based on the National Research Council's recommended dietary allowances for a young, moderately active man. Some foods within a group have more of a nutrient, some less; but in a varied diet, which is common in this country, a group is likely to average as shown.

KIND OF FOOD	SIZE OF SERVING (READY-TO-EAT)	PROTEIN	CALCIUM	IRON	VITAMIN A VALUE	B VITAMINS†			VITAMIN C (ASCORBIC ACID)	FOOD ENERGY (IN KILOCALORIES)
						THIAMIN	RIBOFLAVIN	NIACIN		
Milk	1 cup	★	★★★★		★	★	★★			165
Cheese, process Cheddar	1 ounce	★	★★★		★		★			105
Meat, poultry, fish	4 ounces	★★		★★	★	★	★	★★		195
Eggs	1 large egg	★		★	★		★			80
Dry beans and peas, nuts	¾ cup cooked beans	★★	★	★★★		★	★	★		170
Whole grain or enriched products	2 slices bread	★	★	★		★	★	★		120
Citrus fruits	½ cup								★★★★★	50
Other fruits	½ cup			★	★				★	60
Tomatoes, tomato juice	½ cup			★	★★★			★	★★★	25
Dark-green and deep-yellow vegetables (except sweet potatoes)	½ cup		★	★	★★★★★		★		★★★★	40
Sweet potatoes	1 medium		★	★	★★★★★	★	★	★	★★★	170
Light-green vegetables¹	½ cup		★	★	★				★★	35
Potatoes	1 medium			★		★		★	★★★	90
Other vegetables	½ cup			★					★	40
Butter, margarine	1 tablespoon				★					100
Other fats	2 tablespoons									220
Sugar, all kinds	2 teaspoons									35
Molasses, sirups	2 tablespoons			★★						110

★★★★★ More than 50 per cent of daily need.
★★★★ About 40 per cent of daily need.
★★★ About 30 per cent of daily need.
★★ About 20 per cent of daily need.
★ About 10 per cent of daily need.

¹Includes asparagus, green snap beans, peas, green lima beans, green cabbage, brussels sprouts, green lettuce.
*Family Fare—Food Management and Recipes. Washington, D.C., U.S. Department of Agriculture, Home and Garden Bulletin No. 1, 1960.
†Foods supplying thiamin, riboflavin and niacin are good sources of other members of the B vitamin group.

PROBLEMS AND SUGGESTED TOPICS FOR DISCUSSION

1. How is the normal diet pattern used in the planning of therapeutic diets?
2. Using the foundation of an adequate diet as a pattern, decide whether your patient eats an adequate diet. Consider (a) locality, (b) income level of the individual (c) available foods, (d) food prescription and (e) nutritional variation from the normal due to injury or disease, if any.

SUGGESTED ADDITIONAL READING REFERENCES

Balsley, M.: A look at selected diet manuals. J. Am. Dietet. A., 47:123, 1965.
Bean, W. B.: The clinician interrogates nutrition. Am. J. Clin. Nutr., 13:263, 1963.
Cooper, L. F.: Florence Nightingale's contribution to dietetics. J. Am. Dietet. A., 30:121, 1954.
Darby, W. J.: Basic contributions to medicine by research in nutrition. J.A.M.A., 180:816, 1962.

Hegsted, D. M.: Nutritional requirements in disease. J. Am. Dietet. A., 56:303, 1970.
Jolliffe, N.: Clinical Nutrition. 2nd ed. New York, Harper and Bros., 1962, Chapter 23, Principles of Nutrition Therapy by N. Jolliffe and W. A. Krehl.
Pollack, H., and Halpern, S. L.: Therapeutic Nutrition. Washington, D.C., National Research Council, Publication 234, 1952.
Recommended Dietary Allowances. 7th ed. Food and Nutrition Board, National Research Council, Pub. No. 1694, 1968.
Robinson, C.: Food therapy begins with the normal diet. Am. J. Clin. Nutr., 1:150, 1953.
Sebrell, W. H., Jr.: Adequate therapeutic diets. J. Am. Dietet. A., 30:1256, 1954.
Selye, H.: On just being sick. Nutrition Today, 5:2, 1970.
Seymour, M.: Current practices, research and education in diet therapy. Am. J. Clin. Nutr., 14:233, 1964.
Walker, A. P. R.: Anomalies in the prediction of nutritional disease. Nutr. Rev. 19:257, 1961.
Wohl, M. G., and Goodhart, K. S. (ed.): Modern Nutrition in Health and Disease. 4th ed. Philadelphia, Lea & Febiger, 1968.
Youmans, J. B.: The changing face of nutritional disease in America. J.A.M.A., 189:672, 1964.

Chapter 20
HOSPITAL
HOUSE DIETS

Food served in any institution is not like that to which patients are accustomed and hospitals are no exceptions. Patients come from all walks of life and they bring their food habits and idiosyncrasies with them. Illness with its stress and anxiety affects appetite, taste, digestion, utilization of foods and personalities of individuals. The kind of diet which is suitable for the person's nutritional needs is prescribed by his physician. Related physiological and psychological problems arise with the ability of individuals to ingest food served to them. In administering patient care, an important aspect of the therapeutic measures instituted for the hospitalized person is how well he consumes the foods served.

Food service to patients requires imagination and ingenuity in planning for a variety of foods familiar to them. The appearance of the food on the tray—its color, texture, composition—is important to most people. Seasonings and flavorings are often restricted. The lack of these usually relates to eating problems which one encounters in giving care.

NUTRITIONAL ADEQUACY OF HOSPITAL DIETS

All hospitals and institutions engaged in feeding the sick have specific, basic, routine diets, designed for uniformity and convenience of service. They are commonly termed "house diets." These diets are based on the foundation of an adequate diet pattern (Chapter 11: Table 11–4 and p. 163), which, in turn, is formulated from the Recommended Daily Dietary Allowances, as outlined and discussed in previous chapters. It must be remembered that these recommendations apply to normal, healthy individuals and are not designed to meet the needs of acutely or chronically ill, injured, or convalescent patients. Therefore, house diets must be carried a step further to cover the increased metabolic demands created by stress or illness.

According to Pollack and Halpern, with the collaboration of the Committee on Therapeutic Nutrition of the Food and Nutrition Board, National Research Council,[1] "It is current practice to calculate the hospital diet on the basis of the nutritional requirements of healthy individuals and to *neglect the additional demands created by disease.*" The interpretation of the house diets for the individual patient must be a liberal one.

TYPES OF HOUSE DIETS The types of house diets are generally referred to as *general, light, soft,* and *liquid.* These diets are used routinely for patients not requiring a therapeutic diet, depending upon their food tolerance and physical condition. It is important for the nurse to be familiar with the principles and contents of the various house diets, since they serve as a foundation for the diversified therapeutic diets.

FOOD INTAKE An important observation for the nurse to make is that the food *served* does not necessarily represent the *food intake* of the patient. In a hospital food intake study conducted by one of the authors (unpublished data), a week's survey of the general diets, as served, showed a daily variation in patient's intake between 1900 and 3200 kcalories, with the average patient's intake approximating 2570 kcalories. When the patients in semiprivate rooms selected food from a menu of approximately 2500 to 3000 kcalories, about 25 per cent of the bread, butter and vegetables, and 37 per cent of the salads were not eaten. The ward patients on a nonselective, general diet of approximately the same number of calories left between 5 and 10 per cent of the food uneaten.

In another hospital food intake study[2] it was

---

[1]Pollack, H., and Halpern, S. L. Therapeutic Nutrition. Washington, D.C., National Research Council, Publication 234, 1952.

[2]Ahart, H. E.: Assessing food intake of hospital patients. J. Am. Dietet. A., 40:114, 1962.

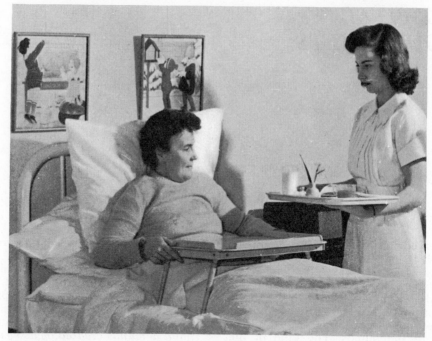

Figure 20–1   To serve a good diet is not sufficient. Consumption of the food by the patient must be assured. (Cornell University photograph. Reprinted from Health News, monthly publication of the New York State Department of Health.)

observed that patients eating from trays appeared to consume diets of higher nutritive value than did ambulatory patients eating in a dining room. However, possible food consumption outside of regular meals was not observed or known. The *average* figures showed a food intake approximating the Recommended Dietary Allowances for the healthy subject, but *individual* records indicated that the food selection and consumption of some patients would not provide sufficient nutrients to meet the standard. Most noticeable was the low intake of fruits and vegetables by some patients, which resulted in a large number of intakes below recommendations for ascorbic acid and vitamin A.

Regardless of the type of diet prescribed for a patient, it is important to check both the food served and the food left on the tray to obtain an accurate indication of the patient's calorie and nutrition intake. This factor is of major importance and it should not be overlooked. (See Fig. 20–1.)

THE GENERAL OR ADEQUATE NORMAL DIET

In some hospitals the general diet is also known as "regular," "full" or "house" diet. The general diet is a basic adequate normal diet of approximately 2000 to 2500 kcalories and contains 70 to 80 gm. of proteins, 80 to 100 gm. of fats and 200 to 300 gm. of carbo-

hydrates. All the protective foods outlined in the foundation of an adequate diet pattern which includes the basic four food groups (p. 18) – meat, milk, eggs, citrus fruits, vegetables, whole grain or enriched bread and cereal – are included. Additional foods or more of the same foods, such as butter or fortified margarine, desserts, salad dressing, crackers and sugar, are added to increase calories and to make the diet more palatable. There are no particular food restrictions. However, foods which may cause digestive disturbances, such as cooked cabbage and fried pork, are used with discretion.

An example of an average general diet is shown in Table 20–1.

THE LIGHT DIET

The light diet (Table 20–2) is an adequate diet. Generally speaking, it is used for a limited period or until the patient is ready to accept a general diet. It is considered a transitional diet, and the limited contents may become monotonous for long-term consumption.

The composition of a light diet is similar to the general diet. The chief difference is the very simple preparation of the foods allowed in the diet. Fried foods, highly seasoned foods, rich pastries, fatty foods such as roast pork, and coarse foods such as bran, celery, melon, and apple are omitted.

TABLE 20-1   GENERAL OR ADEQUATE NORMAL DIET

MEAL PLAN	SAMPLE MENU	SERVINGS Weight Grams	Household Measure
	BREAKFAST		
Fruit	Fresh grapefruit	100	one half (no skin)
Cereal	Cooked oatmeal (cooked weight)	118	½ cup
Egg	Soft cooked egg	50	1
Bread	Whole wheat toast	23	1 slice
Butter	Butter or fortified margarine	7	1 pat
Milk	Milk	244	1 cup
Cream	Cream	60	2 ounces
Sugar	Sugar	15	3 teaspoons
Coffee	Coffee	200	2 coffee cups
	LUNCHEON		
Soup	Beef broth with rice	125	½ cup
Crackers	Saltines	8	2
Entrée	Macaroni and cheese	110	½ cup
Vegetable	Cooked asparagus	96	6 spears
Salad	Tomato and watercress	100	1 serving
Salad dressing	French dressing	15	1 tablespoon
Bread	Whole wheat roll	30	1 average
Butter	Butter or fortified margarine	7	1 pat
Milk	Milk	244	1 glass
Fruit	Stewed Royal Anne cherries	100	10 with juice
	DINNER		
Meat	London broil	85	3 ounces
Potato	Stuffed baked potato	150	1 medium
Vegetable	Savory green beans	75	½ cup
Bread	Rye bread	23	1 slice
Butter	Butter or fortified margarine	7	1 pat
Dessert	Strawberry ice cream	62	1 average dipper (3½ oz.)
Milk	Milk	244	1 glass

TABLE 20-2   LIGHT DIET

MEAL PLAN	SAMPLE BREAKFAST	SERVINGS Weight Grams	Household Measure
	BREAKFAST		
Fruit	Orange juice	124	½ cup
Cereal	Cooked oatmeal (cooked weight)	118	½ cup
Egg	Soft cooked egg	50	1
Bread	Toasted enriched bread	23	1 slice
Butter	Butter or fortified margarine	7	1 pat
Milk	Milk	244	1 cup
Cream	Cream	60	2 ounces
Sugar	Sugar	15	3 teaspoons
Coffee	Coffee	200	2 coffee cups
	LUNCHEON		
Soup	Beef broth with rice	125	½ cup
Crackers	Saltines	8	2
Entrée	Macaroni and cheese	110	½ cup
Vegetable	Cooked wax beans	75	½ cup
Salad	Tomato and lettuce	100	1 serving
Salad dressing	French dressing	15	1 tablespoon
Bread	Light rye bread	23	1 slice
Butter	Butter or fortified margarine	7	1 pat
Fruit	Canned peaches	117	2 halves and 2 tbsp. syrup
Milk	Milk	244	1 glass
	DINNER		
Meat	Lamb chops, broiled	137	1 thick, with bone
Potato	Mashed potato	98	½ cup
Vegetable	Buttered beets	83	½ cup
Bread	Light rye bread	23	1 slice
Butter	Butter or fortified margarine	7	1 pat
Dessert	Vanilla ice cream	62	1 average dipper (3½ oz.)
Milk	Milk	244	1 glass

FOODS INCLUDED

Milk: Milk beverages, buttermilk, cream.

Eggs: Hard or soft cooked, poached, scrambled.

Meat, fish, poultry: Prepared by boiling, broiling or roasting – ground or tender beef, lamb, veal; liver; fish; poultry; and bacon. Meat is frequently limited to lamb, chicken and fish.

Cheese: Cottage, pot, cream, and mild American-Cheddar.

Breads: Plain or toasted fine whole wheat, rye without seeds, and enriched white; refined white crackers.

Cereals: Refined or finely ground (enriched).

Cereal products: Macaroni, spaghetti, noodles, rice.

Fats: Butter, fortified margarine, and oil.

Vegetables: Cooked vegetables of low fiber – asparagus, beets, carrots, green beans, young peas, potatoes, spinach, and squash – which are either boiled, mashed, creamed, baked or scalloped; lettuce and tomato salad.

Fruits: Cooked without skin or seeds (no pineapple), fruit juices, and ripe banana.

Soups: Clear soup broths, strained vegetables, and strained cream soups.

Desserts: Plain puddings, cakes, cookies, and frozen desserts prepared without nuts.

Beverages: All liquids.

FOODS OMITTED

Salads with the exception of lettuce and tomato, raw fruits with the exception of bananas and fruit juices, coarse vegetables, rich pastries, nuts.

THE SOFT DIET

The soft diet (Table 20–3) is used as a transition diet. Since the present trend in diet therapy is toward a more liberal interpretation of diet and foods allowed, the soft and light diets are frequently combined. In other words, the hospital will have either a *soft diet* or a *light diet.* The very limited diets are not used so much nor are they so acceptable to hospital regimen and management.

The soft diet is an adequate diet with the characteristic of being moderately low in cellulose and connective tissue. Fried foods are omitted. The soft diet is planned for conditions where mechanical ease in eating or digestion, or both, is desired plus supplying a diet low in residue. It is a good diet for patients who have no teeth, only a few teeth or ill-fitting dental plates.

The average composition of the soft diet is 1800 to 2000 kcalories. However, the calories as well as the protein, fat, and carbohydrate allowances are adjustable according to the individual's needs based on activity, height, weight, sex, age, and any specific demands made by disease.

TABLE 20–3   SOFT DIET

MEAL PLAN	SAMPLE MENU	Weight Grams	Household Measure
		SERVINGS	
BREAKFAST			
Fruit	Orange juice	124	1/2 glass
Cereal	Cooked farina (cooked weight)	119	1/2 cup
Egg	Poached egg on toast	50	1
Bread	Toasted bread (enriched)	23	1 slice
Butter	Butter or fortified margarine	7	1 pat
Cream	Cream	60	2 ounces
Milk	Milk	244	1 cup
Sugar	Sugar	15	3 teaspoons
Coffee	Coffee	200	2 coffee cups
LUNCHEON			
Soup	Tomato consommé	120	1/2 cup
Entrée	Baked macaroni and cheese	110	1/2 cup
Vegetables	Cooked asparagus tips or purée	96	6 spears
Bread	Light rye bread	23	1 slice
Butter	Butter or fortified margarine	7	1 pat
Fruit	Applesauce	127	1/2 cup
Milk	Milk	244	1 glass
DINNER			
Meat	Sliced chicken	85	3 ounces
Potato	Mashed potato	98	1/2 cup
Vegetable	Buttered spinach purée	90	1/2 cup
Bread	Light rye bread	23	1 slice
Butter	Butter or fortified margarine	7	1 pat
Dessert	Chocolate ice cream	62	1 average dipper (3½ oz.)
Milk	Milk	244	1 glass

Some hospitals limit the use of vegetables in the soft diet to purées and do not allow any meats. This procedure is practiced if a *soft* and a *light diet* are included in the hospital regimen.

However, the current trend in diet planning fosters liberal interpretation. Vegetable purées are notoriously unpopular and patients refuse to eat them. To prove the point one large hospital[3] omitted vegetable purées from the soft diet in favor of cooked low-fiber vegetables. The result was a more palatable diet. The response was noticeable in happier patients who benefited from eating vegetables which previously had been refused. The number of vegetable purée servings for luncheon and dinner was reduced from seventy to twenty.

The hospitals following the trend of more liberal diet interpretation and planning serve fine whole grain or enriched bread and cereals on soft diets.

FOODS INCLUDED

Milk: Milk beverage, buttermilk, cream.

Eggs: Soft or hard cooked, poached, scrambled.

Meat, fish, poultry: Prepared by boiling, broiling or roasting—ground beef, lamb, veal, liver; fish; poultry without skin; bacon. (Some hospitals omit all meats on the diet.)

---

[3]Krause, Marie V.: Some modern concepts concerning hospital diets. J. Am. Dietet. A., 20:610, 1944.

Cheese: Cottage, pot, and cream cheese; other cheese may be used for flavoring in cooking, such as American-Cheddar of a mild variety.

Breads: Plain or toasted fine whole wheat, rye without seeds, enriched white; white crackers.

Cereals: Enriched, refined or finely ground.

Cereal products: Macaroni, spaghetti, noodles, rice.

Fats: Butter, oil, fortified margarine.

Vegetables: Cooked vegetables of low fiber—asparagus, beets, carrots, green beans, young peas, potatoes, spinach, and squash—which are boiled or steamed, mashed, creamed, baked, or escalloped; vegetable purées; vegetable juices. (Some hospitals do not serve any whole vegetables on the *soft diet.*)

Fruits: Cooked without skin or seeds (no pineapple), cooked fruit purées, fruit juices, and ripe banana.

Soups: Clear soup broths, strained vegetables and strained cream soups.

Desserts: Plain puddings, cakes, cookies, and frozen desserts prepared without nuts.

Beverages: All liquids.

FOODS OMITTED

Salads, raw fruits with the exception of bananas and fruit juices, coarse vegetables, coarse breads and cereals, rich pastries, nuts.

TABLE 20–4   FULL LIQUID DIET

| | | SERVINGS | |
MEAL PLAN	SAMPLE MENU	Weight Grams	Household Measure
	BREAKFAST		
Fruit	Strained orange juice	124	½ cup
Cereal	Cooked thin farina gruel (cooked weight)	120	½ cup
Cream	Cream	60	2 ounces
Sugar	Sugar	15	3 teaspoons
Coffee	Coffee	200	2 coffee cups
	10:00 A.M.		
Milk beverage	Milk	244	1 glass
	LUNCHEON		
Soup	Tomato consommé	120	½ cup
Fruit juice	Grape juice	254	1 cup
Dessert	Vanilla ice cream	62	1 average dipper (3½ oz.)
	3:00 P.M.		
Milk beverage	Vanilla malted milk	270	1 cup
	DINNER		
Soup	Strained cream of pea soup	122	½ cup
Dessert	Raspberry gelatin	60	¼ cup
Beverage	Tea	200	2 teacups
Sugar	Sugar	10	2 teaspoons
	8:00 P.M.		
Milk beverage	Eggnog	233	1 cup

Note: To increase the calories for the daily diet, add sugar, cream, and butter or fortified margarine whenever possible.

LIQUID DIETS

Liquid diets are commonly ordered for patients with conditions requiring easily digested and easily consumed nourishment, free from mechanical irritants and irritating condiments. The two varieties of liquid diets are classified as full liquid diet and clear or restricted liquid diet.

FULL LIQUID DIET

The full liquid diet (Table 20-4) contains all foods which are liquid at room and body temperature. For example, ice cream is considered a liquid.

The diet may be considered adequate for maintenance requirements. The average composition of the diet is approximately 1300 to 1500 kcalories, 45 gm. of protein, 65 gm. of fat, and 150 gm. of carbohydrate. By careful planning, the diet can be increased in protein and caloric value to more nearly approach the normal diet and even a high calorie diet. Increasing the protein and calories in a liquid diet is necessary when a patient must remain on such a diet for an indefinite period. Protein and vitamin supplements (Ch. 43) can be added to the liquids to increase the protein and vitamin intake.

FOODS INCLUDED

Milk: Milk and milk beverages, cream.
Soups: Clear broth, strained cream soups, strained vegetable soups.
Cereals: Cereal gruel.
Fruits: Strained fruit juices.
Vegetables: Strained vegetable juice and vegetable water.

Beverages: Tea, coffee, albuminized beverages, carbonated beverages, eggnog, malted milk beverages.
Desserts: Plain gelatin dessert, ice cream without seeds or nuts, ices, sherbet, milk-rennet pudding, soft custard.
Sweets: Sugar.
Fats: Butter, fortified margarine, oil.

CLEAR OR RESTRICTED LIQUID DIET

The clear or restricted liquid diet (Table 20-5) is frequently ordered for postoperative patients to furnish non-gas-forming fluid and nourishment. It is an inadequate diet composed chiefly of water and carbohydrates; therefore, it is used a very short time. The average *clear* or *restricted liquid diet* contains 400 to 500 kilocalories, 5 gm. of protein, no fat, and 100 to 120 gm. of carbohydrate.

The liquid is served at frequent intervals to supply the tissues with fluid and to relieve thirst. As the name would indicate, the diet consists of clear liquids such as tea, broth, carbonated beverages, and strained fruit juice. Milk and liquids prepared with milk are omitted. Fats are omitted. Some patients become distended and very uncomfortable if given fruit juice, especially orange juice. Carbonated beverages, especially ginger ale, seem to be tolerated by the majority of the patients. Fruit juices which do not agree with the patient are omitted from the diet. As usual, the diet is planned with due consideration to the patient's food idiosyncrasies.

TABLE 20-5 CLEAR OR RESTRICTED LIQUID DIET

MEAL PLAN	SAMPLE MENU	SERVINGS Weight Grams	Household Measure
	BREAKFAST		
Fruit juice	Orange juice (strained)	124	1/2 cup
Beverage	Coffee (decaffeinated)	200	2 coffee cups
Sugar	Sugar	10	2 teaspoons
	10:00 A.M.		
Fruitade	Lemonade	240	1 cup
	LUNCHEON		
Soup	Consommé	120	1/2 cup
Fruit juice	Grapefruit juice (strained)	123	1/2 glass
Tea	Tea	200	2 teacups
Sugar	Sugar	10	2 teaspoons
	3:00 P.M.		
Carbonated beverage	Ginger ale	230	1 cup
	DINNER		
Soup	Chicken broth	125	1/2 cup
Gelatin	Raspberry gelatin	60	1/4 cup
Tea	Tea	200	2 teacups
Sugar	Sugar	10	2 teaspoons
	8:00 P.M.		
Fruit juice	Orange juice (strained)	248	1 cup

TABLE 20-6   SUMMARY OF BASIC HOSPITAL DIETS

TYPE OF FOOD ALLOWED	GENERAL OR ADEQUATE NORMAL DIET	LIGHT DIET	SOFT DIET	FULL LIQUID DIET	CLEAR LIQUID DIET
Milk, cream, buttermilk	Included	Included	Included	Included	Not included
Eggs	Raw and cooked	Included	Included	In beverages	Not included
Cheese	All varieties	Cottage, pot, cream, mild American Cheddar	Cottage, pot, cream; American Cheddar as flavoring	Not allowed	Not included
Fats	All kinds	Butter, fortified margarine, oil, mayonnaise and French dressing	Butter, fortified margarine, oil	Butter, fortified margarine, oil	Not included
Meat, fish, poultry	All included	Ground and tender beef, lamb, veal, liver; bacon; fish; poultry.	Ground beef, lamb, veal, pork, liver; fish; poultry without skin; bacon.	Not allowed	Not included
Vegetables	All included	Cooked vegetables of low fiber; lettuce and tomato salad; potatoes boiled, mashed, baked, creamed, scalloped	Vegetable purée, vegetable juices, sometimes choice of low fiber vegetables; potatoes boiled, mashed, baked, creamed, scalloped	Vegetable juices; vegetable purée used in soups	Vegetable water
Fruits	All included	Fruit juices, ripe bananas, cooked fruit without skin or seeds	Fruit juices, ripe bananas, cooked fruit without skin or seeds	Fruit juices, fruitades	Strained fruit juices, fruitades
Breads	All varieties	Fine whole grain, rye without seeds, enriched white, refined crackers	Fine whole grain, rye without seeds, enriched white, refined crackers	Not allowed	Not included
Cereals	All varieties	Refined; finely ground	Refined; finely ground	Cooked gruel	Not included
Cereal products	All varieties	Cooked macaroni, spaghetti, noodles, rice	Cooked macaroni, spaghetti, noodles, rice	Not allowed	Not included
Soups	All varieties	Clear broth, consommé, strained cream and vegetable soups	Clear broth, consommé, strained cream and vegetable soups	Clear broth, consommé, strained vegetable and cream soups	Clear broth and consommé
Beverages	All kinds	All kinds	All kinds	Tea, decaffeinated coffee, albuminized, carbonated, eggnog	Tea, decaffeinated coffee, carbonated beverages
Desserts	All kinds	Plain puddings, simple cakes and cookies; frozen desserts without nuts; custard; gelatin; milk-rennet pudding	Plain puddings, simple cakes and cookies; frozen desserts without nuts and seeds; custard; gelatin; milk-rennet pudding	Plain gelatin dessert, ice cream without nuts and seeds, ices, sherbets, milk-rennet pudding, soft custard	Plain gelatin desserts and ices

FOODS INCLUDED

Fruits: Strained fruit juices and fruitades.

Soups: Clear soup broths.

Beverages: Tea, coffee (decaffeinated), carbonated beverages.

Desserts: Plain gelatin, plain fruit ice made with strained fruit juices.

Sweets: Sugar, lactose.

See Table 20–6 for a summary of the diets previously discussed.

PSYCHOLOGICAL FACTORS IN FEEDING THE SICK

Throughout the text an effort has been made to bring out the psychological factors in feeding the sick. It is suggested that the part dealing with The Care and Feeding of Patients, outlined in Chapter 1, be reviewed at this point.

Attractive service, contrast in textures and color of food have been previously stressed, but the psychological importance bears mentioning again. The manner in which the tray is presented to the patient may influence acceptance or rejection of the meal. (Review Psychological Factors of Food Digestion in Chapter 7.)

If the nurse will take the time and thought to be pleasant to the patient and show interest in the food on the tray, the result will often be most rewarding. A patient's acceptance of a diet is closely related to the nurse's attitude toward it. There is no more need to try to convince the patient that he *likes* his diet than there is to try to convince him that he *likes* an unpalatable medication. There is every need, however, to approach the patient and win his confidence to accept the diet. The nurse who is convinced that the diet contributes toward restoration of her patient's health will communicate this conviction to him by her actions, her facial expressions, and by her conversation. The patient who understands that his diet is related to the benefit he is deriving from medical or surgical therapy will usually accept the diet more willingly. In this capacity the nurse is serving as an interpreter of the therapeutic diet.

When patients need to adhere to a therapeutic dietary program indefinitely, the nurse may need to confer with the dietitian, the social worker or the community health nurse or bring the members of the health team together to help the patient resolve his concerns. In this role the nurse is a coordinator. During the course of nursing care the nurse comes in contact with many individuals who do not require a therapeutic program. Actually informal opportunities for discussing nutrition principles with all patients are present and especially with those individuals receiving regular diets. With most of these patients the nurse is the only member of the team who is available to discuss the normal nutrition. In this role the nurse is a teacher. A dietary evaluation of the person's customary food intake and eating pattern points out the areas needing improvement. These areas form the nucleus for discussion. Unfortunately many nurses have a negative attitude about their own nutrition. A study[4] showed not only the negative attitude in responses of nurses but also that nurses closest to the patient placed the least priority value on nutrition in patient care. Attitudes about nutrition would improve if the health team would become more "people centered" in teaching nutrition.

PROBLEMS AND SUGGESTED TOPICS FOR DISCUSSION

1. What dietary adjustments necessary for the sick are frequently overlooked?
2. What is meant by routine house diets, and what purpose do they serve? What are the (a) advantages, and (b) disadvantages or limitations?
3. Compare the house diets served in the hospital where you are located with those outlined in this chapter. If there are any differences between the diets, justify the discrepancy.
4. Plan a Full Liquid Diet for a 46-year-old female patient requiring 2000 kcalories. Check with Recommended Allowances for adequacy.
5. List the foods usually allowed on a Clear Liquid Diet. How adequate is a clear liquid diet? Why is it not necessary that the diet meet requirements for nutritive adequacy?
6. Discuss the conditions (diagnosis of patient and hospital management) when it is advantageous to use the Soft Diet.
7. Discuss the advantages and disadvantages of the current trend for more liberal treatment and management of various dietaries.
8. List the psychological factors to be considered when feeding the sick. How can the nurse help?

SUGGESTED ADDITIONAL READING REFERENCES

Ahart, H. E.: Assessing food intake of hospital patients. J. Am. Dietet. A., 40:114, 1962.

Babcock, C. G.: Problems in sustaining the nutritional care of patients. J. Am. Dietet. A., 28:222, 1952.

Babcock, C. G.: Comments on human interrelations. J. Am. Dietet. A., 33:871, 1957.

Burton, B. R. (ed.): Heinz Handbook of Nutrition. 2nd ed. New York, McGraw-Hill Book Company, 1965, Chapter 23, Diets in disease.

English, O. S.: Psychosomatic medicine and dietetics. J. Am. Dietet. A., 27:721, 1951.

Fogelman, M. J., and Crasilneck, H. B.: Food intake and hypnosis. J. Am. Dietet. A., 32:519, 1956.

Hildreth, H. M.: Hunger and eating. J. Am. Dietet. A., 31:561, 1955.

Hodges, R. E.: The effect of stress on ascorbic acid metabolism in man. Nutrition Today, 5:11, 1970.

Mayo Clinic Diet Manual. 4th ed. Philadelphia, W. B. Saunders Company, 1971.

Moore, H. B.: Psychologic facts and dietary fancies. J. Am. Dietet. A., 28:789, 1952.

Selye, H.: On just being sick. Nutrition Today, 5:2, 1970.

Turner, D.: Handbook of Diet Therapy. 5th ed. Chicago, University of Chicago Press, 1970.

[4]Newton, M. C., et al.: Nutritional aspects of nursing care. Nurs. Res., 16:46, 1967.

Chapter 21

NUTRITION OF THE CHRONICALLY ILL AND DISABLED PATIENT

"The way to live a long life is to contract a chronic disease—and take care of it."

Sir William Osler

Chronic diseases are not likely to be caused by one specific factor, but rather are a result of multiple factors usually operating over a long period of time. Chronic disease is most commonly found in the age group over 60. With steadily increasing longevity it is only natural that there will be an increase in persons chronically ill. It should be stressed, however, that not all chronically handicapped individuals are in the geriatric age group. Figures reveal that some one third to one half of those with long-term illness are under 45 years of age; about 16 per cent of all known persons with chronic disease are under age 24. At any one of the stages in growth and development an individual may experience the stress of a disabling physical condition or mental illness. Any individual may have a crippling injury or illness.

Insurance statistics, based on male risks, give information on the incidence and prevalence of sickness by age group. Although these statistics are not representative of the entire population, they provide some indication of the relative frequency and duration of sickness.

Older persons do not have many more sicknesses than the younger adults, but the average duration of disability is much longer. An increase in the incidence of chronic illness with advancing age occurs. Thus, the prob-lems in feeding and nutrition frequently encountered in the aged apply, to a large extent, to the chronically ill as well. (See Chapter 18, Nutrition and Aging.)

The most prevalent chronic diseases are those associated with circulatory impairment, metabolic dysfunction, the arthritides, neuromuscular impairments, neoplasms and addiction to drugs and alcohol. In spite of various handicaps imposed by illness, effort should be made to meet the normal nutritional requirements, as well as any specific demands made by disease. Halpern[1] points out that the basic dietary requirements of the chronically ill person are essentially the same as those of the well individual. However, the physiological stress of prolonged illness requires quantitative and, at times, qualitative modifications. Although the destructive phase is not so great in the chronically ill as in the seriously ill patient, the net result may be the same because of the prolonged inadequate intake of essential nutrients.

Good nutrition plays a role in the prevention of many chronic illnesses and it is important in the rehabilitation of the individual whether a cure is imminent or not.

CALORIES   The calorie requirement of the individual is of prime importance and is adjusted from time to time according to energy needs. The energy requirement in the acute febrile disease phase or following bone fractures or other types of accidents is usually

---

[1]Halpern, S. L.: Nutrition and chronic illness. Health News, 32:15, 1955.

high. There is a loss of weight due largely to anorexia and the failure of food intake and the catabolic response on the part of the body to the noxious or toxic or mechanical agents which produced the condition. In the chronic phase and when weight has reached the ideal level the calorie intake is adjusted. The amount of calories depends upon the activity expended. For instance, during physical therapy, which is often required for the rehabilitative process, hard work is involved and calories should be sufficient to furnish the energy for metabolic demands. Excessive calorie intake causes obesity. A patient with hemiplegia, quadriplegia or other type of paralysis has a tendency to gain weight. His need for satisfaction probably accounts for excessive calorie intake. Once the patient becomes obese it is difficult to get him mobile again. There is the possibility of recurrence in the hemiplegic of another hemiplegia attack if the patient becomes obese. Weight loss is necessary to effect control over the hypertension and the cardiac decompensation (whichever is the basic cause) or to relieve the load on the muscles during physical rehabilitation and mobilization of the patient.

PROTEIN Protein requires special attention. Halpern states that "insufficient protein in the diet leads to delay in convalescence, poor wound healing, poor antibody formation, impaired tissue and organ growth and repair, increased susceptibility to superimposed infections and lowered resistance to complicating diseases, reduction of enzyme activity, liver injury and other impaired organ functions and to hypoproteinemia with anemia, weight loss, edema and bed sores." Protein depletion of stroke patients can be reduced by programed exercise and ambulation. The loss continues, however, if the calorie intake falls short of the energy expenditure.[2] Any type of restriction of caloric intake will put the patient into negative nitrogen balance during the rehabilitation process. Therefore it is important to make sure that the quality of protein is optimum for the individual. A minimum of 70 to 100 gm. of protein per day is recommended for the average patient, while many patients will require as much as 150 gm. The presence of kidney damage associated with nitrogen retention would be, however, an indication for restricting protein intake.

CARBOHYDRATE AND FAT Sufficient carbohydrate and fat are necessary to provide energy and to prevent loss of nitrogen. Stress following an injury causes an increase in activity of pituitary and adrenal gland which inhibits the proper functioning of the cellular enzyme systems. Inadequate phosphorylation and oxidation of glucose results. To provide energy more breakdown of tissue protein and fat takes place.

VITAMINS AND MINERALS Optimum dietary intake of vitamins and minerals is essential. When a vitamin supplement is indicated the ones that are needed should be chosen to meet the need and to prevent deficiency. Iron supplements are often indicated. It has been observed that patients with chronic illness or under stress lose potassium, a mineral important to muscle contraction and strength. (See Chapter 8.)

THE EFFECT OF PROLONGED IMMOBILIZATION ON NUTRITIONAL REQUIREMENTS

Prolonged bed rest can result in the development of negative nitrogen balance. Immobilization of a healthy person leads to increased nitrogen loss of an appreciable magnitude. Nitrogen losses in healthy, immobilized subjects average about 55 gm. over a 6-week period or as much as 2 to 3 gm. of nitrogen per day when the diet would normally be adequate in protein and calories. To replace 2 to 3 gm. of nitrogen lost, an additional 15 to 20 gm. of protein is needed (N lost × 6.25). On the other hand, debilitated, chronically ill patients will be in positive nitrogen balance (2 to 3 gm. per day) when consuming the same diet at bed rest. During hospitalization prevention of skin breakdown, decubitus ulcers, infection and negative nitrogen balance requires optimum protein in quantity and quality, sufficient calories and ascorbic acid. Helping the immobilized patient to avoid skin breakdown is a challenge to nursing care. Adequate dietary management and the turning and positioning of the patient and providing passive exercise for him during nursing care will help to prevent adverse metabolic effects of immobility.

Calcium is lost following a fracture and during prolonged periods of bed rest. Normally bone integrity and homeostatic balance are maintained by weight-bearing and muscle tension and are produced by normal motion and activity. A diet, liquid or regular, of milk or milk products containing an equivalent amount (800 mg.) of calcium is recommended. The increase in milk for calcium will also contribute substantially to meeting the increased protein needs. However, high calcium intake and/or demineralization of the skeleton with resulting hypercalcemia and hypercalciuria due to immobilization may be complicated by renal calculi. In this instance the calcium content of the diet is reduced to about 400 or

---

[2]Albanese, A. A.: Nutritional and metabolic effects of physical exercise. Food and Nutrition News, National Live Stock and Meat Board, Chicago, Ill., 38:No. 8, May, 1967.

500 mg., depending upon the individual's need.

Patients requiring 10 or more days of hospitalization, or bed rest, will often have sufficient metabolic insult to require larger amounts of protein and calcium than the normal, healthy adult requires. The nurse can play a very important part by noting the length of time a patient is on bed rest, and observing the dietary intake and reporting her findings to the doctor and dietitian.

In the paralyzed patient calcium and nitrogen losses may precipitate the formation of urinary calculi (see Chapter 32). Poor bladder function may cause urinary infection and may influence the formation of urinary calculi by alkalinizing the urine. An acid-ash diet is used to help keep the urine acid. Acid ash diet is described in Chapter 32. A high fluid intake is necessary in the prevention and treatment of infection and urinary calculi. Diminished thirst sensation has been observed in these patients. Therefore close attention is necessary to be sure that the person has sufficient fluid intake.

During bladder training fluid is given at regularly spaced intervals throughout the day and recording the time, type and amount must be a routine procedure. (All fluids during the night are prohibited.) During bowel training, a high fiber diet served at regular intervals is desirable. Too much fiber may cause fecal impaction. Foods causing watery stools should be avoided, since they are apt to cause irregular defecation. A regular time should be set for defecation. With some individuals, prune juice in large amounts given at a certain time may be helpful.

The nutritional status of drug addicts and alcoholics is known to be very poor. Both would rather get high or intoxicated than eat. They differ in that the drug contains no calories and alcohol does. With the latter the amount of alcohol consumed may supply sufficient calories for energy needs. Both suffer from malnutrition because of irregular and inadequate intake of the nutrients and calories. When a person goes on methadone his appetite increases and he usually gains weight rapidly. The nurse should be aware of the fluctuation in the person's weight. A rapid weight loss may indicate the use of diet pills or amphetamines. Craving for fruit juices seems to prevail with persons on methadone and constipation seems to be a problem. Occasionally a patient develops increased appetite for sweet foods while using marihuana. No adequate explanation is available.[3] Amphetamine may cause elevations of metabolic rate, plasma corticosteroids and immunoreactive growth hormone.[4] The chronic alco-

[3]Weil, A. T., et al.: Clinical and psychological effects of marijuana in man. Science, 162:1234, 1968.
[4]Besser, G. M., et al.: Influence of amphetamine on plasma corticosteroids and growth hormone levels in man. Brit. Med. J., 4:528, 1969.

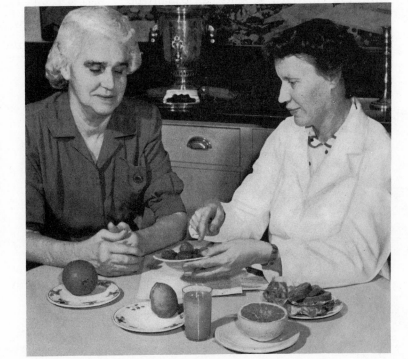

Figure 21–1   Careful attention to the details of diet is essential to ensure the adequacy of diets planned for treatment of specific illnesses and to avoid iatrogenic malnutrition. (S. L. Halpern: Nutrition and Chronic Disease; reprinted from Health News, monthly publication of the New York State Department of Health, October, 1955.)

holic needs counseling at regular intervals to encourage him to eat an adequate diet at regular intervals. The cause of the drug and alcoholic addiction is related to the cause of malnutrition in this group of individuals.

PROBLEMS IN FEEDING THE CHRONICALLY ILL PATIENT

All the suggestions of ways and means to attract the appetite and provide the essential nutrients apply here. The psychology of feeding is especially important, since most chronically ill individuals are limited in activity and, hence, have a greater amount of leisure time to focus attention on the meals. Planning the dietary pattern with the patient around his customary pattern usually attracts his interest and motivation. A review of his food intake periodically discloses how well the person is following the principles of therapy recommended. (See Figure 21-1.)

One of the aims in the rehabilitation of the person is to help him become as self-sufficient and productive as possible. The training process usually begins in the hospital or rehabilitation center, depending upon the nature of the illness or injury. His follow-up nursing care in the home is supervised by the community health nurse. The importance of nutrition is stressed from the onset. Persons who have difficulty feeding themselves and in swallowing are often depressed because of this handicap. Food placed on the unaffected side of the mouth and beyond the tip of the tongue in paralyzed patients can usually be tasted and swallowed. If unable to swallow or ingest enough food, tube feedings are available to supply adequate calories and nutrient. Mechanical devices are available for those individuals who have difficulty in using ordinary eating utensils. Kitchens have been renovated to heights that are convenient for those homemakers in wheelchairs. Guides for streamlining kitchen tasks are available.

PROBLEMS AND SUGGESTED TOPICS FOR DISCUSSION

1. How does feeding the chronically sick patient differ from feeding the acutely ill patient?
2. Why is the number of chronically ill patients increasing?
3. List the most prevalent chronic diseases.
4. Discuss the effect of prolonged immobilization on nutritional requirements.

SUGGESTED ADDITIONAL READING REFERENCES

Albanese, A. A.: Nutritional and metabolic effects of physical exercise. Food and Nutrition News, National Live Stock and Meat Board, Chicago, Ill., 38:No. 8, 1967.

Germain, L. D.: Dietetic aspects of nursing care. J. Am. Dietet. A., 29:906, 1953.

Goodman, J. I.: Nutrition in the treatment of the chronically ill. Am. J. Nursing, 51:165, 1951.

Goodman, J. I., and Dowdell, W.: The specter of malnutrition in chronic illness. Ann. Int. Med., 43:1241, 1955.

Hirschberg, G. G., et al.: Rehabilitation: A Manual for the Care of the Disabled and Elderly. Philadelphia, J. B. Lippincott Co., 1964.

Howard, M. S.: Energy-saving kitchen. J. Am. Dietet. A., 39:201, 1961.

Klinger, J. L., Frieden, F. H., and Sullivan, R. A.: Mealtime Manual for the Aged and Handicapped. New York, Essandess Special Edition. Div. of Simon & Schuster, Inc., 1970.

Weir, D. R., and Houser, H. B.: Problems in the evaluation of nutritional status in chronic illness. Am. J. Clin. Nutr. 12:278, 1963.

Wohl, M. G. (ed.): Long-Term Illness. Management of the Chronically Ill Patient. Philadelphia, W. B. Saunders Company, 1959, Nutrition in chronic diseases, pp. 552–567.

Wynder, E. L., and Day, E.: Some thoughts on the causation of chronic disease. J.A.M.A., 175:997, 1961.

Chapter 22
DIET IN FEBRILE DISEASES

Fever, which may be defined as an elevation of body temperature above normal, is the most important sign of an infection. Modern drug therapy, with the use of sulfonamides, penicillin and the newer antibiotics, has revolutionized the treatment of febrile diseases. The control achieved over the infectious diseases ensures that, in the years to come, fewer people entering the older ages will have serious organic impairments of infectious origin. These products also help to reduce the mortality rate, shorten the period of disability, and relieve the congestion in the hospitals.

DIET AND RESISTANCE TO INFECTIONS

Laboratory, clinical, and field observations have demonstrated that the severity and outcome of infection is frequently worsened by malnutrition. Studies have shown how it is possible to influence the body's susceptibility to disease through diet. During the early part of the century it was established that severe bacterial infections such as typhoid fever, pneumonia, malaria, and tuberculosis cause severe and prolonged loss of nitrogen as a result, chiefly, of the toxic destruction of intracellular protein. Studies[1] have shown that mild and asymptomatic viral invasion such as that produced by yellow fever vaccine, or mild chickenpox in children, will produce adverse nitrogen balance effects, even when the patient is receiving an apparently adequate protein intake. With anorexia, which results in a decreased food intake during fever and infection, protein intake is bound to be lowered, with further loss of nitrogen.

When diets inadequate in protein are fed, it is very likely that lowered resistance to infection will develop. This will interfere with the production of antibodies which play an important role in both natural and acquired immunity. For example, during periods of war and the consequent famine, epidemics of disease and pestilence usually occur because the underfed people do not eat sufficient calories and proteins to build protective antibodies. More studies are needed to determine the practical importance and general applicability of the observations concerning nutritional deficiencies and reduced capacity to form antibodies.

In animal experiments and clinical studies, deficiencies of protein and vitamins have been found to reduce the phagocytic activity of white blood cells and to lower resistance. The greatest phagocytic activity seems to occur at levels of vitamin intake greater than those needed for good growth. The correlation of phagocytic activity and protein intake appears so striking that the effects of vitamin deficiencies are thought to be dependent upon this factor, either through functional disturbance of protein metabolism or by a possible decreased protein intake coincident with the vitamin deficiency.

No doubt future research will support current evidence showing why people with inadequate diets have a decreased or lowered resistance to bacterial infection. The mechanisms whereby nutritional deficiencies influence resistance to infectious diseases are the subject of considerable controversy.

EFFECT OF INFECTION AND FEVERS ON THE BASAL METABOLIC RATE AND CALORIC REQUIREMENT

According to DuBois,[2] there is an elevation of approximately 13 per cent in the metabolic

---

[1]Scrimshaw, N. S.: Malnutrition and infection. Borden's Rev., 26:No. 2, 1965.

[2]DuBois, E. F., and Chambers, W. H.: Calories in Medical Practice. Handbook of Nutrition. Chicago, American Medical Association, 1943. pp. 55–70.

rate for each rise of 1° Centigrade in body temperature or 7.2 per cent for each degree Fahrenheit.

In health the normal temperature of the body is regulated at approximately 37° Centigrade or 98.6° Fahrenheit. When an infection gives rise to fever, the temperature regulating center seems to adjust at a different level, sometimes fairly constant, but usually fluctuating 2 to 3° C. during the day. *A disturbance in the balance normally maintained between heat production and heat elimination leads to fever;* that is, the body's heat production exceeds its heat loss. When the temperature regulating center is set suddenly at 40° C. (104° F.), the body finds itself 3° too cool, and therefore calls into play the mechanism of increased heat production. If the patient has attained a high temperature of 40° C. (104° F.) and the heat regulating center is adjusted suddenly to the normal of 37° C. (98.6° F.), the body finds itself 3° too warm (5.4° F.), which calls into play the mechanism of heat loss, and heat is lost rapidly through perspiration.

There is a rise in metabolism during fever; sometimes the increase is as much as 40 per cent when a patient has a temperature of 40° C. or 104° F. If the patient is restless, delirious or coughing, the total energy need is affected because of increased activity.

An easy method to determine the metabolism of a patient with fever, suggested by DuBois, is: Calculate the normal basal rate and then add 13 per cent for each degree Centigrade or 7 per cent for each degree Fahrenheit of elevation of temperature; when there is great toxic destruction of body tissues, add another 10 per cent; if the patient is very restless, add another 10 per cent or even as much as 30 per cent. This method will give a sufficiently accurate caloric allowance or energy requirement for a patient with fever.

TYPES OF INFECTIONS

Infections may be classified as (1) acute, (2) chronic and (3) recurrent. The acute infections are of stormy but short duration, and they occur along with colds, pneumonia, influenza, measles, chickenpox, scarlet and typhoid fever. The duration of most acute infectious diseases has been markedly decreased by the use of various antibiotics. Chronic infections may continue for months and stretch into years. Tuberculosis is an outstanding example. An example of recurrent infection of primary importance is malaria.

CHARACTERISTICS   The chief characteristics of acute or chronic infection are (1) an increase in metabolism, which, except in pulmonary tuberculosis, parallels with considerable uniformity the rise in temperature,

(2) a destruction of tissue protein by bacterial invasion, which causes an increased protein metabolism, (3) an accumulation of toxic products, and (4) a disturbance of the water balance of the body. Digestive disturbances, diarrhea, and abdominal distention are also frequent complications.

ACUTE INFECTIONS

"Starving a fever" leads to a prolonged convalescence and to precipitation of acute deficiency diseases. The *protein* and *calorie* content of the diet should be adequate to counterbalance the increased metabolism and losses of nitrogen that are characteristic of febrile illnesses. The Committee on Therapeutic Nutrition[3] recommends an increase of protein to 2 gm. per kg. of body weight (125 to 150 gm. total) in febrile diseases of more than transient nature, and an increase in the energy requirement may be 50 percent or more with a total of 3000 to 4000 kcalories daily.

FLUIDS   Fluids are of major importance in the treatment of infections. Any fluids that appeal to the patient are satisfactory. As a rule, very sweet liquids are not appealing and frequently cause gastric disturbance besides distention in the abdominal region. Carbonated beverages (ginger ale) and not too sweet lemonade seem to be favorites. If the patient is nauseated and vomiting, and too ill to take fluids by mouth, liquid may be given parenterally. Often *three* to *four* quarts of liquids are required daily to facilitate the elimination of toxins and to replace water lost through excessive perspiration.

CARBOHYDRATES   Carbohydrates in the form of sugar (cane sugar, glucose, corn syrup and lactose) are added to the liquids as soon as possible to replenish glycogen stores, to maintain the ketogenic and antiketogenic ratio and to increase calories. Lactose is less sweet than cane and corn syrup and may be taken in greater amounts. It dissolves more slowly than the other sugars and may cause diarrhea due to increased fermentation in the small intestine. Glucose is readily absorbed. Milk is an excellent liquid food, providing calories, protein, certain vitamins, minerals and fluid. When the patient has received insufficient fluids and carbohydrates, acidosis may occur.

FATS   Such fats as cream, butter, margarines increase the energy intake. Improperly fried foods and rich pastries may delay digestion of fats.

VITAMINS   Fevers increase vitamin requirements, especially B-complex, ascorbic

---

[3]Therapeutic Nutrition. Washington, D.C., National Research Council, Publication 234, 1952.

acid and vitamin A. As the calorie need increases, thiamin, riboflavin and niacin requirements increase. Antibiotics and drugs may interfere with the intestinal synthesis of the B-complex vitamins. Vitamin supplements are usually advised during the illness and convalescence.

MINERALS   Loss of sodium and potassium during fevers may be considerable during the acute phase of illness. Unless contraindicated, salty broth, soups and additional amounts in foods usually replenish the loss. A full liquid or regular diet, when eaten, supplies enough potassium. An inadequate intake of food may be supplemented by fruit juices and milk, which are good sources of potassium.

MEAL PLAN   Frequent small liquid feedings are usually best tolerated in the beginning. Occasionally, tube feedings (p. 384) may be necessary if the patient has no appetite. The full liquid diet (Table 20–4) is served to the patient as soon as it is tolerated. Such a diet contains food which is easily and quickly digested. Protein supplements may be added in varying amounts to fruit juice, milk, and soup. See Chap. 43 for protein supplements plus suggested ways to use them. The liquid diet is followed by the soft diet, with increased protein and calories, and stepped up progressively to the general diet as quickly as possible. Many patients do better when they eat a regular diet, with protein and calorie adjustments to meet the individual requirements. They experience less anorexia, nausea and vomiting. (See Chapter 20, Hospital House Diets.) See Table 22–1 for increased protein content of the daily meal plan; see Table 29–4 for suggestions to increase calories.

The dietary and fluid intake are important concerns of the nurse who cares for patients with febrile diseases. Observations by the nurse help to determine the type of diet that best meets the individual needs of the patient.

Typhoid Fever

Typhoid fever is an infectious disease caused by *Salmonella typhosa*. The infection is usually transmitted by drinking water or milk contaminated with intestinal contents. Improved hygiene and prophylactic public health measures have greatly reduced the incidence, while the use of antibiotics has shortened the course of the disease from what used to be a chronic fever to one of short duration. However, the length of convalescence is to a large extent still dependent upon nutritional therapy.

Peyer's patches (ulceration of the intestinal tract, which may hemorrhage) and diarrhea are early involvements and may interfere with absorption. In addition, if not controlled in the early stages, there are often extensive changes in the liver, with complicating diseases of the gallbladder and bile passages.

During the height of the fever the metabolic rate may increase 40 or even 50 per cent above normal. The protein destruction is great, approximating three times that which occurs during normal health.

DIETARY TREATMENT   The dietary treatment outlined under acute infections is followed with levels of protein 100 gm. or more (Table 22–1). In addition, the foods introduced into the diet should be low in fiber content (p. 341) to prevent intestinal irritation. Large quantities of milk (one to two quarts daily) form the basis of the diet. Three to six eggs daily, served soft cooked or in soft custards, are well tolerated. The milk and eggs provide calories, proteins, minerals and vitamins. Cooked cereals (low in fiber), milk toast, white toast with butter or margarine, honey, jelly, ice cream, cream, gelatin desserts and lactose may be included in the diet when tolerated. To prevent overburdening of the stomach, frequent small feedings are recommended.

Most patients do not have an appetite, and experience an unpleasant taste in the mouth. To help counteract this disturbing factor, the mouth should be cleansed both before and following any feedings.

Rheumatic Fever

Rheumatic fever is a disorder of unknown etiology with relatively high incidence among underprivileged children. The streptococcic organism is considered to be the cause since in most cases a respiratory disorder, in which the germ was implicated, preceded the rheumatic manifestations. The joint symptoms are similar to those of early rheumatoid arthritis, a disease with which it is frequently confused.

Although it is a disease of childhood and adolescence, adults do not escape it. Rheumatic fever is one of the leading causes of chronic illness in children. If it is not recognized and treated early, permanent damage to the heart ensues. (See Chap. 36.)

Rheumatic fever may develop for a long period before it is recognized. Those known to have the disease are advised to take every precaution against infections of all types. In the presence of a cold there is always the danger that organisms will gain access to the circulation and invade the heart valves, causing permanent damage to the heart.

DRUGS   Lowered incidence and a decrease of severity characterizes rheumatic fever in the 20th century.[4] Protection of pa-

---

[4]Editorial: Acute rheumatic fever—a changing disease. J.A.M.A., *182*:1035, 1962.

TABLE 22-1   INCREASED PROTEIN CONTENT OF THE DAILY MEAL PLAN*

DAILY MEAL PLAN *To increase the protein content of the day's meals from 100 grams to 125 or 150, use the allowances of dried milk solids indicated in columns 2 and 3.*	PROTEIN CONTENT IN GRAMS		
	(1) 100 grams approx.	(2) 125 grams approx.	(3) 150 grams approx.
BREAKFAST			
Fruit juice, citrus, ½ cup	.5	.5	.5
Cereal, enriched, ½ cup, cooked or prepared	2.5	2.5	2.5
½ cup whole milk	4.2	4.2	4.2
Plus 2 tablespoons dried nonfat milk solids	—	6.0	6.0
Egg, 1	6.5	6.5	6.5
Bread (white, enriched, or whole wheat) 1 slice	2.5	2.5	2.5
Butter or enriched margarine (as desired)			
Whole milk, 1 cup	8.5	8.5	8.5
LUNCH			
Meat, poultry, fish, 2 oz. cooked; or cheese	15.2	15.2	15.2
Salad, ½ cup (with dressing)	.5	.5	.5
Cooked vegetable, green or yellow, ½ cup	2.0	2.0	2.0
Bread (white, enriched, or whole wheat) 1 slice	2.5	2.5	2.5
Butter or enriched margarine (as desired)			
Simple dessert,† *fruit*	.5	.5	.5
Whole milk, 1 cup	8.5	8.5	8.5
Plus 2 tablespoons dried nonfat milk solids	—	6.0	6.0
MIDAFTERNOON SNACK			
Whole milk, 1 cup	—	8.5	8.5
Plus 2 tablespoons dried nonfat milk solids	—	—	6.0
Graham crackers, 2	—	—	2.5
DINNER			
Meat, poultry, fish (liver once a week); or cheese— 4 oz. raw weight; 3 oz. cooked	22.8	22.8	22.8
Cooked vegetable, ½ cup	2.0	2.0	2.0
Potato	2.0	2.0	2.0
Plus 2 tablespoons dried nonfat milk solids	—	6.0	6.0
Bread (white, enriched, or whole wheat) 1 slice	2.5	2.5	2.5
Butter or enriched margarine (as desired)			
Simple dessert,† *pudding*	4.5	4.5	4.5
Plus 2 tablespoons dried nonfat milk solids	—	—	6.0
Whole milk, 1 cup	8.5	8.5	8.5
EVENING SNACK			
Whole milk, 1 cup	8.5	8.5	8.5
Plus 2 tablespoons dried nonfat milk solids	—	—	6.0
Total Grams of Protein	104.7	131.2	151.7

If additional calories are needed to maintain body weight, concentrated foods may be added, such as sugar, jelly, sauces, and salad dressings.

*Sources of calculations: Turner, D. F.: Handbook of Diet Therapy. Chicago, University of Chicago Press.

†Desserts—custards, puddings, plain ice cream, fruit.

Note: To make these meal plans low in sodium content, omit all salt in cooking and at the table; omit the cheese; substitute unsalted butter or fortified margarine; and replace all or part of the whole milk and dried nonfat milk solids with low sodium milk, available in fresh fluid and canned forms, and in powdered whole milk (Lonalac, Mead Johnson and Co., Evansville, Ind.) and powdered skim milk (Cellu, Chicago Dietetic Supply House, Chicago). Protinal (The National Drug Co., Philadelphia), a protein supplement very low in sodium content, can also be used to increase the protein content of a diet. (See Table 43–1, Approximate Values of Some Protein Supplements.)

tients, isolation of carriers, chemotherapy, and antibiotics have all played a part. In patients suffering an acute attack, cortisone and corticotropin (ACTH) have been reported to shorten the period of acute illness, lessen its severity, and decrease the likelihood of cardiac involvement. These two drugs tend to cause retention of sodium and fluids, which may require the use of a sodium-restricted diet.

DIET SUGGESTIONS   During the acute stage of rheumatic fever the diet outlined for any acute infection (page 000) should be followed. Research findings would indicate that it is advisable to increase the intake of ascorbic acid by administering pure ascorbic acid or citrus fruit juices (orange, lemon, grapefruit, and tomato).

The diet is increased gradually as outlined under dietary treatment for acute infections to an adequate normal diet high in iron, ascorbic acid, and protein, with calories to maintain desired weight. The rate of increase will depend on the patient's temperature, weight and general progress in health. Since absolute bed rest is paramount for many weeks or even months, the appetite often lags. Thus, it may be advisable to restrict concentrated sweets to encourage the intake of foods containing the essential nutrients. If carditis develops, the diet must be restricted in sodium to avoid sodium and fluid retention. (See Chapter 30.)

Poliomyelitis

Poliomyelitis is a generalized virus infection, which, in a small percentage of cases, affects the central nervous system. If skeletal muscles become paralyzed, it is called *spinal poliomyelitis*. If the brain nerve cells become involved, producing impairment or paralysis in swallowing, it is termed *bulbar poliomyelitis*. In about 10 per cent of the cases, permanent handicap results. With the introduction of the Salk vaccine in 1955 and now the oral vaccine for prevention, the future looks promising. Infants, children and young adults are the usual victims.

DIETARY TREATMENT   During the acute febrile stage, a liquid to soft diet is indicated. As the patient improves, a high protein, high calorie, high vitamin diet is needed to compensate for the rapid tissue destruction. Protein supplements usually are better tolerated than milk in the acute stage. Vitamin supplements are indicated, especially when the food intake is necessarily restricted.

The most difficult dietary problem occurs in the bulbar poliomyelitis patient with dysphagia. Vomiting is a common symptom in the acute stage, and there is grave danger of choking or aspiration. The first nourishment, which consists of glucose and fructose solutions, protein hydrolysates, and electrolyte solutions, is given parenterally.

Seifert[5] has devised a feeding program which he divides into four stages.

Stage I   Following the initial feeding by the parenteral route, tube feedings are given by way of a plastic tube through the nose and into the stomach. The tube feedings vary in amount and concentration of calories and/or protein, depending upon what is needed at the time. They consist of milk and cream, Karo, orange juice, and egg mixtures in varying amounts, with or without protein concentrates and fat emulsions; or a skim milk formula with sugar and eggs. To each of the tube feeding formulas is added the daily requirement of vitamins in a soluble multiple-vitamin preparation. The quantity given at each feeding is small to start with (30 to 50 ml.), alternating every 2 hours with water, but is stepped up as rapidly as tolerated (150 to 200 ml.).

Stage II   Tube feedings and vitamin supplements are continued. In addition, minute quantities (1 to 2 teaspoons) of a liquid, such as grape juice, are tried. If swallowing is successful (as observed through the tracheotomy opening), dilute strained citrus fruit juices, apple juice, clear broth, tea with sugar, and flavored gelatin are cautiously tried. Milk and cream are not well tolerated at this stage, as they seem to produce mucus.

Stage III   As soon as the liquids are well tolerated, a soft, low fiber diet of easily digested foods is begun. Foods such as potatoes (prepared any style) and cheese will tend to stick in the throat, and must be avoided. The tube feeding intake is decreased proportionately as the oral intake is increased. The foods allowed in addition to Stages I and II include:

Soup: Bouillon or strained meat broth.
Beverages: Water, tea with sugar, coffee.
Cereals: Cream of Wheat, farina with large amount of sugar and little milk.
Eggs: Poached or soft cooked.
Meats: Strained or well cooked.
Fats: Butter or margarine as desired.
Fruits: Strained, cooked or canned (without seeds, skin or fiber).
Vegetables: Strained or well cooked.
Desserts: Flavored gelatins, sherbet or custard.

Stage IV   As soon as the patient can swallow the soft foods from Stage III, he is allowed more solid foods, such as ground meat, bread and milk products. The diet is gradually increased to include a general high protein, high calorie, high vitamin diet. The duration of each feeding stage varies with the patient from days to weeks and, occasionally, to months.

In general, the appetite is very poor, and it is of utmost importance, in all stages, for the food to be appetizing in appearance and attractively served. Nursing care in relation to the diet is of great importance. Patients who have extensive loss of muscle formation require special encouragement and may need assistance in the mechanics of eating. Dishes on the tray should be placed carefully, so the foods can be reached easily by the patient.

Cholera

Cholera outbreaks in Asiatic countries are common. It is an infection of the intestine which produces sudden and massive diarrhea, with the resultant loss of electrolytes and water. Shock and death occur within a few hours. It has been reported[6] that rehydration intravenously, followed by oral administration of a solution of electrolytes, glucose and an antibiotic, saves lives of infected individuals. The glucose aids in the reabsorption of sodium and water from the intestinal tract and stool, and the antibiotic combats the bacterial infection.

[5]Seifert, M. H.: Poliomyelitis and the relation of diet to its treatment. J. Am. Dietet. A., 30:671, 1954.

[6]Medical News, World Wide Report, May 15, 1967.

CHRONIC INFECTIONS

CALORIES AND PROTEIN In chronic infections *caloric* and *protein* requirements will depend upon the presence or absence of fever. An attempt must be made to repair losses resulting from increased energy and protein metabolism. In the absence of fever 2500 to 3000 kcalories is considered to be a desired level which will insure optimum utilization of dietary protein. About 150 gm. of protein daily is desirable. The diet must be modified to meet these increased needs of the body and to maintain weight at the optimum level.

MINERALS AND VITAMINS The *mineral* and *vitamin* intake must also be maintained at an optimum level. The mixed diet containing the essential foods (see Chapter 11) will contain adequate amounts of calcium, phosphorus, iron and other minerals. It is fairly well established that some of the avitaminoses have reduced natural resistance to various bacterial infections. The reason for this is still obscure. Blood levels of vitamin A are reduced in infections. Considerable research has been carried on to note the relation between vitamin A and the common cold, pulmonary tuberculosis, rheumatoid arthritis, and other infectious diseases. Apparently, a deficiency may play a role in reducing natural resistance, but the administration of vitamin A during the course of an infection has little, if any, beneficial effect unless a deficiency is present.

Ascorbic acid deficiency is believed to be responsible for a reduction in natural resistance to infection and may have some bearing upon the progress and prognosis of such diseases as pulmonary tuberculosis and rheumatoid arthritis.

The Committee on Therapeutic Nutrition recommends giving vitamin supplements to ensure efficient metabolism of the ingested foods.

CARBOHYDRATE Similar to the suggested diets for acute fevers, every effort should be made to keep the diet high in *carbohydrate* content to replenish the glycogen stores and to avoid acidosis. Fluids are forced; but fluids which cause distention are eliminated in the early stage of fever.

FOODS Even though a high calorie diet is necessary, it is usually desirable for the patient to start on simple, easily digested foods, and then gradually increase to foods on the general diet. Such a procedure helps to prevent gastric upsets besides preventing the patient from becoming discouraged at the overabundance of food. The liquid diet can be stepped up in caloric value by adding cream to the milk; margarine, butter or oil to soups and broth; and sugar to fruit juices and other beverages. Protein can be increased by adding protein concentrates (Chaps. 34 and 43) and eggnog mixtures, using dried skim milk and dried eggs.

Since most patients with fevers have poor appetites, it is important that special attention be given to the selection of food. An attempt should be made to appeal to the appetite through the careful choice of color, temperature and texture of different foods. Oftentimes the person can suggest a food(s) that would appeal to him. The foods should be easily digested and of concentrated food value, such as cereal, whole-grain or enriched bread, potatoes, ice cream, custards, butter, margarine, cream, eggs, fruit juices and jelly. Meat, leafy green and yellow vegetables should be included as soon as tolerated. The average high calorie diet contains approximately 3000 kcalories. However, it may be necessary to provide as many as 5000 kcalories if the patient is very restless and there is great toxic destruction along with high temperature. The old aphorism to "starve a fever and feed a cold" has been proved to be false.

The basic house diets (liquid diet, soft diet, light diet, and general diet, Chapter 20) are used as the basis or pattern for the increased calorie diets, depending upon the stage of illness. Additional foods or increased amounts of the basic foods will provide the additional daily calories. In-between feedings are recommended, such as high calorie beverages, which furnish calories and protein, along with additional fluids. Examples are hot chocolate and malted milk with whipped cream, eggnogs, and fruit juices with added sugar or lactose.

To increase the daily protein and caloric intake in 500 kcalorie steps, the plan in Table 29-4 (p. 437) is suggested. The additional milk, eggs and bread will increase the protein intake as well as the calories. Additional meat may be served, when practical and advisable. For example, the normal basic general house diet for an individual is calculated to be approximately 2000 kcalories. If a diet of 2500 kcalories is desired, a step-up of 500 kcalories is added; or if 3000 kcalories are desired, then two such supplements are added. The choice of food for the addition of calories will be governed by the preference, tolerance and reaction of the patient. When the appetite is very poor, small meals and a concentrated supplement is tolerated best. Patients are often overwhelmed by the quantity of food served on the high calorie, high nutrient content diets.

Tuberculosis

Tuberculosis is still the most dreaded of the chronic infectious diseases, and still is among the leading causes of death throughout the world. The incidence is on the increase, especially in adolescence. The disease particularly affects people in areas of poverty, poor sanitation, poor education and malnutrition. It is characterized in the acute stage by a marked rise of body temperature, constant fatigue, flushed face, loss of weight, cough following a cold, and a general run-down condition.

The increase in metabolism is not so marked as the amount noted in typhoid fever. If the temperature goes above 39° C. (102.2° F.) there may be an increase of 20 to 30 per cent above the normal metabolic rate. Compared with typhoid, the protein destruction is not so great; however, due to the length of the illness, wasting of the body tissues may be considerable.

Since the early 1950's the drugs isoniazid, streptomycin, pyrazinamide, ethionamide, capreomycin, and other antibiotics have contributed a great deal in helping to bring the disease under control. The duration of necessary hospital stay has been reduced by about 50 per cent. Preliminary studies were done on advanced cases and a remarkable improvement has occurred, especially in appetite and body weight. The antituberculosis vaccine, BCG, is being used to some extent in persons with a negative tuberculin test who are likely to be exposed to the tubercle bacillus. This group includes nurses, medical students and children in tuberculous families. In a study of teen-agers, the incidence of tuberculosis was reduced by 80 per cent in the vaccinated.

Rest, antibiotics and fresh air, along with nourishing food, are the four important factors necessary to promote recovery from tuberculosis.

DIETARY TREATMENT As in other acute fevers, a high protein, high calorie fluid regimen is given during the acute phase of tuberculosis, when the fever is high; the normal diet is begun as soon as improvement is noted. Forced feedings or "stuffing" the patient to gain weight in excess of normal is known to be more harmful than advantageous. It has been observed that too much food, especially fats, frequently causes gastric upsets and diarrhea. Now it is realized that the caloric intake should be sufficient to maintain body weight at the normal level or slightly above normal. A diet of 3000, then reduced to 2500, kcalories is usually sufficient to gain weight or maintain weight desired. The diet should be adequate, containing approximately the same type of foods that are found in the normal diet. The food should be simple, easily digested, and well prepared. Because there is lack of appetite, the foods should be made tempting.

The diet should supply a liberal quantity of protein, vitamins and minerals. Johnston[7] found that there is a good correlation between healing and maintenance of an adequate nitrogen balance. Conversely, spreading of the disease took place, even with weight gain, without nitrogen storage. Serum albumin value tends to be low. The daily amount of protein should be slightly above normal — 75 to 100 gm. Brewer[8] and coworkers found a greatly increased need for calcium (1.22 gm.) in a study of women with active tuberculosis, in order to maintain calcium balance and provide for the calcification of the tuberculous lesions. Increased need of iron may be present if there has been hemorrhage. Studies show low ascorbic acid levels of the blood stream in the tuberculous patient, which indicates that vitamin C is required in much larger quantities than ordinarily needed by the normal person. Vitamin A requirement is also believed to be increased. Carotene appears to be poorly converted to vitamin A in tuberculosis. The diet should contain the foods providing vitamin A (liver, eggs, butter, whole milk) as such.[9] Vitamin D is considered to be essential to tuberculous patients of all ages for the absorption and the metabolism of calcium. No doubt the tissue destruction increases the demand for other vitamins too. Specific vitamin concentrates may be indicated in some individuals who need to supplement the vitamins supplied by foods in the diet.

Milk has always been an important food in the treatment of the tuberculosis patient. A minimum of one quart of milk daily is advocated. Vitamin D fortified milk will assure an adequate intake of the vitamin. Milk is an excellent source of calcium, vitamins, proteins, and calories. It is possible to use milk as a beverage, in cooking as in soups, custards and puddings, or in cultured form as yoghurt, buttermilk, or acidophilus milk. Eggs, meat, fish, and poultry for protein should be used in liberal amounts. Liver and dark green and deep yellow vegetables for iron and citrus fruit for ascorbic acid should be used freely. The normal diet, plus additions to help the patient maintain normal weight or gradually gain weight if indicated, is recommended. The 500 kcalories additions described (Ch. 29) are useful when planning daily meals and nourishments for the tuberculosis patient.

Emphasis placed on the need to adhere to an adequate diet and to maintain ideal weight for prevention of recurrence is an integral part of teaching the person with tuberculosis. Those in contact with the person should have

[7]Johnston, J. A.: Nutrition in tuberculous adolescence. J. Am. Dietet. A., 33:1273, 1957.

[8]Brewer, W. D., et al.: Calcium and phosphorus metabolism of women with active tuberculosis. J. Am. Dietet. A., 30:21, 1954.

[9]Getz, H. R.: Problems in feeding the tuberculosis patient. J. Am. Dietet. A., 30:17, 1954.

benefit of counseling in order to prevent the spread of the disease to members of the family or community.

Isoniazid (INH), the antibiotic commonly used in treatment, usually contains B_6, since it was found that INH causes rapid excretion of pyridoxine. The deficiency of vitamin B_6 results in peripheral neuritis.

RECURRENT INFECTIONS

Malaria

Malaria is an example of a *recurrent* infection caused by a parasite carried by the mosquito. The WHO has worked to eradicate the disease from malaria ridden regions. While eradication of malaria as an endemic disease has been accomplished in the United States, there is always the possibility that, until global elimination is achieved, it can be reintroduced surreptitiously. A high incidence of malaria was found among members of the Armed Forces during World War II and Viet Nam conflict. Effective new specifics in the treatment of this disease are now available.

DIETARY TREATMENT   During an attack of malaria with chills and fever, the calorie, protein and vitamin requirements are increased. Fluids and salts may be lost. Since the patient will usually not eat very much during the attack, the diet should be regulated during the quiescent period to maintain nutrition at the desired level. The Committee on Therapeutic Nutrition recommends the diet outlined for acute febrile illnesses, with an increase of calories to bring the total to an average of 4000 to 5000 daily. Because the liver is frequently enlarged and its function impaired following malaria, the high protein, high carbohydrate, moderate fat diet is indicated. (See Chapter 25.)

The role of the diet was highlighted during the research experiments with the anti-malaria drug Atabrine. When given to rats which were on a low protein diet, the drug had a definite toxic effect; the rats lost weight, developed diarrhea, their hair became disheveled and their whiskers encrusted. When large single doses of Atabrine were given to one group of rats fed a stock diet and two groups fed different fasting diets, all of the rats on the stock diet lived, while 22 per cent of one group on fasting diet died overnight, and 48 per cent of the other group on fasting diet died 36 hours later. Each rat in the two groups fed fasting diets had developed severe liver injury. The slow rate of growth of rats receiving suboptimal amounts of protein and riboflavin was retarded further when Atabrine was added to their diet.

Studies have shown that chicks and ducks whose diets are deficient in biotin are more susceptible to malaria than those whose diets are normal. It has been suggested that various malarial parasites require different optimal concentrations of biotin in the blood. If biotin levels exceed these concentrations, the multiplication of the parasite is reduced and the acute infection ended.

Although these experiments cited show some relationship between malaria and nutrition, there is need for intensive research before all of the answers to the numerous questions are known.

Emphysema

Securing an adequate diet may be difficult for the person with emphysema because of the symptoms associated with it. Depending upon the severity of the condition, he may not have the energy required to purchase, prepare or go to a restaurant for the food he needs. Shortness of breath, chewing and swallowing require further effort and the person is unable to eat sufficient amounts of food. Weight loss, tissue wasting and malnutrition follow. Persons with emphysema may complain of abdominal distress, and peptic ulcers frequently develop.

A soft diet high in calories with small frequent feedings of concentrated foods is indicated. Fibrous fruits, vegetables and meats require energy for chewing. These persons often experience difficulty in eating breakfast. They are especially short of breath in the morning after a night's sleep.[10] Swallowing of air while eating can cause discomfort.

PROBLEMS AND SUGGESTED TOPICS FOR DISCUSSION

1. Explain the body needs for diet nutrients during an infection with fever. How can the body's susceptibility to disease be influenced through diet?
2. Correlate the care of a tuberculosis patient with the planning of his meals. With the patient, compare his plan with the recommendations of the basic food groups.
3. What are the principles involved in feeding a patient with fever of short duration? What are the principles involved in feeding a patient with fever of long duration?

SUGGESTED ADDITIONAL READING REFERENCES

Andrews, J. M.: Perspective on malaria today. J.A.M.A., 184:873, 1963.
Cannon, P. R.: The importance of proteins in resistance to infection. J.A.M.A., 128:360, 1945.
Editorial. Nature of rheumatic heart disease. J.A.M.A., 175:230, 1961.

[10]Wilson, N. L.: Protein intakes in pulmonary emphysema and tuberculosis. J. Am. Dietet. A., 47:194, 1965.

Edwards, H. R., and Turner, J.: Diet suggestions for the tuberculous on low income. Pub. Health Nursing, 43:681, 1951.

Getz, H. R.: Problems in feeding the tuberculous patient. J. Am. Dietet. A., 30:17, 1954.

Grifone, J. W.: Active rheumatic heart disease in patients over sixty. J.A.M.A., 154:1341, 1954.

Schwartz, W. S.: Developments in treatment of tuberculosis and other pulmonary disease. J.A.M.A., 178:43, 1961.

Schwartz, W. S.: Management of common pulmonary diseases. J.A.M.A., 181:134, 1962.

Scrimshaw, N. S.: Nutrition and Infection. National Live Stock and Meat Board. Food and Nutrition News, 32:1, No. 8 May, 1960.

Scrimshaw, N. S.: Malnutrition and Infection. Borden's Review of Nutrition Research, 26(No. 2), April-June, 1965.

Stollerman, G. H.: Factors determining the attack rate of rheumatic fever. J.A.M.A., 177:823, 1961.

Welsh, D. E.: Recommendations for feeding tuberculous patients. Hospitals, 3:68, 1957.

Wilson, N. L., et al.: Nutrition in tuberculosis. J. Am. Dietet. A., 33:243, 1957.

Wilson, N. L., et al.: Nutrition in pulmonary emphysema. J. Am. Dietet. A., 45:530, 1964.

Wilson, N. L.: Protein intakes of pulmonary emphysema and tuberculosis. J. Am. Dietet. A., 47:197, 1965.

Wolstenholme, G. E. W., and O'Connor, M.: Nutrition and Infection. Boston, Little, Brown and Company, 1968.

Zagala, J. G., and Feinstein, A. R.: The preceding illness of acute rheumatic fever. J.A.M.A., 179:863, 1962.

Gastric diseases are usually classified as (1) organic and (2) reflex or functional. The latter are the more common. An organic disease of the stomach is one in which a definite pathologic change has taken place in the structural tissues. Peptic ulcer and cancer are examples. A reflex or functional disorder of the stomach is a disturbance of the nerve center of digestion, either sensory, motor, or secretory in origin.

ORGANIC DISEASES OF THE STOMACH

GASTRIC AND DUODENAL ULCERS

An eroded lesion in the gastric or intestinal (duodenum) mucosa is termed an *ulcer* (see Fig. 23–1). The location of the ulcer determines its nomenclature. That is, if the ulcer is located in the stomach, it is a *"gastric" ulcer*; if it is located in the duodenum, it is called a *"duodenal" ulcer*. Often both types are grouped together under the general term *"peptic" ulcer*. Since the treatment for both types is essentially the same, their diet care will be considered together. Duodenal ulcers are much more common than gastric ulcers, and both kinds occur in the male more frequently than in the female, usually in people who are naturally *tense*, hard-working and hard-worrying.

It is reported that approximately 10 per cent of our population is or has been afflicted with gastric or duodenal ulcer. Sometimes during routine x-ray examination scars are found, although the individual never knew that the disorder existed. This would seem to indicate that healing sometimes takes place spontaneously.

Predisposing Causes

The cause of peptic ulcer is unknown. However, many theories pertaining to possible causes have been suggested. Too much secretion of gastric juice is believed to be the basic cause of peptic ulceration. Normally the mucosa of the stomach is protected from the strongly acid digestive juices by the mucus that is secreted by mucous glands beginning at the lower esophagus to the upper duodenum. The duodenum is protected by the alkalinity of the small intestines, which contain large quantities of sodium bicarbonate that neutralize the hydrochloric acid in the gastric juice. The pepsin is thereby inactivated to prevent digestion of the mucosa. Irritation of the stomach mucosa by excess gastric juice prevents neutralization of the gastric juices by the secretions of the small intestine, and an ulcer develops.

A rather high incidence of moderate hypoproteinemia in peptic ulcer cases has been reported in humans. This may be a causal effect of inadequate dietary buffering of the strongly acid gastric secretion, or it may result from the insufficient quantity of protein supplied by the limited diets frequently used in ulcer treatment.

Faulty dietary habits, excessive smoking, and *excessive indulgence in alcohol* are believed to be contributing factors to the development of peptic ulcer. Rushing through meals, improper selection of food, and irregular meals are poor nutrition and eating habits which should be discouraged.

Heredity has been mentioned as a possible factor in ulcers. It has been observed that patients with type O blood have ulcers more often than do persons with other blood types.

When the body has been overtaxed physically and *low resistance* results, ulcers may occur. Therefore, inadequate sleep and rest

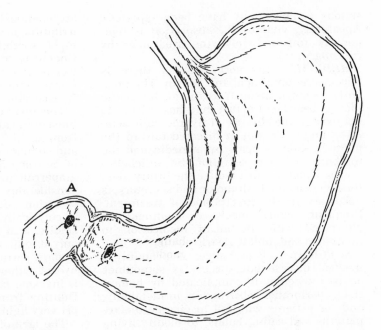

Figure 23–1   Diagram showing stomach and duodenum with eroded lesions. *A,* duodenal ulcer; *B,* gastric ulcer.

may be predisposing factors in their development.

Emotional conflicts, stress, nervous strain or *psychic trauma* cause a disturbance of the nerves which control the blood supply to the lining of the stomach and the duodenum, thus weakening it and permitting the juices to attack. It is believed that most instances of peptic ulcerations result from excessive stimulation of the dorsal nucleus of the vagus by impulses originating in the cerebrum.[1] Dragstedt[2] advanced the concept that an increase in the corrosive properties of the gastric content as a result of hypersecretion, rather than a local decrease in mucosal resistance, is the chief cause of peptic ulcer in most patients. Succeeding publications support this concept. Evidence has been presented to suggest that hormones and humoral agents which arise in the gastrointestinal tract may play a significant role in ulcerogenesis.[3]

Then again, peptic ulcers may develop with no apparent cause. They usually occur between the ages of 15 and 40 years after a prolonged digestive disturbance, especially when the digestive disturbance is accompanied by hypersecretion of acid.

Although chronic ulcer usually follows a typical course and produces characteristic symptoms, occasionally the symptoms are either nil or indefinite and hemorrhage or perforation is the first signal of the illness.

Treatment

The objectives of treatment are relief of pain, healing of the ulcer, and prevention of recurrences and complications. Unfortunately for the patient, there is no cure-all for gastric and duodenal ulcers. Because resistance must be kept at a high level, physical and mental rest are important. If the ulcer is moderately advanced, bed rest, either at home or in the hospital, may be advocated for a period of one to three weeks. An equal period of convalescence is prescribed, particularly for the business man, who should stay away from disturbing office situations. In mild cases the patient can usually continue his regular routine work activities while following the diet and rest treatment. If the atmosphere and surroundings at home or office are unpleasant and cause emotional upsets, the patient may be advised to consider a complete change.

The reports of *gastric freezing*[4] are highly promising; however, further corroborative studies are required before the procedure can be generally accepted. Intractable duodenal ulcer is the current principal indication for gastric freezing. Side effects and sometimes

[1]Guyton, A. C.: Textbook of Medical Physiology. 4th ed. Philadelphia, W. B. Saunders Company, 1971, p. 777.

[2]Dragstedt, L. R.: Cause of peptic ulcer. J.A.M.A., *169*: 203, 1959.

[3]State, D.: Gastrointestinal hormones in the production of peptic ulcer. J.A.M.A., *187*:410, 1964.

[4]Gastric freezing. J.A.M.A., *185*:811, 1963; *187*:1032, 1964; *188*:409, 1964.

serious complications have been reported.[5] Apparently, vitamin B_{12} absorption is temporarily impaired following treatment by freezing.[6]

MEDICAL   In most patients there is hypersecretion of acid and pepsin. The presently accepted medical treatment for peptic ulcer is based on the fact that these ulcers do not exist in the absence of hydrochloric acid. Accordingly, therapy is directed toward the neutralization of acids by antacids and the inhibition of acid secretion by anticholinergics, which in turn reduce the injury. Rest for the stomach, both motor and secretory, is necessary in the first period of treatment. Frequent, regular meals (or feedings) are alternated with the alkali medication to neutralize and inhibit gastric acidity.

SURGICAL   Peptic ulcer is primarily a medical disease but surgery is sometimes advised when it is complicated by hemorrhage, perforation, obstruction, intractability, and for patients who fail to change dietary patterns and eating habits, to modify living conditions or to adhere to the medication regimen.

CURRENT CONCEPTS IN ULCER DIETARY.[7]   The traditional methods are being challenged by some physicians who question their effectiveness in the treatment of peptic ulcers. An expert committee composed of members of the American Medical Association and of the American Dietetic Association appointed to study the question of diet as related to gastrointestinal function reported that knowledge in this particular field is exceedingly meager despite the long and sometimes successful use of the empirical regimens.

The basic difficulty with diet therapy as related to gastrointestinal structure and function was concluded to be "ignorance as to what happens to an individual food item in the gut, as to its effect on the alimentary tube, and as to the real explanation of symptoms that might follow its ingestion." Many of the diets used are a result of deep-rooted practice, without a true scientific justification.

It is known that sight, smell, taste, water and practically anything taken into the stomach stimulate gastric secretions to a greater or lesser degree. Those foods which are chemically, mechanically and thermally irritating to the mucosa and those believed to be soothing have not been determined. Chemical composition and physical properties of foods before ingestion are available. Correlations between the nature of a food and its gastrointestinal effects are unknown.

The effect of acidic food on gastric contents must be evaluated. The pH of foods ranges from about 2 in lime juice to 8 in egg whites and Graham crackers. Most foods have a pH of between 5 and 7. The pH of orange and grapefruit juice is about 3.2 to 3.6, which is considerably less acid than normal gastric secretion. Gastric secretion is about 1.6. Theoretically on the basis of their immediate acidity, acid fruit juices are contraindicated only to oral, esophageal and possibly gastric lesions, particularly if the stomach is achlorhydric. Otherwise the pH of a food before it is ingested has little therapeutic importance. Diluting fruit juices with water affects the pH very lightly.

The lack of knowledge and the many factors influencing intestinal gas makes it unwise to classify foods on the basis of their gas-forming properties. Data on laxative properties in foods are very sparse. It is not known what foods do or can have laxative properties or on what part of the intestines they act or how they function. The laxative property said to be present in prune juice is di-hydroxyphenyl isatin. It appears to have some effect on the small bowel.

Gastric secretion is not affected by most spices in any major or consistent way. Black pepper, chili powder, cloves, nutmeg and mustard seed have been thought to cause a slight reddening of the mucosa. Black pepper has been shown to be an irritant causing a specific and localized hyperemia, whereas other spices are apparently innocuous in this respect. Caffeine and alcohol are known to stimulate gastric juices when consumed by themselves.

Pepsin secretion in response to the intake of different foods tends to parallel the gastric acid secretion. The production of mucus in response to various foods is not known. Secretory or motor activity increases gastric mucosal vascularity.

A dietary regimen that reduces and controls the daily total gastric acid output varies with individuals. With some individuals an hour-to-hour program—frequent and regular meals—is probably more important than the type of food ingested. Protein foods have a dual role related to gastric content and secretions. They act as a buffer. Milk is an especially good buffer but the buffering action is temporary. Fats apparently inhibit gastric secretion. No experimental observations were

[5]Karacadag, S., et al.: Side effects and complications of gastric freeze. J.A.M.A., *188*:1151, 1964.

[6]Temporary impairment of vitamin B_{12} absorption. Another side effect of therapeutic gastric freezing. J.A.M.A., *190*:779, 1964.

[7]Weinstein, L., et al.: Diet as related to gastrointestinal function. J.A.M.A., *176*:935, 1961; and J. Am. Dietet. A., *38*:425, 1961; Odell, A. C.: Ulcer dietotherapy—past and present. J. Am. Dietet. A., *58*:447, 1971.

found by the Committee to indicate that dairy fats traditionally recommended to the ulcer patient are more effective in depressing the gastric secretions than are animal fats or fried foods.

Shull[8] and others suggest that specific food intolerances and their influence on motor and secretory function of a given patient are the important factors; whether or not a food will be tolerated by an ulcer patient is best determined by trial. It is assumed that the intelligent individual will avoid any food which from experience caused indigestion, pain or other digestive symptoms. Wolf,[9] a strong supporter of a liberal diet regimen, considers it important to recommend frequent feedings so that the stomach will not be empty and that the feedings should contain milk and cream, which promote neutralization and inhibition of gastric function. Doll et al.[10] observed 121 patients with peptic ulcer on a controlled dietary regimen and reported that a conventional bland diet does not increase the healing rate. Todd[11] states that there is no proof that the avoidance of certain foods customarily considered irritating is beneficial unless these foods cause immediate distress. He believes that the therapeutic ulcer diet has no proven virtue over and above that of diminishing the stomach acid. Roth's[12] study indicated that a rigid dietary regimen is difficult for the patient. He reported that the majority of patients given the traditional ulcer diet did not understand the regimen and were apt to be more restrictive than necessary. These patients seemed to associate from the diet what foods were good and bad for the ulcer. They believed that they should adhere to a diet for under six months to over five years or indefinitely.

The application of the liberal concept centers around the person rather than the diet and around normal nutritional needs rather than a special regimen. Regularity and frequency of meals and moderation in eating habits are important in the long-term management of patients proved to have peptic ulcers. An understanding common sense approach to the dietary treatment which considers the patient as a whole will provide for the essential nutritional needs and acid-reducing features that are therapeutic to the individual. For example: What changes does the patient need to make in his present dietary pattern to provide the calories and nutrients that he needs? What changes does he need to make in his eating habits? How will he implement the changes?

TRADITIONAL ULCER DIETARY   Since the traditional treatment remains widely used, the conventional diet outline is presented.

Food   Foods included in the conventional ulcer diet should be of a soft consistency with a minimum amount of fiber. Any foods which are believed to stimulate gastric secretion are omitted. In 1915 Sippy introduced a progressive regimen. Milk, or milk and cream, is the basis of the diet and is conventionally used for its acid-buffering capacity; the fat in cream inhibits gastric secretion. Current criticism of the conventional diet is that it may predispose to myocardial infarction because of the high content of saturated fats. Some physicians recommend substituting polyunsaturated for saturated fats; others reduce the total fat content of the diet. The neutralizing effects of cream, whole milk, and skim milk are identical. The delayed emptying time of the stomach produced through the use of cream can generally be duplicated by prescribing anticholinergic drugs. Enriched, refined or finely ground whole grain cereals are included early in the diet. Eggs are usually added to the diet during the same period when bread and cereal are provided. Fruits and vegetables are cooked to soften fiber. Chicken, fish and meat are withheld until the convalescent stage is approached. Meat extracts (broth, soups and gravies), tea, coffee, cocoa, concentrated chocolate, alcohol, condiments, and spices are avoided because they tend to stimulate gastric activity. Fried foods are traditionally excluded. Although sweets in concentrated form are thought to be somewhat irritating, custard, simple puddings, gelatin desserts, and vanilla ice cream are well tolerated, and may be added to the diet near the beginning of the treatment.

Protein and Calories   Because the normal protein requirements are increased during the healing stage in the ulcer patient, large quantities of milk plus eggs and soft cheeses must be consumed to meet the protein demands in the early stages of treatment. Although the extractives of meat may stimulate gastric secretion to some extent, the excellent neutralizing action of meat proteins is so effective, the more easily digested meats are added as soon as possible. Any ulcer represents tissue loss, and protein is required for rebuilding. If the protein supply is inadequate,

[8]Shull, H. J.: Diet in the management of peptic ulcer. J.A.M.A., *170*:124, 1961.

[9]Wolf, S.: Critical appraisal of dietary management of peptic ulcer and ulcerative colitis. Am. J. Clin. Nutr., 2:1, 1954.

[10]Doll, R., et al.: Dietetic treatment of peptic ulcer. Lancet, *1*:5, 1956.

[11]Todd, J. W.: Treatment of peptic ulcer. Lancet, *1*:113, 1952.

[12]Roth, H. P., and Caron, H. S.: Patients' misconception about their peptic ulcer diets: Potential obstacles to cooperation. J. Chron. Dis., 20:5, 1967.

the various needs of the body must compete and several will be unsatisfied. Co Tui, conducting research at New York University, observed that a more striking remission of gastroduodenal ulcers followed treatment with a high protein, high calorie diet than followed the conventional diet treatment. The protein in his diet was given by mouth as a protein hydrolysate. The calories were calculated for 40 to 50 calories per kilogram of body weight.

The Committee on Nutrition[13] recommends a minimum of 100 gm. of protein per day (see page 330). To accomplish this, as well as adequate calorie intake, the addition of protein concentrates to the milk or milk-cream feedings is suggested. Milk powder and other oral protein preparations will prevent protein and caloric deficiency, as well as provide the desired buffer action, and they are preferred over protein hydrolysates (see Chaps. 26 and 43).

Feeding Intervals   Small meals or feedings are served at intervals of one, two or three hours, depending upon the acuteness of the condition of the patient. Food should always be present in the stomach to combine with hydrochloric acid and decrease the amount of free acid.

Amount of Food   To reduce pressure and maintain neutrality of the gastric contents of the stomach, frequent feedings are advocated. It is customary to start the diet treatment with 3- to 4-ounce feedings of milk or milk and cream given at one- to two-hour intervals from 7:00 A.M. through 9:00 or 10:00 P.M. (and during the night if awake), and alternated with alkaline powder or nonabsorbable antacid for a period of approximately one week. When additional food is allowed, small feedings of soft fiber foods are added to or substituted for some of the milk or milk and cream feedings, and the number of feedings increased until a total of six feedings are served. The next stage is an ambulatory ulcer diet which consists of low fiber foods divided into six small meals or three meals with milk served between meals. The foods allowed in each stage of increased feedings are outlined below. The physician prescribes the diet treatment best suited to meet the individualized condition of the patient. Usually, surgical patients who have had gastric resections tolerate small amounts of food fed regularly. Medical patients who are ambulatory seem to get along well on the schedule of three meals plus milk served midmorning, midafternoon, and at bedtime.

[13]Therapeutic Nutrition. Washington, D.C., National Research Council, Publication 234, 1952.

Four-Stage Peptic Ulcer Diet Therapy
Following are typical stages in the conventional treatment of peptic ulcer.

First Stage   For the active, acute peptic ulcer, 3 to 4 ounces of milk or milk and cream (half and half or one-third cream and two-thirds milk) are served at one- to two-hour intervals from 7:00 A.M. through 9:00 or 10:00 P.M. (and during the night when awake) until pain disappears or about one week. When whole milk alone is ordered, with fifteen hourly 4 ounce feedings, the diet contains approximately 68 gm. protein, 68 gm. fats, 90 gm. carbohydrates, and 1245 kcalories. When milk and cream (half and half) are prescribed, the diet contains approximately 60 gm. proteins, 210 gm. fats, 83 gm. carbohydrates, and 2460 kcalories. Sometimes pain may not entirely disappear even after three or four days on this feeding schedule. These patients will usually react favorably to continuous intragastric drip of the same milk and cream mixture for a few days.

Second Stage   As pain disappears, small feedings of soft fiber foods are added to or supplemented for some of the milk or milk and cream feedings. The initial feedings of 3 to 4 ounces served at frequent and regular intervals throughout the waking hours are gradually increased, and the interval between feedings is lengthened until the patient is established on a schedule of five feedings daily. Thorough mastication of all foods to promote mixing with saliva in preparation for gastric digestion is important.

Foods allowed in the supplementary feeding are selected from the following list:

Milk toast.
Egg, poached or soft cooked.
Cereal: enriched Cream of Wheat, farina, boiled rice or oatmeal.
Strained cream soup.
Toasted enriched white bread and butter or margarine.
White crackers and butter or margarine.
Dessert: rennet-milk pudding, custard, gelatin dessert, vanilla ice cream, bread pudding, tapioca pudding, plain sugar cookies.

Third Stage: Six-feeding Diet for Patient with Peptic Ulcer   When six feedings are ordered, the sixth feeding is added at bedtime, and the service of food closely follows the customary meal pattern (Table 23–1). The diet contains approximately 100 gm. of protein, 140 gm. of fats, 240 gm. of carbohydrates and 2620 kcalories. If fewer calories or reduction of serum lipids is desired, cream may be omitted from the diet, or the amount of cream may be reduced or replaced by milk, or even skim milk, and milk served exclusively.

TABLE 23–1   SIX-FEEDING DIET FOR PEPTIC ULCER PATIENT

MEAL PLAN	SAMPLE MENU	Weight Grams	Household Measure
	SERVINGS		
	BREAKFAST		
Fruit	Strained, diluted orange juice (taken at end of meal)	124	½ cup
Cereal	Cooked farina	119	½ cup
Milk and cream	Milk and cream	181	1 glass (6 oz.)
Cream	Cream (for cereal)	60	2 ounces
Sugar	Sugar (for cereal)	10	2 teaspoons
	10:00 A.M.		
Egg	Poached egg	50	1
Bread	Toasted enriched white bread	46	2 slices
Butter	Butter or margarine	7	1 pat
Milk	Milk	244	1 cup
	LUNCHEON		
Soup	Strained cream of pea soup	128	½ cup
Crackers	Soda crackers	11	2
Cheese	Cottage cheese	56	2 ounces
Vegetables	Baked potato	99	1 medium
Bread	Enriched white bread	23	1 slice
Butter	Butter or margarine	14	2 pats
Dessert	Strawberry gelatin	120	1½ cup
	3:00 P.M.		
Dessert	Milk-rennet dessert	100	½ cup
Milk	Milk	244	1 cup
	DINNER		
Vegetable	Strained, diluted tomato juice (taken in middle of meal)	120	½ cup
Meat	Broiled beef patty	57	2 ounces
Cereal product	Noodles, buttered	80	½ cup
Bread	Enriched white bread	23	1 slice
Butter	Butter or margarine	7	1 pat
Dessert	Baked custard	124	½ cup
Milk and cream	Milk and cream	121	½ cup
	8:00 P.M.		
Crackers	Soda crackers	11	2
Milk beverage	Eggnog	244	1 cup

FOODS INCLUDED

Milk or Milk and Cream: Four to 8 ounces with each meal, the amount depending upon the need.

Eggs: Poached or soft cooked.

Meats: Ground or tender beef, lamb, pork,* liver; fish; minced chicken. (Prepare by boiling, broiling or roasting methods.)

Cheese: Cottage or cream.

Breads: Enriched white bread, plain white rolls, soda crackers. (Serve plain or toasted.)

Cereals: Enriched refined varieties (cooked or ready-to-eat).

Cereal products: Macaroni, spaghetti, noodles or rice. (Serve cooked without sauce.)

Fats: Butter, margarine or oil.

Vegetables: White potatoes (baked and skin removed, boiled, mashed or creamed); cooked vegetable; tomato juice.

Fruits: Cooked fruit; fruit juices.

Soups: Cream soups.

Desserts: Simple puddings; custards; gelatin desserts; milk-rennet pudding; unfrosted, plain white cake; plain white sugar cookies, vanilla ice cream.

FOODS OMITTED

Improperly fried foods, condiments (such as black pepper, chili powder, cloves and mustard seed), pickles, coffee, tea, cocoa, concentrated chocolate, soft drinks, beer, alcohol, salads, raw high fiber vegetables, raw fruits, candy, nuts, pastries, hot cakes, hot breads, gravies and very hot or very cold foods.

Fourth Stage: Low Fiber Diet for Ambulatory Peptic Ulcer Patients. This diet may be prescribed either in six meals or three meals with milk served between meals. Such a diet contains approximately 100 gm. of protein, 100 to 110 gm. of fats, 230 to 250 gm. of carbohydrates, and 2300 kcalories. Cream is no longer added to the milk. The cooked vegetables are of low fiber content, depending

---

*Pork is a highly nutritious food and should not be eliminated from low fiber diets.

upon the individual's tolerance. The taste, preferences and condition of the individual patient are considered. Soups are limited to creamed vegetable soups, from which the patient advances to cooked whole vegetables of low fiber content.

FOODS INCLUDED

Milk: Milk, skim milk, milk beverages, buttermilk, cream.

Eggs: Poached, soft or hard cooked, scrambled in double boiler or as eggnog.

Meat, fish and poultry: Ground or tender beef, veal, pork or lamb; tender liver; fresh fish; sweetbreads; canned tunafish and salmon; and turkey or chicken (no skin).

Cheese: Cottage, cream cheese, and other mild cheeses for flavoring.

Bread: Plain or toasted enriched white; white crackers.

Cereals: Enriched refined, ready-to-eat, and cooked.

Cereal products: Macaroni, spaghetti, noodles, and rice (cooked and served with *mild* cheese sauce, if desired).

Fats: Butter, fortified margarine, oil.

Vegetables: Vegetable juices; cooked vegetables of low fiber content (asparagus tips, beets, carrots, green beans, immature peas, potatoes—boiled, mashed, creamed and baked without skin—pumpkin, spinach, winter squash). If still greater reduction in fiber is needed, these vegetables are puréed, or the juice only is given.

Fruits: Fruit juices; strained prunes; peeled, cooked or canned peaches, pears, apples, apricots and plums; ripe bananas. If still greater reduction in fiber is needed, these fruits are puréed.

Soups: Strained soups. If it is desirable to restrict the extractives, limit to cream soups.

Desserts: Bread, cream, rice and tapioca pudding; arrowroot cookies; custard; gelatin desserts with allowed fruit; milk-rennet pudding; unfrosted sponge or angel food cake; vanilla ice cream, sherbets.

Beverage: Postum or decaffeinated coffee, if desired. Tea, coffee, cocoa, chocolate malted or milk shake, carbonated beverages as ordered.

Sweets: Sugar, honey, jelly in moderate amounts.

Condiments: Cinnamon, allspice, mace, thyme, sage, paprika, caraway seeds.

FOODS OMITTED

Meat and Fish: Smoked, dried, pickled or salted meats and fish.

Condiments: Black pepper, chili pepper, cloves, mustard seed, nutmeg.

Miscellaneous: Coconut, rich gravies, alcoholic beverages, nuts, candy, pickles, salads, rich sauces, soft drinks, jams, highly seasoned foods, and improperly fried foods.

Maintenance Diet for Healed Peptic Ulcer Patient   The patient who has had an ulcer should adopt an adequate diet and establish regular eating habits. Individuals with a past history of ulcers are predisposed to new ulcer formations. The reason for this is not known, just as the cause of ulcers is unknown. A basic diet pattern to follow is the low fiber diet (p. 341 and Table 23–2) to which may be added fine whole grain bread and cereals; meat soups and gravy; raw fruits and vegetables in moderation, as tolerated.

Complications and Adequacy of the Diet Over a long period the large amount of alkali administered may lead to alkalosis. As previously stated, calorie and protein deficiencies frequently accompany ulcers, especially during the initial treatment, interfering with the healing of the lesions. Avitaminosis may develop unless vitamin supplements or specific vitamin rich foods are added. Before accurate vitamin information was available,

TABLE 23–2   LOW FIBER DIET

BREAKFAST	SAMPLE MENU* LUNCH	DINNER
Strained orange juice	Cream of asparagus soup	Tender roast beef
Cooked cream of wheat	Cottage cheese	Buttered noodles
Poached egg	Baked potato (no skin)	Cooked young peas
Toasted enriched white bread	Buttered carrots	Enriched white bread
Butter or margarine	Enriched white bread	Butter or margarine
Milk	Butter or margarine	Vanilla ice cream
Cream	Applesauce	Milk
Decaffeinated coffee	Milk	
Sugar		

*Milk may be served between meals (10:00 A.M., 3:00 P.M. and 8:00 P.M.) when indicated, or the diet may be served in six small meals. Usually, the egg and toast listed for breakfast are served at 10:00 A.M.; the dessert and bread designated for luncheon are saved for the 3 o'clock feeding; and the dessert from dinner is served at 8:00 P.M.

TABLE 23-3   TYPICAL REGIMEN FOR DIETARY MANAGEMENT OF PEPTIC ULCER

	8 A.M.	10 A.M.	12 NOON	3 P.M.	6 P.M.	8 P.M.
Second Stage Supplementary feedings added as tolerated (6 to 8 oz.)	1 feeding Farina with cream and sugar		Milk toast		Baked custard	
	2 feedings Boiled rice with cream and sugar				Gelatin and cream	
	3 feedings Farina with cream and sugar				Vanilla ice cream with sugar cookies	
	4 feedings Oatmeal with cream and sugar	Poached egg on toast	Cream soup with white crackers			
	5 feedings Cream of wheat with cream and sugar	Soft cooked egg with 1 slice toast	Boiled rice with cream and sugar	Bread pudding with cream	Cream soup with croutons	
Third Stage (Six feedings) (10 to 12 oz.)	As long as indicated Strained orange juice (end of meal) Farina with cream and sugar Milk and cream (6 oz.)	Poached egg on toast Milk (8 oz.)	Creamed pea soup Crackers Cottage cheese Baked potato (no skin) Enriched white bread and butter Strawberry gelatin	Milk-rennet pudding Milk (8 oz.)	Tomato juice Broiled beef patty Buttered noodles Enriched white bread and butter Baked custard Milk and cream (4 oz.)	Eggnog with cinnamon Soda crackers
Fourth Stage Low fiber diet for ambulatory patient	Strained orange juice (end of meal) Cream of wheat with cream and sugar Soft cooked egg Buttered enriched white toast Milk (8 oz.) Decaffeinated coffee with cream and sugar	Milk (8 oz.)	Cream of spinach soup Crackers Cottage cheese Baked potato (no skin) Asparagus tips Enriched white bread and butter Canned peaches Milk (8 oz.)	Milk (8 oz.)	Tender roast beef Boiled rice Cooked beets Enriched white bread and butter Vanilla ice cream Milk (8 oz.)	Milk (8 oz.)

First Stage: 3 to 4 oz. milk or milk and cream (half and half) are served every 1 to 2 hours on the hour, 7 A.M. through 9 P.M. and during the night if necessary.

it was not unusual to see patients in the hospital medical wards with typical symptoms of ascorbic acid deficiences, such as areas of bluish skin (weakened capillary walls which may lead to hemorrhages) and bleeding gums. Today, when signs of avitaminosis are detected they may be attributed to neglect, carelessness, lack of knowledge or insufficient income for an adequate diet.

Secondary anemia may develop in the ulcer patient during the early phase of the diet treatment when only milk or milk and cream are fed. Although egg yolk is a good source of iron, not enough is consumed to provide the day's requirement. Meat, another source of iron, is often added near the conclusion of the diet treatment. It should also be recalled that iron absorption depends upon an acid medium; thus, neutralization of gastric acids interferes with iron absorption (see p. 106).

There has been concern among physicians[14] because the conventional peptic ulcer diet therapy requires an excessive fat intake, resulting in elevation of serum lipids. Actually, increased amounts of fats are not required over and above the normal diet, as milk, or even skim milk, can be used in place of cream as previously pointed out. The use of frequent feedings of protein in the form of gelatin dishes, pot and cottage cheese in the early stages, and fish, poultry and meat added as soon as tolerated, will serve to control gastric acidity and ulcer pain.

Patients receiving restricted ulcer diets need careful supervision. Whenever there is doubt about the adequacy of the diet, protein, vitamin and iron supplements should be added. X-rays show that complete healing takes from 14 to 100 days, with an average

of 40. This is why medical treatment is sometimes continued for six to seven weeks before changes are made in the medication and diet.

Bleeding Ulcer

DIETARY TREATMENT   Whether it is advisable to prescribe food for a patient with a bleeding ulcer remains controversial. The conservative method of dietary treatment withholds all food by mouth for a period of 24 to 72 hours after hemorrhage has stopped. Glucose is given intravenously. When food is allowed orally, milk and cream are offered at hourly intervals. The supplementary feedings outlined in Table 23–3 are added, as tolerated.

Meulengracht Diet[15]   In 1935 the Meulengracht diet for treatment of bleeding ulcer was introduced. It consists of an abundant "purée diet," given on the first day of hemorrhage. Foods allowed are similar to the low fiber diet outlined previously (p. 341 and Table 23–2), with the exception that all fruits and vegetables are puréed, bread is limited to the refined varieties, and tea is permitted. The dietary objective is to neutralize the gastric acidity, prevent digestion of the newly formed clot, and to maintain nutrition.

Andresen Diet[16]   The Andresen diet, to be used following gastric surgery or for treatment of bleeding ulcer, was presented in 1927 and generally ignored until years later. It consists of a simple mixture of milk, cream, gelatin, and glucose given at frequent intervals to supply fluid, the major classes of nutriment, and calories in satisfactory amounts. (See Tables 23–4 and 23–5.) This treatment takes advantage of the fact that

[14]Berkowitz, D., and Glassman, S.: Serum lipid and fat tolerance determinations in patients receiving Sippy diets. J.A.M.A., *181*:176, 1962.

[15]Meulengracht, E.: Treatment of hematemesis and melaena with food. Lancet, 229:1220, 1935.
[16]Andresen, A. F. R.: The peptic ulcer problem. New York J. Med., *49*:2811, 1949.

TABLE 23–4   FORMULA FOR GELATIN-MILK FEEDING, ANDRESEN DIET FOR GASTRIC HEMORRHAGE

FOOD	AMOUNT	CARBO-HYDRATE (gm.)	PROTEIN (gm.)	FAT (gm.)	KILOCALORIES
Gelatin	50 gm.	...	45	...	180
Dextrose	60 gm.	60	...	...	240
Cream (20 per cent)	100 ml.	3	3	18	180
Milk	900 ml.	36	27	27	550
Total		99	75	45	1150 per L.

Milk, cream, and dextrose mixed and kept in refrigerator. Gelatin in paper cup at bedside. Stir teaspoonful into small amount of warmed milk mixture and mix with remainder of a 6-ounce feeding. Flavor with tea, vanilla, or cocoa if desired; serve cool or warmed.
First 4 days: 6 ounces every 2 hours. Nothing else by mouth.
Fifth, sixth days: Add to each of 3 or 4 feedings one of the following: 1 egg; 3 ounces cereal; custard, jello, or ice cream. Allow water in 3-ounce quantities between feedings.
Seventh, eighth days: 2 of above foods with each feeding.
Ninth day: Ulcer diet.

TABLE 23–5   FORMULA FOR GELATIN-WATER FEEDINGS*

FOOD	AMOUNT	CARBOHYDRATE (gm.)	PROTEIN (gm.)	CALORIES
Gelatin	50 gm.	......	45	180
Dextrose	90 gm.	90	......	360
Juice of 3 oranges		30	......	120
Water to	1000 ml.	......	......	......
Total		120	45	660 per L.

*Used for patients intolerant of or allergic to milk. Mixture without gelatin kept in refrigerator. Add gelatin and serve as with milk mixture. Tables 23–4 and 23–5 from Andresen, A. F. R.: Management of gastric hemorrhage. New York State J. Med., 48:603, 1948.

the stomach with food in it is a quieter stomach, and that any clot-digesting tendency will be counteracted by the acid-neutralizing effect of the protein in the diet.

Postoperative Peptic Ulcer Treatment

The preferable treatment for some types of gastric and duodenal ulcers (namely, old ulcers of five or more years' duration; the calloused and obstruction-producing kind; the very large and cancer-suspicious type; the perforating ulcer; and those which show a persistent tendency to bleed) is surgery.

Sometimes in surgery only a small portion of the stomach needs to be resected, while at other times large sections are removed. As a rule, the stomach heals quickly, and the progression of the diet advances rapidly. When a large portion of the stomach has been resected, the patient is more comfortable if small meals are served frequently for a period of several months. (See Andresen diet, Tables 23–4 and 23–5.) Although the ulcer has been removed, the patient should be informed that permanent dietary discretion is essential since an operation is no cure-all. Frequent recurrences of ulcer have been observed following both medical and surgical treatment.

Postoperatively parenteral feedings are continued for several days along with clear liquids. Then 2 to 3 ounces of milk are given every 2 hours. Food is added as soon as tolerated. The program similar to the second stage ulcer regimen is instituted and progressed to full dietary. See Chapter 26, Diets in Surgery and Surgical Conditions, for further discussion of diet following gastric surgery and for the "dumping syndrome."

ACUTE GASTRITIS

Acute gastritis is an inflammation of the gastric mucosa, sudden and sometimes violent in onset, but the term is often applied to any stomach discomfort. Attacks very often follow errors in the diet, such as overeating, the eating of specific foods to which the individual is sensitive, bolting of food, or eating when overtired or emotionally upset. The employment of too much alcohol, tobacco, and highly seasoned foods may also contribute to the cause.

The possibility of ingestion of certain toxic substances, such as spoiled food (as with staphylococcal toxin) or drugs such as salicylates and ammonium chloride, is another factor. Also, the toxin of an infectious disease, germs from the teeth, tonsils or sinuses may bring on an attack of gastritis.

The initial treatment is to get rid of the offending substance as soon as possible. It may be necessary to empty the stomach by induced vomiting, lavage or both. Irrigation of the colon and the administration of a laxative may also be of value in hastening the cleansing process.

DIETARY TREATMENT   To allow the stomach to rest and heal, food is usually withheld for from 24 to 48 hours. Even the water taken by mouth is restricted, with the exception of cracked ice which may be held in the mouth to relieve thirst. Fluids are given intravenously or by proctoclysis.

Following the fast period, low fiber liquid foods are added as tolerated. Milk is usually the best food to start the diet. Small amounts of milk toast, cereal, and cream soups are fed at intervals of 30 to 45 minutes. Stimulating broths and highly seasoned food should be avoided. The amount of food and the number of feedings are increased according to the patient's toleration until the full regular diet is reached. A discussion of the patient's customary dietary pattern and eating habits is indicated and areas of improvement noted.

CHRONIC GASTRITIS

The cause of chronic gastritis is vague. The attacks follow the same type of conditions described for acute gastritis. Chronic gastritis often accompanies organic gastric lesions such as cancer and ulcer, or it may be due to an antral defect which closely resembles these diseases. It may also be related indirectly to diseases such as tuberculosis, myocardial failure, and nephritis. The same dietary indiscretions listed for acute gastritis seem to be frequent causes. The stomach seems to be long-suffering, willing and capable of accepting neglect, abuse, and ill treatment. But there comes a time – sooner in some, later in others – when the stomach rebels. Chief among the manifestations is pain which may be mild at times but severe and cutting at intervals.

Physicians have a relatively simple way of ascertaining the true state of affairs. The electric gastroscope can be passed down the esophagus into the stomach and the appearance of the stomach mucosa viewed and studied. If there are erosions or ulcerations, they can be seen. Changes in the blood vessels, with the destruction of surface cells, will be evident. This should be amplified by chemical, histological, and clinical findings before a true diagnosis of gastritis can be made.

Even without this instrument and laboratory determinations, one can adopt a careful, hygienic regimen and make certain, first of all, that the diet is well balanced, containing all of the essential nutrients, vitamins, and minerals.

DIETARY TREATMENT Because the conception of chronic gastritis is vague, the dietary management must follow general principles. The diet should be adequate in calories and nutrients, soft in consistency, and food eaten at regular intervals and chewed well. Highly seasoned foods are not usually well tolerated. Excess liquids with meals has a tendency to cause discomfort. The low fiber diet outlined on page 341 is advised when the cause is likely to be improper eating or drinking. In some cases start with cream soups and toast and proceed to the low fiber fruits and vegetables listed. The important factor is to determine the cause for the discomfort and then to prescribe the treatment.

CARCINOMA OF THE STOMACH

The etiology of carcinoma of the stomach is unknown and is believed by some authorities to include a number of causes rather than a single cause. Symptoms are so slow to manifest themselves and the growth of the tumor so rapid that frequently carcinoma of the stomach is overlooked until it is too late for an effective cure. Because it is a disease of middle age, any unusually prolonged gastric discomfort appearing at that stage in life should be investigated, even though it is seemingly slight. Loss of appetite, loss of strength, and loss of weight frequently precede other symptoms. Extreme hypochromic anemia is associated with cancer of any part of the alimentary tract. Achylia gastrica or achlorhydria has been shown to exist for years preceding the onset of gastric carcinoma. However, in some cases increased secretory activity is evident, especially when cancer develops on the site of an old ulcer.

Periodic physical examinations or checkups are encouraged for middle-aged people. X-ray examinations aid in the very early diagnosis, a period when surgical treatment is likely to be successful.

Speculation as to the role of diet in the etiology of cancer of the stomach has been growing.[17] Numerous experts consider it significant that decrease in incidence has coincided with changes in food habits in the United States. During the past 50 years, there has been an increased use of citrus fruits and lettuce and a decreased consumption of potatoes, cabbage and wheat flour. In addition, larger amounts of beef, milk and green vegetables have been included in diets, especially in high income groups. Studies indicate that stomach cancer occurs more frequently among low income persons than among those with a higher income. Compared to other countries, the United States has a very low rate of stomach cancer incidence and deaths.

Methods of food preparation and preservation have also been suggested as having a bearing on cancer of the stomach. For example, a relationship was suggested between the high incidence in rural Ireland and the practice of eating smoked meat and fish kept in smokehouses for long periods. Cancer investigators believe that diet must be at least partially responsible for the downward trend in incidence of stomach cancer in the United States.

DIETARY ADJUSTMENT The dietary regimen for carcinoma of the stomach can be determined somewhat by the location of the cancer, the nature of the functional disturbance, and the stage of development. The patient with advanced, nonoperable cancer should receive a diet adjusted to provide comfort. His food preferences, unless definitely harmful, usually are granted, because his days are numbered, and living should be made as bearable as possible. In the later stages of the disease the patient may tolerate only a liquid diet, and it may be necessary to resort to parenteral fluids or transfusions. Anorexia is almost always present from the early stage throughout the entire course. The patient who is encouraged to select his own menu and who suggests foods which have an appeal usually ingests more than when he is not involved in the selection or when force is applied.

---

[17]Cancer of the Stomach. U.S. Department of Health, Education, and Welfare, Public Health Service Pub. No. 1237, Health Information Series No. 120, 1964.

When the gastric secretion is depressed or lacking, the diet discussed for *hypochlorhydria* (below) is used; when the gastric secretion is increased, the diet outlined for *hyperchlorhydria* (below) or *ambulatory ulcer* (p. 341) is indicated.

Surgery   When an operation has been performed, the diet outlined for gastric surgery (Chap. 26) is usually prescribed.

REFLEX OR FUNCTIONAL DISEASES OF THE STOMACH

INDIGESTION

Indigestion or dyspepsia is an indefinite term frequently used to describe any discomfort occurring from a disorder of the digestive tract. The core of the trouble may be in the stomach or it may be a reflex symptom of a derangement of some other organ, such as the colon, gallbladder disease, renal calculus, chronic appendicitis or diabetes. Indigestion as manifestation of psychoneurosis is frequently encountered. The association between emotional and gastrointestinal disturbances is so frequent, the relationship cannot be denied. Many people complain of a "nervous stomach" which they attribute to the eating of certain foods. Besides the psychic disturbance, other avoidable causes of indigestion are rapid eating, poor mastication, overindulgence in rich foods, and a poor diet.

DIETARY TREATMENT   Before dietary treatment begins, the cause of indigestion must be determined. The symptoms may be a warning of a more serious illness. A therapeutic diet for simple indigestion is seldom necessary. A well-balanced diet plus correct eating habits is usually sufficient. However, many patients will feel more comfortable if they follow for a short time the low fiber diet outlined on page 341. Gradually, the patient advances to the normal adequate diet. To treat the cause, whether mental or physical, is the important factor. Emphasis in the teaching is placed on the improvement of the patient's customary dietary and eating habits.

SLIDING HIATAL HERNIA

Sliding hiatal hernia is an abnormal situation in which there is loss of the sling-like support of the lower esophagus and herniation of the upper portion of the stomach into the thoracic cavity. The pain is described as burning or pressing. Tight abdominal garments and activity which requires bending or lifting are to be avoided.

DIETARY TREATMENT   The patient is usually placed on a six-feeding ulcer regimen (p. 340 and Table 23–1) or low fiber diet (p. 341 and Table 23–2) divided into six small meals, and antacid medication to maintain acid neutralization. If the patient is obese, weight reduction is important. The development of bleeding is sometimes treated as described for treatment of bleeding ulcer (p. 344). If symptoms persist, surgery may be advised in order to prevent bleeding and/or stricture.

HYPERCHLORHYDRIA

Hyperchlorhydria is a condition in which the gastric juice as secreted by the stomach glands contains an excess of hydrochloric acid. Normally, an excess amount of acid is promptly neutralized, either by regurgitation of bile from the small intestines or by the mucus produced through the gastric mucosa. It is not known whether hyperchlorhydria is the result of a failure of the mechanism for the regulation of acid or of an increased secretory activity of the gastric glands. Excess free hydrochloric acid may be very irritating to the mucous lining of the stomach, and may bring discomfort and pain to the patient.

DIETARY TREATMENT   Authorities seem to agree that if hyperacidity recurs constantly the condition may indicate peptic ulcer, and the diet regimen outlined in this chapter is recommended. Fats are included in the diet to retard gastric secretion, and other foods are selected to combine with the hydrochloric acid in the stomach. Sometimes the low fiber diet (p. 341 and Table 23–2) is adequate. Either dietary treatment usually brings comfort to the patient. Usually an adequate diet, regularity of meals and an environment conducive to better eating habits are indicated. Teaching centers around the patients' need for change in his customary pattern.

HYPOCHLORHYDRIA

Hypochlorhydria is a condition in which the gastric juice secreted by the stomach glands contains a diminished amount of hydrochloric acid, although some free hydrochloric acid is present. As a result, proteins are not digested properly in the stomach, carbohydrates ferment very readily, and the gastric mucosa is hypersensitive. The lack of sufficient hydrochloric acid in the gastric juices lowers resistance to bacterial action, both fermentative and putrefactive. Diarrhea is a common symptom. Disturbances may occur anywhere along the digestive tract.

To avoid confusion two other conditions similar to hypochlorhydria deserve mentioning. *Achlorhydria* is a condition in which free hydrochloric acid is not found, but combined acid is present. *Achylia gastrica* is a condition in which neither free nor combined acid is present.

These conditions often accompany other diseases such as pernicious anemia, sprue, carcinoma, diabetes, nephritis and chronic gastritis.

DIETARY TREATMENT Every precaution should be taken to prevent the introduction of bacteria into the digestive tract and to avoid foods that will favor their development. Milk, one of the chief offenders, must be selected carefully or treated to keep the bacterial count low. Cultured milk preparations are favored. A low fiber diet is advised, as fibrous foods have a tendency to delay the emptying of the stomach, and thus favor bacterial activity. The low fiber diet (p. 341 and Table 23–2) is especially recommended when diarrhea is present. In cases of severe diarrhea it may be advisable to boil the drinking water.

Because fats inhibit the secretion of hydrochloric acid and retard the emptying of the stomach, the amount in the diet should be restricted to a minimum. Fried foods and rich desserts should be avoided. Iced and very cold beverages and foods are contraindicated.

Because broth and clear soups stimulate gastric secretion, they may be included in the diet. Because carbohydrates in the form of starch are less likely to ferment, they are preferred to the sugar type of carbohydrates. Cooked fruits and vegetables (or fruits and vegetables of low fiber content) are recommended.

TESTS FOR DIAGNOSIS

Tests to determine gastric acidity and emptying time of the stomach are often helpful in establishing a definite diagnosis. Those used most frequently are described.

EWALD'S TEST MEAL If an analysis of the gastric contents is required, a test meal is usually given in the morning before the patient has received any other type of food. The Ewald's test meal consists of:

4 large soda crackers or arrowroot cookies
Approximately 400 ml. or 2 glasses of weak tea or water (no cream or sugar)

After 45 minutes to 1 hour, the meal is extracted and examined for total acidity and free hydrochloric acid.

Rehfuss and his associates advise the *fractional method* for determining the degree of acidity. Samples of the gastric contents are withdrawn at half-hour intervals with the aid of a stomach tube. A chemical analysis is made of the samples. The frequent withdrawals of gastric contents are recommended in preference to a single sample because of the opportunity to check results more accurately.

HISTAMINE TEST Histamine is a drug which stimulates gastric secretion; therefore, it is used in gastric function tests to check the ability of the stomach to secrete acid and pepsin. It is administered subcutaneously following a 12-hour fast and aspiration of the contents of the stomach.

Samples of gastric contents are removed every 15 minutes during the period of active secretion and then titrated for total and free acidity. This is of aid in differentiating between a true and a false achlorhydria.

BARIUM TEST MEAL Barium sulfate or bismuth is given in buttermilk or malted milk after a 12-hour fast, usually in the morning before breakfast. Radiography of the stomach is then possible. The progress of the barium sulfate may be observed through the entire digestive tract and any defects or abnormalities detected.

MOTOR MEAL The motor meal consists of a meal including substances such as tea leaves, raisins, jam, or berries with seeds. The contents of the meal remain in the stomach for a 12-hour period, and they are then withdrawn. The purpose of the test is to determine whether the motor processes are impaired, which is indicated by the rate at which the food leaves the stomach.

PROBLEMS AND SUGGESTED TOPICS FOR DISCUSSION

1. Discuss the A.M.A. and A.D.A. Committee findings concerning diet therapy as related to gastrointestinal function.
2. Classify gastric diseases as to (1) organic and (2) functional.
3. What are the principles of the dietary treatment for peptic ulcer? List a food to illustrate each principle.
4. Compare the medical dietary treatment for ulcers used in your hospital with the dietary treatment outlined in this chapter.
5. Study the eating habits of three ulcer patients of different nationalities who are in the hospital wards. Check for adequacy.
6. Obtain the diet history of a patient with peptic ulcer admitted to the hospital ward. Follow up the prescribed treatment and plan the necessary diet with the patient. If possible, follow the patient's progress in the outpatient clinic. Check his diet for adequacy.
7. List six dietary factors that might produce indigestion.
8. Obtain a dietary history from a patient who complains of indigestion. How adequate is his dietary pattern? Indicate where improvement is needed. How will he implement the changes?
9. How would a patient suffering with hypochlorhydria modify his dietary and eating habits?
10. In your hospital, study the feeding programs for patients suffering with carcinoma of the stomach. What part does the diet take in treatment?
11. What is the rationale for liberal peptic ulcer diet therapy?

SUGGESTED ADDITIONAL READING REFERENCES

Allison, P. R.: Reflux esophagitis, sliding hiatal hernia and the anatomy of repair. Surg. Gynec. Obstet., 92:419, 1951.

Bachrach, W. H.: Abdominal distention and gas pains. Ann. West. Med. Surg., 6:445, 1952.

Brown, M., Bresnahan, T. J., Chalke, F. C. R., Peters, B., Poser, E. G., and Tougas, R. V.: Personality factors in duodenal ulcer. Psychosom. Med., 12:1, Jan.–Feb., 1950.

Buchman, E., et al.: Unrestricted diet in the treatment of duodenal ulcer. Gastroenterology, 56:1016, 1969.

Co Tui, et al.: The hyperalimentation treatment of peptic ulcer with protein hydrolysates and dextrimaltose. Gastroenterology, 5:5, 1945.

Doll, R., et al.: Dietetic treatment of peptic ulcer. Lancet, 1:5, 1956.

Dragstedt, L. R.: Why does not the stomach digest itself? J.A.M.A., 177:758, 1961.

Duncan, G. G.: Some nutritional hazards of the hospitalized patient. J. Am. Dietet. A., 25:330, 1949.

Foltz, E. L.: Neurophysiological mechanisms in production of gastrointestinal ulcers. J.A.M.A., 187:413, 1964.

Guyton, A. C.: Textbook of Medical Physiology. 4th ed. Philadelphia, W. B. Saunders Company, 1971, p. 775.

Ham, G. C.: Psychosomatic investigation and management of gastrointestinal disorders. New York J. Med., p. 2250, Sept. 15, 1952.

Hartroft, W. S.: The incidence of coronary artery disease in patients treated with the Sippy diet. Am. J. Clin. Nutr., 15:205, 1964.

Hock, C. W.: Peptic ulcer – A curse of modern civilization. Am. J. Clin. Nutr., 15:223, 1964.

Ingegno, A. P.: Observations regarding therapy of bleeding peptic ulcer. New York J. Med., page 2187, Oct. 1, 1953.

Johnson, A.: Some dietary principles in digestive diseases. Am. J. Digest. Dis., 17:161, 1950.

Kirsner, J. B.: Facts and fallacies of current medical therapy for uncomplicated duodenal ulcer. J.A.M.A., 187:423, 1964.

Kramer, P., and Caso, E. K.: Is the rationale for gastrointestinal diet therapy sound? J. Am. Dietet. A., 42:505, 1963.

Laureta, H. C., et al.: An appraisal of the management of peptic ulcer including comparative studies of the value of a polyunsaturated fat nutritional preparation in the management of gastric hypersecretion. Am. J. Clin. Nutr., 15:211, 1964.

Lewisohn, R.: Basic principles in the surgical treatment of duodenal ulcers. J.A.M.A., 149:423, 1952.

Lipp, W. F., and Phillips, J. F.: An appraisal of the end-results of treatment in carcinoma of the stomach. J.A.M.A., 174:1683, 1960.

McIlrath, D. C., and Hallenbeck, G. A.: Review of gastric freezing. J.A.M.A., 190:715, 1964.

Moeller, H. C.: Conventional dietary treatment of peptic ulcer. Am. J. Clin. Nutr., 15:194, 1964.

Morson, B. C.: Precancerous lesions of upper gastrointestinal tract. J.A.M.A., 179:311, 1962.

Odell, A. C.: Ulcer dietotherapy past and present. J. Am. Dietet. A., 58:447, 1971.

Pallette, E. C., and Harrington, R. W.: Long-term results in surgical treatment of peptic ulcer. J.A.M.A., 168:20, 1958.

Roth, J. A., Ivy, I. C., and Atkinson, A. J.: Caffeine and peptic ulcer. J.A.M.A., 126:814, 1944.

Rubin, H.: The Ulcer Diet Cook Book. New York, M. Evans and Company, Inc., 1963.

Seymour, C. T.: Emotion and gastric activity. J.A.M.A., 171:1193, 1959.

Sippy, B. W.: Gastric and duodenal ulcers: medical cure by an efficient removal of gastric juice erosion. J.A.M.A., 64:1625, 1915.

Shull, H. J.: Diet in the management of peptic ulcer. J.A.M.A., 170:124, 1959.

Snorf, L. D.: Emotional factors in gastrointestinal disorders. J.A.M.A., 162:857, 1956.

State, D.: Gastrointestinal hormones in the production of peptic ulcer. J.A.M.A., 187:410, 1964.

Symposium: Clinical management of peptic ulcer. Am. J. Clin. Nutr., 15:191 and 235, 1964.

Todd, J. W.: Treatment of peptic ulcer. Lancet, 1:113, 1952.

Weinstein, L., et al.: Diet as related to gastrointestinal function. J.A.M.A., 176:935, 1961.

Wirts, C. W., Rehfuss, M. E., Snape, W. J., and Swenson, P. C.: Effect of tea on gastric secretions and motility. J.A.M.A., 155:725, 1954.

Wohl, M. G., and Goodhart, R. S. (ed.): Modern Nutrition in Health and Disease. 4th ed. Philadelphia, Lea & Febiger, 1968. Chapter on Nutrition in diseases of the stomach.

Zollinger, R. M., and Ellison, E. H.: Nutrition after gastric operations. J.A.M.A., 154:811, 1954.

Chapter 24
DIET IN INTESTINAL DISEASES

PHYSIOLOGY AND FUNCTIONS OF THE INTESTINES

The absorption of food is practically completed in the small bowel. Food is emptied from the stomach into the duodenum where the breaking down process continues. Secretions from the intestine, the pancreas, and the liver have prepared the gastric contents for the work to be completed in the remainder of the small bowel.

The food material is now ready for absorption, which is the function of the lower part of this structure. Digestion and absorption do

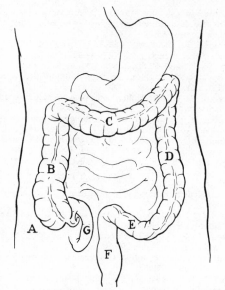

Figure 24–1   Normal colon, *A,* cecum; *B,* ascending; *C,* transverse; *D,* descending; *E,* sigmoid; *F,* rectum; *G,* ileum.

not always proceed in orderly fashion. Each person has encountered, at some time, a mild digestive upset. Such disturbing experiences are relieved usually through correction of eating or drinking habits.

The large intestine or colon takes up considerable space in the abdomen. The structure is about 1.5 meters long and starts with the cecum. From this segment projects the appendix. From the lower right side of the abdomen, the tube extends upward (ascending), crosses (transverse) underneath the liver and stomach to the spleen, and turns downward (descending) on the left side. It is connected with the rectum by a small part called the sigmoid. (See Fig. 24–1.)

The main functions of the colon are (1) the absorption of water and crystalloids, and (2) the transfer of feces from the ascending colon to the descending colon, and then via the rectum to the exterior. This latter function is accomplished largely by periodic, relatively frequent, intervals of progressive mass peristalsis. The sigmoid sphincter prevents the passage of fecal material into the rectum until a desire for a bowel movement arises. Normal rectal sensibility is needed for the desire for evacuation; and regularity of habit and ample roughage are prime requisites for proper functioning of the colon.

The mechanism of the entire alimentary tract is controlled by the nervous system. When an individual becomes tense or overfatigued, the tube may go into a single or series of spasms. The constriction may be associated with alternating constipation and diarrhea.

This brief review has been presented as a basis to better understanding of the various diseases in the intestinal region, and their dietary treatment. A review of Chapter 7, Digestion, Absorption and Cell Metabolism, is recommended.

CONSTIPATION

DEFINITION   Constipation may be defined as a retention of the feces in the colon beyond the normal length of emptying time. It is a condition of stasis in the large intestines. Under normal conditions the residue of food eaten one morning will reach the large bowel (but not the rectum) the following morning. Defecation takes place normally within 12 to 72 hours, or longer, after the intake of food. The type of diet eaten is believed to influence in some degree the length of time before defecation takes place; that is, a diet high in fiber content (nondigestible carbohydrates) resists enzymatic digestion or absorbs liquids in its passage along the intestinal tract and thereby produces bulk, a stimulant to defecation. The opposite is true of a diet low in residue.

Many people believe it is necessary to have a daily bowel movement and become disturbed when this does not occur. For comfort and health, the majority of persons should have a daily bowel movement; however, there are individuals who require an evacuation only every second or third day, and sometimes the intervals may be longer.

ETIOLOGY   The causes of constipation are numerous and varied. The strain and speed of the present modern life with resulting poor habits of hygiene are contributing factors. Repeated lack of response to the urge for defecation and failure to establish a regular time for defecation, lack of exercise, which causes a loss of tone in the intestinal musculature, use of cathartics for a long period, nervous strain, and worry are the most common causes. The chief cause may be attributed to either an inadequate diet or improper food habits. Insufficient fiber in the diet may cause constipation because there is little residue reaching the colon, lack of vitamin B and insufficient intake of water.

Regularity in eating is equally essential. A missed meal may temporarily disrupt the habit, and on the next day there is no movement. Constipation that occurs because of lack of exercise as in illness or while traveling is on this basis. With the return to the normal pattern of living, the condition will usually be corrected.

Chronic constipation may result from an organic disorder such as a physical defect, obstruction, or constriction associated usually with some debilitating disease, or it may be functional in origin as occurs in old age.

TREATMENT In the treatment of constipation, the aim is to relieve the cause. If a faulty diet is the cause, then the diet regimen to be prescribed depends upon the nature of the constipation. There are three types of constipation generally recognized, namely: (1) atonic, (2) spastic or irritable colon syndrome, and (3) obstructive.

ATONIC CONSTIPATION

Atonic constipation is sometimes called the "lazy bowel" constipation because of loss of rectal sensibility; the rectum is full of feces but the urge to defecate is lacking (Fig. 24–2). The peristaltic waves which are normally strong become weak and fecal matter moves slowly and accumulates. This type of constipation is often observed in older people whose body processes are slowing down. It also occurs during obesity, accompanying fevers, following operations and during pregnancy. Inadequate diet, irregular meals, insufficient liquids and failure to establish a regular time for defecation are the most frequent causes of atonic constipation.

TREATMENT The current trend in treatment is to develop regularity of habit through a bowel training program regimen and established good health habits: regular meals, adequate diet providing ample fiber, regular time for elimination, rest, relaxation, adequate intake of fluids and exercise.

Dietary Treatment The adequate or normal diet is used for patients with atonic constipation. It includes adequate bulk (vegetables, fruit, and whole grain cereal products), so that the cellulose residue left in the bowel after digestion is completed will be sufficient to favor the onward movement of the intestinal contents and to stimulate periodic evacuation. It is necessary to include approximately 800 gm. of fruits and vegetables to produce a daily normal bowel movement. Raw and cooked fruits and vegetables and cereals including their skins and bran will provide the cellulose. If the amount is dropped to 600 gm., there will be many complaints of constipation.

Prunes and prune juice have been found to stimulate intestinal motility by pharmacologic means.[1] The laxative principle found to be active is identified as dihydroxyphenyl isatin. Other foods may have this same quality but to date data on pharmacologically laxative principles in food are very sparse.

Because water is absorbed by the colon, a habitual intake of 8 to 10 glasses of fluid daily is necessary. If the fluid intake is less, constipation is likely to result. To some people milk is believed to be "constipating." Usually the cause for the constipation may be found in other factors which contribute to it. Buttermilk or an acid preparation milk may be suggested.

Bran should be used in moderation. Excessive amounts may irritate a sensitive alimentary tract, and large quantities may cause an intestinal block.

The use of mineral oil is discouraged except for occasional lubrication to provide ease of evacuation in cases of stubborn constipation. It has been found that mineral oil interferes seriously with absorption of the fat-soluble vitamins, especially vitamins A and K.

Florence H. Smith of the Mayo Clinic found a high fat diet to be of value in combating the constipation of patients who were too sick or uncomfortable to consume an adequate amount of vegetables and fruits. The diet contains approximately 164 gm. of carbohydrates, 66 gm. of proteins, and 224 gm. of fat, totaling 3026 kcalories. The diet is particularly suitable for undernourished patients. Diarrhea may result if too much fat is included in the diet; therefore, such a diet is reserved for selected cases. Each patient must be treated individually. An obese patient needs more fresh fruits and vegetables (bulk); a thin patient needs more fats.

The typical high fiber diet suggested for use in the average cases of atonic constipation is an adequate normal diet with an increase in or emphasis on the amount of whole-grain cereal products, fruits, and vegetables (Table 24–1).

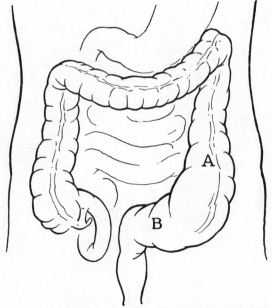

Figure 24–2 Atonic constipation. *A*, distended descending colon; *B*, distended sigmoid colon.

[1]Baum, H. M., et al.: The occurrence of diphenyl isatin in California prunes. J. Am. Pharm. A., 40:348, 1951.

TABLE 24-1   HIGH FIBER DIET

MEAL PLAN	SAMPLE MENU	SERVINGS	
		Weight Grams	Household Measure
BREAKFAST			
Fruit juice	Orange Juice (unstrained)	248	1 glass (8 oz.)
Fruit	Stewed prunes	135	1/2 cup
Cereal	Cooked oatmeal	118	1/2 cup
Egg	Poached egg	50	1
Bread	Toasted whole wheat bread	23	1 slice
Butter or margarine	Butter or margarine	7	1 pat
Milk	Milk	122	1/2 glass (4 oz.)
Coffee	Coffee	200	1 pot
Sugar	Sugar	15	3 teaspoons
LUNCHEON			
Soup	Vegetable soup	125	1/2 cup
Protein dish/meat	Macaroni and cheese	110	1/2 cup
Vegetable	Cooked green beans	63	1/2 cup
Salad	Sliced tomato salad	100	1 medium
Bread	Whole wheat bread	23	1 slice
Butter or margarine	Butter or margarine	7	1 pat
Milk	Milk	244	1 glass (8 oz.)
Fruit	Mixed fruit cup	128	1/2 cup
DINNER			
Meat, fish, poultry	Roast beef	85	3 ounces
Potato	Baked potato	99	1 medium
Vegetable/large serving	Cooked spinach	135	3/4 cup
Salad	Head lettuce salad	50	1/6 head
Bread	Whole wheat bread	23	1 slice
Butter or margarine	Butter or margarine	7	1 pat
Milk	Milk	244	1 glass (8 oz.)
Fruit	Fresh pear	182	1 medium

IRRITABLE COLON SYNDROME OR SPASTIC CONSTIPATION

The irritable colon syndrome or spastic constipation (also known as *spastic colitis* or *mucous colitis*) is directly opposite to the atonic type of constipation. It is caused by an overstimulation of the intestinal nerve endings which results in irregular contractions of the bowel. Evidence[2] suggests that there is excessive or incoordinated sigmoidal motility and loss of rectal sensibility. It is accompanied by abdominal pain, and sometimes nausea, constipation or diarrhea, which may alternate. Mucus may be found in the stool. Because of the spasms there are irregular movements of the mass along the intestinal tract (Fig. 24-3). Attacks are almost always associated with an emotional upset or a prolonged period of stress. Contributing causes are varied and include excessive use of cathartics, laxatives and tobacco, eating very coarse foods, drinking too much tea, coffee, and alcohol, stressful or emotional disturbance, previous gastrointestinal illness, antibiotic therapy, enteric infections and poor hygiene (sleep, rest, fluid intake and evacuation.) Patients complain of heartburn, distention, flatulence and a full feeling and mild or severe cramping pain.

TREATMENT   A therapeutic regimen must include helping the patient to cope with stressful situations and to relieve pent-up emotions. Good habits of personal hygiene must be established, with adequate time allowed for a bowel movement.

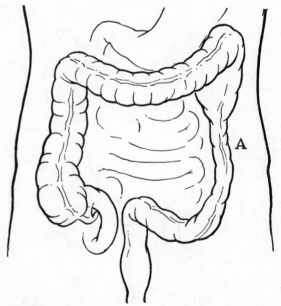

Figure 24-3   Spastic constipation. A, pinched descending colon.

[2]Almy, T. P.: Experimental studies on the irritable colon. Am. J. Med., 10:60, 1951.

Dietary Treatment   Persons suffering with spastic constipation are frequently underweight and tense and upset. Because of past experiences they are afraid to eat, fearful of additional pain. The aim of the dietary treatment is to relieve the condition, nourish the patient and bring the weight of the patient to normal.

The normal diet is recommended with emphasis on soft fiber foods which are believed not to irritate the mucous membrane of the intestinal tract. The foods included in the diet are directly opposite to the kind included in the diet for atonic constipation. Sometimes it is necessary to begin the dietary treatment with a low fiber diet (p. 341 and Table 23–2) containing smooth, nonirritating foods, such as milk, eggs, refined bread and cereals, butter, oil, finely ground meat, fish or poultry and simple desserts. Fruit and vegetable juices are allowed in limited amounts *only*, in the beginning, in order to avoid the fibrous content of these foods. They will be increased to creamed soups and whole cooked (allowed on diet) as the condition improves. Fats (oils, butter, and margarine) are especially advocated, and large amounts are recommended because of the calorie contribution and lubricating effects. Vitamin supplements are indicated, especially if the restricted diet is prolonged. The return to the normal diet is gradual. During stressful situations the low fiber program is recommended.

"Fiber," "Roughage," "Residue" and "Bland" Diets   Sometimes there are confusion and misunderstanding in the definition of terms and diets, particularly in the meaning of bland, low residue, low fiber, and low roughage diets. It should be clarified that, in this text, "low residue" describes the form of the food when it has reached the large intestine. "Roughage" and "fiber" include the indigestible organic tissues of plants or animals, consisting chiefly of nondigestible carbohydrates (hemicellulose and cellulose) found principally in fruits and vegetables. Frequently, the "low roughage," "low fiber" and "low residue" diets are used as synonymous terms. For the purpose of liberalization, simplification and uniformity, the "bland" and "low fiber" foods are combined into one diet in this text, as was adapted in the Handbook of Diet Therapy,[3] prepared for the American Dietetic Association, and termed the low fiber diet. All foods have some residue. Even if no food is eaten, there is residue in the intestinal tract from the normal body metabolism or processes of life. Milk and fats seem to increase the bulk of stools although they are actually low in fiber content. Milk, while reported and considered by many to be a high residue food, should be classified as medium residue on the basis of fecal studies reported (Table 24–2). Thus, while a food might be low (or high) residue because of its fiber content, it does not necessarily follow that a low-fiber food is also low residue.

Low Fiber Diet   The low fiber diet (p. 341 and Table 23–2) follows the normal diet pattern, with modifications in consistency. Turner[3] defines it as "a diet which contains a minimum of indigestible carbohydrates and no tough connective tissue." Hosoi[4] et al. studied the amount of residue produced by certain foods in dogs with ileorectal anastomosis. From their experiments, they concluded that the foods which give the least residue are gelatin, sucrose, dextrose, Karo, concentrated broth, hard cooked egg, meat, liver, rice, farina, and cottage cheese. Among those which give the largest residue are fruits, potatoes, bread, lard, butter, Swiss cheese, soft boiled egg, raw egg albumin, milk and lactose. The applicability of this

---

[3]Reprinted from Turner, D.: Handbook of Diet Therapy. 2nd ed. 1952, p. 202, and 5th ed., Chicago, Univ. of Chicago Press, 1970. By permission of the University of Chicago Press.
[4]Hosoi, K., Alvarez, W. C., and Mann, F. C.: Intestinal absorption: A search for a low residue diet. Arch. Int. Med., *41*:112, 1928.

TABLE 24–2   FOOD RESIDUE*

DIET	QUANTITY TAKEN PER 24 HR.	WET WEIGHT (gm.) PER 24 HR.	DRY WEIGHT (gm.) PER 24 HR.
Mixed	–	100–150	20–30
Meat	1,435 gm.	64.0	17.2
White bread	1,237 gm.	109.0	28.9
Dark bread	1,360 gm.	815.0	115.8
Potato	3,078 gm.	635.0	93.8
Peas	960 gm.	927.1	124.0
Milk	3,075 gm.	174.0	40.6
Milk	3 qt.	114.5	25.3
Milk	1,680 gm.	–	21.5
Cabbage (raw)	210 gm.	700 (approx.)	–

*J. Am. Dietet. A., 38:425, 1961.

study to human dietetics, however, has been questioned. Since most of these foods found to be high in residue are usually included in the typical "low residue" diet; "low fiber" seems to be a more appropriate term to use. The Joint Committee[5] states that: "In general, foods may be listed in order of increasing residue production, as follows: proteins, fats, milk, digestible carbohydrates, and carbohydrates with indigestible material."[6] (See Table 24–2.)

OBSTRUCTIVE CONSTIPATION AND CANCER OF BOWEL

In obstructive constipation, an obstruction or closure hinders the passage of intestinal residue. The obstruction may be complete or partial. Adhesions, cancer (Fig. 24–4), a tumor or an impaction usually causes the obstruction. Surgical treatment is frequently indicated.

DIETARY TREATMENT   The diet recommended is the same type advised for spastic constipation (p. 353). Residue is kept to a minimum, the amount related to the size of the obstruction. If the obstruction is very extensive, a liquid diet may be necessary. In such cases the liquids should provide ample nutrients and include such foods as cream, malted milk, oil, sugars, and fruit juices. Vitamin concentrates are used as supplements. Sometimes it may be more desirable to administer foods and fluids parenterally. Regardless of the type of diet, attention should be directed toward insuring sufficient calories, proteins, electrolytes, vitamins and fluids. All nutrients may be provided by intravenous hyperalimentation when patient is unable to ingest food orally. (See Chapter 26.)

The dietary regimen following intestinal resections and colostomy will be discussed in

---

[5]Report: Diet as related to gastrointestinal function. J. Am. Dietet. A., 38:429, 1961.

[6]Report of the Joint Committee on Diet as Related to Gastrointestinal Function of the American Dietetic Association and The American Medical Association: Diet as related to gastrointestinal function. J. Am. Dietet. A., 38:425, 1961.

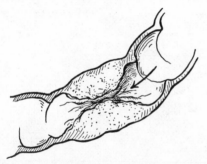

Figure 24–4   A bowel obstruction resulting from cancer.

Chapter 26, Diets in Surgery and Surgical Conditions.

DIVERTICULITIS

In persons past middle age and in cases following the excessive use of cathartics for constipation, an aging bowel frequently exhibits outpocketings (*diverticula*). Symptoms may not be encountered unless constipation induces irritation. If many pockets are present without symptoms, the condition is known as *diverticulosis*. The diverticula may occur anywhere along the intestinal tract but are most frequently observed in the colon. The accumulation of fecal matter in the pockets often results in infection, and sometimes causes ulceration or even perforation. This is *diverticulitis*. Surgery is sometimes advised, especially if perforation occurs. Approximately 10 to 15 per cent of patients with diverticulosis develop diverticulitis.

DIETARY TREATMENT   If the problem is medically treated, a low fiber diet (p. 341 and Table 23–2) usually is prescribed, depending upon the severity of the patient's condition. There may be many or few diverticula. If an acute attack of pain occurs, accompanied by tenderness and fever, a fast of 24 to 48 hours may precede the dietary treatment. Nonstimulating liquid foods are served prior to the beginning of the low residue diet regimen. In the beginning the fruits and vegetables should be restricted to limited amounts of juice; then as the condition improves purées are added. Most people prefer puréed vegetables in cream soups and puréed fruits in fruit whip or jello. One gradually proceeds to the full low fiber diet. Any food known to cause discomfort should be eliminated. Adequate water or liquids (8 to 10 glasses) is advised to prevent constipation. If the diagnosis of diverticulosis has been made, but symptoms are absent, the patient is advised to follow a restricted residue diet (avoidance of skins, seeds, bran and strings) to avoid irritation and accumulation of fecal matter in the pockets. When the food intake is inadequate in vitamins, supplements should be added.

HEMORRHOIDS

Hemorrhoids are ruptured blood vessels located around the anal sphincter. They may be either external or internal; and they may or may not cause pain and discomfort (Fig. 24–5). It is important for the patient with hemorrhoids not to become constipated because the pressure from the dry hard feces often causes bleeding and severe pain. Surgery usually is advised if the condition of the hemorrhoids becomes progressively worse. Some of the

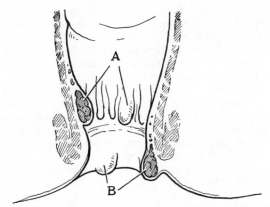

Figure 24–5   Hemorrhoids. A, internal hemorrhoids; B, external hemorrhoids.

causes of hemorrhoids are constipation, prolonged and continued use of cathartics or enemas, childbearing; sometimes they appear without apparent cause.

DIETARY TREATMENT   Diet is not used as treatment of the condition but to provide comfort for the patient. The low fiber diet (p. 341 and Table 23–2), with the soft cooked or whole cooked fruits and vegetables listed, plus 8 to 10 glasses of water or liquids, is usually adequate to avoid constipation and reduce possible irritation from too much roughage. Fats may be added to the diet (suggested in the diet outline for spastic constipation) if the constipated condition becomes troublesome. Whatever foods are known by the patient to be irritating (such as highly seasoned foods) should be avoided. A discussion of a normal diet and regular eating and elimination habits with the patient is indicated.

DIARRHEA

Diarrhea is more a symptom than a disease, manifested by frequent liquid stools. The passage of foods through the intestines is abnormally rapid and impairs complete digestion and absorption. The fecal matter passes through the colon so rapidly there is no chance for the fluid to be absorbed. Because of this idiosyncrasy, replacements are necessary. Diarrhea is the direct opposite of constipation, in which the fecal matter remains dormant and becomes hard and dry.

CLASSIFICATION   Diarrhea is classified as *functional* and *organic* in origin. The functional type is less severe than the organic and may occur in any normal person whose intestines are exposed to an irritant. In organic diarrhea there is a demonstrable lesion of the intestinal mucosa which is not present in functional diarrhea.

ETIOLOGY   The causes of diarrhea are many and varied. Some of the major causes of functional or simple diarrhea are overeating or eating the wrong foods, putrefaction in the intestinal tract, fermentation caused by incomplete carbohydrate (starch) digestion, habitual use of cathartics, nervous irritability, endocrine disturbance, and diarrhea associated with diseases such as sprue and pellagra. During periods of stress and strain adults may have diarrhea. Adolescents may have loose bowel movements preceding the excitement of a dance or football game. In children, fright may cause diarrhea. One of the most obstinate varieties of diarrhea is exhibited during hysteria. During hot weather diarrhea occurs frequently. Food poisoning is a common culprit. Food spoilage caused either by poor refrigeration or unsanitary handling may produce diarrhea if enough food is ingested, the decomposition or fermentation creating toxins. (See Chapter 14.)

Organic diarrhea may be caused by external poison, bacterial and protozoan invasion, and may accompany certain diseases such as tuberculosis, amebic dysentery, typhoid fever, viral hepatitis, chronic ulcerative colitis, regional ileitis, and enteritis, or by enzyme deficiencies which result in impaired digestion and absorption of carbohydrates.

DIETARY TREATMENT   For all types of diarrhea the dietary treatment is similar regardless of the cause. The aim of the medical treatment is to remove the cause. The diet generally adopted is one which will leave very little residue in the intestinal tract. The low fiber diet (p. 341 and Table 23–2) is a typical example.

ACUTE DIARRHEA

In the beginning of the dietary treatment for severe diarrhea a fast of 24 to 48 hours is often prescribed to provide rest for the gastrointestinal tract. The nature and severity of the diarrhea determine the duration of the rest. Lost nutrients and fluid must be replaced parenterally. The losses of electrolytes, especially potassium and sodium, should be corrected early with saline solutions. Glucose, ascorbic acid and B vitamins are added to the intravenous solutions to help minimize protein losses and to prevent ketosis. If the parenteral feeding must be continued for longer than 48 hours, protein hydrolysates should be added. As soon as possible, foods should be given by mouth to provide calories not possible to obtain in intravenous parenteral feedings. Simple foods are served at first, such as broth, gruel, dry toast and tea. The amount of food allowed gradually proceeds to the low fiber diet, high in calories (45 kcal./kg./day), high in protein (1.5 to 2 gm./kg./day), and served frequently in small amounts. Vitamin supplements are frequently prescribed. To achieve the high protein and high calorie level, protein concentrates such as dry skim milk powder can be added to milk beverages, desserts and creamed dishes (see Ch. 43, protein supplements); and suitable carbohydrates, such as glucose and lactose, can be added to beverages. Furthermore, increased intake of cereals, custards, simple puddings, and jelly will increase the protein and calorie level; and emulsified fats, such as butter and cream, can be added to foods as tolerated. In the beginning only the vegetable and fruit juices will be included, then creamed vegetable soup and, finally, the selected whole cooked foods, as listed on the diet. Diet changes are always guided by the patient's condition and toleration for foods. The return to the normal diet is gradual.

Pectin has value in the treatment of diarrhea, and it is included in diets for children. Scraped raw apple or liberal amounts of applesauce may be given every 2 to 4 hours, as tolerated, for their pectin content.

CHRONIC DIARRHEA

Chronic diarrhea may be associated with a number of nutritional deficiencies. Except for certain types of neurogenic diarrhea, impaired absorption resulting from abnormal anatomic changes or mucosal alterations of the small bowel is a common feature in most nutritional complications of diarrhea.

Diarrheal disorders can cause impaired absorption and heavy loss of electrolytes, vitamins, minerals, and protein which will need to be replaced. There is excessive fecal excretion of electrolytes and the increased water volume loss demands increased amounts of sodium and potassium to maintain physiologic tonicity of the bowel fluid. Potassium is probably the most important electrolyte loss, reflecting tissue depletion rather than specific changes in the circulating plasma levels. The loss of potassium alters bowel motility, encourages anorexia, and can introduce a cycle of bowel distress. Loss of iron may be severe enough to cause anemia. Protein is poorly digested and absorbed. Vitamins are lost. If antibiotic therapy is used, intestinal synthesis of some of the B vitamins is impaired. Deficiencies of folic acid, vitamin B_{12} and niacin have been reported.

DIETARY TREATMENT In diseases with chronic diarrhea, low fiber diets may have to be used for months. Careful attention needs to be given to maintain adequate intake of calories and protein to avoid great loss of body weight and tissue protein. It may be necessary to provide up to 4000 kcalories and 150 gm.

protein daily for several months to correct protein deficits and achieve clinical remissions. If inadequate amounts of food are ingested, frequent tube feedings of small amounts of liquid foods, and parenteral injections of vitamin supplements may be resorted to. Isotonic saline for electrolyte and fluid depletion is sometimes necessary. Large quantities of fluid (2 to 3 quarts daily) are required in an attempt to replace loss of body fluids in the stools. Food sources with a high potassium content (Appendix Table 9), such as fruit juices and bouillon preparations, can be included in the diet.

STEATORRHEA

Steatorrhea is a diarrhea characterized by an excess of fat in the stool, and is generally accepted as indicative of serious organic disease. The excessive amount of exogenous fat in the stool may result from (1) failure of proper digestion, such as in pancreatitis, diseases of the liver or biliary system (Chapter 25), and following gastric resection (Chapter 26); and (2) failure of normal absorption after digestion, such as in sprue (Chapter 34), resection of over half of the small intestines, and in regional enteritis. Lactose has been shown to cause steatorrhea in lactose deficient patients with ulcerative colitis, regional enteritis, and after partial gastric or small intestinal resection. Normally, the fecal fat amounts to about 2 to 5 gm. daily, but when there are defects in absorption or digestion, food fat appears in the stool in amounts as great as 60 gm. daily.

TREATMENT Since steatorrhea is a symptom and not a disease, the underlying disorder must be determined and treated. Weight loss is universally present, requiring increased caloric intake. Dietary protein should be high, with carbohydrates and fats as tolerated to meet individual needs. Multiple vitamin deficiencies are common, making supplemental vitamin therapy necessary, with special emphasis on vitamins D and K. Foods high in iron and calcium are recommended, plus medication as necessary. Other hematopoietic factors such as B_{12} and folic acid should be included when macrocytic anemia is present (Ch. 31). Potassium is increased in the diet and, in some cases, is required as medication.

Some conditions of faulty digestion and absorption of fat respond to medium chain triglyceride therapy (MCT). Medium chain triglycerides apparently are absorbed without first being hydrolyzed and absorption takes place in the absence of pancreatic juice and bile. Resynthesis of free fatty acids into triglycerides within the mucosal cell is not necessary with fatty acids of eight or less carbon atoms. Following absorption, the short and medium chain fatty acids enter the portal venous blood and are transported to the liver directly without being resynthesized into triglycerides. MCT is available in oil and dry power preparations. The dry power formula supplies protein and carbohydrate as well as fat and is supplemented with minerals and vitamins.

ENTERITIS

Enteritis is an inflammation or irritation of the bowel of varying degree. It may result from many disorders, such as food or chemical poisoning, the consumption of indigestible material, or overeating. It has been stated that anything which irritates the intestinal mucosa, whether mechanical or chemical, can produce enteritis. However, in most cases bacterial invasion causes the disease; in the advanced state it is known as *bacillary dysentery* (Ch. 36) There is also a form of enteritis involving primarily the lower ileum, known as *regional enteritis* or *regional ileitis.*

Acute attacks must be well managed because, if neglected, the ailment may become chronic. When inflammation persists the patient may complain of loss of weight, fatigue, cramping, and diarrhea. Mucus is present in the stools, and frequently blood and pus. Fat in the stools (steatorrhea) may be a factor. At times the discharge may be firm, dry and shiny, at other times the character of the stool may be watery.

DIETARY TREATMENT   The diet should be low in residue; high in caloric value, liberal in animal proteins, and rich in vitamins and minerals. In regional enteritis with malabsorption steatorrhea, there is usually improvement when fats are moderately restricted (25 per cent of calories); sometimes severe restriction (10 per cent of calories) is necessary. Improvement may be manifested by the use of medium chain triglycerides. Ideally, a loss of stool fat should be kept below 10 gm. daily.

For bacillary dysentery see amebic dysentery (p. 359) for diet treatment.

ULCERATIVE COLITIS

Ulcerative colitis is an organic disease of inflammation and ulceration of the mucosa of the large intestine. (See Fig. 24-6.) The etiology is unknown although a number of theories have been offered by medical authorities. The four most common theories are as follows: (1) It is of infectious origin, (2) it is a deficiency state in which certain vitamins, especially vitamin B, and possibly protein of high biologic value are lacking, (3) it is an allergic condition, and (4) it is due to psychogenic disturbances. That these individuals are frequently depressed, irritable, and emo-

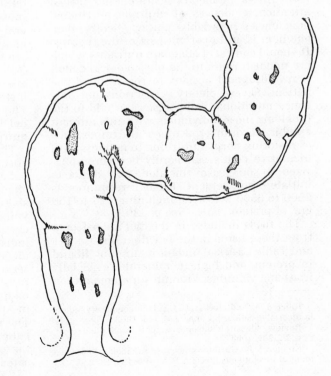

Figure 24-6   The large intestine showing ulceration of the mucosa.

tionally unstable is a common observation. A combination of multiple causal factors probably is involved.

The general characteristics are rectal bleeding, diarrhea accompanied by pain and spasm, fever, ulcerative lesions in the intestinal mucosa of the large intestine, nutritional edema, negative nitrogen balance, avitaminosis, dehydration, electrolyte imbalance, anorexia, and malnutrition. Anemia may be present as a result of blood loss. It usually occurs in young people (below the age of 40 to 50 years), though no age is exempt. Chronic ulcerative colitis has a striking tendency to exacerbations and remissions.

Elimination test diets are sometimes employed as a method of diagnosis when a food allergy is suspected (see Chapter 27). Milk, eggs, oranges, wheat, spinach, and tomatoes are the foods most frequently found as the cause of the allergy. Rider and Moeller[7] obtained good clinical results by removing from the diet foods which produced a hypersensitivity type of reaction when injected intramucosally. Others have reported dramatic results on withholding milk from the diet.[8]

If medical treatment fails to produce results, surgery may be advised. Surgery is reported to be required for 20 to 30 per cent of patients with chronic ulcerative colitis.

DIETARY TREATMENT   Ulcerative colitis is a chronic disease and the frequent stools, which are characteristic of the disease, tend to limit absorption of the nutrients in the diet. Unless the dietary treatment has special attention, evidences of multiple nutritional deficiencies invariably appear. Dietary management is an important part of the therapy. It should consist of adequate nutrients which are nondisturbing to the physiological condition and appeal besides to the taste of the patient. Severe dietary restrictions not only cause nutritional deficiencies but add to the problems most individuals with this ailment exhibit. According to Kirsner[9] the importance of restoring normal nutrition in patients with ulcerative colitis can hardly be overemphasized; in some cases this alone may suffice to initiate improvement. Kirsner recommends 2500 to 3500 kcalories, including 125 to 150 gm. of protein, daily. (See p. 330.)

The foods included in the diet are selected from those listed in the low fiber diet (p. 341 and Table 23–2), abundant in amount, liberal in protein, and high in minerals (especially iron) and vitamins. Vitamin supplementation

by medication is recommended. In severe cases fruits and vegetables may have to be temporarily omitted or restricted to juices and purées. The dietary treatment outlined for chronic diarrhea (p. 356) is followed. If anemia or hypoproteinemia develops, periodic whole blood transfusions may be required in addition to increased iron and protein in the food intake. Severe diarrhea causes excessive losses of potassium, sodium, and chloride, and dehydration which may need correction by intravenous solutions.

Unless the patient is allergic to or has an idiosyncrasy for milk, it is advisable for him to consume, if possible, the equivalent of 2 quarts of milk daily. Milk is an excellent source of protein besides containing essential minerals and vitamins. The milk allowance adds an appreciable amount of calories to the total sum of calories needed. Dry skim milk powder and protein supplements can be added to the milk for additional protein and calories. In cases of severe diarrhea boiled milk or evaporated milk is agreeable. If milk is not tolerated, calcium salts will be required and the nutrients contained in milk supplied by other foods.

Other protein foods to include in liberal amounts are eggs, cheese (if tolerated), tender meat, fresh fish, and poultry. See Chapter 43 for high protein recipes and suggested ways to use protein supplements. Treatment varies from clinic to clinic and from patient to patient, depending upon the severity and duration of the disease. While the treatment must necessarily be individualized, the general principles of rest and diet, with particular attention to the patient's state of nutrition, are followed.

Frequent small feedings are advised and are usually more acceptable to the individual instead of the customary three meals a day. The frequent small feedings are more beneficial, permitting better absorption of the nutrients in the diet.

The nurse can be of great help by giving encouragement and understanding to these patients who are frequently described psychiatrically as dependent, immature, obsessive and hostile. These individuals are highly vulnerable to the ordinary events of life. Understanding their emotional difficulties is indispensable to the effective treatment of ulcerative colitis. Attention to the attractive service of food, cheerful surroundings, efforts to inspire confidence, and encouragement to eat the diet prescribed are of uppermost importance to effective total therapy. The nurse has an opportunity to explore the patient's eating habits and to assist him with the changes or improvements that are indicated for his customary dietary. Emphasis on

[7]Rider, J. A., and Moeller, H. C.: Hypersensitivity factors in ulcerative colitis. J.A.M.A., *183*:545, 1963.

[8]Review. Idiopathic ulcerative colitis and milk. Nutr. Rev., 22:262, 1964.

[9]Kirsner, J. B.: Current concepts of the medical management of ulcerative colitis. J.A.M.A., *169*:433, 1959.

the patient's need is more apt to bring a change in eating habits than sessions on the diet (do's and don't's). As with all patients, especially those with intestinal diseases, the dietary regimen should be individualized. It is unrealistic to expect a person to adhere to a theoretical plan indefinitely. (A strict regimen in the acute phase is stressful to most patients.)

AMEBIASIS AND AMEBIC DYSENTERY

Amebiasis is an inflammation of the intestines, especially the colon. It is an infectious disease acquired by consuming contaminated food or drink and is spread chiefly through unsanitary water supply, flies and insects, and careless food handlers. Leafy vegetables become carriers of the disease if they are grown where human waste is used as fertilizer or where they are washed in polluted water. Following World War II, a survey was made of the Americans returning from the Far East. *Entamoeba histolytica,* the parasite which produces ulceration in varying degree in the intestinal mucosa of the lower bowel, was found in 25 per cent of the passengers studied. No doubt the unsanitary conditions which prevailed in the concentration camps account for the high incidence. The disease can occur in mild or severe form. In its severe forem, amebiasis is known as *amebic dysentery.* Severe cases are more frequent in the tropics, and less common in temperate zones. The disease does occur, however, in every section of the United States.

DIETARY TREATMENT   During the acute stage of the disease nothing is given by mouth except broth, tea, barley water, and strained fruit juice. Boiled milk may be cautiously added as tolerated. The parenteral alimentation and diet, outlined under dietary treatment in acute diarrhea, should be followed. Large quantities of fluids are encouraged to make up for the loss through watery stools. When the symptoms subside, foods low in fiber or residue content are gradually added to the diet. It may be necessary for the patient to follow an adequate diet low in fiber content for many months until evidences of intestinal irritation have disappeared. Unless careful attention is given to maintaining an adequate intake of calories and protein, considerable body weight may be lost, and tissue depletion may follow. See dietary treatment for chronic diarrhea (p. 356).

DIET AND CANCER PRODUCTION

Natural food ration in an experiment on female rats was shown to contain a factor not present in highly purified diets that protects animals from tumor development after X-irradiation.[10] Other studies have indicated the protective effect of natural food diet on animals fed toxic doses of various chemical hormones and drugs. It is believed that a natural food ration may contain a higher concentration of certain antioxidants that prevent excessive peroxide formation and may provide a protective effect against the development of cancer. More research to identify protective factors in food is needed before conclusive evidence can be made.

Burket[11] believes from a survey of the incidence of cancer in various parts of the world that refined carbohydrates such as sugar and white flour play a major role in the pathogenesis of cancer of the colon and rectum. The incidence of cancer of the colon and rectum is greater in the highly industrialized countries using more refined carbohydrates than in the rural underdeveloped areas. The high residue fibrous diet of the simpler cultures, Burket believes, affects the behavior of the bowel and contains a protective factor against the development of colonic cancer. Further research in this area is needed before application can be made.

TEST DIETS FOR DIAGNOSIS

To facilitate the diagnosis of diseases of the intestinal tract, test diets are sometimes employed. The following diet is the one used most frequently.

SCHMIDT INTESTINAL TEST DIET

The Schmidt test diet is used to diagnose diarrhea. The diet consists of easily digested foods which are low in residue. Physical examinations of the stool are made to determine the ability of the intestine to digest the content of the diet. Separate analyses of the stools are made to determine the ability of the intestine to digest protein, fats and carbohydrates.

The food served in the diet is generally weighed. The suggested restricted diet is served for 3 days, which is considered ample time for a diagnosis.

Sometimes the test diet is used therapeutically for fermentative diarrhea.

A typical diet schedule is outlined in Table 24–3.

---

[10]Ershoff, B. H., et al.: Comparative effects of purified diets and a natural food stock ration on the tumor incidence of mice exposed to multiple sublethal doses of total-body X-irradiation. Cancer Res., 29:780, 1969.

[11]Burket, D. P.: Modern diet may play a role in cancer of the bowel. J.A.M.A., 215:717, 1971.

TABLE 24–3   SCHMIDT INTESTINAL TEST DIET

FOOD	WEIGHT GRAMS
BREAKFAST	
Milk or cocoa made with milk	488
Vienna roll	45
Butter or margarine	8
One egg, soft cooked	50
10:00 A.M.	
Thick oatmeal gruel, cooked with milk	150
Sugar	10
DINNER OR LUNCHEON	
Cream of potato soup	120
Scraped beef, slightly browned in pan	115
3:00 P.M.	
Milk	488
Vienna roll	45
Butter or margarine	8
SUPPER	
Thick oatmeal gruel, cooked with milk	150
Sugar	10
Two eggs, soft cooked	100
Vienna roll	45
Butter or margarine	8

PROBLEMS AND SUGGESTED TOPICS FOR DISCUSSION

1. Describe the physiology and function of the intestines.
2. Classify foods into low and high fiber types.
3. Differentiate between the low fiber diet and low residue diet. List the foods which are good sources of cellulose. Why does cellulose form residue? What is the difference between residue and roughage? List foods low in fiber.
4. When is a diet low in fiber used? A diet high in fiber?
5. Plan a high protein, high calorie, low fiber diet for a patient with amebic dysentery. The patient is a 40-year-old male, 20 pounds underweight, who works in a factory and carries his lunch.
6. Plan menus for a 2 week period for a patient with (a) ulcerative colitis and (b) atonic constipation. The patient is a 25-year-old female who lives alone, clerks in a store, and eats lunch and dinner in a restaurant. Check for adequacy.
7. What are the principles of a diet for chronic diarrhea? Differentiate between diarrhea and steatorrhea.

SUGGESTED ADDITIONAL READING REFERENCES

Berry, R. E. L.: Diagnosis and treatment of acute intestinal obstruction. J.A.M.A., 148:347, 1952.

Burket, D. P.: Modern diet may play a role in cancer of the bowel. J.A.M.A., 215:717, 1971.

Clifton, J. A.: Intestinal absorption and malabsorption. J. Am. Dietet. A., 39:449, 1961.

Editorial. Amebiasis. J.A.M.A., 160:392, 1956.

Editorial. Is there a rationale for the bland diet? J. Am. Dietet. A., 33:608, 1957.

Editorial. Ulcerative colitis. J.A.M.A., 157:1312, 1955.

Engel, G. L.: Studies of ulcerative colitis. III. The nature of the psychologic processes. Am. J. Med., 19:231, 1955.

Ershoff, B. H., et al.: Comparative effects of purified diets and a natural food stock ration in the tumor incidence of mice exposed to multiple sublethal doses of total-body X-irradition. Cancer Res., 29:780, 1969.

Felsen, J., and Wolarsky, W.: Acute and chronic bacillary dysentery and chronic ulcerative colitis. J.A.M.A., 153:1069, 1953.

Flood, C. A., and Lepore, M. J.: Medical management of chronic ulcerative colitis. New York J. Med., p. 2265, Sept. 15, 1952.

Frohman, L. P.: Constipation. Am. J. Nursing, 55:65, 1955.

Fullerton, D. T., Kollar, E. J., and Caldwell, A. B.: A clinical study of ulcerative colitis. J.A.M.A., 181:463, 1962.

Gardner, F. H.: Nutritional management of chronic diarrhea in adults. J.A.M.A., 180:147, 1962.

Hoppert, C. A., and Clark, A. J.: Digestibility and effect on laxation of crude fiber and cellulose in certain common foods. J. Am. Dietet. A., 21:157, 1945.

Johnson, D.: Naming the Diets. J. Am. Dietet. A., 30:1010, 1954.

Kalser, M. H.: Laboratory aids in diagnosis of steatorrhea. J.A.M.A., 188:37, 1964.

Kern, F., and Struthers, J. E.: Intestinal lactose deficiency and lactose intolerance in adults. J.A.M.A., 195:143, 1966.

Kirsner, J. B., and Palmer, W. L.: Ulcerative colitis. J.A.M.A., 155:341, 1954.

Kirsner, J. B.: Current Therapeutic considerations in chronic ulcerative colitis. J. Iowa M. Soc., 45:119, 1955.

Kirsner, J. B.: Current concepts of the medical management of ulcerative colitis. J.A.M.A., 169:433, 1959.

McDermott, W.: Diverticulitis. Am. J. Nursing, 54:1231, 1954.

McNealy, R. W., and Wolfe, F. D.: Diverticulitis of the colon. J. Internat. Coll. Surgeons, 17:92, 1952.

Review. Idiopathic ulcerative colitis and milk. Nutr. Rev., 22:262, 1964.

Rider, J. A., and Moeller, H. C.: Hypersensitivity factors in ulcerative colitis. J.A.M.A., 183:545, 1963.

Ruffin, J. M., and Tyor, M. D.: Steatorrhea in adults. J.A.M.A., 172:2045, 1960.

Streicher, M. H.: Management of chronic constipation. Am. J. Digest. Dis., 13:1, 1946.

Wikoff, H. L., Marks, B. H., Caul, J. F., and Hoffman, W. F.: Some effects of high lipid diets on intestinal elimination. Am. J. Digest. Dis., 14:58, 1947.

Wohl, M. G.: Long-Term Illness. Philadelphia, W. B. Saunders Company, 1959, pp. 289–301.

Wohl, M. G., and Goodhart, R. S.: Modern Nutrition in Health and Disease. 4th ed. Philadelphia, Lea & Febiger, 1968, Chapter on Nutrition in disease of the intestinal tract.

Wolf, S.: A critical appraisal of the dietary management of peptic ulcer and ulcerative colitis. J. Clin. Nutr., 2:1, 1954.

Chapter 25
DIET IN DISEASES OF THE LIVER AND BILIARY SYSTEM

PHYSIOLOGY AND FUNCTIONS OF THE LIVER

In the metabolism of food, the liver is one of the most important of the body organs. (See Fig. 25-1.) It is the largest glandular organ of the body, comprising between 2.5 and 3 per cent of the body weight.

The liver also has the largest and most varied functions of any organ in the body. Most of the end-products of the digestion of food are transported directly to the liver. Compounds which it manufactures or stores are sent to other parts of the body as needed. Poisons which enter the body through food or are produced in other parts of the body are detoxified in the liver. The liver has many functions in the metabolism of all major nutrients. A brief summary of the role of the liver in this metabolic process follows.

CARBOHYDRATE METABOLISM The hepatic cells serve as a storehouse for glyco-

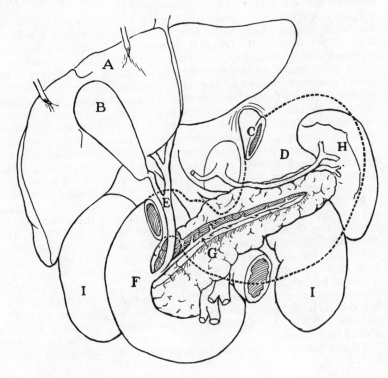

Figure 25-1 Schematic drawing showing relationship of organs of the upper abdomen. *A*, liver (retracted upward); *B*, gallbladder; *C*, esophageal opening of stomach; *D*, stomach (shown in dotted outline); *E*, common bile duct; *F*, duodenum; *G*, pancreas and pancreatic duct; *H*, spleen; *I*, kidneys.

gen which it forms from the glucose, fructose and galactose received from the portal circulation (glycogenesis). When glucose is needed by the body, glycogen is converted to glucose (glycogenolysis) and returned to the blood stream to maintain blood levels of glucose. When glucose concentration in the blood begins to fall below normal, conversion of protein and fat to glucose (gluconeogenesis) occurs in the liver and it is sent to the blood stream to maintain normal blood glucose level.

FAT METABOLISM   The liver synthesizes fat from fatty acids, deaminized amino acids and carbohydrates. It synthesizes cholesterol and converts about 80 per cent of it into bile salts; the remainder is transported as lipoproteins in the blood. Phospholipids from fatty acids and the phospholipid lecithin synthesized in the liver are transported in the lipoproteins to adipose tissue and stored. Oxidation of fatty acids to acetoacetic acid and then to acetyl-CoA occurs in the liver. This in turn can enter the Krebs cycle and be oxidized to liberate energy. About 60 per cent of all initial oxidation of fatty acids in the body takes place in the liver.

PROTEIN METABOLISM   In the metabolism of proteins deamination of the amino acids must take place in the liver cells before they can be used for energy or before they can be converted to carbohydrate and fats. Conversion of amino acids into other amino acids (non-essential) occurs in the liver through several stages of transamination in the liver. They are released from the liver to maintain normal blood levels of each amino acid. Other important chemical compounds (purines and pyrimidines, etc.) are synthesized from amino acids through transamination. Formation of urea by the liver removes ammonia. It is excreted and the carbon residues are converted into fatty acids or glucose for energy or storage. Most all of the plasma proteins (albumin, globulin, fibrinogen, prothrombin and heparin) are synthesized by the hepatic cells. A reserve of these proteins is maintained in the liver to replenish serum proteins as needed.

MINERALS AND VITAMINS   The greatest portion of the body's iron is stored in the liver in the form of ferritin until needed by the body. Copper is stored in the liver and is necessary for the production of hemoglobin. Iron is an integral part of hemoglobin, and vitamin B_{12} which also is stored in the liver brings about the maturation and release of red blood cells in the bone marrow. The iron from old discarded red blood cells is recovered and stored by the liver.

All the fat-soluble vitamins are present in the liver. Considerable vitamin A, D and K are stored in the liver. The liver converts carotene into vitamin A and vitamin K into prothrombin. It also stores appreciable amounts of ascorbic acid and the B complex vitamins.

DISEASES OF THE LIVER RELATED TO DIET

The type of diet used in diseases of the liver is related directly to the functions of the liver. An understanding of the metabolic functions is necessary to determine the character of the diet for any hepatic disturbance. An organ that performs so many varied activities will manifest many types of pathologic conditions (functional and organic). Fortunately, the liver has the characteristics of great power of reserve and compensation and responds to treatment under adverse conditions.

OBJECTIVES OF DIETARY TREATMENT The important role of diet in the treatment of liver diseases is recognized. Improvement in diseases of the liver is observed as the result of diet therapy. The diet should have two objectives: first, to provide adequate calories and nutrients and, second, to enable the organ when damaged to function as easily and efficiently as possible. The principles of dietary treatment are similar for all of the hepatic disturbances.

VIRAL HEPATITIS

Hepatitis is an inflammation of the liver. During World War II, as well as in previous and present wars, many men and women in service became ill with viral hepatitis, which is believed to be caused by a virus, toxins or drugs (chloroform, carbon tetrachloride). It has been called *catarrhal jaundice* or *infectious hepatitis*. The disease, common among children and young adults, is mildly contagious and is readily transmitted through contaminated drinking water, food or sewage. In the acute phase there are symptoms such as nausea, vomiting, anorexia, elevation of temperature, headache, and abdominal discomfort that relate to the dietary treatment of these individuals.

DIETARY TREATMENT   Since there is no proven antidote, every attempt is made to spare the liver. Complete bed rest is essential. In severe cases, accompanied by vomiting, 5 to 10 per cent solution of glucose is administered intravenously and protein hydrolysates are added if prolonged parenteral feeding is indicated or protein solutions, such as concentrated human plasma and albumin, may be used. Concentrated liquid

TABLE 25–1   HIGH PROTEIN (100 GRAMS), HIGH CARBOHYDRATE (400 GRAMS), MODERATE FAT (100 GRAMS) DIET, TOTAL KILOCALORIES 2900

| | | SERVINGS | |
MEAL PLAN	SAMPLE MENU	Weight Grams	Household Measure
	BREAKFAST		
Fruit	Orange juice	124	1/2 glass (4 oz.)
Cereal	Cooked oatmeal	177	3/4 cup
Eggs	Poached eggs	100	2
Bread	Toasted whole wheat bread	46	2 slices
Butter or margarine	Butter or margarine	7	1 pat
Jelly	Jelly	20	1 tablespoon
Coffee	Coffee	200	1 pot
Cream, 20%	Cream, 20%	60	2 ounces
Sugar	Sugar	12	1 tablespoon
	MID-MORNING		
Fruit juice	Lemon and pineapple juice	248	1 glass (8 oz.)
with lactose	with lactose	16	2 tablespoons
	LUNCHEON		
Soup	Broth	120	1/2 cup (4 oz.)
Meat	Cold sliced turkey	85	3 ounces
Vegetable	Cooked green snap beans	63	1/2 cup
Salad	Sliced tomato salad	150	1 medium
Bread	Whole wheat bread	46	2 slices
Butter or margarine	Butter or margarine	7	1 pat
Jelly	Jelly	20	1 tablespoon
Dessert	Mixed fruit cup	128	1/2 cup
Beverage	Milk	244	1 glass (8 oz.)
	MID-AFTERNOON		
Fruit juice	Grapefruit juice	246	1 glass (8 oz.)
with lactose	with lactose	16	2 tablespoons
	DINNER		
Meat	Roast lamb	85	3 ounces
Potato or alternate	Boiled potato with parsley butter	122	1 medium
Vegetable	Baked winter squash	103	1/2 cup
Bread	Whole wheat bread	46	2 slices
Butter or margarine	Butter or margarine	7	1 pat
Jelly	Jelly	20	1 tablespoon
Dessert	Bananas and strawberry gelatin	194	1 sauce dish
Beverage	Milk	244	1 glass (8 oz.)
	BEDTIME		
Fruit juice	Orange juice and lemon juice	247	1 glass (8 oz.)
with lactose	with lactose	16	2 tablespoons

formulas orally or by tube feeding provide essential nutrients and sufficient calories and should be given until the person is able to consume an adequate diet. Fruit juices with sugar added, hard candies, jelly, honey, cereals, and bread products should be given at frequent intervals. The same type of diet as outlined for cirrhosis of the liver is prescribed. The diet should supply about 3000 kcalories or more, be high in carbohydrates (300 to 400 gm.) and proteins (100 to 120 gm.) and it is usually supplemented with vitamins B (especially thiamin and B_{12}) and K and ascorbic acid. (See Table 25–1.) At one time it was believed that fat in the diet should be low to prevent deposit in the liver, but the various studies have shown no adequate rationale for fat restriction. Alcohol is forbidden. As a result of controlled studies by Chalmers[1] on the treatment of the disease, the Armed Forces Epidemiological Board recommends a diet consisting of approximately 3000 kcalories containing about 150 gm. each of protein and fat. During the stage of severe anorexia, frequent small feedings are advised. In cases with impending hepatic coma or fulminating disease, a maintenance quantity of protein is prescribed.

While most attacks are not serious in children, it may be severe in older persons. If liver damage is severe in older patients, fatty infiltration of the liver may occur and hepatic coma may develop. Hepatitis is usually severe if it develops in the third trimester of pregnancy.

[1]Chalmers, T. C., et al.: The treatment of acute infectious hepatitis. J. Clin. Invest., 34:1163, 1955.

SERUM HEPATITIS

The symptoms of serum hepatitis are similar to infectious hepatitis but it is transmitted through transfusions of blood or serum from a donor who is a carrier of the virus, or through improperly sterilized medical instruments, dental drills, tattooing needles, or any other skin-puncturing instrument which has come in contact with contaminated blood.

The dietary treatment is the same as outlined under viral hepatitis.

CIRRHOSIS

Cirrhosis is the most serious, or final, stage of liver injury and degeneration. The normal liver tissue is gradually destroyed and fibrous connective tissue replaces the liver cells following fatty degeneration of long standing. In contrast to the enlarged fatty liver, the cirrhotic liver is contracted and has lost most of its function. There is a reversible and an irreversible stage in the development of cirrhosis. Once dense vascular and fibrous bands have formed, scarring is reported to be permanent. It is now listed as the fifth most common cause of death in the United States.

ETIOLOGY   Until recent years chronic alcoholism was considered the most common cause. This theory has been questioned, and it is now thought that protracted nutritional deficiencies may be a contributory factor. It is generally accepted that there is an association between liver disease, chronic alcoholism, and malnutrition, but the relationship is controversial. Chronic alcoholics usually have a long-standing inadequate food intake which may lead to malnutrition and to necrosis of liver tissue (with eventual replacement by scar tissue) and cirrhosis. Studies by Lieber[2] indicate that an intake of 11 to 12 ounces of 86 proof whiskey per day can lead

[2]Lieber, C. S.: The prolonged cocktail hour and liver disease. J.A.M.A., *185*:419, 1963.

to the development of fatty liver in man regardless of maintenance of an adequate diet intake. When rats were fed this amount of alcohol, a fatty liver could be produced within 2 to 6 weeks, even though a well-balanced and controlled dietary intake was maintained. Whether a more prolonged intake of these amounts of alcohol can lead to hepatic cirrhosis in humans who are maintaining an adequate diet has not been determined with controlled studies. It is possible for man to obtain maintenance energy needs in the alcohol calories consumed and be malnourished because of inadequate intake of the nutrients. Fibrosis of the liver has been demonstrated both in man and animals as a result of gross dietary inadequacy, especially of protein. (See Fig. 25–2.) The liver is more vulnerable to injury from various toxic agents when there is a nutritional deficiency.

Cirrhosis may also be due to various toxic and infectious agents which cause destruction of the liver cells, such as is seen in infectious hepatitis, and ultimately lead to fibrosis of the liver. Regardless of the origin, malnutrition is the common denominator. To spare the liver and prevent further change, infections throughout the body must be eliminated and constipation combated.

DIETARY TREATMENT   Results of research indicate that in man the most important protective factors for the liver in an adequate diet are animal protein, choline, and methionine (a dietary precursor of choline). These nutrients are present in adequate amounts in the average well balanced diet. However, under some circumstances, such as failure to absorb methionine and choline in the food ingested, supplements may be justified.

Serious undernutrition is frequently seen in patients with cirrhosis because of inadequate intake or interference with gastrointestinal functions. Protein deficiency is likely to be present because it is probable that most of the components of the plasma are synthesized in the liver. The specific

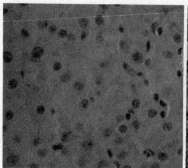 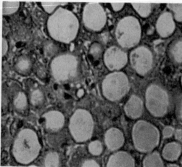

Figure 25–2   Fatty changes occur in the liver when a diet devoid of animal proteins is superimposed on a diet which is already nutritionally inadequate in other respects. (Halpern, S. L.: Nutrition and chronic disease. Reprinted from Health News, monthly publication of the New York State Department of Health, September, 1955.)

Normal liver   Fatty infiltration of liver

manner in which liver damage involves protein metabolism is not known. However, it is believed that the serum albumin level is maintained with difficulty in patients with advanced cirrhosis.

On the basis of the observations of various research workers, the diet should be high in calories, high in carbohydrates, high in protein (about 1.5 gm./kg. body weight), with moderate fats and an abundance of vitamins, especially B-complex. This diet is designed to prevent further degeneration of the liver cells, and to regenerate the tissue which has not been too seriously damaged.

Calories   Jolliffe[3] states that "provision of adequate calories appears to be just as important as adequate vitamins and minerals." Since there is often extreme weight loss, a high calorie diet with at least 45 to 50 kcalories per kg. desired body weight daily is indicated.

High Carbohydrate   Increased carbohydrate in the diet for patients with liver disease is well tolerated and seems to have a definite therapeutic value. The carbohydrate content of the diet protects and supports hepatic function. Three hundred to 400 gm. is recommended to spare the protein and to aid in recovery. A 5 to 10 per cent solution of glucose is frequently administered intravenously in acute and severe cases. Liquids and solid foods such as fruit juices with sugar or lactose added, hard candies, jelly, honey, bread, cereals, potatoes, vegetables and fruits or a concentrated formula supplement are given by mouth as soon as is feasible.

High Protein   A liberal protein intake offers protection in cirrhosis of the liver and is essential for the repair of hepatic cells and the formation of cholic or cholalic and other bile acids. A daily intake of 1.5 gm./kg./ desired body weight or 100 to 150 gm. daily (p. 330) is usually adequate. A cause for exception to the high protein intake is hepatic coma (p. 366). Both the quality and quantity of protein are important. It should be of high biologic value and rich in the lipotropic factors methionine and choline which mobilize liver fat and thus counteract fatty infiltration and degeneration of the parenchyma. Meat, fish, poultry, eggs, milk, dry skim milk powder, and cottage cheese are good sources of proteins to include in the diet prescribed for cirrhosis.

Concentrated Oral and Parenteral Protein   If a patient is too ill, or has a typically poor appetite, he may experience difficulty in consuming the large quantity of protein food required. In such cases concentrated protein may be included, such as a calcium caseinate, dried milk, soybean flour, and dried yeast. (See Chapter 34.) Tube feeding is contraindicated for patients who have esophageal varices. Intravenous administration of protein hydrolysates, carbohydrates, and water-soluble vitamins may be prescribed if the oral consumption is inadequate.

High Vitamins   Large doses of dried brewer's yeast (50 gm. daily), or an equivalent therapeutic vitamin preparation, a good source of the vitamin B-complex and amino acids, are frequently administered and found to be very effective. All of the vitamins should be supplied in abundance to fortify the liver against stress and to repair damage already done. Vitamin supplements including vitamin E are prescribed, with the addition of vitamin K if evidence of hypoprothrombinemia exists.

Moderate Fat   The low fat diets at one time recommended are not necessary.[4] Food is more palatable and easier to prepare when moderate amounts of fat are allowed. In addition, inclusion of fats increases calories, and supplies certain essential unsaturated fatty acids and fat-soluble vitamins. One hundred to 150 gm. or more are frequently allowed. The best types of fats to include in the diet are milk, salad oil, egg, and fortified margarine.

Liver Extract and Folic Acid   The development of iron deficiency and macrocytic anemia is a fairly common complication of cirrhosis of the liver, probably as a result of gastrointestinal bleeding and the failure of the damaged liver to store the erythrocyte maturation factor. In such cases, liver extract and folic acid are given parenterally.

Fluids and Sodium   Fluids are forced unless edema and ascites are present, in which event sodium and fluids are restricted according to the individual needs (1000 to 1500 ml.). Patients with ascites and edema should receive a low sodium, high calorie, high vitamin diet. Dried, low sodium milk products are recommended to help provide the necessary protein and calories in this diet. Eggs, meat and milk are relatively high in sodium. Therefore, when sodium is restricted, these protein foods as well as the table salt, will have to be limited. (See sodium restricted diets in Chapter 30.) Restriction of sodium to approximately 200 mg. daily usually halts ascites formation. Foods known to disagree and excessive use of condiments and alcohol are prohibited.

[3]Jolliffe, N.: Clinical Nutrition. 2nd ed. New York, Harper & Brothers, 1962, p. 245.

[4]Crews, R. H., and Faloon, W. W.: The fallacy of a low-fat diet. J.A.M.A., *181*:754, 1962.

DIET PRESCRIPTION The diet should contain a daily minimum of 2500 to 3000 kcalories to include 100 gm. protein, 400 gm. carbohydrate, and 80 to 100 gm. fat (Table 25-1). Since hepatic damage also leads to faulty vitamin metabolism, a daily supplementary therapeutic vitamin capsule is recommended, plus 25 to 50 gm. of brewer's yeast. Additional vitamin K must be given if the prothrombin time is found to be prolonged.

FOODS TO INCLUDE DAILY

Milk: 1 pint of milk; 2 ounces cream, 20%.

Eggs: 2 poached, hard- or soft-cooked.

Meats, fish, poultry: 6 ounces of meat, fish, or poultry which is lean or medium fat.

Cheese: Pot or uncreamed cottage cheese, as desired.

Bread: 6 slices whole grain or enriched white bread.

Cereals: 1 serving enriched or whole grain cereal.

Cereal products: Macaroni, spaghetti, noodles, and rice as an alternate for potato.

Fats: 3 pats of butter or fortified margarine.

Vegetables: 4 to 5 servings, including 1 to 2 servings potato or equivalent, 1 serving green leafy or yellow vegetable, 1 to 2 servings other vegetables.

Fruits: Fresh and canned fruits as tolerated; at least 1 serving of citrus fruit daily; 2 servings of other fresh fruits or sweetened canned fruit.

Soups: Clear soups.

Desserts: Cake, pie, gelatin sherbets, ice cream and ices as desired.

Beverages: Tea, coffee, Postum, carbonated beverages, fruit juices.

Sweets: Sugar, lactose, jelly, honey and syrup (at least 9 tablespoons daily).

FOODS OMITTED

Foods known to cause discomfort, salty foods if sodium is restricted, rich gravies, fried foods improperly prepared, alcohol.

PROBLEMS IN FEEDING Great care should be taken to have the patient select food attractive to him whenever possible. This cannot be overemphasized, since food for these patients is the most important single therapeutic measure. The appetite is almost always poor, and much difficulty is frequently encountered in maintaining nutritional intake. The division of meals into six to eight small feedings per day is usually more inviting than three large meals. The patient's understanding of the importance of the nutritional therapy helps him to ingest the food he selected. Guidance from the nurse in assisting the person to make the right choices is indicated. Appetite tends to improve as the patient eats more food. Establishing a regular eating pattern is often the problem these patients have to resolve.

HEPATIC COMA

In patients having severely impaired liver function, particularly those having advanced cirrhosis or vascular shunts between the portal and caval venous systems, ammonia gains access to the general circulation, raising the blood ammonia and causing intoxication of the central nervous system. Following ingestion of protein or following an episode of bleeding into the gastrointestinal tract, the liver is unable to convert ammonia to nontoxic urea, and absorption of nitrogenous catabolites from the gastrointestinal tract produces the toxic symptoms. The accumulation of blood in the gastrointestinal tract has the same effect as the ingestion of a high protein meal because of the very high protein content of blood.

DIETARY TREATMENT While generous quantities of protein are essential in the treatment of liver diseases, excessive amounts (over 2 gm./kg./body weight) should be avoided in impending hepatic coma. When signs and symptoms of ammonia intoxication are manifested, the dietary intake of protein must be markedly reduced (30 gm.) or even eliminated completely. With improvement, the dietary protein is gradually increased until a normal or high protein intake is tolerated. Protein intake as low as 30 to 40 gm. daily (using protein of high biologic value) will permit nitrogen balance in an otherwise adequate diet supplying adequate calories.

A diet of 30 to 40 grams of protein for the day consists of the following:

Meat, fish or poultry (2 to 3 ounces)
= approx. 14–21 gm. of protein

Milk (8 ounces)
= approx. 8 gm. of protein

Bread and cereals (3 servings)
= approx. 6 gm. of protein

Vegetables (2 to 3 servings)
= approx. 4 gm. of protein

Non-protein food: sufficient to supply calories needed — (sugar, jelly, fruit, oil, salt free butter)

Vitamin and mineral supplements —

Total 32–39

A diet[5] providing no protein and supplying

---

[5]Cream salt free butter or margarine and sugar. Add flavor extract if desired. Chill. Form into small balls. Keep refrigerated. Give to patient during the day or night. (May add water to the above amount of fat and sugar to use as a beverage or thicken with cornstarch to make a soup.)

approximately 2600 kcalories consists of the following:

Fat (salt free butter,
    margarine or oil) (200 gm.) = 1800 kcal.
Sugar   (200 gm.) = 800 kcal.
                                  2600 kcal.

Vitamin and mineral supplements

PHYSIOLOGY AND FUNCTION OF THE GALLBLADDER

The gallbladder is shaped like a pear (Fig. 25–1), the large end pointing upward. It is attached to the right side of the undersurface of the liver. Variations in shape and position are not unusual. Diseases of the biliary tract and gallbladder are so closely associated with liver disorders that they are usually grouped together.

FUNCTION   The main task of the gallbladder is to store the bile secreted by the liver. The bile is an excretion, composed of bile salts and acids, color pigments, lipids, mucin, and water. Table 25–2 shows the composition of bile as it is secreted by the liver and then as it has been concentrated in the gallbladder. During the concentration process water and electrolytes are reabsorbed by the gallbladder mucosa. Other constituents, particularly the bile salts, and lipid substances such as cholesterol are not reabsorbed. They become highly concentrated in the gallbladder bile. Approximately one quart of bile is produced daily.

Bile assists in the digestion and absorption of fats, and the absorption of fat-soluble vitamins A, D, E and K and the minerals iron and calcium. In addition it has a slightly laxative action and is believed to retard fermentation.

The rate of secretion of bile is directly related to the type of food digested. The rate is increased when a meat diet is consumed and is less when the diet is composed chiefly of carbohydrate foods. Fatty foods excite the secretory activity. A high percentage of the bile salts which pass into the intestines is

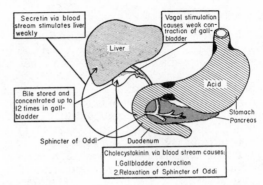

Figure 25–3   Mechanisms of liver secretions and gallbladder emptying. (From Guyton: Textbook of Medical Physiology. 4th ed. W. B. Saunders Company, 1971.)

reabsorbed into the portal vein and returns to the liver to be secreted again into bile. This circulation of the bile salts stimulates the liver to further secretion. The bile is a carrier of waste products, such as bile pigments, which are finally excreted with the feces.

The gallbladder is ordinarily full and relaxed between meals, with the sphincter of Oddi closed. During the course of digestion as food, especially food fat or fatty acids, reaches the duodenum, its presence initiates the production of the hormone *cholecystokinin* in the intestinal mucosa. When brought to the gallbladder by the blood stream, this hormone instigates the gallbladder to contract and the sphincter of Oddi to relax, thus releasing the concentrated bile into the duodenum via the common duct.

DISEASES OF THE GALLBLADDER

Peptic ulcer is found to occur more frequently in men, but women are more often the subjects of gallbladder disease. It is a disease which occurs most frequently in obese women over 40 years of age.

TABLE 25–2   COMPOSITION OF BILE*

	LIVER BILE	GALLBLADDER BILE
Water	97.3 gm. %	92 gm. %
Bile salts	1.1 gm. %	3 to 10 gm. %
Bilirubin	0.2 gm. %	0.6 to 2.0 gm. %
Cholesterol	0.1 gm. %	0.3 to 0.9 gm. %
Fatty acids	0.12 gm. %	0.3 to 1.2 gm. %
Lecithin	0.24 gm. %	0.1 to 0.4 gm. %
Na^+	145 mEq./liter	130 mEq./liter
K^+	5 mEq./liter	9 mEq./liter
Ca^{++}	5 mEq./liter	12 mEq./liter
Cl^-	100 mEq./liter	75 mEq./liter
HCO_3^-	28 mEq./liter	10 mEq./liter

*Taken from Guyton, A. C.: Textbook of Medical Physiology. 4th ed. Philadelphia, W. B. Saunders Company, p. 863, 1971.

JAUNDICE

CLASSIFICATION   Jaundice is the symptom of various diseases of the biliary tract rather than a disease in itself. The types of jaundice may be classified as (1) *obstructive* and (2) *hepatocellular*. The obstructive type is the result of a complete or partial obstruction caused by stones, tumor, or inflammation within the common bile duct (Fig. 25–1) or duodenum or is caused by external pressure. This type usually needs surgical treatment or may be the result of postoperative traumatic stricture of the bile ducts. The hepatocellular type includes *catarrhal* and *hemolytic* jaundice. Catarrhal jaundice is synonymous with infectious and viral hepatitis (p. 362). Hemolytic jaundice is characterized by excessive hemolysis such as occurs in pernicious anemia. It is generally hereditary in character.

ETIOLOGY   Through the bile the liver helps to remove poisons and waste products from the body.

Much of the pigment which gives the bile its greenish color is derived from the ingredients of old, broken-down, red corpuscles. Should the biliary tract become obstructed by stone or inflammation, bile is no longer able to reach the intestine, the coloring matter undergoes changes and returns to the circulation. The overflow of bile from the bile ducts into the general circulation causes the yellow pigmentation of the skin and discoloration of the eyes, which are typical of jaundice.

DIET AND OBSTRUCTIVE JAUNDICE   Vitamin K plays an important role in controlling the bleeding in individuals afflicted with certain types of jaundice. Vitamin K is not used by the system unless bile salts are present in the digestive tract. Patients who bleed profusely find surgery hazardous. In many cases vitamin K is of considerable help in controlling bleeding.

Although the obstructive jaundiced patient may eat foods containing vitamin K, absorption is usually inadequate because none of the secretions from the liver pass the obstruction. To counteract the shortage, vitamin K is now administered hypodermically or fortified with bile salts when taken by mouth. After vitamin K is absorbed, it is transported to the liver, helping to produce prothrombin which is necessary to clot blood.

Since steatorrhea is generally present in chronic obstructive jaundice, malnutrition due to loss of calories, protein, minerals and vitamins results. Thus, to prevent ill effects, the diet should be high in calories and protein (1.5 to 2.0 gm./kg./day). Fat is poorly tolerated and absorbed and should be restricted to about 40 gm. daily. If bone lesions exist, vitamin D

therapy is indicated, plus increased use of skim milk, nonfat buttermilk, and other high calcium-containing foods. In severe cases, supplemental calcium may be required. The presence of anemia is treated with increased iron-containing foods plus vitamin B-complex medication and may also require supplemental iron. The fat soluble vitamins, A and K, are generally given prophylactically.

DIET AND HEPATOCELLULAR JAUNDICE   The diet for hepatocellular jaundice is described under viral hepatitis on page 362.

BILIOUSNESS

Biliousness may be defined as an acute hepatic congestion. Bilious "attacks" are almost as popular in the layman's diagnosis as indigestion. The condition is usually caused by overindulgence in eating or drinking, especially in consumption of rich and fatty foods. However, the condition may have a direct relationship to a diseased liver or biliary tract. Constipation is another cause.

DIETARY TREATMENT   No food is given during the acute attack, which usually lasts 1 or 2 days. Simple foods which are low in fat content are served first, such as fruit juices, ginger ale, tea, and skim milk. Later, toast, baked potato and cereal are added to the simplified diet, with a gradual return to the normal diet.

BILIARY DYSKINESIA

Indigestion may result when normal movements of the gallbladder are disturbed or become sluggish in the presence of inflammation or stones. An indefinite condition, *biliary dyskinesia* produces vague abdominal complaints. In the past, physicians often referred to the condition as a "sluggish liver." X-rays reveal that the gallbladder fills and empties poorly, but there is no history of colic or acute inflammation.

CHOLECYSTITIS

Inflammation of the gallbladder is known as *cholecystitis*.

Gallbladder infection is fairly common. Bacteria may stray from any part of the body such as the tonsils, teeth, sinuses, or even the appendix and travel via the blood stream to the gallbladder. Other elements influencing abnormal functioning include overweight, pregnancy, constipation, constricting clothes, improper diet, and digestive upsets. The walls of the gallbladder become red and swollen, and sometimes pus collects, which causes distention. During such episodes, the patient is aware of pain in the region of the gallbladder, which is accompanied by nausea, vomiting, flatulence, and soreness in the upper right side of the abdomen. Jaundice may appear.

GALLSTONES (CHOLELITHIASIS, CHOLE-CYSTOLITHIASIS AND CHOLEDOCHOLITHI-ASIS)   Stones develop in a sluggish, diseased gallbladder. It is generally believed that gallstones form as a result of infection, stagnation of the bile, or changes in the chemical composition of the bile. Overeating and poor eating habits contribute to their formation. A combination of infection and stones is known as *cholecystolithiasis*. The formation of gallstones without infection is called *cholelithiasis*. *Choledocholithiasis* develops when stones slip into the common bile duct, producing obstruction and cramps. The existence of stones may cause no symptoms and the patient may be unaware of their presence. On the other hand, if the stones start to travel, the bile pathways may be obstructed and a typical colic results. In most cases the stones remain stationary and the symptoms are similar to chronic inflammation. If the gallbladder and stones are removed by surgery, the majority of patients are cured completely.

Gallstones are usually the cause of the obstruction of the common duct or neck of the gallbladder in about 95 per cent of the cases. They are composed of *cholesterol* crystals, or bile salt and pigment, or both. Most of the stones are found to contain a high percentage of cholesterol. Therefore, the stones are probably caused by stagnation of the bile, with the formation of calculi, plus a change in the colloidal state of the bile. It has been suggested that a diet low in cholesterol is indicated. However, more recent observations and studies indicate that the cholesterol levels in the blood and the tissues have little relationship to the cholesterol content of the food ingested. The Council on Foods and Nutrition of the American Medical Association[6] states, "There is no good evidence that the appearance of 'insoluble cholesterol' in the bile is retarded in any way by a low-fat or low-cholesterol diet."

DIETARY TREATMENT   The gallbladder patient learns through experience that he is more comfortable if he eats plain, simple foods, and avoids rich pastries, nuts, chocolate, fatty, fried and gas-forming foods. Easily digested soft fiber foods are recommended. Condiments, highly seasoned and high residue foods frequently cause distention and increase peristalsis, which ultimately results in irritation to the gallbladder. However, the disturbance varies with the individual patient and the dietary management is individualized.

When the patient experiences discomfort or is under emotional stress, high residue foods are often not well tolerated.

The fats and fatty acids in the foods are most active in stimulating the gallbladder and bile duct contractions, and it has been learned through experience that patients are more comfortable when fat is restricted in their diet. Acute attack almost always occurs in connection with an obstruction. At this time the gallbladder should be kept as inactive as possible. No visible fat in the dietary treatment is given. An all liquid diet of 2 to 3 liters/day and parenteral supplementation may be required. The protein (30 to 40 gm.) is supplied by skim milk and carbohydrate (200 to 300 gm.) is obtained in sweetened fruit juices, fruit nectars and gelatin. As soon as tolerated, toast, cereal, potatoes, rice, cooked vegetables, lean broiled or roasted meat, fish or poultry and a limited amount of fat are added. The patient is advised to adhere to a low fat diet until it is known whether surgical removal of the gallbladder is indicated. An example of a 50-gm. fat diet is shown in Table 25-3. Basically a combination of foods which contain about 50 gm. of fat are as follows:

Lean meat, fish or poultry (3 ounces)	15 gm. of fat
Egg (1 ounce)	5 gm. of fat
Butter, margarine or oil (2 tablespoons)	30 gm. of fat
Total	50 gm. of fat

Skim milk, cream-free cottage cheese, cereals, breads, vegetables, fruits, ices, jello and puddings made with skim milk. Sweets are taken in amounts that will supply calories and nutrient for an adequate diet. A regimen free of visible fat would restrict the protein foods to skim milk, cream-free cottage cheese and egg whites only. No fat of any kind would be allowed in the cooking or added to food.

For the dietary treatment of patients with chronic cholecystitis it is desirable to keep diet low in fat. Too strict limitation, however, is undesirable, since fat in the intestines is an effective stimulus of contraction and drainage of the biliary tract. Many patients with cholecystitis are overweight. Attention would be given to weight reduction. The intake of fat may vary from 40 to 70 gm. per day or approximately 25 per cent of the total calories.

The protein allowance is kept at the normal requirement, or high, and the carbohydrate allowance is normal, decreased or increased to maintain the patient's weight at the desired level. Increasing the amount of carbohydrates serves as a therapeutic measure in cases complicated with jaundice.

Individuals differ considerably as to the foods which are "gas-forming" or cause discomfort. It is best to determine for oneself the foods which cause disturbance and then to eliminate the offending ones from the dietary.

[6]Council report. J.A.M.A., *181*:417, 1962.

TABLE 25-3   LOW FAT (50 GRAM) DIET

MEAL PLAN	SAMPLE MENU	SERVINGS Weight Grams	Household Measure
	BREAKFAST		
Fruit	Grape fruit	285	1/2 medium
Cereal	Cooked oatmeal	118	1/2 cup
Egg	Poached egg	50	1
Bread	Toasted whole wheat bread	46	2 slices
Jelly	Jelly	20	1 tablespoon
Milk	Milk (skim)	244	1 glass (8 oz.)
Coffee	Coffee		1 cup
Sugar	Sugar	12	1 tablespoon
	LUNCHEON		
Soup	Clear broth	120	1/2 cup (4 oz.)
Vegetable	Broiled tomato	75	1/2 tomato
Vegetable	Cooked asparagus	96	6 spears
Salad	Orange and cottage cheese salad	{ 100 56	{ 1/2 orange 2 oz. cottage cheese
Bread	Whole wheat bread	46	2 slices
Butter/margarine	Butter or fortified margarine	10	1 pat
Jelly	Jelly	20	1 tablespoon
Beverage	Milk (skim)	244	1 glass (8 oz.)
Dessert	Canned peaches	117	2 halves and 2 tbsp. syrup
	DINNER		
Meat	Roast beef	90	1 slice (3 oz.)
Potato or substitute	Boiled potato	122	1 medium
Vegetable	Cooked carrots	73	1/2 cup
Salad	Head lettuce	75	1/6 head
Bread	Whole wheat bread	46	2 slices
Butter/margarine	Butter or fortified margarine	10	1 pat
Jelly	Jelly	20	1 tablespoon
Dessert	Strawberry gelatin	120	1/2 cup
Beverage	Tea		1 cup
Sugar	Sugar	10	2 teaspoons

Foods are prepared without the addition of any kind of fat. Fat of meat removed before broiling or roasting.

Usually if they are cooked properly, and not overcooked, little if any distress is experienced. A survey of hospitalized gallbladder patients failed to show any more incidence of specific food intolerances than patients without gastrointestinal disorders.[7] The following lists of vegetables and fruits are most often referred to as gas-forming.

VEGETABLES

Beans, kidney	Onions
Bean, lima	Peas, split, black eye
Beans, navy	Peppers, green
Broccoli	Pimento
Brussels sprouts	Radishes
Cabbage	Rutabagas
Cauliflower	Sauerkraut
Corn	Scallions
Cucumbers	Shallot
Kohlrabi	Soybeans
Leeks	Turnips
Lentils	

FRUITS

Apple (raw)	
Avocados	Cantaloupe
	Honeydew melon
	Watermelon

[7]Koch, J. F., and Donaldson, R. M.: A survey of food intolerances of hospitalized patients. New Eng. J. Med., 271:657, 1964.

The low fat diet   The low fat diet shown in Table 25-3 is typical. It contains approximately 80 gm. of protein, 50 gm. of fats, 275 gm. of carbohydrates, and 1870 kcalories. If the patient is overweight, or further reduction of fat is indicated, skim milk may be substituted for whole milk, with vitamin A given as a supplement to avoid deficiency of vitamin A and sweets may be eliminated.

FOODS LIMITED

Milk, skim milk: 2 cups (1 pint) daily.
Eggs: 1 poached, hard- or soft-cooked, daily.
Meats, fish or poultry: 3 ounces of meat, fish or poultry, lean and free from all visible fat, and skin of chicken, daily.
Fats: 2 pats (4 level teaspoons) of butter or fortified margarine daily.

FOODS INCLUDED

Cheese: Pot cheese or uncreamed cottage cheese.
Breads: Whole grain or enriched white preferred.
Cereals: Whole grain preferred, except the very coarse varieties.
Cereal products: Macaroni, spaghetti, noodles, rice.

Vegetables: As tolerated (to include 1 serving green leafy or yellow vegetable daily).

Fruits: As tolerated (to include at least 1 serving citrus fruit daily). Fruit juices.

Soups: Clear soups with fat removed or soups made with skim milk.

Desserts: Angel food cake, gelatin desserts with fruits as tolerated, sherbets, and ices.

Beverages: Tea, coffee, Postum, carbonated beverages.

Sweets: Sugar, jelly, honey, hard candy, and syrup.

FOODS OMITTED

Meats, fish or poultry: Fat of meat, skin of chicken, bacon, scrapple, cold cuts, sausages, fatty fish (mackerel), duck, goose, fish canned in oil.

Fats: All fat except butter or fortified margarine oil.

Desserts: Except those included.

Miscellaneous: Chocolate, peanut butter, cream, nuts, pastries, fried foods, highly seasoned foods, pickled foods and pickles, rich gravies and cream sauces.

Postoperative cholecystectomy diet   If the patient has surgical removal of the gallbladder, it is still advisable to continue the low fat diet regimen for several months following the operation to permit the inflammation to subside. When the gallbladder is removed, the bile is stored in the large common duct connecting the liver and small intestine. The tube stretches to perform its new function.

PHYSIOLOGY AND FUNCTION OF THE PANCREAS

The pancreas is located deep in the upper abdomen, behind the stomach (Fig. 25–1). Some of its cells manufacture insulin; others secrete powerful enzymes that aid in the digestion of protein, fats and carbohydrates in the intestine (see Table 7–1, page 91). The duct leading from the pancreas joins a common tube through which both bile and pancreatic juices drain into the duodenum.

PANCREATITIS

The common bile duct offers gallbladder and intestinal infection a direct route to the pancreas. For example, some bile may be forced back into the pancreatic duct by stones in the common duct or by spasm of the sphincter. The presence of bile may cause inflammation of the pancreatic tissues or *pancreatitis*. Jaundice, in varying degrees, is usually present.

Mild inflammation does not present a serious problem. However, if the pancreas becomes engorged and congested, the ferments escape into the pancreas and digest the cellular structures. Sometimes the caustic juices escape into the abdominal cavity and produce severe pain and shock. Profound emotional reactions frequently occur.

DIETARY TREATMENT   The liberation and activation of the potent pancreatic digestive enzymes is brought about by a strong stimulus such as food or alcohol. In addition, fatty foods excite the secretory activity of bile (p. 367). Thus, the dietary treatment of pancreatitis must be adjusted to consist of foods which will not stimulate these systems into action.

During severe, acute attacks of pancreatitis, all oral feeding is withheld. In less severe attacks, easily digested, nonstimulating foods, very low in fat (25 to 30 gm.), with increased carbohydrate and protein, should be given. The meals are better tolerated if divided into six small meals rather than the usual three. The low fat diet (Table 25–3) can be used.

Chronic pancreatitis ensues when inflammation fails to subside or recurs at intervals. The patient is almost always a feeding problem because food provokes nausea and vomiting which make it difficult to maintain a good nutritional status. Pancreatin may be administered orally *after* each meal to facilitate digestion of carbohydrate, protein and fats, and polysorbate given orally *with* each meal to promote absorption of fats. Effort should be made to cater to the patient's tolerances and preferences insofar as the diet prescription permits. In the interval phase, the low fat diet may be used, using the fruits and vegetables allowed on the low fiber diet. Alcohol is prohibited, as it acts as an intestinal irritant and encourages recurrences.

PROBLEMS AND SUGGESTED TOPICS FOR DISCUSSION

1. List the various functions of the liver and then determine the relationship of each function to the metabolism of food.
2. Take a dietary history of a patient with cirrhosis of the liver. Identify the areas of his dietary which need improving. How will the patient implement the changes?
3. Under what conditions does hepatic coma appear? Why is a low protein diet used?
4. Adjust the diet in problem 2 to limit the sodium to 200 mg. When would such a diet be required in cirrhosis of the liver?
5. Plan a diet containing 30 gm. protein for a patient with hepatic coma. The patient is a 40 year old male requiring 2600 calories. Why is it important to maintain adequate calorie intake?
6. Obtain the diet history of a patient with gallbladder disease. What adjustments need to be made to restrict the diet to 40 gm. of fat? Adjust the protein and carbohydrate to meet the individual's caloric needs. Why does a patient with gallbladder disease experience pain on the ingestion of fat?

7. What is the rationale for using a high protein diet in viral hepatitis?
8. What are the principles of diet for chronic pancreatitis? Plan a diet and meal pattern for a patient with chronic pancreatitis who is 50 years old and requires 2300 kcalories.

SUGGESTED ADDITIONAL READING REFERENCES

Anderson, M. C., et al.: Chronic interstitial pancreatitis. J.A.M.A., *179*:560, 1961.

Bartholomew, L. G., and Cain, J. C.: Medical management of pancreatitis. J.A.M.A., *175*:299, 1961.

Brown, H. B., and Spodnik, M. J.: Meat for low-fat diets. J. Am. Dietet. A., 38:540, 1961.

Burton, B. T. (ed.): Heinz Handbook of Nutrition. 2nd ed. New York, McGraw-Hill Book Company, Inc., 1965, Chapter 27, Nutrition and diet in diseases of the liver; Chapter 28, Nutrition and diet in diseases of the biliary tract.

Child, C. G., and Kahn, D. R.: Current status of therapy of pancreatitis. J.A.M.A., *179*:363, 1962.

Crews, R. H., and Faloon, W, W.: The fallacy of a low-fat diet. J.A.M.A., *181*:754, 1962.

Davidson, C. S.: Cirrhosis in alcoholics – Protein nutrition and hepatic coma. J.A.M.A., *160*:390, 1956.

Dreiling, D. A.: The pathological physiology of pancreatic inflammation. J.A.M.A., *175*:183, 1961.

Eisenstein, A. B., et al.: An epidemic of infectious hepatitis in a general hospital. J.A.M.A., *185*:171, 1963.

Farquhar, J. D., Stokes, J., Jr., and Schrack, W. D.: Epidemic of viral hepatitis apparently spread by drinking water and by contact. J.A.M.A., *149*:991, 1952.

Gabuzda, G. J.: Clinical and nutritional aspects of lipotropic agents. J.A.M.A., *160*:969, 1956.

Guyton, A. C.: The textbook of Medical Physiology. 4th ed. Philadelphia, W. B. Saunders Company, 1971.

Harper, H. A.: Protein intake in liver disease. J. Am. Dietet. A., 38:350, 1961.

Herbert, V., et al.: Correlation of folate deficiency with alcoholism and associated macrocytosis anemia and liver disease. Ann. Intern. Med., 58:977, 1963.

Iber, F. L.: In alcoholism the liver sets the pace. Nutrition Today, 6:2, 1971.

Jolliffe, N.: Clinical Nutrition. 2nd ed. New York, Harper & Brothers, 1962, pp. 240 to 245, 815.

Kater, R. M. H., et al.: Relationship of serum tocopherol to beta-lipoprotein concentrations in liver diseases. Am. J. Clin. Nutr., 23:913, 1970.

Kaufmann, G. G., et al.: Outbreak of infectious hepatitis – Presumably food-borne. J.A.M.A., *149*:993, 1952.

Krugman, S., et al.: Infectious hepatitis. J.A.M.A., *174*:823, 1960.

La Londe, J. B., et al.: Hepatic regulation of sodium and water in ascites. J.A.M.A., *187*:117, 1964.

Leevy, C. M., et al.: B-Complex vitamins in liver disease of the alcoholic. Am. J. Clin. Nutr., *16*:339, 1965.

Leevy, C. M.: Nutritional factors in liver disease in man. Am. J. Clin. Nutr., 7:146, 1959.

Leone, N. C., et al.: Clinical evaluations of high-protein, high-carbohydrate, restricted-fat diet in treatment of viral hepatitis. Ann. New York Acad. Sci., 57:948, 1954.

Nefzger, M. D., and Chalmers, T. C.: The treatment of acute infectious hepatitis. Ten year follow-up study of the effects of diet and rest. Am. J. Med., 35:299, 1963.

Okey, R.: Cholesterol content of foods. J. Am. Dietet. A., 21:341, 1945.

Reader, G. G., et al.: Practitioners' Conference. Acute and Chronic Hepatitis, New York Medicine, p. 16, July 5, 1952.

Review. Council report on dietary fat regulation. Nutr. Rev., 21:36, 1963.

Review. Nutritional cirrhosis of the liver. Nutr. Rev., 21: 175, 1963.

Rindge, M. E., et al.: Infectious hepatitis. J.A.M.A., *180*:33, 1962.

Sborov, V. M.: Diet and nutritional aids in liver disease. Am. J. Digest. Dis., N.S. 3, p. 94, 1958.

Sparberg, M., and Kirsner, J. B.: Feature: Pancreatitis. World-Wide Abstracts of General Medicine. Warner-Chilcott Lab., Vol. 8, No. 3 and 4, 1965.

Wohl, M. G.: Long-Term Illness. Philadelphia, W. B. Saunders Company, 1959, pp. 267–288.

Wohl, M. G., and Goodhart, R. S. (ed.): Modern Nutrition in Health and Disease. 4th ed. Philadelphia, Lea & Febiger, 1968. Chapters on Nutrition in liver disease and in pancreatic insufficiency.

Chapter 26
DIETS IN SURGERY AND SURGICAL CONDITIONS

The dietetic treatment before and after surgery plays an important role in the success of the operation, as well as in the welfare and comfort of the patient. The duration of disability, which follows surgery, can be significantly shortened, complications fewer, wound healing improved, and mortality reduced by providing adequate nutrition. General rules besides the individual characteristics of the patient must be considered.

PREOPERATIVE DIETS

The actual preoperative dietary treatment given a patient will depend largely upon the situation, whether the operation is an emergency or is elective. If it is an emergency operation, there is little or no time for preliminary dietary treatment. In elective cases the patient can be brought to the best possible nutritional state for the operation. Illness and disease prior to surgical intervention may cause patients to restrict their food intake for days or weeks, predisposing nutritional depletion; for these cases it is advisable for them to improve their nutritional state to the best level possible. In some instances, vomiting, diarrhea, and bleeding may have contributed further to the patient's depletion, with marked losses of sodium, chloride, potassium and iron. In some individuals where there is excessive adipose tissue it is advisable for the patient to lose some weight with a diet adequate in all the nutrients. Patients who are extremely overweight or underweight are frequently poor operative risks. Diabetes needs to be under good control in the diabetic patient before surgery. Patients with anemia need increased amounts of iron and protein in their diets preceding surgery. Each case must

be considered individually and treated accordingly. The individual who appears well nourished deserves an evaluation of his dietary practices as well as those who overtly need counseling. The aim is to obtain the calories and nutrients needed by the individual to place him in as good a nutritional state as possible before surgery.

The type of operation, whether major or minor, will further determine the type of preoperative diet treatment to prescribe. A serious operation in which there is considerable risk needs more preliminary treatment than a minor operation involving little or no risk.

DIETARY MANAGEMENT In emergency cases it may be necessary to administer glucose or some other suitable parenteral solution preoperatively.

CALORIES

Carbohydrate and Protein In elective surgery it is advisable to administer a diet adequate in calories, high in carbohydrate (300 gm.) content, with ample proteins (150 gm.) for a period of 7 to 14 days prior to the operation. The length of the time of preparation is observed to be in direct proportion to weight loss. In extreme malnutrition, preoperative preparation up to a month may be advisable. The extra amount of carbohydrate spares the proteins and enables the liver to store glucose and glycogen, an action which exerts a protective function on the liver and helps to prevent postoperative ketosis and vomiting. The added protein improves the postoperative physiologic status and helps to avoid the use of stored body fat.

Vitamins and Minerals Selection of foods to provide the minerals (calcium and iron) and the vitamins (fat-soluble and water-soluble) is important. However, therapeutic doses of vitamins are also recommended during this period. Ascorbic acid deficiency predisposes to poor wound healing, vitamin K deficiency interferes with normal blood clotting, and the B-complex vitamins play a role in carbohydrate and protein metabolism.

Food   It is important that the stomach should be empty of food at the time of the operation. If food remains in the stomach there is danger of aspiration of vomitus during the induction of anesthesia, or upon awakening. In elective cases no food is allowed by mouth for at least 6 hours prior to the time of the operation. This is usually managed routinely by allowing a light meal the night prior to the operation and nothing by mouth from midnight on. In emergency cases it is advisable to perform gastric lavage to remove the stomach contents before starting the anesthesia.

In intestinal surgery it is desirable to have the colon free of residue content to prevent postoperative distention. This is usually accomplished by giving low fiber foods for 2 to 3 days preceding the operation and by giving the patient an enema a few hours before he goes to the operating room.

Fluids   It is of utmost importance to the safety of the patient that no operation should be attempted when a state of dehydration exists. In an emergency case, if there is insufficient time to administer fluids orally, fluids can be given parenterally.

Nutritional Depletion   Patients who have had an inadequate diet prior to surgery frequently manifest poor wound healing, develop complications, and convalesce slowly. In addition, when a person is bedridden for days or weeks prior to an operation, a rapid tissue protein breakdown takes place, as indicated by increased nitrogen excretion in the urine (see p. 324). Every effort must be made to correct the nutritional deficiencies. When time and the patient's ability to take food by mouth permit, complete nutritional rehabilitation should be given to reduce the operative risk. Tube feeding (p. 384) may have to be resorted to. When adequate oral or tube feeding is impossible, parenteral feeding of nutrients (glucose, vitamin preparations, amino acids) and/or repeated blood and plasma transfusions may be necessary.

In general, infusions (preoperative, during operation, and postoperative) are administered to maintain fluid and electrolyte balance. The presence of a needle in the vein during operation also permits the immediate administration of blood in the event of serious hemorrhage. Otherwise, transfusion might be delayed owing to technical difficulties associated with the collapse of veins which accompanies hemorrhage and shock. In cases in which deficiency of specific stores may be present (as in malnutrition), it is important to supplement the infusion appropriately. This is especially true in vitamin C and K deficiencies. Glucose may be required if the liver stores are inadequate, as in alcoholic patients. Glucose is also used to avoid insulin shock in diabetic patients. (See Chapter 28.)

Calorie and Protein Concentrates   When a sufficient quantity of food is not eaten, calorie and protein concentrates can be administered in in-between meal drinks. Powdered dried skim milk is approximately 35 per cent protein of high biologic value. Casein and lactalbumin can be added to the dried skim milk powder to increase its protein content at low cost. This type of preparation has a low lactose content, which minimizes gastrointestinal disturbances. Other forms of concentrated protein which can be used are powdered whole eggs and powdered dried egg albumin. By the use of these low bulk protein concentrates, it is possible to give orally as much as 300 gm. of protein per day in 2000 ml. of total fluid. (See Table 43–1, Protein Supplements Commonly Used.) Instant tube feedings are available which provide 1 kcalorie per milliliter. Gerber's Tube Feeding Formula 1 is an example.[1]

POSTOPERATIVE DIETS

The dietary treatment of a patient following surgery varies. It is individualized and is related to the type of surgery. For example, a patient who had a major stomach operation receives a different diet program from that given to a patient who underwent a limb amputation.

Whereas the importance of adequate postoperative nutrition is well recognized, evidence indicates that oral feeding in the first 24 to 28 hours following operation can precipitate vomiting and subsequent ileus. Blood, fluids, and electrolytes are lost from the body during surgery. Further loss may occur through vomiting and drainage. To prevent dehydration and shock during the immediate postoperative period, fluid and electrolytic balance are maintained by intravenous, subcutaneous and rectal infusion.

GENERAL DIETARY MANAGEMENT

Many surgeons prefer to give daily postoperative diet orders for their patients. Some physicians have formulated their own diet program, based on past experiences. How-

---

[1]Gormican, A.: Prepackaged tube feedings. Hospitals, 44: Sept. 1, 1970.

ever, there are some general principles applicable to most of the postoperative diets. In general, adequate nutrition of the patient will usually reduce the time of convalescence, infections, and complications.

CALORIES AND PROTEIN   The important role nutrition plays in wound healing and convalescence following injury or surgery is well established. Moderate or severe tissue damage, caused by either injury or surgery, leads to an increased excretion of nitrogen and often to considerable loss of body protein. The nitrogen wastage is due to the body's effort to meet the needs for repair and maintenance. If the diet does not provide sufficient calories and the essential protein, the body must use its own reserve. About 150 gm. per day are indicated postoperatively as well as preoperatively. Co Tui[2] found the amount of protein necessary to overcome negative nitrogen balance in postoperative patients to be proportional to the severity of the operation. (See p. 330.)

As soon as injury or disease occurs, malnutrition, especially loss of proteins, almost always begins. This is the result of either an increased destruction of the tissues or the diminished intake of foods because of an inability or disinclination of the patient to consume needed foods.

If there are not enough carbohydrates and fats to supply calories in the diet, protein must be broken down through the metabolic processes to carbohydrate and fat to provide energy needs. If there are exudates or discharges such as occur in peritonitis or open wounds, much nitrogen may be lost daily (6.25 gm. of protein is required to replace 1 gm. of nitrogen lost). There may be some loss of nitrogen through hemorrhage or the excretion from the kidneys. Nitrogen loss is associated with fractures or infected wounds. Insufficiency of protein in the diet or loss in exudates may not be the reasons. The toxic destruction of protein can be alleviated only by the effective treatment of the injury or disease which causes it. However, adequate nutrition will minimize this toxic reaction besides promoting and shortening the process of repair.

Depletion of body protein is very serious. It causes edema, inhibits wound healing, renders the liver more liable to toxic damage, impedes regeneration of hemoglobin, prevents resumption of normal gastrointestinal activity, and delays the return of muscular strength. It is largely responsible for postoperative weakness.

Protein Hydrolysates (predigested proteins) are now frequently used to supplement the

diet in cases of surgical convalescence. They have no nutritional advantage over intact, whole protein and are, therefore, indicated only for parenteral feeding or in cases of pancreatic disease when the digestive tract is incapable of properly digesting whole protein. They are more expensive than whole protein, have an objectionable taste, and may cause nausea and diarrhea. Commerical preparations of protein hydrolysates are available. (See Chapter 34, p. 510, for a discussion of concentrated protein.)

VITAMINS   Ascorbic acid is associated with the delay or prevention of wound healing. It is required for the formation of collagen precursors and collagen. Vitamin K deficiency is characterized by a decrease in prothrombin content of the blood, with resultant defect in clotting. It is, therefore, of particular interest in surgery. The B vitamins (thiamin, riboflavin and niacin) provide essential coenzyme factors to metabolize carbohydrate and protein. Other members of the B-complex vitamins have important metabolic roles in stress conditions. A healthy person having minor surgery usually does not require vitamin supplements. Patients having major surgery, especially those poorly prepared for surgery, usually require therapeutic amounts of the vitamins. Vitamin A is of surgical interest in that a deficiency may interfere with normal epithelization.

FLUIDS   Directly following an operation each patient should be supplied with sufficient fluids to maintain normal water and electrolyte balance. At this time, the patient experiences more or less difficulty with the intake of large quantities of water by mouth, and fluids are usually administered by intravenous instillations, except in certain cases of cardiac disease when fluids are given subcutaneously so as not to overload the circulation too abruptly. In many instances, fluids are given by mouth as soon as the patient has recovered from the anesthesia. Some institutions still favor the administration of fluids by proctoclysis.

FOOD   The introduction of food following surgery will depend upon the condition of the patient's gastrointestinal tract. To meet the all-important calorie, protein and carbohydrate needs, generous amounts of high quality protein foods such as milk, meat and eggs and simple carbohydrate foods are needed. When adequate amounts of such foods cannot be tolerated, protein in the form of hydrolysates or other protein compounds, which also provide adequate minerals, vitamins and calories, should be available. Sustacal, made by Mead Johnson Laboratories, Evansville, Indiana (47721), is an example of a commercial protein-vitamin-mineral product. One 12-ounce can, ready-to-eat mixture

[2]Co Tui: Clinical experiences with oral use of protein hydrolysates. Ann. New York Acad. Sci., 47:359, 1946.

TABLE 26–1   FORMULAS FOR USE IN TUBE FEEDING

	GRAMS	KILOCALORIES PER FLUID OZ.
I*		
Water	1000	45
Sustagen (Mead Johnson Co.)	500	
Pour the required amount of warm water (120° F.) into a pan of suitable size. Add the required amount of Sustagen to the surface of the water. Allow the powder to absorb the water. Mix until blended and smooth. Strain.		
II*		
Whole milk	1000	30
Meritene (Dietene Co.)	150	
Pour milk into a covered jar, mixer or beater. Add Meritene and shake, mix or beat until smooth.		
III*		
Whole milk	1000	48
Egg yolks 4 yolks		
Heavy cream, 40 per cent	240	
Karo syrup	100	
Yeast: 2 cakes dissolved in 200 ml. hot water. Mix all together and cook in a double boiler. Cool, strain and add orange juice	200	
Cod liver oil	16	
IV*		
Water	1000	38
Skim milk powder	225	
Whole milk powder	200	
The water in this formula is used to reconstitute the skim milk.		
Low Sodium†		
Water	670	45
Lonalac, dry (Mead Johnson Co.)	150	
Casec, dry (Mead Johnson Co.)	25	
Eggs (two)	100	
Dextrose	120	
Vitamin supplement (ml.)	.5	
This formula contains 155 mg. sodium and 1,400 mg. potassium.		
Blended Formula†		
Water	250	30
Strained meat (beef)	100	
Strained vegetable (peas)	100	
Strained fruit (pears)	100	
Evaporated milk	410	
Eggs (two)	100	
Dextrose	25	
Vitamin supplement (ml.)	0.5	

APPROXIMATE ANALYSIS

	KILO-CALORIES	PRO-TEIN GM.	FAT GM.	CHO. GM.	CA. GM.	FE. MG.	VIT. A I.U.	ASCOR-BIC ACID MG.	THIA-MIN MG.	RIBO-FLAVIN MG.	NIA-CIN MG.
Formula I*	2035	118	18	323	3.5	8	2778	167	5.5	5.5	56.0
Formula II*	1205	84	40	131	2.6	22	9550	136	3.8	8.1	34.0
Formula III*	2321	54	158	183	1.5	7	7270	110	0.9	2.9	10.2
Formula IV*	1798	132	56	193	4.8	3	2890	28	1.4	7.3	3.9
Low Sodium†	1495	75	55	175	1.7	2.6	7260	50	2.09	2.66	24.6
Blended†	1005	60	45	90	1.0	6	8310	57	1.97	2.45	25.6
Recommended	2800	65			0.8	10	5000	60	1.4	1.7	18.0

Recommended allowances for a 65 kg., 25 year old man, moderately active, are used for comparison. For some patients it may be advisable to give certain vitamins and iron by medication to prevent deficiencies.

*Adapted from Wohl, G. W., and Goodhart, R. S.: Modern Nutrition in Health and Disease. 2nd ed. Philadelphia, Lea & Febiger, 1960.
†Clinical Center Diet Manual, Nutrition Dept., The Clinical Center, National Institutes of Health, U.S. Dept. of Health, Education and Welfare, Public Health Service Pub. No. 989, 1963.

contains 21.7 gm. protein, 8.3 gm. fat, 49.6 gm. carbohydrate, and 360 kcalories or 1 kcalorie per ml. It can be used as an in-between meal supplemental feeding[3] and may be served hot or cold. A mixture of puréed meat, vegetables and fruit may be added to juices, milk, milk powder, cream, eggs and sugar put through a blender and may be used to supply the calories and nutrients needed. (See Table 26–1.)

ROUTINE DIET REGIMEN

PARENTERAL FEEDING   Fluid balance and prophylaxis against nutritional depletion should be started during the first 24 hours after major surgery. Blood transfusions are no longer used routinely because of the danger of hepatitis but are given if there is excessive blood loss. As a general rule, each postoperative patient should receive a minimum of from 2500 to 3500 ml. of fluid daily, provided there is normal kidney function and no excessive or abnormal loss of fluid or electrolytes. Sodium and water have a tendency to be retained directly following surgery or trauma, and excessive sodium chloride should be avoided the first 48 hours postoperatively. There is also an increase in potassium and nitrogen excretion in the urine the first 24 to 48 hours, and if the patient is unable to take fluid orally in 24 hours, potassium should be added to the basic intravenous fluid. A sample routine is to give 5 to 15 per cent glucose in physiologic saline solution or water with added vitamins, especially ascorbic acid and the B-complex, plus 5 per cent protein hydrolysate in 5 to 10 per cent glucose solution. This preparation can satisfy the fluid and electrolytic needs as well as part of the caloric and protein requirements. Whenever there will be need for parenteral nutrition for longer than 3 to 4 days' duration, adequate quantities of all the essential nutrients should be supplied in the parenteral fluids, starting with the first postoperative day. A sample schedule suggested by the Committee on Therapeutic Nutrition,[4] is shown at the top of the page.

Elman[5] recommends oral feeding as soon as possible, as intravenous feeding does not and cannot compete with oral feeding; it competes only with starvation.

ORAL FEEDING   Bits of ice or sips of water as tolerated are usually the first thing given by mouth. Although it is advisable to

ADEQUATE PARENTERAL FEEDING FORMULA

700 ml. 15 per cent glucose in saline (after the first 24 hours, add 2.23 gm. potassium chloride if urinary output is normal) and 2 ml. of the recommended parenteral vitamin mixture,* plus 2000 ml. of 5 per cent protein hydrolysate in 5 per cent glucose solution. This will apply:

Water	2700 ml.
Amino acids	100 gm.
Nonprotein calories	820
Total calories	1220
Sodium chloride	6 gm.
Potassium	30 mEq.
Ascorbic acid	300 mg.
Thiamin HCl	5 mg.
Riboflavin	5 mg.
Niacinamide	100 mg.
Calcium pantothenate	20 mg.
Pyridoxine	2 mg.

*Each 2 ml. contains: 5 mg. thiamin, 5 mg. riboflavin, 100 mg. niacinamide, 20 mg. calcium pantothenate, 2 mg. pyridoxine hydrochloride, 300 mg. ascorbic acid, 1 mcg. vitamin B_{12} and 1.5 mg. folic acid.

avoid a period of starvation immediately after an operation, it is important not to increase the quantity of the diet too rapidly. Nondistending fluids, such as tea, ginger ale and clear broth, are the first foods allowed. Milk and orange juice are invariably distending to the patient and should be avoided the first 2 to 3 postoperative days.

The usual diet routine, especially for major abdominal operations, is to place the patient on a restricted or clear liquid diet on the second postoperative day, then allow the full liquid diet on the third to fourth postoperative day. Usually by the fourth to fifth day a soft diet is well tolerated. On the fifth to sixth postoperative day a general diet is prescribed. (Review Chapter 20.)

There is an increasing trend to feed solid foods earlier.[6] However, this calls for considerable individualization in terms of both the patient and the kind of surgery done.

Any diet increase must be adjusted to the condition of the individual patient. The return to the normal diet is the aim in the treatment of surgical cases, but the return must be gradual to avoid gastric upsets and discomfort to the patient. The patient's diet should receive attention throughout convalescence. The Recommended Daily Dietary Allowances (Table 11–1, p. 158) for normal, healthy people should probably be exceeded by about 100 per cent (except for calories), with the protein intake, especially, kept high (150 gm. per day).

DIET FOLLOWING GASTROINTESTINAL SURGERY

Patients undergoing gastrointestinal surgery frequently suffer nutritional depletion

[3]Artz, C. P., et al.: Some recent developments in oral feedings for optimal nutrition in burns. Am. J. Clin. Nutr., 4:642, 1956.

[4]Pollack, H., and Halpern, S. L.: Therapeutic Nutrition. Washington, D. C., National Research Council, Publication 234, 1952.

[5]Elman, R.: Protein needs in surgical patients. J. Am. Dietet. A., 32:524, 1956.

[6]Hayes, M. A.: Postoperative diet therapy. J. Am. Dietet. A., 35:17, 1959.

for some time prior to the operation (p. 373). Every effort should be made to correct the nutritional state and to bring the patient into positive nutritional balance prior to surgery when possible. When it is desirable to keep the gastrointestinal tract empty in preparation for surgery, and then postoperatively until the alimentary tract can function normally, parenteral feeding may be used to forestall nutrition and fluid depletion. The postoperative convalescent period is shortened and complications reduced when protein, calories and general nutrients are adequate. Low fiber, mild flavored, foods should be given, with a gradual return to the normal diet as tolerated.

Diet Following Gastric Surgery

After gastric surgery, such as partial or total gastrectomy (for cancer or peptic ulcer), all fluids and foods by mouth are withheld for 24 to 48 hours. An adequate parenteral feeding formula, as outlined under parenteral feeding on page 377, is administered the first few days and gradually reduced as oral feeding is resumed. The first types of fluids allowed by mouth are ice, which is held in the mouth, or infrequent sips of water. Some patients tolerate warm water better than iced or cold water. When vomiting ceases, larger amounts of fluids may be served. The feedings can be chosen from those outlined in Chapter 23 under the second and third stages of dietary treatment for peptic ulcer, and gradually increased to a six-feeding diet regimen.

The purpose of the diet is to provide simple, easily digested, mild flavored foods to give the gastrointestinal tract a chance to perform its normal functions. Nutritional impairment frequently occurs after gastrectomy and many patients have difficulty regaining normal preoperative weight due to either (1) inadequate food intake related in most instances to the dumping syndrome, (2) malabsorption of ingested food, specifically fat and protein, (3) increased metabolic requirements, especially of protein, or (4) a combination of all these factors. Patients who have had total or nearly total gastrectomy often have difficulty in taking large amounts of food and may need to continue dividing their meals into six, instead of three, indefinitely. All patients with any gastric resections are usually advised to continue to take nourishment (milk or milk and cookies) between meals and not to eat large amounts of raw, coarse or highly seasoned foods.

The loss of intrinsic factor which follows a gastrectomy results in a depletion of vitamin B_{12} stores, and macrocytic anemia may develop several years later unless the vitamin deficiency is compensated for. (See p. 468.)

THE DUMPING SYNDROME   The dump-

ing syndrome is a complex physiological response to the presence of undigested food in the jejunum. Following gastric surgery some patients who have had two-thirds or more of the stomach removed and have advanced to the full diet regimen may experience the dumping syndrome. After food is swallowed, it is "dumped" into the jejunum about 10 to 15 minutes after ingestion instead of being gradually released in small amounts and without benefit of the stomach's participating in the digestive process. Most patients who undergo this type of surgery develop a new pouch through nature's stretching of the remaining stomach tissue. The ingested foods and liquids are prepared for absorption in the gastric pouch exactly as in the original stomach. However, in a number of these patients, symptoms develop.

Symptoms   Some individuals complain of abdominal fullness, nausea and, at times, crampy, abdominal pain followed by diarrhea within 15 minutes after eating. Others feel warm, dizzy, weak and faint; their pulse races and they break into a cold sweat. Lying down immediately after eating lessens these symptoms because food remains longer in the stomach pouch. Because of these symptoms, patients tend to eat very sparingly, with resultant malnutrition and loss of weight.

A *summary of changes* occurring in the dumping syndrome as proposed by Vanamee[7] is demonstrated in Figure 26-1 and is as follows:

"(1) Rapid hydrolysis of ingested nutrients in the jejunum leads to a hypertonic intestinal content. (2) This hypertonic material is rapidly diluted by fluid drawn from the plasma and extra-cellular fluid, leading to a sharp drop in circulating blood volume. (3) Drop in blood volume, decrease in cardiac output, and perhaps dilatation of the jejunum lead to decreased pancreatic secretion and a sympathetic vasomotor response producing sweating, tachycardia, electrocardiographic changes, and weakness. Changes in effective circulatory volume may be modified further by splanchnic pooling as well as autonomic discharge." Serotonin, a vasoconstrictor released into the circulatory system, accompanies the dumping syndrome. It may produce symptoms of flushing and sweating and may stimulate the gastrointestinal tract. The hypermotility may be the cause of the cramps and diarrhea.[8]

Rapid emptying of the stomach contents into the jejunum causes some of the symp-

[7]Vanamee, P.: Nutrition after gastric resection. J.A.M.A., 172:2045, 1960.

[8]Stemmer, E. A., et al.: A physiological approach to the surgical treatment of the dumping syndrome. J.A.M.A., 199:159, 1967.

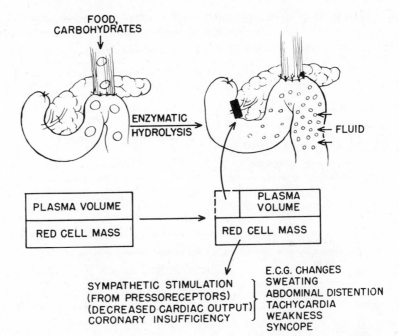

Figure 26–1   Changes occurring in dumping syndrome. (Courtesy of Dr. Parker Vanamee and J.A.M.A.)

toms as explained above. These symptoms occur within minutes after eating. Other symptoms which are related to concentrated carbohydrate, especially sugar intake, occur from 1 to 2 hours after the meal is ingested. The glucose rapidly enters the blood stream and causes a postprandial elevation in blood glucose. The glucose load stimulates an overproduction of insulin which results in hypoglycemia. Symptoms resembling a mild hypoglycemic reaction result.

Dietary Treatment   Jordan[9] points out that dietary management is the basic factor in treatment of the dumping syndrome. Protein and fats are better tolerated than carbohydrates because they are hydrolyzed into osmotically active substances more slowly. Solid foods are better than liquids as they enter the jejunum less rapidly. Evidence indicates that fats of large molecular weight in the naturally occurring state are better tolerated than the homogenized fats, particularly those fat solutions containing carbohydrates.

Some patients learn through experience that certain foods such as milk and sweets are likely to produce symptoms. Sweets should be eliminated, and milk as well as other liquids should be taken between meals. Small amounts of milk are apt to be tolerated better than large amounts. Dried, skim milk or various commercial food concentrates, designed to meet the needs, may be used and well tolerated. It is important to note that meals should be eaten without fluids. Fluids may be taken up to 45 minutes to 1 hour before eating, and resumed 45 minutes to 1 hour after eating. Each diet must be adjusted to the individual requirements of the patient, based on a *careful dietary history* (p. 19).

Good results have been reported[10, 11] when using a diet high in fat. Pittman and Robinson recommend a high fat, high protein, low carbohydrate routine with frequent feedings (six) and the omission of all liquids at mealtime. Each serving of food or beverage is indefinitely limited to about 4 or 5 ounces or less until the patient's alimentary capacity is compensated for. Rich gravies and sauces are omitted. Artificial nonnutritive sweeteners (Chap. 43) can be substituted for sugar. Multiple vitamin supplements are prescribed routinely, and iron when indicated. A sample menu of a six-feeding dry diet containing approximately 3000 kcalories, 150 gm. protein, 225 gm. fat and 100 gm. carbohydrate is shown in Table 26–2.

DIET FOLLOWING GALLBLADDER AND COMBINED ABDOMINOPERINEAL RESECTIONS

Following surgery such as removal of the gallbladder or combined abdominoperineal

---

[9]Jordan, G. L.: Treatment of the dumping syndrome. J.A.M.A., *167*:1062, 1958.

[10]Pittman, A. C., and Robinson, F. W.: Dumping syndrome—Control by diet. J. Am. Dietet. A., *34*:596, 1958; and *40*:108, 1962.

[11]Scott, H. W., et al.: The dumping syndrome. Gastroenterology, 37:194, 1959.

TABLE 26–2   SIX-FEEDING, HIGH PROTEIN, LOW CARBOHYDRATE, HIGH FAT DRY DIET
FOR PATIENTS WITH DUMPING SYNDROME SYMPTOMS[11]

(Approximately 3000 Kcalories, 150 Gm. Protein, 225 Gm. Fat, 100 Gm. Carbohydrate)

SAMPLE MENU

BREAKFAST	LUNCHEON OR SUPPER	DINNER
2 eggs prepared with 1 tbsp. butter or margarine 2 strips of bacon 1 thin slice of bread 2 tsp. butter or margarine	4 ounces of chicken 1 serving A vegetable* 1 serving B vegetable† 4 tsp. butter, margarine or mayonnaise	4 ounces of beef 1 small potato or substitute 1 serving A vegetable* 3 tbsp. butter, margarine or mayonnaise
MID-MORNING	**MID-AFTERNOON**	**LATE EVENING**
2 ounces cottage cheese with 2 tbsp. cream 1 thin slice of bread 2 tsp. butter or margarine	2 ounces meat, fish, poultry or cheese 2 thin slices of bread 2 tsp. butter, margarine or mayonnaise	Same as mid-afternoon

No sugar, jelly, jams, candy, malts, pastries, cookies, sweetened milk products, sweetened carbonated beverages or alcohol permitted.

Fluids (tea, coffee, broths) may be taken one hour before or after meals. May have 4 to 6 ounces of tomato or V-8 juice and 8 ounces of milk daily.

*A vegetables—Select a cooked vegetable from List II A, page 402.
†B vegetables—Select a cooked vegetable from List II B, page 403.

[11]Scott, H. W., et al.: The dumping syndrome. Gastroenterology, 37:194, 1959.

resections, oral feedings are usually resumed early. A sample schedule, as suggested by Pollack and Halpern, is as follows:

1st day (day of operation): Necessary transfusions and the adequate intravenous feeding formula, outlined on page 377, are given.

2nd day: Add small amounts of liquids (tea, clear broth, gelatin, and ginger ale), without milk or fruit juice, ad libitum.

3rd day: Liquids, including skim milk and fruit juices, as tolerated. The intravenous feeding is continued, except that glucose in water, plus vitamins, is substituted for part of the saline solution.

4th day: Small amounts of high protein liquid mixture are added as tolerated. On this day 1 liter of the protein hydrolysate can be omitted from the intravenous feeding schedule.

5th day: Increase food as tolerated. At least 70 to 100 gm. protein should be provided in the oral feeding. Furthermore, oral vitamin capsules should be started. All intravenous feedings can usually be discontinued.

6th day: Usually the General Diet (p. 316) can be taken. The Recommended Dietary Allowances on nutrients for normal, healthy individuals should probably be increased about 100 per cent (except for calories) throughout convalescence, with the protein intake especially high.

Some patients who have had the gallbladder removed may be more comfortable on the low fat diet for several weeks, or even months,

following the operation since there is the possibility, when large amounts of fat are eaten, of pain from contractions of the tissues irritated and inflamed by surgery. (See p. 370 and Table 25–3.)

DIET FOLLOWING INTESTINAL RESECTIONS (COLOSTOMY, ILEOSTOMY)

Patients who undergo small or large bowel resection for treatment of cancer, diverticulitis, ileitis, local abscess, perforation or obstruction are denied all oral feedings for a limited period. The parenteral feeding outline under Routine Diet Regimen (p. 377) is continued throughout the period of restricted oral intake. As food by mouth is gradually resumed, the amounts of intravenous feedings are proportionately reduced.

The oral feedings should be sufficient in calories, high in protein, low in residue, and low in fat. Fats are added to the diet as tolerated, which is of special significance in the patient with total or partial ileectomy since a considerable amount of fat absorption is believed to be restricted to the ileum. The less ileum remaining, the less absorption area, and dietary fat may need some restriction. In addition, certain other nutrients such as vitamin B_{12} may be absorbed mainly in the ileum and thus require parenteral administration. Multiple vitamin supplementation and iron medication are frequently given to maintain adequate nutrition. The dietary management progresses to a regular diet as soon as possible. During this period, the patient with a colostomy should observe the stools to determine which foods to eliminate in order to have good control of movements. Each person must learn which foods he should avoid. The list differs with individuals. Usually corn and dried beans are not tolerated by most people. The nurse is of great assistance in helping these people establish good eating habits and an adequate dietary regimen.

Patients with a colostomy or an ileostomy require considerable sympathetic understanding from the nurse and the entire medical, surgical, and dietary team. It is difficult for the person to accept his condition and the problems involved in maintaining bowel regularity. Plans to have these patients meet other people who have undergone similar surgery will help them to adjust to the new problems by comparing and discussing the difficulties involved.

DIET FOLLOWING RECTAL SURGERY

Following rectal surgery such as hemorrhoidectomy, feedings can usually be resumed within 24 hours or sooner, depending upon whether a general anesthetic has been administered. Postoperative regimen varies. Some surgeons prefer to give a low fiber diet, with limited residue, to discourage early bowel movements. Others permit a normal diet and encourage defecation facilitated by mineral oil or a stool softener. Prolonged use of the mineral oil is discouraged because it interferes with the absorption of fat-soluble vitamins. In either case, a normal diet is resumed when tolerated and the patient instructed in a diet to avoid constipation. (See p. 350.)

DIET FOLLOWING GENERAL SURGERY

The diet prescribed for patients who have undergone orthopedic surgery or tooth extractions, or who have been involved in minor accidents, can usually advance at a much faster rate than the slower paced diet program after gastrointestinal surgery. Frequently, the patient can tolerate the full liquid diet by the second day, the soft diet on the third day, and the general diet on the fourth day or he may go from a liquid diet to a general diet by the second day. The patient's condition determines the diet order. Attention must be directed toward supplying adequate calories and liberal amounts of protein to compensate for losses. Vitamin supplements may or may not be indicated.

DIET FOLLOWING FRACTURES AND OTHER MECHANICAL TRAUMA

Following fractures of the long bones there is an increase in protein breakdown in well-nourished individuals, which is aggravated still further by prolonged immobilization in bed. The loss in protein (loss of nitrogen) is accompanied by loss of potassium, phosphorus and sulfur. Development of osteoporosis will coincide with loss in calcium due to immobilization. Severe functional imbalance and loss of fluids and electrolytes may take place.

DIETARY TREATMENT   Replacement of the losses is the aim of diet therapy. Proteins, calories and all nutrients need to be supplied in liberal amounts. About 150 gm. of protein, plus 3000 kcalories is recommended. Moderate restriction of calories and protein 100 to 150 gm. is indicated for overweight patients. Replacement of fluids and electrolytes is also required. If the patient cannot eat an adequate amount at meals, high protein, high calorie beverages can be served between meals as calorie allowance permits (see p. 374).

Fractures heal poorly when the tissues are depleted. Liberal protein in the diet favors deposition of calcium in the bones and formation of good callus.

DIET FOLLOWING TONSILLECTOMY

Following a tonsillectomy, very cold and very mild flavored foods bring the most comfort to a patient, and offer the most protection to prevent bleeding of the surgical area. Because the convalescent period is comparatively short, the nutritional adequacy of the diet is not so important.

For the first 24-hour postoperative period, these foods are recommended:

> Cold milk
> Milk beverages, such as malted milk and eggnogs
> Chocolate and vanilla ice cream
> Fruit ice
> Iced coffee
> Iced tea
> Pear, peach or prune juice

The following foods are usually added to the diet by the second day. Warm fluids and food may be started and cautiously replaced by hot foods as healing progresses.

> Strained soups
> Jellied consommé
> Enriched refined cooked cereals
> Soft-cooked or poached egg
> Milk toast (no crust)
> Soft puddings, custard, milk-rennet puddings and gelatin desserts
> Mashed potatoes and strained vegetables

Finely ground chicken or meat in broth or gravy; creamed fish
Fruit purée (whips)

The patient will gradually return to the normal diet within a week to ten days.

DIET FOLLOWING SURGERY OF THE MOUTH OR THE ESOPHAGUS

After extensive surgery of the mouth or esophagus, parenteral feedings are usually administered in the beginning, followed by tube feedings given by nasogastric tube or by direct feeding into the jejunum or stomach (p. 384), depending on the operative area. Since the patient may have to stay on such a schedule for a long period, or even permanently, it is of utmost importance that the formula be adequate in all nutrients. Either as a tube feeding or as a liquid diet, variety can be obtained by liquefying normally solid foods, such as potatoes, chopped meat, vegetables and fruit purées, in a food blender, or by forcing them through a sieve and adding liquids. (See Formulas for Use in Tube Feeding, Table 26–3, p. 383.) Commercial preparations of strained baby foods are widely available for use when labor and/or special devices needed for preparation are lacking.

Psychology of feeding, as previously outlined in Chapter 20, should be reviewed and put into practice here. The success of getting adequate nourishment into these patients is largely dependent upon the attention and encouragement given to them. Attractive dishes and service are important to stimulate the appetite.

DIET FOLLOWING BURNS

Severe burns are usually a surgical problem and frequently present a difficult problem in nutritional therapy. Vast quantities of protein are lost, the amount depending upon the extent and depth of the burn. If infection develops, the losses increase even further. Following severe burns there may be a daily negative nitrogen balance. In addition to losses of protein, much fluid and electrolytes (especially potassium and sodium chloride) are lost through exudation and must be replaced. Anemia may be an additional problem.

FLUIDS AND ELECTROLYTES   Therapy must be directed to counteract shock and to maintain life. Formerly, standard routine consisted of administering whole blood and plasma immediately. Recent reports, however, recommend giving less blood or no blood at all in the early fluid replacement therapy of the severely burned patient. Within the first few hours following severe thermal injury, the loss of fluids and electrolytes far overshadows that of red blood cells. The hemoglobin and hematocrit levels increase greatly within the first 24 to 48 hours after thermal injury. The addition of blood to that already sludged may do more harm than good. On the other hand, the provision of adequate fluid and electrolytes during the first few hours helps to prevent the development of shock. Individualized fluid therapy to maintain or to establish adequate urinary excretion is considered the most important consideration in the early resuscitation of the individual with extensive burns.[12] Current thinking is that blood therapy plays a role during the ensuing weeks and months of convalescence when there is chronic loss of erythrocytes and plasma through extensive burn sites. The anemia from severe burns does not respond well to administered iron; therefore, fairly frequent transfusions of whole blood or red blood cells may be necessary. Prevention of tissue depletion is essential for successful skin grafting.

DIETARY TREATMENT   An individualized high protein, high calorie, high vitamin diet is needed throughout convalescence. As much as 300 to 400 gm. of protein are sometimes necessary, and sufficient calories must be given to spare the existing body protein and to enhance the utilization of the new protein. As much as 3500 to 5000 kcalories a day, or more, may be indicated. Supplementary between meal beverages, high in protein and calories, are frequently necessary (see Chapter 43 for protein supplements and high protein recipes), as the patient is usually unable to take an adequate amount of the usual foods. Tube feedings (see Tables 26–1 and 26–3) are given if the patient is unable to eat or drink the large quantity of food required. Hyperalimentation therapy may be indicated in order for the person to obtain adequate nutrition. Vitamins should be supplied in quantities to meet the increased requirements. At least 1 gm. of vitamin C is needed daily.

Supportive nursing care is extremely important in carrying out a successful rehabilitation program in cases of severe burns. Anorexia and depression are problems with which the nurse has to cope in caring for these patients. It is important to keep a record of the calories and protein especially consumed by these patients and to find ways of involving the person in the selection of foods that appeal to him.

STERILE FOOD

Cancer patients undergoing chemotherapy are highly susceptible to infection. Regular

---

[12]Feller, I., and DeWeese, M. S.: A reappraisal of fluid therapy in the burned patient. J.A.M.A., *181*:361, 1962.

TABLE 26-3 FORMULA OF HIGH NUTRITIVE CONTENT FOR USE IN TUBE FEEDING*

(115 Gm. Protein; 3000 Calories)

DAILY FOOD INTAKE (Blenderized and strained)	QUANTITY		FOODSTUFFS				MINERALS		VITAMINS				
	Weight (Gm.)	Approximate Measure	KILO-CALORIES	Carbo-hydrate[1] (Gm.)	Protein (Gm.)	Fat (Gm.)	Ca (Gm.)	Fe (mg.)	A (I.U.)	Ascorbic Acid (mg.)	Thia-min (mg.)	Ribo-flavin (mg.)	Niacin Equiv. (mg.)
Milk, whole[2]	488	1 pint	330	24	17	19	0.58	0.4	780	5	0.18	0.84	4.6
Cream, 20 per cent	480	1 pint	1,000	19	14	96	0.47	0.2	3,960	6	0.14	0.68	4.4
Calf liver, raw, ground	120	4 oz. E.P.	170	5	23	6	0.01	12.7	27,000	43	0.25	3.74	25.0
Eggs	216	4 medium	300	trace	24	24	0.12	5.2	2,200	—	0.20	0.56	7.0
Brewer's yeast, dried	13	5 level teaspoons	385	5	5	—	0.01	2.4	—	—	1.27	0.72	6.2
Sucrose, glucose, lactose	100	½ cup	385	100	—	—	—	—	—	—	—	—	—
Milk powder, whole	128	1 cup	630	49	33	34	1.22	0.7	1,790	8	0.39	1.87	8.8
Applesauce[3]	60	4 level tablespoons	45	12	—	—	—	—	20	1	0.01	0.01	0.2
Orange juice	123	½ cup	55	14	1	—	0.02	—	230	61	0.10	0.03	0.2
TOTAL[4]			2,950	228	117	179	2.43	21.6	35,980	124	2.54	8.45	56.4

*Reprinted from Turner, D.: Handbook of Diet Therapy. 3rd ed. By permission of the University of Chicago Press, 1959, Chicago.

[1] Calories have been rounded off to nearest 5.

[2] Or milk equivalents.

[3] Apple powder or pectin may be added to prevent diarrhea.

[4] The mineral, vitamin, and protein content of this diet will exceed the Recommended Dietary Allowances for the normal adult. To meet additional caloric needs, further amounts of the above foods may be used and/or other sugars, starches and fats.

hospital food is not free of pathogenic organisms. It is unsuitable for patients who require a sterile environment to protect them from infection while undergoing treatment. Procedures for preparation and serving of sterile food have been developed.[13] These methods of preparation include autoclaving, baking in a dry oven and 300° F. "aseptic" cooking and "dipping" sterile canned foods in antiseptic solutions. Special procedures are followed to make sure that no food is contaminated before reaching the patient. Procedures in autoclaving foods and the foods suitable for germ-free environments are listed in the report by Watson and Bodey.[13]

ARTIFICIAL METHODS OF FEEDING

TUBE FEEDINGS   Tube feedings are most frequently employed in the nutritional therapy of surgical patients. When the patient is unable to take food by mouth following surgery, accidents, unconsciousness, or when part of the body has to be resected as in carcinoma of the esophagus, adequate nutrition must be supplied by a liquid meal which can be put through a tube. Such feedings may vary from a mixture of the foods served in the adequate normal diet finely homogenized in a mechanical blender and strained to ensure passage through the tube, to food combinations planned to meet specific therapeutic needs.

[13]Watson, P., and Bodey, G. P.: Sterile food service for patients in protected environments. J. Am. Dietet. A., 56:515, 1970.

A typical highly nutritious, high caloric combination of foods which may be used in a tube feeding, supplying approximately 115 gm. of protein, 180 gm. of fats, 230 gm. of carbohydrates, and 3000 calories is outlined in Table 26–3.

The amount of the feeding is designated by the physician's diet prescription. Additional calories may be supplied through the addition of oil, lactose, or heavy cream. The milk may be supplanted by all cream. Additional protein may be supplied through use of protein concentrates. Substitution of whole milk for cream will lower the fat content (and calories). To further reduce the fat (and calories), skim milk may be substituted for the whole milk and cream. If diarrhea is present, the addition of apple powder, pectin, Kaopectate or Kanana-Banana flakes may frequently furnish effective control.

There are a number of commercial tube feeding formulas available, designed to provide the variations in feeding content to meet the individual patient's needs or tolerances. These save time in preparation but are generally more expensive. Krehl[14] reported a study in which nine patients developed diarrhea while being given the usual skim milk-based formula. He replaced the formula with a soy bean preparation made by dilution of a can of the ready-prepared soy bean milk (Mull-Soy, Borden Co.) with an equal amount of water and fortification with vitamins. The bowel movement pattern returned to normal

[14]Krehl, W. A.: Tube feeding, J.A.M.A., 169:1153, 1959.

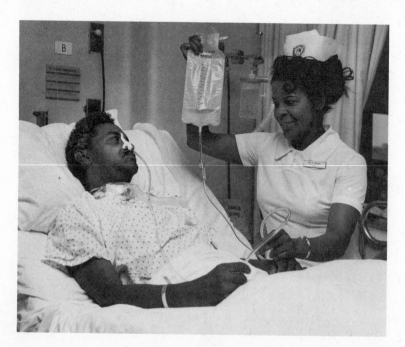

Figure 26–2   Tube feeding administered through a nasogastric tube. (Courtesy of Graduate Hospital of the University of Pennsylvania.) (Photo by Paul Axler.)

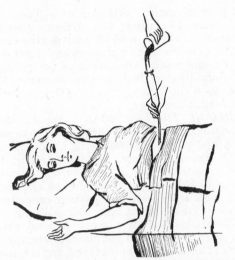

Figure 26-3   Fluid flows into the stomach by gravity. (McClain and Gregg: Scientific Principles in Nursing. The C. V. Mosby Company.)

limits in seven of the nine patients. Soy bean milk fortified with vitamins meets the recommended dietary allowances except for iron, which should be added if the formula must be used for a prolonged period of time. Table 26-1 contains six suggested formulas, with an approximate analysis of each, for use in tube feeding. The types of foods used can be readily obtained and easily prepared in the average home.

Tube feedings are usually administered through a nasogastric tube (Fig. 26-2). However, when the normal continuity of the esophagus is not intact, as in cancer of the esophagus, a gastrostomy is performed and a catheter is secured to the abdominal wall through which fluid nourishment may be given into the jejunum or stomach. The fluid flows into the stomach by gravity (Fig. 26-3). These patients need a great deal of en-

TABLE 26-4   ADULT HYPERALIMENTATION SOLUTION PREPARATION*

Unit Preparation of Base Solution		
Bulk Method (Pharmacy)		
165 gm anhydrous dextrose USP + 860 ml 5% dextrose in 5% fibrin hydrolysate		
Sterilization through 0.22μ membrane filter under laminar-flow filtered-air hood		
Volume	1,000	ml
Calories	1,000	kcal
Glucose	208	gm
Hydrolysates	43	gm
Nitrogen	6.0	gm
Sodium	8	mEq
Potassium	14	mEq
Single Unit Method (Ward or Pharmacy)		
350 ml 50% dextrose +		
750 ml 5% dextrose in 5% fibrin hydrolysate		
Aseptic mixing technique under laminar-flow filtered-air hood		
	1,100	ml
	1,000	kcal
	212	gm
	37	gm
	5.25	gm
	7	mEq
	13	mEq
Additions to Each Unit of Base Solution (Average Adult)		
Sodium (chloride)	40–50	mEq
Potassium (chloride)	30–40	mEq
Magnesium (sulfate)	4–5	mEq
Additions to Only One Unit Daily (Average Adult)		
Vitamin A	5,000–10,000	USP units
Vitamin D	500– 1,000	USP units
Vitamin E	2.5–5.0	IU
Ascorbic acid	250–500	mg
Thiamin hydrochloride	25–50	mg
Riboflavin	5–10	mg
Pyridoxine hydrochloride	7.5–15	mg
Niacin	50–100	mg
Pantothenic acid	12.5–25	mg
Optional Additions to One Unit (as indicated by serum studies)†		
Phytonadione	5–10	mg
Cyanocobalamin	10–30	μg
Folic acid	0.5–1.5	mg
Iron (dextriferron)	2.0–3.0	mg
Calcium (gluconate)	4.5–9	mEq
Phosphate (potassium acid salt)	4–10	mEq

*Micronutrients such as zinc, copper, manganese, cobalt, and iodine are present as contaminants in hydrolysate solutions, but may be given in plasma transfusion once or twice weekly if desired.

†Alternatively may be given intramuscularly in daily or weekly dosages.

From Dudrick, S. J., and Rhoads, J. E.: New horizons for intravenous feeding. J.A.M.A., *215*:943, 1971.

couragement to adjust to the situation. When administering the nourishment, the nurse can be of great assistance in establishing pleasant associations with the feedings and food. The tube feeding should be in an attractive pitcher placed on a neat clean tray with a napkin and tray cover. To avoid diarrhea and aid digestion, the tube feedings should be heated over hot water to body temperature and administered slowly. See Chapter 43 for beverages and protein supplements that could be used for tube feeding.

INTRAVENOUS HYPERALIMENTATION Positive nitrogen balance can be attained by providing all nutrients intravenously. It can be sustained for prolonged periods of time by the continuous infusion of complete intravenously administered diet. It is used for individuals severely debilitated and malnourished who are unable to obtain adequate nutrition orally or by peripheral intravenous feedings. Rehabilitation is hastened in such instances. Hyperalimentation may be useful for the treatment of such conditions as anorexia. Intravenous solutions formulated according to the nutrient requirement of an adult (Table 26–4) are fed through polyvinyl or siliconized rubber catheters inserted into the superior vena cava via a subclavian vein or an external

or internal jugular vein and are infused continuously by pump. The solution contains approximately 20 to 25 per cent dextrose, 4 to 5 per cent fibrin hydrolysates and 5 per cent additional solute consisting of all required vitamins, minerals and trace elements. Figure 26–4 shows a patient receiving hyperalimentative feeding.[15]

BLOOD TRANSFUSIONS   Whole blood transfusions play an important part in supplying food to the body following major surgery with excessive blood loss, in cases of hyperthyroidism, severe hemorrhage, certain cases of blood dyscrasia, and types of poisoning which decrease the oxygen capacity of erythrocytes (carbon monoxide poisoning).

Blood plasma or serum may be more easily prepared, stored and combined without danger of clotting than whole blood, and it is more widely used because typing or classification is not necessary. Blood plasma or serum is adequate to meet the needs of protein depletion which occurs in cases of burns and shock. If hemorrhage occurs to the extent of depleting the oxygen carrying capacity of the blood, red blood cells must be administered either in the form of whole blood or red cell suspension. Blood plasma or serum does not correct the anemia following hemorrhage or severe burns.

[15]Dudrick, S. J., and Rhoads, J. E.: New horizons for intravenous feeding. J.A.M.A., 215:939, 1971.

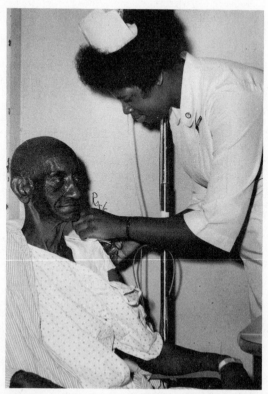

Figure 26–4   A patient receiving intravenous hyperalimentation. (Courtesy of Graduate Hospital of the University of Pennsylvania.) (Photo by Paul Axler.)

PROBLEMS AND SUGGESTED TOPICS FOR DISCUSSION

1. List the principles of diet treatment for a preoperative patient; a postoperative patient.
2. Give reasons for emphasis on (a) adequate protein therapy, (b) adequate fluid therapy, (c) adequate electrolyte therapy for a preoperative patient; a postoperative patient.
3. Keep a record of the food ingested in one day by a patient hospitalized for a colostomy. How adequate is his intake of food? What change will he make?
4. How will he need to modify his usual dietary pattern after postoperative phase is past?
5. How will the patient whom you have interviewed modify his regimen following gastrectomy?
6. Become familiar with the various types of tube feedings which are used for patients. What do they contain and determine whether what the patient actually receives meets his nutritional needs?
7. If you had the care of a severely burned patient what problems would you have in helping the patient receive the nutrients he needs?
8. Under what conditions would intravenous hyperalimentation be indicated?

SUGGESTED ADDITIONAL READING REFERENCES

Artz, C. P.: Recent development in burns. Am. J. Surg., 108:649, 1964.

Artz, C. P., et al.: Some recent developments in oral feedings for optimal nutrition in burns. Am. J. Clin. Nutr. 4:642, 1956.

Barker, H. G.: Supplementation of protein and caloric needs in the surgical patient. Am. J. Clin. Nutr., 3: 466, 1955.

Biggar, B. L., et al.: Nutrition following gastric resection. J. Am. Dietet. A., 37:344, 1960.

Bisgard, J. D.: Subtotal gastric resection for acute perforated peptic ulcers. J.A.M.A., 160:363, 1956.

Blocker, T. G., Jr., et al.: The care of patients with burns. Nursing Outlook, 6:382, 1958.

Crandon, J. H.: Nutrition in surgical patients. J.A.M.A., 158:264, 1955.

Dudrick, S. J., and Rhoads, J. E.: New horizons for intravenous feeding. J.A.M.A., 215:939, 1971.

Eagle, J. F., et al.: Parenteral fluid therapy of burns. J.A.M.A., 174:1589, 1960.

Editorial. Dumping syndrome. J.A.M.A., 168:1229, 1958.

Elman, R.; Protein needs in surgical patients. J. Am. Dietet. A., 32:524, 1956.

Fason, M. F.: Controlling bacterial growth in tube feedings. Am. J. Nurs., 67:1246, 1967.

Feller, I., and DeWeese, M. S.: A reappraisal of fluid therapy in the burned patient. J.A.M.A., 181:361, 1962.

Hayes, M. A.: Postoperative diet therapy. J. Am. Dietet. A., 35:17, 1959.

Jordan, G. L.: The postgastrectomy syndromes. J.A.M.A., 163:1485, 1957.

Jordan, G. L.: Treatment of the dumping syndrome. J.A.M.A., 167:1062, 1958.

Krehl, W. A.: Tube feeding. J.A.M.A., 169:1153, 1959.

Machella, T. E.: Postsurgical problems of the gastrointestinal tract. J.A.M.A., 174:2111, 1960.

Magruder, L., et al.: Gastric resection: Nursing care. Am. J. Nursing, 61:76, 1961.

Mecray, P., Jr.: Nutrition and wound healing. Am. J. Clin. Nutr. 3:461, 1955.

Pareira, M. D., et al.: Therapeutic nutrition with tube feeding. J.A.M.A., 156:810, 1954.

Pearson, E., et al.: Metabolic derangements in burns. J. Am. Dietet. A., 32:223, 1965.

Pittman, A. C., and Robinson, F. W.: Dietary management of the dumping syndrome. J. Am. Dietet. A., 40:108, 1962.

Postoperative distention and fruit juices: Questions and answers. J.A.M.A., 194:244, 1965.

Review. Burns and negative balances. Nutr. Rev., 17:164, 1959.

Robinson, F. W., and Pittman, A. C.: Dietary management of postgastrectomy dumping syndrome. Surg. Gynec. and Obst., 104:529, 1957.

Schwartz, P. L.: Ascorbic acid in wound healing—A review. J. Am. Dietet. A., 56:497, 1970.

Scribner, B. H., et al.: Long term parenteral nutrition. J.A.M.A., 212:457, 1970.

Smith, A. V.: Nasogastric tube feedings. Am. J. Nursing, 57:1451, 1957.

Vanamee, P.: Nutrition after gastric resection. J.A.M.A., 172:2045, 1960.

Watson, P., and Bodey, G. P.: Sterile food service for patients in protected environments. J. Am. Dietet. A., 56:515, 1970.

White, D. R.: I have an ileostomy. Am. J. Nursing, 61:51, 1961.

Williams, R. D., and Zollinger, R. M.: Principles of surgical nutrition. Am. J. Clin. Nutr., 3:449, 1955.

Willis, M. T., and Postlewait, R. W.: Dietary problems after gastric resection. J. Am. Dietet. A., 40:111, 1962.

Wohl, M. G., and Goodhart, R. S. (ed.): Modern Nutrition In Health and Disease. 4th ed. Philadelphia, Lea & Febiger, 1968, Chapter on Nutrition in the care of the surgical patient.

Zollinger, R. M., and Ellison, E. H.: Nutrition after gastric operations. J.A.M.A., 154:811, 1954.

UNIT TEN
DISEASES OF
ALLERGY AND
THE SKIN

Chapter 27
*NUTRITION IN
DISEASES OF
ALLERGY AND
THE SKIN*

ALLERGY

DEFINITION   Allergy may be defined as a condition of exaggerated specific susceptibility to a substance which is harmless in similar amounts to the majority of persons. The allergies are many and varied. In this text the discussion will be limited to food allergy. It is estimated that allergies affect about 10 per cent of the population.

CLASSIFICATION   The offending substance, the *allergen*, may gain access to the body by *ingestion, inhalation, direct contact,* or by *injection* (drugs, serums). Allergic individuals are believed to have groups of body cells known as "shock organs" which are susceptible to allergens. These may be located in almost any tissue of the body. It is postulated that much of the allergic symptomatology is due to histamine being released from the tissues in response to the irritating agent, as after the eating of certain foods or contact with offending materials.

MANIFESTATIONS   The tendency to allergy is possibly inherited, although the inheritance is seldom specific. Several manifestations of allergy may appear in the same individual, varying from a minor reaction of slight eye or nose itching or rash to a severe gastrointestinal attack. Stunted growth and malnutrition have been traced to an allergy. Bronchial asthma, hay fever, dermatitis, urticaria, eczema, acne, migraine, and cardiovascular disorders are some of the observed manifestations of an allergy which may be caused by foods. Anorexia and food aversion may be due to an allergy to one or more common foods.

COMMON FOOD ALLERGIES

A person may become allergic to a food or other allergen at any age. Children are frequently attacked; however, there is a higher incidence in adults than in children. (Allergy in children is discussed in Chapter 17.) The sensitiveness may wear off or the patient may become desensitized. In later life individuals may be entirely free from the disturbance that affected them in childhood. Foods that belong to the same botanic group may produce a similar allergic reaction; for example, cabbage and cauliflower; orange and grapefruit. Furthermore, an allergic individual who experiences a reaction to a given food may on another day eat the same food without reaction. This may be due to his general physical condition. An allergic response may occur only when the individual is fatigued or emotionally upset. These are some of the numerous observations that baffle allergists.

PROTEIN   Any food can produce the allergic manifestations. However, it is believed that protein is the important factor in food allergy, although the offending food may contain only a minute amount of protein. Among the *most common offenders are wheat, milk, eggs, fish, shellfish, strawberries, tomatoes,* and *chocolate.* Others to be considered are pork, oranges, spices, condiments, nuts, corn, asparagus, spinach, cabbage, celery, onion, garlic and rhubarb. The ingestion of the smallest quantity of an offending food may produce symptoms or reaction; therefore, it is necessary for the allergic individual to analyze prepared foods and food combinations before eating them. For example, sausage may contain wheat, and the small amount of wheat could cause an allergic disturbance.

It has been found that 30 per cent of the persons who suffered from an idiosyncrasy to some foods were uncomfortable after taking milk and cream. This is important for the nurse to know since she helps to feed and care for the sick. When a patient says he cannot drink milk, he should not be told he is "imagining things" . . . "milk is a health food" . . . he "must drink at least a pint a day." Although milk is an excellently nutritious food, a patient may be allergic to it! If milk is the offender, then cheese, ice cream and any product made with milk must also be omitted. However, thoroughly boiled milk or evaporated milk, having had the offending proteins denatured, may sometimes be consumed without evoking symptoms in individuals who are allergic to raw or pasteurized milk.

In some cases of food intolerance, allergy may not be the basic cause. For example, some patients with an intolerance for milk have been found when tested to have a lack of hydrochloric acid in the stomach, which is necessary for the proper digestion of milk. When given hydrochloric acid along with the meals, they are able to tolerate milk and develop a natural taste for it. In other individuals an intolerance for milk may be caused by rapid emptying of the stomach, the partially digested milk curd going into the small intestine and causing cramp-like pains.

FOOD HISTORY   A carefully detailed food history (see p. 19) should be taken of every individual suspected of having an allergy. The food history often discloses specific food allergies through the listing of disliked foods or foods that disagree.

FOOD DIARY   If a patient writes a food diary, recording the foods eaten preceding the appearance of allergic symptoms, the data will be useful for diagnosis.

ALLERGENS OTHER THAN FOOD

Most persons allergic to one or more foods are usually sensitive to one or more of the common inhalants. House dust, feathers, animal hair, horse dander, pollens, molds, grain dust, silk, wool, bacteria, plant oils or resin, orris root, drugs, cosmetics, and tobacco smoke are potent allergens. Many of them are met in everyday living and are difficult to avoid. Asthma and hay fever seem to be caused by one or more of the inhalants.

TESTS FOR ALLERGY

In addition to the food history and food diary, other aids employed to establish a diagnosis of a food allergy are (1) skin tests and (2) elimination diets.

SKIN TESTS   The most popular and well known of the skin tests is the *scratch test*. A series of scratches are made on the arm or back of the patient and a solution containing the suspected offending allergen is dropped into each scratch. If the person is allergic to any of the solutions used, welts or wheals surrounded by a red or inflamed area may develop within a few minutes, or there may be a delayed reaction which will not manifest itself for a day or so. The greater the area of the reaction, the more potent is the allergen to the patient. Because some foods do not react well to the skin tests and may produce negative skin tests in some individuals, or vice versa, that is, a food may exhibit a positive skin test without causing allergic symptoms, the scratch test cannot be relied upon for complete accuracy. However, when properly interpreted, it may throw some light on the diagnostic problem.

Another skin test, the *patch test*, is administered by applying the suspected antigen on a filter paper and placing it on a certain patch of skin and then covering with cellophane; readings are made in from 2 to 4 days.

In the *intradermal test* a solution of food extracts is injected into the superficial layers of the skin. The interpretation and the accuracy of the reactions are similar to those described for the scratch and patch tests.

ELIMINATION TEST DIETS   An elimination diet may be defined as an allowance of foods which have rarely produced sensitivity in human patients. Because of the fallibility of skin tests, the use of trial diets for suspected food allergy is considered the most reliable test. The elimination test diets most frequently used are those devised by Rowe,[1] outlined in Table 27-1. He has devised a series of four different test diets which are based on a few carefully selected foods chosen from those which have been found least likely to cause allergic symptoms. Besides, each diet contains none of the foods found in the other three diets. The patient is placed on one of the diets which, on the basis of diet history, food diary, and/or skin tests, is least likely to produce allergy symptoms. The diet is followed for a period of 1 to 3 weeks, unless severe adverse reactions occur in the meantime. If there is no change in symptoms and no positive reaction, another diet is tried for a similar period until all diets have been used. If at the end of the trial diets, no change in symptoms and no new reaction appears, all foods on the combined diets may be used and the allergy is probably other than food in origin. However, should relief of symptoms appear while the patient is on any one of the trial diets, he is kept on the diet for another week or so. Gradually other foods are added to the basic diet. Wheat, eggs, and milk are the foods added at the conclusion of the test because these three foods have been found to cause allergy symptoms most frequently. If the patient shows allergic symptoms following the addition of a specific food to the basic diet, that food (or foods) is suspected of causing the allergy.

TREATMENT OF ALLERGY

Removal of the offending food or foods from the diet, or desensitization are two possible methods of treatment for allergy. In patients with severe allergic manifestations,

[1]Rowe, A. H.: Elimination Diets and the Patient's Allergies. Philadelphia, Lea & Febiger, 1944.

TABLE 27-1   ROWE ELIMINATION DIETS*

DIET 1	DIET 2	DIET 3	DIET 4
Rice	Corn	Tapioca	Milk‡
Tapioca	Rye	White potato	Tapioca
Rice biscuit	Corn pone	Breads made of any combination of	Cane sugar
Rice bread	Corn-rye muffins	soy, lima bean, and potato starch	
	Rye bread	and tapioca flours	
	Ry-Krisp		
Lettuce	Beets	Tomato	
Chard	Squash	Carrot	
Spinach	Asparagus	Lima beans	
Carrot	Artichoke	String beans	
Sweet potato or yam		Peas	
Lamb	Chicken (no hens)	Beef	
	Bacon	Bacon	
Lemon	Pineapple	Lemon	
Grapefruit	Peach	Grapefruit	
Pears	Apricot	Peach	
	Prune	Apricot	
Cane sugar	Cane or beet sugar	Cane sugar	
Sesame oil	Mazola	Sesame oil	
Olive oil†	Sesame oil	Soybean oil	
Salt	Salt	Salt	
Gelatin, plain or flavored with	Gelatin, plain or flavored with	Gelatin, plain or flavored with	
lime or lemon	pineapple	lime or lemon	
Maple syrup or syrup made	Karo corn syrup	Maple syrup or syrup made	
with cane sugar flavored with	White vinegar	with cane sugar flavored with	
maple	Royal baking powder	maple	
Royal baking powder	Baking soda	Royal baking powder	
Baking soda	Cream of tartar	Baking soda	
Cream of tartar	Vanilla extract	Cream of tartar	
Vanilla extract		Vanilla extract	
Lemon extract		Lemon extract	

Sample Menus for Rowe Elimination Diets

DIET 1	DIET 2	DIET 3
BREAKFAST	**BREAKFAST**	**BREAKFAST**
Grapefruit half	Stewed prunes	Grapefruit half
Cooked rice with maple syrup	Corn flakes	Soybean biscuit with peach
Sautéed lamb liver (using oil	Bacon	marmalade
allowed)	Rye toast with apricot jam	Bacon
LUNCHEON OR SUPPER	**LUNCHEON OR SUPPER**	**LUNCHEON OR SUPPER**
Lamb patties	Cold sliced chicken	Beef liver and bacon
Carrots	Asparagus tips vinaigrette	Lima beans
Spinach with lemon slices	(made with allowed oil and	Sliced tomatoes
Rice bread with grapefruit mar-	vinegar)	Potato flour biscuit with apricot
malade	Corn-rye muffin with apricot	jam
Lime gelatin	jam	Lime gelatin with sliced peaches
Lemonade	Fresh peach slices	Lemonade
	Apricot juice	
DINNER	**DINNER**	**DINNER**
Roast leg of lamb	Chicken roasted with prunes	Boiled beef with carrots, potato
Baked sweet potato	Baked squash	and peas
Head lettuce with allowed oil	Pickled beets and artichoke	Grapefruit sections with allowed
and lemon juice	hearts	oil and lemon juice
Rice biscuit with grapefruit	Ry-Krisp with apricot jam	Apricot tapioca
marmalade	Pineapple gelatin	
Baked pear	Apricot juice	
Grapefruit juice		

*Rowe, A. H.: Elimination Diets and the Patient's Allergies. 2nd ed. Philadelphia, Lea & Febiger, 1944.
†Allergy to it may occur with or without allergy to olive pollen. Mazola may be used if corn allergy is not present.
‡Milk should be taken, up to 2 or 3 quarts a day. Plain cottage cheese and cream may be used. Tapioca cooked with milk and milk sugar may be taken.

the hormones, corticotropin and cortisone, have been found to be highly efficient drugs for the symptomatic *control* of all types of allergies. They are not used to replace treatment directed against the cause of the allergy, but to relieve severe symptoms. The symptoms return promptly upon cessation of the drug.

DESENSITIZATION   To develop tolerance for the offending food, the food allergen is excluded from the diet for an indefinite period. The length of time to build up the tolerance varies with the individual; it may be weeks, months or years, or it may never occur. Following the period of complete abstinence from the offending food, tiny amounts are given by mouth, and the size of the servings gradually increased until average food portions are tolerated by the patient.

A patient will more likely develop an immunity to a mild allergen rather than to a food which has produced severe symptoms. If the offending allergen is a protective food, such as milk, meat or eggs, desensitization is important. Seasonal foods, such as strawberries, may not be worth the bother of immunization to the patient.

ELIMINATION DIET TREATMENT   The importance of elimination diets in the diagnosis of an allergy has been discussed. Elimination diets are also prescribed in the treatment of an allergy. Some patients may find it necessary to avoid continuously certain foods to which they are hypersensitive. Following are outlined the more common food allergy diets,[2] listing the foods to avoid for each.

MILK-POOR DIET

Avoid
Milk, buttermilk, cream, as such and in prepared foods, as ice cream, sodas, milk sherbet, Bavarian cream mousses, custards, gravies, cream sauces, soups, chowders.
Prepared flour mixes for home cooking.
Malted milk, hot chocolate or cocoa prepared with milk.
Cheese.
Evaporated, powdered, condensed milk (bakery products, as pies, breads and cakes containing small amounts of cooked milk can often be tolerated).
Butter and oleomargarine can usually be permitted in modest amounts. (Traces of milk are present.)
Study the label on packaged foods for evidence of milk or milk products content.

EGG-POOR DIET

Avoid
Eggs: Fresh, frozen, powdered, cooked in any form.
Egg-containing foods, such as:
Soups, broths made with egg.
Prepared flour mixes for home cooking.
Waffles, doughnuts, pretzels.

Pancakes, griddle cakes, pastries, French toast.
Macaroons, meringues, frostings.
Cakes, cookies, unless known to be egg-free.
Breads with glazed crust.
Foods breaded with egg mixture.
Sausages, croquettes, meat cakes, containing egg as binder.
Poultry, especially chicken, if fricasseed or in broth.
Salad dressings, unless known to be egg-free; Hollandaise, mayonnaise, and egg sauces.
Ice cream and sherbets, unless known to be egg-free.
Custards, cream candies, fondants, Bavarian cream.
Marshmallows.
Baking powder containing egg white.
Prepared drinks containing egg or egg powder for insomnia or underweight.
Study the labels on packaged foods for evidence of egg in any form.
Avoid virus vaccine made in egg, as for influenza, spotted fever, yellow fever.

SEAFOOD-FREE DIET

Avoid
Fish, shellfish, fresh, canned, smoked, pickled; fish liver oils, and concentrates in vitamin preparations.
Fish and shellfish stews, bisques, broths, soups, salad, hors d'oeuvres, caviar.
Avoiding licking labels, which may contain a fish glue adhesive.
Avoid injections of fish origin in the treatment of varicose veins.

WHEAT-POOR DIET

Avoid
White, whole wheat, cracked wheat flour in breads, waffles, griddle cakes, doughnuts, muffins, pastries, pies, cakes, crackers, spaghetti, macaroni, dumplings, pretzels, zwieback, noodles.
Corn bread, unless known to be wheat-free.
Soy bread, unless known to be wheat-free.
Rye bread, unless known to be wheat-free.
Gluten bread.
Breakfast cereals, dry or cooked, containing wheat, whole wheat, cream soups, Farina or bran.
Custards, gravies, sauces, containing wheat.
Breaded foods prepared with wheat.
Coffee substitutes containing wheat; beer; ale.
Prepared meats, as sausages, frankfurters, meat loaf, croquettes made with wheat.
Prepared mixes for biscuits, muffins, pastries, pie crusts, cookies.
Study the label on prepared foods for evidences of wheat or wheat product content.

NUT-POOR DIET

Avoid
Nuts, of all types, also peanuts (although a member of the bean family), cottonseed meal in health and laxative breads, soybean bread.
Nut crumbs on cookies, cake icings, ice cream.
Candies containing nuts.
Salad oils, lard substitutes, margarines made of cocoanut, soybean, cottonseed or peanut oils (many are so made). (Olive oil permitted.)

Individuals highly sensitive to nuts are often allergic to seeds, such as cottonseed, flaxseed, mustard (by external application in poultices, as well as when ingested as food), beans, peas. Legumes, such as peas, beans, lentils, are often allergenic factors in the patient sensitive to nuts, but some patients tolerate legumes, such as peanuts, despite high degrees of nut sensitivity.

[2]Wohl, M. G., and Goodhart, R. S.: Modern Nutrition in Health and Disease. 3rd ed. Philadelphia, Lea & Febiger, 1964, pp. 970–971. Used by permission.

INSTRUCTING THE PATIENT   Patients who follow an elimination diet program for a long period require careful supervision. It is not sufficient to instruct the patient to omit specific offending foods. The essential, nutritious foods should be included in the diet if possible. If foods such as milk, meat or eggs are eliminated from the dietary, adequate substitutions or supplements must be made. Malnutrition must be guarded against from self-inflicted, but often unjustified, curtailment of the diet.

A number of procedures have been advocated for the treatment of foods to render them less antigenic. One of these procedures is the denaturation of food. This is done by chemical treatment or by heat and is both simple and useful. For example, denatured milk (boiled, evaporated, and powdered) is valuable prophylactically. Milk substitutes, such as soybean milk or meat base milk, may at times be useful to serve the same purpose. Patients who are allergic to wheat can substitute rice or barley.

Rowe has emphasized the importance of well-planned menus and recipes to protect the patient's state of nutrition during a restricted diet program. Bizarre and unbalanced diets which result in deficiency diseases are frequently encountered when careless instructions are given and followed. Vitamin and mineral supplements are often necessary. For example, if milk must be omitted from the diet, there must be proper substitution of other foods, and probably calcium given by supplemental medication to maintain adequate nutrition. (See Chapter 43 for allergy recipes.) Additional wheat-, milk-, and egg-free recipes are available in a booklet, "Allergy Recipes," from the American Dietetic Association, 620 North Michigan Avenue, Chicago, Illinois, 60611.

PROGNOSIS

The prognosis for allergy varies with the individual. Some patients are cured, others are improved, while still others receive very little aid through treatment. The patient must be impressed with the fact that continuous adherence to the program is necessary to expect beneficial results. The duration of the treatment depends upon the individual; it may be weeks, months or years.

Careful, frequent checkups of the patient are essential to avoid the unnecessary exclusion of foods and to ingest an adequate diet to correct mistakes. Psychosomatic medicine enters into the treatment of allergy since some patients prefer clinging to symptoms rather than getting well; others develop the emotional tension typical of any recurrent disease.

SKIN DISEASES

NUTRITION AND SKIN DISEASE   Persons with skin diseases which result in unattractive complexions frequently succumb to the bewitching promises of advertisements and the quackery of food faddists. Many erratic diets, in various combinations, have been used and eventually discarded, in the treatment of skin disorders. Needless restrictions are often enforced without adequate proof of their usefulness.

While dietary inadequacy, whether primary or conditioned, may be associated with dermatologic lesions which can respond to proper therapy, probably most do not respond to specific therapy with vitamins or diet. Specific therapy directed toward the skin disorder without attention to the patient's nutritional status as a whole can be of definite harm. Nutritional deficiencies are discussed in Chapter 34.

Krehl[3] and Lorincz[4] point out that dermatoses are the most common problem in the United States and are often associated with obesity. The obese person has excessive fat folds which foster conditions leading to intertrigo. Decreased caloric intake with exercise is required therapy. In technically underdeveloped countries, the general dermatologic changes associated with undernutrition are extremely common, and improvement of the protein intake, both as to quality and quantity, seems to be the big problem. Any skin disorder is a problem for the physician or specialist to solve, not the beautician or food faddist. Only a few of the more prevalent skin diseases, in which diet has been extensively involved in their management, will be discussed.

PSORIASIS

Psoriasis attacks both the young and old, and it has no regard for sex or social status. In about 80 per cent of cases, there is a family history of the disorder. Because it comes and goes, it is doubtful whether therapy is valuable or whether improvement coincides with the normal course of the malady. Sun seems to benefit the condition, as most victims improve in the summer. The most prevalent theory is that it is caused by a disturbance in fat metabolism. Since the etiology is unknown, the cure is unknown. However, relief is often possible. ACTH (adrenocorticotrophic hormone) and cortisone control the lesions, but the effect is temporary.

[3]Krehl, W. A.: Skin disease and nutritional therapy. J. Am. Dietet. A., 35:923, 1959.
[4]Lorincz, A. L.: Nutrition in relation to dermatology. J.A.M.A., *166*:1862, 1958.

Good health must be maintained and nervousness alleviated. Many diets have been tried with varying results. Citrin, made from fresh lemons, and sarsaparilla preparations have been reported favorably as constituents of the diet treatment. Vitamins A, D and ascorbic acid are given credit, too. For years a diet free from fat, or one very low in protein, has been used with moderate effectiveness. Currently, the role of sulfur amino acid metabolism is being investigated.

ACNE VULGARIS

Acne vulgaris appears most frequently during adolescence (Fig. 27–1), but may present itself at any age. It is a chronic, inflammatory disease of the sebaceous glands, resulting from blocking of the secretions and the formation of blackheads. Its unsightliness affects the personality because the lesions appear at a time in life when boys and girls want to look attractive. In addition, severe acne leaves scars.

Until recently, most authorities believed the condition resulted from an intolerance to carbohydrates. In 1933 Wise and Sulzberger advanced the theory from their observations that the acne skin reaction may be due to an idiosyncrasy toward specific carbohydrate items rather than to the high carbohydrate intake. They believe chocolate and white bread to be the greatest offenders. Also, these research workers advise against the use of iodine and bromine. Iodized salt is avoided but sodium chloride is given in tablet form to facilitate the excretion of the offending chemicals.

In 1936 Crawford and Swartz placed ten patients suffering with acne vulgaris on a high carbohydrate diet supplemented with daily intravenous injections of dextrose. They observed distinct improvement in five (50 per cent) of the cases; two were questionable as to improvement, and three were unchanged.

Other authorities believe that fats tend to bring about acne vulgaris and advocate the restriction or exclusion of fatty and fried foods.

The treatment is variable. Baird[5] suggests no rigid diet restrictions be enforced but advises against excess carbohydrates, especially candy and soft sweetened beverages; also that fatty foods such as chocolate, fried foods, nuts and peanut butter be omitted from the diet. The diet should be generous in lean meat, fruits and vegetables. Milk should be consumed in adequate amounts, but not in excess. The diet should be simple but adequate, balanced to avoid excess of calories and excess gain in weight.

PROBLEMS AND SUGGESTED TOPICS FOR DISCUSSION

1. What are the most common allergenic foods? List suitable substitutions that can be made for each of these foods to keep the diet nutritionally adequate.
2. What are the common methods used to diagnose a food allergy? What is the procedure for using the Rowe Elimination Test Diets?
3. Plan menus for 1 week for a patient instructed to follow Rowe's Elimination Diet No. 2. Check for adequacy.
4. If a patient is allergic to milk, what foods in what amounts will supply 800 mg. calcium?
5. Obtain a dietary history of a patient suspected of having a food allergy who is in the hospital ward or in the outpatient clinic.
   (a) List the foods to which he may be hypersensitive.
   (b) Have the patient plan 3 days' menus.
   (c) Analyze the nutritional adequacy of the menus, considering calories, proteins, calcium, iron and the vitamins.
   (d) How could the patient desensitize himself to the allergen?
6. Study the relationship of dietary treatment to skin diseases besides those described in the text. For example, study the skin diseases seborrheic eczema and urticaria.
7. Interview a boy or girl with acne vulgaris. How adequate is their diet? What changes are they willing to make in their present pattern?

SUGGESTED ADDITIONAL READING REFERENCES

Cooke, R. A.: Diagnosis and management of allergy in general practice. New York J. Med., p. 3025, Dec. 15, 1952.

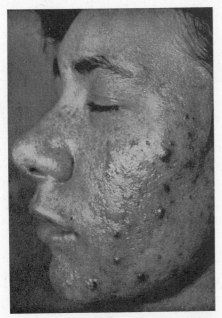

Figure 27–1   Acne vulgaris. Note oily seborrhea scars and pustules. (From Andrews: Diseases of the Skin.)

[5]Baird, J. W.: Acne. A new approach to an old problem. J. Pediat., 52:152, 1958.

Cooke, R. A.: The scope of allergy. New York J. Med., p. 3141, Nov. 1, 1955.

Cormia, F. E.: Acne vulgaris. Am. J. Nursing, 57:198, 1957.

Criep, L. H.: The march of allergy. J.A.M.A., 166:572, 1958.

Feinberg, S. M., and Feinberg, A. R.: Allergy—As it is and as it might be. J.A.M.A., 162:529, 1956.

Fries, J. H.: Milk allergy—Diagnostic aspects and the role of milk substitutes. J.A.M.A., 165:1542, 1957.

Hubler, W. R.: Unsaturated fatty acids in acne. A.M.A. Arch. Derm., 79:644, 1959.

Kessler, W. R.: Food allergy. Pediatrics, 21:523, 1958.

Krehl, W. A.: Skin disease and nutritional therapy. J. Am. Dietet. A., 35:923, 1959.

Lorincz, A. L.: Nutrition in relation to dermatology. J.A.M.A., 166:1862, 1958.

Pratt, E. L.: Food allergy and food intolerance in relation to the development of good eating habits. Pediatrics, 21:642, 1958.

Ratner, B., et al.: Allergenicity of modified and processed foodstuffs. Ann. Allergy, 10:675, 1952.

Review. Food Allergy. Nutr. Rev., 9:83, 1951.

Rowe, A. H., et al.: Bronchial asthma due to food allergy alone in 95 patients. J.A.M.A., 169:1158, 1959.

Speer, F.: Food allergy in childhood. Arch. Pediat., 75:363, 1958.

Withers, O. R., and Hale, R.: Food allergy—A review of the literature. Ann. Allergy, 14:384, 1956.

Wohl, M. G., and Goodhart, R. S. (ed.): Modern Nutrition in Health and Disease. 3rd ed. Philadelphia, Lea & Febiger, 1964, Chapter 28, Nutrition in the allergies; and Chapter 30, Nutrition and diseases of the skin.

Zohn, B.: Prophylaxis in allergy. New York J. Med. p. 1527, May 1, 1958.

Chapter 28

UNIT ELEVEN
DISEASES OF
METABOLISM AND
THE ENDOCRINE
GLANDS

*METABOLIC
DISORDERS
RELATED TO
NUTRITION*

DIABETES MELLITUS

Diabetes mellitus is generally considered to be an inborn error of metabolism in which the body is unable to utilize sugars completely. Manifestations may appear in youth, referred to as juvenile-onset type (ketosis-prone), or in later life, as maturity-onset type (ketosis-resistant). In some instances, the diabetic clinical manifestations may remain latent even though the inherent pattern can be demonstrated by laboratory methods. The clinical syndrome is characterized by (1) an impaired ability to metabolize carbohydrates, (2) an increased concentration of glucose in the circulating blood (hyperglycemia), and (3) the excretion of varying amounts of glucose in the urine (glycosuria). The etiological development of diabetes mellitus is unknown, but it is fairly well established that the entire endocrine system is involved, particularly the pancreas. (See Figure 28–1.) The pancreas has microscopic islet cells scattered throughout, known as the islands of Langerhans, which secrete the hormone *insulin,* necessary in the utilization of the carbohydrates.

CONTRIBUTORY FACTORS   Any serious disturbance of the pancreas which interferes with the production of a sufficient amount of insulin predisposes to clinical manifestations of diabetes. Two contributing factors are (1) overweight and (2) an inheritance of the disease. Before the condition has become evident, most adult diabetics are overweight. It becomes apparent that a normal or slightly underweight person is less prone to develop the disease. Poor, inadequate diet habits plus overeating and lack of physical activity may be predisposing factors preceding diabetic symptoms. Some physicians claim that diabetes is a disease of mental rather than of physical workers. With nervousness an element, mental strain, excitement or worry may help to aggravate the disease.[1]

[1]Slawson, P. F., et al.: Physiological factors associated with the onset of diabetes mellitus, J.A.M.A., *185*:166, 1963.

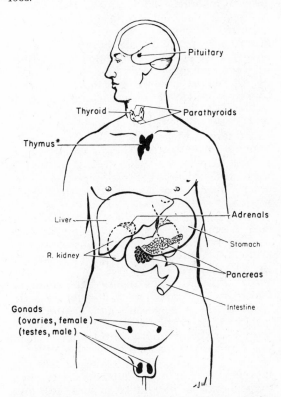

Figure 28–1   Location of principal endocrine glands. (Brooks: Basic Facts of General Chemistry. W. B. Saunders Company, 1956.) *Function unknown. The thymus is present only up to puberty.

TABLE 28–1   METABOLIC AND VASCULAR CHANGES IN VARIOUS STAGES OF DIABETES

| DIABETIC STAGE | CARBOHYDRATE TOLERANCE | | | INSULIN-LIKE ACTIVITY AND SYNALBUMIN ANTAGONIST* | VASCULAR CHANGES |
	FASTING BLOOD SUGAR	GLUCOSE TOLERANCE	CORTISONE-GLUCOSE TOLERANCE		
Prediabetes	Normal	Normal	Normal	May be increased	+
Subclinical	Normal	Normal (Abnormal during pregnancy)	Abnormal	Increased	+
Latent	Normal or Increased	Abnormal	Test not necessary	Increased	++
Overt	Increased	Test not necessary	Test not necessary	Increased	+++

*Test used for screening large numbers of people. From Waife, S. O. (ed.): Diabetes Mellitus. 7th ed. Indianapolis, Lilly Research Laboratories, Eli Lilly & Company, 1970, p. 9.
+ = degree of vascular change present.

Infectious diseases such as influenza, pneumonia and scarlet fever, or accidents, may help to precipitate symptoms of diabetes. Diseases of the liver, gallbladder, thyroid, pituitary, and pancreatic glands are frequently associated with diabetes.

Arteriosclerotic changes in the coronary arteries and associated cardiovascular disease, peripheral vascular disease, retinopathy, neuropathy and nephropathy appear more frequently in diabetics than in non-diabetics. Heredity seems to be the significant factor. Diabetes begins at conception. The time between conception and the development of overt diabetes varies from months to years. The progression of the disease is shown in Table 28–1. The tendency to diabetes is believed to be inherited as a Mendelian recessive characteristic. This means that if a diabetic marries a true non-diabetic the children may not get diabetes but will carry the strain. If these children and their children's children consistently marry nondiabetics, the carrier tendency will eventually disappear. If both parents have diabetes, then the children of such a union will almost invariably develop the disease. If one parent has diabetes and the other does not but is a carrier, the children of this marriage may develop it.

INCIDENCE   The reported incidence of diabetes is increasing. It is impossible to evaluate the reason, although greater food consumption, reduction in physical exercise, more obesity, the improved methods of diagnosis, increased longevity, and concentrated efforts of the medical profession to seek out individuals with it undoubtedly contribute.

Frequently a silent type of sickness, presenting without symptoms, it is more prevalent in the over 45 age group. In about two thirds of the number of diabetics the condition manifests itself after 40 years of age. The American Diabetes Association has established that one out of four Americans may be a carrier of diabetes. It is diagnosed in all ages. One in 2500 juveniles under age 15 has diabetes. The younger the individual in whom clinical symptoms appear, the more serious the condition. (Diabetes in children is discussed in Chapter 36.) The lack of clinical symptoms is indicated dramatically by the fact that 78 per cent of the selectees in World War II who were found to have diabetes did not know they had it. The estimated number of diabetics in the United States is 4,200,000 based on an estimated population of 200,000,000 as of July, 1967. Of these, approximately 1,600,000 are undiscovered diabetics. An additional 5,600,000 persons are potential diabetics. Approximately one in twenty has diabetes or is a potential diabetic person. According to various estimates the prevalence of diabetes is 2 to 16 per cent of the population.[2]

SYMPTOMS   When symptoms are present, they usually are increased thirst (polydipsia), increased urination (polyuria), increased appetite (polyphagia), failing strength and loss of weight. Pruritus vulvae, skin infection or irritation and visual disturbances are frequently present. Excessive urinary output and the failure to balance it by fluid intake causes dehydration and electrolyte imbalance. Inability of tissues to heal and degenerative changes occur, especially in advanced cases. Acidosis or ketosis is a symptom of accumulation of fatty acid in the blood. The failing strength and loss of weight are from starvation because the body is unable to utilize food. Glycosuria is not necessarily diagnostic of diabetes mellitus, because it may appear through some harmless causes, such

[2]Sharkey, T. P.: Diabetes-mellitus—present problems and new research. J. Am. Dietet. A., 58:201, 1971.

as emotional upset, overeating, pregnancy, or peculiar function of the kidneys.

There are four types of other carbohydrates which may appear in the urine without creating any suspicion of the disease: pentose, galactose, fructose, and lactose. Glucose is the specific sign in the urine of the diabetic.

PHYSIOLOGICAL DISTURBANCES   In order to understand the controls for maintaining normal blood glucose levels and the impairment of these controls in diabetes, intermediary metabolism should be reviewed (Chapter 7) as well as carbohydrate, lipid and protein metabolism (Chapters 4, 5 and 6).

Glucose from dietary carbohydrate, protein and fat and from liver glycogen (glycogenolysis) maintains blood glucose levels. Normally glucose combines with a carrier substance in the cell membrane and is transported to the inside of the membrane where it is released to the interior of the cell in most tissues of the body. An exception to this is the brain in which the glucose transport is more dependent on diffusion through the blood-brain barrier than through the cell membrane. Insulin influences the rate of glucose through the membrane of cells. Glucose is handled normally by the body in different ways: (1) it may be utilized for energy at once (cell oxidation), (2) it may be converted to glycogen for storage in the liver (glycogenesis), (3) it may be converted to fat for storage in adipose tissue (lipogenesis), and (4) it may be converted to muscle glycogen (see Chapter 4). Non-diabetics dispose of the glucose in these ways as rapidly as it enters the blood stream. This rapid disposition prevents the concentration from rising above the threshold established by the kidneys. The diabetic, with little or no insulin activity, has lost the ability to perform these functions completely. Glucose cannot cross the cell membrane and be oxidized through the glycolytic pathway in the cell to supply energy and it cannot be converted or stored. Hyperglycemia and glycosuria follow.

The normal renal threshold averages 160 to 180 mg. per 100 ml. of blood. The non-diabetic may, however, have a normally low threshold. If so, glucose may be excreted from the kidneys but this does not mean that he has diabetes. Whether the person has a low or high renal threshold is determined by the glucose tolerance test.

Fatty acid synthesis decreases and fatty oxidation increases in diabetes. The glycogen stores are depleted. Excess amounts of ketone bodies are released into the blood stream. Ketone bodies, beta-hydroxybutyric acid and acetoacetic acid, combine with basic ions and are excreted in the urine. Acetone is excreted by the lungs and gives a "fruity" odor to the breath. Acidosis develops when the basic ions are depleted, diabetic coma ensues and, if not treated, death occurs.

In the absence of insulin the lipoproteins-triglycerides, cholesterol and phospholipids increase in the blood. These high concentrations have been suggested as factors in the development of arteriosclerosis in persons with diabetes.

Protein synthesis is affected by insulin. It promotes the transport of amino acids through the cell membrane in much the same carrier transport system as glucose is transported. Normally the total quantity of protein stored in the tissues of the body is increased by insulin.

In diabetes there is an increase in protein breakdown. Amino acids are deaminized, and the non-nitrogenous part of the molecule forms glucose and fatty acids. This leads to an increase of glucose and incompletely oxidized fatty acids in the blood and an increased excretion of nitrogen and potassium in the urine.

It has been noted previously that glucose in the body is derived from other food sources besides carbohydrate in the diet. It should be remembered that carbohydrates are estimated to yield approximately 100 per cent, proteins, 58 per cent, and fats 10 per cent of their weight as available glucose in the body.

INSULIN   Insulin, a hormone produced by the beta cells of the islands of Langerhans in the pancreas, is concerned with the metabolism of carbohydrate. It functions in the conversion of glucose to glycogen in the liver and its storage in the liver and in the oxidation of glucose in the tissues. With insulin in the blood stream, the glucose is utilized economically by the tissues or stored for future use and the glucose in the blood is kept delicately balanced at approximately 0.1 per cent. The pancreatic gland of the non-diabetic produces and excretes sufficient insulin, which varies with the amount of available glucose in the blood.

A diabetic secretes either insufficient insulin or none. In either case, he frequently has to resort to commercial insulin preparations; he must inject a fixed amount of the hormone into his body each day. Because the amount of the daily injection is fixed and constant, he cannot have the same freedom in the intake of food as the non-diabetic. A balance must be maintained between the insulin and the glucose received from food. Unusual exercise increases the ability to utilize carbohydrates which can temporarily increase the need for greater carbohydrate intake. For example, an office worker who takes an afternoon off to play golf may need to take some form of carbohydrate about halfway round the course to avoid an insulin reaction.

Commercial Insulin   Insulin is a protein

TABLE 28-2   TYPES OF INSULIN AND CHARACTERISTICS OF INSULIN AVAILABLE
IN THE UNITED STATES

TYPE OF INSULIN	APPEAR-ANCE	ACTION	DURATION (Hours)	ZINC CONTENT (mg./100 Units)	BUFFER	PROTEIN Type	PROTEIN mg./100 Units
Regular Crystalline	Clear	Rapid	5 to 7	0.016–0.04	None	None	—
Semilente®	Turbid	Rapid	12 to 16	0.2 –0.25	Acetate	None	—
Globin	Clear	Intermediate	18 to 24	0.25 –0.35	None	Globin	3.8
NPH	Turbid	Intermediate	24 to 28	0.016–0.04	Phosphate	Protamine	0.5
Lente®	Turbid	Intermediate	24 to 28	0.2 –0.25	Acetate	None	—
Protamine Zinc	Turbid	Prolonged	36+	0.2 –0.25	Phosphate	Protamine	1.25
Ultralente®	Turbid	Prolonged	36+	0.2 –0.25	Acetate	None	—

From Waife, S. O. (ed.): Diabetes Mellitus. 7th ed. Indianapolis, Lilly Research Laboratories, Eli Lilly & Company, 1970, p. 41.

extracted from the pancreas of animals and is packaged in crystalline form. In 1964, the synthesis of insulin was completed – another step forward in scientific achievement. A standardized unit of insulin provides for the use of 1.5 to 3.0 gm. of glucose.

There are three general types of commercial insulin: (1) the quick-acting regular crystalline or unmodified insulin, (2) the slow-acting protamine zinc insulin and (3) the intermediary insulin. The types and characteristics of the insulins available in the United States are summarized in Table 28–2. The diabetics response to the insulin determines the kind and amount which the physician will prescribe.

Injections of insulin must be continued during the period the pancreas is unable to function adequately. Very often improvement occurs, in which event the amount of insulin is either reduced or omitted. For example, an obese person who requires insulin at first may, after sufficient weight loss, be able to control his diabetes by diet alone, or by diet plus one of the oral hypoglycemic agents. The *severity* and the *nature* of the diabetes determine whether insulin must be continued.

Administration of Insulin   The insulin preparations currently available require parenteral administration because of the destructive effects of the digestive juices. Insulin, a protein, would be digested.

Insulin is best injected where the skin is loose. The sites of injection should be frequently changed or rotated. Because the nurse most often has the responsibility of teaching the use and administration of the insulin to a patient, she should become very familiar with the technique used in her institution. Other procedures are given in diabetic manuals. (See list on p. 421.)

Special care is required in the handling, storage and administration of insulin. In-

sulin, regardless of the source, is sold in standard potencies. The different concentrations may be recognized easily by the legends and colors of the labels and by the colors of the rubber stoppers.

ORAL HYPOGLYCEMIC AGENTS   A recent development in the treatment of diabetes is the oral administration of hypoglycemic agents, the sulfonylurea and phenethylbiguanide compounds. The sulfonylurea compounds lower the blood sugar level and reduce glycosuria in certain diabetic patients. Current results indicate that these drugs act by stimulating the pancreatic beta cells to secrete endogenous insulin. These compounds are effective only in diabetics who have beta cells which can respond to the stimulus. This insulin appears to exercise its main effect in the liver by promoting a decrease in the output of glucose from the liver glycogen into the blood stream. Results to date have generally not been satisfactory in young diabetics, or in treating such complications as infection, surgery or acidosis, but satisfactory results have been reported in mild or moderately severe and stable diabetics of the older age group who have a residual insulin supply (require less than 20 units daily), and in whom onset took place after age 40. The current available hypoglycemic compounds are shown in Table 28–3.

The phenethylbiguanide, *phenformin* (DBI), has been reported to have hypoglycemic activity when used in mild cases, the elderly, and the obese if used alone or in combination with sulfonylurea. In addition, when it has been used as a supplement to insulin in certain young diabetics, it has been possible to reduce the insulin dosage significantly. The mode and site of action of the biguanides are different from those of the sulfonylureas but are not clearly understood. Long term obser-

TABLE 28–3   AVAILABLE ORAL HYPOGLYCEMIC COMPOUNDS

COMPOUNDS	MAXIMUM RECOMMENDED DAILY DOSE	DURATION OF ACTION (*Hours*)
Sulfonylureas Tolbutamide (Orinase)	2–3 gm.	6 to 12
Acetohexamide (Dymelor) ®	1.5 gm.	12 to 24
Chlorpropamide (Diabinese)	0.5 gm.	up to 60
Tolazamide (Tolinase)	0.75 gm.	12 to 24
Phenethylbiguanides Phenformin (DBI)	200 mg.	4 to 6
Phenformin (long-acting)	200 mg.	8 to 12

From Waife, S. O.: Diabetes Mellitus. 7th ed. Indianapolis, Lilly Research Laboratories, Eli Lilly & Company, 1970, p. 125.

vations have been made and more are needed for evaluation of the full usefulness and potential toxicity of the oral hypoglycemic agents.[3–7]

DIAGNOSTIC TESTS

To make a definite diagnosis of diabetes mellitus certain laboratory tests are used.

URINE   The urine is tested for total volume, specific gravity, glucose and fatty acids. Although glucose in the urine does not necessarily mean diabetes mellitus, with the exception of mere traces it may be indicative of the disease. Tests are available in which the concentration of glucose in the urine is read colorimetrically: (1) by indicator paper (Tes-Tape), (2) by paper stick (Clinistix), (3) by addition of a powder to urine (Gala-test), or (4) by adding a tablet to urine (Clinitest).

Ketonuria, the presence of fatty acids (ketone bodies) in the urine, indicates the incomplete oxidation of fats. This is considered a serious condition and requires immediate adjustment of diet and insulin.

BLOOD   The oral *glucose tolerance test* indicates the ability of the patient to utilize a specific amount of glucose calculated at the rate of 1.75 gm. per kg. of body weight. (Glu-

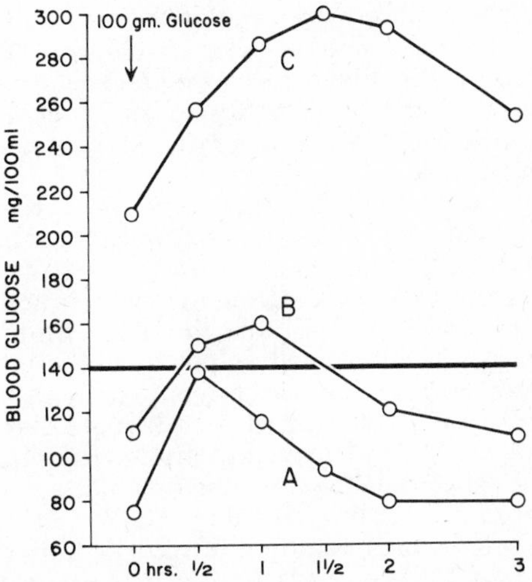

[3]Beaser, S. B.: Critical appraisal of sulfonylurea therapy of diabetes mellitus. J.A.M.A., *174*:1233, 1960.

[4]Camerini-Dávalos, R. A., and Marble, A.: Incidence and causes of secondary failure in treatment with tolbutamide. J.A.M.A., *181*:1, 1962.

[5]Editorial. Oral hypoglycemic agents in diabetes. J.A.M.A., *181*:43, 1962.

[6]DeLawter, D. E., and Moss, J. M.: A five-year study of tolbutamide in the treatment of diabetes mellitus. J.A.M.A., *181*:156, 1962.

[7]Maha, G. E., et al.: Acetohexamide. Preliminary report on a new oral hypoglycemic agent. Diabetes, *11*:83, 1962.

Figure 28–2   Glucose tolerance curves. *A* depicts a normal glycemic response of an adult to the oral administration of 100 gm. of glucose. The rise is rapid but the peak does not exceed 150 mg./100 ml., and the mild degree of hyperglycemia has subsided by 1½ hours. In *B* the fasting blood glucose value is slightly above normal but the peak at 1 hour exceeds 140 and the 2-hour value exceeds the upper border of normal (100 mg./100 ml.) as seen in mild diabetes. *C* depicts the fasting hyperglycemia with values far exceeding 140 mg. at 1½, 2 and 3 hours as seen in uncontrolled diabetes, which is identifiable by finding glycosuria and a hyperglycemia *without resorting to a glucose tolerance test.* Glycosuria usually occurs when the blood sugar level is maintained for varying periods above 140 mg./ml. as indicated by the heavy black line. (From Duncan, G. G. (ed.): Diseases of Metabolism. 5th ed. Philadelphia, W. B. Saunders Co., 1964.)

cose flavored with lemon or glucola are commonly used.)

A blood sugar estimate is made before the glucose preparation is served and again ½ hour, 1 hour, 2 hours and 3 hours after the glucose preparation has been taken. Figure 28–2 illustrates the difference in the glucose tolerance curve between a normal person (*A*) and diabetics (*B, C*). The normal level is 70 to 100 mg. per 100 ml. of blood. Additional tests and procedures can be found in the various diabetic manuals. (See page 421.) The intravenous glucose tolerance test, the cortisone-glucose tolerance test and the oral and intravenous tolbutamide tolerance tests are also used in the diagnosis of diabetes.

DIETARY MANAGEMENT

The diet of a diabetic is a normal diet. It consists of sufficient calories for his activity and the maintenance of ideal weight and is adequate in carbohydrate, protein, fat, minerals and vitamins. The dietary treatment of diabetes consists essentially of reducing and systematizing the intake of carbohydrate in order to place as little strain as possible on the impaired blood glucose-regulating mechanism Treatment with exogenous insulin more or less restores the regulating mechanism, and dietary management currently being prescribed for diabetics corresponds closely in composition and quantity to those deemed optimal for healthy nondiabetic persons of similar age.

The role of the diet in diabetes is (1) to provide sufficient calories to maintain ideal body weight; (2) to adjust the food ingestion to the available insulin, allowing (a) small amounts or no glucose to spill into the urine, and permitting (b) the blood sugar to rise slightly above normal; (3) to prevent acidosis and shock; and (4) to furnish an adequate diet for good health and normal activity. Among 60 per cent of the diabetics, the diet alone is capable of controlling the abnormality. Though the secretion of insulin is diminished, there is enough to take care of his dietary needs. Other diabetic patients need specific food restrictions plus the administration of insulin or an oral hypoglycemic agent. To these individuals, insulin or the oral drug makes it possible for an individual to have the essential nutrients and sufficient calories to sustain a normal life.

CLINICAL CONTROL   The methods by which adequate control of diabetes may be accomplished have been the subject of much study and debate. On the one hand, the patient may be treated by permitting him to eat what he likes so long as he is free from clinical symptoms, maintains or gains weight (as necessary), and is free from ketosis and hypoglycemia. This is known as clinical control. Insulin dosage under these circumstances must be adjusted frequently. Continuous glycosuria and hyperglycemia are permitted so long as the patient maintains his normal weight and shows no ketone bodies in the urine. Concentrated sweets such as sugar, candy, syrup, jelly, and sweet desserts are omitted or limited.

CHEMICAL CONTROL   In contrast, many physicians use a measured diet, and insulin, when indicated, regulated to control the blood sugar within normal limits and the urine free or nearly free of sugar. By this means an adequate intake of calories, protein, minerals, and vitamins is assured, while the amount of carbohydrates and calories is limited. With this type of regulation, a constant insulin requirement is more readily established, and normoglycemia may be maintained for long periods. This is known as chemical control.

The question arises as to whether or not it is true that the meticulous control involving the regulated diet with nearly perfect insulin balance will minimize the incidence of complications throughout the years. The group advocating a liberal diet feels that glycosuria is not incompatible with well-being, and intimates that vascular damage is perhaps in-evitable and not delayed by strict regimen. Many years of study and observation are needed for the complete answer. The Committee on Therapeutic Nutrition[8] states that "until it is proved that permitting glycosuria and hyperglycemia is not harmful to the organism, the diet and insulin administration should be regulated to prevent them." Caution should be exercised, however, against putting emphasis on "the diet" rather than on the person with the diabetes.

CALORIC ALLOWANCE   The same procedure used to plan the normal diet is followed when computing a diet prescription for a diabetic patient. First, the caloric allowance is determined, based on the patient's height, weight, age, sex, and occupation or activity. Details for calculating a diet have already been given (Chapter 19). Most authorities consider it advisable to keep the weight of the diabetic slightly below average (about 10 per cent). It is a well-established fact that when the caloric value of the food intake is kept below normal over an extended period, the basal metabolic rate is lowered, thereby decreasing the body's food requirement. However, at the lower equilibrium the individual is often incapable of a full, active, healthy life, and will fatigue easily, have decreased resistance to infection, and suffer mental apathy and depression. The diet should supply sufficient energy to achieve and maintain the desired weight while allowing for full activity.

PROTEIN ALLOWANCE   Next, the protein allowance is determined, which is essentially the same as that for the normal individual and may vary from 0.9 to 1.5 gm. of protein per kg. of desirable body weight.

Untreated or poorly regulated diabetics excrete large quantities of nitrogen in the urine, the result of the increase in the conversion of proteins to carbohydrates. Because of this (or ketosis) a large protein deficit may occur. It is advisable to allow 1.5 gm. of proteins during the beginning few weeks of the treatment to correct the deficit. Later in the course of treatment, 0.9 gm. per kg. of desirable body weight or a minimum of 65 gm. of proteins daily may be sufficient for an adult. However, current practice is to prescribe from 80 to 100 gm., because there is less available glucose in protein, and the metabolism to glucose is slower. Reserve protein is needed during episodes of ketosis, whether very mild or severe.

It has been reported that high protein diets will help to prevent neuritis, a frequent complication in diabetic patients. Protein foods

[8]Pollack, H., and Halpern, S. L.: Therapeutic Nutrition. Washington, D.C., National Research Council, Publication 234, 1952.

METABOLIC DISORDERS RELATED TO NUTRITION   401

are generally good sources of vitamin B-complex, including thiamin. The lack of thiamin is believed to predispose to neuritis. In addition, many forms of the degenerative diseases seen in the diabetic patient may be nutritional in origin.

CARBOHYDRATE ALLOWANCE   The carbohydrate allowance is the next determination of the diet. The estimation is guided by the patient's blood sugar, urinalysis, and available insulin. Carbohydrates provide 45 to 50 per cent of the total calories in the diet of most Americans. In diabetics, a moderate restriction of carbohydrate calories to about 40 per cent, with the avoidance of highly concentrated sugars, appears to be reasonable. An amount less than 100 gm. is inadvisable, since a low level frequently leads to ketosis and an amount over 300 gm. may overtax the metabolic capacity of the diabetic.

FAT ALLOWANCE   To balance the caloric requirement, the remaining calories in the diet are supplied by the fats. The amount is determined after the protein and carbohydrate calories are totaled. The difference between the total calories supplied by protein and carbohydrate and the calories computed as necessary for the diet will be supplied by fat. Thus, the energy requirement of an individual will largely determine the proportion of fat in the diet, and some authorities recommend that the fat should contain mostly polyunsaturated fatty acids as a preventative measure against atherosclerosis (p. 459).

MINERALS AND VITAMINS   Vitamin and mineral requirements of patients with well controlled diabetes do not differ significantly from those of normal subjects. There is no necessity for mineral and vitamin supplements when the diet is adequate and the glycosuria is controlled.

WEIGHED VERSUS MEASURED DIETS   Dietary control is highly desirable, though strict arithmetical standards do not seem warranted. With the exception of rare cases, it is no longer considered necessary to weigh the food on a gram scale. Measured amounts of the foods using the available and familiar household measures of teaspoon, tablespoon and measuring cup, will suffice.

MEAL PLANNING WITH EXCHANGE LISTS   In 1950 the American Diabetes Association, working jointly with the U.S. Public Health Service and the American Dietetic Association, published a simplified, widely used method of calculating a diabetic diet and planning the diabetic's meals. An effort was made to reclassify and standardize food values and reduce the complexity of diabetic diets. This material was revised in 1956.[9] The booklet,

"Meal Planning with Exchange Lists," and nine complete meal plans varying in carbohydrate, protein and fat content, based on this material, are available at small cost to use in meal planning.[10] These meals provide 40 per cent of the calories as carbohydrate, with varying protein and fat content. The total calories range from 1200 to 3000. Printed instructions for modifying the "exchange lists" to permit sodium restriction and for bland, low fiber diets have been prepared and are also available from the same sources. It should be remembered that these are printed diet lists. Going over one of these standardized diet sheets with the patient and assuming that a change in his dietary pattern will take place is not teaching. (See Chapter 2.) The approximate composition of a person's dietary may be calculated in the following way according to the simplified method.

1. To determine the basal calories expended for 24 hours, the patient's ideal weight in pounds is multiplied by 10.
2. If the person is young, tall, and male, 100 to 200 calories are added to the basal calorie requirement.
3. If the person is elderly, short, and female, 100 to 200 calories are subtracted from the basal calorie requirement.
4. Light activity requires 30 per cent added to the calculated basal calories. Greater activity requires an addition of 50 to 75 per cent of the calculated basal calories.
5. To estimate the protein allowance, the patient's ideal weight in pounds for his height and age is divided by two.

The Diet

The dietary pattern of the patient is obtained and evaluated for the presence of the protective food groups which are the same as for a non-diabetic. Appropriate dietary practices are noted and become the foundation for planning the revised pattern with the patient. It should include meat, eggs, milk, vegetables, fruits, and whole grain or enriched cereals and breads, butter or fortified margarine. (See Application of Dietary Allowances, p. 161.)

The first objective in planning the dietary regimen with the patient is to determine the approximate number of calories needed to maintain ideal weight.

The foods to meet the carbohydrate allowance are determined before the protein and fat requirements are considered. The analysis of some carbohydrate foods shows that they contain fat and protein. For example, using

---

[9]Diabetes Guide Book for the Physician. New York, American Diabetes Association, revised 1956.

[10]Meal Plans 1 to 9, The American Dietetic Association, 620 No. Michigan Ave., Chicago, Ill., 60611, and the American Diabetes Association, 18 East 48th Street, New York, New York, 10017.

the Exchange List, 8 ounces of milk contains 12 gm. carbohydrate, 8 gm. protein and 10 gm. fat. A vegetable in list II B contains 7 gm. carbohydrate and 2 gm. of protein.

The protein foods, meats, eggs, cheese, are identified. Most of the protein foods contain a percentage of fats. For example, 3 ounces of meat contains 21 gm. protein and 15 gm. fat.

The fat allowance is the last adjustment made in the diet. Because butter, fortified margarine, oil, and mayonnaise are consid-ered pure fats, their inclusion or exclusion from the diet can be easily and simply ad-justed to meet the fat requirement.

In the simplified method of calculating the diabetic diet, *food exchanges are basic*. The principal foods allowed the diabetic are classi-fied into six groups, determined by the com-position of the food. Each group contains sim-ilar kinds and amounts of food according to the nutritional value of carbohydrate, protein and fat. The groups are:

---

*These vegetables have high vitamin A content; use at least one serving of one each day.

	WEIGHT IN GRAMS	APPROX. MEASURE	COMPOSITION FOR 1 EXCHANGE OR 1 SERVING	CALORIES
List I	240	1 cup	Milk (carbohydrates, 12 Gm.; proteins, 8 Gm.; fats, 10 Gm.)	170
List II A	—	As desired	Vegetables (II A: negligible C, P, and F in amounts ordinarily used)	—
II B	100	½ cup	Vegetables (II B: C, 7 Gm.; P, 2 Gm.)	36
List III	Exchange varies		Fruit (C, 10 Gm.)	40
List IV	25 (varies)	1 slice	Bread exchanges (C, 15 Gm.; P, 2 Gm.)	68
List V	30 (varies)	1 oz.	Meat exchanges (P, 7 Gm.; F, 5 Gm.)	73
List VI	5 (varies)	1 tsp.	Fat exchanges (F, 5 Gm.)	45

Other items vary

Adapted from Diabetes Guide Book for the Physician. New York, American Diabetes Association, 1956, second edition, 1 East 45th Street, New York City, pp. 25–26.

FOOD EXCHANGES

The following exchange lists are adapted from Meal Planning with Exchange Lists, The American Dietetic Association, 620 N. Michigan Ave., Chicago, 11, Ill., and from Diabetes Guide Book for the Physician, New York, American Diabetes Association, 2nd ed., 1956, pp. 27–34.

List I. Milk

Carbohydrate, 12 Gm.; protein, 8 Gm.; fat, 10 Gm.; calories 170 per serving.

FOOD	APPROX. MEASURE (1 exchange)	WEIGHT IN GRAMS
Milk, whole (plain or homogenized)	1 cup (8 oz.)	240
Milk, evaporated	½ cup	120
Milk, powder, whole	¼ cup (3 tbsp. level)	35
*Milk, powder, skim (non-fat dried milk)	¼ cup (3 tbsp. level)	35
Buttermilk (made from whole milk)	1 cup	240
*Buttermilk (made from skim milk)	1 cup	240
*Milk, skim	1 cup	240

* Add 10 Gm. fat (2 fat exchanges).

Table continued on opposite page.

LIST II. VEGETABLES

One or more fat exchanges from the diet allowance may be used to season the vegetables.

A. Vegetables—negligible carbohydrate, protein and fat in amounts ordinarily used. If more than one cup in cooked form is used at one meal, it should be calculated as one serving of a Group B vegetable. Limit tomatoes to one per meal.

Asparagus	Lettuce	*Watercress
*Broccoli	Mushrooms	*Greens:
Brussels sprouts	Okra	Beet greens
Cabbage	*Pepper, green	Chard
Cauliflower	Radish	Collards
Celery	Rhubarb	Dandelion
*Chicory	Sauerkraut	Kale
Cucumber	String beans, young	Mustard
*Escarole	Summer squash	Spinach
Eggplant	*Tomatoes	Turnip greens

B. Vegetables—carbohydrate, 7 Gm.; protein, 2 Gm.; fat negligible; calories 36 per serving.
   1 exchange = ½ measuring cup = 100 Gm.

Beets	Peas, green	*Squash, winter
*Carrots	Pumpkin	Turnip
Onions	Rutabagas	

* These vegetables have high vitamin A content; use at least one serving of one each day.

LIST III. FRUITS

Fresh, cooked, canned or frozen *unsweetened*.
Carbohydrate, 10 Gm. per exchange; protein and fat negligible; calories 40 per serving.

FRUIT	APPROX. MEASURE (1 exchange)	WEIGHT IN GRAMS
Apple, 1 small	2 in. diameter	80
Applesauce (cooked without sugar)	½ cup	100
Apricots, fresh	2 medium	100
Apricots, dry	4 halves	20
Banana	½ small	50
Berries (blackberries, raspberries and *strawberries)	1 cup	150
Blueberries	⅔ cup	100
*Cantaloupe	¼ (6 in. diameter)	200
Cherries	10 large or 15 small	75
Dates	2	15
Figs, dried	1 small	15
Figs, fresh	2 large	50
*Grapefruit	½ small	125
*Grapefruit juice	½ cup	100
Grapes	12	75
Grape juice	¼ cup	60
Honeydew melon	⅛ (7 in. diameter)	150
Mango	½ small	70
Nectarines	1 medium	100
*Orange	1 small	125
Orange juice	½ cup	100
Papaya	⅓ medium	100
Peach	1 medium	100
Pear	1 small	100
Pineapple	½ cup, cubed	80
Pineapple juice	⅓ cup	80
Plums	2 medium	100
Prunes, dried	2 medium	25
Raisins	2 tbsp. level	15
Rhubarb	(See List II A)	
*Tangerine	1 large	125
Watermelon	1 cup diced	175
	1 slice 3 in. × 1½ in.	

* These fruits are rich sources of vitamin C; use at least one serving each day.

Table continued on following page.

List IV. Bread Exchanges

Carbohydrate, 15 Gm.; protein, 2 Gm.; fat negligible; calories 68 per serving.

FOOD	APPROX. MEASURE (1 exchange)	WEIGHT IN GRAMS
Bread, baker's	1 slice (3½ in. × 4 in. × ½ in.)	25
Biscuit, roll	1 (2 in. diameter)	35
Muffin	1 (2 in. diameter)	35
Cornbread	1 (1½ in. cube)	35
Cereals, cooked	½ cup, cooked	100
Cereals, dry (flakes, puffed and shredded varieties)	¾ cup	20
Flour	2½ tbsp.	20
Rice, macaroni, noodles, spaghetti, grits	½ cup, cooked	100
Crackers:		
Graham	2 (2½ in. × 2¾ in.)	20
Oyster	20 (½ cup)	20
Saltines	5 (2 in. square)	20
Soda	3 (2½ in. × 2½ in.)	20
Round, thin varieties	6–8 (1½ in. diameter)	20
Vegetables:		
Beans, peas, dried (cooked) Includes limas, navy, kidney beans, blackeyed, cowpeas and split peas, etc.	½ cup	90
Baked beans, no pork	¼ cup	50
Corn	⅓ cup or ½ ear	80
Parsnips	⅔ cup	125
Potatoes:		
White, baked, boiled	1 (2 in. diameter)	100
White, mashed	½ cup	100
Sweet or yam	¼ cup	50
*Ice cream	⅛ qt.	70
Sponge cake, no icing	1 (1½ in. cube)	25

* Omit 2 fat exchanges from total allowance for day.

List V. Meat Exchanges

Carbohydrate negligible; protein, 7 Gm.; fat, 5 Gm.; calories 73 per serving. Note: All items expressed in cooked weight. Bones and extra fat should not be counted in the total weight; a 3-oz. serving of cooked meat is about equal to 4 oz. of raw meat. One or more fat exchanges from the diet may be used to cook or season these foods.

FOOD	APPROX. MEASURE (1 exchange)	WEIGHT IN GRAMS
Meat:		
Beef, fowl, lamb, veal (medium fat), liver, pork, ham (lean)	1 oz.	30

Table continued on opposite page.

LIST V. MEAT EXCHANGES (*Continued*)

Coldcuts:		
Salami, minced ham, bologna,	1 slice	45
cervelat, liver sausage,	(4½ in. diameter × ⅛ in.)	
luncheon loaf		
Frankfurter (8—9 per lb.)	1	50

Fish:		
Cod, haddock, halibut, herring, etc.	1 oz.	30
Salmon, tuna, crabmeat, lobster	¼ cup	30
Shrimp, clams, oysters	5 small	45
Sardines	3 medium	30

Cheese:		
Cheddar type	1 oz.	30
Cottage	3 tbsp. level	45
*Peanut butter	2 tbsp.	30
Egg	1	50

* Limit to one serving per day unless adjustment is made to balance carbohydrate content

LIST VI. FAT EXCHANGES

Carbohydrate and protein negligible; fat, 5 Gm.; calories 45 per serving.

FOOD	APPROX. MEASURE (1 exchange)	WEIGHT IN GRAMS
Butter or margarine	1 tsp.	5
Bacon, crisp	1 slice	10
Cream, light, sweet or sour—20%	2 tbsp.	30
Cream, heavy—40%	1 tbsp.	15
Cream, cheese	1 tbsp.	15
French dressing	1 tbsp.	15
Mayonnaise	1 tsp.	5
Nuts	6 small	10
Oil or cooking fat	1 tsp.	5
Olives	5 small	50
Avocado	⅛ (4 in. diameter)	25

BEVERAGES, SEASONINGS, CONDIMENTS, AND FOODS ALLOWED AS DESIRED*

The following may be used as desired, unless the physician finds a special reason to limit them. The foods listed have no appreciable carbohydrate, protein or fat content if used in ordinary amounts.

Coffee	Rennet tablets	Garlic	Parsley seasoning
Tea	Rhubarb	Lemon	Pepper
Clear broth	Cranberries,	Mint	Saccharine, Sucaryl and
Bouillon,	unsweetened	Mustard	other noncaloric
without fat	Celery seasoning	Nutmeg	sweeteners
Gelatin,	Cinnamon	Onion seasoning	Vinegar
unsweetened			Pickles (sour or
			unsweetened dill)

* Adapted from Diabetes Guide Book for the Physician. American Diabetes Association, Inc., 2nd ed., 1956, p. 34.

TABLE 28–4   EXAMPLE OF A METHOD FOR PLANNING A DIABETIC DIET

Diet prescription: Calories, 2180; C, 200 grams; P, 120 grams; F, 100 grams.

FOOD	AMOUNT	LIST	C GRAMS	P GRAMS	F GRAMS
			TOTAL DAY'S FOOD		
Milk, whole	1 pint	I	24	16	20
Vegetables	as desired within limits	II A			
Vegetables	1 serving	II B	7	2	
Fruits	3 servings	III	30		
			61 (total)		
Bread exchanges	9 servings	IV	135	18	
				36 (total)	
Meat exchanges	12 servings	V		84	60
					80 (total)
Fat exchanges	4 servings	VI			20
Totals:			196	120	100

Determine the number of servings of bread, meat and fat exchanges required to complete the diet prescription in the following way:

1. Subtract the carbohydrate grams (61) furnished by the milk, vegetables, and fruit from the grams of carbohydrate prescribed (200); and divide the result by 15, which is the amount of grams of carbohydrate in one bread exchange (List IV).

   200 — 61 = 139; 139 ÷ 15 = 9 servings *bread* exchanges

2. The protein grams in a diet are adjusted by the addition of one or more meat exchanges (List V).

   120 — 36 = 84; 84 ÷ 7 = 12 servings *meat* exchanges

3. The fat grams in a diet are adjusted by the addition of one or more fat exchanges (List VI).

   100 — 80 = 20; 20 ÷ 5 = 4 servings *fat* exchanges

Ease and simplicity are features of the simplified method of calculating the diabetic diet. The basic protective foods are included to assure nutritive adequacy. See Table 28–4.

MEAL PLANNING

The need for insulin is the determining factor which decides how the foods of the diet should be distributed among meals. Also, the *kind* of insulin employed by the patient affects the meal planning. For the satisfaction of the patient and the physician, some convenient methods of distributing the required foods into meals have been evolved, Some of them will be discussed.

USING NO INSULIN   When no insulin is prescribed, the daily carbohydrate allowance usually is divided equally into three meals.

Breakfast	1/3
Luncheon	1/3
Dinner	1/3

In some patients, the blood sugar is higher in the morning, and for these individuals a smaller amount of carbohydrate is given for breakfast, for example, 1/5, breakfast; 2/5, luncheon; and 2/5, dinner.

USING REGULAR (CRYSTALLINE) INSULIN   When regular, quick acting (crystalline) insulin is employed, the carbohydrate allowance is divided equally into three meals, following the same proportions suggested when using no insulin. Regular insulin is little used today except for diabetics undergoing surgery or those with an infection.

USING PROLONGED ACTING INSULIN   Protamine zinc insulin, for example, has a prolonged activity of approximately 24 hours. When arranging meal schedules to synchronize with insulin injections, Pollack and Dolger[11] originally demonstrated that it is important that the maximum availability of glucose from foods should coincide with the maximum availability of insulin. Thus, when protamine zinc insulin is administered, an

[11] Pollack, H., and Dolger, H.: Advantages of prozinsulin (protamine zinc insulin) therapy: Dietary suggestions and notes on the management of cases. Ann. Int. Med., *12*: 2010, 1939.

evening feeding (bedtime) is usually required to prevent insulin shock during the night or early morning. For a correct distribution of *carbohydrates*, the amount planned for the bedtime feeding (when ordered) is deducted from the total daily carbohydrate allowance, and the remaining carbohydrates are then divided into the three daily meals as follows:

Breakfast	1/5
Luncheon	2/5
Dinner	2/5

Bedtime 25 to 30 gm. (when indicated), deducted from the total carbohydrate allowance before division into meals.

USING REGULAR AND PROTAMINE ZINC INSULIN
When regular insulin and protamine zinc insulin are employed together, the daily carbohydrate allowance is frequently divided into three meals following these proportions.

Breakfast	2/5
Luncheon	1/5
Dinner	2/5

The larger proportion of carbohydrates served at breakfast will synchronize with the regular insulin availability if it is injected before breakfast.

USING INTERMEDIARY ACTING INSULINS
The intermediary acting insulins have an action which is intermediate in duration and intensity. When an insulin of intermediate action (globin zinc insulin, NPH and lente insulin) is given before breakfast, a late afternoon nourishment (3:30 to 4:00 P.M.) is frequently required to counteract any hypoglycemic tendency at this time. This is particularly characteristic of globin. A bedtime feeding often is unnecessary when intermediate insulin preparations are used. The carbohydrate allowance may be divided as follows:

Breakfast	1/6
Luncheon	2/6
Afternoon nourishment	1/6
Dinner	2/6

If a midafternoon feeding is not given, the carbohydrate deducted from breakfast is added to the noon meal. With NPH and lente insulins, the division of carbohydrate is frequently apportioned as described for protamine zinc insulin.

Protein Allowance Divided into Meals

There are some authorities who like to divide the *protein* allowance of the diet among the meals in a manner similar to that described for carbohydrate. Because of the present trend of liberalizing the diabetic diet, however, a more liberal procedure is to subdivide only the *carbohydrate* allowance. It should be remembered that an adequate meal contains a complete protein.

Pollack and Dolger established that it is advisable to include about one-half of the proteins in the evening and bedtime meals if protamine zinc insulin is used, thereby allowing a continuous flow of glucose during the night. The other half is divided to include one-sixth for breakfast and one-third at noon. They state: "When the patient consumes one half to two thirds of the daily protein allowance (meat) at supper time, it is rare to find nocturnal hypoglycemic episodes, the reason for this being that about one half of the protein consumed is converted into available carbohydrate. This conversion is slow.... The slow rise in blood sugar concentration, and the absence of any tendency to rapid fluctuations after the ingestion of meat, establishes its usefulness without question."

When using insulin of intermediate action, protein in the night meal and/or feeding also helps to prevent early morning hypoglycemia.

Special Diabetic Foods

Contrary to popular belief, the purchase or preparation of special diabetic foods is not necessary. The diabetic patient can and should eat the same variety of foods as the rest of the family, with the exception of sugar and foods prepared with sugar. Canned and frozen fruits present the greatest problem because of the syrup in which they are prepared. However, waterpacked fruits, both canned and frozen, are quite widely available, and are becoming more equitable in price. As a diabetic person becomes less accustomed to sugar, sweetened foods are no longer enticing. Presenting the diet in meal patterns makes it much easier for the diabetic patient to select foods available at home, or in a restaurant, to fit into his personally prescribed plan. Every patient should know the food equivalents to encourage variety in the selection of foods.

The diabetic diets in Tables 28–5 and 28–6 are examples of (1) a diabetic diet for a patient using regular insulin or no insulin, and (2) a diabetic diet for a patient using protamine zinc insulin or an intermediary acting insulin.

Food Values

The composition and classification of the most frequently served foods will be found in

TABLE 28–5   AN EXAMPLE OF MEAL PLANNING FOR AN ADULT USING REGULAR INSULIN OR NO INSULIN

Diet Prescription: Calories, 2140; proteins, 110 grams; fats, 100 grams; carbohydrates, 200 grams. The carbohydrates are divided approximately as follows:

Breakfast	⅓	67 Gm.
Luncheon	⅓	67 Gm.
Dinner	⅓	69 Gm.

TOTAL DAY'S FOOD

FOOD	AMOUNT	LIST	C GRAMS	P GRAMS	F GRAMS
Milk, whole	1 pint	I	24	16	20
Vegetables	as desired within limits	II A	—	—	—
Vegetables	2 servings	II B	14	4	
Fruits	3 servings	III	30		
Bread exchanges	9 servings	IV	135	18	
Meat exchanges	10 servings	V		70	50
Fat exchanges	6 servings	VI			30
			203	108	100

SAMPLE MEAL PLAN

		LIST
Breakfast:	Fruit, 1 serving	III
	Bread exchanges: 3 servings	IV
	Eggs: 2 or 2 other meat exchanges	V
	Milk: 1 glass (8 ounces)	I
	Butter: 2 level teaspoons, or 2 other fat exchanges	VI
	Tea or coffee, as desired	
Luncheon:	Meat exchanges: 2 servings	V
	Bread exchanges: 3 servings	IV
	Butter: 2 teaspoons, or 2 other fat exchanges	VI
	Vegetables (as desired within limits)	II A
	Fruit: 1 serving	III
	Milk: 1 glass (8 ounces)	I
Dinner:	Meat exchanges: 6 servings	V
	Vegetables (as desired within limits)	II A
	Vegetables: 2 servings	II B
	Bread exchanges: 3 servings	IV
	Butter: 2 level teaspoons, or 2 other fat exchanges	VI
	Fruit: 1 serving	III
	Tea or coffee, as desired	

SAMPLE MENU

Breakfast:	Orange juice	½ cup
	Poached egg	2
	on toast	2 slices
	Butter	2 teaspoons
	Cornflakes	¾ cup
	Milk, whole	6 ounces
	Coffee	as desired
	Evaporated milk	1 ounce
Luncheon:	Sandwich:	
	Ham	2 ounces
	Rye bread	2 slices
	Butter	2 teaspoons
	Lettuce and tomato salad	
	Apple	1 small
	Graham crackers	2
Dinner:	Roast lamb	6 ounces
	Browned potato	2 (2 inches in diameter)
	Green peas	1 cup
	Celery and radishes	
	Muffin	1 (2 inches in diameter)
	Butter	2 teaspoons
	Honeydew melon	⅛ (7 inches in diameter)
	Tea with lemon	

Diet Prescription: Calories, 2180; proteins, 120 grams; fats, 100 grams; carbohydrates, 200 grams.
The carbohydrates and proteins are divided approximately:

	CARBOHYDRATES			PROTEINS	
Breakfast	1/5	37 Gm.		1/6	24 Gm.
Luncheon	2/5	70 Gm.		1/3	36 Gm.
Dinner	2/5	62 Gm.		1/2	60 Gm. (including bedtime)
Bedtime feeding		27 grams (subtracted from total carbohydrates)			

The Total Day's Food is calculated in Table 28–4.

SAMPLE MENU PLAN		LIST
Breakfast:	Fruit: 1 serving	III
	Bread: 1 serving	IV
	Butter: 1 level teaspoon or 1 other fat exchange	VI
	Eggs: 2 or 2 other meat exchanges	V
	Milk: 1 glass (8 ounces)	I
	Coffee or tea, as desired	
Luncheon:	Meat exchanges: 4 servings	V
	Vegetables: as desired within limits	II A
	Bread exchanges: 4 servings	IV
	Butter: 1 level teaspoon or 1 other fat exchange	VI
	Fruit: 1 serving	III
	Tea or coffee, as desired	
Dinner:	Meat exchanges: 5 servings	V
	Vegetables: as desired within limits	II A
	Vegetables: 1 serving	II B
	Bread exchanges: 3 servings	IV
	Butter: 2 level teaspoons or 2 other fat exchanges	VI
	Fruit: 1 serving	III
	Tea or coffee, as desired	
Bedtime: *	Bread exchanges: 1 serving	IV
	Meat exchanges: 1 serving	V
	Milk: 1 glass (8 ounces)	I

* If an intermediary-acting insulin is used, the bedtime feeding may be given in the afternoon
(3:30–4:30 P.M.).

SAMPLE MENU		
Breakfast:	Banana	1/2 small
	Eggs	2 soft boiled
	Toast	1 slice
	Butter	1 teaspoon
	Milk	1 glass (8 ounces)
	Coffee or tea	as desired
Luncheon:	Meat balls	4 ounces
	Boiled spaghetti	1 1/2 cup
	Mixed green salad with	1 teaspoon olive oil and vinegar
	Red raspberries	1 cup
	Plain sponge cake	1 1/2 inch cube
	Tea or coffee, as desired	
Dinner:	Tomato juice	small glass
	Broiled liver	5 ounces
	Crisp bacon	1 slice
	Baked potato	1 (2 inches in diameter)
	Carrots	1/2 cup
	Celery hearts	
	Whole wheat bread	1 slice
	Butter	1 teaspoon
	Applesauce, without sugar	1/2 cup
	Graham crackers	
	Tea or coffee, as desired	
Bedtime:	Bread	1 slice
	Peanut butter	2 tablespoons
	Milk	1 glass (8 ounces)

Appendix Tables 1 and 2. The classifications of fruits and vegetables according to their carbohydrate content are offered in Appendix Table 11. These tables may be useful if a system other than the method described in this text using "exchange lists" is employed. The "exchange lists" have been emphasized because of their more universal use and greater simplicity. However, other systems have certain merits that probably warrant their continued use. Space does not permit a description of others.

The total value of the ingredients makes up the nutrient value of any prepared dish. For example, when a custard is analyzed for its nutrient value, the ingredients of the custard are listed, namely milk or cream, sweetening, egg, and flavoring. The nutrient value of the custard is the total of the nutrients. Recipes based on exchange lists can be found in Chapter 43.

DIABETES IN PREGNANCY AND CHILDHOOD

The diet of the pregnant diabetic woman was discussed in Chapter 15, Nutrition for Pregnancy and Lactation. The diabetic child's diet will be discussed in Chapter 36, Diet Therapy in Diseases of Infancy and Childhood.

DIABETES AND SURGERY

If the diabetic patient's condition has been kept under control, he may undergo needed surgery without any unusual risk. When the surgery is an emergency, preoperative preparation is impossible. In emergency surgery cases, the regulation of insulin, intravenous fluids, and glucose is begun during the actual operation and carried on after its completion. Frequent urinalyses and necessary insulin injections for a sugar-free urine are carried out.

In elective surgery, it is advisable to plan a preoperative program for the patient, following the same principles suggested for the nondiabetic. To prevent dehydration large amounts of fluids are administered by mouth or parenterally, especially the day preceding the operation. Additional carbohydrates are prescribed to allow an adequate storage of glycogen, and sufficient insulin is given to enable the patient to oxidize the carbohydrates, thereby guarding against acidosis. Food is permitted until 4 or more hours prior to the operation and resumed as soon as possible postoperatively. The degree of severity of the surgery will help to guide the pre- and postoperative diet treatment.

To maintain fluid and electrolyte balance, abundant amounts of saline fluids are administered parenterally immediately after the operation. Glucose is usually given in the fluid, with adequate injections of insulin to metabolize the glucose.

Food in liquid form is usually the first type of food permitted orally. After minor surgery, the patient may be given his usual diet immediately. The diet advances in similar procedure as described for the nondiabetic. If fruit juices cause gas and bring discomfort to the patient, ginger ale or glucose solution is prescribed. The blood sugar determination and urinalysis govern the amount and type of insulin injections.

DIABETIC DIETS IN EMERGENCIES

Sometimes a diabetic patient may become too ill to eat the foods prescribed. When such a condition occurs, a soft or liquid diet is indicated. It is most important that the calculated carbohydrate allowance should be consumed daily even on a limited calorie diet, that is, if the quantity of insulin injected remains the same. If necessary, the protein and fat allowances may be sacrificed for the emergency and the amounts limited to coincide with the comfort of the patient.

The advantages of the soft or liquid diet are that the foods included in the diet are easily ingested and digested and contain a limited amount of bulk.

Here are some suggested adjustments which may be made to the regular prescribed diabetic diet:

Fruit juices and ginger ale may be served instead of whole fruits.

The cooked cereal may be diluted with the milk allowance in the diet to make a soft gruel which is usually enjoyed by a sick diabetic patient. Soft cooked cereal may be substituted for the potato or bread included in the diet.

Some of the bread and milk allowance can be served as milk toast.

Eggs and/or cottage cheese may be substituted for the meat allowed in the diet. Use the eggs for an eggnog or custard and blend with the milk allowed in the diet.

The cooked vegetables may be puréed and then diluted with some of the milk allowance in the diet to make a vegetable-milk soup.

Consult the lists of food substitutions and equivalents for diabetics which will suggest further possibilities. See also recipes in Chapter 43.

DIABETIC COMA Uncontrolled diabetes, which results in ketosis, is followed by coma. It is brought about either by overeating, deliberate or unavoidable omission of pre-scribed insulin injections, an infection, a surgical operation, or is the result of undiag-nosed and long untreated diabetes. The in-crease of glucose in the blood and urine in a controlled diabetic is indicative that the pa-tient's metabolism demands additional in-sulin. If this urgent need is not recognized and the insulin supplied immediately, the patient may go into a diabetic coma.

The warning symptoms are: thirst and dry mouth, flushed face, progressive drowsiness, nausea, vomiting, abdominal pain, cold and dry skin, characteristic acid breath, difficult breathing, headache, dizziness, pain in back and legs, and extreme weakness. When one of the symptoms occurs, it may not indicate anything is seriously wrong, but when several or all of the symptoms appear, it is cause for alarm. The urine will contain large amounts of sugar.

Treatment   Coma caused by ketone aci-dosis may prove fatal if not treated promptly and efficiently. Speed in treatment is essen-tial. The treatment consists of (1) insulin, (2) electrolytes, and (3) fluids. In severe keto-acidosis, fluid and electrolyte replace-ment usually requires the intravenous route and consists of normal saline solution. As hyperglycemia and glycosuria diminish, 5% glucose is added. If there is no nausea or vomiting, oral replacement may be attempted, using salty broth with supplementary water and tea. Later, carbohydrates are added such as fruit juice (orange juice), ginger ale, and gruel. Sufficient sugar must be present for metabolizing purposes. Potassium is given after 4 to 6 hours, preferably with electrocar-diogram control; urinary output must be adequate.

Diabetic patients should have frequent physical examinations and checkups by a physician to avoid complicating symptoms. The patient should keep on the alert for the symptoms of coma and report their occur-rence to the physician.

INSULIN REACTIONS (INSULIN SHOCK). Insulin reactions occasionally experienced by diabetics result from the sudden decline of the percentage of glucose in the blood (hypo-glycemia). The early symptoms are usually sweating, impatience, double vision, hunger, pallor, trembling, palpitation, headache, faint-ness, and an "all-gone" feeling. Although fleeting, these reactions can be relieved by the immediate consumption of an easily digested carbohydrate such as a fruit juice, Life Savers, sugar water or loaf sugar.

An insulin reaction from regular insulin is rapid and requires immediate recognition and treatment; with a slow acting insulin the onset is more gradual. When the reaction occurs from protamine zinc insulin, it may be necessary to repeat for several hours the administration of the rapidly absorbed car-bohydrate plus a more slowly absorbed food such as crackers and milk. Some authorities prefer the serving of a more slowly digested and absorbed carbohydrate, such as bread, combined with a rapidly digested carbohy-drate, such as jam, for a reaction from prota-mine zinc insulin. When severe reactions re-sult in unconsciousness, the patient receives glucose intravenously or by stomach tube. Assuming that the insulin is given before breakfast, reactions from regular unmodified insulin often occur before lunch (between 3 and 6 hours after injection); reactions from intermediary acting insulins (globin, NPH, lente) are apt to occur in the afternoon before the evening meal; and reactions from pro-tamine zinc insulin occur later. Reactions may be caused by an unusual amount of exer-cise, a delay in eating, the omission of a meal or of the prescribed amount of food, or by an error in the administration of an excessive amount of insulin, or by a decreased need for insulin.

If reactions occur too frequently the insulin dose should be adjusted to prevent permanent brain damage. Patients taking insulin are ad-vised to carry lump sugar or Life Savers for such emergencies. To avoid dangerous delays, diabetics should carry cards of identification. More than one staggering diabetic afflicted with an insulin reaction has been shunned as being intoxicated. Glucagon produced in the alpha cells of the islands of Langerhans may be used in the treatment of hypoglycemic re-actions. Subcutaneous injection of 1 or 2 mg. is used. Glucagon stimulates glycogenolysis in the liver and glucose is released rapidly into the blood stream.

COMPLICATIONS OF DIABETES MELLITUS

Diets for control of diabetes should be designed not merely to avoid signs and symp-toms but also to minimize the development of complications. The modern treatment of the diabetic patient has as its primary goal the prevention of vascular degenerative compli-cations. Evidence is accumulating that early control of diabetes can postpone and mini-mize the onset of such complications as reti-nopathy, neuropathy, severe atherosclerosis, and renal vascular disease.

DEGENERATIVE VASCULAR COMPLICA-TIONS   The increased life span of the diabetic made possible by improved control of the disease has brought a steady increase in the incidence of vascular complications in these patients. Atherosclerosis is commonly associated with diabetes, especially if the diabetic patient is elderly. The relationship between the two diseases is not clear, but it is known that they frequently appear together and the atherosclerosis generally develops at an earlier age than in nondiabetics. Any damage to the skin of the diabetic patient who has atherosclerosis either heals very slowly or never heals. Very often a gangrenous condition develops at the site of the injury. The diabetic patient should learn about the condition and function of the blood vessels. Atherosclerosis or complications in the blood vessels may affect the diabetic's eyes, causing partial or complete blindness; his heart and coronary arteries, causing impairment of physical activities; and his limbs, which are frequently the site of degeneration of the arteries, from a mild to an extreme degree, resulting in gangrene of one or both legs.

For the diabetic patient with atherosclerosis, a reduction of dietary cholesterol to 200 mg.; moderate reduction of total fat to 30 per cent of total calories with polyunsaturated oils in amounts of 60 to 90 ml. daily in place of saturated fats is recommended. (See dietary management of hyperlipoproteinemia (Chapter 30). It has been postulated that insulin, endogenous or exogenous, interferes with the action of several hormones which activate a fat hydrolyzing lipoprotein lipase normally present in the endothelial lining of the arterial wall, resulting in accumulations of fat in atheromatous foci.[12]

INFECTIONS   The diabetic is highly susceptible to infection. Uncontrolled diabetes favors uncontrollable infections. The nurse must be aware of this and be alert to any signs. The span of life of a diabetic depends to a large part upon the continuation of adequate treatment to assure freedom from complications of the disease.

OVERWEIGHT AND UNDERWEIGHT The diabetic should determine his ideal weight, and maintain it under authoritative guidance, measured by the gain or loss of weight. (See Chapter 29, Overweight and Underweight.)

Because the basal food needs decrease with the advancement of age, the older person should eat less to maintain an ideal weight. The "fat forties" is an apt expression, showing the results of constant or increased food intake during a period when food requirements have decreased. (See Chapter 18, Nutrition and Aging.)

Approximately 82 per cent of all adults with diabetes are 5 per cent or more overweight prior to the detection of the disorder. Middle-aged prediabetics frequently gain weight before sugar begins to appear in the urine. This happens so often that overweight is regarded as a precipitating factor. Indirectly, overeating may be an early symptom, because the increased consumption of food overtaxes the pancreas and, in time, too little insulin is secreted. Karam, et al.[13] observed that obese subjects appear to require increased amounts of insulin to maintain normal glucose levels. Obesity is an added burden to the proper functioning of the body. The overweight diabetic is adding "insult to injury." This should serve as an important lesson to an obese person, especially one with a family history of the disease; he is considered a potential diabetic.

Uncontrolled diabetics will often lose weight, especially during the onset of the disease, because of the body's inability to utilize glucose. The underweight condition is more prevalent in diabetic children than in adults. Children have the additional physiologic stress of body growth and development. (See Chapter 36 for discussion of diabetes mellitus in children.)

EDUCATION OF THE PATIENT

Every person with diabetes should know how to calculate and plan his own diet. He or a member of his family should be given an opportunity to learn how to do it. If for any reason this is not possible, he should be involved in the planning of the program which he can reasonably follow. Changes in eating habits and dietary pattern are not easily attained and frequent adjustments are necessary until an acceptable pattern evolves. He usually has to experience the steps or phases in the process of learning before he adopts a program.

The first step in the teaching-learning process is to begin with the patient's customary dietary patterns and eating habits and retain as many of them as possible if he is to eat at the family table and at favorite restaurants. (See Chapter 2.) The more familiar he becomes with the food values the better he is able to meet changing situations. Timing and spacing of meals, so important in the treatment, should be planned with the person to conform with his living conditions.

At each follow-up visit to the clinic, hospital or doctor's office the interview should begin with a determination of the pattern the patient is now following. If there has been a change in weight and/or abnormal blood and urine tests, the well-informed diabetic usually

[12]Starkey, T. P.: Diabetes mellitus—present problems and new research. Part IV. J. Am. Dietet. A., *158*:340, 1971.

[13]Karam, J. H., et al.: Excessive insulin response to glucose in obese subjects as measured by immunochemical assay. Diabetes, *12*:197, 1963.

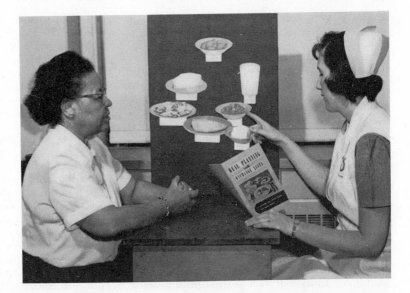

Figure 28–3   In all programs of therapeutic nutrition, the patient must receive sound dietary instructions to help him develop good food habits. Here the nurse is giving instructions to a diabetic patient using the booklet "Meal Planning with Exchange Lists." (S. L. Halpern: Nutrition and chronic disease. Health News, New York State Department of Health, October, 1955.)

knows the reason. Many times he needs assistance in adjusting to life's changing conditions.

Standardized diet sheets are seldom applicable to the person's needs. Distributing and going over them with the person requires little preparation and could be done by a clerk. It is the role of the professional interviewer (nurse, dietitian, physician) to involve the diabetic person in planning his own program. The time thus spent will be rewarding to all concerned.

Most people resist changes in diet. Furthermore, they resist being different from their fellow men. The nurse can help to develop a healthy mental attitude in the patient. Her daily association at mealtime, during the administering of insulin, and during the bath offers an opportunity to help the patient to accept his handicaps. Available teaching aids to demonstrate the importance of substituting foods equal in caloric, protein, carbohydrate, fat, mineral and vitamin content should be made use of. (See Figure 28–3.) An understanding of the function of foods, the relationship of the diet to health, the purpose of insulin administration, body care, and the testing of urine for sugar content will abolish fear. A dread of the injection needle will send many diabetics in search of an easy cure, an insulin substitute that can be taken by mouth, without benefit of a physician's advice.

The diabetic patient requires skillful care and thoughtful guidance to help him gain confidence. The cooperation of the physician, dietitian, nurse, and patient is important. If there is failure in the control of the diabetic condition, it may be attributed to ignorance of the complications and consequences. To the diabetic patient "knowledge is freedom."

Programs[14] for patients with diabetes are developing throughout the United States, sponsored by various health agencies, dietetic associations, hospitals and clinics. The aim is to give practical and continuing education, guidance and support to the diabetic.

The bimonthly magazine published for diabetics by the American Diabetes Association contains helpful information about the disease, diets, and recipes based on the Exchange Lists, plus interesting and pertinent stories. The Diabetes and Arthritis Program of the U.S. Public Health Service has a booklet, "Taking Care of Diabetes," to use in patient education.

HYPERINSULINISM (SPONTANEOUS HYPOGLYCEMIA)

Hyperinsulinism is a disorder of metabolism characterized by excessive insulin secretion which results in hypoglycemia. This may occur in the presence of a tumor of the pancreas, but often the origin is obscure. The liver may be implicated, and there may be a glandular disturbance and malnutrition. Hyperinsulinism is the direct opposite of diabetes mellitus. In diabetes mellitus there is not enough insulin to promote the metabolism of carbohydrates. It was noted that the diabetic who receives too much insulin or too little food has the same blood picture and symptoms as the patient with hyperinsulinism. Hyperinsulinism occurs less often

[14]Kaufman, M.: Newer programs for patients with diabetes. J. Am. Dietet. A., *44*:277, 1964; Programmed instruction materials on diabetes. J. Am. Dietet. A., *46*:36, 1965.

than diabetes. However, Briedahl and associates[15] working at the Mayo Clinic reported that family histories indicated a positive relation to diabetes. In 76 of 91 cases, which ranged in age from 9 to 72 years, an actual tumor of the islet cells of the pancreas was found and removed.

The patient usually experiences symptoms within 2 to 4 hours after nourishment is taken. This peculiar timing is attributed to the rapid absorption of sugar into the circulation although the carbohydrates are ingested along with the other nutrients. If tests were made at this stage, a marked elevation of the blood sugar would be noted. When the rise in blood sugar occurs, the pancreas is signaled to produce sufficient insulin to utilize the excessive amount. In the healthy person, the pancreas furnishes the correct quantity of insulin, and the blood sugar falls to the normal level; in hypoglycemia the initial glucose level in a glucose tolerance test is low and the increase after ingestion of glucose is slight. A six-hour glucose tolerance test is often given. In hypoglycemia the blood glucose level is below normal at the 5th and 6th hours.

DIETARY TREATMENT   Surgery to remove the tumor is the preferred treatment when the diagnosis is established definitely. Some patients refuse to have an operation, and others, with mild symptoms, may prefer to try medical regimens, including diet. The basic principles of the diet treatment for hyperinsulinism are focused upon the quick utilization of the carbohydrates, which stimulates the islet cells of the pancreas to secrete insulin and draw glucose from the blood. Because the sugars (dextrose) in fats and proteins are released and liberated into the blood stream evenly and more slowly, causing no stimulation to arouse the secretion of insulin, a diet rich in proteins and fats, and low in carbohydrates is recommended.

The diet for hyperinsulinism is calculated in a procedure similar to that used to plan the diabetic diet and the Exchange Lists (p. 402) may be employed. The diet may be divided into five or six meals, with a protein in each meal in order to reduce the rate of carbohydrate absorption. A small snack between meals will relieve the symptoms temporarily, but unless the patient eats within a short time, a recurrence of the symptoms may be expected.

The calories for the diet are based upon the normal requirements of the patient. The procedure has been discussed previously. When the total calories are known, the amounts of proteins and carbohydrates are determined. A high protein content of 90 to 130 gm. is

average; and a low carbohydrate content of 75 to 120 gm. is the usual range. After deducting these two requirements, the balance of the calories is allotted to fats. Caution must be exercised to prevent the development of any dietary inadequacies. Calcium and riboflavin may be very low because of the limited amount of milk permissible on a low carbohydrate diet. In such cases it is often advisable to prescribe the necessary calcium and riboflavin by medication as a supplement to the diet.

Since concentrated sweets are rapidly digested and absorbed and they stimulate insulin production, sugar and sweetened desserts; jelly, jams, honey, syrups, candy; sweetened fruits and fruits high in carbohydrates; vegetables high in carbohydrates; and soft drinks are omitted or used sparingly. The low carbohydrate fruits and vegetables and a limited amount of breads, cereals and potatoes should comprise the carbohydrates in the diet.

ADRENAL CORTEX INSUFFICIENCY

Addison's disease is a rare metabolic disorder in which there is adrenal insufficiency of the hormones of the adrenal cortex, either because of an infection such as tuberculosis, or a tumor, or general wasting or atrophy following removal of the pituitary gland in the treatment of cancer (hypophysectomy). The adrenals, two small glands of vital importance, are deeply imbedded in the back tissues near the kidneys. (See Fig. 28–1.) They consist chiefly of two parts. The central portion (medulla) contains cells originating from nerve structures which secrete *epinephrine*. The outer shell (cortex) secretes *aldosterone*, a mineralocorticoid which controls water and electrolyte balance; the glucocorticoids, cortisol and cortisone, which function in gluconeogenesis; and the androgenic hormones, which stimulate protein synthesis and the formation of sex hormones.

MINERALOCORTICOID   DEFICIENCY In Addison's disease the lack of aldosterone decreases sodium reabsorption and allows the excretion of sodium ions, chloride ions and water in the urine in excessive quantities. A greatly decreased extracellular fluid volume results; acidosis develops due to failure of hydrogen ions to be excreted in exchange for sodium reabsorption; potassium retention is increased; potassium in blood rises sharply; blood volume falls and cardiac output decreases. A crisis develops in a few days.

GLUCOCORTICOID DEFICIENCY   In Addison's disease the lack of cortisol secretion makes it impossible for the person to maintain normal blood glucose levels between

---

[15]Breidahl, H. D., et al.: J.A.M.A., 160:198, 1956.

meals because he cannot synthesize sufficient amounts of glucose by gluconeogenesis. Rapid glycogen depletion occurs and hypoglycemia follows. Severe hypoglycemia may be experienced in a person without food for 10 or more hours. Mobilization of fats and protein from tissues is reduced and many other metabolic functions are depressed. Most persons with Addison's disease have a melanin pigmentation of the skin of a deep tan or bronze. The cause is believed to be due to an excessive secretion of melanocyte-stimulating hormone (MSH) by the pituitary to exert an inhibiting effect when the adrenal steroids are lacking. These people frequently experience abdominal discomfort, diarrhea, nausea, vomiting and anorexia. The prognosis for Addison's disease is grave, but up-to-date therapy has improved the outlook.

TREATMENT   Supplying the missing adrenal cortex hormone to the patient has proved advantageous. A synthetic product, *desoxycorticosterone*, has largely superseded the natural substance and has revolutionized the treatment of Addison's disease. The patient is kept under close supervision because overdosage may cause palpitation, elevated blood pressure, chest pain, and edema. The underlying cause of the disease also must receive attention.

The more recent method of hormone replacement therapy causes release of serum potassium and retention of salt and water, with the sodium and potassium reaching or approaching a normal concentration level. However, 4 to 6 gm. of additional salt daily is often advised to spare the hormonal needs and thus reduce the expense of the treatment. In a few cases, sodium chloride therapy alone is sufficient to relieve the symptoms for years. If electrolyte balance is not thus achieved, then active cortical extracts or aldosterone is given.

Dietary Treatment with Hormones   Because of the tendency to hypoglycemia and the extreme weakness experienced by patients with Addison's disease, frequent feedings of an adequate diet, high in protein and low in carbohydrate—similar to that described under hyperinsulinism (p. 413)—are indicated. The individual with Addison's disease must understand the symptoms of hypoglycemia and carry crackers and a protein (such as cheese) with him to control attacks if they occur frequently. He should have a fairly substantial meal at bedtime in order to prevent an early morning hypoglycemic reaction. Because the sufferer is frequently dehydrated, a generous intake of fluids is required. Vitamins, particularly ascorbic acid and those of the B-complex which function as components of metabolic enzymes, should be given in liberal amounts to provide for the increased metabolism. An acceptable procedure to provide some of the necessary vitamins would be to prescribe concentrated vitamin supplements. Foods rich in potassium (Appendix Table 9) are avoided. However, extreme restriction of potassium may be harmful.

Prior to the introduction of desoxycorticosterone acetate, dietary treatment consisted of a diet low in potassium and high in sodium, in an attempt to correct the faulty mineral metabolism. Such a diet is difficult to prepare and is not very acceptable to the patient.

ADRENOCORTICOTROPIC HORMONE THERAPY

The steroids of the adrenal cortex and the adrenocorticotropic hormone of the anterior pituitary gland (ACTH) are used for the treatment of a variety of disorders. The effect of long-term usage on metabolism is important to note here.

ELECTROLYTE AND WATER METABOLISM   ACTH induces renal reabsorption of sodium in an ion exchange for potassium and water. Sodium restriction is indicated for many patients. Potassium is provided by an adequate intake of fruits, fruit juices, vegetables, whole-grain cereals, meat and broth.

PROTEIN METABOLISM   A large amount of cortisone given to a person may result in a negative nitrogen balance. An equilibrium may be maintained with a diet sufficient in calories, high in protein and liberal in carbohydrate to exert maximum protein-sparing effect.

CARBOHYDRATE METABOLISM   Therapeutic quantities of cortisone given may produce hypokalemia and hypochloremic alkalosis may result. Cortisone therapy increases the storage of glycogen by stimulating gluconeogenesis. Insensitivity to insulin is manifested and diabetics taking cortisone require additional insulin.

ASCORBIC ACID   Considerable amounts of ascorbic acid are present in adrenal tissue. ACTH depletes the adrenal tissue of this vitamin. A supplement of ascorbic acid is indicated in ACTH therapy.

OTHER MANIFESTATIONS   Adrenocortical steroid therapy increases hydrochloric acid secretion. Peptic ulceration may develop and if not treated may result in hemorrhage. Frequent feedings are indicated.

DIETARY MANAGEMENT   A diet adequate in calories, high in protein (100 gm.) and carbohydrate (200 to 300 gm.), low in sodium (1000 mg.) and an ascorbic acid supplement may be indicated when ACTH therapy is given over an extended period of time.

HYPERTHYROIDISM (EXOPHTHALMIC GOITER, THYROTOXICOSIS, BASEDOW'S DISEASE OR GRAVES' DISEASE)

Hyperthyroidism is a condition in which the thyroid gland is overactive, with a consequent increase in the rate of metabolism. Disorder of carbohydrate metabolism (with glycosuria and abnormal blood sugar curves), increased protein metabolism, calcium imbalance, and disorder of creatine metabolism are frequently present. There are also changes in the liver and destruction of the muscle tissue. It is also referred to as exophthalmic goiter, thyrotoxicosis, Basedow's disease or Grave's disease. In many cases, a subtotal thyroidectomy is performed. However, even following a successful operation, many symptoms remain. Therefore, the medical treatment is of paramount importance. (See Fig. 28–4.)

Shorr observed that patients who develop Graves' disease have a constitutional predisposition with characteristics similar to those who develop peptic ulcer. Also there is a strong familial tendency. Shorr believed that the patient's environment and capacity for mental adjustment to life's situation play an outstanding role in the causation of the disease. Emotional upsets are precipitating factors. Lack of adequate iodine, infections, the unstabilizing influences which occur in the endocrine system during puberty, menopause and pregnancy are other factors. Hence, women make up the predominating number of patients with Graves' disease.

DIETARY TREATMENT   In hyperthyroidism all the metabolic processes in the body are accelerated. A high calorie diet is indicated to prevent the destruction of the body tissue and rapid loss of weight.

Calories   The increase of calories over normal allowances should be in accordance with the elevation of the metabolic rate. In mild cases the increase may be from 15 to 25 per cent above the normal allowance, while in severe cases an increase from 50 to 75 per cent is required. A diet containing 4500 to 5000 kcalories or more is frequently prescribed.

Protein   The protein allowance should be liberal but not high, because a high protein intake increases the specific dynamic energy and influences calorie waste. It should be sufficient to meet the increased need for nitrogen. By supplying sufficient calories through carbohydrates and fats, an allowance of 100 gm. of protein will usually be adequate to maintain nitrogen balance.

Carbohydrate   Carbohydrate intake

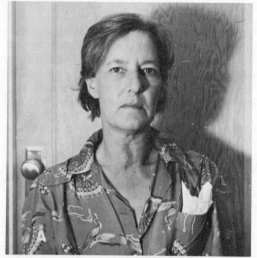

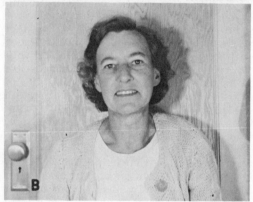

Figure 28–4   Before and after 2½ months treatment for severe hyperthyroidism (without exophthalmos). An antithyroid drug was administered. Patient was later treated with I¹³¹ and made a complete recovery despite a stormy course. Note weight loss, enlarged thyroid (goiter) and tense expression before treatment. (Courtesy of Dr. R. H. Hoffman.)

should be increased to compensate for the disturbance in the carbohydrate metabolism and to supply an excellent source of easily assimilated energy food. The increase in carbohydrates will spare the proteins in the diet.

Minerals and Vitamins   The diet should be abundant in all essential food nutrients, especially calcium, phosphorus, B vitamins, and vitamins A and C. At least one quart of milk a day should be included in the diet to maintain a positive calcium balance. Vitamin supplements should be a regular part of any diet program to meet the greatly increased demand. The high calorie diet discussed and outlined in Chapter 29, Overweight and Underweight, can be used as a basic diet.

Iodine   Iodine administration plays a significant role in the treatment of Graves' disease. Iodine is an essential component of the thyroid hormone *thyroxin,* the active principle of the thyroid gland. Cases of *simple goiter* can be prevented and sometimes improved by the administration of iodine. (See Chapters 8 and 34.) In hyperthyroidism there is a disturbance in creatine metabolism, which is similar to the symptoms seen in muscle dystrophy. If this disturbance is allowed to continue uncorrected, it will result in muscle destruction. It is impossible to correct this metabolic defect by diet; however, iodine specifically has been demonstrated to relieve the symptoms.

Stimulants   The stimulating effect of tea, coffee, tobacco, and alcohol is limited or avoided, as indicated and as ordered by the physician.

Psychology of Feeding   The psychological aspect of hyperthyroidism is important and should be considered seriously in the dietetic treatment of the condition. When the person is involved in planning the dietary regimen, successful adoption of the prescribed amount of food is apt to occur. Physical rest and peace of mind are essential in the successful treatment of these patients.

Drugs   Two measures in the management of Graves' disease mark an encouraging advancement in the nonsurgical treatment: (1) the use of radioactive iodine and (2) thiouracil. Both need longer periods of treatment and more extensive clinical trial before their ultimate value can be determined. (See Fig. 28–4.)

DIAGNOSTIC TEST DIET   The *low creatine-creatinine* diet is used sometimes as a test diet for cases of Graves' disease and diseases of the muscles. The purpose of the diet is to aid in determining the creatine content of the patient's blood.

All meats, meat products, fish, poultry, cranberries, plums, prunes, and gelatin are omitted from the regular diet. This same diet may be prescribed as a therapeutic diet when indicated.

HYPOTHYROIDISM (MYXEDEMA OR GULL'S DISEASE)

Hypothyroidism is an endocrine condition characterized by the deficient activity and lessened secretion of *thyroxin,* the thyroid gland hormone. In adults, the medical term for the advanced stage of this difficulty is myxedema or Gull's disease. A similar disorder in children, termed cretinism or infantile myxedema, develops in fetal life or early infancy if the mother has severe hypothyroidism. (See Fig. 28–5.) It will be discussed in the chapter on diseases of childhood.

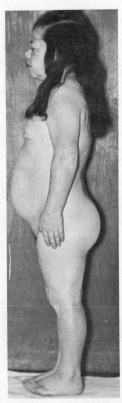

Figure 28–5   Hypothroidism before full maturity results in cretinism. The cretinous dwarf above shows effects of retardation in growth, infantile proportions persisting. (Courtesy of the Endocrine Clinic of the Beth Israel Hospital, Boston.)

In myxedema (Gull's disease) the thyroid undergoes a slow, progressive, specific type of atrophy. The cause is unknown. Symptoms may develop slowly and proceed unrecognized.

Because of the lowered basal metabolic rate (ranging from 15 per cent to 30 per cent, or more), there is rapid increase in weight, and elevated blood cholesterol value. Myxedema is more frequent in the female than the male (See Fig. 28–6.)

TREATMENT   Treatment consists of the administration of thyroid extract, preferably by mouth, and regulation of the diet. Because most of the patients suffering with myxedema are overweight, a low calorie diet is indicated. The amount of decrease in calories under normal requirement should be in accordance with the low metabolic rate and the degree of overweight. Principles of calorie reduction described in Chapter 29, Overweight and Underweight, are adequate. The low calorie diet with increased protein is usually the most effective treatment in cases of myxedema because protein increases specific dynamic energy.

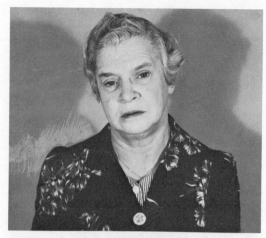

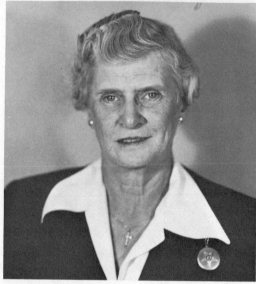

Figure 28-6   Upper, Severe case of myxedema prior to therapy. Lower, Same case following adequate thyroid therapy. (Courtesy of Arnold S. Jackson, M.D., Jackson Clinic, Madison, Wisconsin, and J.A.M.A., *165*:122, 1957.)

TETANY (SPASMOPHILIA)

Tetany is a condition caused by abnormal calcium metabolism manifested by convulsions, cramps or muscle twitching. It is commonly classified as (1) hypocalcemic tetany, the result of parathyroid hypofunction, and (2) alkalosis, the result of vomiting or the ingestion of alkaline salts.

Hypocalcemic tetany (low blood calcium), most frequently observed in children, is usually associated with rickets, acute infections and gastrointestinal disease. In adults it occurs as a result of injury of the parathyroids during a thyroidectomy, pregnancy, severe gastrointestinal disease, osteomalacia or kidney disease. Vitamin D or calcium intake or absorption deficiency may also cause the disease.

DIETARY TREATMENT   A normal adequate diet, emphasizing the foods rich in calcium and vitamin D, is prescribed, particularly when the blood calcium is low (hypocalcemic tetany). (See Table 19–4 and Appendix Table 7, for foods high in calcium content.) Milk and cheese are excellent sources of calcium, and at least one to one and one-half quarts of milk should be included in the daily diet. In addition to foods rich in calcium, medicinal calcium may be administered. Vitamin D is given to promote the absorption and utilization of calcium. Vitamin D enriched milk is an excellent source of calcium and the vitamin.

Tetany occurring from *alkalosis* is treated by administering large doses of an acid-producing salt or hydrochloric acid. The ketogenic diet (Table 33–1) is sometimes used as a part of the acid therapy.

GOUT

Gout is one of the oldest diseases recorded in medical history. Even Hippocrates mentioned gout in his writings. It is a disorder of purine metabolism, in which an excess of uric acid appears in the blood and the sodium urates are deposited as *tophi* in the small joints (Fig. 28–7) and the surrounding tissues; their most common site in chronic gout is the helix of the ear (Fig. 28–8). For some unknown reason, individuals with gout have trouble eliminating uric acid, an end product of purine metabolism formed in the breakdown of nucleoproteins, chiefly of animal origin. The normal person eliminates 700 mg. of uric acid daily via the kidneys. The body maintains a reserve pool of at least 1000 mg. in solution in body fluids. In gout, not only is there overproduction of uric acid, so that the amount in the pool increases from 3 to 15 times normal, but excretion is decreased.

CHARACTERISTICS   The disease resembles arthritis. Sudden pain in the great toe, with the pain continuing up the leg, is characteristic of the disease.

Gout usually occurs after the age of 35 and is characterized by specific heritable metabolic defects. The ailment comes in attacks. In the beginning the attacks last but a few days then disappear for a period of months. With the advancement of the disease, the symptoms occur more frequently and are more prolonged. Trivial injury or unaccustomed exertion may encourage the episodes. It is now questioned whether the attacks are related to excessive eating, drinking and exercise. There are, however, individual food allergies which will bring on an acute attack regardless of purine content of these foods. Occasionally, the disturbance is a sequel to an

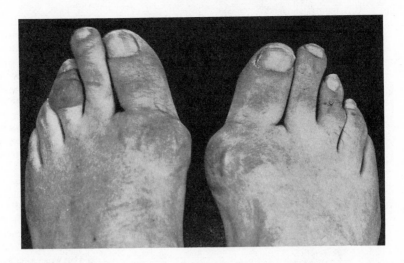

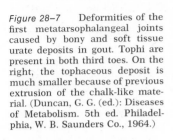

Figure 28–7   Deformities of the first metatarsophalangeal joints caused by bony and soft tissue urate deposits in gout. Tophi are present in both third toes. On the right, the tophaceous deposit is much smaller because of previous extrusion of the chalk-like material. (Duncan, G. G. (ed.): Diseases of Metabolism. 5th ed. Philadelphia, W. B. Saunders Co., 1964.)

operation or the administration of liver extract. Obesity is usually associated with a gouty condition.

PRINCIPLES OF DIETARY TREATMENT
The emphasis that should be placed on purine restriction in the diet is debatable. Drugs have largely replaced the need for rigid restriction of purine in the diet of patients with gout. From a practical point of view, it is almost impossible to plan a diet which is devoid of purine bodies. All foods have some traces of nucleoprotein from which purines are de-

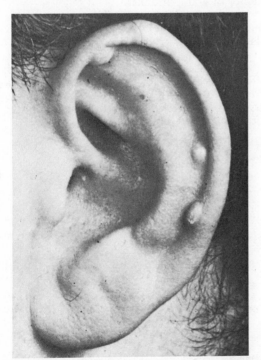

Figure 28–8   Tophi on the ear of a patient who had had gout for many years. (Courtesy of Dr. John H. Talbott, from Seminar Report, Fall, 1956, Merck, Sharp and Dohme, Div. of Merck and Co., Inc.)

rived. However, a number of foods are almost purine free (Table 28–7). Robinson[16] points out that *exogenous* sources of uric acid can be decreased by a diet eliminating foods high in preformed purine; however, the *endogenous* formation of uric acid is apparently influenced very little by dietary regulation. Purines are synthesized in the body from simple metabolites, which are constantly available from dietary carbohydrate, fat and protein as well as from endogenous purine breakdown. Thus, it is unlikely that avoidance of foods high in purine content will significantly decrease the uric acid pool. However, since purine metabolism is disturbed, restriction of foods containing nucleoproteins, which give rise to purines, is indicated. Excessive use of fats should be avoided, since fats are believed to prevent the normal excretion of urates. Protein should be adequate but not excessive. The calories should be maintained with carbohydrates, which have a tendency to increase uric acid excretion.

Acute Stage   Rigid restriction of foods containing purines (Table 28–7) is generally recommended in the acute stage of gout so as not to add exogenous purines to the already existing high uric acid load. Usually a soft diet, relatively high in carbohydrate, moderate in protein and low in fat is indicated. Fluids, such as water and fruit juice, should be forced to assist the excretion of uric acid and to minimize the possibility of calculi formation.

Interval Stage   Dietary management during intervals between attacks is regulated along with uricosuric drugs (such as probenecid) to achieve negative uric acid balance to control the urate deposits and serum uric acid. The current dietary treatment for pa-

[16]Robinson, W. D.: Nutrition and joint disease. J.A.M.A., *166*:253, 1958.

TABLE 28–7   FOODS GROUPED ACCORDING TO PURINE CONTENT

GROUP 1: HIGH PURINE CONTENT
(100 to 1,000 mg. of Purine Nitrogen per 100 gm. of Food)

Anchovies	Meat extracts
Bouillon	Mincemeat
Broth	Mussels
Consommé	Partridge
Goose	Roe
Gravy	Sardines
Heart	Scallops
Herring	Sweetbreads
Kidney	Yeast, baker's
Liver	and brewer's
Mackerel	

Foods in this preceding list should be omitted from the diet of patients who have gout (acute and remission stages).

GROUP 2: MODERATE PURINE CONTENT
(9 to 100 mg. of Purine Nitrogen per 100 gm. of Food)

*Meat and Fish
(except those on
     Group 1):*

Brains	*Vegetables*
Fish	Asparagus
Poultry	Beans, shell
Meat	Lentils
Shellfish	Mushrooms
	Peas
	Spinach

One serving (2 to 3 ounces) of meat, fish or fowl or 1 serving (½ cup) vegetable from this group is allowed each day or five days a week (depending upon condition) during remissions.

GROUP 3: NEGLIGIBLE PURINE CONTENT

Bread,	Fruit
enriched white	Gelatin desserts
and crackers	Herbs
Butter or fortified	Ice cream
margarine	Milk
(in moderation)	Macaroni products
Cake and cookies	Noodles
Carbonated	Nuts
beverage	Oil
Cereal beverage	Olives
Cereals and	Pickles
cereal products	Popcorn
(refined and	Puddings
enriched)	Relishes
Cheese	Rennet desserts
Chocolate	Rice
Coffee	Salt
Condiments	Sugar and sweets
Cornbread	Tea
Cream	Vegetables
(in moderation)	(except those in
Custard	Group 2)
Eggs	Vinegar
Fats	White sauce
(in moderation)	

Foods included in this group may be used daily.

---

intake and limitation of protein to 50 to 75 gm. daily, given insofar as possible in the form of plant and dairy protein products, may be helpful (Table 28–7). Protein intake is limited because it has been shown that endogenous uric acid biosynthesis may be accelerated in both normal and gouty patients by a high protein intake. Most of the proteins in the therapeutic diet come from cheese, eggs and milk, which are low in nucleoproteins. Fluids should be adjusted to produce a normal urinary output (2000 ml.).

It is now believed that mild or moderate use of alcohol by the patient with gout will not necessarily induce an acute attack, unless the patient has an allergy to alcohol. However, "Lactic acid, which appears during the metabolism of ethanol, has a demonstrable effect on the metabolism of uric acid."[17] Additional studies are needed to establish the need for abstention. For the remainder of the patient's life, certain dietary restrictions may be necessary.

Obesity   It is advisable that the obese patient should reduce and maintain a body weight which is 10 to 15 per cent below the calculated normal weight. However, weight loss should not be drastic but rather gradual over a period of several months. A sudden drastic reduction of calories that results in a metabolic state comparable to fasting or a high fat diet is recognized as a precipitating factor of acute attacks.

Low Purine Diet   Foods grouped according to purine content are listed in Table 28–7. The normal diet contains from 600 to 1000 mg. of purines daily. In cases of severe or advanced gout the purine content of the daily diet is restricted to approximately 100 to 150 mg. The diet may be prescribed according to these groupings, allowing for considerable individualization among patients.

LOW PURINE DIET

Foods Included Daily:

> *Milk:*   2 to 3 cups.
> *Cheese:* 1 or 2 ounces.
> *Eggs:*   1 or 2.
> *Lean meat, fish or poultry:* 2 to 3 ounces.
> †*Vegetables:* 4 servings including 1 serving potato, 1 to 2 servings green leafy or yellow variety, 1 serving other vegetable.
> *Fruit:* as desired, including 1 serving citrus fruit.
> *Bread, cereals and cereal products (enriched):* 4 to 6 servings or as desired.
> *Fat:* in moderation.
> Omit all foods in Group 1, Table 28–7
> Omit for low fat diets: Pastries, chocolate, nuts, olives Cream, ice cream, cream cheese Whole milk (use skim milk)

*Omit during the acute phase.
†Omit vegetables in Group 2, Table 28–7 in acute phase.

---

tients who are maintained on probenecid is a normal adequate diet adjusted to the *desired* weight, moderate in protein (70 to 80 gm.), increased in carbohydrate and relatively low in fat, avoiding foods of high purine content such as liver, kidney, sweetbreads, meat extracts, smoked meat, anchovies, sardines and leguminous vegetables. In the majority of patients, further dietary restriction does not seem to be justified. However, in severe or advanced cases, a further restriction of purine

[17]Editorial. Ethyl alcohol in the pathogenesis of gout. J.A.M.A., *183*:203, 1963.

Sample Menus

Remission Stage

BREAKFAST
Half grapefruit
Cream of Wheat with milk and sugar
Poached egg on toast
Butter or fortified margarine if allowed
Coffee with milk and sugar

LUNCHEON OR SUPPER
Macaroni and cheese
Lettuce and tomato salad
Chocolate pudding
Milk (whole or skim)

DINNER
2–3 ounces roast beef or hamburger
Baked potato
Mashed yellow squash
Enriched white bread and butter, and jelly
Fruit gelatin dessert and cookie
Milk (whole or skim)
Coffee or tea

BEDTIME
Milk or fruit juice

Acute Stage

BREAKFAST
Orange juice
Cream of Wheat with milk and sugar
Poached egg on toast
Coffee with milk and sugar

LUNCHEON
Macaroni and cheese
Broiled tomato
Chocolate pudding
Milk (whole or skim)

DINNER
Scrambled eggs or jelly omelet
Baked potato
Mashed yellow squash
Enriched white bread and preserves
Fruit gelatine dessert
Milk (whole or skim)
Coffee or tea

BEDTIME
Milk (whole or skim) or fruit juice

Fruit juice and carbonated beverages between meals

Use of Drugs   Most patients require continuous administration of a urate eliminant such as probenecid (Benemid). It decreases the uric acid level in the blood by increasing the elimination of the acid through the kidneys, and it aids in preventing recurrences. It is frequently used with colchicine. Colchicine has proved helpful in reducing the urates in the circulation and relieving the joint pains of gouty arthritis but has no effect on uric acid metabolism. It is of more value during the acute stage but may be needed during symptom-free periods as a preventive. In some instances, use of ACTH (adreno-corticotropic hormone) during the acute stage is reported to be beneficial.

PROBLEMS AND SUGGESTED TOPICS FOR DISCUSSION

1. What is diabetes mellitus? Give the possible contributing factors. What tests are used to diagnose the disease?
2. List the symptoms of an untreated diabetic. How can they be controlled?
3. What is the purpose of insulin? Describe the different kinds, and point out how they differ.
4. Describe the oral hypoglycemic agents and explain their use in the treatment of diabetes mellitus.
5. Describe diabetic acidosis or ketosis. What is the cause and treatment?
6. What is an insulin reaction? How is it treated?
7. What percentage of *each* – carbohydrate, protein and fat – is possibly metabolized as glucose in the body?
8. Interview a patient with diabetes and show how his present dietary pattern can be modified for diabetic management.
9. Plan the menu guide with the patient, using the Exchange Lists.
10. Check the planned menus for nutritional adequacy.
11. Compare the differences and similarities of chemical regulation and clinical regulation of diabetes mellitus.
12. Study the diabetic diets used in your institution, and analyze the characteristics.
13. (a) Calculate a diet for a patient with hyperinsulinism containing daily: 75 gm. carbohydrates, 100 gm. proteins and 180 gm. fats.
    (b) Determine the total calories.
    (c) Plan a meal pattern.
14. (a) Interview a patient with Addison's disease and obtain a diet history.
    (b) Plan a menu pattern with the patient.
    (c) Check for adequacy of calcium, protein, iron, vitamins and calories.
15. (a) Interview a patient in the hospital ward suffering with Graves' disease and obtain the average daily food intake.
    (b) Estimate the amount of proteins and calories.
    (c) Estimate the *normal* daily calorie and protein requirements for the patient and compare with the estimated intake.
    (d) Determine the patient's *present* daily calorie and protein requirements. What is the percentage of increase in calories over the normal requirements?
    (e) Plan a meal pattern using household measures to determine the amount of food per serving.
    (f) Check the nutritional adequacy of the menus, particularly for minerals and vitamins.
16. (a) Obtain the diet history of a patient suffering with myxedema.
    (b) Determine the patient's *normal* calorie requirements per day.
    (c) Estimate his average calorie intake for the day.
    (d) Determine his *present* daily calorie requirements; then compare with the calculations made for the patient's calorie intake and normal calorie requirements.
17. What is tetany and how may it be treated?
18. Interview a chronic gouty patient in the interval stage requiring protein to be restricted to 70 gm., fat to 60 gm. and purine moderately restricted daily.

DIABETIC MANUALS

A.D.A. Forecast (published bimonthly) and the A.D.A. Meal Planning Booklet. American Diabetes Association, Inc., 18 East 48th Street, New York, New York, 10017.

Behrman, Sister Maude: A Cookbook for Diabetics. New York, The American Diabetes Association, Inc., 1959.

Danowski, T. S.: Diabetes as a Way of Life. New York, Coward-McCann, 1964.

Duncan, G. G.: A Modern Pilgrim's Progress for Diabetics. 2nd ed. Philadelphia, W. B. Saunders Company, 1967.

Gormican, A.: Controlling Diabetes with Diet. Springfield, Illinois, Charles C Thomas, 1971.

Joslin, E. P.: A Diabetic Manual. Philadelphia, Lea & Febiger, 1959.

Pollack, H., and Krause, M. V.: Your Diabetes, A Manual for the Patient. New York, Harper and Brothers, 1951.

Rogers, F. L., et al.: Your Diabetes and How to Live with It. Lincoln, Neb., University of Nebraska Press, 1961.

Rosenthal, H., and Rosenthal, J.: Diabetic Care in Pictures. 4th ed. Philadelphia, J. B. Lippincott Company, 1969.

SUGGESTED ADDITIONAL READING REFERENCES

DIABETES MELLITUS

Allen, F. A.: Education of the diabetic patient. New Eng. J. Med., 268:93, 1964.

Beaser, S. B.: Oral treatment of diabetes mellitus. J.A.M.A., 187:887, 1964.

Bierman, E. L., et al.: Obesity and diabetes: the odd couple. Am. J. Clin. Nutr., 21:1434, 1968.

Bortz, W. M., II, and Bortz, E. L.: Surgery of the diabetic patient: Changing concepts. Am. J. Clin. Nutr. 3:494, 1955.

Camerini-Dávalos, R. A., and Marble, A.: Incidence and causes of secondary failure in treatment with tolbutamide. J.A.M.A., 181:1, 1962.

Caso, E. K.: Diabetic meal planning—A good guide is not enough. Am. J. Nursing, 62:76, 1962.

Cervantes-Amezcua, A., et al.: Long-term use of chlorpropamide in diabetes. J.A.M.A., 193:759, 1965.

Cohn, C.: Meal-eating, nibbling, and body metabolism. J. Am. Dietet. A., 38:433, 1961.

Conn, J. W.: The dietary management of spontaneous hypoglycemia. J. Am. Diet. Assoc., 23:108, 1947.

Danowski, T. S. (ed.). Diabetes Mellitus. Diagnosis and Treatment. New York, American Diabetes Associate, 1964.

DeLawter, D. E., and Moss, J. M.: A five-year study of tolbutamide in the treatment of diabetes mellitus. J.A.M.A., 181:156, 1962.

Diabetes Mellitus: A Guide for Nurses. U.S. Public Health Service, Pub. No. 861, 1962.

Duncan, G. G. (ed.): Diseases of Metabolism. 5th ed. Philadelphia, W. B. Saunders Company, 1964. Chapter 14.

Editorial. Inborn errors of metabolism. J.A.M.A., 175:1814, 1959.

Editorial. Oral hypoglycemic agents in diabetes. J.A.M.A., 181:156, 1962.

Hamwi, G. J.: Treatment of diabetes. J.A.M.A., 181:124, 1962.

Hinkle, L. E., Jr.: Customs, emotions, and behavior in the dietary treatment of diabetes. J. Am. Dietet. A., 41:341, 1962.

Joslin, E. P.: A renaissance of the control of diabetes. J.A.M.A., 156:1584, 1954.

Joslin, E. P., Root, H. F., White, P., and Marble, A.: The Treatment of Diabetes Mellitus. 11th ed. Philadelphia, Lea & Febiger, 1969.

Kaufman, M.: Newer programs for patients with diabetes. J. Am. Dietet. A., 44:277, 1964.

Kaufman, M.: Programmed instruction materials on diabetes. J. Am. Dietet. A., 46:36, 1965.

Kaufman, M.: The many dimensions of diet counseling for diabetes. Am. J. Clin. Nutr., 15:45, 1964.

Karam, J. H., Grodsky, G. M., and Forsham, P. H.: Excessive insulin response to glucose in obese subjects as measured by immunochemical assay. Diabetes, 12:197, 1963.

King, L. S.: Empiricism, rationalism, and diabetes. J.A.M.A., 187:521, 1964.

Kinsell, L. W.: The case for routine use of diets high in polyunsaturated fat for diabetics. Diabetes, 11:338, 1962.

Krysan, G. S.: How do we teach four million diabetics? Am. J. Nurs., 65:105, 1965.

McDonald, G. W., and Kaufman, M. B.: Teaching machines for patients with diabetes. J. Am. Dietet. A., 42:209, 1963.

Pollack, H.: Dietary management of diabetes mellitus. Am. J. Med., 25:708, 1958.

Pollack, H.: Fat content of the diabetic diet. Diabetes, 9:145, 1960.

Sharkey, T. P.: Diabetes mellitus—present problems and new research. J. Am. Dietet. A., 58:201, 336, 442 and 528, 1971.

Singer, D. L., and Hurvitz, D.: Long-term experience with sulfonyl ureas and placebo. New Eng. J. Med., 277:450, 1967.

Skiff, A. W.: Programmed instruction and patient teaching. Am. J. Pub. Health, 55:409, 1965.

Stone, D. B.: A rational approach to diet and diabetes. J. Am. Dietet. A., 46:30, 1965.

Stowers, J. M.: Nutrition in diabetes. Nutr. Abst. Rev., 33:1, 1963.

Tani, G. S., and Hankin, J. H.: A self-learning unit for patients with diabetes. J. Am. Dietet. A., 58:331, 1971.

Thrush, R. S., and Lanese, R. R.: The use of printed material in diabetes education. Diabetes, 11:132, 1962.

Waiffe, S. O. (ed.): Diabetes Mellitus. 7th ed. Lilly Research Laboratories, Eli Lilly Company, Indianapolis, 1970.

Wilder, R. M.: Adventures among the islands of Langerhans. J. Am. Dietet. A., 36:309, 1960.

Williams, F. F., et al.: Dietary errors made at home by patients with diabetes. J. Am. Dietet. A., 51:19, 1967.

Williams, R. H.: Oral therapy for diabetes mellitus. J.A.M.A., 193:829, 1965.

Williams, T. F., et al.: The clinical picture of diabetic control studied in four settings. Am. J. Pub. Health, 57:441, 1967.

Wilson, J. L., et al.: Controlled versus free diet management of diabetes. J.A.M.A., 147:1526, 1951.

Winter, F. C.: Diabetic retinopathy. Degenerative vascular complications of diabetes and discussion of clinical aspects of the disease. J.A.M.A., 174:143, 1960.

Wohl, M. G., and Goodhart, R. S. (ed.): Modern Nutrition in Health and Disease. 4th ed. Philadelphia, Lea & Febiger, 1968.

MISCELLANEOUS METABOLIC DISORDERS

Astwood, E. B.: Management of thyroid disorders. J.A.M.A., 186:585, 1963.

Beeuwkes, A. M.: The dietary treatment of functional hyperinsulinism. J. Am. Dietet. A., 18:731, 1942.

Breidahl, H. D., Priestly, J. T., and Rynearson, E. H.: Clinical aspects of hyperinsulinism. J.A.M.A., 160:198, 1956.

Carpenter, T. M.: The historical development of metabolism studies. J. Am. Dietet. A., 25:837, 1949.

Conn, J. W., and Seltzer, H. S.: Spontaneous hypoglycemia. Am. J. Med., 19:460, 1955.

Duncan, G. G. (ed.): Diseases of Metabolism. 5th ed. Philadelphia, W. B. Saunders Company, 1964, Chapter 10, Chapter 12, and Chapter 17.

Dunn, J. P., et al.: Social class gradient of serum uric acid levels in males. J.A.M.A., 185:431, 1963.

Editorial. Control of gout. J.A.M.A., 175:1127, 1955.

Editorial. Ethyl alcohol in the pathogenesis of gout. J.A.M.A., *183*:203, 1963.

Gutman, A. B., and Yu, T. F.: Prevention and treatment of chronic gouty arthritis. J.A.M.A., *157*:1096, 1955.

Hoffman, W. S.: Metabolism of uric acid and its relation to gout. J.A.M.A., *154*:213, 1954.

Jackson, A. S.: Hypothyroidism. J.A.M.A., *165*:121, 1957.

Jay, A. N.: Hypoglycemia. Am. J. Nursing, *62*:77, 1962.

Krane, S. M.: Selected features of the clinical course of hypoparathyroidism. J.A.M.A., *178*:472, 1961.

Kupperman, H. S., and Epstein, J. A.: Oral therapy of adrenal cortical hypofunction. J.A.M.A., *159*:1447, 1955.

Murlin, J. R.: Historical background for the nutritional treatment of metabolic diseases. J. Am. Dietet. A., 24:381, 1948.

Review. Relationship between thyroid hormone and vitamin B_{12}. Nutr. Rev., *19*:274, 1961.

Talbot, J. H., and Ricketts, A.: Gout and gouty arthritis. Am. J. Nursing, *59*:1405, 1959.

Thomas, H. M.: The treatment of hyperthyroidism, medical or surgical. New England J. Med., *248*:760, 1953.

Watkins, E., et al.: Incidence and current management of post-thyroidectomy hypoparathyroidism. J.A.M.A., *182*:140, 1962.

Wohl, M. G., and Goodhart, R. S. (ed.): Modern Nutrition in Health and Disease. 4th ed. Philadelphia, Lea & Febiger, 1968, Chapter on Gout.

UNIT TWELVE
IMBALANCE OF
BODY WEIGHT

Chapter 29
OVERWEIGHT AND UNDERWEIGHT

OVERWEIGHT OR OBESITY

Obesity in the United States is recognized as a medical problem of growing concern. Society has created an abundant food supply while physical activity continues to diminish. Because overweight is definitely detrimental to health and tends to shorten life, it is a public health problem. More educational programs directed toward prevention of overweight are needed. It is estimated that approximately 20 per cent of the population in the United States are overweight as a result of imbalances between food calorie intake and calorie expenditure.

DEFINITION Overweight or obesity is a condition of the body in which there is an excessive deposit of fat. The condition may be either slight (overweight) or gross (obese). However, 10 per cent above the desirable weight in the normal individual is considered overweight; a deviation of 25 per cent above this weight is indicative of obesity. In heart disease, nephritis, diabetes or gout, a body weight that exceeds the desirable weight by 10 per cent is considered excessive and constitutes obesity. For optimum health, all individuals more than 10 per cent overweight should reduce their body weight to the desired weight for age, height and body build.

CLASSIFICATION AND ETIOLOGY Obesity is generally accepted to be always the result of excess caloric intake over energy output, and may result from any combination of increased caloric intake or decreased energy expenditure. Obesity may be classified as (1) simple or (2) glandular. The simple type may be (a) exogenous or alimentary, developed through an excessive food intake and low activity level and (b) endogenous or constitutional, that is, the result of some metabolic or other physiologic disorder or psychological instability. The measurable metabolic processes of most obese persons are not abnormal and do not account for

obesity. Newburgh[1] found that these people expend more total energy in performing work and produce more total heat in the basal state than those of normal weight. Gaylor[2] presents evidence that certain types of obesities in man may be metabolic in origin.

Heredity is believed to influence the endogenous or constitutional type. Genetic characteristics of heavy bone structure and muscle mass may influence the weight to vary from the "ideal" weight standards. The observations of Seltzer and Mayer[3] that, as a group, obese adolescent girls differ from the nonobese population in morphological features other than their greater adiposity, are of special significance. It would appear that there are constitutional factors operating in the predisposition to obesity. Many authorities do not recognize the endogenous type, believing that overindulgence in food is the basic cause of obesity. The cause of overeating varies with the individual. In many cases, family traits are blamed for overweight, thereby allowing some obese persons to indulge in overeating without attempting to correct the situation. Generally, it is believed that children of obese parents gain weight because they eat the same foods and are exposed to the same eating habits.

An endocrine basis for obesity is uncommon. Obesity may involve a disturbance in the functioning of one or more of the ductless glands, either the thyroid or the pituitary, but usually an excessive food intake is a contributing factor. In persons in whom endocrine factors play a role, they facilitate the weight imbalance but do not cause it. Cor-

---

[1]Newburgh, L. R.: Obesity. Arch. Int. Med., 70:1033, 1942.

[2]Gaylor, J. L.: Metabolic obesity. New York J. Med., 62:3801, 1962.

[3]Seltzer, C. C., and Mayer, J.: Body build and obesity— Who are the obese? J.A.M.A., 189:677, 1964.

rection of the hormonal deficiency does not obviate the need for dietary restriction.

Studies reported[4] indicate that human obesity is accompanied by a marked increase in adipose cell number. A decrease in cell size can be achieved by weight loss while cell number remains high. Early onset of obesity may be associated with greater increases in cell number than when obesity begins later in life. It is not yet known whether the stimuli that increase adipose cell number are nutritional, endocrine, behavioral, genetic or some mixture of these. Further investigations in these areas may lead to a more rational approach to the prevention and treatment of human obesity than is at present available.

The widely accepted reasons for overeating and obesity are summarized as: (1) emotional, when compulsive eating becomes a compensation for emotional problems; (2) regulatory, when the brain's appetite control center is not functioning properly; and (3) cultural, when parents overeat and children learn the same habit.

DANGER OF OVERWEIGHT   Excessive overweight can become a menace to health. If the vitality and functioning of the body are to be kept at a maximum level of efficiency, a normal weight must be maintained.

Statistics show that obesity decreases life expectancy. Only 60 per cent of obese people reach the age of 60, compared with 90 per cent of slim persons. Thirty per cent of the obese reach the age of 70, while 50 per cent of the slim reach 70. The age of 80 is reached by only 10 per cent of the obese compared with 30 per cent of the thin, a ratio of one to three.

Overweight is often a dangerous complication or the forerunner of another disease (see Fig. 29–1). As described in Chapter 28, Metabolic Disorders Related to Nutrition, individuals with a diabetic tendency, or whose family history reveals the disease, should strive to maintain a normal or slightly below normal weight. These individuals are considered "potential diabetics" and must avoid obesity in an attempt to prevent or at least to delay the development of the disease. Fat people are greater operative risks and, if feasible, should lose weight before elective surgery, with care to maintain the protein reserves.

Obesity encourages circulatory disorders, and patients with cardiovascular disease should maintain a body weight approximately 10 per cent below the computed normal weight to lessen the work of the heart and circulatory system. (See Chapter 30,

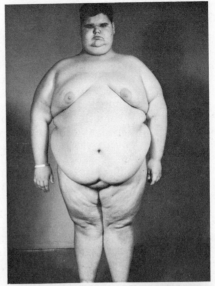

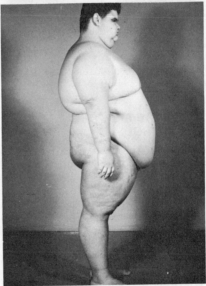

Figure 29–1   Overweight is deleterious and is associated with premature death. The obese individual is prone to develop diabetes, hypertension and degenerative cardiovascular disease. Above is a 13-year-old boy diagnosed as having exogenous obesity, developed through an excessive food intake. (Courtesy of Burtis B. Breese, M.D., Rochester, New York.)

Cardiovascular Diseases.) Arthritis, gout and nephritis are some of the other diseases in which it is necessary to maintain normal weight. Even without disease symptoms, the obese patient is advised to reduce for optimum health conditions. Years ago a fat person was considered healthy, but present medical knowledge and life longevity statistics have proved such beliefs false. It is interesting to note that fashion has followed the path of medical knowledge.

[4]Hirsch, J., and Knittle, J. L.: Cellularity of obese and nonobese human adipose tissue. Fed. Proc., 29:1516, 1970.

STANDARDS OF DESIRABLE WEIGHT

A fixed set of desirable weight standards (i.e., weights associated with lowest mortality) based on height and bodily frame (the latter designated as small, medium and large) for men aged 25 and over and women aged 18 and over, was compiled (1959) by the life insurance actuarial societies. (See Appendix Table 13 and 14.) These standards represent data gathered by twenty-six insurance companies between the years 1935 and 1953. Because of individual variations, the figures given as desirable or normal standards must be used only as a guide. Height-weight standards for children will be discussed in Chapter 38.

Body composition is important also in determining the desirable weight of an individual. Measures for variations in body composition include thickness of subcutaneous tissue determined by calipers; anthropometric measurement of body contour and size of body frame; underwater weight measures fat content of body; x-ray shadows measure fat surrounding organs; radioactive potassium count measures amount of body leanness.

LOW CALORIE DIETS FOR WEIGHT CONTROL

Regardless of the type or cause of obesity, the overweight individual must curtail his food intake. The safe and best way for an individual to lose weight is to adopt a regimen that is adequate in the essential nutrients. During the course of losing weight, the reduction of calorie intake enables the body to deplete its adipose tissue stores. The allure of fashion and glamour and to some extent life insurance statistics have played a role in making people diet conscious.

FADDIST DIETS   Periodically, new diets for weight reduction become popular. Some of these may be followed effectively for short periods, whereas others are nutritionally inadequate to support good health. A drastic reduction diet should be followed only with the consent or advice of a physician. In the overanxious desire to lose the pounds which were so easily put on by uncontrolled eating habits, different varieties of reducing diets have been followed indiscreetly. An endless number of low calorie diets, with emphasis on first one and then another dietary component, with and without special medication, have been proposed, tried, abandoned, and resurrected. It is not surprising that the reduction diet is the most abused and ridiculed! Nutritionists advocate a diet which is adequate but low in calories.

FORMULA DIETS   Formula diets for reducing weight come into vogue periodically. They are supplied by pharmaceutical, dairy, and food companies, and are liquid, powder or solid (wafers, etc.) in form. The recommended daily quantity supplies approximately 900 calories and consists of 30 per cent protein, 20 per cent fat, and 50 per cent carbohydrate.

The use of the formula diets is simple since they require no meal planning and no decisions. However, since weight reduction is usually a long-term procedure, the individual through the process of change in behavior strives to adopt better eating habits and an adequate dietary pattern. The change is best accomplished by building the diet around customary foods. Liquid formulas soon become monotonous and are discarded often in favor of another fad. The person will most likely return to previous dietary habits and regain the pounds lost.

Formula diets may be of value in the early treatment of obesity, or for those individuals who watch the scales and use formulas occasionally to lose a few pounds, but should be restricted to a limited period. On the long-term basis, they may be useful as a substitute for one meal per day. They also have a limited use for patients with a serious medical disorder which requires immediate weight reduction, or patients requiring surgery whose obesity poses a hazard, or patients who have become discouraged after many futile attempts at dieting. The formula diets are not a panacea for overweight, and the best approach to excessive weight still is a combination of reduced calories and increased exercise, carefully balanced to meet the individual's nutritional needs in terms of his sociological, cultural, economic, physiological, and psychological requirements.

STARVATION AND OBESITY   Fasting as a treatment for obesity has recently gained popularity. "Physicians in many areas have found that fasts, lasting from 48 hours to two weeks or more, produced virtually no hunger, were usually well tolerated, and seemed to be safe."[5] Loss in weight of 4 to 8 pounds in 24 hours in the early days of the fast are not rare. Some of this is water and sodium diuresis, which is usual during the first day or two. As the treatment progresses, the nitrogen loss tends to increase while the loss of salt and water decreases.

Starvation treatment should be done in a hospital under strict medical supervision as severe complications may develop such as gouty arthritis; normochromic, normocytic

---

[5]Editorial. Starvation and obesity. J.A.M.A., *187*:144, 1964.

anemia; and orthostatic hypotension. Individuals with a history of gout, cardiac, renal, cerebral, or hepatic disorders are not suitable candidates for this strenuous treatment. Fasting is used chiefly for extremely obese individuals so that normal weight can be achieved in a reasonable length of time. Vitamin supplements are given to meet the recommended allowances. Some physicians allow limited amounts of such low calorie foods as lettuce, celery and tomatoes plus black coffee or tea. Water intake is liberal (2 liters/day) to prevent dehydration. Normal exercise is encouraged. How effective this method of reducing weight will prove to be in large numbers of patients over a period of many years remains to be seen. A point of concern is the lay person who might overextend his starvation period for extra weight loss, provoking serious complications.

Duncan[6] advises one day of total fasting in every 7 or 10 days for those patients who are unable to adhere to a low calorie diet. This regimen permits a more liberal diet during nonfasting intervals. For those patients who are extremely obese, 2 fast days in 10 are advised.

Safe limits of weight reduction of 1 to 2 pounds per week can be achieved on nutritionally adequate diets of 1200 to 2000 kcalories per day.

THE DIET PLAN

CALORIES Calorie restriction is the only positive method of weight reduction. The number of calories is decreased to the point where fat is no longer deposited in the tissues, but the body is forced to draw on some of its own fat stores to meet energy needs. When this stage is reached the individual will lose weight. This is true on any regimen when a reduction in calorie intake occurs. The calorie value of body fat is 3500 kcalories per pound. This is the figure on which weight loss depends. Thus to lose one pound a week 500 fewer kcalories must be ingested each day. The number of calories a person ingests can be estimated by determining his basal needs and adding the activity increment. The basal needs for an adult male are 1 kcal. per kg. per hr. (see Chapter 3). The estimated activity needs are listed also in Chapter 3. For example a man engaged in sedentary activity weighing 253 lb. (115 kg.) needs approximately 3000 kcalories to maintain his weight at 250 lb.

$$115 \ (253 \ \text{lb.}) \times 1 \times 24 = 2760$$
$$+ \quad \text{activity increment} = \quad 225$$

$$\text{Total kcalories} = 2985$$

His desirable weight for his height and age is 165 lb. To maintain this weight at 165 lb. he needs approximately 2000 kcalories. The difference is 1000 kcalories. If he elects to reduce his present intake by 1000 kcalories per day (to lose 2 pounds per week), it would take him about 247 days or approximately 8 and a half months to lose 85 pounds.

If a person is currently consuming 4000 calories and his work includes a great deal of activity, then a reduction diet of 2000 to 3000 kcalories could be instituted at first and later reduced to the number of calories that will maintain weight at the desired level.

Because it may be injurious to the health of the patient, rapid weight reduction is not generally advocated. It should be accomplished only under careful medical supervision.

PROTEIN Protein in the diet is kept at the maximum amount permitted by the regimen, although exceptions may be made in certain cardiovascular and renal conditions in which high protein is contraindicated. (See Chapters 30 and 32.) Frequently the protein ranges from 0.9 gm. to 1.5 gm. or more per kilogram of body weight. Animal protein foods, such as eggs, milk, and meats, have high satiety value. In contrast, carbohydrate foods, such as fruits and vegetables, are emptied quickly from the stomach. The person gets hungry about two hours after ingestion of a meal composed largely of carbohydrate foods. From a socioeconomic viewpoint, however, a high protein diet is not always practical.

CARBOHYDRATES AND FATS After the protein allowance is determined, the remaining calories in the diet are divided between carbohydrates and fats.

The apparent superiority of low calorie diets composed chiefly of protein and fat in contrast to the usual protein-carbohydrate, low calorie diets has been reported.[7, 8] Subjects maintain that the fats eliminate the hunger and fatigue commonly experienced when fat is greatly limited. The efficacy of these plans has been attributed to the fact that no change in basal metabolic rate occurs on the low calorie, fat-protein diet. When the same number of calories is provided by a carbohydrate-protein diet, however, there

[6]Duncan, G. G.: Obesity—Some considerations of treatment. Am. J. Clin. Nutr., 13:199, 1963.

[7]Thorpe, G. L.: Treating overweight patients. J.A.M.A., 165:1361, 1957.
[8]Young, C. M.: Weight reduction using a moderate fat diet: Clinical response and energy metabolism. J. Am. Dietet. A., 28:410, 1952.

appears to be a compensatory drop in the basal metabolic rate which apparently allows the body to adapt to the lowered calorie intake, preventing any significant weight loss.

Bortz reports that the relative composition of the diet in terms of protein, fat and carbohydrate contents and the timing of meals are of little long-range consequence. Weight loss occurs when there is a deficit of calories.[9]

MINERALS AND VITAMINS   The foods selected for the diet should supply an adequate amount of minerals and vitamins. If the diet has an extremely low caloric value (800 kcalories), vitamin and mineral supplements are necessary.

WATER BALANCE   When a person reduces his calorie intake drastically he may experience a large weight loss during the first week. This is due to loss of water.

However, during the period of weight reduction there may be a week or 10 days when a plateau is reached and no weight loss is experienced. The body reconstitutes the early large fluid loss. However, during this time the patient may lose large amounts of adipose body tissue before he shows a reduction in weight.

Because water weighs more than fat, the scales may show a gain in the patient's weight during the period of fluid retention. However, water intake is not restricted in the diet unless complications occur. In such cases, salt (sodium) is also restricted to allow the release of fluids from the tissues and to avoid thirst. Weight gain can be deceptive because of the water retention. After a period of no loss or a gain due to fluid balance, the patient will usually experience a sudden substantial weight reduction.

FOODS TO INCLUDE   The calorie-restricted diet plan is basically the same as any well-balanced normal diet. It must meet the standards for adequate nutrition. To be certain of this, the protective foods are included (Chapter 11 and Tables 11–3 and 19–4). To give a satisfied feeling, sufficient bulk should be included. The low calorie diet is a modification of the normal adequate, or general hospital diet (Chapter 20). Amounts and kinds of individual foods are adjusted for weight loss. A faulty diet program would result in the development of a nutritional deficiency. (See Chapter 43 for low calorie recipes.) The lower the calorie intake, the more necessary it is to eat a diet of high quality. This is because when the food intake is large, there is greater probability of obtaining all necessary nutrients. When the intake is low, food choices become important.

[9]Bortz, W. M.: Predictability of weight loss. J.A.M.A., 204:99, 1968.

Sample Low Calorie Diets

Examples of two low calorie diets are given. Both provide 1200 kcalories and 80 to 85 gm. of protein. The first is a low fat (30 gm.), moderate carbohydrate (150 gm.) diet for an adult. The second example for an adult has a moderate fat (55 gm.), low carbohydrate (100 gm.) content. (See Tables 29–1 and 29–2.)

Caloric Value of Foods

The caloric value of foods varies within specific limitations. Fats offer the highest caloric value. Protein and carbohydrates contain less than one-half as many calories as equal grams of fats. Butter, margarine, oil, bacon, and mayonnaise are examples of foods which are primarily fat. Meats, eggs, milk and cheese are protein foods. Fruits and vegetables are composed chiefly of carbohydrates. Food values are discussed in Chapter 28, Metabolic Disorders Related to Nutrition and may be found in Appendix Tables 1 and 2.

The calculation figures for the two low-calorie diets in this chapter (Tables 29–1 and 29–2) are based upon the Food Exchange Lists in Chapter 28. However, the nutritive value of specific foods varies. For example, apples vary from 12 to 35 per cent in their carbohydrate content, depending upon the kind and the conditions of growth. In the nutritive analysis of an apple most authorities list the average carbohydrate content as 15 per cent. The cited example is applicable to many foods. Some of the foods listed in the tables have been analyzed in the uncooked form, while in reality cooked foods are eaten. The method of cooking may reduce the caloric value as much as 50 per cent. Therefore, these minor variations may be discounted.

ALCOHOL   Alcohol is relatively high in calorie content. One gram of alcohol yields about 7 calories or 200 kcalories per ounce—almost as much as fat! In addition, sugar or some form of carbohydrates is frequently added to alcoholic beverages (see Appendix Table 3) and they are taken along with a "snack" (Appendix Table 3).

A pint of beer, 4% alcohol, yields about 200 kcalories; a glass of wine, 10% alcohol, has about 75 kcalories, and an ounce of distilled liquor, such as whiskey, brandy, gin or rum, yields from 75 to 80 kcalories.

One Martini has about the same number of calories as 2½ slices of bread (a bread slice averages 60 to 75 kcalories). One whiskey highball has the same number of calories as six teaspoons of sugar, and an old-fashioned totes up the same number of calories as 17 teaspoons of cream. Tack on potato chips at the rate of 100 kcalories for 8 to 10 of them; or peanuts, 10 of them around 50 kcalories;

TABLE 29–1   1200 KCALORIE DIET FOR AN ADULT (HIGH PROTEIN, LOW FAT, MODERATE CARBOHYDRATE)

Diet Prescription: Kcalories, 1200; proteins, 85 grams; fats, 30 grams; carbohydrates, 150 grams. Calculation based on Food Exchange Lists, pp. 402–405. All diets are calculated with a leeway of 3 to 5 grams above or below the diet order.

FOOD	NUMBER EXCHANGES	LIST	CARBO-HYDRATE (gm.)	PROTEIN (gm.)	FAT (gm.)
Milk, skim	2	I	24	16	
Vegetables	As desired within limits	IIA			
Vegetables	1	IIB	7	2	
Fruits	4	III	40		
Bread	5	IV	75	10	
Meat,* lean	8	V		56	24
Fat	1	VI			5
			146	84	29

Sample Meal Plan

BREAKFAST	LIST
Fruit, 1 exchange	III
Bread, 2 exchange	IV
Meat, lean, 2 exchange	V
Milk, skim, 1 exchange	I

LUNCHEON OR SUPPER	
Vegetables, 1 serving	IIA
Bread, 2 exchanges	IV
Meat, lean, 3 exchanges	V
Fruit, 1 exchange	III
Milk, skim, 1 exchange	I

DINNER OR SUPPER	
Meat, lean, 3 servings	V
Vegetable, 1 serving	IIA
Vegetable, 1 exchange	IIB
Bread, 1 exchange	IV
Fat, 1 exchange	VI
Fruit, 2 exchanges	III

Sample Menu

BREAKFAST
½ grapefruit (small)
½ cup plain cottage cheese
2 slices whole wheat toast
1 glass (8 oz.) skim milk
Coffee or tea as desired

LUNCHEON
5 small oysters with catsup and horseradish
Sandwich:
  2 slices rye bread
  2 oz. cold sliced tongue
2 stalks celery and
3 radishes
1 peach (medium)
1 glass (8 oz.) skim
  buttermilk

DINNER
Bouillon
1 parsley potato
  2 in. diameter
3 ounces roast veal, lean
½ cup peas and carrots
Lettuce and tomato salad
1 teaspoon mayonnaise
1 cup applesauce
  unsweetened
Tea or coffee as desired

*Lean meat with visible fat removed, is used, reducing the fat content from 5 to 3 gms. per Meat Exchange. Limit eggs to 1 per day and omit peanut butter.

TABLE 29–2   1200 KCALORIE DIET FOR AN ADULT (HIGH PROTEIN, MODERATE FAT, LOW CARBOHYDRATE)

Diet Prescription: Kcalories, 1200; proteins, 85 grams; fats, 50 grams; carbohydrates, 100 grams. Calculation based on Food Exchange Lists, pp. 402–405. All diets are calculated with a leeway of 3 to 5 grams above or below the diet order.

FOOD	NUMBER EXCHANGES	LIST	CARBO-HYDRATE (gm.)	PROTEIN (gm.)	FAT (gm.)
Milk, skim°	2	I	24	16	
Vegetables	As desired within limits	IIA			
Vegetables	2	IIB	14	4	
Fruit	3	III	30		
Bread	2	IV	30	4	
Meat, lean	9	V		63	27
Fat	5	VI			25
			98	87	52

Sample Meal Plan

BREAKFAST

	LIST
Fruit, 1 exchange	III
Bread, 1 exchange	IV
Meat, 2 exchanges	V
Milk, skim, 1 cup (8 oz.)	I
Fat, 1 exchange	VI
Coffee	

LUNCHEON OR SUPPER

Meat, 3 exchanges	V
Vegetables, 1 serving	IIA
Vegetable, 1 serving	IIB
Fat, 2 exchanges	VI
Fruit, 1 exchange	III
Milk, skim, 1 cup (8 oz.)	I

DINNER

Meat, 4 exchanges	V
Bread, 1 exchange	IV
Vegetable, 1 exchange	IIB
Vegetable, 1 serving	IIA
Fruit, 1 exchange	III
Fat, 2 exchanges	VI
Tea or Coffee	

Sample Menu

BREAKFAST

½ cup orange juice
2 eggs (omit 1 tsp. fat)
1 slice whole wheat toast
8 ounces skim milk
Coffee or tea as desired

LUNCHEON

3 oz. broiled halibut
½ cup cooked
   turnip greens
Dried prunes, 2
½ cup carrots
2 teaspoons butter
1 glass (8 oz.) skim milk

DINNER

4 oz. lean roast beef
½ cup cooked rice
½ cup baked
   winter squash
Mixed green salad
   with 1 teaspoon oil
   and vinegar
1 teaspoon butter
Strawberries (1 cup)
Tea or coffee

°If whole milk is used, substitute 6 oz. lean meat with visible fat removed for 6 Meat Exchanges allowed.

TABLE 29–3   ENERGY EQUIVALENTS OF FOOD CALORIES EXPRESSED IN MINUTES OF ACTIVITY

		ACTIVITY				
FOOD	CALORIES	Walking*	Riding Bicycle†	Swimming‡	Running#	Reclining◖
		min.	min.	min.	min.	min.
Apple, large	101	19	12	9	5	78
Bacon, 2 strips	96	18	12	9	5	74
Banana, small	88	17	11	8	4	68
Beans, green, 1 c.	27	5	3	2	1	21
Beer, 1 glass	114	22	14	10	6	88
Bread and butter	78	15	10	7	4	60
Cake, 1/12, 2-layer	356	68	43	32	18	274
Carbonated beverage, 1 glass	106	20	13	9	5	82
Carrot, raw	42	8	5	4	2	32
Cereal, dry, ½ c., with milk and sugar	200	38	24	18	10	154
Cheese, cottage, 1 Tbsp.	27	5	3	2	1	21
Cheese, Cheddar, 1 oz.	111	21	14	10	6	85
Chicken, fried, ½ breast	232	45	28	21	12	178
Chicken, "TV" dinner	542	104	66	48	28	417
Cookie, plain, 148/lb.	15	3	2	1	1	12
Cookie, chocolate chip	51	10	6	5	3	39
Doughnut	151	29	18	13	8	116
Egg, fried	110	21	13	10	6	85
Egg, boiled	77	15	9	7	4	59
French dressing, 1 Tbsp.	59	11	7	5	3	45
Halibut steak, ¼ lb.	205	39	25	18	11	158
Ham, 2 slices	167	32	20	15	9	128
Ice cream, 1/6 qt.	193	37	24	17	10	148
Ice cream soda	255	49	31	23	13	196
Ice milk, 1/6 qt.	144	28	18	13	7	111
Gelatin, with cream	117	23	14	10	6	90
Malted milk shake	502	97	61	45	26	386
Mayonnaise, 1 Tbsp.	92	18	11	8	5	71
Milk, 1 glass	166	32	20	15	9	128
Milk, skim, 1 glass	81	16	10	7	4	62
Milk shake	421	81	51	38	22	324
Orange, medium	68	13	8	6	4	52
Orange juice, 1 glass	120	23	15	11	6	92
Pancake with sirup	124	24	15	11	6	95
Peach, medium	46	9	6	4	2	35
Peas, green, ½ c.	56	11	7	5	3	43
Pie, apple, 1/6	377	73	46	34	19	290
Pie, raisin, 1/6	437	84	53	39	23	336
Pizza, cheese, 1/8	180	35	22	16	9	138
Pork chop, loin	314	60	38	28	16	242
Potato chips, 1 serving	108	21	13	10	6	83
Sandwiches						
Club	590	113	72	53	30	454
Hamburger	350	67	43	31	18	269
Roast beef with gravy	430	83	52	38	22	331
Tuna fish salad	278	53	34	25	14	214
Sherbet, 1/6 qt.	177	34	22	16	9	136
Shrimp, French fried	180	35	22	16	9	138
Spaghetti, 1 serving	396	76	48	35	20	305
Steak, T-bone	235	45	29	21	12	181
Strawberry shortcake	400	77	49	36	21	308

*Energy cost of walking for 70-kg. individual = 5.2 calories per minute at 3.5 m.p.h.
†Energy cost of riding bicycle = 8.2 calories per minute.
‡Energy cost of swimming = 11.2 calories per minute.
#Energy cost of running = 19.4 calories per minute.
◖Energy cost of reclining = 1.3 calories per minute.
From Konishi, F.: Food and energy equivalents of various activities. J. Am. Dietet. A., 46:187, 1965.

or almonds, 100 kcalories to the dozen. The amount and nutritional quality of the food consumed help to determine how much a person will weigh.

FOODS TO AVOID OR LIMIT IN AMOUNT
WHILE PATIENT IS REDUCING CALORIE INTAKE

Alcohol	Ice cream (made
Beer	with cream)
Cake	Jelly
Candy	Mayonnaise
Cereals	Nuts
Cocktails	Oil
Crackers	Potatoes
Cream (sweet	Sauces
and sour)	Soft drinks
Desserts	Spaghetti
Fried foods	Sugar
Gravy	Wine

"SNACK" FOODS AND BEVERAGES People need to learn about food values. In Appendix Table 3 is a list of foods and beverages commonly consumed between meals. This table is included for the purpose of showing how easy it is to add calories, especially "empty" calories. A few snacks taken during the day can equal or exceed the entire day's calorie allowance!

ACTIVITY EQUIVALENTS OF FOOD CALORIES The energy equivalents of various activities in relation to energy value of common foods is shown in Table 29–3.

FOODS ALLOWED AS DESIRED Foods that have little or no caloric value and can be taken in unrestricted amounts by diabetic and obese patients, unless the diet order specifies to the contrary, are listed on page 405 in Chapter 28.

MENTAL HEALTH AND OBESITY

Some overweight individuals eat to satisfy an inner need; gorging overcomes their emotional problems. "Overindulgence in food compensates and substitutes in significant measure for the disagreeable affective elements generated by the intrapsychic conflicts."[10] Frustrations, depressive reactions, worry, guilt, shame, hopelessness, feelings of isolation and unusual stress seek compensations in eating. To the obese patient, food may represent love, security, or satisfaction, and provide a means of relieving the ever-present nervous tension. A compulsive pattern becomes established, and frequently the underlying causes are overshadowed by habit and addiction. It is not unusual for individuals to gain weight after giving up cigarette smoking. This aspect of weight control has assumed relatively greater importance in view of the recent campaign emphasizing the health hazards of cigarette smoking. The gain in weight is actually due to the substitution of eating for smoking and is not related to any alteration in basic metabolic processes. Obesity once established is sometimes clung to as a defense against feared social contact. In other instances, the obese patient may take the attitude that excessive food and weight are a sign of wealth, prosperity or success in life, which is unrelated to the physiologic sense of satiety.

Moore and co-workers[11] studied the relationship between obesity and mental health, using data obtained from 1660 persons selected as representative of 110,000 inhabitants of a residential area of New York City. The previously noted relationship that obesity increases with increasing age was confirmed. In addition, analysis revealed a striking relationship between obesity and socioeconomic status. The prevalence of obesity was seven times higher among women in the lowest social class category as compared with those in the highest category. Scores made by the obese respondents on nine mental health indices were compared with scores made by individuals of average weight. The obese group made more pathological scores on eight of the nine measures; on three of these—immaturity, rigidity, and suspiciousness—the difference was statistically significant. Often there is an inner conflict between desire to lose weight and enjoyment of the attention gained through failing to cooperate with treatment. Usually the causes of obesity are multiple. An adequate explanation of the physiological and psychological factors of excessive appetite awaits further research.

Psychology of Weight Reduction

The overweight person first of all must be aware that he needs to lose weight. Many times attention to the need is given in the hospital or in the physician's office. In the hospital the patient is introduced to the regimen through the meals served to him. In the physician's office most likely he is given a diet list to follow.

It is of utmost importance to utilize the principles of learning in assisting patients with the dietary program to lose weight. The plan is individualized to his needs and in terms of how he perceives his task and is developed from the dietary history.

The person may be *aware* of his need to change but not interested in losing weight. One who is *interested* in losing weight is usually ready to learn how the task can be

[10]Simon, R. I.: Obesity as a depressive equivalent. J.A.M.A., *183*:209, 1963.

[11]Moore, M. E., et al.: Obesity, social class, and mental health. J.A.M.A., *181*:962, 1962.

achieved. He *evaluates* possible solutions and becomes involved in planning his regimen. He then gives the plan a *trial*. Satisfaction may or may not occur and adjustments are necessary before complete satisfaction with the program and its adoption take place. These are the stages[12] which an individual undergoes to change former eating habits and dietary patterns. Some people do not progress beyond the awareness stage. They may "go on diets" but never become involved in a change of eating habits and dietary pattern.

Eating habits are acquired. The person who is overweight, regardless of age, in most instances has poor food habits. If the past food habits have caused overweight, then the patient must change eating habits and not just restrict calories for a limited period of time. The overweight patient needs nutritionally adequate meals. The number should be determined. If the patient is accustomed to eating large quantities of food at irregular hours of the day, the habit to eat regardless of hunger is established. If this factor is explained to the hospitalized person on a restricted calorie intake he is likely to experience less craving for food and more satisfaction in the program. The greatest hurdle for the patient is to lose the first few of the accumulated pounds. The task seems quite hopeless if the excessive weight amounts to 70 to 80 or more pounds. Even for those individuals, the loss of 3 to 5 pounds will arouse enthusiasm and encourage him to continue to reach the goal.

The overweight patient should be reminded that it took time to accumulate his excessive weight and that the effective changes occur gradually. He should understand the reasons for losing weight and become familiar with the role of food and food habits. Good habits acquired during weight reduction should be those which can well be continued for an indefinite time. The best motivating force to reach and maintain desired weight is the possibility of improved health, appearance and efficiency. His motivation and ability to bring about change in food habits and not return to former habits and obesity means success.

The process of re-education on the part of the individual is difficult. He has to make the necessary changes and adopt a pattern that he can reasonably follow.

The correction of obesity poses dual problems: (1) the balance between calorie intake and output; and (2) the dependence upon food for satisfactions. Attempts at weight reduction are futile if a large share of food — and satisfaction — is denied and there is no compensatory replacement. Attention to other activities (away from eating) helps some individuals. (See Table 29–3.)

INDIRECT APPROACHES   The essence of weight reduction is decreased caloric intake. Various indirect approaches have been popularized. These include administration of thyroid extract for more complete caloric utilization; administration of drugs to produce anorexia, most of which have adverse side effects; and administration of bulk agents to satisfy the appetite. Microcrystalline cellulose added to some foods ordinarily limited in most reduction regimens has been acceptable to overweight individuals.[13] Each of these crutches may have some use in individual cases but, in general, such methods defeat the purpose by submitting to the all important factor of will power. The control of obesity almost always demands control of will power, and the indirect approach must of necessity leave something to be desired.

MORALE   Regular follow-up contacts are reassuring to the patient and serve as a stimulus to continue the diet treatment. Organizations such as Weight Watchers and Take-Off-Pounds-Sensibly help individuals during the period of adjustment in calorie intake. The person is encouraged with a weekly record showing his progress. A full length mirror will reflect the results, too.

EXERCISE   The activity of the patient is also considered. If the patient is inactive, exercise is prescribed to promote the oxidation of body fat. It aids in restoring muscle tone, good posture, and a feeling of well-being. Brisk walking, not strolling, is recommended. This can be done even by the very heavy person who may find other forms of exercise impossible because of his awkward bulk. Daily gymnastic exercises, golf and swimming are advised, too. The type and amount of exercise must be prescribed for the individual patient. The amount of exercise for patients who have complications of cardiovascular diseases and arthritis must be very limited or withheld. Good judgment must be used when exercises are prescribed, keeping in mind the age and physical condition of the patient. Because the increased activity may inspire the appetite, the amount of food consumed must be kept under strict control.

Modern living is conducive to more rest and less physical activity. Labor-saving devices and electronic equipment have eliminated much of the daily exercise. A man who lives

---

[12]Craig, D. G.: Guiding the change process in people. J. Am. Dietet. A., 58:22, 1971.

[13]Pratt, D. E., et al.: Bulking agents in foods. J. Am. Dietet. A., 59:120, 1971.

two and one-half miles from work burns up 17 calories driving his car according to Pollack et al.[14] Cycling would utilize 122; walking, 210. Thus, 193 more calories are burned by walking than by riding. The typist working a mechanical typewriter burns up 450 more calories than the girl who operates an electric typewriter for a 5 day week; in 10 weeks this can be equivalent to 1 pound of weight, assuming a constant intake.

In general, it should be stressed that the approach to weight reduction is through caloric restriction. The amount of weight that can be lost by active or passive exercise is proportionately negligible. A definite distinction must be drawn between weight loss due to temporary dehydration and that following an adequate period of caloric restriction. The patient may find that he has lost several pounds after a brisk session in the gymnasium and he feels free to compensate by overindulgence at the next meal. Perhaps the greatest misunderstanding on the part of the patient concerns the distinction between water balance and caloric balance.

MALNUTRITION

Malnutrition may be defined as "a condition of the body resulting from an inadequate or

[14]Pollack, H., et al.: Metabolic demands as a factor in weight control. J.A.M.A., 167:216, 1958.

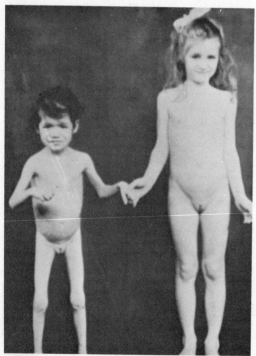

Figure 29–2   Two children of the same age. The one on the left suffers from malnutrition. (Courtesy of Burtis B. Breese, M. D., Rochester, New York.)

excessive supply, or impaired utilization, of one or more of the essential food constituents."[15] In malnutrition there is a lack of the normal amount of adipose tissues or else the tissue is of poor quality (Fig. 29–2). Undernutrition is the major problem affecting the health of mankind in the developing countries of the world today. Obesity, like underweight, is malnutrition. Malnutrition is further discussed in Chapter 34.

UNDERWEIGHT

Almost eclipsed by all the attention focused on obesity in the United States is the effort of some persons to gain weight. Underweight is a form of malnutrition important to the health of those needing to gain weight. The term underweight is applicable to persons who are 10 to 15 per cent or more below the normal accepted weight standard or desired weight. Because underweight is often a symptom or predisposing cause of a disease, it should receive medical investigation. In underweight individuals the resistance to disease is lowered, the growth during childhood and adolescence is retarded, and efficiency is impaired. The person who is seriously underweight often tires easily, is sensitive to cold, and complains of feeling weak. (See Fig. 29–3.)

ETIOLOGY   Underweight may be caused by (1) an insufficient intake in the quantity and quality of food to meet the needs of the person's activity; (2) poor absorption and utilization of the food consumed; (3) poor choice of food consumed; (4) a wasting disease such as tuberculosis or hyperthyroidism which increases the metabolic rate; and (5) the psychological reason of mental strain and worry, or psychological abnormality (anorexia nervosa). Elkinton and Huth[16] report that it is becoming well recognized that undernutrition itself may lead to multiple endocrine disturbances. Undernourished individuals may show signs of underfunction of the pituitary, thyroid, gonads and adrenals.

TREATMENT   Before starting a program to gain weight, it is necessary to determine the basic cause of the underweight of the patient. If a wasting disease is the cause, then the disease must be treated and the diet becomes part of the treatment. Information on the budgeting of foods, marketing, meal planning and preparation may be needed by the patient. If the problem is psychological, the meals are consciously limited by the pa-

[15]Turner, D.: Handbook of Diet Therapy. 5th ed. Chicago, University of Chicago Press, 1970.

[16]Elkinton, E. J., and Huth, E. J.: Metabolism: Clinical and Experimental, Part 1 (July), 1959.

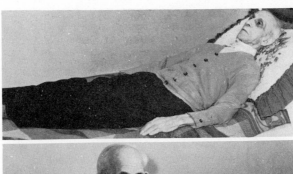

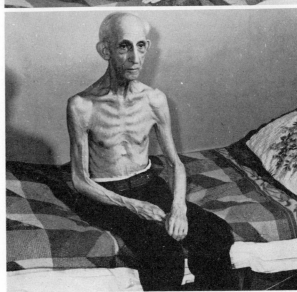

Figure 29–3   Underweight. Resistance to disease is lowered in underweight individuals. (S. L. Halpern: Nutrition and chronic disease. Health News, New York State Department of Health.)

tient to attract attention and sympathy. The advice of the psychiatrist is needed to direct the interests of the patient. In cases of anorexia nervosa, the basic fears and anxieties need to be discovered and removed; at the same time, maximal food intake is encouraged. Faulty absorption of food is a medical problem. Probably the most common cause of underweight is an inadequate food intake.

It is frequently more difficult for an underweight individual to gain weight than it is for an obese patient to lose weight. The selection and service of food is important. The appetite of the underweight person must be teased with eye-appealing, nutritious meals. Well planned meals at scheduled hours, instead of hastily planned, bolted meals, is advised. Mealtimes should be periods of leisure and relaxation. If upset about something, the person should postpone his meal until he is calmed down. Nervous tension is often part of the problem circle of underweight individuals.

HIGH CALORIE DIETS FOR WEIGHT GAIN

Before a diet is planned with the person, a careful dietary history of the patient should be taken. This history of the food intake should reveal the good and poor dietary habits and inadequacies.

The Diet Plan

CALORIES   The food allowance must provide sufficient calories to meet the total energy requirement of the body plus an allowance of 500 to 1000 additional calories for storage of fat in the adipose tissues. An acceptable method of determining the patient's daily caloric requirement is simply to calculate his needs on the basis of his ideal or desirable weight. If a hospitalized person normally needs 2800 kcalories to maintain desirable weight, his dietary needs would be 2800 to 3000 kcalories to gain weight. The intake should be gradually increased to avoid gastric discomfort and periods of discouragement. When a person is offered or expected to ingest more food at a time than he can take, he is apt to be overwhelmed by the amount and is unable to eat very much. The amount of food that could be ingested at one meal should be determined and the rest of the calories supplied in a concentrated form.

It has been found through experiences with patients of both sexes and different ages that men seem to prefer the additional calories through extra portions of the usual foods served at meals; children and adolescents prefer between meal nourishment; and women seem to favor more concentrated foods, such as the addition of cream to milk when it is served as a beverage. The secret of a successful diet program is to *individualize* the treatment for each patient and to include foods which the patient really enjoys.

PROTEIN In the average high calorie diet for the underweight, the daily protein allowance is maintained at the optimum level. High protein intake of 100 gm. or more is reported as necessary for replacement and repair of the body tissues.[17] In cases of severe malnutrition caused by the patient's inability to take sufficient foods, crystalline amino acids are sometimes given orally or parenterally. It has been found that, after a certain period of malnutrition, the gastrointestinal tract is incapable of digesting a sufficient amount of protein foods, especially if edema of the gastrointestinal tract is present, and vomiting or diarrhea may result. Sparing digestion by giving amino acids (protein hydrolysates) will frequently alleviate the difficulty.

CARBOHYDRATES AND FATS The amount of fuel foods, carbohydrates and fats, is increased in the high calorie diet. The concentrated calorie foods, such as butter, fortified margarine, cream, cereals, bread, potatoes, and high calorie desserts, are especially advised. A moderate fat allowance is made to increase palatability of the diet and increase the caloric value without dulling the appetite. Carbohydrates are digested easily and when taken in excess of body needs are readily converted into body fat.

MINERALS AND VITAMINS The mineral and vitamin allowances should be maintained at an optimum level. Supplements of vitamins, especially the B vitamins, are given to stimulate the appetite and meet the requirement when calories are increased.

For the high calorie diet this food pattern provides about 3000 kcalories, 130 gm. protein, with generous amounts of vitamins and minerals. The normal protective diet, outlined in Tables 11–3 and 19–4, is the basis or pattern for the high calorie diet. Increase in the amounts of the basic foods increases the intake of daily calories, minerals and vitamins. Additional foods, such as desserts, candy, and special dishes, may be enjoyed by the patient if the protective foods are not sacrificed. Eating between meals is encour-

aged but should not interfere with the patient's appetite for regular meals. Candy is usually served at the conclusion of a meal.

To increase the patient's daily calorie intake, the 500 kcalorie step-up is suggested. For example, the general hospital menu or adequate normal diet of an individual (Table 20-1) is calculated to contain 2500 kcalories. If a diet of 3000 kcalories is desired, then a step-up of 500 kcalories is added, or, if an increase of 1000 kcalories is desired, then two 500 kcalorie step-ups are added (Table 29–4). The high calorie diet is the adequate normal diet with increased calories. A 500 kcalorie increase over the daily caloric requirements should allow for a gain of a pound a week.

Suggestions for Increasing Calories in the Diet

Serve heavy cream instead of light cream.

Include cereal in the breakfast menu with a banana or other fruit because sugar, cream and cereal offer additional calories.

Butter breakfast toast when it is hot because more butter or margarine can be used. Cinnamon toast, griddle cakes, waffles, and French toast are good alternates for breakfast toast.

Serve jelly and jam along with bread and butter. Also, add jelly, jam and preserves to cheese cake, puddings and other desserts.

Add cream or undiluted evaporated milk to milk beverages. Malted milk and eggnogs can replace milk beverage.

Add skim milk powder to milk, milk beverages, soups, puddings and on hot cereal.

Add ice cream or whipped cream to desserts and milk beverages.

Serve cream soups instead of clear bouillon.

Eat dried fruits between meals because they are high in calories besides being good sources of minerals and vitamins.

Serve mayonnaise, oil and salad dressings whenever possible with sandwiches, salads and vegetables.

Serve gravy on meat and potatoes.

Add sauce to desserts such as puddings, molded gelatins, custards, rennet puddings, cakes, and ice creams.

Consume at least one quart of milk daily. When possible substitute cream for one half of the milk, or add nonfat dry milk solids if fat is not well tolerated.

Potatoes, spaghetti, rice, macaroni, and noodles may be served twice every day.

Along with the breakfast egg, serve bacon, sausage or ham.

Eat nuts between meals. They are high in fat content besides good protein and calorie additions.

---

[17]Seifrit, E.: The high calorie diet. Am. J. Clin. Nutr., *12*:66, 1963.

TABLE 29–4   SUGGESTIONS FOR INCREASING CALORIC INTAKES IN STEPS OF 500 KCALORIES*

	WEIGHT IN GRAMS	KCALORIES	PRO-TEIN
PLUS 500 KCALORIES:			
Additional foods (served between meals and/or before retiring):			
1. 1 cup (8 ounces) half milk and half cream (20%)	242	325	8
1 slice bread	23	60	2
2 pats butter or fortified margarine	14	100	
		Total 485	10
2. 3 cups milk (3/4 quart)	732	Total 480	27
3. 4 slices bread	92	240	8
1 serving II B. vegetable (p. 403)	100	36	2
1 egg	50	80	6
1 cup milk (8 ounces)	244	160	9
		Total 516	25
PLUS 1000 CALORIES:			
Additional foods (beverage served between meals and/or before retiring):			
1. 3 cups milk nourishments (3/4 quart), eggnogs and malteds	810	840	39
1 tablespoon jelly	20	55	
2 pats butter or fortified margarine	14	100	
		Total 995	
2. 3 slices bread	69	180	6
2 servings potato or equivalent	244	160	4
1 egg	50	80	6
3 cups milk (3/4 quart)	732	480	27
2 tablespoons jam	40	110	
		Total 1010	43
PLUS 1500 CALORIES:			
Additional foods (some served between meals and/or before retiring):			
1. 2 cups (1 pint) milk nourishment, eggnogs and malteds	540	560	26
2 cups (1 pint) half milk and half cream (20%)	484	650	16
1 baked custard	248	285	13
		Total 1495	55
2. 2 cups (1 pint) milk nourishment (malted milk, etc.)	540	560	26
3 cups milk (3/4 quart)	732	480	27
1 glass fruitade (8 ounces)	240	65	
3 slices bread	69	180	6
1 serving II B. vegetable (p. 403)	100	36	2
2 servings potato or equivalent	244	180	6
		Total 1501	67

Plan a definite eating schedule and then adhere to it. The benefits derived from an improved physical condition will more than repay the effort.

See Appendix Table 3 for additional suggestions.

It may be more difficult for an underweight person to gain one pound a week than for an obese person to lose a pound a week. It is not an easy task for the underweight person to add 500 kcalories to his daily intake of food. He should be involved in planning what and how much additional food he will take at one time and how often he will eat. He usually can suggest what can be added to make the plan appealing.

PROBLEMS AND SUGGESTED TOPICS FOR DISCUSSION

1. Define (a) overweight; (b) obesity.
2. Why is obesity becoming a recognized public health problem?
3. Classify obesity and list (a) the direct cause, and (b) factors that may influence obesity.
4. What are the principles of a low calorie diet?
5. Describe various reducing regimens and give the one most generally accepted.
6. Should all overweight individuals reduce? Explain. (See Young, C. M.: J.A.M.A., 186:903, 1963.)
7. Assist a person who is overweight with the necessary changes in her present dietary pattern to lose one pound per week. Permit her to indicate the changes that she will make.
8. Interview a patient who is obese. How many calories is he consuming to maintain his present weight? How many excess calories is he consuming. How can he improve his dietary? Try to follow the patient's progress in the outpatient clinic.
9. How would you help a person who is underweight gain weight? How will he implement the changes?
10. Take a food-consumption history of an underweight patient who is in the hospital ward or in the outpatient clinic. Calculate the calories. How many calories does he need to reach his ideal or desired weight? How long will it take him to reach the desired weight?
11. List the foods that should be stressed or added to the normal diet to make it a high calorie diet.

SUGGESTED ADDITIONAL READING REFERENCES

Alexander, M. M.: Have formula diets helped? J. Am. Dietet. A., 40:538, 1962.

Bayles, S., and Ebaugh, F. G.: Emotional factors in eating and obesity. J. Am. Dietet. A., 26:430, 1950.

Berkowitz, D.: Metabolic changes associated with obesity before and after weight reduction. J.A.M.A., 187:399, 1964.

Berryman, G. H., et al.: Desire vs. attrition in long-term weight reduction. J. Am. Dietet. A., 40:532, 1962.

Bortz, W. M.: Predictability of weight loss. J.A.M.A., 204:99, 1968.

Bullen, B. A., Reed, R. B., and Mayer, J.: Physical activity of obese and nonobese adolescent girls appraised by motion picture sampling. Am. J. Clin. Nutr., 14:211, 1964.

Bulletin. Food and Your Weight. U.S. Department of Agriculture Home and Garden Bulletin No. 74, Washington, D.C., 20402, Supt. of Documents. U.S. Gov't Printing Office.

Cedarquist, D. C.: Comments on "fad" dieting. J. Am. Dietet. A., 40:535, 1962.

Council Statement. Formula diets and weight control. J.A.M.A., 176:439, 1961.

Coursin, D. B.: Undernutrition and brain function. Borden's Rev. of Nutr. Research, 26, No. 1, Jan.–Mar. 1965.

Drenick, E. J., et al.: Prolonged starvation as treatment for severe obesity. J.A.M.A., 187:100, 1964.

Dudleston, A. K., and Bennion, M.: Effect of diet and/or exercise on obese college women. J. Am. Dietet. A., 56:126, 1970.

Duncan, G. G.: Obesity—Some considerations of treatment. Am. J. Clin. Nutr., 13:199, 1963.

Duncan, G. G. (ed.): Diseases of Metabolism. 5th ed. Philadelphia, W. B. Saunders Company, 1964, Chapter 8, Undernutrition, and Chapter 9, Obesity.

Duncan, G. G., et al.: Correction and control of intractable obesity. Practicable application of intermittent periods of total fasting. J.A.M.A., 181:309, 1962.

Editorial. Obesity. J.A.M.A., 186:65, 1963.

Editorial. Starvation and obesity. J.A.M.A., 187:144, 1964.

Fabry, P., and Tepperman, J.: Meal frequency—a possible factor in human pathology. Am. J. Clin. Nutr., 23: 1059, 1970.

Gaylor, J. L.: Metabolic obesity. New York J. Med., 62:3801, 1962.

Goldberg, M., and Gorden, E. S.: Energy metabolism in human obesity. J.A.M.A., 189:616, 1964.

Goldblatt, P. B., et al.: Social factors in obesity. J.A.M.A., 192:1039, 1965.

Hashim, S. A., and Van Itallie, T. B.: Clinical and physiologic aspects of obesity. J. Am. Diet. A., 46:15, 1965.

Hirsch, J., and Knittle, J. L.: Cellularity of obese and nonobese human adipose tissue. Fed. Proc., 29:1516, 1970.

Jolliffe, N. (ed.): Clinical Nutrition. New York, Harper and Bros., 1962, Chapter 4, Caloric deficiency and starvation; Chapter 26, Obesity.

Lew, E. A.: New data on underweight and overweight persons. J. Am. Dietet. A., 38:323, 1961.

Lewis, K. J., and Doyle, M. D.: Nutrient intake and weight response of women on weight-control diets. J. Am. Dietet. A., 56:119, 1970.

Mayer, J.: The physiological basis of obesity and leanness. Part II. Nutrition Abstr. & Rev., 25:871, 1955.

Mayer, J.: Obesity: Causes and treatment. Am. J. Nursing, 59:1732, 1960.

Mayer, J.: Obesity: Physiologic considerations. Am. J. Clin. Nutr., 9:530, 1961.

Medical News. Obesity: Part I, Prevention. J.A.M.A., 186:Nov. 9, 1963; Part II, Treatment and hazards, 186:Nov. 16, 1963.

Montague, A.: Obesity and evolution of man. J.A.M.A., 195:149, 1966.

Moore, M. E., Stunkard, A., and Srole, L.: Obesity, social class, and mental illness. J.A.M.A., 181:962, 1962.

Patterson, M. I., and Marble, B. B.: Dietetic foods. Am. J. Clin. Nutr., 16:440, 1965.

Pollack, H.: Protein therapy in emaciation. J. Am. Dietet. A., 23:410, 1947.

Prugh, D. E.: Some psychologic considerations concerned with the problem of overnutrition. Am. J. Clin. Nutr., 9:538, 1961.

Review. Adipose tissue and obesity. Nutr. Rev., 22:84, 1964.

Review. Are all food calories equal? Nutr. Rev., 22:177, 1964.

Review. Glucagon and insulin in starvation. Nutr. Rev., 21:332, 1963.

Seifrit, E.: The high calorie diet. Am. J. Clin. Nutr., 12:66, 1963.

Seltzer, C. C., and Mayer, J.: Body build and obesity—Who are the obese? J.A.M.A., 189:677, 1964.

Shipman, W. G., and Plesset, M. R.: Predicting the outcome for obese dieters. J. Am. Dietet. A., 42:383, 1963.

Simon, R. I.: Obesity as a depressive equivalent. J.A.M.A., 183:208, 1963.

Stock, A. L., and Yudkin, J.: Nutrient intake of subjects on low carbohydrate diet used in treatment of obesity. Am. J. Clin. Nutr., 23:948, 1970.

Straus, B. V.: Emotions and obesity. New York J. Med., p. 2497, 1955.

Stunkard, A., and Mendelson, M.: Disturbances in body image of some obese persons. J. Am. Dietet. A., 38:328, 1961.

Swendseid, M. E., et al.: Nitrogen and weight losses during starvation and realimentation in obesity. J. Am. Dietet. A., 46:276, 1965.

Westerfeld, W. W., and Schulman, M. P.: Metabolism and caloric value of alcohol. J.A.M.A., 170:197, 1959.

Wohl, M. G., and Goodhart, R. S. (ed.): Modern Nutrition in Health and Disease. 4th ed. Philadelphia, Lea & Febiger, 1968, Chapter 31A, Obesity; 31B, Undernutrition.

Young, C. M.: Weight reduction using a moderate fat diet: Clinical response and energy metabolism. J. Am. Dietet. A., 28:410, 1952.

Young, C. M.: Planning the low calorie diet. Am. J. Clin. Nutr., 8:896, 1960.

Young, C. M.: Management of the obese patient. J.A.M.A., 186:903, 1963.

Young, C. M.: Some comments on the obesities. J. Am. Dietet. A., 45:134, 1963.

Young, C. M.: Effects of frequency of eating. Food and Nutrition News. National Live Stock and Meat Board, Chicago, 42:No. 7, 1971.

Young, C. M., et al.: Frequency of feeding, weight reduction and body composition. J. Am. Dietet. A., 59:466, 1971.

Chapter 30
CARDIO-
VASCULAR
DISEASES

UNIT THIRTEEN
DISEASES OF THE
CIRCULATORY
SYSTEM, BLOOD,
AND
BLOOD-FORMING
ORGANS

The United States is reported to have the highest death rate from cardiovascular diseases of any country in the world. Coronary disease takes first place, with stroke in second place; combined they account for three-fourths of all deaths from cardiovascular diseases. Proper functioning of the cardiovascular apparatus depends upon good nutrition, and dietary regulation plays an important role in the management of heart disease.

CARDIAC DISEASES

CLASSIFICATION   The diseases of the heart may be classified according to the type of disorder, whether acute or chronic and whether compensated or decompensated. Cardiac disease may attack persons of any age although it is most common in the older age group. *It causes the highest percentage of deaths* in the United States today and is, therefore, a primary public health consideration. (See Fig. 30-1.) The decrease in the death rate from infectious diseases has allowed a greater percentage of men and women to reach the age at which heart attacks are likely to occur.

DRUGS   Today, antibiotic drugs play an important role in the treatment of certain infectious types of heart conditions: for example, bacterial endocarditis, often a sequel to rheumatic heart disease or congenital heart disease. In addition, steroids and penicillin have had a salutary effect on the course of rheumatic heart disease. (See Chapter 22 for discussion on rheumatic fever.)

CARDIAC SURGERY   Although diseases of the heart and circulatory system lead in the

cause of death in this country, great advances have been made in conquering many of them. Many forms of congenital disturbances of the heart and blood vessels are now helped or cured by surgery to the extent that the pa-

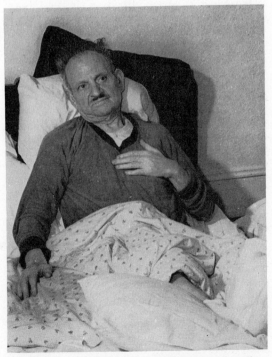

Figure 30-1   There are millions of persons with cardiac disease in the United States. Duration of life and freedom from symptoms in these individuals are often influenced by the diet consumed. (S. L. Halpern: Nutrition and chronic disease. Health News, New York State Department of Health.)

tient frequently returns to a completely normal life. In severe mitral stenosis, the valve between the left ventricle and auricle is so small that the flow of blood is interfered with, causing congestion and heart failure. Improvement or cure is often feasible through intracardiac surgery.

More recently, the surgical approach to coronary artery disease has produced encouraging results.

However, not all patients with cardiac diseases are amenable to surgery. Ideal candidates for surgery must be screened from sufferers who cannot be helped by these operations or for whom the risk is too great. For such less fortunate patients, therapeutic diet and drugs are relied upon to prolong life and give greater comfort.

PRINCIPLES OF DIET   The purpose of the diet in cardiac disease is to give adequate nourishment with the least possible work effort and muscular strain on the heart and to prevent or eliminate edema.

Energy   Loss of weight results in less work for the heart and improved cardiac efficiency. The patient who is obese in bed usually is given a 1000 to 1200 kcalorie diet. Those patients whose weight is normal are permitted calories sufficient to maintain weight slightly below the desired weight level.

Protein   The normal intake of protein (0.9 gm. per kilogram of body weight or about 60 to 70 gm. daily) is adequate for maintenance of body tissues.

Carbohydrate and Fat   The relative proportions of carbohydrate and fat are determined according to the nature and amount of fat and carbohydrate to be included in the diet. (See discussion on atherosclerosis.)

Minerals   All minerals should be provided in normal amounts except when sodium restriction is indicated. The average daily dietary provides 2800 to 6000 mg. sodium (2 to 6 gm.), although a liberal intake of salty food and/or a high content in drinking water may result in considerably higher sodium levels. Each molecule of salt contains approximately 40 per cent sodium; one teaspoon of salt contains approximately 2400 mg. sodium. In geographical areas of the country where iodine intake is largely dependent on iodized salt, the diet should be carefully evaluated for adequate iodine content when prolonged sodium restriction is required. (See page 116.) Supplemental iodine may have to be provided if the iodine content of the diet and local drinking water is inadequate.

Vitamin   The selection of food to include all vitamins is important. In instances when the intake of deep yellow and dark green vegetables is restricted, the vitamin A intake may be below recommended allowance. Also when fat such as butter, whole milk or margarine is omitted, the intake of vitamin A is low. A vitamin supplement may be indicated. Foods soft in consistency, easily digested and requiring little chewing are usually best tolerated during periods of decompensation. As his condition improves the patient may return to foods of normal consistency. Frequently, the patient tolerates five or six small meals a day much better than the usual three regular meals. Foods commonly considered bulky, gas-forming (p. 370), easily fermented, and indigestible are generally restricted to avoid pressure on the heart from the stomach, a situation which can cause distress or an acute attack. The cardiac patient should not eat when upset, under stress or in a hurry, because at that time there may not be a sufficient supply of blood in the digestive organs to carry on good digestion. Each patient is an individual. The dietary management should be planned according to his individual needs.

ACUTE CARDIAC DISEASE

In acute cardiac disease, which occurs in certain acute infections resulting in endocarditis or carditis and in cardiac failure, the diet is reduced to the minimum nutritional requirements. Dyspnea and chewing are incompatible in the patient with severe congestive heart failure. They often have to breathe through their mouths. Initially, these individuals should be given soft or liquid food which does not require chewing. The frequency of feeding is also important; more frequent and smaller feedings are obviously indicated. The *Karrell diet,* which consists of 800 ml. of milk (given in four equal feedings) is a well known diet. This diet provides about 600 calories and 500 mg. of sodium. For patients who cannot tolerate milk, variations have been devised, most of them containing 800 ml. of fluids and no free salt. Because these diets are nutritionally inadequate, they are prescribed for a short period of 4 to 7 days. As cardiac compensation increases, salt (sodium) and the diet can be liberalized.

CHRONIC CARDIAC DISEASE

In chronic cardiac disease the myocardium and valves of the heart are most likely to be involved. The condition may be (1) *compensated* or (2) *decompensated.* In compensated heart disease the organ is able to maintain almost normal circulation, through its own efforts, by an enlargement of the heart and by an increased pulse rate. In decompensated heart disease the heart is unable to compensate for its disturbance; it is unable to maintain normal circulation to supply nutrients and oxygen to the tissues or to carry away the waste products.

DIETARY TREATMENT FOR COMPENSATED HEART DISEASE The patient's weight should be normal or 10 per cent underweight to help improve the functional state of the vascular system. Slight underweight lessens the burden on the heart and thereby improves its efficiency. If the patient is overweight, it will be necessary to reduce calorie intake. The well compensated heart may not require any diet modification other than to avoid obesity. However, mild restriction of sodium (p. 442) is sometimes prescribed to maintain some control of sodium intake during periods of compensated heart failure.

DIETARY TREATMENT FOR DECOMPENSATED HEART DISEASE In decompensated heart disease a rigid diet treatment is usually planned to relieve the present strain and prevent further damage to the organ. These patients, if obese, will experience symptomatic relief following weight reduction, which will also serve as an inducement for them to adhere to additional diet restrictions in their supervised regimens should this become necessary.

There is often an increased metabolic rate in patients with chronic heart disease, particularly if the patient is dyspeptic. In such cases, a mild degree of weight loss may be prescribed, even for the individual of normal weight, in an effort to depress the metabolism. The protein is kept at the normal (60 to 70 gm.) allowance. Carbohydrates should furnish the bulk of the remaining calories, with fat adjusted to type and calorie allowance. Vitamins and minerals (except, perhaps, sodium) are given in normal amounts but may

need some supplementation. The diet is increased gradually to a more liberal program as tolerated.

Sodium and Fluids Edema is often present, the result of impaired cardiac function causing sodium and, therefore, fluids to accumulate in the tissues (dropsy). (See Figure 30-2.) Therefore, salt (sodium) and sometimes fluids are restricted and adjusted to the patient's individual needs (1000 to 1500 ml. daily). Current medical concepts regarding dietary control of fluid balance emphasize the restriction of sodium, and there is an increasing trend not to limit the fluid intake. When the sodium intake is limited, the formation of edema fluid can be prevented, since the mechanisms which usually regulate the sodium concentration in extracellular fluid do not permit the retention of water without sodium. The effect of electrolytes upon the fluid balance is related primarily to the sodium ion, rather than to the chloride ion, and dietary recommendations should refer to total sodium, rather than to salt.

SODIUM RESTRICTED DIETS FOR CARDIOVASCULAR DISEASES

NOMENCLATURE The past few years have brought significant changes in the so-called "low salt" diets. Diets restricted in salt, specifically sodium, for congestive cardiac failure, arteriosclerotic heart and hypertension are commonly used. Since it has been determined that the retention of sodium is the main factor causing retention of fluids and edema, the *salt restricted diets* have been replaced by *sodium restricted diets*. (To convert a specified weight of sodium chloride to

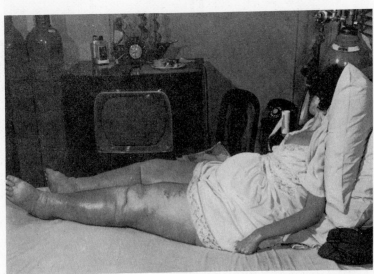

Figure 30–2 The rapidity with which this patient's dropsy will be cured will be influenced by her therapeutic diet. (S. L. Halpern: Nutrition and chronic disease. Health News, New York State Department of Health.)

TABLE 30–1   TABULATION OF NUTRITIVE VALUE OF BASIC DIET PATTERN FOR THE SODIUM-RESTRICTED DIET[1]

FOOD	MEASURE*	WEIGHT GM.	KCALORIES†	PROTEIN GM.	FAT GM.	CARBOHYDRATE MG.	MINERALS Na‡ Mg.	MINERALS Ca Gm.	MINERALS Fe Mg.	VITAMINS A I.U.	VITAMINS Thiamine Mg.	VITAMINS Riboflavin Mg.	VITAMINS Niacin Mg.	VITAMINS Ascorbic Acid Mg.
Milk	2 cups (1 pint)	488	335	17	19	24	244	0.58	0.4	780	0.18	0.84	0.6	6
Meat, fish, or poultry	5 ounces (raw)	120 (cooked)	365	28	27		104	0.01	3.5	2280§	0.30	0.40	6.9	1
Egg	1 medium	54	75	6	6		70	0.03	1.3	550	0.05	0.14	tr.	0
Whole-grain or enriched cereal°	1 serving	20	75	2	tr.	16	tr.	0.01	0.6	0	0.11	0.03	0.7	0
Whole-grain or enriched bread (without added sodium)	3 slices	90	250	8	1	47	27	0.07	1.6	0	0.22	0.14	2.0	0
Potato	1 medium	150	125	3	tr.	29	4	0.02	1.0	30	0.14	0.05	1.5	21
Leafy, green, or yellow vegetable¶	1 serving	100	30	2	tr.	6	9	0.05	0.9	880	0.08	0.07	0.7	26
Other vegetable#	1 serving	100	35	1	tr.	8	4	0.02	0.6	770	0.06	0.06	0.7	17
Citrus fruit	1 serving	100	45	1	tr.	12	1	0.03	0.4	120	0.07	0.03	0.2	47
Other fruit**	2 servings	200	125	1	1	32	5	0.02	1.0	120	0.08	0.08	0.8	18
Butter, unsalted	2 tablespoons	30	215		24		3			990				
			1675	69	78	174	471	0.84	11.3	6520	1.29	1.84	14.1	136
Recommended Dietary Allowances:‡ Woman (35–55 years)			1850	55				0.8	18	5000	1.0	1.5	13*** equiv.	55
Man (35–55 years)			2600	65				0.8	10	5000	1.3	1.7	17*** equiv.	60

* Average values for each food group have been computed according to the percentage distribution of food supplies as described in "Planning Food for Institutions," Agriculture Handbook No. 16, Washington, D.C.: U.S. Dept. of Agriculture, 1951. Food values used are those published in "Composition of Foods—Raw, Processed, Prepared" by Bernice K. Watt and Annabel L. Merrill, Agriculture Handbook No. 8, Washington, D.C.: U.S. Dept. of Agriculture, 1950.

† Calories have been rounded to the nearest 5. The total calories should be adjusted to the patient's needs by using more or less of cereal foods, bread, potatoes, or unsalted fat. Sugar and jelly may be used when there is no calorie restriction.

‡ Values for sodium are those naturally occurring in food before any additions have been made through processing and cookery.

§ This vitamin A value is reduced to 0 if average of 1 ounce liver per week is omitted.

° Includes farina, rolled oats, rolled wheat, wheat meal, puffed wheat, puffed rice, shredded wheat. Quick-cooking cereals and other dry cereals omitted because of high sodium content.

¶ Includes asparagus, green Lima beans (not frozen), snap beans, broccoli, Brussels sprouts, lettuce and escarole, okra, peas (not frozen), peppers, pumpkin, winter squash, turnip greens and products packed without added sodium. Excludes carrots, kale, beet greens, chard, spinach.

Includes cauliflower, corn, cucumber, eggplant, onion, parsnip, radishes, summer squash, rutabagas, tomatoes and products packed without added sodium. Excludes beets, celery, white turnips.

** Includes all fruits other than citrus—fresh, canned, or frozen according to consumption data.

*** Niacin equivalents include sources of the preformed vitamin and the precursor, tryptophan. 60 mg. tryptophan equals 1 mg. niacin.

‡ From Recommended Dietary Allowances. Washington, D.C.: National Research Council, Publication 1684, 1968.

[1] From Sodium-Restricted Diets. A Report of the Food and Nutrition Board. National Research Council. Washington, D.C.: National Research Council, Publication 325, 1954.

TABLE 30-2   BASIC 500 MG. SODIUM DIET

MEAL PLAN	SAMPLE MENU	Weight in Grams	Household Measure	Na (mg.)
			SERVINGS	
BREAKFAST				
Fruit	Grapefruit (half)	285	½ medium (with skin)	2
Cereal	Cooked oatmeal	118	½ cup	5
Egg	Soft cooked egg	50	1	70
Bread (Low Na)	Toasted whole wheat bread (Low Na)	19	1 slice	5
Butter (Low Na)	Sweet butter or margarine	7	1 pat	—
Coffee	Coffee	200	1 cup	—
Milk	Milk	122	½ cup (4 oz.)	60
Sugar	Sugar	15	3 teaspoons	—
LUNCHEON				
Meat	Sliced cold chicken	58	2 ounces	50
Vegetable	Cooked asparagus	100	6-7 spears	9
Bread (Low Na)	Whole wheat bread (Low Na)	23	1 slice	5
Butter (Low Na)	Sweet butter or margarine	7	1 pat	—
Fruit	Baked Apple	150	1 medium	2
Milk	Milk	244	1 cup (8 oz.)	120
DINNER				
Meat	Roast lamb	58	2 ounces	50
Potato	Parsley potato	122	1 medium	8
Salad	Lettuce and tomato	50	1 serving	9
Bread (Low Na)	Whole wheat bread (Low Na)	23	1 slice	5
Butter (Low Na)	Sweet butter or margarine	7	1 pat	—
Fruit	Fresh or stewed pear	182	1 medium	8
Milk	Milk	122	½ cup (4 oz.)	60

Note: All foods are cooked and prepared without salt; and no salt is served with any of the meals.

sodium, multiply by 0.393. In other words, 10 gm. of sodium chloride contains 3.93 gm. of sodium.)

THE BASIC SODIUM RESTRICTED DIETS

The physician prescribes diets representing varying degrees of sodium restriction, depending upon the severity of the cardiac or vascular disease, and the amount of edema or fluid retention present.

Table 30-1 shows the nutritive value of a basic normal dietary pattern, providing approximately 500 mg. of sodium daily. The foods included provide nutrients at levels, which, except for total iron content for young women, equal or exceed those of the Recommended Dietary Allowances for the normal healthy adult. The iron content can be increased by using sources which contain insignificant amounts of sodium such as green leafy vegetables (except beet greens, kale, dandelion, mustard greens, spinach), dried fruit, dried beans, or dried lentils. Adjustments and substitutions can be made from this basic pattern for the individual requirement and eating habits.

The calorie content of this basic diet can be increased or decreased to meet the individual requirements by using more or less of the foods low in sodium, such as unsalted cereal foods, bread, potatoes, and fat. Sugar and jelly may be used as desired within the calorie allowance. None of these additions will significantly offset the sodium level of the diet. Refer to Table 30-2, a sample meal plan and menu of the basic diet pattern (Table 30-1). See Appendix Table 12 for sodium content of foods.

Degrees of Sodium Restriction   Diets based on three levels of sodium restriction are classified as follows:

1. *Mild Sodium Restriction.* Containing 2400 to 4500 mg. (100 to 200 mEq.) sodium daily.

2. *Moderate Sodium Restriction.* Containing 1000 mg. (43 mEq.) sodium daily.

3. *Strict Sodium Restriction.* Containing 500 mg. (23 mEq.) sodium daily. (See Table 30-1, Basic Sodium-Restricted Diet.)

Diet booklets explaining these three sodium restriction levels have been prepared by a special group working with the American Heart Association's Nutrition Committee and are available on prescription at local heart association offices, to distribute to patients as indicated. The sodium-restricted dietary patterns are based on the Exchange Method such as the one used for diabetic dietary patterns (Chapter 28). In each booklet, the appropriate calorie level for the patient can be selected from among three levels—1200 kcalories, 1800 kcalories, and unrestricted calories. These diet levels are illustrations and when used as supplementary aids will help the person in planning his regimen. Variety in food selection is possible through food unit lists or "exchanges" based on the sodium content per

(Text continues on page 449.)

TABLE 30-3 SODIUM CONTENT OF FOOD EXCHANGES
(PROCESSED OR PREPARED WITHOUT THE ADDITION OF SALT)†

MILK

LIST 1

GROUP A
REGULAR MILK

GROUP B
LOW-SODIUM MILK

Each unit in both groups contains about 170 kcalories, 8 grams protein, 10 grams fat, and 12 grams carbohydrate. Group A units contain 120 milligrams sodium, whereas group B units contain 7 milligrams sodium.

1 cup	Evaporated whole milk (reconstituted)	4 tablespoons	Low-sodium dry milk (powder)
2 fat units and 1 cup	Nonfat buttermilk (unsalted – ask dairy)	1 cup	Low-sodium dry milk (reconstituted)
2 fat units and 3 tablespoons*	Nonfat dry milk (powder)	2 fat units and 3 tablespoons*	Low-sodium nonfat dry milk (powder)
2 fat units and 1 cup	Nonfat dry milk (reconstituted)	2 fat units and 1 cup	Low-sodium nonfat dry milk (reconstituted)
2 fat units and 1 cup	Skim milk	1 cup	Low-sodium whole fresh milk
1 cup	Whole milk		
1 cup	Whole milk buttermilk (unsalted – ask dairy)		

Note: Two units from the meat list may be substituted for not more than one milk unit a day.

*Use the amount specified on package for making one cup of milk – usually 3 or 4 tablespoons.

DO NOT USE: Any kind of milk not on list.

Any commercial foods made of milk: ice cream, sherbet, milk shakes, chocolate milk, malted milk, milk mixes, condensed milk.

VEGETABLES

LIST 2

USE FRESH, FROZEN, OR DIETETIC CANNED VEGETABLES ONLY

GROUP A

Each unit contains about 9 milligrams sodium and negligible calories, protein, fat, and carbohydrate.

GROUP B

Each unit contains about 9 milligrams sodium, 35 kcalories, 2 grams protein, negligible fat, and 7 grams carbohydrate.

GROUP A UNITS

Each unit is a ½-cup serving

Asparagus
Broccoli
Brussels sprouts
Cabbage
Cauliflower
Chicory
Cucumber
Eggplant
Endive
Escarole
Green beans
Lettuce
Mushrooms
Okra
Peppers, green or red
Radishes
Squash, summer
(yellow, zucchini, etc.)
Tomato juice (low sodium dietetic only)
Tomatoes
Turnip greens
Wax beans

GROUP B UNITS

Each unit is a ½-cup serving

Onions
Peas (fresh or low-sodium dietetic canned only)
Pumpkin
Rutabaga (yellow turnip)
Squash, winter
(acorn, Hubbard, etc.)

Note: Two units from Group A may be substituted for one unit from Group B.

(*Table continued on opposite page.*)

TABLE 30–3   SODIUM CONTENT OF FOOD EXCHANGES
(PROCESSED OR PREPARED WITHOUT THE ADDITION OF SALT)† *(Continued)*

VEGETABLES

LIST 2

USE FRESH, FROZEN, OR DIETETIC CANNED VEGETABLES ONLY

GROUP C

Each unit contains about 5 milligrams sodium, 70 kcalories, 2 grams protein, negligible fat, and 15 grams carbohydrate.

DO NOT USE:

Canned vegetables or vegetable juices except low-sodium dietetic.

Frozen vegetables if processed with salt. (Watch out especially for frozen peas and lima beans.) *Read the label.*

Do not use these vegetables in any form:

GROUP C UNITS

½ cup cooked	Beans, Lima or navy (fresh or dried)
¼ cup	Beans, baked (no pork)
⅓ cup or	
½ small ear	Corn
½ cup cooked	Lentils (dried)
⅔ cup	Parsnips
½ cup cooked	Lentils (dried)
⅔ cup	Parsnips
½ cup cooked	Peas, split green or yellow, cowpeas, etc. (dried)
1 small	Potato, white
½ cup	Potatoes, mashed
¼ cup or	
½ small	Sweet potato

Artichokes
Beet greens
Beets
Carrots*
Celery*
Chard, Swiss
Dandelion greens
Hominy
Kale
Mustard greens
Sauerkraut
Spinach
Turnips, white

do not use
salt or MSG in
cooking or
at the table

Note: One unit from the bread list, page 447, may be substituted for one unit from Group C.

*Note: Even though carrots and celery are high in sodium to be used as vegetables, you may use them sparingly to season (for example, one stalk of celery and/or carrot to a pot of stew) or as decorations.

FRUIT

LIST 3

USE FRESH, FROZEN, CANNED, OR DRIED FRUIT

Each unit contains about 2 milligrams sodium, 40 kcalories, negligible protein and fat, and 10 grams carbohydrate.

DO NOT USE:

Crystallized or glazed fruit.
Maraschino cherries.

FRUIT UNITS

1 small	Apple
⅓ cup	Apple juice or apple cider
½ cup	Applesauce
4 halves	Apricots (dried)
2 medium	Apricots (fresh)
¼ cup	Apricot nectar
½ small	Banana
1 cup	Blackberries
⅔ cup	Blueberries
¼ small	Cantaloupe
10 large	Cherries
1 tablespoon	Cranberries (sweetened)
⅓ cup	Cranberry juice (sweetened)
2	Dates
1 medium	Fig
½ cup	Fruit cup or mixed fruits
½ small	Grapefruit
½ cup	Grapefruit juice

12	Grapes
¼ cup	Grape juice
⅛ medium	Honeydew melon
½ small	Mango
1 small	Orange
½ cup	Orange juice
⅓ medium	Papaya
1 medium	Peach
1 small	Pear
½ cup diced or 2 small slices	Pineapple
⅓ cup	Pineapple juice
2 medium	Plums
2 medium	Prunes
¼ cup	Prune juice
2 tablespoons	Raisins
1 cup	Raspberries
2 tablespoons	Rhubarb (sweetened)
1 cup	Strawberries
1 large	Tangerine
½ cup	Tangerine juice
1 cup	Watermelon

Note: Read labels on packages of dried and frozen fruit. Sometimes sodium sulfite has been added to dried fruit and salt to frozen fruit.

do not use
salt or MSG in
cooking or
at the table

Note: Fresh lemons and limes (and their juice) may be used as desired. They do not count as a unit. Unsweetened cranberries and cranberry juice, and unsweetened rhubarb, may also be used as desired.

(Table continued on following page.)

TABLE 30–3   SODIUM CONTENT OF FOOD EXCHANGES
(PROCESSED OR PREPARED WITHOUT THE ADDITION OF SALT)† *(Continued)*

BREAD

LIST 4

LOW-SODIUM BREADS, CEREALS, AND CEREAL PRODUCTS

Each unit contains about 5 milligrams sodium, 70 kcalories, 2 grams
protein, negligible fat, and 15 grams carbohydrate.

BREAD UNITS

Breads and rolls (yeast) made without salt.

1 slice	Bread
4 pieces (3½″ × 1½″ × ⅛″)	Melba toast (unsalted)
1 medium	Roll

Breads (quick) made with sodium-free baking powder or potassium bicarbonate and without salt, or made from low-sodium dietetic mix

1 medium	Biscuit
1 cube (1½″)	Cornbread
2 three-inch	Griddle cakes
1 medium	Muffin

Cereals (cooked), unsalted
Each unit is a ½-cup serving

Farina
Grits
Oatmeal
Rolled wheat
Wheat meal

Cereals (dry)

¾ cup	Puffed rice
¾ cup	Puffed wheat
⅔ biscuit	Shredded wheat

(You may use other dry cereals—¾-cup serving—*if the label states*
that there are no more than 6 milligrams of sodium to each 100 grams
of cereal.)

1½ tablespoons uncooked	Barley
2 tablespoons	Cornmeal
2½ tablespoons	Cornstarch
5 two-inch-square	Crackers (low-sodium dietetic)
2½ tablespoons	Flour
½ cup cooked	Macaroni
1 five-inch-square	Matzo (plain, unsalted)
½ cup cooked	Noodles
1½ cups	Popcorn
½ cup cooked	Rice, brown or white
½ cup cooked	Spaghetti
2 tablespoons uncooked	Tapioca
1 three-inch-square section	Waffle, yeast or low-sodium baking powder, and/or your egg for the day

Note: One unit from the vegetable list, Group C, page 445, may be
substituted for one bread unit.

DO NOT USE:

Yeast breads or rolls made with salt, MSG, or from commercial mixes

Quick breads made with baking powder, baking soda, salt, MSG, or
made from commercial mixes

Quick-cooking and enriched cereals which contain a sodium compound.
Read the label.

Dry cereals except for those listed as allowed

Self-rising cornmeal

Graham crackers or any other crackers except low-sodium dietetic
Self-rising flour

Salted crackers
Salted popcorn
Potato chips
Pretzels

Waffles containing salt, baking powder, baking soda

---

do not use
salt or MSG in
cooking or
at the table

(Table continued on opposite page.)

TABLE 30–3 SODIUM CONTENT OF FOOD EXCHANGES
(PROCESSED OR PREPARED WITHOUT THE ADDITION OF SALT)† *(Continued)*

MEAT

LIST 5

MEAT, POULTRY, FISH, EGGS, AND LOW-SODIUM CHEESE AND PEANUT BUTTER

Units allowed per day will average about 25 milligrams sodium, 75 kcalories, 7 grams protein, 5 grams fat, and negligible carbohydrate.

MEAT UNITS

Meat or poultry (fresh, frozen, or canned low-sodium dietetic)

1 ounce, cooked, of any of the following is a unit

beef	quail
chicken	rabbit
duck	tongue (fresh,
lamb	cooked without salt
liver (beef, calf,	turkey
chicken, pork)	veal
pork	

(Beef or calf liver allowed not more than once in two weeks.)

Fish or fish fillets (fresh only)

1 ounce, cooked, of any of the following is a unit

bass	eels	salmon
bluefish	flounder	sole
catfish	halibut	trout
cod	rockfish	tuna

1 ounce	Canned low-sodium dietetic fish (tuna or salmon)
¼ cup	Cottage cheese (unsalted)
1	Egg (limit is 1 a day)
1 ounce	Low-sodium dietetic cheese
2 tablespoons	Low-sodium dietetic peanut butter

DO NOT USE:

Brains or kidneys

Canned, salted, or smoked meat: bacon, bologna, chipped or corned beef, frankfurters, ham, meats koshered by salting, luncheon meats, salt pork, sausage, smoked tongue, etc.

Frozen fish fillets

Canned, salted, or smoked fish: anchovies, caviar, salted and dried cod, herring, canned salmon,* sardines, canned tuna,* etc. Shellfish: clams, crabs, lobsters, oysters, scallops, shrimp, etc.

Cheese*

Salted cottage cheese

Regular peanut butter

*unless it is low-sodium dietetic.

Guide to Buying Meat, Poultry, and Fish

An average serving of meat, poultry, or fish is three ounces. This is equal to three units.

Because these foods shrink during cooking, you will have to buy more than three ounces for a three-ounce serving.

To have a three-ounce serving of fish or lean meat without bone—for example, liver or ground beef—you will need to start with four ounces, raw.

For meat with bone or fat, you will need to buy five to six ounces of raw meat to give you three ounces of lean cooked meat.

Here are some examples to guide you when you shop. One of these will usually give you three meat units:

> 1 pork chop
> 2 rib lamb chops
> leg and thigh of 3-pound chicken
> half breast of chicken
> 2 meat patties, 2″ diameter, ½″ thick
> 2 thin slices roast meat, each 3″ × 3″ × ¼″

> do not use
> salt or MSG in
> cooking or
> at the table

(Table continued on following page.)

TABLE 30–3   SODIUM CONTENT OF FOOD EXCHANGES
(PROCESSED OR PREPARED WITHOUT THE ADDITION OF SALT)† *(Continued)*

FAT

LIST 6

Each unit contains negligible sodium and about 45 kcalories and 5 grams fat.

FAT UNITS		DO NOT USE:
⅛ of four-inch	Avocado	
1 teaspoon	Butter, unsalted	Salted butter
(1 small pat)		Bacon and bacon fat
1 tablespoon*	Cream, heavy	Olives
	(sweet or sour)	Salt pork
2 tablespoons*	Cream, light	Commercial French or other dressing*
	(sweet or sour)	Salted margarine
1 teaspoon	Fat or oil for	Commercial mayonnaise*
	cooking, unsalted	Salted nuts
1 tablespoon	French dressing,	
	unsalted	
1 teaspoon	Margarine, unsalted	
1 teaspoon	Mayonnaise, unsalted	
6 small	Nuts, unsalted	

*Limit is 2 tablespoons a day because cream contains more sodium than the other fats.

*unless it is low-sodium dietetic.

MISCELLANEOUS FOODS

LIST 7

Each food listed contains small amounts of sodium.

DO NOT USE:

Sugar, white or brown
Syrup, honey, jelly, jam, marmalade

Alcoholic beverages
Cocoa, made with milk from diet
Coffee, regular and instant
Coffee substitute
Tea
Postum

Candy, homemade without salt
Cornstarch
Gelatin

Cream of tartar
Sodium-free baking powder
Potassium bicarbonate
Yeast

Bouillon cube (Low-Na)
Spices
Chives
Flavorings
Vinegar
Wine

Saccharin
Molasses
Instant cocoa mixes
Beverage mixes, including fruit-flavored powder
Fountain beverages: Malted milk and their milk preparates
Commercial candies
Commercially sweetened gelatin desserts
Regular baking powder
Regular baking soda
Barbecue sauce
Regular bouillon cubes
Catsup and sauces
Celery, onion, and garlic salts
Meat sauces, extracts and tenderizers
MSG salt
Soy or Worcestershire sauce
Salt substitutes, unless recommended by physician
Mustard, prepared
Olives, pickles, relishes
Celery leaves, dried or fresh
Cooking wine
Horseradish

†Refer to Exchange List, Chapter 28. From Your 500 Milligram Sodium Diet, American Heart Association, New York, 1970, pp. 38–53, and Appendix Table 12.

serving in the unit. Table 30–3 gives the average sodium values of the food exchanges.

Mild sodium restriction: 2400 to 4500 mg. sodium daily For the patient with only moderate heart damage when some control of sodium intake is indicated, a *limited* amount of salt is allowed in cooking: however, no salt is allowed on the tray or at the table; salty foods such as those listed from one through six in Table 30–4 should be omitted.

Moderate sodium restriction: 1000 mg. sodium daily For the patient with edema or a tendency to develop edema when following only mild sodium restriction: no salt is added during the preparation of food or at the table, with the exception of either allowing ¼ teaspoon salt daily or measured amounts of such foods as regular bakery bread (1 slice contains 150 mg. sodium) and salted butter (2 teaspoons contains 100 mg. sodium) to make the diet more palatable and no salty foods such as listed in Table 30–4 are allowed. A diet providing these restrictions will usually increase urine output.

Strict sodium restriction: 500 mg. sodium or less daily (Table 30–1) If edema and pulmonary congestion persist despite drugs, medication, and moderate sodium restriction, sodium should be reduced to 500 mg. (0.5 gm.) or less daily. For strict sodium restriction no salt is added during the preparation of food or at the table; and foods listed in Table 30–4 are avoided.

Severe sodium restriction: 250 mg. sodium daily Further reduction in sodium content of this basic diet pattern (Table 30–1) can be accomplished by substituting appropriate amounts of low sodium whole or nonfat milk (14 mg. sodium per pint) for the regular whole or skim milk (244 mg. sodium per pint). For a diet containing 250 mg. sodium, substitute low sodium milk for the regular milk allowed on the basic 500 mg. sodium diet.

Sodium deficient milk has been processed to remove most of the naturally occurring sodium. It is usually prepared in powder form which can be reconstructed. However, a fluid milk preparation is available. Thus, the dietary adequacy is maintained so long as the sodium deficient milk contains the other nutrients usually present in regular milk. For those who object to the taste of this milk, flavorings such as chocolate, honey, lemon, vanilla, maple, and coffee can be added. The milk can also be used in preparing such dishes as soups, custards and puddings.

Severe sodium restriction is intended primarily for the hospitalized patient whose sodium tolerance is unusually low. Caution should be employed to avoid sodium depletion

TABLE 30–4   DIETARY SUBSTANCES GENERALLY TO BE AVOIDED IN SODIUM RESTRICTION

1. Smoked, processed or cured meats and fish, such as ham, bacon, corned beef, cold cuts, frankfurters, sausage, tongue, salt pork, chipped beef, and anchovies.
2. Meat extracts, bouillon cubes, and meat sauces.
3. Salted foods, such as potato chips, nuts, and popcorn.
4. Prepared condiments, relishes, Worcestershire sauce, catsup, pickles, mustard and olives.
5. Vegetable salts and flakes, such as onion, garlic or celery salt; celery and parsley flakes.
6. Sodium in any form, such as sodium benzoate as a preservative, and monosodium glutamate as a flavoring aid.
7. Bread or bakery products unless prepared without salt and other souces of sodium.
8. Frozen fish fillets and shellfish, except oysters.
9. Prepared flours, flour mixes, baking powder, and baking soda.
10. Frozen peas and lima beans; sauerkraut in any form.
11. All canned meat and vegetable products unless prepared without salt (dietetic pack).
12. Canned pears, figs, and applesauce unless prepared without salt (dietetic pack).
13. Butter, cheese, and peanut butter unless prepared without salt.

azotemia which may develop with this regimen. Harmful results may follow drastic and prolonged restriction of sodium intake (see Chapter 8), and it is important that the patient be watched carefully for evidence of sodium depletion. Grave danger may exist in severely restricting sodium intake in cases of renal insufficiency in which the kidneys cannot excrete dilute urine. However, the possibility that the low sodium syndrome may occur does not contraindicate the use of a sodium restricted diet when therapeutically indicated.

Malnutrition may be a factor in unresponsiveness of cardiac failure to therapy. Edema often masks emaciation except in the pectoral muscles and upper extremities.

Sources of Sodium In their natural state, the majority of foods contain varying amounts of sodium, but the main source of sodium in the diet is salt in food preparation, food preservation and processing, and added at the table, and other sodium compounds in leavening agents (baking powder, baking soda), disodium phosphate (used in some cereals and cheeses), monosodium glutamate (used to enhance food flavor), sodium alginate (used in some ice creams and chocolate milks), sodium benzoate (a preservative), sodium hydroxide (used in food processing), sodium propionate (used to inhibit growth of mold), and sodium sulfite (used to bleach certain fruits and as a preservative).

The sodium content of water supplies must be known before it is possible to design effective sodium restricted diets. The amount of sodium in drinking water may vary widely in different localities and is apt to be relatively high where "softening" treatment is employed. Beverages and processed foods also reflect the sodium content of the drinking water where they are manufactured. Various synthetic detergents used as dishwashing aids contain a much higher proportion of sodium than do true soaps, and the residue on dishes should be removed by rinsing. It may be necessary to use distilled or a natural water, low in sodium, when sodium intake is restricted.

The animal protein foods, namely, milk, cheese, eggs, meat, poultry and fish, are relatively high in sodium. Thus, while nutritionally essential, these foods must be used in measured amounts (unless processed foods are used, such as milk and meat that have had most of the natural occurring sodium removed. See Chap. 43.) Fruit is low in natural sodium. Certain vegetables—beets, beet greens, celery, kale, dandelion greens, carrots, chard, white turnips and spinach—are relatively high in natural sodium (50 to 80 mg. per serving). Prepared foods such as breads, desserts, cakes, and cookies vary appreciably in amounts of sodium. In these foods salt must be omitted, an appropriate leavening agent chosen, and allowances made for milk and eggs used. Cream of tartar, sodium-free baking powder, potassium bicarbonate and yeast are leavening agents that may be used. Appendix Table 12 gives the sodium content of certain common basic foods.

Incidental sources of sodium In addition to the sodium in food and water, incidental amounts may be ingested in the form of medicines and dentifrices. Barbiturates, sulfonamides, antibiotics, cough medicines, stomach alkalizers, laxatives, tooth pastes and powders, and mouthwashes may contain large amounts of sodium. Labels on these items should be read carefully.

Availability of Special Low Sodium Foods Many of the more important food items are available as specially prepared low sodium products. These include:

Low sodium milk (whole and skimmed)
Unsalted canned meat
Unsalted canned vegetables
Unsalted cheese (cottage, cheddar)
Unsalted butter and margarine
Unsalted bakery products (bread, crackers, cake, cookies)
Low sodium baking powder

Caution should be employed to read the manufacturer's label on the product. The term "salt free" does not imply necessarily that the product is low in sodium. Processing, which removes the natural sodium from foods, also may remove other nutrients, and may require that the diet be appropriately supplemented.

Commercial Salt Substitutes Most salt substitutes are mineral bases consisting of salts other than sodium compounded to simulate sodium chloride in taste. Potassium chloride and ammonium chloride are used, but it is conceivable that the administration of a substitute containing large amounts of potassium to patients with renal insufficiency, or of ammonium to patients with severe liver disease, is harmful.

Other products classified as vegetized salts are available. They range somewhere between condiments and salt substitutes. Most products have powdered dehydrated vegetables as a base and varied additional ingredients. However, they may contain considerable quantities of sodium and should, therefore, not be used. Salt substitutes should be used only when recommended by a physician for a particular patient. Generally, it is advisable for the patient to learn to avoid the salt substitutes and to employ other methods such as the use of herbs and spices in making the sodium restricted diet more palatable.

SUGGESTIONS FOR MAKING THE SODIUM RESTRICTED DIET PALATABLE Every possible means should be used toward making the sodium restricted diet palatable. The preparation of food for the sodium restricted diet need not be complicated, but ingenuity should be exercised in developing flavorings which will compensate for the lack of salt. A number of recipe manuals and cooking suggestions are available and are listed at the end of this chapter. See also sodium restricted recipes in Chapter 43. In general, as in the case of the diabetic diet, the recipes must be related to the daily food allowances from the diet especially when calories are limited. For example, the milk and egg used in a custard will be deducted from the total day's food allowance.

Many spices, herbs and other seasonings can be used to improve the flavor of low sodium foods. According to Elvehjem and Burns,[1] "Most of the values (of sodium in spices) are below 0.05%, and all are below 0.1% with the exception of allspice, celery seed, dehydrated celery flakes, whole mace, and dehydrated parsley flakes. These figures indicate that, with the exception of celery flakes and parsley flakes, the amount of sodium contributed through the usual amount of spices used is insignificant, and that most spices can be used safely in low sodium diets." See Chap. 43 for a list of seasonings and sug-

---

[1]Elvehjem, C. A., and Burns, C. H.: Sodium content of commercial spices. J.A.M.A., *148*:1033, 1952.

gestions for making the food more palatable without adding significant amounts of sodium to the diet.

VASCULAR DISEASE

Chronic passive congestion of the viscera, including the stomach, may interfere with digestion. *Heartburn* is associated with such congestion. Patients may take large quantities of sodium bicarbonate to relieve the distress, only to defeat the physiologic purpose of low sodium diets. Easily digested foods are more properly recommended for cases of indigestion. (Consult Chapter 23.) In fact, when there is impairment of renal function due to venous congestion, relief is achieved by *reduction* of salts and fluids. Anorexia and nutritional edema may result from impairment of the assimilation of proteins by the gastrointestinal tract. In such cases the amount of proteins in the diet is increased, but the sodium intake is kept as low as possible.

ATHEROSCLEROSIS

Atherosclerosis is a form of arteriosclerosis, or thickening of the walls of the arteries. Normally, the blood vessels are smooth-lined tubes. In atherosclerosis small yellow flakes appear on the inner lining of arteries and arterioles which represent early deposits of fatty-like materials containing *cholesterol* and *phospholipids*. (See Chapter 5, Lipids.) These deposits gradually harden into tough, fibrous bulges called *plaques*. As the plaques in these patches become more numerous, the arteries become roughened and narrowed, the elasticity is lost, and the flow of blood through the vessels is curtailed. (See Fig. 30–3). The arteriosclerotic process does not develop at a uniform rate in all arteries.

Atherosclerosis is generally recognized as the leading cause of death today, and one of the greatest contributors to physical and mental incapacity. It interferes with the circulation, chiefly to the heart, kidneys and brain. These organs need blood to function efficiently, and when impairment occurs, the effect is noted throughout the system. Atherosclerosis of the coronary arteries—coronary atherosclerosis—underlies most heart attacks. Stroke, or apoplexy, is often caused by the same condition. The problem of preventing or retarding these attacks or diseases is, then, largely one of preventing or retarding atherosclerosis.

Symptoms occur only when the supply of blood to an organ is reduced 70 per cent or stopped completely. Chest pain develops when the coronary arteries are affected.

ETIOLOGY The exact origin of atherosclerosis is unknown. Most researchers hold

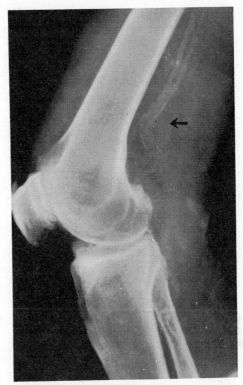

Figure 30–3   Advanced arteriosclerosis in lower extremity. (S. L. Halpern: Nutrition and chronic disease. Health News, New York State Department of Health, September, 1955.)

that a variety of factors must be involved. It is a gradual process that probably begins at birth. Whether it is a disease or a natural process of aging has not been established. Heredity plays a role in that some individuals inherit the tendency to develop atherosclerosis at an earlier age. Evidence indicts cholesterol and lipoproteins as a cause. Studies[2] have shown that members of countries and races that consume large amounts of fat have more coronary and aortic atherosclerosis than those of comparable age who eat less fat. In contrast, many populations in parts of the world—for example, large groups in Africa, Asia and Latin America—eat food containing barely 15 per cent of the total calories in fat. The concentration of serum cholesterol is low and heart attacks are correspondingly fewer. Increasing evidence suggests blood cholesterol levels are directly related to exercise, favoring a long-continued, active life of muscular work. Sex and hormones have also been mentioned as playing a role. The disease is more common in young males than young females. During the childbearing years women have relatively little cardiovascular

[2]Scrimshaw, N. S.: Progress in solving world nutrition problems. J. Am. Dietet. A., 35:441, 1959.

disease and the blood fat levels are relatively low. After menopause there is a greater frequency of such disorders and higher blood cholesterol levels. This suggests that the female sex hormones are a protective factor. Studies have shown that a positive relationship exists between cigarette smoking and coronary heart disease and between cigarette smoking and elevated serum lipids.[3] Brief repeated insults resulting from fever, infection, intense emotional upsets, fatigue, stress[4] and obesity are also claimed to be contributing factors. Moreover, in certain diseases such as hypertension of long-standing, nephrosis, diabetes, and xanthoma, there is more cholesterol in the blood than normally, and atherosclerosis frequently is associated with these conditions.

HYPERCHOLESTEREMIA AND HYPER-LIPOPROTEINEMIA[5] Increased concentrations of lipids in the plasma, specifically cholesterol or triglycerides, are associated with increased susceptibility to atherosclerosis. See Table 30-5 upper limits of normal plasma cholesterol and triglycerides.

All the blood lipids, cholesterol, phospholipid, and triglyceride, bound to specific proteins circulate in the plasma. These proteins transport the lipids into and out of plasma. Normally four major lipoprotein families are in the plasma. These lipoproteins may be identified by paper electrophoresis or ultracentrifugation. Each lipoprotein family defined by these methods contains cholesterol, phospholipid, triglyceride and protein in different proportions. The plasma lipoproteins are (1) chylomicrons, (2) pre-β-lipoproteins (very low density proteins – VLDL), (3)

β-lipoproteins (low density lipoproteins – LDL), (4) α-lipoproteins (high density lipoproteins – HDL). Normally most of the plasma cholesterol is found in β-lipoprotein and most of the triglycerides are in the pre-β-lipoproteins.

Chylomicrons consist mostly of triglyceride, 80 to 95 per cent of dietary or exogenous origin, with 2 to 7 per cent cholesterol, 3 to 6 per cent phospholipids, and 1 to 2 per cent protein. Normally synthesized in the intestines, chylomicrons transport dietary triglycerides from the intestines into the plasma. They give a milky appearance to normal plasma after a fatty meal.

The pre-β-lipoproteins (VLDL) are composed largely of triglycerides (60 to 80 per cent) and function to transport triglycerides of endogenous origin largely from the liver. An increased concentration of plasma (VLDL) in the absence of chylomicrons is correlated with plasma levels of triglycerides.

The function of β-lipoprotein (LDL) which normally carries from one half to two thirds of the total plasma cholesterol is not clear. It apparently represents the plasma residue of VLDL catabolism. By weight LDL is about 45 per cent cholesterol and 25 per cent protein.

The fourth and smallest of the lipoprotein family is α-lipoproteins (HDL). They contain about 45 to 50 per cent protein, 20 per cent cholesterol and 30 per cent phospholipid and their function is not clear. No known genetic abnormality resulting from an increased HDL concentration has been described.

Classification of Hyperlipoproteinemias. Many different genetic and metabolic factors control lipoprotein concentrations and many abnormalities may cause hypercholesteremia. Five lipoprotein types have been described in the hyperlipoproteinemias (see Table 30-6). Each is classified in terms of the abnormal accumulation in plasma of one or more lipoprotein families.

Dietary Management.[6] The dietary management of the five types of hyperlipoproteinemias has been carefully formulated and is available upon request through the physician from the U.S. Department of Health, Education and Welfare Public Health Science National Institutes of Health. Appropriate suggestions for using, buying and cooking foods are included. The person for whom any one of these dietary programs is prescribed should maintain weight at the desired level. (See Table 30-7.)

---

[3]Kershbaum, A., and Bellet, S.: Cigarette smoking and blood lipids. J.A.M.A., *187*:32, 1964.

[4]Luongo, E. P.: Health habits and heart disease – Challenge in preventive medicine. J.A.M.A., *162*:1021, 1956.

[5]Lees, R. S., and Wilson, D. E.: The treatment of hyperlipidemia. New Eng. J. Med., *284*:186, 1971; and Levy, R. I., et al.: Dietary management of hyperlipoproteinemia. J. Am. Dietet. A., *58*:406, 1971.

TABLE 30-5   UPPER LIMITS OF NORMAL PLASMA CHOLESTEROL AND TRIGLYCERIDES

AGE	PLASMA TOTAL CHOLESTEROL	PLASMA TRIGLYCERIDES (mg. per 100 ml.)
1 to 19	230	140
20 to 29	240	140
30 to 39	270	150
40 to 49	310	160
50 and above	330	190

From Fredrickson, D. S., et al.: The Dietary Management of Hyperlipoproteinemia: A Handbook for Physicians. National Heart and Lung Institute, Bethesda, Md., 1970.

[6]Fredrickson, D. S.: Dietary Management of Hyperlipoproteinemia: A Handbook for Physicians. National Heart and Lung Institute, National Institutes of Health, Bethesda, Md., 1970.

TABLE 30–6   THE FIVE TYPES OF PRIMARY HYPERLIPOPROTEINEMIA

FEATURES	TYPE I	TYPE II	TYPE III	TYPE IV	TYPE V
Incidence	Very rare	Common	Relatively uncommon	Common	Uncommon
Appearance of plasma	Cream layer over clear infranate on standing	Clear	Clear, cloudy or milky	Slightly turbid to cloudy, unchanged with standing	Cream layer over turbid infranate on standing
Cholesterol	Normal or elevated	Elevated	Elevated	Normal or elevated	Elevated
Triglyceride	Markedly elevated	Normal	Usually elevated	Elevated	Elevated to markedly elevated
Clinical presentation	Lipemia retinalis, eruptive xanthomas, hepatosplenomegaly, abdominal pain	Xanthelasma, tendon and tuberous xanthomas, juvenile corneal arcus, accelerated atherosclerosis	Xanthoma planum; eruptive, tuberous and tendon xanthomas; accelerated atherosclerosis of coronary and peripheral vessels	Accelerated coronary vessel disease, abnormal glucose tolerance, hyperuricemia	Lipemia retinalis, eruptive xanthomas, hepatosplenomegaly, abdominal pain, hyperglycemia, hyperuricemia
Origin; possible mechanism	Genetic recessive; deficiency in lipoprotein lipase	When genetic, dominant, sporadic; decreased catabolism of beta-lipoprotein	When genetic, recessive; sporadic?	When genetic, dominant, sporadic, excessive endogenous glyceride synthesis or deficient glyceride clearance?	Probably genetic sporadic
Age of detection	Early childhood	Early childhood (in severe cases)	Adulthood (over age 20)	Adulthood	Early adulthood
Conditions to be excluded	Dysgamma-globulinemia, diabetes, pancreatitis?	Dietary cholesterol excess, porphyria, myxedema, myeloma, nephrosis, obstructive liver disease	Myxedema, dysgamma-globulinemia	Diabetes, glycogen storage disease, nephrotic syndrome, pregnancy, Werner's syndrome	Myeloma and macroglobulinemia, insulin-dependent diabetes mellitus, nephrosis, alcoholism, pancreatitis

From Levy, R. L., and Fredrickson, D.: The current status of hypolipidemic drugs. Postgrad. Med., 47:132, 1970.

TABLE 30–7   SUMMARY OF DIETS FOR TYPES I TO V HYPERLIPOPROTEINEMIA

TYPE	DIET	DRUG OF CHOICE
I	1. Restriction of fat to about 25–35 gm per day 2. Supplementation with medium chain-length triglycerides	None effective at present
II	1. Low-cholesterol diet (less than 300 mg per day) 2. Increased intake of polyunsaturated fats	1. Cholestyramine, 16 to 32 gm per day 2. D-Thyroxine 3. Nicotinic acid
III	1. Reduction to ideal body weight 2. Balanced diet (40 per cent of calories fat, 40 per cent carbohydrate 3. Low-cholesterol diet (less than 300 mg per day, 20 per cent protein)	1. Clofibrate, 2 gm per day 2. D-Thyroxine 3. Nicotinic acid
IV	1. Reduction to ideal body weight 2. Increased intake of polyunsaturated fats 3. Modest restriction of carbohydrates (most concentrated sweets eliminated) 4. Moderate restriction of cholesterol (300–500 mg)	1. Clofibrate, 2 gm per day 2. Nicotinic acid, 3 to 6 gm per day
V	1. Reduction to ideal body weight 2. Increased intake of protein 3. Reduction of fat to 30 per cent of calories 4. Restriction of carbohydrates 5. Moderate restriction of cholesterol (300–500 mg)	1. Nicotinic acid, 3 to 6 gm per day 2. Clofibrate

Adapted from Levy, R. L., and Fredrickson, D.: The current status of hypolipedemic drugs. Postgrad. Med., 47:133, 1970.

Type I indicates an inability to clear chylomicrons. A diet low in fat results in clearing of the hyperglycemia. Triglycerides of medium chain length (MCT) may be used as a supplementary fat. Medium chain triglycerides are absorbed directly into the portal vein. They are transported to the liver without requiring chylomicron formation for transport.

SAMPLE MENU FOR THE ADULT WITH TYPE I
1700–2000 KCALORIES[7]

DAILY FOOD PLAN	SAMPLE MENU PATTERN
1 quart skim milk (fortified with vitamins A and D)	*Breakfast:* Citrus fruit or juice Whole-grain or enriched cereal
5 ounces cooked poultry, fish or lean trimmed meat	Whole-grain or enriched toast Jelly and sugar Skim milk Coffee or tea if desired

5 servings of vegetable and fruit, including
  1 serving citrus fruit
  1 serving dark green or deep yellow vegetable
	Lunch:
	2 oz. cooked poultry, fish or lean meat or 2 eggs or plain cottage cheese
	Potato, rice, spaghetti or noodles

6 or more servings whole wheat or whole grain	Dark green or deep yellow vegetable Whole-grain or enriched bread
1 or more servings potato, rice, noodles, grits	Jelly and sugar Fruit Allowed dessert Skim milk
Desserts*	*Dinner:* 3 oz. cooked poultry, fish or lean meat
Sugars, sweets	Potato, rice or noodles Vegetable Whole-grain or enriched bread
Beverages (non-dairy)	Sugar and jelly Allowed dessert Skim milk
	Between-Meal Nourishment: Skim milk Fruit or allowed dessert

*Made with skim milk; jello, fruit, fruit ices and medium chain triglycerides (MCT) may be used if prescribed by a physician, in which instance adjustment in calories is necessary.

Type II or hyperbetalipoproteinemia is characterized by an increase in beta lipoprotein. It is thought to be transmitted as an autosomal dominant trait. The treatment involves lowering the intake of cholesterol to less than 300 mg. per day and modifying the fat intake to a high polyunsaturated to saturated fatty acid ratio (P/S approximately 2). (See cholesterol content of food listed in Appendix Table 4 and polyunsaturated foods in Chapter 5.) The distribution of calories varies with individual needs: protein, 10 to 20 per cent; fat, 25 to 40 per cent; and carbohydrate, 40 to 65 per cent. Lean meat including fish and poultry (without skin) is limited to not more than 9 ounces per day, and beef, lamb, ham

and pork is limited to a 3-ounce portion three times a week. An intake of at least 1 teaspoon of oil high in polyunsaturated fat is recommended for every ounce of meat. When beef, lamb or pork is selected, 2 teaspoons of oil is recommended for each ounce of meat. Recipes are available for low fat cooking and cooking with oil.

Some liquid vegetable fats are more unsaturated than others – safflower and corn oil are more unsaturated than olive and peanut oils. Coconut oil or hydrogenated oils are saturated fats and as such are eliminated from the diet.

SAMPLE MENU FOR THE ADULT WITH TYPE II
1700–2000 KCALORIES[8]

DAILY FOOD PLAN	SAMPLE MENU PATTERN
1 pint or more skim milk Cooked poultry, fish or lean trimmed meat†	*Breakfast:* Citrus fruit or juice* Whole-grain or enriched cereal** Whole-grain or enriched toast†
5 servings of vegetable and fruit; including 1 serving dark green or deep yellow vegetable	Allowed fat Jelly and sugar Skim milk Coffee or tea if desired
7 or more servings of bread or cereal	*Lunch:* Poultry, fish or lean meat Potato or substitute Dark green or deep yellow vegetable**
1 or more servings of potato, rice, etc.	Other vegetable Whole-grain or enriched bread Allowed fat
Fat‡	Fruit or allowed dessert Skim milk
Desserts and sweets made with skim milk, egg whites, oil; jello, fruit, fruit ices§	*Dinner:* Poultry, fish or lean meat Potato or substitute Vegetable Whole-grain or enriched bread Allowed fat Fruit or allowed dessert Skim milk
	Between-Meal Nourishment: Fruit Skim milk

*One serving of citrus fruit is recommended daily to provide adequate ascorbic acid.
**Enriched cereal or bread should be included in the diet to provide adequate vitamin B complex and iron.
†One dark green or deep yellow vegetable is recommended daily to provide adequate vitamin A.
‡To restrict the saturated fat, the meat, which is the principal source of saturated fats, must be limited to not more than 9 ounces (well trimmed, cooked) per day.
Limit beef, lamb and pork to 3-ounce portions 3 times per week.
Fish and poultry without skin are naturally lower in fat and should be used in place of meat as often as possible.
For each 3 ounces of cooked meat consume 3 teaspoons of polyunsaturated fat.
§To maintain calories at this level, it will be necessary to omit additional desserts and sweets.

Type III is a pattern associated with the presence of an abnormal form of beta-lipoprotein in the plasma. This type is usually familial and apparently transmitted as a recessive trait. The initial diet therapy is a reduction in weight to the desired level. The cholesterol

[7]Fredrickson, *op. cit.*

[8]Fredrickson, *op. cit.*

intake is maintained at less than 300 mg. per day. The amount of fat is limited to not more than 40 per cent of the total calories. The polyunsaturated fat, vegetable oil and special margarine are recommended. The amount of carbohydrate is restricted to not more than 40 per cent of the total calories. Sugars and starches as used in desserts and sweets are eliminated. The dietary plan is similar in form and food groups to the diabetic pattern.

SAMPLE MENU FOR THE ADULT WITH TYPE III
1700–2000 KCALORIES[9]

Daily Food Plan*	List	Sample Menu Pattern
2 to 3 ounce servings of poultry, fish or lean trimmed meat	V	*Breakfast:* 1 serving citrus fruit or juice 2 servings whole-grain or enriched cereal or toast
3 servings skim milk	I	3 servings allowed fat 1 serving skim milk
8 servings bread, cereal	IV	
15 servings allowed fat**		*Lunch:* 1 serving poultry, fish or lean trimmed meat
3 servings fruit, unsweetened	III	1 serving potato or substitute dark green or deep yellow vegetable
Vegetables (as desired)	IIA IIB	Other vegetable 2 servings whole-grain or enriched bread 6 servings allowed fat 1 serving fruit 1 serving skim milk
		Dinner: 1 serving poultry, fish or lean trimmed meat 1 serving potato or substitute vegetable 2 servings whole-grain or enriched bread 6 servings allowed fat 1 serving fruit 1 serving skim milk

---

*Use Exchange List for calculation, Chapter 28.
**Avoid saturated fats.

300 to 500 mg. per day. The fat is restricted to approximately 30 per cent of the total calorie needs and the polyunsaturated fats are emphasized, especially if large amounts of meat are consumed. Concentrated sweets and empty calories are eliminated in the diet.

SAMPLE MENU FOR THE ADULT WITH TYPE IV
1700–2000 KCALORIES[10]

Daily Food Plan*	List	Sample Menu Pattern
2 to 3 ounce servings poultry, fish or leaned trimmed meat Egg, cheese, shellfish**	V	*Breakfast:* 1 serving citrus fruit or juice 2 servings whole-grain or enriched cereal or toast Allowed fat 1 serving skim milk
3 servings skim milk	I	*Lunch:*
8 servings bread, cereal, etc.	IV	1 serving poultry, fish or lean trimmed meat
15 allowed fat polyunsaturated***	VI	1 serving potato or substitute dark green or deep yellow vegetable Other vegetable
3 servings fruit	III	2 servings whole-grain or enriched bread
Vegetables, (as desired)	IIA IIB	Allowed fat 1 serving fruit 1 serving skim milk
		Dinner: 1 serving poultry, fish or lean trimmed meat 1 serving potato or substitute vegetable 2 servings whole-grain or enriched bread Allowed fat 1 serving fruit 1 serving skim milk

---

*Use Exchange List for calculation, Chapter 28.
**Egg allowance – 3 egg yolks per week. Include egg yolk in cooking or baking;
or 2 ounces of shellfish (oysters, lobsters, scallops, shrimp, clams or crab) in place of 1 egg yolk;
or 2 ounces of liver, heart or sweetbreads for 1 egg yolk;
or 2 ounces of cheddar-type cheese for 1 egg yolk.
***All vegetable oil (except coconut), special margarine, salad dressings without sour cream or cheese, mayonnaise.

Type IV is a common lipoprotein pattern and is often associated with diabetes mellitus and possibly premature atherosclerosis. It is characterized by an increase in endogenous glyceride, pre-beta-lipoprotein (VLDL). About 50 per cent have abnormal glucose tolerance tests. Diet therapy stresses reduction in weight to the desired level. At the desired weight the individual nearly always has lower or normal triglyceride concentrations than when he was heavier. Carbohydrate and alcohol restrictions are recommended, since an excess of either tends to increase endogenous triglyceride concentrations. The cholesterol content of the diet is moderately restricted to

Type V pattern is familial trait and is usually secondary to acute metabolic disorders such as diabetic acidosis, pancreatitis, alcoholism and nephrosis. It is characterized by a mixed hyperlipidemia. Both exogenous (chylomicrons) and endogenous glyceride (pre-betalipoproteins) accumulate in the fasting plasma. Plasma triglycerides are markedly elevated and abnormal glucose tolerance is frequently associated with this type pattern. Diet therapy stresses caloric restriction and maintenance of desired body weight. The amount of fat is restricted to 25 to 30 per cent of the calories, with unsaturated fats predominating; protein is high, 20 to 25 per cent of

---

[9]Fredrickson, *op. cit.*

[10]*Ibid.*

the calories, and carbohydrate is modified to 40 to 50 per cent. Concentrated sweets and empty calories are eliminated and alcohol is not recommended. Cholesterol is restricted to 300 to 500 mg. per day. Restriction of fat and carbohydrate is recommended for the following reasons:

(1) An increase in plasma triglycerides of exogenous origin may occur in persons who eat too much fat.

(2) An increase in plasma triglycerides of endogenous origin, VLDL, frequently occurs in persons with Type V who eat excessive carbohydrate.

SAMPLE MENU FOR THE ADULT WITH TYPE V 1700–2000 KCALORIES[11]

Daily Food Plan*	List	Sample Menu Pattern
2 to 3 ounce servings of poultry, fish or lean trimmed meat, egg, cheese, shellfish**	V	*Breakfast:*
		1 serving citrus fruit or juice
		3 servings whole-grain or enriched cereal or toast
		2 servings allowed fat
4 servings skim milk	I	1 serving skim milk
10 servings bread, cereal, etc.	IV	*Lunch:*
6 to 9 servings allowed fat***	VI	1 serving poultry, fish or lean trimmed meat
3 servings fruit	III	1 serving potato or substitute dark green or deep yellow vegetable
Vegetables (as desired)	IIA	Other vegetable
	IIB	2 servings whole-grain or enriched bread
		2 servings allowed fat
		1 serving fruit
		1 serving skim milk
		Dinner:
		2 servings poultry, fish or lean trimmed meat
		1 serving potato or substitute vegetable
		2 servings whole-grain or enriched bread
		2 servings allowed fat
		1 serving fruit
		1 serving skim milk
		P.M. Snack:
		1 serving skim milk
		1 serving from breads and cereals group

*Use Exchange List for calculation, Chapter 28.
**Egg allowance—3 egg yolks per week. Includes egg yolks in cooking or baking;

    or   2 ounces of shellfish (oysters, lobster, scallops, shrimp, clams or crab) for 1 egg yolk;

    or   2 ounces of liver, heart or sweetbreads for 1 egg yolk;

    or   2 ounces cheddar-type cheese for 1 egg yolk.

***All vegetable oil (except coconut), special margarine, salad dressing without sour cream or cheese, mayonnaise.

Reduction in risk, it is believed, can be attained when the aim of prevention as well as treatment is to maintain normal plasma concentration of cholesterol and triglycerides. Obesity resulting from overeating contributes

to hyperlipidemia in our population. Excessive intake of sucrose and concentrated sweets in many dietaries usually take the place of or exclude foods high in the nutrients thus contributing to inadequate intake of essential nutrients. Reduction of calories in an otherwise adequate dietary must be the first consideration in prevention and therapy.

It is not good practice to omit or restrict fats or cholesterol or carbohydrate indiscriminately to prevent or treat atherosclerosis. By means of tests mentioned above the physician determines the type and treatment indicated. To try to eliminate all exogenous cholesterol when it is produced endogenously by many cells and tissue is to deprive the body of essential nutrients found in these foods. Egg yolks, for example, are not only good sources of protein, iron and vitamin A but are also rich in lecithin (phospholipid) which serves to protect against cholesterol deposition. Evidence indicates that high cholesterol levels per se do not cause atherosclerosis unless accompanied by relatively low levels of phospholipids in the blood. The most desirable ratio between phospholipid and cholesterol levels in blood is believed to be 1:2:1.[12]

Plasma cholesterol and triglyceride concentrations are only two factors related to development of atherosclerosis. Cardiac patients tend to show a deficiency in vitamin B_6. The requirements of vitamin B_6 may not be met in those individuals who consume considerable fat. Vitamin B_6, an essential co-catalyst, is necessary for the endogenous production of polyunsaturated fatty acids. Vitamin B_6 is found in the whole grains. Most of the vitamin is lost in the milling of white flour and cereals. Enrichment does not put it back.[13]

Experimental animals fed diets which ordinarily induce atherosclerosis do not develop atherosclerosis when given high levels of magnesium. Magnesium deficiency in experimental animals results in calcification in the areas affected by coronary heart disease and is thought to be a factor in all human atherosclerotic plaques.

The function of vitamin E in ischemic heart disease is not clear. It primarily functions as a fat-soluble antioxidant which inhibits the destruction of unsaturated fatty acids, vitamin A and coenzyme Q. In various experimental animals a deficiency of vitamin E has been shown to produce heart and/or blood vessel lesions. Vitamin E is believed by some investigators to play a role in the prevention of ischemic heart disease.[14]

[11]Frederickson, *op. cit.*

[12]Williams, R. J.: Nutrition and Ischemic Heart Disease. Borden's Review of Nutrition Research, *31*: No. 2, 1971, p. 18.

[13]*Ibid.*

[14]*Ibid.*

In a study of elderly people with chronic arteriosclerosis given folic acid in the amount of 5 mg. daily, improved vision, increased capillary blood flow and heightened skin temperatures were observed.[15]

Thiamin deficiency affects the heart; ascorbic acid deficiency may cause severe heart damage and apparently a deficiency of coenzyme Q is a factor in heart disease.

Deficiencies of single nutrients are uncommon. In all probability several mild deficiencies occur in an individual at the same time.

In order to prevent ischemic heart disease from the nutrient standpoint, it is important to avoid all nutritional deficiencies.[16]

TEACHING THE PATIENT   The diagnostic tests administered by the physician determine the type hyperlipoproteinemia therapy required for the patient. The modifications from the normal dietary are implicit in the sample menus recorded on pages 454–456. However, the teaching centers around the person and not the diet. It is a waste of time and energy to "go over" the diet list with the person. Learning begins with the present eating and dietary practices from which the necessary modifications and improvements evolve. The pattern which develops from this approach would come close to the sample. The patient's understanding of and involvement in the adjustments motivate the action to adopt the changes recommended. The importance of an adequate intake of the essential nutrients cannot be overemphasized. If certain nutrients are lacking because of the necessary therapeutic modifications, appropriate supplements are indicated.

For example, Type I (low fat diet) is low in the fat-soluble vitamins and iron. Dark green and deep yellow vegetables three or four times a week and liver occasionally should be selected.

FATTY ACID AND CHOLESTEROL CONTENT OF THE DIET   It has been demonstrated that by substituting highly unsaturated fats (those with multiple double bonds, such as safflower, corn and cottonseed oil) with high proportions of linoleic acid, derived from vegetables and from some fish oils, for saturated fats (animal or hydrogenated vegetable fats) in human diets, or in some instances by adding sufficient amounts of unsaturated fats to a normal fat intake, the total plasma lipids and serum cholesterol are consistently lowered in a high percentage of cases. Whether the changes are the result of the total fat content of the diet, of a direct action of vegetable (unsaturated) fat alone, or of some unknown factor is not fully understood. The use of polyunsaturated fatty acids offers a convenient and efficient means of reducing the blood lipid level. Evidence suggests that requirements for vitamin E are increased when large amounts of polyunsaturated fats are ingested. Apparently, it is the proportion of saturated and unsaturated fatty acids in the total fat consumed that determines the lipid level and, consequently, the lipid vascular deposition. Appendix Table 4, *Fatty Acid and Cholesterol Content of Foods,* shows the content and ratio of unsaturated to saturated fatty acids in various foods. This table can be used when diets are prescribed with modifications in proportions of fatty acids and cholesterol for individuals with coronary artery disease.

Sebrell[17] points out that protein deficiency may result in a decrease in serum cholesterol. The incidence of atherosclerosis in the different areas of the world can be correlated with the amount of protein, especially animal protein, consumed per person. In kwashiorkor (severe protein malnutrition in infants [see p. 509]), an exceptionally low blood cholesterol level is present as well as decreased lipoprotein, which tends to return to normal on nutritional rehabilitation with fat-free milk powder. Sebrell rationalized that this observation could be explained on the basis that a protein deficiency limits the formation of β-lipoproteins and may thereby depress the blood level. Recently, Bagchi et al.,[18] working with rats and children in India, found a close correlation between the serum cholesterol level and the protein nutritional status.

Hormones   Research in which a high cholesterol diet was fed to animals did not show hardening of the arteries unless the thyroid gland was suppressed. In others, atherosclerosis was inhibited by injecting female hormones. This suggests that the glandular system may play a role and that thyroid extract influences the disorder.

Fat Controlled Diets   Fat controlled diets are used by some physicians to lower patients' serum cholesterol levels. The Council on Foods and Nutrition of the American Medical Association has prepared three groups of diets[19] for reducing serum cholesterol, with three calorie levels in each group—1200, 1800, and 2400 kcalories. *Two* of these groups are designed for reducing fat intake: (1) diets representing severe reduction of dietary fat (10 per cent of total calories), and (2) moderate reduction of dietary fat (25 per cent of

[15]*Ibid.*
[16]*Ibid.*

[17]Sebrell, W. H., Jr.: An over-all look at atherosclerosis. J. Am. Dietet. A., 40:403, 1962.
[18]Bagchi, K., et al.: The influence of dietary protein and methionine on serum cholesterol level. Am. J. Clin. Nutr. 13:232, 1963.
[19]The regulation of dietary fat. J.A.M.A., 181:411, 1962.

TABLE 30–8   FOOD EXCHANGE LISTS*

Milk Exchanges—List 1

Nonfat dried milk	¼ cup
Skim milk	1 cup
Buttermilk (made from skim milk)	1 cup

Vegetable Exchanges—List 2

Vegetable A, As desired

Asparagus	Cauliflower
Beans, string, young	Celery
Broccoli	Chicory
Brussels sprouts	Cucumber
Cabbage	Escarole
Lettuce	Eggplant
Mushrooms	Sauerkraut
Okra	Squash, summer
Pepper	Tomatoes
Radishes	Watercress

"Greens"

Beet greens	Kale
Chard, swiss	Mustard greens
Collard	Spinach
Dandelion greens	Turnip greens

Vegetable B (½ cup per serving)

Beets	Pumpkin
Carrots	Rutabaga
Onions	Squash, winter
Peas, green	Turnip

Fruit Exchanges—List 3

Apple (2 in. diam.)	1
Applesauce	½ cup
Apricots,	
fresh	2 medium
dried	4 halves
Banana	½ small
Blackberries	1 cup
Blueberries	⅔ cup
Cantaloupe (6 in. diam.)	¼
Cherries	10 large
Dates	2
Figs,	
fresh	2 large
dried	2
Grape juice	½ cup
Grapefruit	½ small
Grapefruit juice	½ cup
Grapes	12
Honeydew melon (7 in. diam.)	⅛
Mango	½ small
Orange	1 small
Orange juice	½ cup
Papaya	⅓ medium
Peach	1 medium
Pear	1 small
Pineapple	½ cup
Pineapple juice	⅓ cup
Plums	2 medium
Prunes, dried	2 medium
Raisins	2 tbsp.
Raspberries	1 cup
Strawberries	1 cup
Tangerine	1 large
Watermelon	1 cup

Bread Exchanges—List 4

Bread	1 slice
† Biscuit, Muffin, Roll (2 in. diam.)	1
† Cornbread (1½ in. cube)	1
Cereal, cooked	⅓ cup
dry, flake or puffed	¾ cup
Rice, grits, cooked	½ cup
Spaghetti, noodles, cooked	½ cup
Macaroni, etc., cooked	½ cup
Crackers, graham	2
saltines	5
soda	3
Beans, peas, dried, cooked	½ cup
Corn, sweet	⅓ cup
Corn on the cob, medium ear	½
Potatoes, white (2 in. diam.)	1
Potatoes, sweet	¼ cup
Parsnips	⅔ cup

Meat, Fish, and Poultry Exchanges—List 5

Select meat from this group for 3 meals a week

Beef, eye of round, top and bottom round, lean ground round, lean rump, tenderloin	1 oz.
Lamb, leg only	1 oz.
Pork, lean loin	1 oz.
Ham, lean and well trimmed	1 oz.

Make selections from this group for 11 meals a week

Chicken, no skin	1 oz.
Turkey, no skin	1 oz.
Veal	1 oz.
Fish	1 oz.
Shellfish	1 oz.
Meat substitute, cottage cheese, preferably uncreamed	¼ cup

Eggs—List 6

Four eggs per week allowed in each diet plan at discretion of physician

Fat Exchanges—List 7

50% polyunsaturated

Corn oil	1 tsp.
Cottonseed oil	1 tsp.
Safflower oil	1 tsp.
Mayonnaise made with corn or cottonseed oil	1 tsp.
French dressing made with corn or cottonseed oil	2 tsp.

30%–40% polyunsaturated

Special margarines	1 tsp.
Special shortenings	1 tsp.

Sugar Exchange ‡—List 8

White, brown or maple sugar	1 tsp.
Corn syrup, honey, molasses	1 tsp.
Candy (no chocolate)	
gum drop	1 medium or 6 small
hard-type	6–8 small fruit drops
mints, cream	3–4
marshmallow, plain	1 average
Jelly, jams, all varieties	1 tsp.
Sherbet	1 tbsp.
Carbonated beverages	2 oz.

* Council on Foods and Nutrition, A.M.A.: The regulation of dietary fat. J.A.M.A., *181*:411, 1962.
† Made with corn or cottonseed oil. Diets planned according to ADA Exchange System.
Meat exchanges were calculated as containing 3 gm. fat instead of ADA value of 5 gm.
‡ 1 oz. alcohol = 1 sugar exch. and may be substituted at discretion of physician.

total calories). The *third* group of diets (3) maintains the fat intake at approximately the usual level for this country (35 to 40 per cent of total calories) but modifies the fat in the diet to supply polyunsaturated fat for much of the saturated fat (ratio ranges from 1.1:1 to 1.5:1. The diet will not remove deposited cholesterol in the arteries but is designed to prevent or retard deposits from forming. Studies have shown that diets of this type usually result in serum cholesterol reduction.

The choice and quality of foods in the diets are based on the Meal Planning and Exchange Lists originally designed for diabetic and overweight patients, as described in Chapter 28, Metabolic Disorders Related to Nutrition. The Food Exchange Lists for the fat controlled diets appear in Table 30–8. Two additional Exchange Lists have been added: (1) Fat Exchanges and (2) Sugar Exchanges.

Fat intake reduction   Severe fat reduction (0 to 15 per cent of total calories) is not generally recommended, particularly at the higher calorie levels. Although the low fat intake will probably decrease the serum cholesterol, it is conceivable that the necessary increase in carbohydrate to meet the required calorie allowance may increase the lipoprotein content of the blood. In addition, certain essential fatty acids, as well as fat-soluble vitamins, may be reduced to the critical point unless the patient is provided with an adequate medical supplement.

To achieve the desired reduction in fat, regardless of the caloric level, all separated fats, whole milk, and nuts are omitted; baked products are restricted. Only lean meat, fish, and poultry are permitted; and the use of fruits and low fat vegetables is emphasized. Methods of food preparation need special consideration not to add fat; for example, salad dressing and frying.

Modified fat diets   The Council on Foods and Nutrition of the American Medical Association states that a diet modified to increase the ratio of polyunsaturated fat to saturated fat is the preferred method for treatment of the "usual" hypercholesteremia. Generally, to reduce the saturated fat content of the diet, meats and dairy products are restricted considerably. Only lean meat, fish and poultry are allowed. Milk is nonfat; and eggs are restricted to four per week. Chocolate and caramel-type candies prepared with cocoa butter are not permitted. Commercial bakery products other than bread are not allowed but, when calories permit, homemade products may be made with the fats allowed on the diet.

"Special" table margarines[20] and shortenings are available that have a polyunsaturated fatty acid content and that may be used in cooking and at the table. Lard, butter, hydrogenated shortenings, and coconut oil (saturated fats) are to be avoided and supplemented with corn, peanut, cottonseed, safflower, and soybean oils which are polyunsaturated (linoleic).

The American Heart Association[21] has prepared two booklets on fat controlled diets. They are available to patients, upon a doctor's prescription, from local Heart Associations and the American Heart Association. One booklet is entitled "Planning Fat-controlled Meals for 1200 and 1800 Calories," and is pri-

[20]AMA Council on Foods and Nutrition: Composition of certain margarines. J.A.M.A., *179*:719, 1962.
[21]44 East 23 St., New York, New York, 10010.

TABLE 30–9   MODIFIED FATTY ACID CONTENT*

(Fat, 35 Per Cent to 40 Per Cent of Total Calories)

	1200 KCALORIES	1800 KCALORIES	2400 KCALORIES
Milk	2 exchanges	2 exchanges	2 exchanges
Vegetables			
A group	As desired	As desired	As desired
B group	1 exchange	1 exchange	1 exchange
Fruit	3 exchanges	5 exchanges	5 exchanges
Bread and cereals	4 exchanges	6 exchanges	8 exchanges
Meat, fish, poultry	5 exchanges	6 exchanges	7 exchanges
Eggs†	4 per week	4 per week	4 per week
Fat	5 exchanges	9 exchanges	15 exchanges
Special margarine	1 exchange		3 exchanges
Sugar, sweets		9 exchanges	12 exchanges

*Council on Foods and Nutrition, A.M.A.: The regulation of dietary fat. J.A.M.A., *181*:411, 1962.

†Meat exchanges may be substituted for egg exchanges (1 exch. = 1 egg). Meat exchanges were calculated as containing 3 gm. fat, instead of ADA value of 5 gm.

Ratio of polyunsaturated to saturated fatty acids ranges from 1.1:1 to 1.5:1. Diets planned according to ADA Exchange System and Table 30–8.

marily for use with overweight patients; and the other, "Planning Fat-controlled Meals for Unrestricted Calories." These diets are based on the modified fat diet calculations of the Foods and Nutrition Council, American Medical Association, described above. The diets in both booklets are moderate, rather than low, in fats, and a substantial amount of the fat is in the form of polyunsaturated vegetable oils. About 35 per cent of the day's calories comes from fat; the usual amount in the American diet is from 40 to 45 per cent. The booklets contain suggestions for shopping and cooking and on eating out. In addition, there are sample menus, lists of foods to use and to avoid, and a group of recipes which use vegetable oils.

Table 30–9, Modified Fatty Acid Content, shows the three caloric levels—1200, 1800 and 2400—each containing 35 to 40 per cent fat of total calories. Table 30–10 summarizes the saturated and unsaturated fats in these diets. Table 30–11 contains the 2400 kcalorie diet Meal Plan and Sample Menu in which the dietary fat is modified to provide approximately 45 gm. polyunsaturated fatty acids and 30 gm. saturated fatty acids. The sample menu was planned using the Food Exchange Lists in Table 30–8.

ESSENTIAL HYPERTENSION

Essential hypertension or high blood pressure is not a disease but is a symptom of unknown origin. It occurs during the course of such maladies as toxic goiter, in certain forms of cardiac disease, atherosclerosis, Bright's disease, and during the course of pregnancy. In the majority of cases the origin cannot be found. Dahl[22] reports that sodium plays a primary role in causing essential hypertension. He also suggests that those with a family history of this disease restrict sodium intake to 200 to 400 mg. per day and that all others include a maximum of 2 gm. of sodium per day. Dahl and others recognize the danger of obesity along with a high sodium intake.

The main considerations are the effect of the elevated tension upon the blood vessels, and the reverse reaction. If the arteries become narrowed, the blood pressure readings mount. The lining of the channels becomes thicker as nature protects the walls to withstand the intensified pressure.

Unfortunately, the changes in the vessels or tissues alter the flow of blood to the heart and kidneys and ultimately injure the organs.

INCIDENCE Medicine has greatly advanced the life expectancy of man. Today the proportion of elderly persons among the population is greater than ever before, and a large number of individuals live to an age when arterial degeneration develops. On the other hand, the onset of hypertension in younger individuals is more serious than after middle age. Any attempt to lower the blood pressure level will help to minimize the stress, strain and degeneration of the tissues. Dahl believes that the high sodium intake of overweight people, rather than obesity, accounts for the increased incidence of hypertension in the overweight. The symptoms start gradually and usually develop into a chronic condition.

SURGERY Surgical treatment is another method of management of essential hypertension. Some excellent results have been reported, especially among comparatively young patients during the early phases of the ailment, from treatment by splanchnicectomy. The long-term results available, however, indicate that side effects following splanchnicectomy may be quite disturbing

[22]Dahl, L. K.: Role of dietary sodium in essential hypertension. J. Am Dietet. A., 34:585, 1958.

TABLE 30–10   SUMMARY OF DIETS WITH MODIFIED FAT CONTENT*

TOTAL KCALORIES	TOTAL KCALORIES FROM FAT, %	TOTAL FAT CONTENT, GM.	SATURATED, GM.	LINOLEATE, GM.	RATIO OF LINOLEATE TO SATURATED
1,200	40	49.5	15.0	16.5	1.1:1
	25	33			
	15†	18			
1,800	40	69.5	20.0	26.0	1.3:1
	25	51			
	10	21			
2,400	40	115.5	30.0	45.0	1.5:1
	25	67			
	10	27			

* Council on Foods and Nutrition, A.M.A.: The regulation of dietary fat. J.A.M.A., *181:* 411, 1962.

†15% is probable content at this calorie level.

TABLE 30–11   SUGGESTED 2400 KCALORIE MEAL PLAN AND SAMPLE MENU*
(Total Fat, 115.5 Gm.; Saturated, 30.2 Gm.; Linoleate, 44.8 Gm.)

	BREAKFAST	LUNCH	DINNER	SNACK
Milk	1 exchange		1 exchange	
Vegetables				
A group		As desired	As desired	
B group			1 exchange	
Fruit	1 exchange	1 exchange	1 exchange	2 exchanges
Bread and Cereals	2 exchanges	2 exchanges	2 exchanges	2 exchanges
Meat, Fish, Poultry		3 exchanges	4 exchanges	
Eggs				
Fat		6 exchanges	7 exchanges	2 exchanges
Special Margarine	1 exchange		2 exchanges	
Sugar, Sweets	5 exchanges	3 exchanges	2 exchanges	2 exchanges

Sample Menu

BREAKFAST	LUNCH	DINNER
½ medium grapefruit with 2 tsp. sugar	Sandwich: 3 oz. chicken, 1 tbsp. mayonnaise, 2 slices bread	4 oz. breaded haddock fried in 1 tbsp. oil (bread crumbs from 1 slice bread)
¾ cup dry or ½ cup cooked cereal with 2 tsp. sugar	Lettuce, celery, and green pepper salad with 1 tbsp. oil, vinegar to taste	½ cup rice or potatoes fried in 1 tsp. oil
1 slice toast with 1 tsp. special margarine and 1 tsp. jelly	1 small baked apple with 1 tbsp. sugar	½ cup tomatoes
1 cup skim milk		½ cup peas with 2 tsp. special margarine
		1 tbsp. mayonnaise with relish as tartar sauce
		1 small pear with 2 tsp. sugar
		1 cup skim milk

SNACK

2 slices cinnamon toast with 2 tsp. oil and 2 tsp. sugar
½ cup orange juice
½ small banana

* Council on Foods and Nutrition, A.M.A.: The regulation of dietary fat. J.A.M.A., *181:* 411, 1962.

to the patient, and surgical treatment of hypertension has gradually lost much of its appeal.

DRUGS   Antihypertensive drugs have been successfully used in the treatment of hypertension. Various agents are employed— alone and in combination—including those which act centrally, those which produce ganglionic blockade, and those which exert peripheral sympatholytic and adrenolytic effects. Unfortunately, side effects are common with the use of every agent currently available, but newer agents are appearing and it is hoped that these side effects can be eliminated.

Chlorothiazide (Diuril) and hydrochlorothiazide (Hydro-Diuril) potentiate the action of antihypertensive drugs. However, the continued use of chlorothiazide or hydrochlorothiazide may produce hypochloremia, hyponatremia, hypokalemia, and hyperuricemia.

DIETARY   TREATMENT   In 1944 the *Kempner rice diet*[23] was introduced for treatment of both hypertensive vascular disease and kidney disease. The patient consumes daily 10 ounces of dry rice (approximately 1050 kcalories), which is cooked to suit the personal taste. Twenty minutes of boiling is usually adequate. The remaining 900 to 1000 kcalories are supplied by liberal quantities of sugar and fresh or preserved fruits. Thus, the diet is high in carbohydrate, furnishes about 2000 kcalories, between 15 and 30 gm. of proteins, 4 to 6 gm. of fat, and from 100 to 150 mg. of sodium daily. Salt is strictly forbidden. Fluids are limited to from 700 to 1000 ml. of fruit juices. Tomato juice and vegetable juices are not permitted. Iron and vitamin supplements are given. The diet is somewhat liberalized after reduction of blood pressure and alleviation of the symptoms. However, it is

[23]Kempner, W.: Treatment of kidney disease, hypertensive disease with rice. North Carolina Med. J., 5:125, 1944, and 5:273, 1944.

difficult for a patient to live on this regimen for any length of time. Too, dietary restriction and manipulation may lead to nutritional deficiencies or imbalance.

Kempner[24] utilized this method in 213 patients with high blood pressure who exhibited various stages of the disease. After an average period of 62 days on the strict or modified diet, improvement was noted in 64 per cent of the patients. Subsequent investigations, carried out by other workers using a more liberal diet, adequate in protein but equally low in sodium, amply demonstrated that sodium restriction was the only important factor.

The diet should be adequate and normal with no excessive amounts of foods. Obesity places an added burden on the heart, and there is general agreement that normal weight is important to relieve the symptoms of hypertension. Highly seasoned foods and stimulants like alcohol and coffee are restricted. Proteins are not restricted unless there is renal function impairment. (See Chapter 32.) If cardiac damage has resulted, sodium is restricted as indicated. A diet with sodium restricted to 250 mg. daily may be necessary to insure maximum therapeutic results. A moderate or mild restriction may effectively control the hypertension in some patients. The degree of sodium restriction will depend upon the severity and the course of the hypertension. See Sodium Restricted Diets, pages 443–449.

In hypertensive patients especially vulnerable to potassium deficiency, increased intake of potassium-rich foods (Appendix Table 9) will usually compensate adequately for potassium lost in diuresis.

INSTRUCTION OF THE PATIENT   If a sodium restricted or modified fat diet is prescribed, it is not enough to give the patient a list of foods he must avoid. The instructions should be directed toward the person's securing an adequate diet. He must be given assistance in planning menus, in methods of preparation of foods at home and in selection of food when eating away from home.

The nurse, dietitian and physician can do much to encourage the patient concerning the necessary modifications in his dietary. The success of the diet depends upon the patient's understanding of the therapeutic importance and the need to adhere to the regimen indefinitely.

The patient should be encouraged to experiment with and try new adventures in seasoning and flavoring foods. Suggestions and recipe sources, such as listed at the end of this chapter, will be stimulating and helpful. (See Chapter 43 for sodium restricted, low fat and fat modified recipes.)

PROBLEMS AND SUGGESTED TOPICS FOR DISCUSSION

1. Interview cardiac patients to learn the foods which cause distention. What is your conclusion?
2. Name some substitutes for salt that can be used safely in flavoring salt-poor food.
3. When is salt restricted for a cardiac patient? Study the diet prescribed for cardiac patients in your institution. Determine the amount of sodium present in the food in your diet.
4. Secure a dietary pattern of a person with compensated heart disease and determine the approximate intake of sodium. How may it be modified to the level of 1000 mg.?
5. Obtain a diet history from a patient with decompensated heart disease who is on the medical ward or in the clinic. Determine how much of a sodium reduction the 500 mg. sodium diet he now receives is from his usual pattern.
6. Check the food intake of a patient on the ward who is recovering from an acute heart attack. Is it adequate? Should it be adequate in calories, carbohydrates, proteins, minerals, and vitamins? Give reasons for your answer.
7. Obtain a diet history from a patient who is suffering with hypertension. Calculate the average daily intake of food. Is the amount normal or excessive? Modify the diet to make it correct in all factors.
8. Assist a person with any one of the diets given for hyperlipoproteinemia. What changes did he need to make in his customary habits?

RECIPES AND MEAL PLANNING FOR SODIUM RESTRICTED DIETS

American Heart Association, local or New York, New York. Booklets: Your Sodium-Restricted Diet 500 mg.; 1000 mg.; Mild Restriction.
Field, F.: Gourmet Cooking for Cardiac Diets. New York, Collier Books, 1962. (Paperback.)
Payne, A. S., and Callahan, D.: Low Sodium–Fat Controlled Cookbook. Revised. Boston, Little, Brown and Company, 1960.
Planning Low Sodium Meals: The Nutrition Foundation, Inc., 99 Park Avenue, New York, New York, 10016. (Fifty cents.)

RECIPES AND MEAL PLANNING FOR FAT CONTROLLED DIETS

American Heart Association, local or New York, New York. Booklets: Planning Fat-Controlled Meals for Unrestricted Calories and Planning Fat-Controlled Meals for 1200 and 1800 kcalories.
Cavanna, E., and Welton, J.: Gourmet Cookery for a Low Fat Diet. Revised. Englewood Cliffs, New Jersey, Prentice-Hall, Inc., 1961.
Keys, A., and Keys, M.: Eat Well and Stay Well. Garden City, New York, Doubleday & Co., Inc., 1959.
Payne, A. S., and Callahan, D.: Low Sodium–Fat Controlled Cookbook. Revised. Boston, Little, Brown and Company, 1960.
Stead, E. S., and Warren, G. K.: Low Fat Cookery. 2nd ed. New York, McGraw-Hill Book Co., Inc., 1959.
Rosenthal, S.: Live High on a Low Fat Diet. Philadelphia, J. B. Lippincott Company, 1962.

---

[24]Kempner, W.: N. Carolina Med. J., 6:61 and 117, 1945.

SUGGESTED ADDITIONAL READING REFERENCES

Aherns, E. H., Hirsch, J., Peterson, M. L., Stoffel, W., and Farquhar, J. W.: Symposium on significance of lowered cholesterol levels. J.A.M.A., *170*:2198, 1959.

Albrink, M. J.: Diet and cardiovascular disease. J. Am. Dietet. A., *46*:26, 1965.

American Spice Trade Association: The art of seasoning low sodium diets. Hospital Management, *89*:80, 1960.

Antar, M. A., et al.: Changes in retail market food supplies in the United States in the last seventy years in relation to the incidence of coronary heart disease with special reference to dietary carbohydrate and essential fatty acids. Am. J. Clin. Nutr., *14*:169, 1964.

Bagchi, K., Ray, R., and Datta, T.: The influence of dietary protein and methionine on serum cholesterol level. Am. J. Clin. Nutr., *13*:232, 1963.

Brown, H. B., and Page, I. H.: Lowering blood lipids by changing food patterns. J.A.M.A., *168*:1989, 1958.

Brown, H. B., and Spodnik, M. J.: Meat for low-fat diets. J. Am. Dietet. A., *38*:540, 1961.

Brown, H. B., et al.: Design of practical fat-controlled diets. J.A.M.A., *196*:205, 1966.

Christakis, G., et al.: Effect of the anti-coronary club program on coronary heart disease. Risk-factor status, J.A.M.A., *198*:129, 1966.

Council on Foods and Nutrition, A.M.A.: Low sodium milk. J.A.M.A., *163*:739, 1957.

Council on Foods and Nutrition, A.M.A.: The regulation of dietary fat. J.A.M.A., *181*:411, 1962.

Dahl, L. K.: Role of dietary sodium in essential hypertension. J. Am. Dietet. A., *34*:585, 1958.

Danowski, T. S.: Low-sodium diets – Physiological adaptation and clinical usefulness. J.A.M.A., *168*:1886, 1958.

Dayton, S., et al.: Can changes in the American diet prevent coronary heart disease? J. Am. Dietet. A., *46*:20, 1965.

Dustan, H. P.: Diet and diuretics in the treatment of hypertensive cardiovascular disease. J.A.M.A., *172*:2045, 1960.

Editorial. Cholesterol lowering agents. J.A.M.A., *178*:1158, 1961.

Editorial. Essential hypertension. J.A.M.A., *160*:673, 1956.

Food and Nutrition Board: Dietary fat and human health. Washington, D.C., National Academy of Sciences, National Research Council, Pub. No. 1146, 1966.

Fredrickson, D. S.: Dietary Management of Hyperlipoproteinemia: A Handbook for Physicians. National Health and Lung Institute, National Institutes of Health, Bethesda, Maryland, 20014, and booklets for each of the five types of hyperlipoproteinemias.

Goldsmith, G. A.: Highlights on the cholesterol-fats, diets and atherosclerosis problem. J.A.M.A., *176*:783, 1961.

Green, J. G., et al.: Use of fat-modified foods for serum cholesterol reduction. J.A.M.A., *183*:91, 1963.

Gwinup, G., et al.: Effect of nibbling versus gorging on serum lipids in man. Am. J. Clin. Nutr., *13*:209, 1963.

Hartroft, W. S.: Should the American diet be drastically modified? J. Am. Dietet. A., *41*:13, 1962.

Hashim, S. A.: Medium-chain triglycerides – clinical and metabolic aspects. J. Am. Dietet. A., *51*:221, 1967.

Kempner, W.: Compensation of renal metabolic dysfunction: Treatment of kidney disease and hypertension vascular disease with rice diet. North Carolina M. J., 6:61, 1945; 6:117, 1945.

Kempner, W.: Treatment of heart and kidney disease and of hypertensive and arteriosclerosis vascular disease with the rice diet. Ann. Int. Med., *31*:821, 1949.

Keys, A.: Effect of dietary cholesterol on serum cholesterol in man. Am. J. Clin. Nutr., *9*:126, 1961.

Keys, A.: Blood lipids in man – a brief review. J. Am. Dietet. A., *51*:508, 1967.

Kritchevsky, D.: Cholesterol and atherosclerosis. Am. J. Clin. Nutr., *10*:269, 1962.

Lees, R. S., and Wilson, D. E.: The treatment of hyperlipidemia. New Eng. J. Med., *284*:186, 1971.

Levy, R. I., et al.: Dietary management of hyperlipoproteinemia. J. Am. Dietet. A., *58*:406, 1971.

Master, A. M., et al.: Relationship of obesity to coronary disease and hypertension. J.A.M.A., *153*:1499, 1953.

Mayer, J.: Nutrition and heart disease. Am. J. Pub. Health, *50*:5, 1960.

Meredith, A. P.: Living with the vegetable-oil food pattern. J. Am. Dietet. A., *38*:543, 1961.

Newman, E. V.: Regulation of electrolytes in the management of heart disease. J.A.M.A., *172*:2045, 1960.

Prior, I. A. M.: The price of civilization. Nutrition Today, 6:2, 1971.

Review. Cardiovascular disease – The picture in the U.S. J. Am. Diet. A., *46*:394, 1965.

Review. Diets of men with high and low blood cholesterol levels. Nutr. Rev., *21*:294, 1963.

Review. Fat and cholesterol in the diet. Nutr. Rev., *23*:3, 1965.

Schizas, A., et al.: Medium-chain triglycerides – use in food preparation. J. Am. Dietet. A., *51*:228, 1967.

Sebrell, W. H., Jr.: An over-all look at atherosclerosis. J. Am. Dietet. A., *40*:403, 1962.

Stamler, J., et al.: Approaches to the prevention of coronary heart disease. J. Am. Dietet. A., *40*:407, 1962.

Tripathy, K. H., et al.: Role of protein upon serum cholesterol level in malnourished subjects. Am. J. Clin. Nutr., *23*:1160, 1970.

Trulson, M. F., et al.: Comparison of siblings in Boston and Ireland. J. Am. Dietet. A., *45*:225, 1964.

Van Itallie, T. B., and Hashim, S. A.: Diet and heart disease – Facts and unanswered questions. J. Am. Dietet. A., *38*:531, 1961.

Williams, R. J.: Nutrition and ischemic heart disease. Borden's Review of Nutrition Research, *31*:No. 2, 1971.

Williams, R. J.: Nutrition Against Disease: Environmental Prevention. New York, Pitman Pub. Corp., 1971.

Wohl, M. G., and Goodhart, R. S. (eds.): Modern Nutrition in Health and Disease. 4th ed. Philadelphia, Lea & Febiger, 1968. Chapter 27A, Nutrition in cardiovascular disease; Chapter 27B, Nutrition in relation to atherosclerosis.

Yudkin, J., and Morland, J.: Sugar intake and myocardial infarction. Am. J. Clin. Nutr., *20*:503, 1967.

Zukel, M. C.: Fat-controlled diets. Am. J. Clin. Nutr., *16*:270, 1965.

Zukel, M. C.: Appraising and issuing educational health materials. J. Am. Dietet. A., *54*:25, 1969.

PHYSIOLOGY AND FUNCTION OF THE BLOOD

Blood transports nutrients, oxygen, hormones, electrolytes, cellular excreta and other substances to and from all parts of the body. It is life itself, and any disease or disorder of the blood or blood-forming organs affects the body as a whole. The red and white blood cells and the blood platelets are the constituents usually concerned in diseases of the blood-forming organs.

In the normal healthy individual the blood amounts to approximately 5 to 6 per cent of the body weight. The concentration of red blood cells (erythrocytes) is approximately 4,500,000 per cu. ml. in women and 5,000,000 red blood cells per cu. ml. in men. The white blood cells (leukocytes) are fewer in number than erythrocytes; the ratio is approximately 1 to 500. (Review Formation of Blood, p. 106.)

DIETARY RECOMMENDATIONS FOR BLOOD DONORS The extensive program which involved the general public in donating blood during and following World War II has raised the question of the nutritional requirements for blood regeneration. Repeated blood donations may produce severe iron loss and a consequent anemia. In studying the problem, McKibbin and Stare[1] conclude that "nutrition is of importance in blood regeneration and that good nutrition favors rapid regeneration." In general, the adequate normal diet, with increased emphasis on iron, ascorbic acid and protein foods, as described under Anemias Resulting from Acute Hemorrhage (p. 465), should provide optimum blood regeneration.

Specific dietary recommendations for blood donors have been prepared by a committee of the American Dietetic Association and are available from the Association office for a nominal fee should the reader be interested in pursuing the subject further.

Food is not generally given to a patient during a transfusion. Actually, the patient is not in need of food since plasma containing glucose, salts and nutriment is being given intravenously. However, if the patient complains of hunger, a light meal of easily digested foods, such as milk and crackers or a sweet drink, is usually given.

THE ANEMIAS

Anemia is a condition in which there is a deficiency in the size or number of erythrocytes, or the amount of hemoglobin which they carry. Nutritional factors of greatest importance in anemias are deficiencies of iron, vitamin B_{12}, and folic acid.

CLASSIFICATION Formerly, the anemias were classified into primary and secondary types. Now it is known that anemia is never primary; it is always secondary to some pathological state in the patient. Anemia may be classified in many different ways. A classification made according to cell size and hemoglobin content based on etiology is the following:

ETIOLOGIC CLASSIFICATION OF ANEMIA[2]

I. Loss of blood
    A. Acute posthemorrhagic anemia
    B. Chronic posthemorrhagic anemia

[1]McKibbin, J. M., and Stare, F. J.: Nutrition in blood regeneration. J. Am. Dietet. A., *19*:331, 1943.

[2]From Wintrobe, M. M.: Clinical Hematology. 5th ed. Philadelphia, Lea & Febiger, 1961, p. 427.

II. Excessive destruction of red corpuscles, resulting from
   A. Extracorpuscular causes
   B. Intracorpuscular defects, congenital (see IV, A below) and acquired
III. Impaired blood production resulting from deficiency of substances essential for erythropoiesis
   A. Iron deficiency
      Experimentally, also copper and cobalt deficiencies
   B. Deficiency of various B vitamins. Clinically B_{12} and folic acid deficiencies (pernicious anemia and related macrocytic, megaloblastic anemias); pyridoxine-responsive anemia
      Experimentally, pyridoxine, folic acid, B_{12} and niacin deficiencies; possibly also riboflavin, pantothenic acid and thiamin deficiencies
   C. Protein deficiency
   D. Possibly ascorbic acid deficiency
IV. Faulty construction of red corpuscles
   A. Congenital or hereditary
      1. Sickle cell anemia and related disorders (hemoglobin C disease, etc.)
      2. Thalassemia
      3. Congenital hemolytic diseases
   B. Acquired
      1. Anemia associated with infection
      2. Anemia associated with various chronic diseases (renal, etc.)
      3. Anemia in plumbism; following irradiation; in drug sensitivity (aplastic anemia)
      4. "Myelophthisic" anemias (leukemia, Hodgkin's disease, myelofibrosis, malignancy with metastases, etc.)
      5. Anemia in myxedema and in other endocrine deficiencies
      6. Anemia associated with splenic disorders: "hypersplenism"
   C. Unknown
      Miscellaneous hypersideremic anemias

MICROCYTIC HYPOCHROMIC ANEMIA

Microcytic hypochromic anemia relates to the cell size and relative hemoglobin content and is characterized by small (microcytic), pale (hypochromic) erythrocytes; but the total cell count may be normal. This type of anemia in the adult indicates iron deficiency as a result of blood loss or malabsorption.

ANEMIAS RESULTING FROM ACUTE HEMORRHAGE

Following an acute hemorrhage in a formerly healthy individual, the body replaces plasma within a few days. However, the speed with which the hemoglobin is restored depends largely upon the type of diet ingested. An adequate normal diet rich in foods containing iron, ascorbic acid and proteins is essential. Liquids are mandatory to replace the fluid loss through hemorrhage and consequent loss from the tissues. In case of very serious hemorrhage, restoration of blood volume by transfusion may be necessary.

NUTRITIONAL ANEMIAS

For the normal individual approximately 10 per cent of the food iron is absorbed. From 2 to 10 per cent of iron in vegetables can be absorbed; from 10 to 30 per cent of iron in animal protein can be absorbed. Ascorbic acid increases iron absorption; phytates decrease absorption. The solubility of iron is influenced by the hydrochloric acid, and certain amino acids enhance absorption.

The anemias which result from an inadequate intake of iron, proteins, certain vitamins (B_{12}, folic acid, ascorbic acid), copper and other heavy metals are frequently termed nutritional anemias. The deficiency may be caused by chronic blood loss or hemorrhage, inadequate ingestion, defective absorption, imperfect utilization, injury to the bone marrow, or increased requirement as in pregnancy. The most common types of nutritional or hypochromic anemia seen in this country are due to iron deficiency. However, not infrequently a combined type of anemia is present, presumably dependent on a need for iron, protein, certain vitamins, and possibly copper. For a long period, diet has been recognized as a remedial agent in overcoming nutritional anemia.

Iron Deficiency Anemias

This form of anemia is characterized by a reduced concentration of hemoglobin in the blood. The three causes of iron deficiency anemia are (1) chronic blood loss, such as from a chronically bleeding peptic ulcer, bleeding hemorrhoids, parasites, or malignancy, (2) faulty iron intake or absorption, and (3) increased growth of blood volume, which occurs in infancy, puberty, pregnancy and lactation. In the early stages of iron deficiency iron stores are depleted and iron absorption increases. The transferrin iron-binding capacity rises as iron stores decrease. When iron stores are depleted plasma iron falls. (See Figure 31–1.) During infancy, a close relationship exists between diet and iron deficiency. At puberty, as well as in infancy, there is an acceleration of growth and an increase in the amount of circulating hemoglobin. This type of anemia is often present in growing children or in girls who are losing blood during menstruation when iron intake is inadequate; this latter anemia is called *chlorosis*. In the adult, however, iron deficiency anemia is, with few exceptions, ascribed to blood loss. While loss of blood is a natural process in females, adequate stores of iron should be made available to meet such demands.

During pregnancy, there is an increased need for iron to supply the growing fetus. During lactation, there is a loss of iron which probably is similar in quantity to the loss in the menstrual flow. Unless iron is provided to replace the amount lost or to build new hemo-

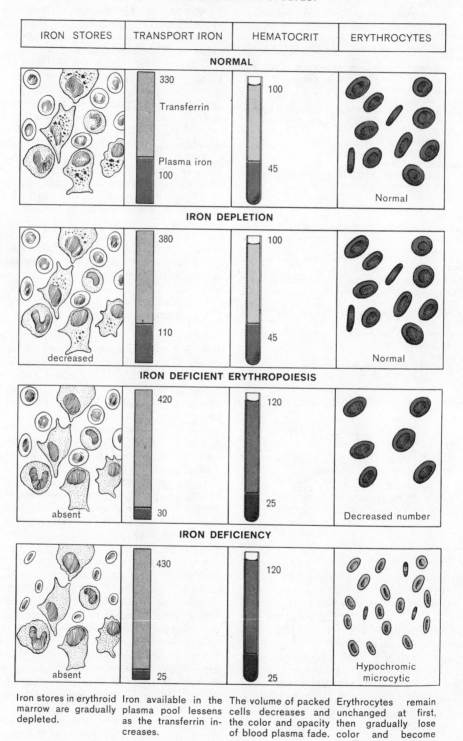

HOW IRON DEFICIENCY EVOLVES:

IRON STORES	TRANSPORT IRON	HEMATOCRIT	ERYTHROCYTES

NORMAL

IRON DEPLETION

IRON DEFICIENT ERYTHROPOIESIS

IRON DEFICIENCY

Iron stores in erythroid marrow are gradually depleted.

Iron available in the plasma pool lessens as the transferrin increases.

The volume of packed cells decreases and the color and opacity of blood plasma fade.

Erythrocytes remain unchanged at first, then gradually lose color and become smaller.

Figure 31–1   How iron deficiency evolves. (From Finch, C. L.: Iron metabolism. Nutrition Today, 4:2, Summer, 1969.)

globin, iron deficiency anemia will develop. Sometimes gastrointestinal disturbances, such as diarrhea, achlorhydria or intestinal disease interfering with the absorption, will prevent iron from entering the blood stream in required amounts, even though the diet contains adequate amounts of iron. When such a condition exists, an individual may maintain a low hemoglobin level for years.

Treatment

Medication Today, the chief treatment consists in oral administration of inorganic iron, preferably ferrous iron, in adequate dosage over a proper time interval. Coleman et al.,[3] recommend parenteral administration of iron for patients with iron deficiency anemias who are unable to take oral iron because of gastrointestinal symptoms or inability to absorb iron, or who need iron reserves. Ascorbic acid greatly increases iron absorption through a capacity to maintain iron in the reduced state.

Diet Treatment In addition, foods which contain a high percentage of iron should be provided, especially when the anemia is caused by faulty ingestion of iron. (See Fig. 31–1.) Liver, kidney, beef, tripe, egg (yolk), dried fruits (apricots, peaches, prunes, raisins), dried peas and beans, nuts, green leafy vegetables (beet greens), molasses, and whole grain bread and cereals rank highest among the iron rich foods. (See Appendix Table 8 for a more complete list; also see Table 19–4, Principal Sources of Food Constituents, and Chapter 8.) The normal or general house diet is recommended with maximal amount of iron-rich foods. If the patient's digestion is impaired, the foods should be simple and easily digested, including those foods which have been suggested and outlined for the soft diet. Anorexia, if present, must be considered when selecting food or planning the diet. Attractive food service and individual preferences should be considered to stimulate a desire for food.

In cases of anemia caused by bleeding ulcer the ulcer regimen is liberalized to include the blood-building foods, such as liver and muscle meats.

Sometimes cobalt is used in treatment of iron deficiency anemia, when iron alone is apparently not effective.

Protein Deficiency Anemia

Protein is one of the essential substances necessary for the proper production of hemoglobin and red blood cells. Because hemoglobin is a protein, one would assume that a rich protein intake should be maintained in patients with anemia. However, a hypochromic or nutritional anemia due to protein deficiency is rare even in cachectic individuals. This is probably due to the fact that hemoglobin formation takes preference over other body protein needs. In some of the underdeveloped areas of the world the anemias may be complicated by deficiencies of iron and other nutrients and by associated infections, parasitic infection and malabsorption. In the anemia of protein malnutrition the defect is believed to be a failure in red blood cell production due to decreased stimulation of the erythroid marrow. Patients usually suffer from multiple deficiencies – such as folic acid and, less frequently, vitamin B_{12} – when their diet is lacking in protein. In such cases, administration of folic acid and/or vitamin B_{12}, along with a normal, well balanced diet, will usually bring good response. An individual on a normal adequate diet usually ingests an adequate amount of proteins. However, in nephrotic conditions in which there is an extensive urinary loss of protein, the amount of food proteins must be increased above the normal requirements. Animal proteins (nucleoproteins) are preferred.

Copper and Other Heavy Metals Deficiency Anemias

While copper and other heavy metals are essential for the proper formation of hemoglobin, the amounts needed are so minute that they are amply supplied by the normal adequate diet. There is probably no justification, except perhaps in foods for infants, to add these substances to the normal diet.

Vitamin Deficiency Anemia

There is an interrelationship between the metabolism of folic acid $\rightarrow$ folinic acid, vitamin B_{12} and ascorbic acid; a deficiency of any one will interfere with the normal development of erythrocytes and lead to anemia. Vitamin B_6 is essential in a number of enzymes involving amino acids. Anemias respond to the therapy of vitamin B_6. Vitamin B_{12} and folic acid (or folinic acid) are essential for the synthesis of nucleoproteins required in the development of erythrocytes. Ascorbic acid is believed to function in the conversion of folic acid to its biologically active state, folinic acid. Ascorbic acid influences the rate of iron absorption and the release of iron from transferrin to the tissues.

FOLIC ACID DEFICIENCY ANEMIA

This is present in tropical sprue (Chapter

---

[3]Coleman, D. H., Stevens, A. R., Jr., and Finch, C. A.: The treatment of iron deficiency anemia. Blood, *10*:567, 1955.

34), in cases during pregnancy (Chapter 15), and in infants born to mothers having the deficiency (Chapter 16), and may respond dramatically to folic acid therapy.[4] Poor eating habits of long duration or faulty absorption and utilization of folic acid are believed to cause the disorder. A folacin deficiency and megaloblastic anemia resulting from poor eating habits over a long period was reported to have responded rapidly to folacin therapy.[5] Inadequate ingestion of folic acid almost always results in a nutritional macrocytic anemia. Administration of vitamin B_{12} has been used to induce a hematologic remission in folic acid deficiency while tissue folate levels remained depleted.[6]

The macrocytic anemia of scurvy may be the result of the ascorbic acid deficiency which interferes with the conversion of folic acid to folinic acid. In such cases, ascorbic acid and folic acid therapy plus an adequate diet high in protein and ascorbic acid are indicated. Not all anemia in scurvy is true macrocytic anemia requiring folic acid therapy. Some scorbutic anemia will respond to ascorbic acid therapy alone, while some may be the result of iron deficiency. (See Folic Acid, p. 139.) The normal adequate diet with increased protein of high biologic value will carry the necessary vitamins unless there is also evidence of vitamin deficiency. In such cases, the deficiency of vitamins must be made up in the adequate diet prescribed. Deep green leafy vegetables and liver are rich sources of folic acid; meat, fish, legumes and whole grains are also good sources. See Chapter 9, Vitamins, for sources of vitamins.

PERNICIOUS AND OTHER MACROCYTIC ANEMIAS

Pernicious anemia is attributed to a deficiency of vitamin B_{12}, and to the lack of the *intrinsic factor,* in the gastric juice, which is necessary for absorption of this vitamin from food[7], resulting in failure of the maturation of red blood cells. Cells are oversized, odd-shaped and have fragile membranes. It is classified as a *macrocytic, hyperchromic* anemia because of the increase in the size of the red cells and in the hemoglobin content. These red cells are released undeveloped into the blood stream and become fewer and larger as the disease progresses. Although the dis-

ease was formerly considered fatal, it can now be treated successfully and controlled.

Pernicious anemia affects not only the blood but the gastrointestinal tract and spinal cord. Treatment, therefore, must not only help the blood count but eliminate symptoms produced by the other structures involved.

TREATMENT In 1926 Minot and Murphy[8] reported the effectiveness of liver therapy in pernicious anemia. Soon after, active concentrates of liver suitable for clinical use were developed, and by 1936 relatively purified extracts of liver were available for intramuscular injection, in addition to those preparations which earlier had been developed for oral administration. *Liver extract* is a specific remedy for deficiency of the intrinsic factor in pernicious anemia. It is also effective in other macrocytic anemias such as the anemia of sprue and macrocytic anemia of pregnancy. The intrinsic factor unites with the extrinsic factor, probably vitamin B_{12} (the principal, if not the sole, antipernicious anemia factor of purified liver extracts), to form an antianemic factor which is stored in the liver until it is needed by the bone marrow for the maturation of red blood cells. Before liver extract was introduced, large quantities of raw and cooked liver were fed daily to the patients. This was most distasteful and difficult to take because the patient afflicted with pernicious anemia has a very poor appetite. The administration of liver extract, or vitamin B_{12}, restores the appetite of the patient in an amazingly short time.

Vitamin B_{12} and liver extract can be used interchangeably. However, vitamin B_{12} has, to a large extent, supplanted the use of liver preparations.

Both liver extract and vitamin B_{12} can be given orally or by way of injection. However, for optimal absorption the preferred method is parenteral administration, except perhaps in the case of pernicious anemia of pregnancy.

Folic Acid In 1946 Spies[9] reported on the therapeutic value of folic acid in certain types of anemia. He found that synthetic folic acid given either parenterally or orally was effective in producing significant hemopoietic response in persons with nutritional macrocytic anemia and with macrocytic anemia of sprue, pregnancy, pernicious anemia, and pellagra. It was found ineffective with aplastic anemia, iron deficiency anemia, and anemia associated with leukemia. It has

[4]Girdwood, R. H.: Folate depletion in old age. Am. J. Clin. Nutr., 22:234, 1969.

[5]Review. Folacin and megaloblastic anemia. Nutr. Rev., 22:3, 1964.

[6]Alperin, J. B.: Effect of vitamin B_{12} therapy in a patient with folic acid deficiency. Am. J. Clin. Nutr., 15:117, 1964.

[7]Darby, W. J.: Present knowledge of human requirements for vitamin B_{12}. Present Knowledge of Nutrition. 3rd ed., New York, Nutrition Foundation, 1967, p. 73.

[8]Minot, G. R., and Murphy, W. P.: Treatment of pernicious anemia by special diet. J.A.M.A., 87:470, 1926.

[9]Spies, T. D.: Effect of folic acid on persons with macrocytic anemia in relapse. J.A.M.A., 130:474, 1946.

since been established that folic acid is not a full therapeutic substitute for vitamin B_{12}. Pernicious anemia frequently is accompanied by gastrointestinal and neurological manifestations which do not respond to folic acid therapy but are cleared up promptly by administration of vitamin B_{12}.

Diet   The normal or general house diet, with increased amounts of proteins, iron and vitamins, is advised for pernicious anemia in addition to vitamin B_{12} and other medication indicated. The high protein diet (1.5 gm. of protein per kg. of body weight) is desirable for both liver function and blood regeneration. Since the green leafy vegetables contain both iron and folic acid, the diet will contain increased amounts of the necessary components. Liver should be included frequently because it carries a good supply of iron, vitamin B_{12}, folic acid and other important nutrients. Meats (especially beef and pork), eggs, milk and milk products are particularly rich in vitamin B_{12}.

Consult Table 19–4, Principal Sources of Food Constituents, page 314, for a listing of foods rich in iron and proteins. Also refer to the foods rich in iron listed in Appendix Table 8 and review the material on folic acid and vitamin B_{12} in Chapter 9.

Anemia patients suffering from malnutrition, especially of those foods which contain vitamin B_{12} (the extrinsic factor), such as liver, muscle meat, eggs, yeast, and wheat germ, may respond to liver extract, vitamin B_{12}, a diet rich in meats, or to large amounts of brewer's yeast. In many of the macrocytic conditions, vitamin B_{12} or liver therapy is only one part of the treatment of the disease. The whole patient must be treated, not only his blood. For example, diarrhea may also be present. Its cause must be determined, and treatment prescribed.

DISEASES OF THE WHITE BLOOD CELLS

Therapy can be successful only if the agent depressing the formation of bone marrow is removed or the causative factor is corrected. Blood transfusions are the chief palliative treatment. Diet therapy has not been found to have direct influence.

Leukemia

Leukemia is the best known example of this condition, with crowding of the erythrogenic tissue, and subsequent anemia. The disease is frequently regarded as a type of cancer of the blood-forming organs. There is an abnormally large production of leukocytes or white blood cells. The normal white count is between 7500 and 10,000; in leukemia it

goes up to 300,000 or more. Many of these cells are abnormal, a sign that the blood-forming organs are overworking. The white cells are manufactured in bone marrow, spleen, lymph glands, and the liver.

ETIOLOGY   The etiology is unknown. Ionizing radiation is one established cause, and a few cases have been attributed to the effects of chemicals, mainly benzol. An unusual incidence of the disease has been recorded among survivors of the atomic bomb in Japan. There appears to be a relation between exposure to x-ray and the development of the disease. Heredity, as well as hormonal abnormalities, is thought to play a role. Recently "clusters" of leukemia cases, primarily among children, have been noticed in a growing number of population centers in all parts of the country, which suggests some validation of evidence favoring virus as a cause.[10] The virus theory is currently being investigated. Little more is understood of the fundamental nature of leukemia than its causes. Leukemia may be classified as (1) acute; (2) chronic myeloid; and (3) chronic lymphatic. The acute variety is most common in children and runs a shorter course than the milder or chronic type, which attacks adults and is more prevalent. The prognosis is almost invariably poor. However, the newer forms of therapy have made life substantially more comfortable and a high percentage who respond to therapy have a remission following treatment.

TREATMENT   Life expectancy has been increased somewhat in the acute form through the use of drug therapy, combined with supportive therapy, for complications such as hemorrhage, infection, and anemia. ACTH, cortisone or the antimetabolite products, amethopterin and 6-mercaptopurine, as well as prednisone and prednisolone, are the most frequently used of the steroid hormones. Remedies are also available for chronic leukemia, including the nitrogen mustard compound, triethylenemelamine (TEM), as well as ACTH, cortisone, radioactive phosphorus, total body radiation (x-ray) and two new specific alkylating agents, chlorambucil (works on lymphocytic tissue) and Myleran (acts on granulocytic tissue). The best results have been with acute leukemia in children.

In addition, transfusions, antibiotics, iron, liver extract, and vitamin B_{12} are given as supportive therapy.

Diet   The patient's individual condition and appetite must be considered as much as possible. Because of the patient's weakness, frequent feedings may be necessary.

---

[10]Editorial. The virus etiology of human leukemia. J.A.M.A., *186*:146, 1963.

Anorexia, lesions in the mouth, and difficulty in swallowing are often present, which must be regarded when selecting foods for the diet. A well-balanced soft diet adequate in protein which is easily digested, and simple foods served attractively are important factors. Highly seasoned and very hot foods and citrus fruits should be avoided when lesions of the mouth are present. Vitamin supplements are usually indicated.

When antimetabolic drugs which interfere with nucleoprotein synthesis are used in the treatment, folic acid or folinic acid may be required by medication.

FAVISM

A large broad bean, *Vicia fava*, is grown in the Mediterranean countries. It is a cheap protein-rich vegetable widely used in many ways—raw, cooked or in bread. In some individuals the eating or inhaling of the pollen causes favism, a serious hemolytic anemia. Death can follow if blood transfusions are not given in time. Children under 4 years of age are especially susceptible and males are affected more frequently than females.

Favism is apparently an inborn error of metabolism associated with a deficiency of enzyme glucose-6-phosphate dehydrogenase (G-6-PD) and glutathione in the red blood cells. Glutathione and G-6-PD are required for the metabolism of glucose. Just how the ingestion of fava beans affects this factor is not clear.[11, 12]

---

[11]WHO Chronicle, 24:29, January, 1970; and Marcus, J. R., and Cohen, G.: Harper's Magazine, June, 1967, p. 98.

[12]Bottini, E., et al.: Favism: Association with erythrocyte acid Phosphatase Phenotype. Science, 171:409, 1971.

PROBLEMS AND SUGGESTED TOPICS FOR DISCUSSION

1. Discuss the functions of hemoglobin.
2. Study the effect of nutritional anemia and pernicious anemia on the metabolic processes of the body. What are the causes of iron deficiency anemia?
3. How much dietary iron, ascorbic acid and protein do you ingest daily? How adequate is your intake of these nutrients?
4. Interview a patient with iron deficiency anemia. How will he improve his dietary?
5. Obtain a dietary history of a person with pernicious anemia or a postgastrectomy patient.
6. What role does vitamin B_{12} play in the treatment of pernicious anemia? How does the treatment of pernicious anemia differ from that of folic acid deficiency anemia?
7. Plan a menu for one day with a patient with leukemia who has sore mouth lesions. What are the main considerations? Why is it often advisable to give folic acid when antimetabolic drugs are used in the treatment of leukemia?

SUGGESTED ADDITIONAL READING REFERENCES

Alperin, J. B.: Effect of vitamin B_{12} therapy in a patient with folic acid deficiency. Am. J. Clin. Nutr., 15:177, 1964.

Bottini, E., et al.: Favism: Association with erythrocyte acid phosphatase phenotype. Science, 171:409, 1971.

Brown, E. B.: The absorption of iron. Am. J. Clin. Nutr., 12:205, 1963.

Burton, B. T. (ed.): Heinz Handbook of Nutrition. 2nd ed. 1965. New York, McGraw-Hill Book Company, Inc., Chapter 33, Nutrition and the Anemias.

Chung, A. S. M., et al.: Folic acid, vitamin B_6, pantothenic acid and vitamin B_{12} in human dietaries. Am. J. Clin. Nutr., 9:573, 1961.

Clinch, C. A.: Iron metabolism. Nutrition Today, 4:2, 1969.

Dairy Council Digest Nutritional Anemias, 40:No. 4, 1969.

Duncan, G. G. (ed.): Diseases of Metabolism. 5th ed. Philadelphia, W. B. Saunders Company, 1964, Chapter 22, Nutritional and Metabolic Aspects of Disorders of the Blood, by Farid I. Haurani and Leandro M. Tocantins.

Editorial. Irradiation and marrow infusion in acute leukemia. J.A.M.A., 178:323, 1961.

Editorial. The function of vitamin B_{12} in metabolism. J.A.M.A., 172:1938, 1960.

Editorial. The virus etiology of human leukemia. J.A.M.A., 186:146, 1963.

Editorial. Vitamins, minerals and anemia. J.A.M.A., 175:1000, 1961.

Ellison, A. B. C.: Pernicious anemia masked by multivitamins containing folic acid. J.A.M.A., 173:240, 1960.

Goldsmith, G. A.: Nutritional anemias with special reference to vitamin B_{12}. Am. J. Med., 25:680, 1958.

Izak, G., et al.: The effect of small doses of folic acid in nutritional megaloblastic anemia. Am. J. Clin. Nutr., 13:369, 1963.

Marcus, J. R., and Cohen, G.: The redale of the dangerous bean. Harper's Magazine, June, 1967, p. 98.

Mueller, J. F., and Will, J. J.: Interrelationship of folic acid, vitamin B_{12}, and ascorbic acid in patients with megaloblastic anemia. Am. J. Clin. Nutr., 3:30, 1955.

Patwardham, V. N.: Nutritional anemias—WHO Research Program. Am. J. Clin. Nutr., 19:63, 1966.

Queries and Minor Notes. Giving food during a transfusion. J.A.M.A., 158:1237, 1955.

Pritchard, J. A.: The response to iron in iron deficiency. J.A.M.A., 175:478, 1961.

Review. Anti-intrinsic factor in pernicious anemia. Nutr. Rev., 22:9, 1964.

Review. Folacin and megaloblastic anemia. Nutr. Rev., 22:3, 1964.

Review. Folacin deficiency and alcoholism. Nutr. Rev., 22:8, 1964.

Review. Gastrointestinal protein loss in iron-deficiency anemia. Nutr. Rev., 21:170, 1963.

Review. Pernicious anemia: Is it an autoimmune disease? Nutr. Rev., 21:205, 1963.

Rundles, R. W.: Hematopoietic effects of folic acid metabolites in the management of megaloblastic anemias. Am. J. Clin. Nutr., 7:385, 1959.

Spies, T. D., et al.: Anti-anemic properties of a reaction product of vitamin B_{12} and the intrinsic factor. South. M. J., 43:206, 1950.

Streiff, R. R., and Little, A. B.: Folic acid deficiency in pregnancy. New Eng. J. Med., 276:776, 1967.

Tandon, B. N., et al.: Protein deficiency and anemias. Am. J. Clin. Nutr., 21:813, 1968.

Wilson, T. H.: Intrinsic factor and B_{12} absorption. Nutr. Rev., 23:33, 1965.

Wintrobe, M. M.: Blood dyscrasias. Am. J. Nursing, 60:496, 1960.

WHO Chronicle—Favism. 24:29, January, 1970.

Chapter 32
NUTRITION IN RENAL DISEASES

PHYSIOLOGY AND FUNCTION OF NORMAL KIDNEYS

The kidneys maintain the chemical homeostasis of all body fluids. Their chief functions are to regulate and to conserve nutrients and water and to excrete waste products. Blood entering the kidneys reaches the arterioles and enters the nephrons. Each nephron is composed of a glomerulus surrounded by a membrane (Bowman's capsule), a convoluted and collecting tubule, and a blood supply through the capillaries. Approximately 1.2 liters of whole blood pass through the nephrons each minute, about one-third of the total cardiac output. The nephrons are arranged close together and in such a pattern that fluid flows from one to the other. Essential chemicals are returned to the venous circulation and elements to be discarded (glomerular filtrate) stay in the kidneys. The glomerular filtrate is virtually protein-free and passes to the proximal convoluted tubules where about 85 percent of the electrolytes, nearly all of the glucose, amino acids and ascorbic acid are reabsorbed into the blood. The filtrate passes through Henle's loop into the distal and collecting tubules where additional water and the remaining electrolytes, sodium, chloride, potassium bicarbonate ions, most of the phosphate and about 57 per cent of the urea are reabsorbed. Ultimately, the waste products proceed into large channels and finally arrive in the funnel-shaped, central edge of the area known as the pelvis of the kidney. Now the waste products are ready to be sent to the bladder for accumulation and in due time to be eliminated as urine. (See Figure 32–1.)

Water is the greatest amount of waste product. The quantity is related to the amount taken into the body and the amount excreted through the skin and lungs in the process of temperature regulation but normally averages 1 to 2 liters daily. Urine normally consists of approximately 95 per cent water and 5 per cent solids. About 60 per cent of the solids is nitrogenous waste and 40 per cent is inorganic salts. Of the nitrogenous wastes, urea predominates; uric acid, creatinine and ammonia are present in small amounts. Of the inorganic salts, sodium chloride predominates; phosphate and sulfate salts of calcium, sodium, potassium and magnesium are present in small amounts. The amount of urea present depends upon the diet. High protein intake increases the urea output and a smaller consumption decreases the urea content. If, for some reason, these normal waste products are not eliminated, they collect in abnormal quantities in the blood.

A minimum urinary volume of approximately 600 ml. (obligatory fluid) is required for the excretion of the average load of solids. More is required for the excretion of increased loads.

A specific transport protein is required for the reabsorption of Na^+ from the distal tubule (Cl^- and HCO_3 passively follow the Na^+). Part of the reabsorbed Na^+ is exchanged for K^+ or H^+ in the distal tube. The synthesis of the specific protein requires the presence of aldosterone, a mineralocorticoid.

Water reabsorption from the distal tubules and collecting duct is controlled by the small peptide hormone, vasopressin or antidiuretic hormone elaborated from the pituitary gland. This peptide hormone is made by the cells of the hypothalamus and stored in the pituitary; when there is a rise in the osmotic pressure of the blood or a fall in the total blood volume, the hypothalamus stimulates the secretion of the antidiuretic hormone which increases the reabsorption of water. The hormone is not released when the osmotic pressure is low. Diuresis takes place.

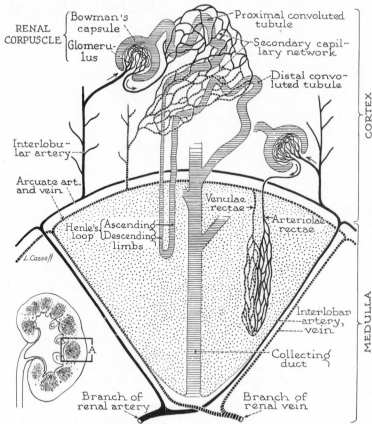

Figure 32–1   Diagram of renal tubule or nephron. Inset A shows the location of the renal tubule in the kidney. (King and Showers.)

Kidneys help to maintain the normal pH in the blood and other fluids and to conserve the alkaline reserve of the body. Foreign substances and drugs are excreted by the kidney.

The kidneys, like any organ of the body, are subject to diseases. Infectious diseases may cause abnormal kidney function. Inflammation of the kidneys may cause kidney degeneration and kidney channels may be blocked by the formation of kidney stones.

OBJECTIVES OF DIETARY TREATMENT The general objectives of dietary treatment in renal disease are: (1) to reduce the work of the diseased organ, (2) to replace the nutritive substances lost to the body in abnormal amounts as a result of impaired kidney function, (3) to exclude substances from the diet which are conducive to retention of nitrogen waste products and sodium in abnormal quantities as a result of impaired excretory function, (4) to maintain nutrition and weight at as nearly a normal level as possible, and (5) to encourage appetite and improve morale.

NEPHRITIS

Nephritis or Bright's disease, named after the English physician who was first to describe the disease, is a general term indicating altered kidney function caused by either a diffuse inflammation or a degenerative change. For a clearer definition, the term Bright's disease is reserved for the varieties of nephritis involving the secretory apparatus in the kidney.

CLASSIFICATION   There are numerous classifications of nephritis. However, the important forms are glomerulonephritis (inflammatory diseases), nephrosis (degenerative diseases), and nephrosclerosis (vascular diseases). Each form may be manifested in acute, subacute or chronic stages.

ACUTE GLOMERULONEPHRITIS (HEMORRHAGIC NEPHRITIS)

ETIOLOGY AND CHARACTERISTICS Acute glomerulonephritis is characterized by inflammation of the capillary loops in the glomeruli of the kidney, with varying degrees of hematuria, edema, hypertension, and nitrogen retention (azotemia). Less urine is excreted (oliguria) and it is highly concentrated. Because of the red blood cells appearing in the urine, the disease is also termed hemorrhagic nephritis. Anorexia and lethargy are present; nausea and vomiting are not unusual. In the more severe cases edema may be noted.

The disorder occurs most frequently in children and young adults, and is often a sequel to an infection in the body, especially of the upper respiratory tract. The causative organisms are numerous, but the streptococcus is the most common offender.

OBJECTIVE AND PRINCIPLES OF DIETARY TREATMENT   The treatment of acute nephritis focuses on an attempt to prevent the disease from becoming chronic by minimizing the work of the kidneys.

Fluid and Electrolyte Balance   The diet should be planned to influence the regulation of water balance and adjustment of the various mineral salts, especially sodium, potassium and the chlorides. Fluid intake is regulated according to the volume of urine. In discussing the therapy of glomerulonephritis, Rantz[1] states that "Restriction of fluids to 700 cc. more than the combined total of urine and vomitus, and of sodium to less than 300 mg. per day, is mandatory in patients with edema and oliguria." After the diuretic phase has passed, edema disappears and the blood pressure is normal; fluids may be given freely.

Low Protein Diet   Regulation of protein content of the diet is important. Authorities differ in their opinions about the amount of proteins to include in the diet for a patient with nephritis. In acute cases, proteins are frequently restricted to an amount below the normal estimated requirement on the theory that an injured kidney will respond more quickly if not pressed into needless action. However, the present trend is to keep a middle course, limiting the protein to 0.5 gm./kg. ideal body weight/day in the beginning to reduce work of the kidneys by reducing nitrogen metabolism and retention; gradually increasing the amount as soon as the kidneys show signs of improving so that by the end of 10 days or 2 weeks the protein allowance is near the normal requirement.

Dietary treatment becomes an individual problem. During the initial stage, with attendant anorexia, nausea, and vomiting, the diet is of necessity limited to fruit juices given at frequent intervals, not to exceed the fluid allowance. Glucose may be added to the fruit juice to add calories and spare tissue protein. As soon as possible or immediately in less severe cases, a low protein (20 to 40 gm. of high biologic value) high carbohydrate, sufficient caloric diet is given. Milk, cereal, toast with butter and jelly, cooked fruit, mashed and baked potato are added as tolerated.

The foundation of an adequate diet for an adult (Table 11–4, p. 163) contains approximately 63 gm. of protein. If the dietary intake of protein is to be reduced to 40 gm., for example, all the meat, poultry and fish or 2 ounces of the meat, poultry, fish and the egg could be omitted. To the diet could be added more carbohydrate foods—jelly, sugar, glucose, fruits, fruit juice, ginger ale—and some fats such as butter and fortified margarine to meet calorie requirements in an attempt to minimize tissue catabolism. Frequent feedings are usually better tolerated than three meals, with protein and carbohydrate taken at the same time to increase the utilization of amino acids.[2] As the condition improves and the protein allowance is increased, eggs and meat are added to the diet.

Salt (sodium) and fluids are restricted when edema is present. However, severe sodium restriction is dangerous in cases of renal insufficiency when the kidney cannot excrete dilute urine. (See Sodium Restricted Diets, in Chapter 30.) One of the first indications of recovery is an increase in the amount of urine excreted. As more urine is excreted, the edema is reduced. The regimen should be maintained until the urine chemistry returns to normal.

CHRONIC GLOMERULONEPHRITIS (CHRONIC HEMORRHAGIC NEPHRITIS)

Should the acute stage of nephritis develop into a chronic form, the disease assumes graveness. However, the majority of patients with chronic glomerulonephritis give no history of having had an acute condition.

The patient usually experiences headaches and frequent urination during the night. Variable amounts of albumin and casts are present in the urine. As the disease progresses, hypertension, proteinuria, lowered serum protein and edema develop. The kidneys are unable to excrete all the urea which is formed. Urea nitrogen is retained in the blood. Eventually uremia becomes a serious complication. Lethargy and anorexia are problems with which the patient has to cope.

OBJECTIVES AND PRINCIPLES OF DIETARY TREATMENT   The primary objectives of the dietary treatment are (1) to maintain good nutritional status, (2) to minimize damage to the kidney, (3) to prevent protein deficiency, and (4) to prevent or correct edema and uremia. Controversy exists among authorities regarding the amount of protein to be permitted during treatment of chronic

[1]Rantz, L. A.: Current status of therapy in glomerulonephritis. J.A.M.A., *170*:948, 1959.

[2]Elman, R.: Time factors in utilization of mixture of amino acids (protein hydrolysate) and dextrose given intravenously. J. Clin. Nutr., *1*:287, 1953.

glomerulonephritis. One group supports a high protein intake to compensate for the loss of serum protein in albuminuria. They recommend intakes ranging from 100 to 150 gm. per day based upon normal optimum protein intake plus that equivalent to the amount lost in the urine. The larger amounts of proteins prevent the body from using its own tissues to supply the necessary nitrogen. A high protein intake aids in the correction of a negative nitrogen balance.

Another group believes that effective therapy is likely to occur when protein intake is reduced, thereby slowing down the degenerative process and avoiding an additional load of nitrogenous products to be excreted by the kidney. This group favors a diet ranging from 40 to 50 gm. protein per day, depending on the individual patient. Further restriction (30–40 gm.) may be necessary if uremia is impending. The minimum protein requirement for metabolic breakdown is considered to be approximately 0.5 gm. per kg. of body weight per day. Increased carbohydrates (300 to 400 gm. daily) are given to spare the proteins. Fat is given in a moderate (80 gm.) amount to complete the calorie requirement. Large amounts may cause nausea and are generally inadvisable.

Sodium and Fluids   Sodium and fluids are reduced while edema is present in relation to the degree of water retention. There is difference of opinion as to whether sodium should be restricted as a prophylactic measure in all cases of chronic nephritis. Danowski[3] and others advise decreasing sodium intake in patients with chronic renal disease without edema by avoiding high salt foods and using salt substitutes. In some patients with severe hypertension, more rigid sodium restriction is prescribed. It should be remembered, however, that to prescribe commercial salt substitutes which contain large amounts of potassium for patients with renal insufficiency may be contraindicated (p. 450). If renal failure is accentuated on this regimen, a more liberal ration of salt is allowed. If severe edema is present fluid intake is generally limited to 1 liter per day; otherwise, an intake of 1 to 2 liters per day is satisfactory.

Vitamins   Vitamin concentrates are frequently prescribed to assure adequate vitamin intake.

High Protein, Sodium Restricted Diets During the course of chronic nephritis, while the body loses proteins through albumin in the urine, the normal diet may be prescribed with an increase in the amount of proteins.

The protein foods in the daily diet may be increased to:

milk: 1 quart
eggs: 3
meat, fish or poultry: ½ pound

If edema is present, the food is prepared and served without the addition of salt. The diet suggested contains approximately 120 gm. of protein and 6 gm. of salt, or 2.36 gm. of sodium (Table 32–1). By replacing the 1 quart of regular whole fluid milk in the diet with modified low sodium milk, the sodium content of the diet is reduced to 1.86 gm. A special low sodium protein supplement, Protinal (The National Drug Company), may be used to increase the protein content of the diet still further. Also see Table 22–1, p. 330, for ways to increase the protein in the daily meal plan.

High Protein, Severe Sodium Restriction Diets   When sodium is restricted to 200 to 300 mg. daily, but the protein intake must exceed 100 gm. a day, it becomes necessary to use larger amounts of sodium deficient milk, since the usual protein foods (regular milk, meat, poultry, fish, eggs) have too high a so-

TABLE 32–1   HIGH PROTEIN, NO FREE SALT DIET

(120 gm. of Proteins; 6 gm. of Salt or 2.36 gm. of Sodium; 2800 Kcalories)

SAMPLE MENU

BREAKFAST

Stewed prunes
Cooked wheatena
Poached eggs, 2
Toasted whole wheat bread, 1 slice
Sweet butter
Milk, 8 oz.
Coffee

LUNCHEON

Cream of pea soup
Cold sliced roast lamb, 4 oz.
Cooked spinach
Sliced tomato salad
Whole wheat bread, 1 slice
Sweet butter
Vanilla ice cream
Milk, 8 oz.

DINNER

Swiss steak, 4 oz.
Mashed potatoes
Baked squash
Whole wheat bread, 1 slice
Sweet butter
Fresh fruit cup
Milk, 8 oz.

BEDTIME

Eggnog
This diet is prepared and served without the addition of salt.

---

[3]Danowski, T. S.: Low-sodium diets—physiological adaptation and clinical usefulness. J.A.M.A., *168*:1886, 1958.

dium content. In such cases unsalted nuts, legumes, low sodium canned meat products, Protinal, and other specially canned low sodium products (p. 450) are valuable adjuncts to the diet. See Chapters 30 and 43 concerning ways in which diets low in sodium can be made more palatable.

Parenteral Protein   In some circumstances, particularly in the presence of pronounced anorexia, nausea and vomiting, oral administration of proteins may not be possible in sufficient amounts to correct the protein deficit. In these cases protein hydrolysates may be employed. A concentrated albumin solution, low in sodium content and fortified with the amino acids tryptophan and isoleucine, is suggested for patients with albuminuria and edema. However, if the nephritic patient has pronounced hypertension and cardiac failure (nephrosclerosis), the intravenous administration of albumin is contraindicated.

Latent Nephritis

During the course of chronic nephritis there is usually a latent period, lasting for several years, when the patient feels well. During this period optimum nutrition should be maintained. To avoid the complication of hyperchromic anemia, the result of blood being lost in the urine (hematuria), an adequate diet emphasizing foods rich in protein, iron and ascorbic acid should be ingested. If hyperchromic anemia appears in the chronic nephritis patient, it usually cannot be remedied either by diet or medication but is treated by blood transfusion.

Urea Nitrogen Retention

If there is nitrogen retention in the blood during the course of chronic nephritis, the protein intake is lowered temporarily. The food protein requirement is balanced against the level of waste products in the blood, known as nonprotein nitrogen. In such cases the normal diet containing adequate but not excessive amounts of protein is prescribed. An optimum protein intake may be attained by increasing the total calories, especially the carbohydrate foods, thus sparing the protein. Proteins of high biologic value are preferred. The amount of sodium and fluid allowed in the diet depends primarily upon the patient's urine output. An adequate consumption of fluids generally aids elimination and prevents acidosis.

Low or Normal Protein, Sodium Restricted Diets   The 70 gm. protein, sodium restricted diets outlined for the treatment of cardiac patients (see Chapter 30) may be followed or adjusted in sodium and protein content as indicated. These diets are planned for patients with mild, moderate, strict and severe sodium restrictions. Also, see Low Protein Diet outlined for acute glomerulonephritis, p. 473.

Renal Hypertension

Hypertension is present in almost all cases of active glomerulonephritis, both acute and chronic. Most authorities believe it is acquired as a result of the kidney disease. Consult Chapter 30 for the diet treatment of essential hypertension.

Terminal Stages of Nephritis

In the terminal stages of nephritis, the end-products of metabolism cannot be eliminated because of kidney failure. Sodium, potassium, fluids, and proteins are all rigidly restricted. In very serious cases, in which the urea in the blood is very high and there are signs of approaching death, the daily intake of proteins is limited to 25 to 35 gm. or omitted altogether. Calories are supplied by sugar and sweet butter.

Tube feeding may be advisable to reduce the physical strain of eating.

THE NEPHROTIC SYNDROME

Lange and co-workers[4] define the nephrotic syndrome as an antigen-antibody reaction comprising forms formerly termed "lipid nephrosis" and the nephrotic stage of subacute glomerulonephritis. There is an increased capillary permeability in the glomeruli and probably throughout the body. Several forms of renal disease may be associated with the nephrotic syndrome. Statistically it is reported to be found in adults most frequently in association with glomerulonephritis. The term nephrosis has caused much confusion in the literature. In 1905 Friedrich Mueller introduced it to describe certain degenerative lesions in the kidneys, which he believed could not correctly be called nephritic, i.e., inflammatory. True nephrosis is a kidney disease accompanied by degenerative changes in the renal glomeruli and tubules and is often termed degenerative Bright's disease. The kidneys usually are able to function adequately in the excretion of urea and other metabolic waste products but there is severe loss of protein in the plasma (hypoproteinemia). It is characterized by marked edema, massive albuminuria and decreased serum albumin, and usually is accompanied by an

[4]Lange, K., et al.: The treatment of the nephrotic syndrome with steroids in children and adults. Arch. Int. Med., 99:760, 1957.

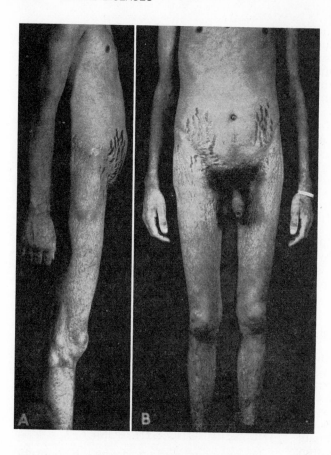

Figure 32–2   Nephrotic syndrome, malnutrition, and "lipoid nephrosis" in 18-year-old male. Photographs show severe tissue wasting and abdominal striae following diuresis and weight loss from 223 to 125 pounds in 6 foot, previously husky youth who had ascites, severe pedal edema, and massive proteinuria. (From Kark, R. M. *In* Wohl, M. G., and Goodhart, R. S. [eds.]: Modern Nutrition in Health and Disease. 3rd ed. Philadelphia, Lea & Febiger, 1964.)

increase in plasma lipids and a low basal metabolic rate. Hypertension and hematuria (bloody urine), although present in nephritis, are absent in the "pure" form of nephrosis. However, the vast majority of cases develop one or more of these signs during their course of illness, and whether true lipoid nephrosis occurs as a distinct entity is a subject of controversy. The protein deficit is sometimes great because of the large amounts of protein lost in the urine, and the results are tissue wastage and malnutrition (Fig. 32–2). Plasma albumin concentrations of less than 1 gm. per 100 ml. are common and account for the massive edema often seen in patients with nephrosis. Nephrosis occurs chiefly in young children; 80 per cent of the cases occur in the age group under 15 years, with the peak incidence at the age of 3½ years. It will be discussed in the chapter on children's diseases (Chapter 36).

OBJECTIVE AND PRINCIPLES OF DIETARY TREATMENT   The chief object of the diet treatment in nephrosis is to replace the albumin (protein) lost from the plasma into the urine. Patients with severe protein deficiency already established, and with continued protein loss occurring, may require months of carefully supervised diet treatment. The diet should provide sufficient proteins to maintain positive nitrogen balance, with a rise in the plasma albumin and disappearance of edema. There are times when the proteinuria is greater in amount than the maximum daily plasma albumin regeneration and, in such cases, it becomes virtually impossible to make up the protein deficit.

The diet is similar to the High Protein Diet outlined (p. 474) for chronic nephritis with albuminuria, although the allowance of proteins is more liberal—150 gm. or more. (See Table 22–1, p. 330.) Chinard[5] recommends a calorie intake of 35 to 50 kcal./kg. ideal body weight/day and a protein intake of 1 to 3 gm./kg. ideal body weight/day. Incidentally, "red meat" may be included in the diet of patients with kidney disease because there is no scientific evidence to substantiate the popular superstition against its use. Red meat is preferred to avoid the anemia which is frequently present in these patients due to the toxemia of the disease.

NEPHROSCLEROSIS

Nephrosclerosis or sclerosis of the kidneys involves the blood vessels of the glomeruli

---

[5]Chinard, F. P.: Current status of therapy in the nephrotic syndrome in adults. J.A.M.A., *178*:312, 1961.

and is associated with hypertension; it usually occurs in the older age group. It may be benign or malignant in form.

OBJECTIVE AND PRINCIPLES OF DIETARY TREATMENT   The diet prescribed for nephrosclerosis should be as near the adequate normal diet (Chapter 11 and Table 11–4) as possible. The obese patient should lose weight gradually until normal weight is reached. The loss in weight is essential to lessen the work of the circulatory system. In cases of moderately severe renal function involvement, the protein allowance is reduced to a low normal amount (50 gm.). Less severe cases are allowed somewhat increased amounts of protein (70 to 90 gm.). In cases of grave kidney involvement with high blood urea nitrogen, indicating failure of the kidney to excrete normal amounts of the end-products of protein metabolism, the daily intake of proteins should be reduced to an average amount of 40 to 50 gm. or less. Foods should be of the simple variety, with high quality protein, and easily digested. Salt (sodium) is moderately restricted, even if there is no edema, to save the work of the kidneys. If edema occurs, the salt is restricted as indicated. These patients should not use salt substitutes containing potassium. See Low Protein Diets with restriction in sodium under discussion of acute glomerulonephritis (p. 473), and under Urea Nitrogen Retention in chronic glomerulonephritis (p. 474). Fluids are forced unless there is kidney retention, in which case they are correlated with output.

The basic sodium restricted diets outlined in Chapter 30 can be adjusted to meet the individual needs of patients who need sodium restriction. Also see discussion under essential hypertension, pp. 460–462.

UREMIA IN KIDNEY FAILURE

Uremia is a toxic condition caused by the retention of urinary constituents in the blood: urea, creatinine, uric acid, and other end-products of protein metabolism. The name indicates that urea is the waste product retained in the greatest amount. The condition is a result of severe progressive loss of renal function, such as nephritis and other kidney diseases, and is characterized by weakness, anorexia, nausea and vomiting, mental disturbances and, if advanced, stupor and coma. The nitrogen retention, urea nitrogen, is an indication of the severity of loss of kidney function. If advanced to the coma stage, the condition is grave and is usually fatal. Both extracorporeal hemodialysis and peritoneal dialysis have enabled physicians to maintain patients with chronic oliguria for extended periods of time.

OBJECTIVE AND PRINCIPLES OF DIETARY TREATMENT   The aim of the treatment for chronic renal failure is (1) to maintain the patient in the best nutritional status possible; (2) to sustain the intake of protein, sodium, potassium and fluids at a desirable level; (3) to maintain a palatable and an attractive diet and a variety of foods; (4) to encourage the patient to ingest the necessary nutrients.

The dietary reduction in protein results in a decrease in production of some nitrogenous waste. The use of potassium exchange resins makes it possible to ingest a greater variety of foods containing potassium. Patients with chronic oliguria are required to rigidly restrict sodium and fluid intake. These patients are unable to excrete acid; control of potassium and protein intake provides for this modification. (See Appendix Table 9 for potassium and sodium content of foods.)

The American Dietetic Association Diabetes Exchange Lists are adapted in similar grouping of foods to the limitations of sodium, potassium and protein intakes.[6] (See Tables 32–2 and 32–3.) All foods used are processed and prepared without salt. The patient's diet may be planned for various levels of sodium content (250 to 2000 or more mg.), depending upon the needs of the individual. Sample menu patterns and recipes are shown in Tables 32–4, 32–5, and 32–6.[7]

The caloric intake should be adequate to provide for energy need, most of which is supplied by carbohydrate and fat. The requirement of protein is met more efficiently by selecting protein foods of high biological value. Sufficient carbohydrate and fat should be ingested simultaneously to provide calorie requirements and to prevent catabolism of endogenous protein. The dietary calcium content of the diet is low. Regulation of the calcium balance may be accomplished by the dializing bath. Iron medication and vitamin supplements, especially the water-soluble vitamins, are indicated. Close medical supervision of these patients is required. Dietary adjustments are frequently indicated, depending upon the observations of body weight, blood urea nitrogen, serum sodium and potassium levels and urinary excretions of nitrogenous sodium and potassium. Fluid restriction varies and is regulated by the excretory ability of the kidneys. The daily intake is limited to the equivalent of insensible losses, in which case the water formed (approximately 400 ml.) from oxidation of food must be counted. (See Chapter 10.) Many patients

---

[6]Mitchell, M. C., and Smith, E. J.: Dietary Care of the Patient with Chronic Oliguria. Am. J. Clin. Nutr., 19:163, 1966.

[7]*Ibid.*

(Text continued on page 482.)

TABLE 32–2   CONTROLLED PROTEIN, POTASSIUM AND SODIUM DIET
(All Foods Prepared Without Salt)

FOODS ALLOWED	SERVING	AVOID THE FOLLOWING	FOODS ALLOWED	SERVING	AVOID THE FOLLOWING
Group I – *Dairy Products*			**Group III – *Fruits and Fruit Juices*** *(Canned except where otherwise specified)*		
———servings allowed/day					
Cream, light	½ cup	Cream, milk and half-and-	**LIST A**		
Cream, heavy	¾ cup	half except in allowed	———servings allowed/day		
Sour cream	½ cup	amounts	Apples, raw		Any dried fruit (peaches,
Half-and-half	½ cup	Buttermilk	Apple juice		apples, prunes, apricots
Milk	½ cup		Applesauce		dates, raisins)
Ice cream	½ cup		Apricots		Cantaloupe, avocado,
Sherbet	½ cup		Apricot nectar		banana, prune juice
Creamed cheese	1 tbs.		Blueberries		
Cream soups prepared with-			Cherries (Bing and		
out the addition of salt	½ cup		Royal Anne)		
			Figs, canned sweet		
Group II – *Vegetables*			Grapes, Concord		
			Cranberries, raw		
LIST A			Cranberry sauce		
———servings allowed/day			Grapefruit sections		
Asparagus	6 spears	Any vegetable prepared	Peaches		
Beans, green or wax	½ cup	with the addition of salt	Peach nectar		
Beets	½ cup	or sodium	Pears		
Carrots	½ cup	Dried vegetables and	Pear nectar		
Lettuce	2 large	legumes	Rhubarb, fresh		
	leaves	Other dark greens	Pineapple		
Onions	1 (medium)	Parsnips and sauerkraut	Pineapple juice		
Peas	½ cup				
Squash, summer (yellow or					
white)	½ cup				
Tomatoes, canned	½ cup				
LIST B			**LIST B**		
———servings allowed/day			———servings allowed/day		
Broccoli	1 stalk (medium)		Blackberries, fresh or frozen	½ cup	Fresh nectarines, mulber-
Brussels sprouts	½ cup		Fruit cocktail	½ cup	ries
Cabbage	½ cup		Grapes (Emperor, Thomp-		Any fruit or fruit products
Corn	½ cup		son or Tokay)	22	which contain sodium
Eggplant	½ cup		Grape juice	⅓ cup	benzoate
Okra	½ cup		Grapefruit juice	½ cup	
Cucumbers	8 slices (⅛ in. thick)		Orange, raw	1 (small)	
Pumpkin	½ cup		Orange juice	½ cup	
Potato	¼ cup		Peaches, raw or frozen	1 (medium)	
Rutabaga	½ cup		Plums, raw or canned	2 (medium)	
Turnips	½ cup		Raspberries	½ cup	
Spinach	½ cup		Strawberries	½ cup	
Squash (acorn & Hubbard)	½ cup		Tangerines	1 (large)	
Tomatoes, raw	1 (small)		Watermelon	½ cup	
Tomato juice	½ cup		Gooseberries	½ cup	

°½ cup = 1 serving

(Table continued on opposite page.)

TABLE 32–2   CONTROLLED PROTEIN, POTASSIUM AND SODIUM DIET *(Continued)*

(All Foods Prepared Without Salt)

FOODS ALLOWED	SERVING	AVOID THE FOLLOWING	FOODS ALLOWED	SERVING	AVOID THE FOLLOWING

Group IV – *Bread and Bread Substitutes*

———servings allowed/day

Bread (salt-free white or Vienna)	1 slice	Whole wheat breads and cereals
Soda crackers	5	"Quick cooking" cereals
Cooked cereal: oatmeal, farina, cream of wheat, cornmeal, cream of rice	1/2 cup	Dry cereals except those listed
Dry cereals: shredded wheat, rice krispies, puffed wheat and rice, cornflakes, wheat flakes, rice flakes	3/4 cup	Pretzels, potato chips, salted popcorn
		Pancake and pastry mixes
Rice, macaroni, noodles or spaghetti, cooked	1/2 cup	Prepared muffins, waffles, cakes
Hominy	1/2 cup	
Popcorn (unsalted)	1 cup	

Group V – *Meat, Fish, Poultry and Eggs*

LIST A

———oz. allowed/day

Egg, prepared any way	1	All cheese except salt-free cheese
Cheese, prepared without addition of salt	1 oz.	All smoked, processed or canned meats
Cottage cheese	1/4 cup	Bacon, ham, sausage, cold cuts, frankfurters, corned beef
Chicken, heart, pork, duck, lobster, shrimp	1 oz.	Any seafood which has had salt added during processing. (It is possible to purchase many seafoods fresh or processed without the addition of salt; check your supermarket)
Clams, fresh	2 or 3	
Oysters, fresh	4	
Tongue, not smoked	1 oz.	
Tuna (without salt)	1/4 cup	Halibut

LIST B

These goods contain higher amounts of potassium and may be substituted ——— times/week for choices from subgroup A

Beef, lamb, liver, rabbit, veal, scallops, cod, fresh salmon, goose	1 oz.	
Peanut butter	1 tbsp.	

Group VI – *Fats and Substitutes*

Butter, margarine, salad dressing, shortening, vegetable oil, lard, cream, sour cream (as specified in group 1)	Bacon fat, meat extracts
	Nuts

Group VII – *Baked Desserts*

———servings allowed/day

1 or 2 crust pie (made with allowed fruit or milk)	1/8 pie	Angel food cake, chocolate
Jello or gelatin (within fluid allowance)		Commercial baked products
Tapioca pudding made with allowed milk or allowed fruit juices		All others not listed
Cookies (plain butter)		
Cake (plain sponge, white, yellow or pound)		
Borden's Fruit Ice (water ice), within fluid allowance		

Group VIII – *Beverages***

Weak coffee or tea	2 servings/day	Coffee and tea except as specified
Gingerale, Seven-Up, R–C Cola, Pepsi Cola, Kool-aide, allowed milk		Malt beverages or cereal beverages
		Milk, except in allowed amounts
		Buttermilk

Group IX – *Condiments and Sweets*

The following spices may be used in the seasoning and preparation of foods:

Allspice	Salt, in any form
Caraway	Baking soda and baking powder
Cinnamon	Anti-acids, laxatives
Coconut	SALT SUBSTITUTES
Curry powder	Prepared mustard, catsup, meat sauces
Garlic	Bouillon or canned soups
Ginger	Olives and pickles
Hard candy	Celery salt, onion salt, garlic salt
Herbs	Accented, salted meat tenderizers
Honey	Prepared horseradish
Horseradish (fresh)	Molasses, chocolate candy and candy bars
Jams, jellies	Jams and jellies which contain sodium benzoate
Lemon juice	
Mace	
Mustard, dry	
Nutmeg	
Paprika	
Pepper	
Peppermint extract	
Sage	
Sugar	
Thyme	
Tumeric	
Vanilla extract	
Vinegar	
Syrup	

Small amounts of the following vegetables may be used for seasoning other foods:

Celery
Cucumber
Green pepper
Mushroom
Onion

**As allowed within fluid restriction.

Adapted from Mitchell, M. C., and Smith, E. J.: Dietary care of patients with chronic oliguria. Am. J. Clin. Nutr., *19*:165, 1966.

TABLE 32–3   AVERAGE PROTEIN, POTASSIUM, SODIUM AND FLUID CONTENT OF ONE SERVING OF VARIOUS FOOD GROUPS*

	FOOD GROUPS	SERVING	PROTEIN (gm.)	POTASSIUM (mg.)	SODIUM (mg.)	FLUID (ml.)
Group I	Dairy Products	½ cup	4	90	60	70
Group II	Vegetables					
	A	½ cup	1	120	9	70
	B	½ cup	2	230	9	70
Group III	Fruits					
	A	½ cup	—	65	2	80
	B	½ cup	—	145	2	80
Group IV	Breads, low sodium and substitutes	1 slice or ½ cup	0.075 to 2	50	5 to 10	10
Group V	Meat, fish, poultry, eggs					
	A	1 ounce	7	70	70	20
	B	1 ounce	7	120	25	20
Group VI	Fats and substitutes	—	—	—	—	1
Group VII	Desserts, special recipes	As specified	2	—	Varies	Varies
Group VIII	Beverages	1 cup	—	5 to 50	Varies	240
Group IX	Condiments, sweets, as indicated		—	—		Varies

*All averages were calculated from figures available for individual items in each group. When more than one value was available, the figures were also averaged.

Adopted from Mitchell, M. C., and Smith, E. J.: Dietary care of patients with chronic oliguria. Am. J. Clin. Nutr., *19*:164, 1966, and Mayo Clinic Diet Manual, W. B. Saunders Co., 1971.

TABLE 32–4   CONTROLLED PROTEIN, POTASSIUM AND SODIUM DIET SAMPLE MENU 1*

FOOD ITEM	CARBO-HYDRATE (gm.)	PROTEIN (gm.)	FAT (gm.)	POTASSIUM (mg.)	SODIUM (mg.)
BREAKFAST					
½ cup oatmeal	15	2	—	50	1
1 tsp. sugar	8	—	—	—	—
½ cup half-and-half	6	2	14	90	65
½ cup grapefruit sections (sweetened)	20	—	—	65	2
LUNCH					
Egg salad (1 egg and salad dressing)	—	7	10	70	63
1 slice salt-free bread	15	2	—	50	10
1 tsp. salt-free butter	—	—	5	—	—
Tossed salad with salt-free vinegar and oil dressing	3	1	5	120	3
Fruit tapioca (pineapple)	31	—	—	65	8
Gingerale (8 oz.)	24	—	—	1	1
DINNER					
2 oz. roast beef	—	14	10	240	42
½ cup rice with 1 tsp. salt-free butter	15	2	5	50	1
½ cup spinach	7	2	—	230	50
Lettuce wedge with dressing	3	1	5	65	3
⅛ of 9 in. apple pie (pie crust and apples)	40	2	10	115	5
8 oz. Seven-Up	24	—	—	8	10
BEDTIME SNACK					
½ cup milk	6	4	5	90	60
3 butter cookies (see recipe)	16	1	7	50	2
Total	233	40	76	1,359	326

*Total kcalories: 1,780.

From Mitchell, M. C., and Smith, E. J.: Dietary care of patients with chronic oliguria. Am. J. Clin. Nutr., *19*:167, 1966.

TABLE 32–5 CONTROLLED PROTEIN, POTASSIUM AND SODIUM DIET
SAMPLE MENU 2*

FOOD ITEM	CARBO-HYDRATE (gm.)	PROTEIN (gm.)	FAT (gm.)	POTASSIUM (mg.)	SODIUM (mg.)
BREAKFAST					
1 egg fried in 1 tsp. oil	——	7	10	70	60
1 slice toast with salt-free butter	15	2	5	50	10
and 1 tsp. jelly	15	——	——	——	2
½ cup canned pears	20	——	——	65	2
1 cup weak coffee	——	——	——	30	1
with 1 tsp. sugar	8	——	——	——	——
LUNCH					
½ cup cream of celery soup, made without the addition of salt	6	4	5	90	60
1 slice toast with 1 tsp. salt-free butter	15	2	5	60	10
Cole slaw with dressing	3	1	5	120	15
½ cup canned apricots	20	——	——	65	2
3 butter cookies	16	1	7	50	2
8 oz. Seven-Up	24	——	——	8	10
DINNER					
2 oz. chicken baked in 1 tsp. salt-free butter	——	14	10	140	30
½ cup buttered noodles	15	2	——	50	2
½ cup buttered corn	15	2	——	230	2
Lettuce wedge with salt-free dressing	3	1	5	120	3
½ cup strawberries on	20	——	——	145	2
1 white cup cake	20	2	——	50	117
8 oz. lemonade	24	——	——	8	——
BEDTIME SNACK					
½ cup ice cream with	15	2	10	90	78
strawberry syrup	10	——	——	——	——
Total	264	40	62	1,431	408

*Total kcalories: 1,774.
From Mitchell, M. C., and Smith, E. J.: Dietary care of patients with chronic oliguria. Am. J. Clin. Nutr., *19*:167, 1966.

TABLE 32–6 RECIPES FOR CONTROLLED PROTEIN, POTASSIUM AND SODIUM DIET

For your convenience, here are some basic recipes with notation on how to exchange them for foods in the diet:

FRUIT TAPIOCA*
2 cups pineapple juice
½ cup water
½ cup sugar
¼ cup tapioca
1 cup crushed pineapple

Blend in a saucepan pineapple juice, water, sugar, and tapioca. Place over double broiler, stirring constantly and cook until mixture slightly thickens. (This takes 5 to 8 minutes.) Remove from heat and cool. Stir in 1 cup crushed pineapple. Chill to serve. Other fruits and juices may be used alone or in combination. (Makes 6 servings.)

PLAIN PASTRY
2 cups sifted all-purpose flour
½ tsp. sugar
⅔ cups salt-free shortening
5 to 6 tbs. ice water

Mix flour and sugar. Cut in shortening. Stir in water, adding just enough to make ingredients adhere together. Pat lightly in hands until dough forms smooth ball. Divide dough in half and roll lightly on floured board. For tender pastry, handle as little as possible. If dough is chilled before rolling, it is easier to handle. (Makes 9 in. 2 crust pie.)

APPLE PIE†
6 medium apples
¾ cup sugar
2 tbs. flour
¼ tsp. nutmeg
1 tbs. salt-free butter or margarine
Add up to 1 tbs. of lemon juice or vinegar if apples are very sweet

Mix flour, sugar and spices. Alternate with layers of sliced apples in pastry-lined pan. Add butter and lemon juice or vinegar. Add top crust. Bake on bottom shelf at 425°F. for 15 minutes. Change to middle shelf and continue baking until apples are tender (about 20–30 minutes).

BUTTER COOKIES‡
1 cup salt-free butter or margarine
1 cup sifted confectioners' sugar
1 tsp. vanilla
2½ cups flour

Mix butter, confectioners' sugar and vanilla thoroughly. Sift flour and stir in. Mix thoroughly with hands. Press and mold into a long smooth roll about 2 in. in diameter. Wrap in waxed paper and chill until stiff. With thin, sharp knife, cut in thin (⅛ to ¹⁄₁₆ in.) slices. Place slices a little apart on ungreased baking sheet. Bake until lightly browned (8 to 10 min.) at 400°F. (Makes 6 doz. 2 in. cookies.)

*1 serving = 1 serving of fruit from group 4, list A.
†⅛ of 9 inch apple pie = 1 baked dessert from group 6, plus 1 serving of fruit from group 4, list A.
‡Three cookies = ½ serving of baked dessert from group 6.
From Mitchell, M. C., and Smith, E. J.: Dietary care of patients with chronic oliguria. Am. J. Clin. Nutr., *19*:168, 1968.

who are maintained by periodic dialysis are anuric. Their intake may need to be restricted (800 to 1000 cc. per day). Persons with chronic renal disease need to understand and be able to plan their dietary and fluid intake with their customary pattern in order to adhere to the necessary dietary restrictions and maintain the best nutritional status possible.

The 20 gm. protein, 1500 mg. potassium modified Giovannetti diet consists of:

1 egg

¾ cup (6 ounces) milk or 1 additional egg or 1 ounce of meat

½ pound low protein bread

Vegetables and fruits selection to provide 3 to 12 gm. of protein and 1300 to 1900 mg. of potassium. (See Groups II and III, Table 32–2.)

Fats, condiments and sweets as desired. (See Groups VI and List IX, Table 32–2, to supply adequate caloric requirements.)

This regimen usually results in a decided fall in blood urea nitrogen and the patient experiences relief of gastrointestinal symptoms, an increased appetite and a feeling of well-being.

Some patients benefit by a protein-free, electrolyte (sodium, potassium)-free diet recommended by Borst.[8] Few foods are available that do not contain varying amounts of protein, sodium and potassium. The mixture, known as butter balls, consists of:

¾ cup sugar 2 tablespoons flour ¾ cup unsalted butter 2 cups water	Mix sugar and flour; add butter and water. Cook to consistency of thin sauce. Flavor with vanilla or any preferred extract. Chill and make into small balls. Roll in sugar. Keep refrigerated until used.

The composition is approximately 160 gm. carbohydrate, 2 gm. protein, 136 gm. fat, and 1872 kcalories. For those patients who cannot tolerate the mixture, liberal servings of rice with unsalted butter and sugar can be tried. Hard candies (sour balls), sucked on throughout the day are sometimes liked. Sugars (glucose, lactose) and melted butter may be added (100 to 200 gm.) to the daily water allowance. A commercial product, Controlyte,[9] provides a high calorie (approximately 1000 kcalories per 7-ounce can), protein-free and minimal electrolytes formula which may be given orally or by tube.

NEPHROLITHIASIS OR RENAL CALCULI

Nephrolithiasis is a condition characterized by the presence of renal calculi. Renal calculi or kidney stones may form in either the kidney or the bladder. They look like pebbles, although their appearance varies, depending upon the constituents. Some have a smooth surface and others are jagged. They vary in size from fine gravel to those which fill the pelvis of the kidney.

ETIOLOGY How renal calculi materialize continues to be a mystery, although many theories have been suggested. Certain diseases seem to favor the precipitation of gravel. These include disorders which bring about increased parathyroid secretion with a loss of calcium phosphate in the urine. If it is excessive the particles of the substance may gather in amounts sufficient to produce a calculus. A deficiency of vitamin A, systemic infections, metabolic disturbances, a hormone, inadequate fluid intake, and lesions obstructing the flow, producing stasis of urine, are considered causative factors. Immobilization favors formation of calcium stones, because of large increases in the excretion of calcium.

TYPES OF STONES Vermooten[10] divides renal calculi into three basic types: (1) organic calculi, such as uric acid, cystine, and xanthine stones, which result from some metabolic disturbance, (2) alkaline earth stones, such as calcium or magnesium ammonium phosphates or carbonates, which are generally secondary to urinary tract infection, and (3) calcium oxalate stones, which usually are not associated with infection. The cause for the formation of kidney stones is not known.

The types of stone which may develop depend largely upon the acidity or alkalinity of the urine. Normally, the urine is slightly acid. The reaction of urine is dependent upon the character of the diet. If the diet consists largely of acid-forming foods, a very acid urine is produced. Diets consisting mainly of base-forming foods yield an alkaline urine. Stones composed chiefly of uric acid and cystine appear most frequently in an abnormally acid urine. Stones appearing in an alkaline urine are composed of phosphates, carbonates and oxalates.

OBJECTIVE AND PRINCIPLES OF DIETARY TREATMENT Although medicine

[8]Borst, J. C. G.: Protein katabolism in uraemia; effects of protein-free diets, infections and blood-transfusions. Lancet, 1:824, 1948.

[9]D. M. Doyle Pharmaceutical Company, Minneapolis, Minnesota.

[10]Vermooten, V.: Some aspects of the medical management of renal calculi. J.A.M.A., 157:783, 1955.

has largely replaced the use of therapeutic diets for the treatment of renal calculi, specific diets are still recognized and advocated by a number of authorities as a preventive measure against the recurrence of stones, especially following surgical removal. Urinary calculi recur in a significant number of patients; therefore, prophylactic programs are desirable.

The type of diet prescribed is determined by the acidity or alkalinity of the urine and upon the variety of stone. Fluids are encouraged (3000 to 4000 ml. or more daily) to prevent concentration of the urine, which is believed to favor precipitation of the stone-forming minerals.

Regardless of the diet prescribed, it must be adequate. Renal calculi are a chronic condition and the diet treatment must be carried on indefinitely.

Calcium-containing Calculi Of all renal calculi 90 to 95 per cent contain calcium salts as the predominant crystalline component. A urine which is high in calcium predisposes to the formation of calcium oxalate and calcium phosphate stones. Conditions which favor calcium stone formation are (1) overindulgence in foods high in calcium, such as large quantities of milk; for example, milk, or milk and cream therapy for patients with peptic ulcer, (2) excessive intake of proprietary antacids which contain calcium salts, (3) excessive vitamin D, which will mobilize calcium and so increase urinary excretion, (4) general body immobilization following fractures or extended bed rest, (5) hyperparathyroidism and (6) osteoporosis. In a study conducted by Boyce et al.,[11] it was concluded that hypercalciuria is one aspect of a metabolic derangement in calculus formation, and that "Until such time as the entire process can be delineated it seems feasible to attempt the prevention of recurrent stone formation by reduction of calcium intake and absorption." They used a low calcium and low vitamin D diet, plus sodium phytate regimen. The sodium phytate forms an unabsorbable complex with calcium in the intestinal tract. When administered orally with the prescribed diet, it effectively reduces the urinary excretion of calcium. Milk, cheese, and other milk products are limited (1–2 cups milk daily). There is some danger of calcium deficiency if the diet regimen is continued indefinitely. Fortified D milk is excluded as well as any other foods fortified with vitamin D (read the labels). See Appendix Table 7.

Aluminum hydroxide gel is also used to combine with the dietary phosphates to form insoluble aluminum phosphate which is excreted in the feces. Calcium is excreted in the urine as calcium chloride and calcium citrate. Calculi are not apt to form.

Recent studies favor limiting the calcium in the food of patients requiring prolonged immobilization in bed, as in fractures of the pelvis or femur, because of large increases in the excretion of calcium. In addition, the protein content of the diet should be high normal in an attempt to promote deposition of calcium in the bones. Acid ash foods to favor production of an acid urine might be a factor in keeping the calcium salts in solution. As soon as the plaster cast is removed, or at least some mobilization of the body is possible, the normal diet should probably be resumed.

Calcium Oxalate Stones When oxalates predominate, the condition is known as oxaluria. There is no generally accepted dietary regimen for patients with recurrent calcium oxalate stones. The diet therapy is to avoid large quantities of foods high in calcium (Appendix Table 7) and high in oxalates. Oxalate stones are extremely resistant to treatment, and clinical experience has demonstrated that oxalate calculi may recur even after strict elimination of dietary oxalate intake. This may be due to the endogenous production, independent of an exogenous food supply. Fluids are forced in order to reduce the concentration of calcium and oxalate ions in the urine.

FOODS OMITTED (BECAUSE OF HIGH OXALIC ACID CONTENT— 0.002 TO 0.9%):

Asparagus	Rhubarb
Beet greens	Raspberries
Spinach	Black tea
Sorrel	Chocolate
Dandelion greens	Cocoa
Cranberries	Coffee
Figs	Gelatin
Gooseberries	Pepper
Plums	

FOODS RESTRICTED (BECAUSE OF MODERATE OXALIC ACID CONTENT):

Milk: 1 pint daily.
Not more than one serving daily of the following foods:

Orange	Brussels sprouts
Pineapple	Potatoes
Strawberries	Tomatoes
Beans	Beets

According to studies by Dr. S. N. Gershoff,[12] Harvard University School of Public Health, vitamin B_6 (pyridoxine) deficiency causes increased production of oxalates. The administration of this vitamin to individuals on diets presumably adequate in vitamin B_6 sharply decreased oxalate production. Experimen-

[11]Boyce, W. H., et al.: Abnormalities of calcium metabolism in patients with "idiopathic" urinary calculi. J.A.M.A., 166:1577, 1958.

[12]Gershoff, S. N., and Prien, E. L.: The effect of daily MgO and vitamin B_6 administration to patients with recurring calcium oxalate kidney stones. Am. J. Clin. Nutr., 20:393, 1967.

tally, calcium oxalate stones have been produced in animals fed a low pyridoxine and magnesium diet, and prevented by increasing the dietary levels of these two nutrients. Magnesium, it is believed, aids in keeping the oxalate in solution and prevents precipitation of oxalates and stone formation. Vitamin B_6 increases citric acid secretion and this may keep oxalates in solution.

Calcium Phosphate Stones   The principles of dietary treatment for calcium oxalate stones are virtually the same for stones consisting largely of calcium combined with phosphate. The diet is the normal adequate diet with moderately low calcium and low phosphorus content. Foods generally considered high in phosphate which should be limited are milk and milk products, eggs, organ meats (brains, heart, liver, sweetbreads, kidney), sardines, fish roe, whole grain bread and cereal, bran, oatmeal, brown and wild rice, wheat germ, nuts, soybeans, and meat in general. (See Table 8–2 for phosphorus content of foods.)

Zinsser,[13] however, warns that in using low phosphorus diets there is a possibility that citrate stones can be formed as a result of a rise in citrate excretion in the presence of inadequate phosphorus intake. Thus, the reduction in phosphorus intake as a panacea for the condition is fraught with hazard.

Uric acid stones   When kidney stones, containing uric acid – an end-product of purine metabolism – have been found to occur in an acid medium, the high alkaline ash diet is sometimes prescribed. While acidifying or alkalinizing agents are more effective and have largely replaced the high alkaline and high acid diets, the diet should support the medication used.

An attempt is made to keep the pH of the urine above 7, or alkaline. If urinary alkalinization alone does not prove adequate, the over-all protein and purine intake restriction may be tried, plus anabolic drugs. Proteins are restricted to 1 gm./kg. ideal body weight. (See Low Purine Diet, p. 420.)

Cystine Stones   If the sulfur-containing amino acid cystine is not broken down in the body and appears in the urine (cystinuria), it may form stones. Cystine stones, an inborn error of metabolism, are very rare.

A low protein diet is sometimes used but has not been shown to be very effective; all protein contains cystine (and methionine from which cystine may be formed) in varying amounts. Zinsser reports encouraging results have been obtained by the use of an amino acid diet containing a low level of sulfur amino acids, adequate in fluids (3500 ml. daily) but not excessive water intake. In addi-

tion, alkalinizing agents and/or the high alkaline ash diet to keep the urine at pH of 7.2 or above is recommended.

ACID AND ALKALINE ASH DIETS
Acid-Base Balance in Foods   When foodstuffs are burned completely outside of the body they may yield either an acid or basic (alkaline) ash. (See Acid-base Balance, in Chapter 8.) The potential acidity or alkalinity of foods means the reaction the food will yield ultimately after being burned in the body. The acids of most fruits and vegetables are utilized in the body and yield an alkaline or basic ash, owing to the high potassium, calcium, and magnesium content. Thus, a diet rich in vegetables and fruits, which contain organic acids such as citric and oxalic, will form bicarbonate and hence decrease urine acidity. On the other hand, a diet containing large amounts of proteins, which in their course of metabolism yield acids such as sulfuric and phosphoric, will increase the urine acidity. Foods which are not acid in taste, such as cereals, meat, fish, egg, and bread, become strongly acid when their end-products reach the blood and urine owing to the high phosphorus, iron, and sulfur content. However, the normal healthy individual always maintains a slightly alkaline reaction in the blood and other tissues regardless of the diet. (See Appendix Table 10 for a listing of alkali-producing, acid-producing, and neutral foods.)

High Acid Ash Diet   The high acid ash diet is sometimes prescribed for patients with stones shown to have been formed in an alkaline medium. The principle of the diet is to endeavor to restrict enlargement of already present stones, or to prevent other calculi from forming. The stones are composed chiefly of calcium salts of *phosphate, carbonate* or *oxalate*.

An attempt is made to keep the urine acid at a pH of 5 to 6. Salt (sodium) is sometimes restricted in the diet because sodium is alkaline and some authorities believe there is a buffer action from the sodium. Baking powder and soda products may also be prohibited. Salt substitutes contain an alkaline radical and cannot be used. Foods high in acid ash are eggs, meat, fish, poultry, bread, cereal, and cereal products. Fruits and vegetables – except prunes, plums, cranberries and corn – are somewhat restricted, as well as milk (1 pint daily) and milk products.

High Alkaline Ash Diet   An alkaline ash diet is sometimes used for uric acid and cystine acid stones. The principle of the diet is to attempt to restrict enlargement of already present calculi which form in an acid medium or to prevent other stones from forming. Foods high in alkaline ash are fruits and vegetables, which should predominate – except prunes, plums, cranberries and corn. Milk, while usually considered alkaline, is

---

[13]Zinsser, H. H.: Urinary calculi. J.A.M.A., *174*:2062, 1960.

limited to 1 pint daily because a considerable amount of the calcium in milk is excreted in the feces while the remainder is excreted in the urine, and its effect on the acidity or alkalinity of urine is controversial. Meat, fish, poultry, eggs, bread, cereal and cereal products are somewhat restricted.

The patient may find it difficult to change his dietary pattern. A person who has been in the habit of eating large portions of meat and the acid-ash-forming foods must learn to like and ingest more vegetables and fruits and much less meat.

PROBLEMS AND SUGGESTED TOPICS FOR DISCUSSION

1. What is the function of the kidneys? Describe the "functioning units." What does the urine from a normal healthy individual contain?
2. Clasify nephritis and give the outstanding characteristic of each type.
3. What are the objective and principles of dietary treatment in acute glomerulonephritis? What is the purpose of the low protein diet?
4. When is fluid restriction indicated? When is salt (sodium) restriction indicated? When is potassium restriction indicated?
5. What salt substitutes are allowed in nephritis? What salt substitutes are not allowed in renal diseases? Why? Using Appendix Table 9, list foods high in potassium and foods high in sodium.
6. What foods are allowed patients with uremia? What are some of the nutrition problems?
7. Obtain a diet history from a patient with chronic glomerulonephritis and outline a meal plan. Assist him in making the necessary adjustments in his dietary pattern.
8. Outline a diet for the following amounts of proteins, in each case keeping the calories to 2000 daily: (a) 20 gm., (b) 40 gm., (c) 60 gm., (d) 100 gm., and (e) 150 gm.
9. Obtain a diet history from a patient with the nephrotic syndrome. Analyze the food history, noting the amount of fats, proteins and calories. What are the objective and principles of diet therapy?
10. Plan a menu pattern with a patient who has kidney stones. A high acid ash diet is prescribed. Observe the daily urine analysis made by the laboratory and note the pH of the urine. Compare with the average normal pH of urine. What are the principles of the dietary treatment?
11. Outline a typical diet for a man with calcium oxalate kidney stones. What is the purpose of the diet?
12. Repeat the procedure in Problem 10 for a patient who requires a high alkaline ash diet.
13. Plan a diet with a person who is receiving hemodialysis. The diet ordered is 60 gm. protein, 800 mg. sodium and 1800 mg. potassium. Fluids are restricted to 1000 ml.
14. Plan a diet for a patient who has recurrent calcium stones. The diet is low in calcium (600 mg.) and not excessive in vitamin D (no vitamin D fortified foods).
15. List foods restricted and foods allowed in a high acid ash diet; list foods restricted and foods allowed in a high alkaline ash diet. When might each diet be used?

SUGGESTED ADDITIONAL READING REFERENCES

Ackerman, G. L., and Flanigan, W. J.: Reversible insufficiency in chronic renal disease. J.A.M.A., 197:95, 1966.

Bailey, G. L., and Sullivan, N.: Selected-protein diet in terminal uremia. J. Am. Dietet. A., 52:125, 1968.

Boyce, W. H., et al.: Abnormalities of calcium metabolism in patients with "idiopathic" urinary calculi. J.A.M.A., 166:1577, 1958.

Burton, B. R. (ed.): Heinz Handbook of Nutrition. 2nd ed. McGraw-Hill Book Company, Inc., New York, 1965, Chapter 30, Nutrition and diet in diseases of the kidney and urinary tract.

Chinard, F. P.: Current status of therapy in the nephrotic syndrome in adults. J.A.M.A., 178:312, 1961.

Compty, C. M.: Long-term dietary management of dialysis patients. J. Am. Dietet. A., 53:439, 1968.

Duncan, G. G. (ed.): Diseases of Metabolism. 5th ed. Philadelphia, W. B. Saunders Company, 1964, Chapter 16, Diseases of the kidney.

Editorial. New dimensions in the study of kidney diseases. J.A.M.A., 177:205, 1961.

Editorial. Renal hypertension. J.A.M.A., 183:132, 1963.

Editorial. The nephrotic syndrome. J.A.M.A., 169:846, 1959.

Gershoff, S. N., and Prien, E. L.: Effect of MgO and vitamin B_6 administration to patients with recurring oxalate kidney stones. Am. J. Clin. Nutr., 20:393, 1967.

Giovannetti, S., and Maggior, Q.: A low-nitrogen diet with proteins of high biological value for severe uraemia. Lancet, 1:1000, 1964.

Hand, J. R.: Infections of the urinary tract. Am. J. Nursing, 57:1008, 1957.

Harlan, W. R., et al.: Proteinuria and nephrotic syndrome associated with chronic rejection of kidney transplants. New Eng. J. Med., 277:769, 1967.

Hughes, J., et al.: Oxalate urinary tract stones. J.A.M.A., 172:774, 1960.

Jordan, W. A., et al.: Basic pattern for a controlled protein, sodium and potassium diet. J. Am. Dietet. A., 50:137, 1967.

Kolff, W. J.: Forced high caloric, low protein diet and the treatment of uremia. Am. J. Med., 12:667, 1952.

Krehl, W. A., and Casimere, D.: Nutritional alterations in the nephrotic syndrome. Am. J. Clin. Nutr., 12:336, 1963.

Kushner, D. S.: Calcium and the kidney. Am. J. Clin. Nutr., 4:561, 1956.

Merrill, A. J.: Nutrition in chronic renal failure. Am. J. Clin. Nutr. 4:497, 1956; J.A.M.A., 173:905, 1960.

Merrill, J. P., et al.: Role of kidney in human hypertension. Am. J. Med., 31:931, 1961.

Mitchell, M. C., and Smith, E. J.: Dietary care of patients with chronic oliguria. Am. J. Clin. Nutr., 19:163, 1966.

Overly, V. A., and Greenwood, M. L.: Developing wafers and biscuits of varying protein content. J. Am. Dietet. A., 45:342, 1964.

Pitts, R. F.: Acid-base regulation by the kidneys. Am. J. Med., 9:356, 1950.

Prien, E. L.: Studies in urolithiasis. III. Physiochemical principles in stone formation and prevention. J. Urol., 73:627, 1955.

Rifkind, D., et al.: Urinary excretion of iron-binding protein in the nephrotic syndrome. New England J. Med., 265:115, 1961.

Shorr, E., and Carter, A. C.: Aluminum gels in the management of renal phosphatic calculi. J.A.M.A., 144:1549, 1950.

Squire, J. R.: Nutrition and the nephrotic syndrome in adults. Am. J. Clin. Nutr., 4:509, 1956.

Trusk, C. W.: Hemodialysis for acute renal failure. Am. J. Nurs., 65:80, 1965.

Wohl, M. G., and Goodhart, R. S. (eds.): Modern Nutrition in Health and Disease. 3rd ed. Philadelphia, Lea & Febiger, 1964, Chapter 25, Some Aspects of Nutrition and the Kidney; Chapter 26, Nutrition in Urologic Diseases.

Zimmerman, H. J.: Nutritional aspects of acute glomerulonephritis. Am. J. Clin. Nutr. 4:482, 1956.

Zinsser, H. H.: Urinary calculi. J.A.M.A., 174:2062, 1960.

Chapter 33
DISEASES OF
THE NERVOUS
SYSTEM AND
MENTAL
ILLNESS

The state of the nervous system is largely dependent upon the state of nutrition of the individual. Minor disturbances, such as forgetfulness, irritability, uneasiness and disorderly thinking, as well as gross mental changes, may develop from poor nutrition. Following prolonged nutrition inadequacy, lesions appear in both the central and peripheral nervous systems.[1] Peripheral neuropathy is reported to be common, especially in deficiency of thiamin.[1, 2]

NEURITIS AND POLYNEURITIS

ETIOLOGY *Polyneuritis* is a term applied to any condition in which there is symmetrical involvement of the peripheral nerves and is usually believed to be the result of some nutritional, toxic, or metabolic disturbance, but may be inflammatory in nature. (See Beriberi in Chapter 34.) Frequently, the cause is unknown and treatment must be in great part symptomatic. *Neuritis* is inflammation of a nerve. It can be caused by pressure, infection, injury, or tumors. In addition, the condition may be a sequel to food inadequacies of long standing, especially the lack of vitamins.

Polyneuropathy may result from a deficiency of any one of three B vitamins: thiamin, pyridoxine (vitamin B_6), or pantothenic acid. This vitamin deficiency is exhibited occasionally by alcoholics, and it may be associated with stomach and liver symptoms. These

individuals neglect to eat, and thereby set the foundation for the vitamin deficiency. Apparently, alcohol requires thiamin to be metabolized, and when large quantities of alcohol are taken, there is a greater demand for this vitamin. By eating an adequate diet, the needs are met, but when meals are replaced by alcohol, the thiamin reserve is exhausted quickly. Consequently, the alcoholic may develop not only neuritis or polyneuritis, but cirrhosis of the liver and other complications, as discussed in Chapter 25.

Deficiency neuritis may also appear in those patients suffering from starvation or from continual vomiting such as during pregnancy. In addition, the malady may accompany uncontrolled diabetes. Such patients describe experiences of intestinal upsets because they have excluded vitamin B foodstuffs from their menus. Polyneuritis, coupled with indigestion, will appear in lead poisoning.

When the absorption of vitamin B and, to a lesser extent, vitamins A, C, D and E is interfered with, the nerves frequently suffer. Replenishing the missing vitamins doesn't necessarily cure the patient, because in many instances either the tissue structures have degenerated beyond repair, or the period of treatment is too short.

Recently, there has been considerable evidence to indicate that polyneuritis is due to disturbances in the enzyme system of the peripheral nerves. Such disorders commonly result in destruction of the myelin of nerve tissue. In line with this concept, it is known that thiamin, niacin, and riboflavin are members of the enzyme system and function as coenzymes. (See Chapter 9.) It has been suggested that in individuals in whom polyneu-

[1]Victor, M.: Alcohol and nutritional diseases of the nervous system. J.A.M.A., *167*:65, 1959.
[2]Pollack, H., and Halpern, S. L.: Therapeutic Nutrition. Washington, D.C. National Research Council, Publication 234, 1952.

ritis develops, there is a constitutional defect in the enzyme system. However, some cases are apparently due to some type of allergic response to an infectious process.

DIETARY TREATMENT   Treatment is dependent on the basic disorder, which must be removed without delay. Regardless of cause, the diet must be adequate and contain liberal amounts of vitamins. Supplementary vitamins, particularly the B-complex, are supplied as indicated. Parenteral vitamin B_{12} is of value in some cases; for example, the neurologic involvement in pernicious anemia. Assuming that many cases are a result of enzyme system disturbance, the administration of thiamin hydrochloride (100 mg. a day) should be beneficial. The mental symptoms of pellagra respond specifically to administration of niacin. The drug dimercaprol has been reported to produce favorable results in a number of cases of neuritis, regardless of the cause.

Establishment of an improved dietary regimen – with high intake of the protective foods – to be carried out through life is the important aim in therapy of any of the neurologic manifestations of nutritional deficiencies. Many of the patients are elderly, with early personality deterioration; some are from poverty-stricken areas and have the further complication of marginal mental ability. Understanding, patience and skill are required to cope with resistance to change in eating habits.

EPILEPSY

Epilepsy is one of the oldest known and most dreaded diseases. The name comes from the Greek word for *seizure,* and in ancient times the seizing was believed to be the work of spirits. It is defined as a chronic functional disease of nervous origin, characterized by seizures or attacks in which there is sometimes loss of consciousness with a succession of tonic or clonic convulsions. The attacks vary in frequency, occurring several times daily in some instances. With other patients, a year or two may elapse between episodes. If severe convulsions appear, the disorder is labeled "grand mal," which is French for "great sickness," or "major attack." When seizures are mild, the condition is called "petit mal," meaning "little sickness," or "minor attack." The attack may last from a few seconds to 20 minutes. Epilepsy may be the result of a variety of lesions of the central nervous system, the most important of which is cerebral trauma. It is estimated that approximately 1 per cent of the total population in the United States have epilepsy. Electroencephalography has aided physicians to a better understanding of the disease.

DIETARY TREATMENT   Anticonvulsant medications have largely superseded diet therapy in treatment of epilepsy. An adequate, well-balanced diet with avoidance of excess food or fluid intake, along with drugs, is the treatment of choice. However, in a few individuals who do not tolerate drugs well, and occasionally for children, a ketogenic diet may be prescribed.

Ketogenic Diet   For many years, the ketogenic diet was used extensively in the treatment of epilepsy. It is a diet constructed to produce a state of ketosis by causing a change in the acid-base balance of the patient. Wilder[3] studied Geyelen's results of fasting diets on epileptic patients and found that acidosis was the common factor which gave relief. Therefore, Wilder arranged the diet to prevent the complete combustion of fats, thus producing this condition. The diet is characterized by being extremely low in carbohydrate content and high in fats, so that a ketogenic-antiketogenic ratio of 3:1 is maintained.

To construct the ketogenic diet prescription, the patient's daily calorie and protein allowance is calculated according to the normal daily requirement. To obtain the desired high ratio of fat, keep the carbohydrate allowance to a low minimum allowance of 15 to 30 gm. Then add the fat allowance to the diet in sufficient amounts to meet the remaining calorie requirement. Details for calculation of the ketogenic diet for children are shown in Chapter 36.

If rapid ketosis is desired, the treatment starts with a period of fasting. During the 3 to 5 days of fasting, the patient is permitted a very restricted daily diet of water, broth, tea and 6 to 8 ounces of orange juice. After the fasting period the prescribed ketogenic diet is given to the patient.

The diet treatment usually starts with an allowance of 75 gm. of carbohydrates, which is decreased gradually until the prescribed low carbohydrate allowance has been reached, or until a state of mild ketosis appears. This development takes approximately 1 week.

If no further attacks are noticed after the prescribed diet has been followed for a period of 3 months, then the carbohydrate intake may be increased gradually in steps of 5 gm., until 50 to 60 gm. of carbohydrates are tolerated daily. Of course, the fats in the diet are reduced proportionately to maintain the desired calories. A state of ketosis must always be maintained, evidenced by diacetic acid and acetone in the urine. Urinalysis will indicate the effectiveness of the diet. The ketogenic diet is sometimes weighed, particularly in the beginning of the treatment.

---

[3]Wilder, R. M.: The effect of ketonuria on the course of epilepsy. Mayo Clinic Bulletin, 2, 1921, p. 307.

TABLE 33–1   KETOGENIC DIET

Diet Prescription: *Kcalories, 2500; proteins, 65 gm.; fats, 240 gm.; carbohydrates, 20 gm. All diets are calculated with a leeway of 3 to 5 grams, above or below the diet order.*

FOOD	WEIGHT IN GRAMS	HOUSEHOLD MEASURE	FOOD CLASS WEIGHT GRAMS		
			Pro-tein	*Fat*	*Carbo-hydrate*
		BREAKFAST			
Fruit, List III*	varies	½ Exchange*			5
Ry-Krisp	6.5	1 piece	1		4
Butter or fortified margarine	10	2 teaspoons		10	
Eggs	50	1	7	5	
Bacon, cooked	32	4 slices	10	16	
Cream, heavy	119	½ eight-ounce cup	2.5	46	3
Coffee		Depends upon fluids allowed			
		Total	20.5	77	12
		LUNCHEON			
Clear broth		Depends upon fluids allowed			
Cheese, Cheddar type	56	2 ounces	14	18	
Vegetables, List II A*	100	1 generous salad	2		3
Fat, List VI*	varies	5 Exchanges*		25	
Gelatin made with saccharin		1 serving			
Cream, heavy to be whipped	79	⅓ eight-ounce cup	2	31	2
		Total	18	74	5
		DINNER			
Meat, List V*	varies	2 Exchanges*	14	10	
Vegetable, List II B*	50	½ Exchange or equivalent	1		3
Fat, List VI*	varies	5 Exchanges*		25	
Egg	50	1	7	5	
Cream, heavy (made into ice cream or custard)	119	½ eight-ounce cup	2.5	46	3
Tea or demitasse		Depends upon fluids allowed			
		Total	24.5	86	6
		Daily Total	63	237	23

*Refer to Food Exchange Lists, pp. 402–405.

Fluids   Sometimes fluids are restricted as it is believed that the convulsive seizures are caused partially by a water metabolism disturbance. Most patients have been observed to have fewer attacks when they are mildly dehydrated.

Stimulants   Stimulants, such as tea and coffee, may be restricted; generally, beer and alcohol are forbidden as they tend to precipitate seizures.

Minerals and vitamins   Great care must be exercised to prevent any nutritional deficiencies, especially in calcium, iron, and the water-soluble vitamins. Medical supplementation of calcium, thiamin, riboflavin and niacin is prescribed as indicated. Ascorbic acid will be adequate if the diet includes sufficient vegetable salads plus a daily serving of citrus fruit.

FOODS ALLOWED IN AMOUNTS TO FIT THE DIET PRESCRIPTION

Cream: 40 per cent cream.
Fats: Butter, fortified margarine, olive oil, vegetable oil, bacon fat.
Meat: Bacon, meat, fish, poultry.
Eggs
Cheese: American Cheddar, cream, Muenster, Swiss, cottage with sour cream.
Vegetables: These may be chosen from Food Exchanges, List IIA and B, Vegetables, p. 402.
Fruits: Especially citrus fruits; all fruits either fresh, canned or frozen prepared without sugar. These may be chosen from Food Exchanges, List III, Fruits, p. 403.
Breads: Ry-Krisp; especially prepared breads without food value such as washed bran muffins.
Desserts: Plain gelatin.

FOODS TO AVOID

Sugar and sweetened desserts; jelly, honey, and candy. Cereals and breads, pastries, cakes, cookies, and pies.

Fruits high in carbohydrate content.

Vegetables high in carbohydrate content.

PRACTICAL POINTS. The ketogenic diet is unpalatable, and it is difficult to induce a patient to keep up the regimen for any extended period.

Hints to make the diet more palatable:

1. For those patients who find it especially difficult to consume the large quantity of butter, oil and fats either in or on the food, it is recommended that they take a "dose" of some oil with each meal as if they were taking medication.

2. Non-caloric sweeteners allowed may be used to sweeten foods. (See Chap. 43.)

3. The cream may be whipped and frozen with small amounts of fruit flavors and non-caloric sweetener incorporated, and served as ice cream.

4. The cream and egg may be baked into a custard or blended into an eggnog.

5. Whipped cream added to fruits (when allowed) makes an attractive dish besides providing a desirable way to serve the cream allowance.

6. Combine the cream and vegetable purée allowed into a cream soup.

7. Use gelatin allowed for making attractive desserts and salads.

8. Serve mayonnaise and oil abundantly on salads.

9. Add butter or fortified margarine to cooked vegetables.

10. It is advisable to include liver once or twice during the week to prevent iron deficiency.

DRUGS

When the ketogenic diet has been used exclusively in cases of epilepsy, it has been reported only partially successful. Several years ago more progress was noted if the sedative phenobarbital was prescribed. Some patients showed more improvement with a combination of the ketogenic diet plus medication.

More recent research has introduced additional drugs which have proved effective and safe when used under medical supervision. Patients who are helped lose the defeatist attitude usually associated with this disease. Dilantin was the first newcomer and since then about 25 other drugs have been introduced. The anticonvulsives are somewhat selective in the way they work. Dilantin, for example, is more effective in controlling convulsions, whereas Tridione, for example, is used to prevent blackouts in petit mal. Each new drug has been used to control seizures in some individuals who were helped only a little or not at all by previous medications. As a result of research, the treatment of epilepsy has advanced farther during the past 25 years than during the preceding 25 centuries. The currently available medications can enable 80 to 85 per cent of epileptics to lead an essentially normal life. Evaluation of the effectiveness of the chemicals continues.

MENIERE'S SYNDROME

Meniere's syndrome is associated with changes in the labyrinth (organ of equilibrium) of the inner ear, and is characterized by pallor, vertigo, nausea, vomiting, and various aural and ocular disturbances. It is named after the French physician who was the first to describe the disease.

ETIOLOGY   Nothing definite is known about the cause of Meniere's syndrome but many authorities suspect the syndrome to be due to an imbalance of the autonomic nervous system leading to spasms in the arterioles with resulting changes in circulation, causing the vestibular apparatus to become swollen. The tiny blood vessels in this area are thought to be influenced by hypersensitivity to certain physical stimuli such as light, heat, cold, physical stress, emotional disturbances, fatigue, toxic substances, and abnormalities in electrolyte metabolism. An ordinary antigen-antibody type of allergy is also suggested as a possible but infrequent cause; others suspect endocrine dysfunction.

TREATMENT   There is no standard treatmen for Meniere's disease. Treatment is aimed at improving circulation by means of vasodilating drugs, such as histamine or nicotinic acid, that act directly on the nerves to control the flow of blood through these vessels.

Salt (sodium) is restricted in an attempt to alleviate the localized edema. (See Chapter 30 for sodium restricted diets.)

Surgical section of the vestibular nerve or its branches is sometimes required in severe cases. Ultrasonic waves have been found[4] to be successfully used, and it is suggested that this treatment may replace both medical and surgical methods now in use. Fowler and Zeckel[5] recommend psychotherapy or analysis to prevent symptoms by removing the conditioned psychic stimulus.

MULTIPLE SCLEROSIS

Multiple sclerosis is a central nervous system disease of unknown etiology affecting the myelinated nerve fibers and the muscles which they innervate. Many theories have been advanced as to cause and include disorder of carbohydrate metabolism, lack of food essentials, high fat intake, infection with a virus, glandular disturbance, or an allergy, but no conclusive evidence for any of these theories has yet been reported. It develops as an acute disease without warning and runs an intermittent course characterized by exacerbations at intervals of weeks, months or years. There is destruction of the fatty myelin sheaths that surround the nerves in different parts of the brain and spinal cord. This insulating material is replaced by scar tissue, and there are many such areas (multiple) of nerve degeneration (sclerosis).

[4]Altmann, F.: Meniere's disease. J.A.M.A., *176*:215, 1961.

[5]Fowler, E. P., and Zeckel, A.: Psychosomatic aspects of Meniere's disease. J.A.M.A., *148*:1265, 1952.

The condition may appear at any age, but usually appears between the ages of 20 to 40. In spite of the handicaps, a normal life expectancy is the rule.

DIETARY TREATMENT   There is no specific treatment. Some authorities recommend the administration of vitamin supplements such as vitamin B_{12} and niacin. The patient should have a well-balanced and adequate diet to meet all the requirements of normal nutrition for the individual's age, activity and desired weight. Because of limited activity, the patient should carefully control his weight. Because of the crippling nature of the disease, every opportunity for rehabilitation should be taken to make life more livable and worthwhile. Present capabilities and potentialities of each patient should be developed to the maximum. The patient should be given feeding aids and taught to use them, rather than be made to feel helpless by being fed (Fig. 33–1). The tray and food should be placed so that it can be reached easily. Swank[6, 7] reported convincing evidence, in a well-controlled study, that a low fat diet (35 gm.: 15 gm. animal fat from meat and eggs — no milk fat; 15 gm. vegetable fat oil; and 5 gm. cod liver oil), maintained over a long period of time, tends to retard the disease process and to reduce the incidence of new attacks. Protein is kept at normal levels (60 to 70 gm.), and carbohydrate is supplied to meet calorie needs. The rationale of this diet is, mainly, the avoidance of increased adhesiveness and aggregation of red blood cells and of increased blood viscosity. Swank[8] suggests that incidence of multiple sclerosis can be correlated with dietary fat intake. In areas of the world where a relatively high fat diet is consumed, the incidence is relatively high; conversely, where much less fat is ingested, the incidence is low. Excessive physical and emotional stress should be avoided. Sawyer[9] reported improvement in symptoms in 6 patients studied when tolbutamide and a low carbohydrate diet were given. Elwell,[10] et al. were unable to confirm these results. Currently, no medication has been proved to be consistently beneficial. Supportive psychotherapy, physical therapy and ancillary service are reported to be beneficial to many.

[6]Swank, R. L.: Treatment of multiple sclerosis with low-fat diet. Arch. Neurol. & Psychiat., 73:631, 1955.

[7]Swank, R. L.: Treatment of multiple sclerosis with a low-fat diet. J. Am. Dietet. A., 36:322, 1960.

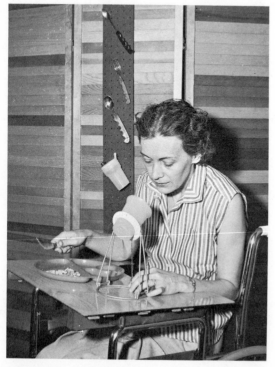

Figure 33–1   Multiple sclerosis patient learning the use of feeding aids at the Treatment Center of the National Multiple Sclerosis Society, Nassau County Chapter, 834 Willis Avenue, Albertson, New York. (Photo by Miyata.)

MENTAL ILLNESS

One out of every two hospital beds in the United States is reported to be occupied by a patient suffering from mental illness. These patients are often in a poor nutritional state and require sympathy and understanding on the part of the entire hospital team — nurse, dietitian and physician — to encourage the ingestion of a balanced diet. Food served in an attractive and pleasant environment will often stimulate the patient to eat. Many psychiatric disorders follow prolonged periods of tension, worry and anxiety. During this time intelligent and adequate food intake was neglected. The patient may be overweight as a result of compulsive eating during anxiety periods, or thin and emaciated from lack of interest in eating. Both require discerning guidance to meet the emotional needs and metabolic requirements. As previously pointed out, mental symptoms such as forgetfulness, confusion, depression, and anxiety may result from dietary inadequacies.

The relation of nutrition to emotional and mental health has been stressed throughout this text. Many nutrients are necessary for the integrity of the nervous system. (Review mental health in relation to: the aged, p. 298; peptic ulcers, p. 337; obesity, p. 432; children, p. 269.) Mental illness deserves as much con-

[8]Editorial. Low-fat diet in multiple sclerosis. J.A.M.A., 177:702, 1961.

[9]Sawyer, G. T.: Treatment of multiple sclerosis with tolbutamide. J.A.M.A., 174:470, 1960.

[10]Elwell, R. H., et al.: Multiple sclerosis: Treatment with tolbutamide and diabetic diet. J.A.M.A., 179:724, 1962.

sideration in treatment as heart disease or gastric ulcers. Methods of therapy, such as the tranquilizers and/or shock treatment, along with psychotherapy, are restoring to a normal life many patients who were once considered hopeless. Spies[11] states that "the tranquilizing drugs certainly are an effective aid in managing severely disturbed, hospitalized psychotics, but special attention should be given to the nutrition of these patients because some of them can be helped by nutritive methods." He reports that vitamin supplements and a good nutritious diet have relieved many patients of symptoms arising from the nervous system. In 1938 Spies[12] et al. found that a lack of niacin in the diet of the pellagrin allowed the mental symptoms to arise; following administration of this vitamin these symptoms disappeared.

Food has many meanings for people. They vary with individuals in health and illness. Ross[13] states that food is the "root of psychopathologies." Food from early childhood continues to form the basis of many motives and behaviors. Feelings are expressed in how one responds to food. Emotional problems may be expressed or acted out through overeating or rejection of foods, defiance, helpless submission, self-contempt, demand for love and affection and many other underlying conditions. Fears and anxieties associated with eating certain foods that will "hurt" or "poison" him, feelings of guilt and unworthiness to eat at the family table, feelings of deprivation are related to the underlying cause of the illness. These feelings may be relieved by permitting the patient to discuss the problem, to participate in the preparation of food or to select his food along with others in whom he has confidence.

Feeding patients "means a good deal more than simply supplying a balanced diet rich in protein, vitamins and balanced in minerals, fats and carbohydrates. It offers a way of reaching them on the level of satisfying a simple human need and thereby also offering them in an unthreatening way the opportunity of rebuilding relationships with their fellowman."[14]

---

[11]Spies, T. D.: Some recent advances in nutrition. J.A.M.A., 167:675, 1958.

[12]Spies, T. D., et al.: The mental symptoms of pellagra. Their relief with nicotinic acid. Am. J. Med. Sci., 196:461, 1938.

[13]Ross, M.: Food in the mental hospital. J. Am. Dietet. A., 40:318, 1962.

[14]Hunscher, M. A.: Nutritional needs of mentally ill geriatric patients. J. Psych. Nurs., 1:220, 1963.

PROBLEMS AND SUGGESTED TOPICS FOR DISCUSSION

1. Obtain a food intake history from a patient suffering with neuritis. Calculate the vitamin content of the food history. Compare the calculation with the Recommended Dietary Allowances issued by the Food and Nutrition Board of the National Research Council. Correct any deficiencies which may occur. What changes are needed to provide foods containing the vitamin B-complex, vitamins A, C, and D?

2. What is the objective of the ketogenic diet for epilepsy? Plan a food prescription for an epileptic patient who is going on a ketogenic diet. The patient is a 14-year-old school girl, who weighs 135 pounds, and her height is 5 feet 2 inches. Using the food prescription as a basis, make out a meal plan.

3. Investigate and then list the various chronic degenerative diseases of the central nervous system. Check those treated with diet. Check those that may have some relationship with diet. Study the experimental work being carried on to show the effectiveness of diet treatment in neurologic conditions.

4. Plan a menu for one day for a 35-year-old woman with multiple sclerosis who has difficulty in chewing and in feeding herself.

5. List typical dietary problems encountered in the mentally ill patient.

SUGGESTED ADDITIONAL READING REFERENCES

Alexander, Leo., et al.: Prognosis and treatment of multiple sclerosis—Quantitative nosometric study. J.A.M.A., 166:1943, 1958.

Altmann, F.: Meniere's disease. J.A.M.A., 176:215, 1961.

Baily, A. A., et al.: Symposium on Epileptic Disorders. Proc. Staff Meet. Mayo Clin., 28:25, 1953.

Cohn, H., et al.: Neurological manifestations in nutritional impairment. Am. J. Digest. Dis., 21:281, 1954.

Council on Mental Health. Program of the A.M.A. Council on Mental Health. J.A.M.A., 181:1080, 1962.

Donahue, H. H.: Some problems of feeding mental patients. Am. J. Clin. Nutr., 5:180, 1957.

Editorial. Low-fat diet in multiple sclerosis. J.A.M.A., 177:702, 1961.

Editorial. Nerve conduction in vitamin B_{12} deficiency. J.A.M.A., 194:189, 1965.

Elwell, R. H., et al.: Multiple sclerosis: Treatment with tolbutamide and diabetic diet. J.A.M.A., 179:724, 1962.

Epilepsy: Hope Through Research. Washington, D.C., U.S. Dept. Health, Education, and Welfare, Public Health Service Pub. No. 938, Health Information Series No. 105.

Gee, D. A.: Effect of psychiatric services on the hospital dietary department. J. Am. Dietet. A., 41:345, 1962.

Horwitt, M. K.: Nutrition in mental health. Nut. Rev., 23:289, 1965.

Kussner, C.: Successful feeding of mental patients. Hospital Management, 80:83, 1955.

Pauli, L., et al.: Minor motor epilepsy: Treatment with corticotropin (ACTH) and steroid therapy. J.A.M.A., 174:1408, 1960.

Ross, M.: Food in the mental hospital. J. Am. Dietet. A., 40:318, 1962.

Rupp, C.: Management of epilepsy. J.A.M.A., 166:1967, 1958.

Sawyer, G. T.: Treatment of multiple sclerosis with tolbutamide. J.A.M.A., 174:470, 1960.

Tower, D. B.: Interrelationships of oxidative and nitrogen metabolism with cellular nutrition and function in the central nervous system. Am. J. Clin. Nutr., 12:308, 1963.

Udenfriend, S.: Factors in amino acid metabolism which can influence the central nervous system. Am. J. Clin. Nutr., 12:287, 1963.

Victor, M.: Alcohol and nutritional diseases of the nervous system. J.A.M.A., 167:65, 1958.

Von Hagen, K. O.: Common neurological diseases seen in general practice. J.A.M.A., 148:1269, 1952.

Wohl, M. G. (ed.): Long-Term Illness. Philadelphia, W. B. Saunders Company, 1964, Chapter 15, Emotional Illnesses Requiring Continued Treatment.

Chapter 34
NUTRITIONAL DEFICIENCY DISEASES

GENERAL DISCUSSION

Scientific progress in research, plus improved economic status, has reduced frank fully developed deficiency diseases in the United States from endemic proportions to a comparative few. However, there are still and probably always will be patients with the traditional forms of nutritional deficiency diseases, and it is important that the medical team be familiar with the manifestations. They are seen among the poor, uneducated, neglected, chronic alcoholics, psychiatric patients or persons consuming bizarre diets. Youmans[1] points out, "There is likelihood of their being missed because of a low index of suspicion, due to unfamiliarity and lack of experience with them. . . . Cases of common nutritional-deficiency disease are being missed because it is assumed that they no longer occur and because their diagnostic features have been forgotten."

DEFINITION A nutritional deficiency disease is usually defined as a pathological condition caused by a diet which lacks one or more of the essential elements. However, this is not always the case. Actually, nutritional deficiency signifies a tissue deficiency of an essential nutrient, not necessarily a dietary inadequacy. Jolliffe[2] classifies nutritional deficiency diseases into two groups: primary (dietary) and secondary (conditioned) in origin. In primary nutritional inadequacy, the deficiency state results from an inadequate intake of nutrients either in amount or kind, or there is an imbalance of nutrients. In secondary or conditioned nutritional inadequacy, the deficiency states

are produced by factors other than inadequate food intake, such as interference with the ingestion, absorption or utilization of nutrients consumed due to a disease or improper dentures. Other secondary factors which may cause malnutrition are: metabolic or functional conditions that increase the requirement for, or cause unusual destruction, or abnormal excretion of nutrients, for example, an increase in the dietary requirement which occurs in certain diseases, during fever, hyperthyroidism and pregnancy; rapid elimination and failure to absorb which may occur in diarrhea, the result of too rapid transit of ingested foods through the intestinal tract; and malutilization, which may result from liver failure.

Multiple deficiencies are present in most individuals who have deficiency conditions. Seldom is an isolated or single deficiency observed in clinical practice. This is apparent when one considers the fact that neither primary dietary failure nor conditioning factors are selective of any particular nutrient.

While classical deficiency diseases, such as rickets, scurvy and pellagra, have long been recognized to be of dietary origin, little was known about the relation of nutrition to other pathological conditions. From the results of research on the various food nutrients, the science of medicine gathers data to correct disease. There are indications that the answer to many medical problems may be found in the field of nutrition. As far back as 1939, Kruse wrote: "Every disease, sooner or later, involves nutrition."

EARLY DIAGNOSIS AND TREATMENT OF NUTRITIONAL FAILURE There are several stages of deficiency disease. Each specific deficiency requires recognition of its velocity, severity, and pathogenesis. Velocity is interpreted as acute, subacute or chronic in duration. Severity refers to mild, moderate or

---

[1]Youmans, J. B.: The changing face of nutritional disease in America. J.A.M.A., *189*:672, 1964.

[2]Jolliffe, N. (ed.): Clinical Nutrition. 2nd ed. New York, Harper & Bros., 1962.

severe. Pathogenesis means whether the deficiency is primary or conditioned. With the present methods and equipment for diagnosis, the terms "clinical" and "subclinical" or "marginal" are used when referring to deficiency diseases. Although the early, mild stages are often below the manifest level, special equipment and procedures are now available for early diagnosis.[3]

Many clinicians assert that they do not see deficiency disease among their patients. This may be attributed to a number of reasons. It is probable that many cases pass unrecognized. The deficiency diseases are present in other forms besides the clearly defined classic picture. Individuals may go along for years in a mild deficiency state in which they are neither acutely ill nor at their most effective and efficient state of nutrition. These are the cases requiring closer, focused attention. (Review Nutritional Status, page 3, and Table 1-1 in Chapter 1.) Gershoff[4] pointed out that "the medical history and physical examination of the patient remain the most important tools of the physician in his provision of medical care" in determining nutritional status. The information thus acquired will often indicate the need for certain laboratory procedures as well as afford evidence of symptoms and physical signs of nutritional failure. The sequence of events that may be supplied to lead to a clinical nutritional deficiency is expressed diagrammatically by Pearson[3] in Figure 34-1.

Many deficiency diseases, particularly in the beginning, show that the levels of essential substances in some of the tissues are lowered or decreased at the expense of others. This results in an inadequate supply of compounds for the maintenance of nutritional balance. This parasitic action is typical and

---

[3]Pearson, W. N.: Biochemical appraisal of the vitamin nutritional status in man. J.A.M.A., *180*:49, 1962.

[4]Gershoff, S. N.: Who is well nourished? Nutr. Rev., *19*:321, 1961.

most noticeable in vitamin deficiency symptoms.

Vitamin deficiencies are usually thought of when nutritional deficiency diseases are discussed. However, protein-calorie malnutrition, nutritional anemia, and simple goiter are a few of the other deficiency diseases.

WORLD NUTRITION DEFICIENCY PROBLEMS   Overt classical nutritional deficiency diseases are uncommon in the United States today. On the other hand, a significant amount of deficiency diseases still remains. Marginal or mild cases are present in a significant segment of the population, particularly children who are not so well fed as they should – or could – be either because of insufficient funds, lack of knowledge or poor dietary habits. There is continued need for better nutritional education, more research, and improved living standards. America has been alerted to the extent of malnutrition within its boundaries. Incidence of hunger and malnutrition has been brought forward in the United States by the Citizens' Board of Inquiry report, "Hunger U.S.A." and by the television program, "Hunger in America." Documentary examples of poverty and malnutrition have been published. The Senate Select Committee on Nutrition and Related Human Needs has been holding hearings for more than a year. Copies of these hearings are available on request. Malnutrition is more prevalent than hunger per se. Physiological impairment from malnutrition is probably common. Iron deficiency, growth impairment and obesity are conditions that are widespread while classical deficiency diseases such as scurvy, beriberi and pellagra are rare. Incidence of goiter and rickets have been reported in alarming proportions.

In early reports of the National Nutrition Survey under the direction of Arnold E. Schaefer, Ph.D., the general impression is that poverty groups in the United States have

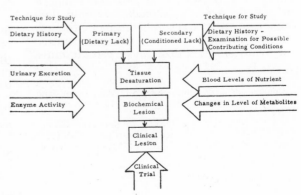

Figure 34-1   Sequence of events leading to clinical nutrition lesion. (From Pearson, W. N.: J.A.M.A., *180*:49-55, 1962.)

signs and indices of malnutrition of essentially the same incidences and severity as found in families of low income in Central America.[5] In the underdeveloped countries where there is overpopulation, poverty and ignorance, millions of people bear, or are acquiring, the stigmata of malnutrition, and hundreds of thousands are dying at an early age as a consequence.

Joint FAO/WHO Expert Committees on Nutrition report a number of nutritional problems of major importance.[6] Figure 34–2 illustrates areas and countries (22) in the world where ICNND nutrition surveys have been conducted and are being planned.[7] In the countries studied to date, ariboflavinosis and goiter were the most prevalent nutritional diseases encountered. However, preventable blindness (vitamin A deficiency), nutritional anemias, beriberi, kwashiorkor, protein and calorie malnutrition, and pellagra occur widely throughout the world. Those who seem to suffer the greatest degree of malnutrition are infants, pregnant and lactating women.

VITAMIN DEFICIENCY DISEASES

The list of vitamin deficiency conditions becomes longer each year. Research is constantly bringing to light new or old diseases attributed to vitamin deficiency. Only those diseases definitely established as being due to vitamin deficiency in human beings will be discussed. Although animal research has indicated there are many others, the evidence still needs to be applied to human nutrition.

An optimal mental and emotional status is dependent upon an adequate supply of all vitamins. The actions of vitamins are closely interrelated, and the lack of any one vitamin may affect the metabolism of the others.

Vitamin deficiency, except in severe injury or illness, is most frequently due to the lack of water-soluble vitamins. The incidence of vitamin A and ascorbic acid deficiency in this country has been noted in Chapter 14. Secondary deficiencies are common in alcoholics or in persons with gastrointestinal or mental disease. Occasionally, vitamin deficiencies arise as a result of antibiotic therapy that destroys the intestinal bacteria required for synthesis or utilization of the vitamins,

especially of the B-complex. When such deficiencies develop, they are usually multiple.

REQUIREMENT IN DISEASE   It is believed that the accepted standards of the Recommended Dietary Allowances for normal healthy persons (Table 11–1) are not always adequate for the sick and injured. As previously stated, it is common practice to administer up to ten times the recommended normal daily allowances under stress situations.

Chapter 9, devoted to a discussion of vitamins, should be reviewed for the chemistry, function and sources of the vitamins.

VITAMIN A DEFICIENCY DISORDERS

Prolonged deficiency of vitamin A may produce skin changes, night blindness and corneal ulcerations. In extreme deficiency states, the mucous membrane of the respiratory, gastrointestinal, and genitourinary tracts may be affected. The relation of vitamin A deficiency to the common cold is controversial. Recent research demonstrates that the vitamin A content of the blood may be decreased in severe acute illness. It is suggested that this may be due to some increased utilization of the vitamin, to interference with conversion of the precursor carotene into vitamin A, or to failure of liberation from the liver.

Night Blindness (Nyctalopia) and Day Blindness (Hermeralopia)

HISTORY   Over one hundred years ago Lewis and Clark, on their exploration of the Northwest, observed a condition of night blindness among the Idaho Indians. Later, in 1865, Gamo Lobo described a similar condition of the eyes of Brazilian natives. For the next fifty years observations of definite symptoms were reported which were unexplainable by the medical knowledge of the time. Then scientists suggested there must be some unrecognized constituent in food. In 1913 the factor was found and named vitamin A.

ETIOLOGY   Night blindness is attributed to functional failure of the retina in the proper regeneration of visual purple. Vitamin A is the precursor of visual purple as well as the product of its decomposition. It is believed that vitamin A unites with a protein in the retina to form visual purple. This is a continuous process and depends upon a sufficient supply of vitamin A.

The ability to perceive details at low levels of illumination is related to tiny nerve endings called rods. These rods are found in the retina, which is made up of rods and cones.

[5]Council on Foods and Nutrition, Malnutrition and Hunger in the United States. J.A.M.A., 213:No. 2, July 13, 1970.

[6]FAO/WHO Report VI, in the series of reports of the Joint FAO/WHO Expert Committee on Nutrition. WHO Technical Report Series No. 245 and FAO Nutrition Report Series No. 32.

[7]Schaefer, A. E.: Nutritional deficiencies in developing countries. J. Am. Dietet. A., 42:295, 1963.

ICNND NUTRITION SURVEYS

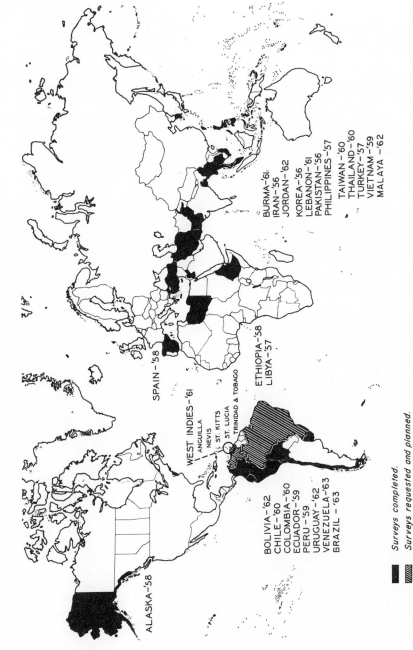

Figure 34–2 World map showing areas and countries in which ICNND nutrition surveys have thus far been conducted or are being planned. (Courtesy of Interdepartmental Committee on Nutrition for National Defense (ICNND), National Institutes of Health, Bethesda, Maryland, and J. Am. Dietet. A., 42:296, 1963.)

The latter are more numerous in the center and are concerned primarily with day sight and the perception of color. The rods are more profuse about the edges and control night vision. Individuals afflicted with night blindness (nyctalopia) cannot see in a dim light or at twilight. Day blindness (hemeralopia) is a condition in which an individual sees better in a dim light than in a bright light. Impairment of dark adaptation, the ability to adapt from a bright light or glare to darkness (encountered in night driving or on entering a dark room from a brightly lighted one), is symptomatic of vitamin A deficiency.

DIAGNOSIS   Special photometric instruments are used in the dark adaptation test to measure vitamin A deficiency. The dependability of the tests has been a provocative topic for discussions.

Xerophthalmia or Xerosis Conjunctivae

Xerophthalmia, one of the serious eye conditions caused by vitamin A deficiency, occurs rarely in the United States but is found throughout much of the Far East and in parts of India, the Near East, Africa and Latin America. It is associated with atrophy of the paraocular glands, hyperkeratosis of the conjunctiva and, finally, involvement of the cornea, leading to softening or keratomalacia (Fig. 34-3) and blindness. Avitaminosis A is reported to be the leading cause of preventable blindness in India and in Southeast Asia today. It manifests itself under unusual circumstances. It appeared in epidemic form in Denmark during World War I, when dairy products were replaced in the diets by fats lacking vitamin A. Although most common

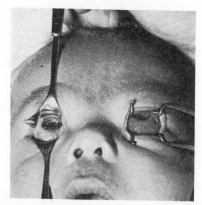

Figure 34-3   Keratomalacia showing the characteristic dry wrinkles, injected conjunctivas and cloudy corneas. (Jolliffe, N. (ed.): Clinical Nutrition. 2nd ed. Harper & Bros., 1962.)

in infants and young children, it may appear at any age.

Cutaneous Changes

Characteristic changes in the skin texture as a result of vitamin A deficiency are the "goose flesh" or "toad skin" (follicular hyperkeratosis) appearance as shown in Figure 34-4, or the "fish skin" or "alligator skin," known as xeroderma, shown in Figure 34-5. The skin becomes dry, scaly and rough. At first the forearms and thighs are affected, but in advanced stages, the entire body may be involved.

Recently, workers have challenged the etiology of follicular hyperkeratosis as being due to vitamin A deficiency, but suggest vitamin B-complex as having a role in its cause.[8] More studies are needed to establish the etiology.

[8]Nutr. Rev., *21*:106, 1963.

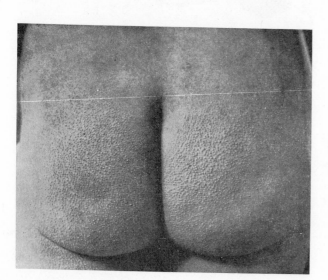

Figure 34-4   Vitamin A deficiency showing early follicular hyperkeratosis resembling "goose flesh." (Reproduced by courtesy of Section of Dermatology and Syphilology, Mayo Clinic.)

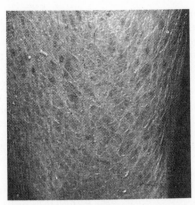

Figure 34–5   Vitamin A deficiency showing advanced xerosis, usually called ichthyosis, resembling "fish skin." (Jolliffe, N. (ed.): Clinical Nutrition. 2nd ed. Harper & Bros., 1962.)

PREVENTION AND TREATMENT OF AVITAMINOSIS A   Evidence exists to substantiate the fact that mild avitaminosis A, such as impairment of the ability to adapt to dark, is currently prevalent in the United States, especially among low income groups. It was also reported in countries where skim milk powder was provided as a relief food for infant feeding without supplementary vitamin A. For a number of years, UNICEF has been including vitamin A supplementation as part of programs in which skim milk is distributed to children whose diets are inadequate in vitamin A activity. FAO and UNICEF have, in addition, encouraged and supported school and home gardens in a number of developing countries as a means of supplying vegetable sources of vitamin A activity.

Although diet alone cannot ordinarily be depended upon to supply the needed vitamin in corrective dosage, a liberal, well-balanced diet is an essential element in the therapy. In any primary deficiency there can be no favorable prognosis unless the patient improves his diet permanently. In the long run, the increased consumption of various green leafy vegetables and yellow fruits and vegetables will correct existing vitamin A deficiencies, unless there is a disturbance of the process of conversion of the precursor, carotene, to vitamin A because of gastrointestinal or liver disease. The administration of a commercial vitamin A preparation such as a fish liver oil concentrate, which is packaged in 5000 and 10,000 I.U. to the capsule, is used when a more potent source is indicated.

The various symptoms of vitamin A deficiency respond to diet and supplementation in about the same order as they appear. For example, night blindness, an early manifestation of vitamin A deficiency, responds very quickly. On the other hand, the skin abnormalities may take several weeks to disappear. Members of vitamin B-complex (riboflavin, thiamin, and niacin) have been reported to be effective in alleviating night blindness and other vitamin deficiency signs when vitamin A failed to bring response.

The production and consumption of carotene food sources must be increased in the developing countries of the world through agricultural and educational guidance. Whenever economically feasible, enrichment with vitamin A of popular fatty or oily foods, such as the predominant vegetable oil of the country, should be considered. Since the most severe forms affect the infant and young child, special attention should be focused on adequate infant and child feeding. (Consult Table 19–4, Principal Sources of Food Constituents, for food sources of vitamin A. Also consult Chapter 9, The Vitamins.)

VITAMIN B-COMPLEX DEFICIENCY DISORDERS

Thiamin Deficiency Disorders

BERIBERI AND ITS CAUSE   From the results of the experimental production of beriberi by diet in 1897, the conception of deficiency disease was formulated. Beriberi is a metabolic disease caused by an extended period of continuous lack or deficiency of vitamin B_1 (thiamin), resulting from faulty diet, faulty utilization, or poor absorption of food. It has been known to the Chinese since 2600 B.C. It occurs during food shortages, famine or war, when the diet is very restricted, or when the staple food is polished rice. In 1880 the Japanese navy suffered a siege of beriberi. When whole barley was substituted for part of the rice rations the disease was controlled. Thus it became known that the lack of a certain food substance caused beriberi. In 1912 the vitamin theory was proposed, and in 1916 vitamin B was isolated. Not until 1926 was it discovered that vitamin B was composed of several vitamins.

Classification   Beriberi is classified into several types. The acute, mixed type of beriberi is characterized by nervous and cardiac symptoms producing neuritis and heart failure. It has been shown that myocardial metabolism is largely dependent upon aerobic glycolysis and that drastic reduction in cardiac pyruvate utilization is caused by thiamin deficiency.[9] There are two other

[9]Akbarian, M., and Dreyfus, P. M.: Blood transketolase activity in beriberi heart disease. J.A.M.A., *203*:77, 1968.

Figure 34–6

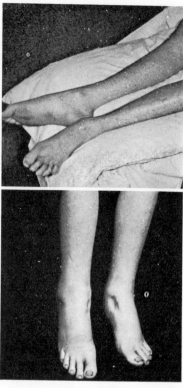

Figure 34–7

Figure 34–6   Advanced polyneuropathy with muscle atrophy and foot and toe drop in a patient with dry beriberi. (Jolliffe, N. (ed.): Clinical Nutrition. 2nd ed. Harper & Bros., 1962.)

Figure 34–7   Edema in a patient with wet beriberi. (Jolliffe, N. (ed.): Clinical Nutrition. 2nd ed. Harper & Bros., 1962.)

types, namely, the "dry" and the "wet" beriberi. In the "dry" type of the disease the nervous manifestations, with loss of function or paralysis of the lower extremities, are predominant; hence the term *polyneuritis* is synonymous (Fig. 34–6). In the "wet" type the edema of heart failure is the most striking sign (Fig. 34–7). Indefinite digestive disorders and emaciation are additional symptoms.

Incidence   This nutritional disease occurs primarily among population groups which subsist on a diet of highly polished rice. The neuritic form is seen most frequently in the United States, with the exception of certain areas in Louisiana where classic beriberi occurs. Infantile beriberi occurs in breast-fed infants of mothers who have the disease. The disease is widespread geographically, occurring endemically or sporadically in all parts of the world. In Thailand, Burma, and Vietnam it is a major cause of death among infants 2 to 5 months of age. Although the most serious form of vitamin

B$_1$ (thiamin) deficiency (beriberi) is rare in the United States, mild and borderline cases are not uncommon.

Relation to Alcoholism   The neuritis of alcoholics is similar if not identical with the polyneuritis of beriberi. (See Chapter 33, p. 486.) Research studies reveal that it is due in part, if not entirely, to a deficiency of thiamin, and in some cases this is conditioned by a damaged gastrointestinal tract. It can be treated with improved diet habits emphasizing an adequate diet supplemented with vitamin B-complex, especially thiamin.

Relation to Other Conditions   Since thiamin requirements are proportional to body weight, metabolism and calorie intake, the allowance should be increased under certain conditions, such as hyperthyroidism, infections, unusual exercise, and during pregnancy. The polyneuritis of pregnancy, resulting from increased metabolic demands, can be treated successfully with a diet abundant in thiamin and, when indicated, administration of thiamin concentrate.

Dietary Treatment   The diet for beriberi and other thiamin deficiencies should be well balanced nutritionally. Foods high in thiamin content, such as whole and enriched grains, vegetables (especially legumes); lean pork, eggs, liver, and milk should be included in abundance. Since most patients suffer from multiple deficiencies, frequently the B-complex concentrate is prescribed. If the damage to the nervous system is not too great, the response to treatment is usually good. In cases where acute heart failure has developed, the outlook is grave.

Prevention of Thiamin Deficiency   Education to prevent deficiencies is of primary importance. People need to learn about the composition of foods and how to prepare foods to preserve the nutrients. Recently, in Burma, Thailand and Vietnam, beriberi has become prevalent because the rice is processed with gasoline-driven mills. Formerly, the grain was hulled by pounding it at home. Thus, it still contained an appreciable amount of thiamin in the form in which it was consumed. Manufacturers of cereals and millers of flour are restoring vitamins to their products, thereby enriching cereals and flours to normal potency. In Japan and the Philippines notably beriberi has practically disappeared as a result of the prophylactic use of thiamin and the enrichment of rice. The daily thiamin intake of predominantly rice eating populations can be increased to adequacy through consumption of undermilled or enriched rice.

Riboflavin Deficiency Disorders

ARIBOFLAVINOSIS   Ariboflavinosis is a disease caused by riboflavin (vitamin B$_2$) de-

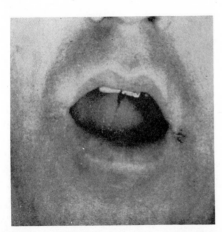

Figure 34-8   A diet lacking in vitamins of the B-complex group may result in lesions of the tongue and oral mucous membranes. Note the angular stomatitis from riboflavin deficiency. (Courtesy of Dr. M. K. Horwitt, reprinted from Health News, New York State Department of Health, September, 1955.)

ficiency, and is usually found in individuals who consume a marginal diet devoid of animal protein sources and leafy vegetables. It is characterized by the development of angular stomatitis, cracks in the skin at the corners of the mouth (cheilosis), a greasy eruption of the skin, a purplish tongue (Fig. 34-8), and by capillary overgrowth around the cornea of the eye.

Dietary Treatment   The diet for ariboflavinosis should include liberal amounts of foods rich in riboflavin. Riboflavin is distributed widely in foods of plant and animal origin, and liver, milk, milk products, eggs, meat, green leaves and buds may be considered the best and most reliable sources for the human dietary. Seeds or whole grain cereals, which are an important source of thiamin, are poor sources of riboflavin unless enriched.

Supplements of the crystalline riboflavin, as well as other B-complex factors, are often prescribed, especially if the underlying cause of the deficiency is faulty utilization or poor absorption of the vitamin.

PREVENTION OF ARIBOFLAVINOSIS
In many developing countries, conditions do not permit use of dairy products and meat. For such areas, an effective remedial step for increasing the riboflavin intake is the enrichment of the basic grain of the country—rice, wheat, or corn.

Niacin Deficiency Disorders

PELLAGRA   Pellagra is a disease caused by a deficiency of the niacin-fraction of the vitamin B-complex or the amino acid tryptophan. Tryptophan is a precursor of niacin, and it has been shown that pellagra can be cured by the administration of tryptophan alone, although the disease is manifested by multiple deficiencies. Pellagra was described originally as occurring in individuals who subsisted on a diet of maize. It was also noted among those people who consumed bad whiskey or had intestinal disturbances of such severity that absorption of food was hindered. The basic factor is an inadequate diet, but there is a possibility that both maize and whiskey give off a toxin which destroys the vitamin.

Incidence   Pellagra occurs most commonly among the people of poor socio-economic status and is usually associated with a diet composed primarily of corn. In the United States most of the cases occur in the Southeastern states during spring and early summer. During the winter, the patient has usually subsisted on cornmeal, salt pork and molasses. Cornmeal has an unusually low niacin and tryptophan content and, whenever this food forms a major part of the diet, pellagra is fairly prevalent.

Prevention of Pellagra   Enrichment of corn with niacin is one solution to the pellagra problem. Goldberger, working among the pellagrins of the South, was the first to demonstrate that the disease was due to a vitamin deficiency. The vitamin was called P-P or pellagra-preventive and later named vitamin B_2 or G. Still later this vitamin proved to have several fractions, one of which was found to be nicotinic acid.

Pellagra is endemic in several countries, particularly Yugoslavia, Egypt, Basutoland and Southern Rhodesia. Vitamin enrichment of the maize and redistribution of cereals within a country are being suggested as aids by FAO in preventing the disease. When the person learns to select enriched corn (and corn products) and other whole or enriched grains along with the food groups (meat-milk-vegetable-fruit) an adequate diet will be obtained.

Symptoms   The early symptoms of pellagra are weakness, lassitude, anorexia, and indigestion, followed by sore ulcerated mouth and tongue (Fig. 34-9) and diarrhea. The typical dermatitis of skin eruptions and scaly skin usually simplifies the diagnosis (Fig. 34-10). Neurological symptoms and mental changes occur in the more advanced cases. The various symptoms, especially the skin lesions, are aggravated by exposure to sunlight. The typical "sore tongue" has suggested to various investigators that the condition is analogous to the disease in dogs called "blacktongue." Both conditions are treated successfully with niacin.

Dietary Treatment   Niacin and/or tryptophan is now used widely in the treatment of pellagra, but it is most effective when used

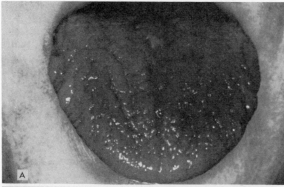
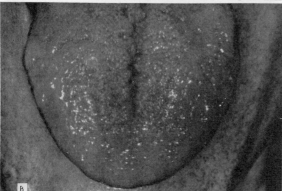

Figure 34-9   Chronic diseases, such as pellagra, may be caused by severe malnutrition. A, Glossitis is an early sign of this disease. B, Same patient after dietary treatment. (S. L. Halpern: Nutrition and Chronic Disease; reprinted from Health News, New, York State Department of Health, September, 1955.)

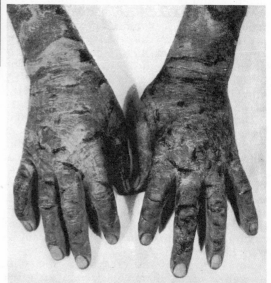

Figure 34-10   A, The lesions on the backs of the hands are typical of pellagra. B, The same patient after two weeks of nicotinamide therapy. (Spies: Rehabilitation through Better Nutrition.)

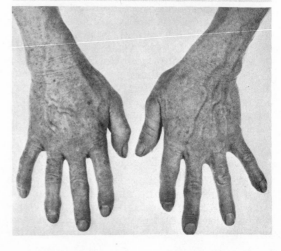

in conjunction with other vitamins, especially thiamin and riboflavin, because pellagrins suffer usually from multiple deficiencies. In severe cases of pellagra, parenteral administration of niacin may be necessary.

A well-balanced diet containing foods high in niacin and tryptophan content is recommended. Liver, whole grains, yeast, lean meats, poultry and canned salmon are rich sources. Vegetables, fruits, milk and nuts are good sources. Because of the sore tongue symptom, it may be necessary to start patients with a liquid diet and progress gradually to a normal diet.

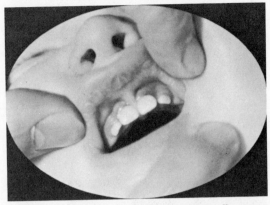

Figure 34–11   Scurvy: Note the bleeding swollen gums. (Courtesy of University of Rochester, Rochester, New York.)

ASCORBIC ACID DEFICIENCY DISORDERS AND SCURVY

HISTORY   Scurvy is a metabolic disease resulting from a deficiency of ascorbic acid. For hundreds of years the malady was known as "the plague of the seas." Men journeying on long voyages, military or exploring expeditions, settlers in new countries, or people in famine areas were afflicted with scurvy. Nothing was known about vitamins, but somehow the Dutch authorities discovered that the feeding of oranges, lemons or limes prevented the dreaded disease. English sailors are called by the nickname "limey," actually a misnomer, since early rations included not limes but lemons as a scurvy preventive. The specific relationship between scurvy, citrus foods and ascorbic acid was not established until the twentieth century. In the 1930's, ascorbic acid was discovered, isolated and synthesized as cevitamic acid. In 1939 the name cevitamic acid was changed officially to ascorbic acid.

INCIDENCE   Few cases of severe ascorbic acid deficiency are seen today. A deficiency may be found among people who consume a diet devoid of fruits and vegetables such as the indigent, the mentally ill, the food faddist, the alcoholic, and patients on restricted therapeutic diets consisting chiefly of milk and cereals (diet for gastric ulcer). Infants who have been taken off breast milk manifest symptoms of ascorbic acid deficiency. Since the introduction of the potato, a source of ascorbic acid, the epidemics of scurvy, which formerly occurred at the end of every winter in Western Europe, have disappeared.

DETERMINATIONS   Ascorbic acid determinations on plasma are useful to determine ascorbic acid subnutrition. Determinations of the level in white cells are made when ascorbic acid deficiency is advanced. Although low blood levels of vitamin C do occur without evident manifestations of scurvy, the result of the determination indicates an intake of ascorbic acid below the amount necessary to maintain the individual's body reserve at the highest level.

SYMPTOMS   Scurvy is characterized by general debility, pallor, poor appetite, sensitivity to touch, pains in the limbs and joints, especially the knee joints; sensitive and swollen gums, with bleeding and loosening of the teeth. (See Fig. 34–11.) In infants, especially those artificially fed, periosteal hemorrhages occurring around the bones of the lower extremities, skeletal changes and failure to grow are manifestations of the deficiency; in adults, petechial hemorrhages in the skin, bleeding in the muscle tissue (Fig. 34–12), and bloody diarrhea are not uncommon signs. Black and blue areas often appear on the surface of the skin because of the hemorrhages. These individuals are classified as bruising easily. Anemia may occur if there is significant blood loss. Many of the symptoms are seen every day in mild cases of ascorbic acid deficiency and are frequently overlooked or ignored.

DIETARY TREATMENT   The treatment for deficiency is the administration of ascorbic acid. In severe cases, ascorbic acid is given in massive doses orally or parenterally. In addition, a well-balanced diet with foods rich in ascorbic acid is recommended. In many mild deficiency cases, the corrective diet is sufficient. Citrus fruits (lemons, limes, oranges, and grapefruit) are excellent sources. Tomatoes, spinach, cabbage, cauliflower, broccoli, berries, and fresh greens are likewise excellent sources, while most of the fresh vegetables and fruits are good sources. Because ascorbic acid is destroyed easily by heat and oxidation, fresh or raw foods are recommended. Fruit juices and tomato juice should be covered when stored in the refrigerator to avoid loss of ascorbic acid through oxidation.

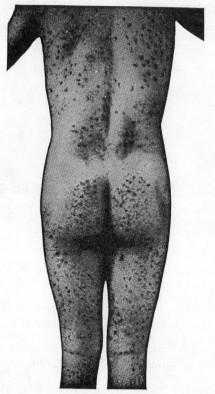

Figure 34–12   A typical case of adult scurvy, showing the numerous petechiae—spots where blood has effused to the skin. (L. J. Harris: Vitamins in Theory and Practice. Macmillan Co.)

Because of sore gums and tongue, the diet may at first be composed of liquids and advanced gradually to solid foods. The administration of the indicated foodstuffs plus ascorbic acid is followed by miraculous improvement, which is most encouraging, both to the patient and the nurse.

PREVENTION OF ASCORBIC ACID DEFICIENCY   In areas where there is evidence of widespread deficiency of ascorbic acid, efforts must be made to increase the production, distribution and availability of fresh fruits and vegetables. Educational efforts should be directed toward helping people make proper selection of foods to supply ascorbic acid.

VITAMIN D DEFICIENCY DISORDERS

Rickets

Rickets is a nutritional and metabolic disease of infancy and early childhood, in which calcification of the bones does not take place normally. It is usually caused by deficiency of vitamin D, with accompanying metabolic disturbances in the calcium-phosphorus ratio. An inadequate, unbalanced diet lacking in sufficient calcium and/or phosphorus may result in rickets. So may poor absorption. Studies[10] confirm early reports that parathyroid overactivity occurs in rickets, and it is postulated that this activity may account for some of the biochemical and skeletal abnormalites in the disease.

Vitamin D is known as the antirachitic vitamin. It is believed that vitamin D controls the utilization of calcium and phosphorus which are important in the formation and proper development of bones. However, the action of vitamin D seems to be concerned chiefly with the intestinal absorption of calcium and phosphorus. It has been reported that one of the first signs of deficiency of vitamin D is the decrease in the amount of calcium in the urine, followed by an increase of calcium in the stool, which progresses until a negative calcium balance exists. The changes in the metabolism of phosphorus differ only in the fact that the urinary excretion of phosphorus is increased. These changes may be reversed with very small doses of vitamin D.

INCIDENCE   The existence of rickets has been noted throughout the world, its frequency and severity varying in different localities. Scientific advances in nutrition and an improved standard of living have almost eliminated the disease as a pediatric problem in North America. However, children with rickets still appear. Rickets in breast-fed infants not receiving a vitamin D supplement and infants receiving non-fortified fluid milk have been a problem in the United States in the past decade. The greatest number of rachitic cases seems to be found in the large cities where poor housing, inadequate diets, and limited exposure to sunshine prevail, and it is observed to occur particularly in children who grow very rapidly. Speaking in general, the disease has been reported to be more prevalent in the north temperate zone and less frequent in the tropical and subtropical areas, where infants and children have more opportunity to be exposed to the sun, even though the mineral content of their diets is not above reproach.

On the other hand, there are a group of cases which belong to a heterogeneous class of patients in whom active rickets persists despite the administration of conventional doses of vitamin D. *Hypophosphatemic vitamin D refractory rickets* of the simple type, resulting from renal tubular dysfunction, is the most common. It may be classified as an

---

[10]Nutritional rickets and parathyroid function. Nutr. Rev., 21:271, 1963.

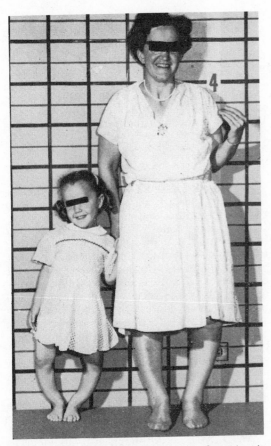

Figure 34–13   Illustration of hypophosphatemic vitamin D-refractory rickets of simple type. Mother and 4-year-old daughter show typical deformities. (Courtesy of Fraser, D., and J.A.M.A., *176*:281, 1961.)

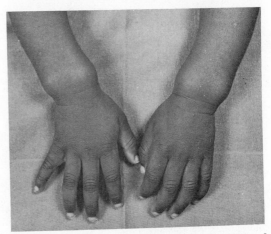

Figure 34–14   Rickets: Note the marked enlargement of wrists. (Courtesy of University of Rochester, Rochester, New York.)

the bones. Because teeth are made up of material similar to bone, it is believed by many authorities that vitamin D has a related effect on the development of teeth.

The beginning visible symptoms of rickets in infants are profuse sweating and restlessness, the sleeping infant moving his head from side to side and rubbing off his hair. Contrary to the usual deficiency disease symptoms, the patient does not become thin or emaciated. Often parents will not recognize the symptoms of rickets until the child starts to walk. The legs will bow because the bones are soft and not strong enough to support the child's weight. A pot belly and beading of the ribs (the rachitic rosary) may pass

inborn error of metabolism and is genetically determined. However, not all examples of vitamin D refractory rickets have an inherited background established. This form of rickets may develop in infancy but not infrequently appears in late childhood, or it may not appear until adult life. Currently, oral administration of massive doses of vitamin D_2 (50,000 to 500,000 I.U. per day) is the treatment of choice. It is rarely completely cured and the stature remains short. (See Fig. 34–13.)

SYMPTOMS   The first adequate description of rickets occurred in 1650. The disease usually develops during the first two years of life. It has the chief characteristic of failure to appropriate or retain calcium in the bones. The softened and deformed bones cause deformities such as pigeon chest, enlarged wrists and ankles (Figs. 34–14 and 34–15), and bowed legs or knock knees. (See Fig. 34–16.) The severity of the condition may be determined chemically through studies of the calcium and phosphorus content of the blood and clinically with roentgenograms of

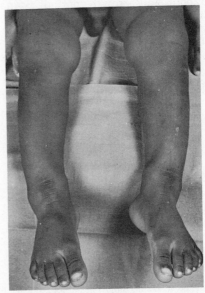

Figure 34–15   Rickets: Note the bowing and increase in width at epiphyses. (Courtesy of University of Rochester, Rochester, New York.)

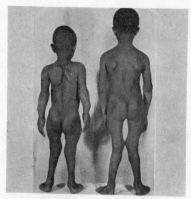

Figure 34–16   Rachitic deformities. Note knock knees and enlarged joints. (Jolliffe, N. (ed.): Clinical Nutrition. 2nd ed. Harper & Brothers, 1962.)

unobserved in a plump, yet malnourished baby. (See Fig. 34–17.) The fat baby is no longer an indication of a healthy infant. If the deficiency appears during the third or fourth month of life, when the skull is growing rapidly, the structure of the head will be larger than normal. The shape is inclined to be square, with bulging on the sides and front. Lesser defects sometimes ensue when the ailment is mild. Swellings may be noted in the wrists and ankles (Figs. 34–14 and 34–15).

PREVENTION AND DIETARY TREATMENT   Vitamin D, when it is converted to the active metabolite, acts to stimulate intestinal absorption of calcium and mobilization of calcium from bone. To prevent rickets in the newborn baby, the importance of starting the administration of vitamin D in appropriate amounts early and continuing throughout the growth period cannot be emphasized too much. If rickets is present, massive doses of vitamin D are given. Vitamin D concentrates of the fish liver oils, such as cod liver oil and viosterol, are often pre-

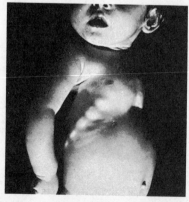

Figure 34–17   Child suffering from rickets. Note rachitic rosary and pot belly (Jolliffe, N. (ed.): Clinical Nutrition. 2nd ed. Harper & Brothers, 1962.)

scribed. Irradiated ergosterol is also an excellent source. However, mothers should be warned against the simultaneous use of several preparations, since it is possible to give too much.

Many foods are being fortified with vitamin D and milk is an example (400 I.U./qt.). Since milk contains calcium and phosphorus, it becomes a good antirachitic food when vitamin D is added.

Osteomalacia

ETIOLOGY AND SYMPTOMS   Osteomalacia is a disease of adulthood similar to rickets in infants and children. It is a nutritional disease usually attributed (1) to defect in renal tubular reabsorption, or (2) to failure to respond to vitamin D, or (3) to deficiency of vitamin D or (4) to inadequate intake of calcium or (5) to loss of excessive amounts of calcium in the feces. In most cases seen in the United States, this condition is associated with steatorrhea. It is characterized by pronounced softening of the bones. The bones become flexible and cause deformities, especially of the limbs, spine, thorax, and pelvis. Typical symptoms are a rheumatic type of pain and general weakness. Although it is seen occasionally in men, it is most often observed in women, especially among those who are pregnant.

INCIDENCE   Although osteomalacia is seldom seen among the people of modern civilization, there are areas where it is a medical problem. It is distributed widely in India, most frequently among the women of the upper and middle classes who practice seclusion or purdah after marriage. It is also prevalent in the Orient, especially among the women, whose diets are extremely low in calcium, who get little sunshine, and who have frequent pregnancies and nurse their infants over extended periods. In the United States, osteomalacia is sometimes encountered among elderly persons living alone, consuming an inadequate diet, and getting inadequate sunshine or other source of vitamin D. It is seldom encountered among the lower classes who wear less clothing and who work outdoors in the sun, or among people who have an abundant diet.

Osteomalacia is frequently confused with a disease having similar symptoms, osteoporosis, discussed in this chapter under Mineral (Calcium and Phosphorus) Deficiencies.

PREVENTION AND TREATMENT   Because the average diet furnishes little vitamin D, it seems reasonable to assume that either the requirement of vitamin D for man is extremely low or his needs are usually provided by exposure to sunlight. Most authorities agree that the normal adult requires only a small amount of vitamin D. For osteomalacia the recommendations are an adequate diet liberal in protein of high biologic value, with an abundance of milk and milk products plus a supplement of vitamin D.

Prevention of rickets and osteomalacia is possible through the supply of adequate and correct proportions of calcium and phosphorus in the diet. Milk or its equivalent is necessary in the diet to provide calcium. In addition vitamin D must be assured from either sunshine, ultraviolet lamp, natural food source, fortified food source, or a concentrated supplement.

MINERAL DEFICIENCIES

Chapter 8, devoted to the subject of minerals, should be reviewed. Function, requirements and sources of minerals will not be repeated.

CALCIUM AND PHOSPHORUS

The relationship and necessity for calcium and phosphorus in the prevention and treatment of rickets, tetany and osteomalacia have been discussed. It has been demonstrated that these diseases can develop when an imbalance or longstanding lack occurs of either or both calcium and phosphorus.

A moderate degree of calcium deficiency is believed to be quite prevalent during pregnancy, and also in childhood; it is usually much worse during adolescence. During the adolescent period the requirement is increased while in contrast too often the intake of calcium-rich foods is decreased. The desire to remain slim is a factor, especially among girls. It is during the adolescent period that dental caries tend to become prevalent, a condition believed to depend on nutritional status and calcium metabolism. Milk and milk products are the best food sources. Calcium salts are considered useful under special circumstances.

OSTEOPOROSIS   Osteoporosis is a metabolic disorder which may be defined as a reduction in the amount of bone without any changes in its chemical composition. That is, the absolute amount has been diminished, but the bone remaining is normal in chemical composition. Osteoporosis (deossification) is frequently confused with osteomalacia (demineralization).

Incidence and Etiology   Osteoporosis is encountered in persons after age 50 and especially in women after the menopause. Practically all people begin to lose bone at about age 55, although the reasons are un-

clear. It is more common in women by a ratio of about four to one. It can be shown by measuring the cortical thickness of the long bones, particularly the fingers.[11] The disease is termed idiopathic, postmenopausal, and senile, depending on the age and/or sex of the patient. The most common type is osteoporosis of aging (senile). It was believed to result primarily from an age-related decline in ratio of anabolic hormone secretion (sex and pituitary glands). Probably, osteoporosis is the result of a variety of factors, of which hormonal change is one.

For a number of years the hypothesis has prevailed that the bony decalcification results from a disorder of the protein matrix in which calcium is deposited, rather than to deficiency of calcium, phosphorus or vitamin D. More recently, however, the protein matrix hypothesis has been questioned, and it has been suggested that osteoporosis results from a prolonged negative calcium balance in individuals with a higher than normal calcium requirement because of excessive loss of calcium via the kidneys or who are unable to adapt to an inadequate intake with a resultant increased bone resorption.[12] Still others believe poor absorption of calcium may be a prime factor, correctable in some cases by the administration of vitamin D.

Lack of exercise of many aging persons may be a factor; there is lack of stimulation to maintain calcium in the bony areas of stress and wear. It may also occur as a result of a deficient protein intake, or whenever the synthesis of protein is impaired, as in Cushing's syndrome, prolonged immobilization, and prolonged semistarvation. Hypercalciuria may occur in the beginning stage, and renal stones frequently develop.

Symptoms   Osteoporosis is acquired slowly, and many years may elapse before the individual is aware of the change. Weakness is the initial manifestation, along with loss of appetite and pain in the back and hips. Fractures often occur easily; for example, individuals may break a hip from tripping over a rug or stepping down a low curb. Involvement of leg bones is followed by pain, tenderness and muscle cramps. Bowing occurs when bone tissue becomes too soft to support the weight of the body. Deformity such as stooped posture is frequently marked, along with decrease in height due to shrinkage of the spine.

Treatment and Prevention   Both male and female hormones are used in the treat-

---

[11]Hegsted, D. M.: Nutrition, bone and calcification. J. Am. Dietet. A., 50:107, 1967.

[12]Nordin, B. E.: Calcium balance and calcium requirement in spinal osteoporosis. Am. J. Clin. Nutr., 10:384, 1962.

ment. Calcium infusions have been used also to improve calcium retention, enhance bone formation and reduce bone resorption. An increase in vitamin D, calcium and protein intake is indicated, as well as exercise to prevent atrophy of bone. The diet should be adequate in all respects to assure normal, or increased, calcium availability. Sufficient vitamin D must be present to permit utilization of the calcium taken into the body. Urist[13] recommends the administration of 1 gm. calcium daily in the form of nonfat milk; of polyvitamin preparations, including vitamin D, 1000 I.U.; and 1 to 2 gm. protein per kg. of body weight daily. An adequate protein intake and positive nitrogen balance are important, as is a positive calcium balance.

Beneficial effects of fluoride have been reported. Its effects are most likely to be on the bone crystal. More perfect crystals are formed which are less soluble and less subject to resorption. It is believed that the effect in bone is similar to that which helps prevent dental caries. These studies also showed that calcified aortas occurred much less often with optimal fluoride intake. If these findings are confirmed, fluoride in some way helps to keep the calcium in the bone and to prevent its deposition in the blood vessel.[14]

IRON

The relationship and necessity for iron in the prevention and treatment of anemias has been discussed in detail in Chapter 31.

ANEMIAS Iron deficiency is the most prevalent type of nutritional anemia and in the adult person is recognized generally by the presence of microcytic hypochromic anemia. Iron deficiency anemia is an important nutritional problem among infants and women of child-bearing age throughout the world, including the United States.[15] Although lack of dietary iron is the basic cause of this disorder, in the United States and the rest of the world other concurrent endemic diseases which contribute to blood loss (hookworm) or interfere with absorption (gastrointestinal diseases) are important contributing factors. Nutrition surveys, such as those made in the United States and by ICNND and the WHO, have disclosed iron deficiency anemia as a major impairment of health and working capacity and, as a consequence, cause of economic loss. As high as 30 to 50 per cent or more of the underdeveloped countries have been found to be affected.

Recent studies suggest that there exists another type of nutritional anemia with a characteristic macrocytic blood picture, primarily among infants and women after pregnancy, distinct from that of iron deficiency anemia. This is usually associated with prolonged consumption of marginal diets poor in protein, vitamin B_{12}, folic acid, and probably other B-complex vitamins, and frequently is combined with iron depletion. See Chapter 31, Diseases of the Blood and Blood-Forming Organs; page 465 for discussion of Nutritional and Iron Deficiency Anemias; Chapter 15 for anemia in pregnancy; and Chapter 36 for anemia in infancy and childhood.

PREVENTION OF IRON DEFICIENCY ANEMIA Careful selection of iron-rich foods in the daily dietary is necessary for all persons. In areas where iron deficiency anemia results from parasitic infections, eradication of the parasites plus the introduction of adequate iron into the diet is the objective for prevention. In acute areas, iron may be supplied in the form of tablets or capsules through the health center distribution program. Iron fortification of other foods besides bread and cereal products is contemplated.

IODINE

Although iodine is distributed extensively throughout the products of nature, the chief storehouse is in the surface soil. Since the amount varies with the local geologic conditions of the soil and water, there is an uneven distribution.

The thyroid gland is the storehouse for iodine in the human body. Iodine is an essential component of thyroxine, the active constituent of the thyroid gland.

SIMPLE OR ENDEMIC GOITER Simple goiter is a state of enlargement of the thyroid gland which develops through a deficiency of ingested iodine. The deficiency may be absolute, especially in areas of subnormal iodine intake, or relative, subsequent to various demands of the body which increase the need for thyroid secretion in the female during adolescence, pregnancy, and lactation.

Incidence The highest incidence in goitrous areas usually occurs in females 12 to 18 years of age and males 9 to 13 years. The incidence of goiter can be correlated with the iodine intake from the water and food of a specific region. In the regions known as the "goiter belt" in the United States (page 507) the soil is iodine poor, producing iodine-poor food. This inadequacy is reflected in a prevalence of goiter among the population. The WHO has estimated that there are approximately 200 million goitrous individuals in

[13]Urist, M. R.: The etiology of osteoporosis. J.A.M.A., *169*:710, 1959.

[14]Hegsted, D. M., *op. cit.*, p. 108.

[15]Council on Foods and Nutrition: Iron deficiency in the United States. *203*:No. 6, 1968.

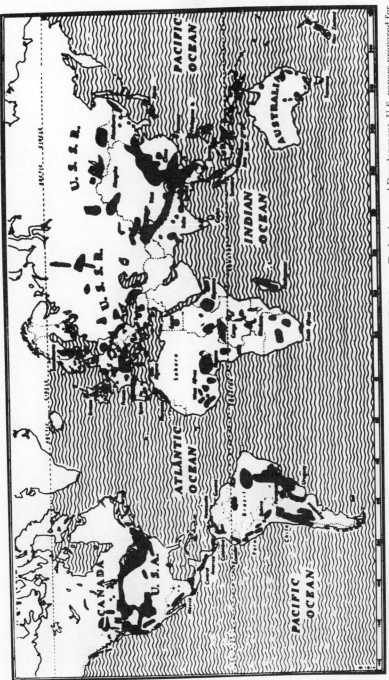

Figure 34-18 Goiter areas of the world. (From Volume III. AGRICULTURE. Science, Technology, and Development, U.S. papers prepared for the United Nations Conference on the application of Science and Technology for the Benefit of the Less Developed Areas, 1962.)

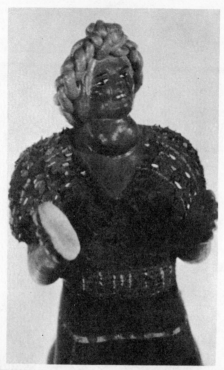

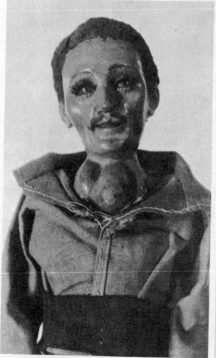
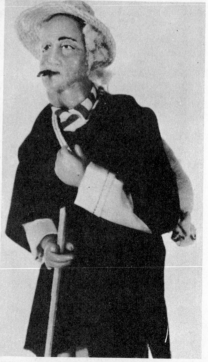

Figure 34-19   Dolls with goiter from the goitrous belt of Middle America. Above, figure of village woman making tortillas, made in local village and purchased in Guatemala City market; lower left figure is old religious statue from Antigua, Guatemala; lower right, doll of recent date manufactured in village in Colombia. All illustrate the acceptance of goiters as a normal physical feature. (From Volume III. AGRICULTURE. Science, Technology, and Development, U.S. papers prepared for the United Nations Conference on the application of Science and Technology for the Benefit of the Less Developed Areas, 1962.)

the world today, and few countries are exempt.

The food iodine is the most important factor determining the goiter incidence in a region. Nutritional iodine is derived essentially from the food and to a lesser degree from supplemented salt or water. The amount of iodine in the local drinking water may be regarded as a measure of the iodine content of the soil and, consequently, of the iodine content of the fruits, grasses, and vegetables grown in the region. However, the iodine content of water is not important as a source of nutritional iodine except in unusual circumstances.

Prevention and Treatment   Simple goiter can be prevented and frequently cured by the administration of iodine. To supply the needed iodine, the use of iodized salt is advised. People residing along the seacoast may obtain iodine from fresh shellfish (rich in iodine) and foods grown in iodine-rich soil. However, even the regional differences in iodine consumption have become less pronounced with the increase in interstate transportation of foods, beverages, vegetables, fruits, and fertilizers. People living in the goiter belt who consume local produce especially should be urged to use iodized salt.

Endemic goiter is still widespread in the underdeveloped areas and a significant number of cases have been found in the United States. (See Figures 34–18 and 34–19.) The international agencies, particularly WHO and ICNND, have addressed a great deal of attention toward effective salt iodization.

MAGNESIUM DEFICIENCY

Magnesium deficiency may develop under conditions of stress and in the course of disease process. A deficiency may precipitate from any condition in which there is a decreased intake or increased loss of magnesium or a shift in electrolyte balance.

The hypomagnesemic tetany syndrome deficiency is reported to be almost identical to hypocalcemic tetany (p. 418) and can be differentiated chemically. Administration of magnesium promptly relieves the symptoms. Patients observed with the deficiency all have a dietary inadequacy. In addition, one or more of the following factors are present: (1) excessive loss of magnesium from persistent vomiting or from removal of intestinal contents by mechanical suction, (2) intestinal malabsorption, or (3) administration of large amounts of magnesium-free parenteral fluids to postsurgical patients. Treatment with intramuscular magnesium sulfate promptly reverses the condition. Conditions in which acute deficiencies may develop are renal disease, diuretic therapy, malabsorption, hyperthyroidism, acute alcoholism, kwashiorkor, diabetes, parathyroid gland disorders, and post-surgical stress.

PROTEIN-CALORIE MALNUTRITION

An inadequate dietary intake of calories and proteins of good quality is the most widespread, serious nutritional problem in technically underdeveloped areas, and is particularly devasting in its effect on children.

In the United States, serious protein-calorie malnutrition, including typical kwashiorkor and marasmus, is observed occasionally in neglected infants brought to large city hospitals and in low income families. The general improvement in the clinical or physical symptoms is usually satisfactory but in many instances there is evident lack of improvement in the functional capacities of the brain.[16] Studies to solve the relationship of nutrition to central nervous system activity are of immense practical and theoretical importance to man. Comparatively recent findings are the profound effects of semi-starvation on the behavior patterns of man.[17]

Protein-calorie inadequacy problems that are secondary to other diseases are many. Serious caloric undernutrition occurs in association with chronic fevers such as tuberculosis, with malignancy, in diseases of the gastrointestinal tract that interfere with intake or absorption of food and in patients with psychiatric problems. Protein deficiency is a complication of numerous pathologic states. Protein may be lost in diarrheas and malabsorption syndromes, or in the urine in certain diseases of the kidney. Trauma of all kinds, including surgery, can result in a negative nitrogen balance; cirrhosis of the liver is commonly associated with protein deficiency.

PROTEIN DEFICIENCY

The simplest, most obvious, common cause of protein deficiency is the lack of adequate protein in the food consumed and inadequate calorie intake. This may be due to one or more of these reasons: inadequate knowledge about sufficient protein intake, ingestion of poor quality protein, poor economic status, unavailability of good quality protein, misinformation, or the existence of some local

---

[16]Coursin, D. B.: Effects of undernutrition of central nervous system function. Nutr. Rev., 23:65, 1965.
[17]Keys, A., et al.: The Biology of Human Starvation. Vol II. Minneapolis, University of Minnesota Press, 1950, pp. 1213–1215.

or generalized disease which results in anorexia and dietary inadequacy. The more general causes of protein deficiency are:

1. Insufficient intake of calories and protein, quantitatively or qualitatively.

2. Impaired digestion or absorption of protein foods—chronic diarrhea, fistula and so on.

3. Inadequate synthesis of plasma protein—liver disease.

4. Increased breakdown of body protein stores: febrile states, elevated basal metabolic rate and the like.

5. Excessive loss of protein, such as nephrotic syndrome, ascites or hemorrhage.

HYPOPROTEINEMIA AND NUTRITIONAL EDEMA

Nutritional edema invariably accompanies periods of famine following war and rapidly disappears when the afflicted are given sufficient food of good quality. Along with the general malnutrition, an inadequacy of proteins appears to be the most important factor in the production of the syndrome. The severe restriction of protein and calories in the diet may lead to the use of body proteins for fuel. If prolonged, large protein deficit may occur in the body with *hypoproteinemia* and *edema*.

In mild cases the edema is usually confined to the lower limbs but when the condition is severe it extends to all parts of the body.

The edema, although in reality a late stage in protein deficiency, is almost the first clinical sign of the deficiency, according to present knowledge. The readiness with which it appears and its clinical picture depend to some extent upon the amount of ingested salt and water. One of the characteristics of the edema is the lack of association with symptoms which suggest other causes of edema, notably heart and kidney disease. Actual loss of weight is usually masked by the edema. In fact, there may be sudden increase in weight, accompanied by weakness and lassitude because of the holding of fluids in the tissues. Subclinical or marginal forms of the hypoproteinemia without edema may occur in debilitating disorders, such as following surgery, severe burns, severe wounds, kidney disease, and in disease with prolonged temperature rise. The most significant and most useful clinical test for protein deficiency is a laboratory test; the measurement of the concentration of the plasma or serum protein.

DIETARY HISTORY The dietary history of the patient is of great importance. (See p. 19.) The inquiry into diet should be made with care because small deficits existing over a long period can cause a deficiency. It is advisable to obtain a record of the kinds and amounts of food eaten during a period of one week or more. From the history a dietary intake can be calculated and an estimate made of the probable intake over a longer period. The calculated intake should be compared with the known standard requirements. Consideration should also be given to the possible deficiency of protein and one or more of the essential amino acids. Thus, the significance of the protein content, quality and utilization, as well as other factors of the diet, such as calorie intake, minerals and vitamins, should be evaluated.

DIETARY TREATMENT In addition to a well-balanced diet, adequate in all the nutritional essentials, proteins of good quality must be provided in abundance. Calories must be adequate to maintain normal weight and to spare body protein. Not only must enough food be available to meet the usual optimal daily requirements, but the body weight and protein deficits produced through years of semi-starvation must be made up.

The return to normal serum protein concentration is slow. Approximately 30 gm. of protein must be deposited in the tissues before 1 gm. is retained in the circulation. Complications, such as severe lesions of the pancreas, may develop with prolonged chronic hypoproteinemia. It also causes an increase in the susceptibility to shock from hemorrhage.

Protein Concentrates Food by mouth is the choice route for the administration of protein. However, for some patients with considerable body protein deficiency, especially if associated with anorexia, it may not be possible to supply sufficient protein orally. Other routes of administration must be used and concentrated protein given by hyperalimentation or stomach tube or parenterally in the form of human plasma, human albumin, gelatin, various hydrolysates of casein, or whole blood. The parenterally administered protein is a useful supplement to the diet but is difficult to give in amounts sufficient to meet the daily requirements.

Supplementary nourishments prepared with protein concentrates are an effective method of increasing the protein intake with limited effort exerted by the patient. The various preparations of hydrolyzed protein rich foods, especially prepared for oral administration, like soybean flours (45 per cent protein), casein (85 per cent protein), dry skim milk (35 per cent protein), wheat germ (35 per cent protein), and "Amigen" (75 per cent protein), can be incorporated into such dishes as puddings, hot cereals, breads, soups, sandwich spreads, and also stirred into milk, fruit juice or tomato juice. They are, however, unpalatable and disturb digestion in some patients. (See also p. 375.)

Kwashiorkor

INCIDENCE The term "kwashiorkor" was given to native children of a certain section of Africa, in whose dialect it means "red boy," because of the resultant depigmentation. It is a comparatively new disease, being first mentioned in literature in 1934 by C. D. Williams, a Jamaican pediatrician working in the African Gold Coast. It is considered the most widespread disease associated with inadequate protein in the tropical and subtropical areas, namely, Africa, Asia, the Middle East, Central and South America. The disease appears among infants and young children in the late breast feeding, weaning and postweaning phases (usually between the ages of 1 and 4 years) wherever children are fed on high carbohydrate, low or poor quality protein diets and, if untreated, has a high mortality; even among children receiving medical and hospital care, mortality still may be as high as 10 to 30 per cent.

ETIOLOGY This disease is caused by insufficient good quality protein, associated with a deficit of calories. It is often aggravated by one or other infectious processes and severe vitamin A deficiency and may result in permanent blindness. In most of the dietary patterns in areas where kwashiorkor is endemic, the intake of animal protein foods is extremely low. The diets are also high in starchy foods and unbalanced in minerals and vitamins. That this disease is, in fact, primarily the result of lack of protein in the diet is supported by the findings of Brock and coworkers.[18, 19] These show that administration of a mixture of amino acids, without supplementary vitamins or other nutrients, is capable of initiating cure.

SYMPTOMS Infants and children afflicted with the disease have a feverish, generally ill condition, accompanied by universal edema, reddish pigmentation of the skin and hair, fatty liver, and loss of the enzymes from the pancreas and intestinal secretions. Additional clinical symptoms are retardation of growth and maturation, weight loss (often masked by edema), diarrhea and a variety of dermatoses. (See Fig. 34–20.)

TREATMENT AND PREVENTION In areas of high prevalence, where economic factors and racial customs limit the variability and availability of proteins, including those of animal origin, prevention is difficult. Treatment and prevention of kwashiorkor lies in education and adoption of infant and preschool child feeding patterns which supply more proteins of relatively high biologic quality when infants are weaned. Until a few years ago the disease was regarded as incurable, but in recent years it has been demonstrated to be easily curable in from 4 to 6 weeks by use of protein-rich foods, such as reconstituted dry skim milk. However, milk is often too costly and/or unavailable where kwashiorkor is prevalent. Thus, the sources of protein must be sought and developed such as a properly selected mixture from available plant or animal sources (mutual supplementation). When economically feasible, powdered dried milk may be included, and this can be extended by judicious mixing with cheaper, locally available concentrates.

A large program for study, evaluation and improvement of children's diets has been carried out for the past several years in cooperation with the government departments of Africa, sponsored jointly by UNICEF, FAO, WHO, and other agencies, particularly the United States Food and Nutrition Board. This program has culminated in the appearance of low cost nutrition foods such as

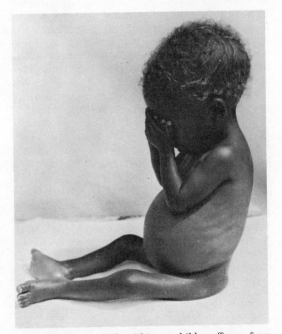

Figure 34–20 A little African child sufferer from kwashiorkor, the regional name for protein malnutrition. Note uncurled graying hair, edema and skin lesions. The condition is common in areas where diets are high in starchy foods and low in protein and can be cured by protein-rich foods or by skim milk. (Courtesy Food and Agriculture Organization of the United Nations. Photo by M. Autret).

[18]Brock, J. F., et al.: Kwashiorkor and protein malnutrition. Lancet, No. 6886:355, 1955.

[19]Brock, J. F., and Hansen, J. D. L.: The role of amino acids in kwashiorkor. Am. J. Clin. Nutrition, 4:286, 1956.

Incaparina evolved by INCAP. This food mixture consists of 29 per cent ground whole maize, 29 per cent ground whole sorghum grain, 38 per cent cottonseed flour, 3 per cent Torula yeast, 1 per cent calcium carbonate, and 4500 units of added vitamin A per 100 gm. The nutritional value of this mixture in infant feeding has been established on practical as well as theoretical grounds. (Also see pp. 78 and 259.)

FAO fostered a survey by Brock and Auret[20] in central and tropical Africa. In their report they suggest long-term measures of prevention of kwashiorkor which include (1) encouragement for increase in the production of protective foods, especially fish, to supplement the present low protein of cereals, cassava and potatoes, (2) storage of food throughout the year to lessen the effect of the hungry months, (3) education, particularly of mothers, in better dietary practices, and (4) the development of a demonstration area, where preventive measures may be introduced, such as the use of dry skim milk. Currently, FAO is encouraging increased protein production for human consumption. It appointed a Protein Advisory Group, which works in close liaison with the staffs of WHO, FAO and UNICEF, and is giving special attention to suitability of such low cost nutritious protein foods as oil seed presscakes, fish meal and soya products for human use. Better utilization of available food supplies is an important part of this program. Also, education in hygiene is needed since infections and parasitic diseases contribute to the development and appearance of this syndrome.

In India where calorie-protein kwashiorkor is prevalent, protein blends containing peanut protein isolate combined with either casein, lysine and methionine or dry skim milk were scientifically tried on groups of children afflicted with the disease. All groups showed satisfactory clinical responses.[21] In Mexico, Peru and Africa fish flour of *high quality* was found to be of considerable value in treatment of convalescent kwashiorkor as a supplement to maize meal diets.[22] Fish flour has a high protein content. In addition, it is a rich source of calcium and phosphorus, and contains considerable magnesium.

Amino acid supplementation of cereal grains and of protein concentrate is of benefit to the people in the cereal-consuming developing countries.[23, 24]

MALNUTRITION

Malnutrition adversely affects the life, development, and health of more people throughout the world than any disease. In certain areas of the United States and in the underdeveloped areas of other parts of the world, malnutrition results from the intake of too few calories, too little high quality protein, and multiple deficiencies of minerals and vitamins. It is complicated further by parasitic, bacterial, and viral infections.

The numerous dietary surveys which have been conducted during the past 10 years show, without exception, that malnutrition is widespread in this country. Although there are relatively few cases of severe malnutrition, there are many mild, chronic cases.

As previously pointed out, malnutrition signifies not a dietary inadequacy but a tissue deficiency of an essential nutrient. (See Table 1–1.)

ETIOLOGY   Probably the most important cause of the tissue deficiency is the failure to eat an adequate diet because of poor food habits, lack of knowledge, or economic status. An adequate diet does not only mean eating enough food to satisfy the appetite but eating the right kinds of food to provide the nutrients that are needed to build, repair, and regulate the body processes.

Sometimes a normal adequate diet is inadequate because factors either interfere with the absorption or utilization of the essential nutrients or increase the destruction, excretion, or requirements for minerals and vitamins. Many people do not eat an adequate diet every day, yet they show no apparent ill effects. This is because their diet is generally good or their requirements are less during the short period of inadequacy. If their diets were faulty for numerous or protracted periods, their bodies would show eventually that they are not getting the proper food.

Formerly, malnutrition was thought of as synonymous with underweight. It has since been demonstrated that weight is an inaccurate yardstick if used as the sole measure to judge the state of nutrition. An overweight person may be malnourished. Judging the nutritional status is not limited to one method

[20]Brock, J. F., and Auret, M.: Kwashiorkor in Africa. FAO Publication No. 8, 1950.

[21]Webb, J. K. G., et al.: Peanut protein and milk protein blends in the treatment of kwashiorkor. Am. J. Clin. Nutr., 14:331, 1964.

[22]Pretorius, P. J., and Wehmeyer, A. S.: An assessment of nutritive value of fish flour in the treatment of convalescent kwashiorkor patients. Am. J. Clin. Nutr., 14:147, 1964.

[23]Howe, E. E., et al.: Amino acid supplementation of cereal grains as related to the world food supply. Am. J. Clin. Nutr., 16:315, 1965.

[24]Howe, E. E., et al.: Amino acid supplementation of protein concentrates as related to the world protein supply. Am. J. Clin. Nutr., 16:321, 1965.

of evaluation. Individualization is of utmost importance in the successful diagnosis and treatment of malnutrition. Malnutrition is frequently associated with several other deficiency diseases which are discussed in this chapter.

MALABSORPTION DEFICIENCIES

There are a number of disorders which interfere with adequate intestinal absorption of essential food elements. Among those discussed elsewhere in this text are celiac disease (Chap. 36), steatorrhea (p. 356), and pancreatitis (p. 371).

SPRUE

Sprue is a disease of unknown etiology believed by many to be a nutritional deficiency disorder. While steatorrhea is the outstanding characteristic of the disease, impaired absorption caused by biochemical or organic disease of the bowel affects all nutrients. A form of anemia, generally of the macrocytic type, is present. The onset of symptoms usually is very gradual, covering a period of months, or years. The patient has loss of appetite and consequent loss of weight, plus emaciation. Osteomalacia and impaired vitamin D absorption resulting in hypocalcemia may occur as a result of calcium losses.

INCIDENCE   Although found in all parts of the United States and Europe (nontropical), it is more common in the Southern states and tropics (tropical); women are affected more frequently than men; and the age group in which it usually occurs is from 20 to 40 years.

DIETARY TREATMENT   Since there is a difference in response to treatment in tropical and nontropical sprue, they will be considered separately.

Tropical Sprue   Folic acid deficiency is believed to be the primary nutritional cause of tropical sprue. Dramatically favorable results have been obtained in patients having tropical sprue with megaloblastic anemia, who were treated with an adequate diet and folic acid.

The diet should be high in protein (120 gm. or more), including liver and lean meat, and low in carbohydrates and fats. Carbohydrates are limited to those from simple sugars, low-starch vegetables, fruits and fruit juices because of faulty absorption. Fats are usually restricted to those which are easily digested and absorbed. Medium chain triglycerides which are absorbed differently from the long chain triglycerides are recommended. Folic acid, frequently 5 to 10 mg. daily, is necessary in addition to the diet. Vitamin supplements, especially vitamin B-complex, calcium and iron should also be administered to help correct the deficiency status.

In the beginning of the treatment, skim milk and ground lean meat are often the only foods tolerated. However, the response to folic acid is usually dramatic, and gradually a more liberal food allowance can be given.

Fatty foods, butter, gravies, cream, oil (especially animal oils), rich desserts, and fats of all kinds must be avoided because they are poorly absorbed. Tolerance to carbohydrates varies with the individual and with the severity of the disease. Bananas, banana preparations (such as flour), and strawberries are the fruits chosen because they are best tolerated by the majority of sprue patients. Orange juice and tomato juice can be taken at an early stage of the treatment, thus providing ascorbic acid. Other nutritional foods are added when improvement indicates. With the gradual addition of foods, the diet reaches normalcy.

Nontropical Sprue (Celiac Sprue)   Concurrent evidence indicates that nontropical sprue is adult celiac disease, identical with idiopathic steatorrhea.[25] Results have not been as favorable in celiac sprue patients, even when adhering to a complete sprue regimen.

The anemia seen in these patients is commonly associated with folic acid deficiency which appears to be caused by unknown interferences with absorption of this vitamin. The problem of therapy in nontropical sprue is complicated by impairment of absorption of multiple nutrients in foods. Therefore, liver extract or vitamin B_{12} or folic acid does not relieve the patient of manifestations of the disease that are unrelated to the deficiency of hemopoietic substances.

The treatment includes reducing or compensating for malfunction of the small bowel and correcting deficiency states. A growing number of investigators suggest that the disease is a manifestation of an abnormal enzyme in the mucosal cell—either a defective or absent enzyme—which fails to digest a toxic peptid contained in gluten which is normally hydrolyzed. Apparently the intestinal epithelium cannot tolerate a glutamine-rich polypeptide contained in gluten. In celiac sprue the polypeptide appears to interfere with normal maturation of the intestinal epithelium, thus injuring the mucosa and causing the pathologic changes which characterize the disease.[26]

[25]Rubin, C. E., et al.: Gastroenterology, *38*:28, 1960; Shiner, M., and Doniach, I.: Gastroenterology, *38*:419, 1960, and Ingelfinger, F. J.: For want of an enzyme. Nutrition Today, 3:2, 1968.

[26]Baker, H., et al.: Mechanisms of folic acid deficiency in nontropical sprue. J.A.M.A., *187*:119, 1964.

Gluten-free Diet   A specific diet[27] omitting the glutamine-bound fraction (glutenin and gliadin) of protein is currently considered the treatment of choice for treatment of celiac sprue disease. In this diet, wheat, rye, barley, and oats are excluded since they all contain a large enough amount of this protein fraction, the toxic substance, to cause symptoms of inability to absorb fat. This means that bakery and packaged foods must be investigated before they are used. The only cereal grains allowed are corn and rice. See Table 34–1 for the diet used and Chapter 43 for recipes. Additional recipes may be found in a booklet by Margaret Abowd, *Low Gluten Diet With Recipes* (Ann Arbor: University Hospital, University of Michigan). Cereal products that can be used as alternates are corn flour, cornmeal, potato flour, rice

flour, soybean flour, and wheat-starch flour (gliadin-free).

Bayles et al.[28] report 6 patients with adult celiac disease who followed the gluten-free diet for 15 months and improved clinically and biochemically, with the histologic appearance of their intestinal mucosa becoming virtually normal. Ruffin[29] reports follow-up observations on 10 patients with celiac sprue treated exclusively with the gluten-free diet for 10 years. Both the immediate and prolonged effect have been satisfactory clinically. Any relapses were due to indiscretions which promptly subsided when gluten was removed from the diet. However, the degree of symptomic and clinical recovery found

[27]Sleisenger, M. H., et al.: A wheat-, rye-, and oat-free diet. J. Am. Dietet. A., 33:1137, 1957.

[28]Bayless, T. M., et al.: Adult celiac disease: Treatment with gluten-free diet. A.M.A. Arch. Int. Med., *111*:83, 1963.
[29]Ruffin, J. M., et al.: Gluten-free diet for nontropical sprue; Immediate and prolonged effects. J.A.M.A., *188*:42, 1964.

TABLE 34–1   WHEAT, RYE, AND OAT-FREE DIET*

This diet is free from cereal proteins, except those found in rice and corn. It is adequate for normal nutrition. The diet for the adult contains approximately 90 Gm. protein, 90 Gm. fat, 200 Gm. carbohydrate, and 2000 kcalories. If a higher caloric diet is desired, a high caloric wheat-, rye-, oat-free diet may be ordered. (All quantities listed are for adults. For children, milk should be increased and size of servings of other foods decreased according to the age of the child.)

FOODS ALLOWED

Milk.........2 glasses or more (more for children); flavored if desired

Eggs.........1 or 2 a day

Meat, fish, and
poultry.....2 medium servings daily (not breaded, creamed, or served with thickened gravy; no bread dressings; otherwise, prepared as desired)

Cheese........as desired

Bread.........made from rice, corn, soy bean, and gluten-free wheat flour only

Cereals.......corn flakes; corn meal; hominy; rice; Rice Krispies; Puffed Rice; pre-cooked rice cereals

Fats..........butter and other fats as desired (note restrictions under *Foods to Be Omitted*)

Vegetables,
potatoes.....as desired, except creamed; include 2 servings green or yellow vegetables and at least 1 raw vegetable daily (the last may be omitted for very young children); rice may be substituted occasionally for potatoes

Fruits.........as desired; 3 servings daily; include citrus fruit once a day

Soups........all clear and vegetable soups; cream soups thickened with cream, cornstarch, or potato flour only

Desserts.......any of the following: gelatin, fruit gelatin; ice or sherbet; homemade ice cream; custard; Junket; rice pudding; cornstarch pudding (homemade); or blanc mange, if thickened with cornstarch

Beverages......milk; fruit juices; ginger ale; cocoa (read label to see that no wheat flour has been added to cocoa or cocoa sirup); for adults, add: coffee (made from ground coffee); tea; carbonated beverages

Sweets........sugar, white or brown; molasses; jellies and jams; honey; corn sirup

FOODS TO BE OMITTED

Meats, fish, and
poultry......meat patties or meat, fish, or chicken loaf made with bread or bread crumbs; croquettes; breaded meats, fish, or chicken; chili con carne and other canned meat dishes; cold cuts, unless guaranteed pure meat; bread stuffings

Gravies, sauces.all gravies or cream sauces thickened with wheat flour

Bread.........all bread, rolls, crackers, cake, and cookies made from wheat or rye; Ry-Krisp; muffins, biscuits, waffles, pancake flour and other prepared mixes; rusks; zwieback; pretzels; any products containing oatmeal, barley, or buckwheat; breaded foods; bread crumbs

Cereals and cereal products.all wheat and rye cereals; wheat germ; barley; oatmeal; buckwheat; kasha; noodles, macaroni, spaghetti, dumplings

Fats..........commercial salad dressings, except pure mayonnaise (read labels)

Vegetables.....any prepared with cream sauce or breaded

Soups........all canned soups, except clear broth; all cream soups, unless thickened with cream, cornstarch, or potato flour

Desserts.......cakes, cookies, pastry; commercial ice cream and ice cream cones; prepared mixes, puddings; all homemade puddings thickened with wheat flour

Beverages......Postum, malted milk, Ovaltine (read labels on instant coffees to see that no wheat flour has been added); for adults: beer, ale

Sweets........commercial candies containing cereal products (read label)

WARNING: *Read labels on all packaged and prepared foods.*

* Sleisenger, M. H., et al., J.Am.Diet.A., *33:*1138, 1957.

had little, if any, correlation with the pathologic picture. The bowel alterations in the small bowel mucosa were unchanged.

Green et al.[30] point out that intestinal function may remain impaired, with steatorrhea persisting, despite good clinical remissions and improved nutritional status after gluten-free dietotherapy. This brings up two points: (1) the possibility that intolerance to gluten is not the ultimate cause of the disease, and (2) if persistence of malabsorption continues, states of nutritional deficiency may develop unless appropriate supplements of vitamins and minerals are added to the gluten-free dietary regimen.

DRUGS Adrenocortical steroids have been observed to facilitate intestinal absorption in the acute stage of the disease in most patients. However, intestinal biopsies taken from these individuals continue to show marked abnormalities despite improvement of symptoms.

---

[30]Green, P. A., et al.: Nontropical sprue. J.A.M.A., *171*: 2157, 1959.

PROBLEMS AND SUGGESTED TOPICS FOR DISCUSSION

1. List the predominating nutrients which are lacking in each of the following deficiency diseases: (1) night blindness, (2) beriberi, (3) ariboflavinosis, (4) pellagra, (5) scurvy, (6) rickets, (7) simple goiter, and (8) tropical sprue. How can a dietary history contribute to the diagnosis?
2. Make a survey of the patients in your hospital who are being treated for deficiency diseases. Obtain diet histories for each type of deficiency disease represented and follow the patients' diets in the hospital. Analyze any typical daily diet obtained from each diet history.
3. In what areas and countries is kwashiorkor prevalent? Why is it found in these areas, and at what age is it most likely to occur? Why? Outline the dietary treatment.
4. Read and prepare a report on recent progress in early recognition and treatment of malnutrition.
5. Discuss the similarities and differences of osteoporosis and osteomalacia. What is the possible cause of each? What segment of the population is usually afflicted? What is the prevention and treatment for each?
6. What is celiac sprue and what is the current treatment? Assist a patient in planning a satisfactory dietary.
7. What adult nutrition deficiency diseases are found in the United States today? What ages and conditions favor deficiency diseases?
8. What is being done in the developing countries to eliminate deficiency diseases?

SUGGESTED ADDITIONAL READING REFERENCES

Autret, M. A., and Behar, M.: Sindrome Policarencial Infantil (Kwashiorkor) and Its Prevention in Central America. Rome, Italy, Food and Agricultural Organization of the United Nations, October, 1954.

Baker, H., et al.: Mechanisms of folic acid deficiency in nontropical sprue. J.A.M.A., *187*:119, 1964.

Bayless, T. M., and Rosensaveig, N. S.: A racial difference in incidence of lactase deficiency. J.A.M.A., *197*:138, 1966.

Bayless, T. M., et al.: Adult celiac disease: Treatment with gluten-free diet. A.M.A. Arch. Intern. Med., *111*:83, 1963.

Bhagavan, R. K., et al.: Use of isolated vegetable proteins in the treatment of protein malnutrition (kwashiorkor). Am. J. Clin. Nutr., *11*:127, 1962.

Bloom, W. L., and Flinchum, D.: Osteomalacia with pseudofractures caused by the ingestion of aluminum hydroxide. J.A.M.A., *174*:1327, 1960.

Brock, J. F., and Autret, M. A.: Kwashiorkor in Africa. Geneva, Switzerland, World Health Organization, Monograph Series No. 8, 1952.

Council on Food and Nutrition: Malnutrition and hunger in the United States. J.A.M.A., *213*:July 13, 1970.

Dairy Council Digest: Nutrition in oral health: Research and practice. 40:No. 6, 1969.

Downs, E. F.: Nutritional dwarfing: A syndrome of early protein-calorie malnutrition. Am. J. Clin. Nutr., 15: 275, 1965.

Duncan, G. G. (ed.): Diseases of Metabolism. 5th ed. Philadelphia, W. B. Saunders Company, 1964, Chapter 7, Vitamins and Avitaminosis.

Follis, R. H.: Some unsolved problems concerning the pathogenesis of human deficiency disease syndromes. Am. J. Clin. Nutr., 6:459, 1958.

Fraser, D.: Clinical manifestations of genetic aberrations of calcium and phosphorus metabolism. J.A.M.A., *176*:281, 1961.

Gershoff, S. N.: Who is well nourished? Nutr. Rev., *19*:321, 1961.

Green, P. A., et al.: Nontropical sprue. J.A.M.A., *171*:2157, 1959.

Hegsted, D. M.: Nutrition, bone and calcified tissue. J. Am. Dietet. A., *50*:105, 1967.

Human pantothenic acid deficiency. Nutr. Rev., *14*:37, 1956.

Ingelfinger, F. J.: For want of an enzyme. Nutrition Today, 3:2, 1968.

Jansen, G. R., and Howie, E. E.: World problems in protein nutrition. Am. J. Clin. Nutr., *15*:262, 1964.

Jolliffe, N.: Diagnosis and treatment of nutritional deficiencies. Am. J. Digest. Dis., *1*:323, 1956.

Jolliffe, N.: Clinical Nutrition. 2nd ed. New York, Harper & Brothers, 1962, Chapter 1, The pathogenesis of deficiency disease; Chapter 2, The clinical signs; Chapter 3, Protein deficiency; Chapter 4, Caloric deficiency and starvation; Chapter 11, Iodine malnutrition; Chapter 13, Vitamin A malnutrition; Chapter 14, Vitamin D and rickets; Chapter 16, Thiamine malnutrition; Chapter 17, Riboflavin malnutrition; Chapter 18, Niacinamide malnutrition and pellagra; Chapter 20, Vitamin C malnutrition and scurvy.

Lutwak, L.: Nutritional aspects of osteoporosis. J. Am. Geriat. Soc., *17*:115, 1969.

Lutwak, L.: Osteoporosis – A mineral deficiency disease? J. Am. Dietet. A., *44*:173, 1964.

McLaren, D. S.: Xerophthalmia. Am. J. Clin. Nutr., *11*:603, 1962.

McLaren, D. S.: Xerophthalmia: A neglected problem. Nutr. Rev., *22*:289, 1964.

Medical News. Fluoride, calcium salts, hormones tried in osteoporosis therapy. J.A.M.A., *188*:27, 1964.

Nizel, A. E., and Shulman, J. S.: Interaction of dietetics and nutrition with dentistry. Recent advances and needs. J. Am. Dietet. A., *55*:470, 1969.

Nordin, B. E.: Calcium balance and calcium requirement in spinal osteoporosis. Am. J. Clin. Nutr., *10*:384, 1962.

Pak, C. Y. C., et al.: The treatment of osteoporosis with calcium infusions. Am. J. Med., *47*:7, 1969.

Pearson, W. N.: Biochemical appraisal of the vitamin nutritional status in man. J.A.M.A., *180*:49, 1962.

Pereira, S. M., and Begum, A.: Prevention of vitamin A deficiency. Am. J. Clin. Nutr., *22*:858, 1969.

Pretorius, P. J., and Wehmeyer, A. S.: An assessment of nutritive value of fish flour in the treatment of convalescent kwashiorkor patients. Am. J. Clin. Nutr., *14*:147, 1964.

Review. A possible role for leucine in niacin biosynthesis

and in the pathogenesis of pellagra. Nutr. Rev., *21*: 334, 1963.

Review. Calcium deficiency in the etiology of osteoporosis. Nutr. Rev., *21*:181, 1963.

Review. Calcium metabolism in osteoporosis. Nutr. Rev., *19*:269, 1961.

Review. Clinical nutritional problems in the United States today. Nutr. Rev., *23*:1, 1965.

Review. Etiology of follicular hyperkeratosis. Nutr. Rev., *21*:106, 1963.

Review. Gluten enteropathy. Nutr. Rev., *21*:300, 1963.

Review. Goiter and iodine deficiency. Nutr. Rev., *22*:169, 1964.

Review. Idiopathic steatorrhea. Nutr. Rev., *21*:168, 1963.

Review. Intestinal calcium and bone formation. Nutr. Rev., *23*:6, 1965.

Review. Nutritional rickets and parathyroid function. Nutr. Rev., *21*:271, 1963.

Ruffin, J. M., et al.: Gluten-free diet for nontropical sprue: Immediate and prolonged effects. J.A.M.A., *188*:42, 1964.

Schaefer, A. E.: Nutritional deficiencies in developing countries. J. Am. Dietet. A., *42*:295, 1963.

Schwartz, M. K., et al.: The effect of a gluten-free diet on fat, nitrogen and mineral metabolism in patients with sprue. Gastroenterology, *32*:232, 1957.

Scrimshaw, N. S.: Synergism of malnutrition and infection. J.A.M.A., *212*:1685, 1970.

Scrimshaw, N. S., et al.: Kwashiorkor in children and its response to protein therapy. J.A.M.A., *164*:555, 1957.

Scrimshaw, N. S.: Progress in solving world nutrition problems. J. Am. Dietet. A., *35*:441, 1959.

Sherlock, P., and Rothchild, E. O.: Scurvy produced by a zen macrobiotic diet. J.A.M.A., *199*:130, 1967.

Shils, M. E.: Experimental human magnesium depletion. I. Clinical observations and blood chemistry alterations. Am. J. Clin. Nutr., *15*:133, 1964.

Smith, R. W., et al.: Determinants of serum antirachitic activity—Special reference to involutional osteoporosis. Am. J. Clin. Nutr., *14*:98, 1964.

Stein, I., and Beller, M. L.: Therapeutic progress in osteoporosis. Geriatrics, *25*:159, 1970.

Tandon, M. I., et al.: Small intestine in protein malnutrition. Am. J. Clin. Nutr., *21*:813, 1968.

Walker, A. R. P.: Osteoporosis and calcium deficiency. Am. J. Clin. Nutr., *16*:327, 1965.

Webb, J. K., et al.: Peanut protein and milk protein blends in the treatment of kwashiorkor. Am. J. Clin. Nutr., *14*:331, 1964.

Whitehead, R. G., and Dean, R. F. A.: Serum amino acids in kwashiorkor. I. Relationship to clinical condition. Am. J. Clin. Nutr., *14*:313, 1964.

Williams, R. R.: Can we eradicate the classical deficiency diseases? J. Am. Dietet. A., *36*:31, 1960.

Wray, J. B., et al.: Bone composition in senile osteoporosis. J.A.M.A., *183*:118, 1963.

Chapter 35

NUTRITION IN DISEASES OF THE MUSCULOSKELETAL SYSTEM

ARTHRITIS

Arthritis may be defined as inflammation of the joints. It has been estimated that at least 4,500,000 persons in the United Stats are afflicted with arthritis of one kind or another. It is one of the diseases which people dread and fear.

The disease may develop into one of many types. Formerly the classification was rather vague but now definite groups have been established. A widely used system of classification[1] is as follows:

1. Arthritis due to specific infectious agents.
2. Arthritis due to direct trauma.
3. Rheumatic fever.
4. Rheumatoid arthritis.
5. Osteoarthritis.
6. Gout.
7. Less common diseases of joints, such as neuropathic arthropathy and tumors.

Arthritis may be acute or chronic. Any acute attack is of short duration but may recur and develop into a chronic condition. When acute arthritis involves multiple joints, rheumatic fever is a likely cause, particularly in a young person. (See Chapter 22, Diet in Febrile Diseases, for discussion of rheumatic fever.) Rheumatoid and degenerative arthritis comprise the most common forms of chronic arthritis, and of these two rheumatoid is the more prominent.

RHEUMATOID ARTHRITIS

The etiology of rheumatoid or atrophic arthritis is unknown. It is a systemic disease

---

[1]Robinson, W. D.: J.A.M.A., *166*:253, 1958. For a more detailed classification officially adopted by the American Rheumatism Association, see J.A.M.A., *171*:1206, 1959.

believed to result from a generalized infection, with joint disturbances only one of the manifestations. These persons are usually underweight and undernourished.

Any joint may be attacked but multiple involvement of the small joints of the extremities, most frequently the proximal interphalangeal joints, hands and feet, is the rule. Pain, stiffness and swelling are the common complaints (Fig. 35–1). The swelling or puffiness is caused by the accumulation of fluid in the lining membranes and inflammation of the surrounding tissues. In severe cases disability may result.

The incidence of rheumatoid arthritis is reported to increase twofold in the later decades, with as high as 15 per cent occurring in females over 60 in some population studies, the average age of onset being 35 years, followed generally by numerous remissions and exacerbations. It occurs much more frequently in females than in males, the proportion averaging three females to one male. While patients with rheumatoid arthritis are frequently underweight, those with osteoarthritis are often overweight. Because of the chronic disability and pain which accompanies arthritis, these individuals are often given unwise or even harmful dietary advice. They become easy prey to the solicitous neighbor, food faddist and charlatan who offer quick and easy cures. The nurse must be alert to this and use every opportunity available to stress good health habits, including a well-balanced diet.

DIETARY TREATMENT Numerous diets have been devised for the treatment of rheumatoid arthritis. At one time or another a low carbohydrate diet, high protein diet, the B-complex vitamins, vitamin C, vitamin A, and sulfur have been advocated.

The use of massive therapeutic doses of

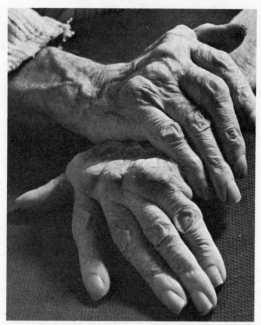

Figure 35–1   A patient with advanced rheumatoid arthritis. Note the twisted hands and the puffiness of the meta-
carpal joints, typical of the disease. (Courtesy of George E.
Pickow, Three Lions, Inc.)

vitamin D has fallen into disrepute largely
because this form of treatment resulted in
severe and sometimes even fatal calcification
of the kidneys. Potent vitamin D preparations
are capable of causing damage because of the
effect of vitamin D on calcium and phosphorus metabolism.

At present, the trend is to treat rheumatoid
arthritis with a normal well-balanced diet,
with calories adjusted to maintain the patient's weight at normal standards. Obesity
should be discouraged. Since the condition is
a chronic disease, measures should be used to
improve the general health of the patient. It is
important to survey the person's dietary pattern and eating habits. The teaching is focused on how the person's dietary may be
improved in order to have a well-balanced
diet and to maintain weight at the desired
level. Many arthritic patients have poor dietaries and eating habits and need to be encouraged to obtain an adequate diet daily and
control weight. Underweight individuals require sufficient calories high in protein, minerals and vitamins to attain the desired
weight. Liver, frequently included in the diet,
will supply vitamin A, vitamin B-complex and
iron. Low blood values for ascorbic acid are
found frequently in rheumatoid arthritis patients. Appropriate vitamin and mineral supplementation may be in order.

It is reported that up to 50 per cent of persons with rheumatoid arthritis overcome the
disease process spontaneously. This means
that the body is capable of building up enough
resistance to the disease. This is encouraged
through a well-directed, daily regimen of
living, including a well-balanced diet.

Hypochromic anemia is found frequently
associated with arthritis, but it does not always respond well to the administration of
iron. However, there is a dramatic response to
the transfusion of whole blood.

HORMONES AND DRUGS   In 1949 rheumatoid arthritis was found to respond dramatically to two hormones, corticotropin
(ACTH) and cortisone. Corticotropin is released by the pituitary gland and acts by stimulating the adrenal cortex to release cortisone,
which relieves pain and stiffness in patients
with rheumatoid arthritis. Since then, several
synthetic variations of cortisone or the
adrenocorticosteroids have been produced
which are more potent and even more effective. Side effects are less common with the
synthetic products because they are effective
in minute amounts. In addition, intravenous
injections of antimalarial drugs are sometimes of benefit in inducing a remission in
younger persons. The drugs hold symptoms in
abeyance, but, when stopped, recurrences
often follow. Most authorities recommend
continued treatment over months or years,
even though the condition has improved.
However, prolonged use of these drugs may
upset sodium metabolism and result in sodium retention and edema. Calcium balance
may be adversely affected, which results in
gradual bone demineralization and bone fracture. (See sodium restricted diets in Chapter
30, Cardiovascular Diseases.)

OSTEOARTHRITIS (DEGENERATIVE, HYPERTROPHIC ARTHRITIS)

Osteoarthritis, also known as hypertrophic
and degenerative arthritis, is more prevalent
among people past 40 years. It probably does
not have a single cause but seems to develop
from the stresses and strains experienced
during the course of one's life. It may follow
injuries and other diseases of the joints and
be influenced by congenital and mechanical
derangements of the joints. Numerous studies
have established that the primary lesion is
degeneration of the articular cartilage.

The joints most likely to be attacked are the
distal interphalangeal joints and the thumb
joint, and especially the joints that bear the
bulk of the weight: the knees, hips, ankles,
and spine. In the beginning there is stiffness,
usually on arising from a chair or after standing. Later definite soreness may be experienced, which is worse when motion is first

attempted but, after warming up, is less noticeable. One or more joints may be affected, and usually symptoms are confined to the afflicted parts. In this respect, the condition differs from rheumatoid arthritis, in which the general health may suffer.

DIETARY TREATMENT   Diet is important in the role of reducing obesity. Excess bulk means an added burden for the weight-bearing joints. Symptoms have been known to disappear completely after the loss of unnecessary pounds. Thus, the main dietary treatment is to direct attention toward acquiring a normal weight. (See Chapter 29 for discussion on losing weight.) Some authorities believe that, in addition to the wear and tear of aging, there is a disturbance of the metabolic process of the body, similar to that which produces atherosclerosis. Obesity, fatigue, injury and stress affect osteoarthritis in much the same way they influence atherosclerosis. Weight reduction and the maintenance of weight at the desired level are indicated in both conditions.

DRUGS   The more potent steroids are used for severe pain and disability but are not so effective as in other types of arthritis.

GOUT

Gout is included in the classification of arthritis because of the frequent occurrence of crippling of the joints. In this textbook it is discussed in Chapter 28, Metabolic Disorders Related to Nutrition; it is caused by an inborn error of metabolism.

LEAD POISONING

ETIOLOGY   Lead poisoning may occur after the prolonged use of salts of lead for medicinal purposes. It may also be introduced into the body through drinking water, food, hair dye, and cosmetics. Workmen who are exposed to the fumes and dust of lead, or who handle metal and paints containing lead, are apt to develop lead poisoning. It is considered the most serious, most frequent, and most insidious of all occupational poisons. It is a typical cumulative one. Lead may enter the body via the skin, the gastrointestinal or the respiratory tract. *Prevention* is the all-important factor.

Most of the lead which enters the body is transferred from the blood stream to the bones where it is stored. It is harmless in the bones. However, if released in large quantities, toxic effects result.

Anemia with diminished platelets and polymorphonuclear leukocytes occurs in both subacute and chronic lead poisoning.

DIETARY TREATMENT   There is considerable difference of opinion as to the value of dietary treatment of lead poisoning at present. A fairly universal treatment during the acute stage consists of a diet high in calcium content plus injections of a calcium chloride solution and administration of vitamin D. The purpose of the additional calcium and vitamin D is to prevent further withdrawal of lead from the bones and to encourage the return of the lead from the blood to the bones. The normal adequate diet, with the inclusion of one to two quarts of vitamin D milk, is favored. Cheese is added to the meals three to four times a week. After the acute stage has passed, a low calcium diet is sometimes given to permit a gradual withdrawal of lead from the bones. Consult Table 19–4, Principal Sources of Food Constituents, for the list of foods containing calcium. Also, consult Chapter 8, and Appendix Table 7. When the poisoning is accompanied by anemia, the diet should contain increased protein of high biologic value and iron-rich foods.

DRUGS   The most recent treatment of severe lead poisoning is the use of intravenous calcium disodium ethylenediaminetetraacetate (EDTA), which removes the lead from the patient's system without causing an exacerbation of symptoms. Orally given, the drug has been used in follow-up therapy and as initial therapy in milder cases. However, oral use is dangerous if there is continued exposure to lead or if lead is present in the gastrointestinal tract. This drug increases urinary excretion of the metal and decreases excretion of porphyrin. Abdominal pain is rapidly relieved when the drug is combined alternately with intravenous calcium gluconate. In this compound the lead replaces the calcium, forming the lead derivative, which is rapidly eliminated in the urine.

DENTAL CARIES

Tooth decay is the most prevalent chronic disease in the United States, and occurs among all populations throughout the world. Some primitive people[2] such as older Eskimos, some Pacific islanders, Greenlanders and South Africans, who live in remote areas of the world under native or natural conditions, are more free from dental caries than civilized man. When these persons come into contact with civilization, they frequently experience increased incidence of tooth decay. The cause is believed to be due, in major degree, to a change in their diets.

ETIOLOGY   Dental caries are characterized by demineralization of the inorganic por-

---

[2]Control of Tooth Decay. National Academy of Sciences – National Research Council, 1953.

tion and dissolution of the organic substance of teeth. Dental caries are recognized as an infection caused by the cariogenic streptococci. The carious process begins with the production of acid by the bacterial enzymatic action of carbohydrates in the dental plaque and the organic acids cause decalcification of the enamel. Proteolytic degradation and demineralization of the dentin follows. It has been shown that three factors must be present simultaneously for dental caries to develop: (1) food must be in contact with the tooth; (2) the specific food is carbohydrate, principally sucrose; and (3) bacteria must be present on the surface of the tooth.[3] The most important relationship of nutrition to dental caries occurs during the development of the teeth. The greatest hope in preventive dentistry lies in the development of teeth with a high resistance to tooth decay. Close adherence to an adequate diet throughout the period of tooth development is of major importance in attaining this end. A review of the reports reveals there is increasing evidence that dental caries is, in part at least, the result of a faulty diet; many theories have been suggested to explain this. No one knows why some individuals are more addicted to dental caries. Hereditary influences have been demonstrated in experimental animals. We know that among humans some families have good teeth, whereas others do not.

Carbohydrates   The current, dominant theory is that decay is caused by a chemical-bacterial action, acting from outside directly upon the enamel and dentin of the teeth. The cariogenic bacteria apparently act upon sucrose to produce an extracellular polyssacharide, dextran and acids. The acids dissolve the calcium in the tooth to form a cavity. Other sugars and starches produce very little or no decay in experimental animals and man.[4] Carbohydrates have been proved mandatory for the metabolism of caries-producing oral flora.[5] Carbohydrate fermentation is a necessary part of the decay process. Fermentable carbohydrate particles adhering to susceptible tooth surfaces or in the crevices of the teeth allow the caries-producing organisms to grow. Bacteria are capable of fermenting carbohydrate to form acid and enzymes, which are generally believed to cause the initial process of tooth decay. Bacterial metabolism and growth lead to destruction of both the tooth enamel and the dentin.

Years ago Bunting and co-workers carried on studies to demonstrate that unrestricted amounts of candy in the diet of a group of 51 children produced an increase in caries in 31 per cent of the group in 5 months and also an increase in the lactobacillus count. Drain and Boyd reported remarkable success in arresting the progress of caries among diabetic patients who were on diets low in carbohydrate content. On the other hand, these same investigators produced arrest of caries with diets which included sweets but also adequate proteins and calories and a high intake of vitamins and minerals.

An extensive experiment, on the relationship between tooth decay and the form in which carbohydrate is taken, was carried on in Vipsholm, Sweden. Under institutional circumstances, patients were given a variety of carbohydrate supplements to the basic, highly nutritious diet. When sucrose in solution was added to the diet over prolonged periods of time, there was practically no increase in the incidence of dental caries. However, when the sugar was fed in the form of sticky candies that adhered to the teeth, the incidence of dental caries increased far above that of tooth decay during the preliminary control period. As soon as these candy supplements were stopped, tooth decay quickly dropped to the control level. In other groups of patients, the sugar was fed in breads, or in less sticky candies. More severe effects were observed than with sugar in solution, but less severe effects than with the sticky candies. A marked increase in caries activity occurs when sweets are consumed between meals. It is logical to conclude from these observations that the longer the carbohydrate is retained in the oral cavity, the greater the possibility of tooth decay. Thus, the physical characteristics of the carbohydrates determine to a large extent their influence on dental caries. In addition, it is generally accepted that carbohydrates must remain in the mouth and must be available to bacteria to cause dental caries. Frequency of eating is an important factor in caries causation, and between-meal eating is to be discouraged, unless noncariogenic foods are consumed. Numerous workers report encouraging results in preventing dental caries with the use of dentifrices containing enzyme inhibitors or substances which prevent the formation of acid on the tooth surface after ingestion of foods, especially sweets. Further research and longer time are needed to evaluate their use.

Minerals   The importance of minerals in the diet, more specifically calcium and phosphorus, has been discussed elsewhere. Since these minerals make up a large percentage of the enamel and dentin of teeth, an ample

[3]Nizel, A. E., and Shulman, J. S.: Dietetics and dentistry. J. Am. Dietet. A., 55:470, 1969.

[4]Massler, M.: Nutrition and dental decay. Food and Nutrition News. National Live Stock and Meat Board, 39: No. 5, 1968.

[5]Bibby, B. G.: Cariogenicity of foods. J.A.M.A., 177:316, 1961.

amount must be supplied in the diet if the teeth are to be sound.

Fluorine   The incidence of dental caries and its relation to the *fluorine* content of the drinking water has been studied. It would appear from the extensive studies of the United States Public Health Service that minute amounts of fluoride taken during the first 8 to 12 years of life—the period when dentin and enamel of the permanent dentition are being formed—will reduce the incidence of dental caries by as much as 65 per cent. This increased resistance is believed to be carried over into later life to an appreciable degree. Fluorine is believed to act systemically or locally by adsorption or in combination in enamel, or in dentin, and more significantly on the tooth surface; it inhibits bacterial invasion or makes the enamel resistant to acid.

Following favorable results from years of water fluoridation in well-controlled studies[6] in Evanston, Illinois, Newburgh, New York, and elsewhere, fluorine is now being added to the drinking water in a number of cities and communities as a prophylactic agent to reduce the incidence of dental caries. The best level considered to be protective is 1.0 to 1.5 parts per million parts of drinking water. When fluorine exceeds 1.5 parts per million, as occurs naturally in some areas, mottling of the enamel is apt to occur (Fig. 8–3). Review Fluorine in Chapter 8.

The addition of fluorine to drinking water found to be free from, or extremely low in, the mineral meets with the approval of the Division of Medical Sciences, National Research Council and WHO, providing it is done under the supervision of the state board of health. Virtually every authoritative public health and medical organization recommends fluoridation, including the American Medical Association, the American Dental Association, and the American Academy of Pediatrics. In reviewing the results of the fluoridation program in 17 countries, the WHO's Expert Committee on the Public Health Aspects of Water Fluoridation found the incidence of dental caries in the permanent teeth of children to have decreased about 60 per cent. Fluoridation also lessens the severity of the caries. In areas with non-fluoridated water, other media used which have demonstrated an appreciable caries-inhibitory effect are milk,[7] prophylactic pastes, fluoride dentifrices, chewing gums, and topical gels. However, water is considered by far the most desirable media.

Vitamins   Many research investigations have been carried on to show the relation between vitamins and the health of the teeth. Research workers have observed that the incisor teeth of rats and guinea pigs are affected by vitamin A deficiency, with a suppression of enamel formation and deformities of the dentin. Similar changes have been reported in the gums of a human infant with vitamin A deficiency. There is no definite evidence that vitamin A is concerned directly with dental caries but it is a vital factor in the formation of dental enamel.

There is no conclusive evidence that lack of any of the B-complex vitamins brings increased susceptibility to decay; however, vitamin B_6 may function in caries control. Painful teeth may be due to a neuritis which is secondary to vitamin B deficiency.

Other research workers have placed great emphasis on ascorbic acid and its relation to both tooth structure and caries. The tooth structure is one of the first parts of the body to show histologic changes when the animal is kept on a vitamin C-free diet. The vitamin is known to be important in building teeth and in maintaining health of gums and other structures. There has not been satisfactory evidence that susceptibility to decay is reduced by giving vitamin C to individuals on a partially deficient C diet. Nor has it been found that scurvy makes a person more subject to tooth decay. In extensive studies on the teeth of 341 children which Hanke made at Moosehart, an institution for children near Chicago, he found that gingivitis disappeared in most of the children and caries was arrested in 50 per cent when one pint of orange

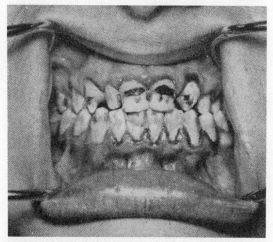

Figure 35–2   Excessive enamel hypoplasia of the anterior teeth of a 16-year-old girl caused by severe malnutrition at the age of 6 months. The marked gingivitis on lower anterior gingiva cleared up quickly as a result of vitamin C therapy. (L. R. Cahn: Pathology of the Oral Cavity. The Williams & Wilkins Co.)

[6]Ast, D. B., and Fitzgerald, B.: Effectiveness of water fluoridation. J. Am. Dent. A., 65:581, 1962.

[7]Rusoff, L. L., et al.: Fluoride addition to milk and its effect on dental caries in school children. Am. J. Clin. Nutr., 11:94, 1962.

juice and the juice of one lemon were added to the adequate daily diet (Fig. 35–2). Changes in the gum tissues are characteristic of scurvy and an improvement of this condition would be expected when ascorbic acid is added to the diet. However, it was not shown that the arrest of caries was due entirely to the addition of ascorbic acid.

Experimenting on several hundred dogs, Mellanby found it possible to modify the calcification of the teeth by varying the amount of vitamin D in the diet, although true caries was not produced. Extending the studies to children in institutions, Mellanby found that an improved diet and the addition of vitamin D prevented the spread of caries. It is known that vitamin D is inseparably linked with the metabolism of calcium and phosphorus, promoting greater absorption of these mineral elements. It is an interesting observation that Mellanby found a greater incidence in the production of caries on a high cereal intake, especially oatmeal, which seemed to interfere with the normal calcium and phosphorus metabolism, increasing the need for vitamin D. One group of investigators found ultraviolet light more effective as a protective agent against dental caries than other sources of vitamin D.

PROPHYLACTIC DIET SUGGESTIONS
There seems to be agreement that diet and the incidence of dental caries are closely related. The adequate normal diet (Chapter 11, and Table 19–1) should be followed, with restriction of foods containing readily adherent, fermentable carbohydrates such as sticky candy or other concentrated sweets. Jams, jellies, candies, sugar, heavily sugared beverages or soft drinks, and all excessive sweets should be discouraged. The intake of nonadherent, rough, coarse foods, such as raw carrots, lettuce, celery, apples and most fruits and vegetables, that clean the teeth by friction is suggested to aid control of dental caries. The longer food is in contact with the teeth, the greater the reaction. Thus, it is claimed that the thicker and more gelatinous foods are more likely to cause dental caries than those of thinner consistency. It has been demonstrated that enamel decalcification occurs during *every* food ingestion as the result of a virtual acid bath from bacterial action on the ingested carbohydrate. The decalcification can be inhibited for the most part if proper oral hygiene is followed and if the "acid bath" exposures are not too frequent. Brushing the teeth and/or rinsing the mouth immediately after each meal or snack will remove the food particles and reduce the reactions. Dentists have discovered that most of the chemical reactions take place within 15 minutes after the meal is started.

The same dietary rules are true for children, and during pregnancy, and lactation. The minerals from the mother's reserve are drawn upon to meet the demands of the growing fetus and later for milk production during the period of lactation. Satisfactory prenatal nutrition is needed for the teeth of the child. The Committee on Dental Health, Food and Nutrition Board, states, "New evidence points toward the dominant importance of building decay-resistant teeth which means a good diet for the mother and for the child from infancy through adolescence."[8]

It has been demonstrated that the early development of the teeth is influenced by the amount of calcium, phosphorus, fluorine, and vitamins in the diet. Consequently, these substances should be supplied in adequate amounts in the diet during pregnancy and of the infant, the growing child, and the adult. An ample supply of vitamin D should be provided daily throughout the period of growth and development. A highly desirable factor in the over-all diet planning for the attainment of maximum caries resistance is the availability of a fluoridated water supply. There is considerable evidence from laboratories and clinics that dental decay can be arrested through an adequate dietary. Reduction in caries has been experimentally produced through the addition of phosphates to the diet. Large scale studies are currently being made on humans.

The status of teeth is often reflected in the general health of an individual. Poorly formed, missing or painful teeth may result in consuming an inadequate diet and in bolting of food, followed by impaired digestion and poor health. Many physicians and dentists believe the poisonous products from decayed teeth to be among the causes of chronic diseases that involve the heart, the kidneys, and the joints.

Denture patients are apt to avoid foods difficult to chew and will resort to soft foods and tend to avoid meat, raw vegetables and fruit and salads. In counseling these patients the person's dietary pattern is obtained; an evaluation of the adequacy of the dietary practice is determined; a plan within his limitations is developed which will enable him to consume a more adequate diet.

[8]Control of Tooth Decay. Committee on Dental Health, Food and Nutrition Board, National Research Council, 1953.

PROBLEMS AND SUGGESTED TOPICS FOR DISCUSSION

1. Make a survey of the wards in your hospital for patients who are suffering with arthritis. Classify the types of arthritis. Obtain a diet history from a patient with rheumatoid arthritis. Analyze the diet history for carbohy-

drates, proteins, fats, calories, minerals (calcium, phosphorus and iron), and vitamins. Calculate a meal plan based on the diet treatment outlined in this text for rheumatoid arthritis.
2. Plan a high calorie diet with an underweight patient who has rheumatoid arthritis with extensive crippling of the hands. Use easy to handle and easy to eat foods.
3. Plan a reduction diet with an obese patient in your hospital who is suffering with osteoarthritis. Follow her progress.
4. Visit the dental clinic in your hospital and obtain a diet history from a patient with severe dental caries. Analyze the diet. Assist the patient with the correct nutritious diet and include suggestions for tooth decay prevention.
5. Find out the fluorine content of the water in your community and give a report. Is it low, adequate or excessive?
6. Outline a suitable diet for a patient who has chronic lead poisoning. What method of treatment is used in your hospital?

SUGGESTED ADDITIONAL READING REFERENCES

Ast, D. B., and Fitzgerald, B.: Effectiveness of water fluoridation. J. Am. Dent. A., 65:581, 1962.

Cohen, A., et al.: Treatment of rheumatoid arthritis with dexamethasone. J.A.M.A., 174:831, 1960.

Committee on Dental Health, Food and Nutrition Board, National Academy of Sciences–National Research Council: Control of Tooth Decay, 1953.

Cox, G. J.: Nutrition and dental health. National Livestock and Meat Board. Food and Nutrition News, 35(No. 5): Feb., 1964.

Dairy Council Digest: Nutrition in oral health: Research and practice. 40:No. 6, 1969.

Editorial. Fluoridation of public water supplies. J.A.M.A., 186:64, 1963.

Fosdick, L. S.: Enzyme inhibitory agents. J. Am. Dent. A., 48:19, 1954.

Holbrook, W. P., et al.: Current status of the treatment of rheumatoid arthritis. J.A.M.A., 164:1469, 1957.

Jaschik, E., and Olsen, C.: Nursing care of the arthritic patient at home. Am. J. Nursing, 55:429, 1955.

Lead poisoning. J.A.M.A., 158:47, 1955.

Massler, M.: Nutrition and dental decay. Food and Nutrition News. National Live Stock and Meat Board, 39: Feb., 1968.

Nizel, A. E., and Shulman, J. S.: Interaction of dietetics and nutrition with dentistry. J. Am. Dietet. A., 55:479, 1969.

Primer on the rheumatic diseases. J.A.M.A., Part I, 171: 1205; Part II. 171:1345, Part III, 171:1680. 1959.

Ragan, C., and Farrington, E.: The clinical features of rheumatoid arthritis. J.A.M.A., 181:663, 1962.

Review. Cariogenic ability of different diets. Nutr. Rev., 21:50, 1963.

Review. The diet of patients with arthritis. Nutr. Rev., 21:203, 1963.

Robinson, W. D.: Nutrition and joint disease. J.A.M.A., 166:253, 1958.

Shaw, J. H.: Nutrition and dental caries. J.A.M.A., 166: 633, 1958.

Shaw, J. H.: Nutrition and tooth decay. National Livestock and Meat Board. Food and Nutrition News, 34(No. 4): Jan., 1963.

Svartz, N.: The rheumatoid factor and its significance. J.A.M.A., 177:50, 1961.

Symposium. Nutrition in Tooth Formation and Dental Caries. J.A.M.A., 177:304, 1961.

Tank, G.: Recent advances in dental caries. J. Am. Dietet. A., 46:293, 1965.

Ursini, D. G.: Preventive dentistry. New York State Society of Dentistry for Children, 6:8, 1955.

Weiss, R., and Trithard, A.: Between-meal eating habits and dental caries experience in preschool children. Am. J. Pub. Health, 50:1097, 1960.

Wohl, M. G., and Goodhart, R. S. (ed.): Modern Nutrition in Health and Disease. 3rd ed. Philadelphia, Lea & Febiger, 1964. Chapter 20, Nutrition in relation to dental medicine; Chapter 29, Nutrition in rheumatism, arthritis and gout.

Zimmer, F. E.: Lead poisoning in scrap-metal workers. J.A.M.A., 175:238, 1961.

DIET THERAPY
IN DISEASES OF
INFANCY AND
CHILDHOOD

The nutritional needs of the child who is ill are the same as or greater than those of the well child of the same age and development. Special consideration should be given to the child on a therapeutic regimen to assist him in meeting his normal nutritional needs for growth and development as well as the particular therapeutic requirements. While the nutritional state of the sick child may not have caused his physical condition, adequate intake of the essential nutrients plays an important part in the control of the disease process and the rate of recovery.

A child's response to illness and hospitalization may lead to undesirable change in eating behavior. Usually this is not serious and when feeling better he will return to his usual eating habits. Food must be served attractively and taste good to the sick child. If the appetite is poor, small meals served more frequently may be helpful. Ingenuity in meal planning and meal preparation may stimulate the appetite. Participation by the nurse in mealtime activities encourages the child to eat (Fig. 36-1). Food whimsies must not become a firmly established habit or it may become a problem. Children are usually interested in learning. They desire to participate in activities. The approach to change a child's dietary habit should be to gain his interest in food and to have him tell you what he knows about food. He can tell the foods that he believes to be good and those he usually ingests. The nurse accepts the child's sugges-

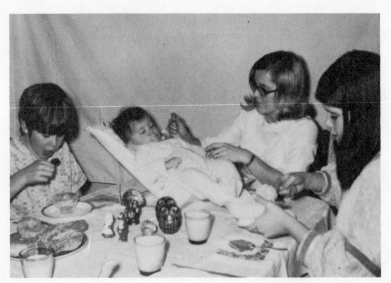

Figure 36-1 These children are obviously enjoying their breakfast under the supervision of an understanding nurse.

tions and reinforces those that are appropriate. This approach tells the nurse how to make suggestions for improvement in his dietary.

Because emotional factors are involved, with the child being separated from parents, and the trauma of medical or surgical treatments, it is difficult to alter food habits or introduce new foods at this time (see Chapter 2).

FEBRILE DISEASES

Chronic and acute infections have been found to influence the growth rate in children. Children seriously ill over a long time grow more slowly than healthy children, even when the food intake is adequate.

Statistics show that the mortality rate of children 5 to 19 years of age has dropped 40 per cent since World War II. This remarkable change is due largely to the further control of infectious diseases, namely, tuberculosis, pneumonia, and rheumatic fever. Medical advances, pure milk and water, general sanitation, disease control, wholesome food, plus improved living conditions in general have all had a part.

ACUTE INFECTIONS

Fever is the most important sign of infection. Children suffering from acute infections of short duration, such as the common cold, measles, pneumonia, or chickenpox, usually have impaired appetite. While it is not essential to insist that the nutritional requirements be met for the few days of the infection and fever, ketosis must be guarded against. (Consult Chapter 22, Diet in Febrile Diseases.) During the first day or two of the illness, it is advisable to serve either small amounts or no food, but fluids are supplied in quantities to meet the child's need. The infant's formula is diluted with water, and when the fever subsides, the regular feeding formula is resumed in order to supply the required calories as soon as possible. The liquid diet prescribed for children includes fruit juices, soups, broth, and milk as tolerated. As the fever subsides, the appetite usually improves and the food intake can be increased accordingly. During convalescence a soft diet, suitable for the age group, is advisable and is increased gradually to the normal diet.

CHRONIC INFECTIONS

It is essential that adequate nutrition be maintained in children who have infections of long duration, such as rheumatic fever and tuberculosis. However, the food can be given in an easily digestible form such as was described in Chapter 22.

Rheumatic fever is a common cause of death among children of school age. It is a leading disease which takes the lives of children between the ages of 5 and 19. Among the number of children who survive, many are left with rheumatic heart disease. Half a million children in the United States have been handicapped by rheumatic fever, with resulting heart damage. Consult the recommended diet for rheumatic fever in Chapter 22. An adequate diet and bed rest are essential for those who have rheumatic fever, a prescription which is often difficult to carry out in the home. As a rule, the patient responds to dietary and medication directed toward the pain and fever and consequently feels good even though tests reveal that the infection is still active.

Drugs such as sulfadiazine and penicillin are used for prophylaxis of streptococcal infections and recurrences of rheumatic fever. In addition, chemoprophylaxis serves to minimize the likelihood of progressive heart damage. In the event that heart disease results from the rheumatic fever, the added diet precautions outlined in Chapter 30, Cardiovascular Diseases, may be prescribed.

In the last fifteen years *primary tuberculosis* mortality in children has been reduced from 20 to 1.5 per hundred cases as a result of the prophylactic plan of treatment with the antituberculosis drugs and an adequate diet. (See Chapter 22.)

Infants and children have benefited from the use of antibiotics for respiratory infections, as demonstrated by the lowered incidence of such infections as bronchiectasis and mastoiditis. However, the widespread occurrence of an increase in the incidence of *staphylococcal* pneumonia and empyema may result from the unavoidable widespread therapeutic—and perhaps sometimes indiscriminate—use of the antibacterial agents. The early use of isoniazid is credited with preventing 80 per cent of the serious complications of the disease in children under 4 years of age. However, isoniazid, an antagonist for vitamin B_6, has led to vitamin B_6 deficiency with convulsive seizures and peripheral neuritis. Vitamin B_6 is given as a supplement when INH is administered. A normal diet and maintenance of weight at the desired level is important not only for the child but for members of the family and those with whom he comes in contact.

GASTROINTESTINAL DISORDERS
PYLORIC STENOSIS

Pyloric stenosis of infancy is not uncommon. The condition is serious and, unless recognized and treated in the early stages, has a high rate of mortality. It usually occurs during the first two months of life.

Mild cases are often treated successfully with continuous gastric suction or frequent lavage. Between aspirations, the infant is given small amounts of formula or is breast-fed. Some infants so affected may require parenteral hyperalimentation to correct dehydration, acid-base balance, and hypoproteinemia. However, if there is no definite improvement, surgery is generally advised.

Babies who are breast-fed are usually fed at intervals of 4 hours. If vomiting occurs and a large part of the feeding is lost, the infant should be refed because refeedings are often retained. The nutritional status of the infant is usually poor because of the nausea and limited food intake. Experience has demonstrated that artificially fed infants show frequent improvement when given thick cereal feedings every four hours. Some formula-fed babies show improvement when fed human milk.

REGURGITATION AND VOMITING

Regurgitation or spitting up is common in infants who overload the stomach or swallow air. Burping should be practiced to give the baby a chance during each nursing to get rid of the air he has swallowed.

Vomiting is a symptom of many disturbances which may or may not be serious. In a baby, vomiting of a whole feeding or a large part of it is often an early sign of an infectious disease. However, it may also be caused by indigestion, by fatigue, or by overexcitement. A child who has eaten a meal while overtired, overexcited, angry or frightened may be unable to digest his food, and vomiting is nature's way of getting rid of the undigested material. Such vomiting is not serious. Sometimes the condition results from an imbalance of food constituents in the formula, particularly from too much fat, which delays normal emptying of the stomach.

Persistent vomiting, especially when accompanied by diarrhea, will cause an imbalance of electrolytes and create a serious condition. The cause should be determined and feedings and fluids adjusted accordingly.

PEPTIC ULCERS

Peptic ulcers occur more frequently in infants and children than was formerly believed. The majority of cases reported are diagnosed only when complications appear. Most cases occur without obvious causes. The stress factors in modern urban society could be a factor in increasing the occurrence of peptic ulcers at an early age, according to a survey of hospital and medical case records of children under 16 years of age made by Dr. H. A. Sultz.[1] In a study by Thomson and Jewett,[2] they found peptic ulceration in infants and children associated with steroid therapy or a serious underlying illness. Some babies are bothered by colic after eating; others vomit after feeding, and the abdomen is tender and distended. Their symptoms are closely allied to those in adult patients: pain in the upper abdomen, more marked when the stomach is empty, which is relieved by food or antacid medication. See Chapter 23 for a discussion and treatment.

DIARRHEA

Occasional diarrheas are common in infancy and childhood. The most frequent causes are contamination or spoilage of food, too much carbohydrates (sugar) or fats in the formula, irritants such as cathartics, and allergic reactions to specific foods. However, the modern safeguards against contamination of foods (especially milk)—refrigeration, improved socioeconomic conditions, public education, and the effects of antibiotic drugs—reflect in fewer cases of infantile diarrhea the year round.

In the developing countries acute diarrheal diseases are commonly associated with the weaning period. Some are identified with a specific organism but the majority are not. The condition is listed among the first five causes of high infant mortality and, in many countries, ranks first in the first and second years of life. Supplementary foods of low nutritive value, prepared under unsanitary conditions, are usually started during the latter part of the first year, and diarrhea follows.

The results of diarrhea are loss of water, electrolytes, and nutrients. Usually, no food is given until the diarrhea subsides. However, water, glucose and electrolytes (sodium and potassium) are given, either by mouth or parenterally, to prevent dehydration and ketosis. When feedings are resumed, the diet is built up gradually, starting with boiled skim milk, cooked cereals, toasted white bread, and fruit and vegetable juices; then a soft diet and, finally, the normal or regular diet for the age and development of the child. Consult Chapter 24, Diet in Intestinal Diseases, for dietary modifications.

Acidified milk is often recommended for infants who are fed formulas. Skim milk is usually recommended, and as the condition

---

[1]Review: Are peptic ulcers on the increase in children? Food and Nutrition News, National Live Stock and Meat Board, 42:2, 1970.

[2]Thomson, N. B., Jr., and Jewett, T. C.: Peptic ulcers in infancy and childhood. J.A.M.A., 189:539, 1964.

improves, whole milk may be used. When the diarrhea has disappeared, the regular formula, including sugar, may be resumed. Also, research has shown that protein milk may be used successfully to combat this condition.

Pectin or apple may be given in the amounts suitable for the age of the child, and low fiber foods described in Chapter 24, The Diet in Intestinal Diseases, are of value in the treatment of diarrhea in children.

BACILLARY DYSENTERY

Bacillary dysentery, as the name implies, is a form of diarrhea produced by a specific organism, such as *Shigella dysenteriae*. Proper diagnosis and treatment are required to avoid a chronic condition.

The dysentery often continues for a considerable length of time, even with antibiotic therapy, before improvement or immunity is established. Therefore, food and fluids must be given regardless of diarrhea. Small frequent feedings are often more successful for the older child than the routine of three meals a day. A diet sufficient in calories to supply energy needs, high in protein and low in fat content, with limited amounts of carbohydrates, is advisable for all ages.

Infants are given fluid and acidified skim milk formulas. Cooked cereal may be given to children who have reached the age when cereal is included in the diet.

The diet for the older child follows the same general principles suggested for adults with diarrhea, which are described in Chapter 24, Diet in Intestinal Diseases. The fat content of the diet is limited, the animal protein increased (skim milk, chicken, lean beef, liver, and pot cheese), and the carbohydrates restricted (sugars).

To avoid dehydration, the quantity of water and juices should be increased to replace the amount lost.

CONSTIPATION AND COLIC

Constipation is a fairly common disturbance of infancy and childhood. As a rule the bottle-fed baby has fewer stools than the breast-fed baby. Human milk is higher in carbohydrate (lactose) than cow's milk (see page 253) and tends to be more laxative. Feces that are hard and expelled with difficulty should be reported to the physician.

Treatment varies with the cause. Constipation is most often caused by restricted or inadequate food intake or poor eating habits. In the case of the formula-fed infant, the sugar can be increased or the type of sugar used in the formula can be changed. The breast-fed infant may have a supplementary bottle of a fruit juice or malt extract in water added to the feeding schedule. In infants with supplementary foods or young children, the diet may include fruit juice (prune, orange), vegetable juice (tomato) fruit purées or fruits (prunes, apricots, applesauce, figs), vegetable purées or vegetables and whole grain cereals, which may be added to or increased in the diet, depending upon the age level. In older children the suggestions outlined in Chapter 24 may be followed.

INTESTINAL COLIC   In infancy this is a fairly frequent result of chronic constipation. Other causes are irritation or inflammation of the digestive tract, swallowing of air (resulting in distention), cathartics and cold. The taking of warm food may give temporary relief, but correction of the diet is necessary to relieve the constipation and distention.

ULCERATIVE COLITIS

Ulcerative colitis is not rare in the pediatric age group. Although chronic ulcerative colitis is basically the same in all ages, the disease is usually more severe and treatment is less satisfactory in children than in adults. Because of its chronic, relapsing nature, its occurrence at a time of active growth, and severe associated complications, the disease requires careful evaluation and active medical treatment, with early surgical intervention when indicated.

These patients are sometimes overweight but are usually underweight and are under emotional stress. Parents of these children may be overprotective, or overaggressive in forcing them to compete beyond their desire and/or ability. Ulcerative colitis may occur after failure to meet a challenge or after an outburst of emotion or severe stress. Care should be directed to assist the person to obtain sufficient calories and an adequate intake of the essential nutrients to provide for growth and to maintain good nutritional status. See Chapter 24 for discussion and dietary treatment.

MALABSORPTION DEFICIENCY

As noted earlier, in malabsorption the products of digestion available to the body are blocked because the absorbing surface of the small intestine is greatly reduced. The microvilli are fewer and misshapen. The structural polarity of the epithelial cells is lost and the intracellular enzymes that are responsible for the metabolism of epithelial cells are destroyed. With too few villi and microvilli, fatty substances other than triglycerides such as phospholipids, cholesterol, and the lipid-soluble vitamins A, D, K, and E are poorly absorbed.

In addition to the inadequacies of the diseased mucosa poor absorption results when triglyceride residues and other lipids hold fatty substances in solution. The vitamins may be given parenterally but the weight loss of patients caused by deficient absorption of fats cannot be controlled by intravenous fat preparations. Medium-chain triglycerides (MCT), which are hydrolyzed more rapidly than long-chain triglycerides, are used to supply the needed calories. The fatty acids enter the epithelial cell and are moved into the portal circulation without change in character. An MCT preparation, Portagen,* (which is made by hydrolysis of coconut oil and the distillation of fatty acids) yields 8.2 to 8.4 kcalories per gram. It may be blenderized with skim milk, fruit juices, and mayonnaise and it can be used in place of table oil in recipes such as cookies, pancakes, and French toast. Foods predominantly MCT are as follows:

> Portagen used as fat
> Skim milk, skim milk cottage cheese
> Egg whites, meringue
> All vegetables and fruit except avocados
> Fat-free bouillon and consommé and gravies made with these
> Angel food cake
> Fat-free desserts
> Gelatin
> Bread, rolls (in limited amounts) and cereals
> Sugar jelly

Schizas et al.[3] lists foods to be restricted and permitted in the diet and gives recipes using MCT.

In such diseases as celiac sprue, protein and carbohydrates also are poorly absorbed, resulting in excessive fecal nitrogen loss as well as steatorrhea. The chyme containing the amino acids and dipeptides, glucose, maltose, sucrose and lactose molecules, cannot be transferred from lumen to blood with inadequate villi, misshapen carriers, and insufficient pumps. Sodium, water, and potassium are apt to stay and accumulate in the lumen.

Screening tests for malabsorption are available. (1) The xylose tolerance test is used in screening for carbohydrate malabsorption. (2) The serum carotene level is used in screening for typical celiac sprue. (3) The vitamin B_{12} absorption test of Schilling is used for screening patients with ileal disease or with extensive bacterial colonization of the small intestine.[4]

CELIAC DISEASE

Holt[5] defines idiopathic celiac disease as "a state of malnutrition induced by a poorly understood chronic functional disorder of intestinal assimilation." It is believed to be a genetically transmitted deficiency. The intestinal epithelium cannot tolerate a glutamine-rich polypeptide derived from gluten. In celiac disease pathologic changes occur in the epithelium and lamina propria affecting the absorption of the nutrients.[6] The absorbing and secretory surfaces of the small intestine are greatly reduced. Celiac disease is a prototype of malabsorption caused by disorder of the absorption tract called enterogenous malabsorption.[7] The chief symptoms are bulky, foamy, pale and foul stools resulting from an excess of unabsorbed fat and carbohydrate fermentation. The patient shows weakness, underweight, malnutrition, retarded growth, bulging distended abdomen, and excessive irritability. (See Fig. 36–2.) The age of onset varies between 4 months and 16 years, with the majority of cases occurring between the first and third years.

Associated with the increased bowel activity is the failure to utilize vitamins and minerals. Rickets complicates the condition, and iron deficiency anemia may be one of the striking symptoms. When the storage of vitamin K is interfered with, bleeding tendencies arise. There is also a vitamin B deficiency which leads to symptoms of red tongue and mouth. Scurvy and hypoproteinemia may also occur.

GLUTEN   Hypersensitivity to the gluten or protein fraction, gliadin, in wheat, oats, barley, and rye flours or cereals was reported in 1950 by two Dutch students, Dicke and Weijers, who presented theses on their observations that wheat flour in the diet of celiac patients aggravated the condition remarkably. Later these and other investigators[8] reported that wheat and rye were responsible for the symptoms of diarrhea and steatorrhea of celiac disease. They found that fat excretion decreased notably when these children were placed on diets free of wheat and rye cereals. The protein-bound glutamine in any given protein is responsible for the symptoms. The gliadin fraction of the protein appears to cause a latent malabsorption syndrome as well. They are high in protein of wheat, rye, barley, and oats, but low in that of rice, corn, and buckwheat.

---

*Mead Johnson & Company, Evansville, Indiana 47721.
[3]Schizas, A. A., et al.: Medium-chain triglycerides—use in food preparation. J. Am. Dietet. A., 51:228, 1967.
[4]Ingelfinger, F. J.: For want of an enzyme. Nutrition Today, 3:8, 1968.

---

[5]Holt, L. Emmett, Jr.: Celiac disease—What is it? J. Pediat., April, 1955.
[6]Ingelfinger, F. J.: For want of an enzyme. Nutrition Today, 3:2, 1968.
[7]Ibid.
[8]Weijers, H. A., and van de Kamer, J. H.: Celiac disease and wheat sensitivity. Pediatrics, 25:127, 1960.

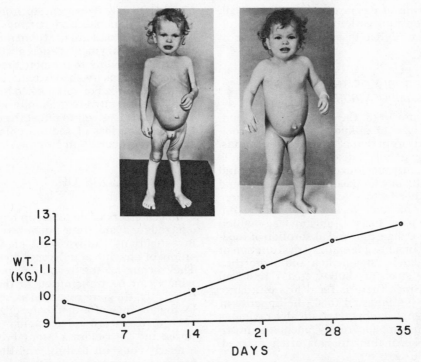

WT.
(KG.)

DAYS

Figure 36–2   Child, age 2½ years, with gluten-induced enteropathy (celiac syndrome) upon admission to the hospital and after 35 days on gluten-free diet. The diagram shows the child's weight gain. (Courtesy P. A. di Sant'Agnese, M.D., and J.A.M.A., *180*:308, 1962.)

DIETARY TREATMENT OF GLUTEN-IN-DUCED ENTEROPATHY   The nutritional needs of the child should be provided. Usually the child requires additional calories and protein and supplemental administration of water-miscible vitamins A and D and iron. The omission of gluten-containing cereals (wheat, oats, barley, and rye) requires careful planning to avoid these in the preparation of foods. Gluten constitutes approximately 10 per cent of the weight of wheat flour. Flour is often contained in frankfurters, gravies, soups and meat loaf. Reading the ingredients on labels is important. The response to gluten restriction is not immediate. The child with very severe celiac disease requires 2 to 6 weeks of treatment before improvement is evident. Usually, appetite returns first, vomiting and diarrhea disappear, and stools become normal in color and consistency. Gradually, deficiency states clear and there is a steady gain in weight (Fig. 36–2). The anemia responds more slowly.

For the child in a state of crisis, treatment may be started with intravenous replacement therapy of fluid and electrolytes. A formula of skimmed milk or protein milk sweetened with glucose, sucrose or banana powder (Probana) is given until diagnosis of gluten-induced enteropathy is established, followed by a soft-fiber, gluten-poor, high-protein, low-fat, low-starch diet as tolerated. Within a few weeks, a normal, high calorie diet excluding gluten is indicated. Supplements of vitamin A, vitamin D, and vitamin K are administered usually. Calcium is prescribed if symptoms of tetany occur. Liver extract may be given intramuscularly.

The gluten-poor diet is generally accepted. Practical suggestions for a diet free from the offending cereal proteins are presented by Sleisinger et al. (Ch. 34). Corn and rice cereal products and flour are used. These workers used the diet for treatment of nontropical sprue in the adult (Ch. 34), believed to be identical with celiac disease. These are probably manifestations of the same disease at different ages of life.

There is no rule of thumb for timing the reintroduction of gluten into the diet of the patient with celiac disease. The severity of the disease usually correlates well with the sensitivity to gluten. The gluten-poor regimen probably should be continued far beyond the point of symptomatic relief in order to reduce the likelihood of malabsorption difficulties later in life. Liberalizing the diet too rapidly may lead to serious and often sudden setbacks which are more difficult to correct than the initial episode. The individual height-weight curve provides a good guide as to the ability to tolerate gluten. Most authorities seem to believe that true cure is rare and prefer to speak of remission in a patient who is able to tolerate gluten. Celiac disease can reappear in adult life.

CYSTIC FIBROSIS OF THE PANCREAS (MUCOVISCIDOSIS)

Cystic fibrosis of the pancreas is a congenital disease of unknown etiology, associated with dysfunction of the exocrine glands. Although generally a disease of children, it is now frequently recognized in adolescents and young adults in whom pancreatic achylia, and perhaps other factors, lead to malabsorption. Deficiency or total lack of pancreatic enzymes – trypsin, lipase, and amylase – which leads to poor digestion and absorption of foodstuffs explains the generalized dysfunction of exocrine glands. Steatorrhea and azotorrhea result. The stools are bulky, greasy, and foul smelling. Since there is fecal loss of a large portion of the ingested food, the appetite of these patients is characteristically ravenous and, despite an apparently adequate nutritional intake, malnutrition is often marked. (See Fig. 36–3.)

Due to the steatorrhea, vitamin A, vitamin K, and possibly vitamin E deficiencies result from the loss of liposoluble vitamins.

DIETARY TREATMENT A diet of simple, easily digested and absorbed foods is prescribed. The carbohydrate is in the form of simple sugars (mono- and disaccharides), since starches are poorly tolerated. The protein should be high – up to 6 to 8 gm./kg. body weight/day – and is often given as a casein hydrolysate. Modified high protein milk is used as the basis. Fat is restricted or eliminated, and liberal amounts of the liposoluble vitamins (in water-soluble form) are usually given to meet the deficiencies and to compensate for those lost in the stools. Calories are high (150/kg. body weight) to promote normal nutrition. Bananas and banana powder are tolerated well and are useful in the treatment. Pancreatic enzymes (pancreatin) are given with each feeding to promote digestion.

Foods such as mashed banana, scraped beef and liver, puréed or soft cooked low fiber vegetables and fruits are gradually added.

Extra salt is given to offset the characteristic excessive loss of sodium chloride in perspiration, especially in summer.

INBORN ERRORS OF METABOLISM

Inborn errors of metabolism have been recognized for a long time, but only recently have investigations thrown light on specific disorders of enzyme activity and dietary control. They occur as the result of mutant genes which can be transmitted to the offspring. Currently, they are regarded as characterized by the absence of a metabolic enzyme. Three such diseases are galactosemia, phenylketonuria, and ketoaciduria. Mental retardation is a nearly constant finding, and the treatment for these disorders is entirely dietary. It has been found that, if diet treatment is started early enough in the infant's life, serious mental and physical deficiencies may be eliminated.

The list of inborn errors of metabolism with important nutritional consequences grows ever longer. More than three hundred errors of metabolism have been discovered. The approximate distribution in man to date may be summarized as follows:[9]

Amino acid metabolism	30
Carbohydrate metabolism	30

[9]Orten, J. M., and Orten, A. V.: DNA and inborn errors of metabolism. J. Am. Dietet. A., 59:339, 1971.

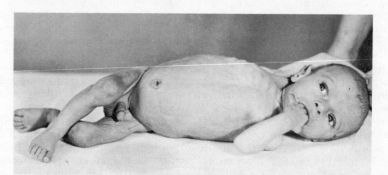

Figure 36–3 Three month old child with cystic fibrosis of the pancreas. He had loose stools, failed to gain weight, was fretful and irritable, but had a good appetite. Although the muscles were well developed, there was complete absence of subcutaneous fat. The abdomen was prominent. No enzymes were found in the duodenal juice. He was first given skim milk, banana powder, dried milk protein and large doses of vitamin A. Later he was given 1 gm. of powder pancreatin before each feeding of evaporated milk formula. He improved rapidly, and at 3 years, after being maintained on a high calorie, low fat diet and pancreatin, he appeared to be relatively normal. (Andersen, D. H.: J. Pediat., *15*:10, 1939.)

Lipid metabolism	12
Abnormal hemoglobins	200
Plasma proteins	10
Miscellaneous (porphyrin, purine, pyrimidine, steroid, and electrolyte)	15
TOTAL	297

GALACTOSEMIA

Galactosemia represents a hereditary disease caused by an inborn error of metabolism in which the body is unable to utilize galactose and lactose normally. In normal infants, sugar derived from lactose in milk is changed enzymatically to glucose in the liver. In galactosemia, an enzyme, galactose-1-phosphate uridyl transferase, is missing, and normal conversion does not take place, resulting in accumulations of the sugar, galactose, in blood and tissues.

The main symptoms of the disease appear when the infant is about 2 weeks old. Jaundice is the first symptom. Later others such as anorexia, nutritional failure, vomiting (and occasionally diarrhea), hepatomegaly, and albuminuria may follow. Sugar in the urine is also indicative of the disease. If the condition remains untreated, the presence of cataracts, mental and physical growth retardation, ascites, and enlarged liver and spleen become apparent with increasing age. The course of the disease may be slow, or death can occur within weeks or months. Guest[10] points out the necessity for early treatment as there is reason to believe that the danger of damage to the central nervous system in galactosemia is greatest during the first few weeks or months of the infant's life, the period of most rapid growth and development of the brain.

A simple sensitivity test (Rorem-Lewis test)[11] for detection of the disease has been developed, making early diagnosis possible, as well as evaluation of dietary control.

DIETARY TREATMENT   Since the missing enzyme cannot be replaced, treatment consists of a galactose-free diet. Milk is the chief source of lactose and galactose; therefore, all milk and milk products, especially human milk with its high galactose content, are withheld from the diet. When galactose is removed from the diet, the level of galactose in the blood falls quickly, proteinuria ceases, and the level of amino acids in the urine decreases to normal amounts. For young infants, liquid formulas are made up with casein hy-drolysate preparations such as Nutramigen.[12] Some investigators[13] have had good results with soy bean products such as Mel-Soy and Sobee. However, Holzel et al.[14] point out that the soy bean contains stachyose, which is a tetrasaccharide with two molecules of galactose and, theoretically, should be avoided. There is considerable controversy concerning soy bean products but Koch et al.[15] (Table 36–1) suggest "these foods can be useful if facilities for monitoring the erythrocyte galactose-1-phosphate content are available."

Galactose-free Diet[16]   The parents and afflicted child need guidance in selection of food for the galactose-free diet to provide adequate calories and essential nutrients for growth and development. Since milk must be omitted from the diet, and the milk substitutions usually have a strong odor and taste, parents need to be cautioned against negative comments and facial expressions when feeding the child. The child should be given as much responsibility as possible concerning his diet at an early age to learn the necessary food habits. It is assumed that dietary restrictions should be enforced for life. (See Chapter 43 for galactose-free diet recipes.)

Table 36–1 is a food plan using Nutramigen as a substitute for milk for those in the family with galactosemia. Calcium, as chloride or gluconate, is prescribed to supplement the low calcium intake of the milk-free diet if Nutramigen or other suitable protein hydrolysate is not used. Fruit juices are selected to augment the potassium intake. (See Appendix Table 9.) Supplemental vitamins are prescribed as indicated.

PHENYLKETONURIA (PKU)

Phenylketonuria is an inborn error involving protein metabolism. The enzyme phenylalanine hydroxylase is missing; accordingly, there is failure to hydroxylate the amino acid phenylalanine to form tyrosine. This results in the accumulation of excessive amounts of phenylalanine in the blood. Phenylpyruvic acid and other abnormal phenylalanine metabolites are excreted in large amounts in the urine.

---

[10]Guest, G. M.: Hereditary galactose disease. J.A.M.A., *168*:2015, 1958.

[11]U.S. Department of Agriculture. Diagnosing galactosemia in infants. Agricultural Research pub. No. *12*:4 (July) 1963.

[12]Mead Johnson and Company.

[13]Zellweger, H. U.: Enzyme deficiency disease. J. Am. Dietet. A., *34*:1041, 1958.

[14]Holzel, A., et al.: Galactosemia. Am. J. Med., *22*:703, 1957.

[15]Koch, R., et al.: Nutrition in the treatment of galactosemia. J. Am. Dietet. A., *43*:216, 1963.

[16]Modified after Koch, R., et al.: J. Am. Dietet. A., *43*:216, 1963. Tested and useful recipes appear in the original article. They are also included in the booklet "Parent's Guide for the Galactose-Free Diet" available from the Bureau of Public Health Nutrition, California State Department of Public Health, 2151 Berkeley Way, Berkeley, California.

TABLE 36-1   FOOD PLAN FOR ALL THE FAMILY MEMBERS*

Food Group	SERVINGS DURING ONE DAY		
	Preschool	School Age	Adults
Milk (Nutramigen for child with galactosemia)[1]	3 to 4 cups	4 or more cups	2 cups
Fruits[2] and vegetables[3]	4 or more small servings	4 or more	4 or more
Meats, fish, eggs, poultry[4]	2 or more small servings	2 or more	2 or more
Breads and cereals (milk free for child with galactosemia)	4 or more	4 or more	4 or more

* From "Parent's Guide for the Galactose-free Diet," published by the California State Department of Health, 2151 Berkeley Way, Berkeley, California.

[1] If Nutramigen is not drunk in these amounts, calcium and vitamin D should be given as supplements.

[2] Include every day a serving of one of these: citrus, tomato, melon, strawberries, broccoli, raw cabbage, green peppers.

[3] Include a deep yellow or dark green, leafy vegetable at least every other day. Omit beets, peas and Lima beans for the child with galactosemia.

[4] Nuts, peanuts and peanut butter are also included in this group.

The excessive accumulation of phenylalanine and its abnormal metabolites prevents normal development of the brain and central nervous system. This process can be arrested but not reversed through the use of the proper dietary management.

The clinical manifestations are a severe mental defect, a lightening in the color of the skin, hair, and eyes. Clinical signs are a strong aromatic odor ("musty") to the urine, vomiting and eczema, which are manifested early in infancy. Irritability of the infant is extraordinary. Varying and numerous unusual mannerisms and automatisms occur. Early diagnosis and treatment are of paramount importance if cerebral damage is to be prevented. Diagnostic tests are available, and intensive detection programs are currently in progress on a national scale in an attempt to treat these patients before serious brain damage occurs.

The incidence of PKU is estimated to be one in every 10,000 infants. It is transmitted by inheritance of an autosomal recessive gene and it is calculated that 1 person in 50 is a carrier of PKU.

DIETARY TREATMENT   The objective of the diet is to lower the abnormally high phenylalanine (15–60 mg./100 ml. serum) in the body to safer levels (2–6 mg.) and still supply an adequate amount for growth and development. All food protein contains appreciable amounts (averaging 5%) of phenylalanine. The basis of the diet is a specially prepared protein substitute from which most of the phenylalanine has been removed and the elimination of all dietary protein foodstuffs. Occasionally, a small supplement feeding of 1 to 2 ounces of milk is necessary for the infant to insure normal serum phenylalanine levels and to prevent growth retardation, anemia, hypoglycemia and cutaneous changes.[17] The amount of phenylalanine required to maintain normal nitrogen balance for growth and development is reported to vary between 10 to 25 mg./pound body weight per day, depending upon the individual child and his age. For accuracy of therapy the phenylalanine in the diet is prescribed in total mg./day or mg./pound per day. Serum level determinations are necessary every 2 to 4 months to detect both excesses and deficiencies of phenylalanine and to make any necessary dietary adjustments.

Special phenylalanine-restricted acid mixtures or milk preparations complete in all constituents other than phenylalanine are available commerically under the trade names, Ketonil, Lofenalac and Enal, and contain minerals and vitamins incorporated with the low phenylalanine casein hydrolysate. These mixtures are rather unpalatable, and their administration frequently meets with considerable resistance. Karle[18] et al. report good results from incorporating Lofenalac powder into puréed foods, low in phenylalanine content (fruits and vegetables except peas and dried legumes).

As soon as the serum phenylalanine returns to normal volume—and this may be several weeks—additional protein, including some phenylalanine, is added. How much phenyla-

17Fisch, R. O., et al.: Responses of children with phenylketonuria to dietary treatment. J. Am. Dietet. A., 58:32, 1971.

18Karle, I. P., et al.: Enzyme deficiency diseases. J. Am. Dietet. A., 34:1051, 1958.

lanine should be added is controversial, and the length of time for administering a phenylalanine-restricted diet has not been established. It is assumed that he will require a low-phenylalanine diet by providing both the protein substitute in amounts adequate to meet the recommended protein requirement for growth and sufficient phenylalanine from natural sources to balance the other essential amino acids in the protein substitute.[19] Reports of results with a phenylalanine-restricted diet have been contradictory. Generally, however, it is agreed that an early diagnosis must be made if cerebral damage is to be prevented. The infant with phenylketonuria is believed to be normal at birth. Unless the deficiency is detected and treated early in infancy, he will be mentally retarded by the end of the first year. However, even if started later in life, diet therapy will help to control the extraordinary irritability and activity, although mental retardation may not improve.

Koch et al.[20] give directions for prescribing and calculating the low-phenylalanine diet for various age groups.

Acosta and Centerwall[21] have evolved a diet using exchange lists, placing comparable foods of approximately the same phenylalanine content together. Recipes are also presented. These exchange lists are reproduced in a comprehensive and informative booklet "Phenylketonuria," Children's Bureau Publication No. 388, available from the United States Department of Health, Education, and Welfare, Washington, D.C., 1961. The State of California, Department of Health, Berkeley, California, also has an excellent booklet available, entitled The Low Phenylalanine Diet. See Table 36–2 for the exchange lists, and Table 36–3 for some samples of low-phenylalanine menus. See Chapter 43 for recipes.

Should the child become mentally retarded, a most helpful guide, focused on nutrition and feeding, has been developed to assist community health nurses working with the mentally retarded child and his family. The bulletin is entitled "Feeding Mentally Retarded Children," U.S. Department of Health, Education, and Welfare, Welfare Administration, Children's Bureau, 1964. For sale by the Supt. of Documents. U.S. Government Printing Office, Washington, D.C., 20402.

As in the case of galactosemia, the parents need conscientious and continued follow-up guidance from the medical team for the child.

Medical centers staffed and equipped for the treatment of phenylketonuria are available throughout the country to follow and evaluate the phenylketonuric children. The treatment includes not only the medical and dietary care but the social counseling and rehabilitation aspects of therapy. Optimal dietary management requires the assistance of the paramedical disciplines of nutrition, community health nursing, social work, and psychology. Again, parents need to be cautioned against comments and derogatory facial expressions concerning the taste or odor when offering the formula or special foods. Parents need reassurance that the child is healthy and to treat him as such. The need for the establishment of normal attitudes for food has been stressed by Umbarger.[22] Normal food habits and an adequate dietary are important. The nutrient needs of the normal infant and child must be considered in order to properly teach good nutrition to parents of the child with phenylketonuria of the same age. The diet must be accepted with a matter-of-fact attitude so as not to focus unnecessary attention upon it. Good discipline in all areas is needed for dietary control of phenylketonuria.

KETOACIDURIA (MAPLE SYRUP URINE DISEASE)

Maple syrup urine disease is an inborn error of metabolism named after the characteristic odor of the urine, and having autosomal recessive characteristics; it was first described in 1954. In patients having this disease there is a metabolic defect occurring in the oxidative decarboxylation of the keto acids derived from transamination of leucine, isoleucine and valine. Elevations of these branched-chain amino acids and respective ketoacids in plasma, cerebrospinal fluid, and urine are marked. The symptoms usually develop in the newborn, although several cases have been reported in late childhood.[23] It is suggested that the disease may be more common than is generally recognized. In most cases the disease results in irritability, retarded growth and development, hypertonicity, convulsions, and death. Pathologic studies reveal severe brain damage similar to that occurring in phenylketonuria.

Treatment consists of a synthetic diet restricting the amino acids leucine, isoleucine, and valine.[24]

[19]Sutherland, B. S.: Growth and nutrition in treated phenylketonuric patients. J.A.M.A., 211:270, 1970.

[20]Koch, R., et al.: Nutrition in the treatment of phenylketonuria. J. Am. Dietet. A., 43:212, 1963.

[21]Acosta, P. B., and Centerwall, W. R.: Phenylketonuria: Dietary management. J. Am. Dietet. A., 36:206, 1960.

[22]Umbarger, B. J.: Phenylketonuria. Treating the disease and feeding the child. Am. J. Dis. Child, 100:908, 1960.

[23]Editorial. Maple syrup urine disease. J.A.M.A., 186:147, 1963.

[24]Hsia, Y. Y.: Inborn errors of metabolism. In Duncan, G. G.: Diseases of metabolism. 5th ed. Philadelphia, W. B. Saunders Company, 1965.

TABLE 36–2　EXCHANGE LISTS FOR LOW PHENYLALANINE DIET*

FOOD	AMOUNT
List I—Lofenalac	
30 Mg. Phenylalanine—2 Equivalents†	
Lofenalac‡ (dry)	4 tbsp.
Lofenalac (reconstituted)	1 c.
List II—Vegetables	
15 Mg. Phenylalanine—1 Equivalent	
Beans, green	
Strained and chopped	1½ tbsp.
Regular	3 tbsp.
Beets	
Strained	2 tbsp.
Regular	3 tbsp.
Cabbage, raw, shredded	4 tbsp.
Carrots	
Strained and chopped	3 tbsp.
Raw	¼ large
Canned	4 tbsp.
Celery, raw	1½ small stalks
Cucumber, raw	⅓ medium
Lettuce, head	2 leaves
Spinach, creamed—strained and chopped	1½ tbsp.
Squash	
Winter	
Strained	3 tbsp.
Chopped	6 tbsp.
Cooked	2 tbsp.
Summer, cooked	4 tbsp.
Tomato	
Raw	¼ small
Canned	2 tbsp.
Juice	2½ tbsp.
List III—Fruits	
15 Mg. Phenylalanine—1 Equivalent	
Apple	2 medium-large
Apricots, dried	4 large halves
Banana	½ med.
Cantaloupe	½ c. diced
Dates, dried	2
Fruit cocktail, canned	2½ tbsp.
Grapefruit	
Sections	⅓ c.
Juice	⅓ c.
Orange	1 medium
Sections	⅔ c.
Juice	3 tbsp.
Grape juice	⅓ c.
Lemon juice	3 tbsp.
Nectarine	1 medium
Peaches	
Raw	1 medium
Canned in syrup	1½ halves
Strained	5 tbsp.
Chopped	7 tbsp.
Pears	
Raw	1⅓ medium
Canned in syrup	3 halves
Strained and chopped	10 tbsp.

FOOD	AMOUNT
Pears and pineapple, strained and chopped	7 tbsp.
Pineapple	
Raw	⅓ c.
Canned in syrup	1½ small slices
Juice	½ c.
Plums, canned in syrup	1½ medium
Plums with tapioca	
Strained	5 tbsp.
Chopped	7 tbsp.
Prunes	
Cooked	2 large
Juice	⅓ c.
Strained	3 tbsp.
Raisins	2 tbsp.
Strawberries	3 large
Tangerine	⅔ small
Watermelon	⅔ c.
List IV—Breads	
30 Mg. Phenylalanine—2 Equivalents	
Barley cereal, Gerber's, dry	2⅓ tbsp.
Biscuits[a]	1 small
Cereal food, Gerber's, dry	2 tbsp.
Cookies, arrowroot	1½
Corn	2 tbsp.
Cornflakes	⅓ c.
Crackers	
Barnum animal	6
Saltines	3
Cream of Wheat, cooked	2 tbsp.
Farina, cooked	2½ tbsp.
Mixed cereal, pablum, dry	1⅔ tbsp.
Oatmeal	
Gerber's strained	1⅔ tbsp.
Pablum, dry	1⅔ tbsp.
Potatoes, Irish	2½ tbsp.
Rice Flakes, Quaker	⅓ c.
Rice Krispies, Kellogg's	⅓ c.
Rice, Puffed, Quaker	½ c.
Sugar Crisps	¼ c.
Sweet potatoes or yams	
Cooked	3 tbsp.
Strained	4 tbsp.
Wafers, sugar, Nabisco	6
Wheat, Puffed, Quaker	⅓ c.
List V—Fats	
5 Mg. Phenylalanine—⅓ Equivalent	
Butter	1 tsp.
Cream, heavy	1 tsp.
Margarine	1 tbsp.
Mayonnaise	1½ tbsp.
Olives, ripe	1 large
List VI—Desserts	
30 Mg. Phenylalanine—2 Equivalent	
Cookies	
Rice flour	2
Corn starch	2

(Table continued on opposite page.)

TABLE 36–2   EXCHANGE LISTS FOR LOW
PHENYLALANINE DIET* *(Continued)*

FOOD	AMOUNT	FOOD	AMOUNT
List VI—Desserts (Continued)		Molasses	—
		Oil	—
Ice cream[a]		Sauces	
Chocolate	⅓ c.	Lemon[a]	—
Pineapple	⅓ c.	White[a]	—
Strawberry	⅓ c.	Syrups	
Vanilla	⅓ c.	Corn	—
Puddings[a]	1 c.	Maple	—
Sauce, Hershey syrup	2 tbsp.	Sugar	
		Brown	—
List VII—Free Foods; Little or No Phenylalanine; May Be Used as Desired		White	—
		Tapioca	—
Candy		**List VIII—Foods to Avoid; High Phenylalanine Content; May Be Used Only Occasionally in Very Small Portions**	
Butterscotch	—		
Cream mints	—		
Fondant	—	Breads, most	—
Gum drops	—	Cheeses of all kinds	—
Hard	—	Eggs	—
Jelly beans	—	Legumes, dried	—
Lollipops	—	Meat, poultry, fish	—
Cornstarch	—	Milk#	—
Guava butter	—	Nuts	—
Honey	—	Nut butters	—
Jams, jellies, and marmalades	—		

*Adapted from "Phenylketonuria," Children's Bureau Pub. No. 388, 1961, U.S. Department of Health, Education, and Welfare, Social Security Adm., Washington, D.C., and Miller, G. T., et al.: Phenylalanine content of fruit, J. Am. Dietet. A., 46:43, 1965. For additional list of vegetables and fruits refer to McCarthy, M. A., et al.: Phenylalanine and tyrosine in vegetables and fruits. J. Am. Dietet. A., 52:131–134, 1968.

†One equivalent may be defined as providing 15 mg. phenylalanine.

‡Mead Johnson & Company.

[a]Special recipe must be used.

#Milk is high in phenylalanine (1 oz. contains 50 mg.), but it may be ordered in infants to keep phenylalanine blood levels up to normal.

Smith and Waisman devised a useful leucine equivalency system for simple and efficient dietary management of patients with branched-chain ketoaciduria.[25] The composition of the semi-synthetic formula low in the branched-chain amino acids fed to a patient at various ages from 4 months to 5 years consisted of (1) homogenized milk (200 to 270 gm.), thus providing an average of 130 mg. leucine per kilogram of body weight per day; (2) mixture of synthetic amino acids in the proportions found in human milk without leucine, isoleucine or valine; these with the cow's milk provided the recommended allowance of protein; (3) dextrimaltose and corn oil provided the balance of calories needed (half the calories by dextrimaltose and half by corn oil); (4) minerals and vitamins to provide the recommended allowances; (5) methyl cellulose to act as a stabilizer; and (6) water to bring the total volume to the amount needed. Juices and solid foods were introduced into the child's diet at the usual times. The composition of the diet was adjusted to conform with the Recommended Allowances for increasing age and with the changing taste preferences.

Histidinemia, another abnormality in the metabolism of amino acids, has been detected in children. High levels of histidine in the blood and urine have been found. Evidence of mental and speech retardation has been reported. Histidinemia is believed to be transmitted by a non-sex-linked recessive gene and is a disease in which the enzyme histidase is absent. Histidase is the catalyst which converts histidine to urocanic acid and it is needed in the synthesis of purines and pyrimidines. Although there is biochemical similarity between phenylketonuria and histidinemia, the only serious harmful effect of the latter seems to be a speech defect. No practical dietary treatment to date has been formulated.

Hyperglycinemia has been described but it has been difficult to determine which metabolic pathway for glycine is abnormal in glycinemia. It has been noted that the conversion of glycine to serine takes place at a slower rate in children with this defect than in normals. The missing enzyme appears to be glycine-serine aldolase.

[25]Smith, B. A., and Waisman, H. A.: Leucine equivalency system in managing branched-chain ketoaciduria. J. Am. Dietet. A., 59:342, 1971.

TABLE 36–3   SOME EXAMPLES OF LOW PHENYLALANINE MENUS*†

Age and weight	Formula	Breakfast	Midmorning	Dinner	Midafternoon	Supper	Bedtime
2 months (10 lbs.)	15 measures Lofenalac 2 oz. milk 26 oz. water	Five or six 5–6 ounce feeding of formula					
8 months (18 lbs.)	22 measures Lofenalac 2 oz. milk 25 oz. water	½ cup chopped peaches 8 oz. formula		½ cup chopped carrots 8 oz. formula		½ cup chopped pears 8 oz. formula	8 oz. formula
2 yrs. (26 lbs.)	26 measures Lofenalac 1 oz. milk 20 oz. water	½ cup dried rice cereal* with 3 oz. formula with sugar ⅓ cup orange sections 6 oz. formula		½ cup cooked carrots 2½ tbsp. mashed potato made with formula and 1 tsp. butter ½ cup apple sauce 6 oz. formula	2 animal cookies 6 oz. formula	3 tbsp. of green beans 3 pear halves 6 oz. formula	
4 yrs. (36 lbs.)	27 measures Lofenalac 25 oz. water	½ cup dried rice cereal* with 2–3 oz. formula 1 small orange 8 oz. formula	wedges of apple	½ cup cabbage and carrot salad with vinegar and oil dressing ½ cup homemade vegetable soup 1 peach half 8 oz. formula	3 animal cookies 4 oz. formula	½ banana ½ cup tapioca pudding made with pineapple juice 8 oz. formula	Synthetic fruit flavored drink

1 measure = 1 tablespoon
16 tablespoons = 1 cup
*Do not use any "protein fortified" cereals.

†From Phenylketonuria. Children's Bureau Publication No. 388. U.S. Department of Health, Education, and Welfare, Social Security Administration, Washington, D.C., 1961.

STARCH INTOLERANCE

Starch intolerance occurs in infancy and is sometimes confused with celiac disease. The stools have the same frothy appearance and foul odor, due to the presence of undigested carbohydrate, but lack the unutilized fat. Other symptoms are abdominal distention, general weakness and weight loss. There is deficient amylase content in the pancreatic juice which probably accounts for the undigested carbohydrate in the stools.

DIETARY TREATMENT   The diet or formula prescribed is low in starch, the carbohydrate being in a simple form such as sugar, honey, corn syrup, dextrose, fruit juices, puréed or cooked soft fiber fruits and vegetables. Starch, such as cereal and bread, is omitted indefinitely. Fats and protein are normal.

DISACCHARIDE INTOLERANCE

In disaccharide intolerance there is a deficiency of the disaccharide splitting enzymes, the disaccharidases. These enzymes are classified as alpha and beta disaccharidases. The alpha disaccharidase, lactase, hydrolyzes lactose. The beta disaccharidases, the maltases and sucrases respectively, split maltose and sucrose into their simple sugars. Normally the disaccharides are absorbed and are digested to their monosaccharide components within or on the surface of the intestinal epithelial cells and enter the blood stream. Cramps and watery diarrhea, bloating, flatulence and voluminous watery, foaming stools are symptoms of intestinal disaccharide intolerance. These symptoms are due to poor absorption of the disaccharides which exerts considerable osmotic pressure, resulting in the passing of much water into the intestines, and the unabsorbed disaccharides cause rapid bacterial fermentation.

Disaccharide intolerance is inherited and is of the autosomal dominant type. (See Chapter 34, Nutritional Diseases, for lactose deficiency in adults.) Inherited lactose intolerance occurs alone in infancy and is usually permanent. A child with an intolerance to sucrose and maltose tends to recover spontaneously when he matures.

DIETARY TREATMENT   In lactose intolerance all forms of milk and cheese and foods containing milk, such as cream soups, creamed casseroles, ice cream and milk chocolate, must be omitted from the diet. Infants and children with lactose deficiency may use the commerical products used in feeding children with galactosemia. In the other disaccharide intolerances the disaccharide which is not tolerated is excluded. Those children intolerant of maltose or isomaltose must exclude all foods containing starch or glycogen. These polysaccharides yield maltose, isomaltose and related oligosaccharides on hydrolysis by salivary and pancreatic amylase. (See Appendix Table 11, Common Carbohydrates in Foods, for planning diets with patients who are intolerant of disaccharides.) Enzyme substitutions using mold disaccharidase preparations are available and are used with the offending disaccharide.

Other intolerances such as sucrose intolerance due to deficiency of the enzyme invertase may be treated by the exclusion of sucrose from the diet. This means the omission from the dietary of granulated sugar, brown sugar, molasses, syrups, jellies, candy, cakes, puddings and some fruits and vegetables high in sucrose content. (See Appendix Table 11.)

MONOSACCHARIDE INTOLERANCE

Fructose intolerance in children is caused by deficiency of the enzyme aldolase in the liver. The condition is transmitted by a recessive gene not related to sex. The treatment consists of the exclusion of all fruits containing fructose and foods containing sucrose. Children are able to absorb and digest glucose, lactose and starch normally and it is possible to obtain an adequate and acceptable dietary.

In glucose-galactose intolerance the infant's symptoms disappear when all sources of carbohydrate except fructose are excluded from the diet. The formula and diet for infants and children with this disorder is given by Linquist.[26]

Essential pentosuria, present almost exclusively in Jewish ancestry, is transmitted by a recessive autosomal gene. An enzyme responsible for the reduction of the pentose L-xylose to xylitol appears to be absent and L-xylose is excreted in the urine. The enzyme has been identified as triphosphopyridine nucleotide xylitol dehydrogenase. There is no treatment of essential pentosuria, since L-xylose is a normal intermediate in the metabolism of hexose sugars. Pentosuria has no relationship to diabetes mellitus and is not harmful to health or longevity.

DEFICIENCY DISEASES

See Chapter 34 for the more detailed discussion of malnutrition as well as additional deficiency diseases of infancy and childhood and their dietary treatment.

---

[26]Linquist, B., and Meeuivisse, G.: Diets in disaccharidase deficiency and defective monosaccharide absorption. J. Am. Dietet. A., 48:307, 1966.

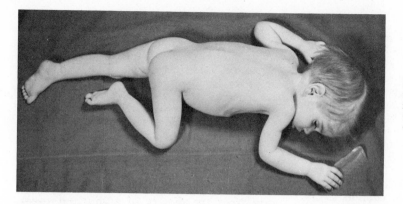

Figure 36–4   This child has general malnutrition of moderate degree, frequently seen in the United States. (Courtesy of University of Rochester, Rochester, New York.)

MALNUTRITION

Malnutrition is usually thought of in reference to children. The malnourished child is not getting adequate food materials needed by his body, either (1) because he does not ingest sufficient food to supply his needs, or (2) because he has faulty digestion, absorption, and/or assimilation. Protein-calorie malnutrition in preschool children is probably the most common and important current nutritional problem in the world. (See Fig. 36–4.)

Over half the world's population are victims of hunger or inadequate nutrition in one form or another, and the principal victims are infants and children. Millions die in their early years because they do not get adequate food, especially protein. When a baby is weaned at about 1 year old to a diet of starchy foods — gruel of rice, sweet potato, maize, or manioc — he invariably is a sick child by 2 years of age. (See Fig. 36–5.) As stated previously, a malnourished child may be either overweight or underweight. In the technically underdeveloped countries, undernutrition is the important factor since insufficient milk and food are available to furnish adequate protein and calories. Emphasis is placed on the prevention and correction of the malnutrition through the provision of protein, minerals, and vitamins and sufficient calories. Nutritional anemia is often present, and is caused by either a lack of sufficient iron rich foods in the diet or poor absorption and utilization.

The current attack on malnutrition by world health organizations such as WHO, FAO, UNICEF, and related organizations helps many infants and children of the present and future to obtain the food needed for normal growth and development. The National Nutrition Survey, USDA Food Consumption Survey and The White House Conference on Food, Nutrition and Health have identified the undernourished and malnourished groups in the United States. Recommendations for action to alleviate the situation are under way. By the passage of the National Child Nutrition Act of 1970 the need for nutrition education along with feeding programs has been recognized.

MARASMUS

Marasmus, or severe malnutrition, is infantile atrophy resulting from semistarvation. It is characterized by gross underweight result-

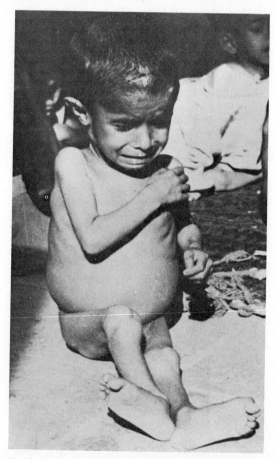

Figure 36–5   Sakeneh, a little Iranian girl, admitted in an advanced stage of malnutrition to a foundling home in Teheran. After 12 months of treatment she became a normal, lively child. (Courtesy FAO.)

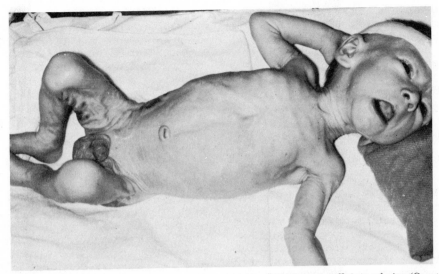

Figure 36–6   Marasmus. This infant shows severe malnutrition resulting from insufficient calories. (Courtesy of Burtis B. Breeze, M.D., Rochester, New York.)

ing from lack of calories rather than from any specific foodstuff. (Fig. 36–6). It is, however, associated with insufficient protein intake as in kwashiorkor. Often it occurs in patients having infectious diseases. Children having kwashiorkor develop rounded cheeks owing to edema, while those having marasmus have shrunken and wizened facies. Anorexia, diarrhea, and/or vomiting frequently accompany marasmus.

DIETARY TREATMENT   Fluid and electrolyte imbalances are corrected appropriately. Caloric deficiency is managed with oral or parenteral glucose as indicated. Once electrolyte balance is established, skim milk in some form is the basis of diet treatment. Sugar is added to approximately 15 kcalories/pound body weight. Solid foods are added when improvement is noted and appetite increases. Foods are added as tolerated with

emphasis on calories and protein. Frequent small feedings are tolerated better than the customary three daily meals. Supplementary vitamins are given as indicated and tolerated. In severe anemia blood transfusion may be necessary. An adequate normal diet to correct the deficiencies is the dietary objective.

CANCRUM ORIS (NOMA)

Cancrum oris is presumably caused by a combination of generally poor nutritional state and infection, and is reported chiefly in South Africa. It looks like hare lip (Fig. 36–7) but actually is a slowly progressive disease in which gangrene of the mouth occurs.

TREATMENT   Good nutrition, antibiotics and surgery are needed. However, the drugs and surgery do not bring on permanent cure unless the diet is corrected (Fig. 36–8). Out-

Figure 36–7

Figure 36–8

Figure 36–7   A child in South Africa suffering with cancrum oris, basically the result of generally poor nutrition complicated by infection. (Courtesy Dr. Robert Alpern.)

Figure 36–8   A child with cancrum oris living in the same area as the child in Figure. 36–7. This one has received drug and diet therapy and the lesion is healing. (Courtesy Dr. Robert Alpern.)

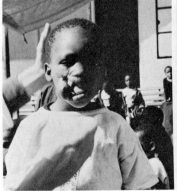

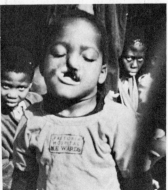

door "soup kitchens" are sometimes provided to prepare nutritionally adequate meals to solve the problem of nutritional deficiency responsible basically for much disease, e.g., cancrum oris.

KWASHIORKOR

Kwashiorkor is protein–calorie malnutrition. This deficiency disease is discussed in Chapter 34, Nutritional Deficiency Diseases.

LINOLEIC ACID DEFICIENCY

Hansen et al.[27] report linoleic acid to be essential in the diet of infants. In a diet adequate except for this fatty acid, dryness of the skin with desquamation, thickening and later intertrigo were the most characteristic features of the deficiency state observed. Unsatisfactory rate of growth was observed in many of the infants. Severe reaction to outbreaks of staphylococcal infection occurred in the hospital. Signs of the deficiency disappeared promptly when 1 per cent or more of the calories were provided as linoleic acid. (See p. 342 and Figure 34–1.)

VITAMIN DEFICIENCY DISEASES

HEMORRHAGIC DISEASE OF THE NEWBORN

This disorder is discussed in Chapter 9 under functions of vitamin K (p. 129). See also p. 256 and Figure 16–1.

PYRIDOXINE DEFICIENCY IN INFANTS

In 1954 a formula deficient in pyridoxine (vitamin B_6) was reported[28] to produce epileptiform convulsions in infants from 8 to 16 weeks of age. The formula producing the convulsions in infants was a liquid commercial formula preparation that had been sterilized by autoclaving, which had destroyed the pyridoxine. When fed another milk formula, or given supplementary vitamin B_6 or foods such as cereals, fruits, meats and vegetables, all of the infants were cured of the convulsions. It was concluded that the convulsions were due to deficiency of pyridoxine. These appear to be the first pyridoxine deficiency states reported in humans and have since been confirmed by other workers. Occurrence of convulsions in rats and pigs fed a diet lacking in this vitamin has been known since 1940. (See pages 136 and 137 for daily allowance and discussion of pyridoxine.)

---

[27]Hansen, A. E., et al.: Role of linoleic acid in infant nutrition. Clinical and chemical study of 428 infants fed a milk mixture varying in kind and amount of fat. Pediatrics, 31:171, 1963.

[28]Molony, C. J., and Parmelee, A. H.: Convulsions in young infants as a result of pyridoxine (vitamin B_6) deficiency. J.A.M.A., 154:405, 1954.

INFANTILE SCURVY

Infantile scurvy occurs usually in artificially fed infants as a result of deficiency in ascorbic acid. Normally the fetus receives the vitamin from the maternal blood supply and is born with a satisfactory supply if the mother had a sufficient amount in her diet. The breast-fed infant receives ascorbic acid which is concentrated in human milk when the mother's diet contains the vitamin. An infant may receive adequate amounts even when the mother's diet and her blood plasma are inadequate. Infants taken off the breast and given a starchy diet devoid of fruits and vegetables may develop classic scurvy. This frequently occurs in the underdeveloped countries. Clinical manifestations appear slowly after the infant has been deprived of an adequate supply of ascorbic acid. The treatment for scurvy for several days is large doses of ascorbic acid – orange juice 90 to 120 cc. or 100–200 mg. ascorbic acid given orally or parenterally. (See Chapter 34, Nutritional Deficiency Diseases, for discussion of scurvy.)

RICKETS

This deficiency disease is discussed in Chapter 34, Nutritional Deficiency Diseases.

METABOLIC DISORDERS

Many diseases overlap in the general classification. For example, the enzyme deficiency diseases are inborn diseases of metabolism, so could be listed correctly here, as well as under deficiency diseases.

DIABETES MELLITUS

Diabetes is likely to be an inborn error of metabolism in children and more severe than in adults. The majority of children are undernourished when the disease is first recognized, and the onset of symptoms is relatively sudden. Dietary management is of major importance, as the nature and severity of the disease are such that insulin therapy is required.

The diabetic child's diet follows the same general treatment suggested for the adult. (Consult Chapter 28.) However, for the child, the calorie and protein requirements per kilogram of body weight are higher to allow for growth and development. The mineral and vitamin requirements are also increased. Therefore, adjustments from time to time to meet the child's changing needs are required. The increase in diet and insulin is calculated in direct proportion to the optimum growth and physical activity needs of the child. Calories should be adequate to maintain the desired weight. The additional foods required for the building of bones and teeth are not neglected. Consult the standards for nutritional adequacy of the nondiabetic child suggested by the Food and Nutrition Board, National Research Council (Table 11–1). Currently, there is almost universal agreement that the maintenance diet of the child with diabetes should be essentially the same as for the child without diabetes. Controversy exists regarding the necessity for strict supervision of the food intake. However, most authorities believe there is a close relationship between control of the diabetes and the development of complications. Consequently, it is advocated that the food intake and insulin distribution be adjusted to avoid insulin reactions, and, insofar as practical, to avoid glycosuria.

Pollack[29] recommends increased protein allowance in the diabetic over the nondiabetic. A negative nitrogen balance occurs during episodes of ketosis, even very mild transient ones, and protein must be present at all times to meet the increased need.

During the initial phase of management, Jackson[30] suggests 1.5 gm. of protein and 35 to 40 kcalories per pound of theoretical body weight to replace the depleted nutritional stores and to rebuild body tissues. Also, vitamin supplementation is recommended when treatment begins. After the initial period, the recommended dietary allowances of the National Research Council are used as guides. Marble[31] suggests 20 per cent of the calories be provided by protein; 35 to 40 per cent by fat; and 40 to 45 per cent by carbohydrate. The distribution of the carbohydrates and calories throughout the day must be relatively uniform to maintain a high degree of control. The interpretation of diets for diabetic children should be particularly liberal. If favorite party dishes are planned occasionally, the child will cooperate more cheerfully and adhere more closely to the established regimen. There are many emotional conflicts in childhood and adolescence which must be considered in the treatment of the diabetic child, requiring sympathetic understanding and tact. Planning the diabetic regimen around the usual dietary pattern of the family helps the child to accept the regimen. He need not appear different from other members of the family at the table. He learns to eat at regular intervals and to live a normal life.

Children are apt students and learn quickly how to plan their own diet under supervision. When possible, it is advisable to give the child responsibility of planning his diet from the family meals. He is able to plan his dietary program to include those foods which he will eat outside of the home. He will appreciate and accept the obligation of the task. It is highly important that the diabetic child and the parents be clearly informed concerning the disease and be guided to face the facts squarely. While there is no known cure at this time, the condition need not interfere with a happy well adjusted life, provided the diabetic receives adequate treatment to control the disorder.

HYPERTHYROIDISM (GRAVES' DISEASE)

A discussion of hyperthyroidism appeared in Chapter 28, Metabolic Disorders Related to Nutrition, and will not be repeated here. The treatment for children follows the same general principles outlined for the adult. However, attention is directed to the need for additional calories for the child to meet the requirements for growth and development as well as the increase in the basal metabolic rate. The amount of protein must be adequate to meet the growth and maintenance needs and the quantity of carbohydrates increased to spare the protein. Fats are increased to meet the calorie requirements. An abundant supply of vitamins and minerals is furnished through the careful choice of foods, and additional vitamins are supplied through medication as indicated. An active adolescent boy may require 6000 calories daily.

HYPOTHYROIDISM (CRETINISM AND JUVENILE MYXEDEMA)

Hypothyroidism, which develops in fetal life or early infancy, is referred to as *cretinism* (Fig. 36–9). The two main causes for cretinism are insufficient thyroid in the newborn because (1) the structure is defective or (2) the iodine intake of the mother has been inadequate. In this country, even in the "goiter belts," the latter is seldom encountered. Distribution of foods which contain iodine and the use of iodized table salt have minimized the danger. In certain provinces of Ecuador, however, the prevalence of endemic goiter as a result of iodine deficiency among school children is 100 per cent. (See Fig. 36–10.) Incidence of goiter in the United States has increased in areas where iodized salt was not generally used.

Hypothyroidism, acquired prior to adolescence, is known as juvenile myxedema (Fig. 36–11). It usually is suspected in an older child when he begins to lag or drop behind in school, loses interest, tires easily, and has definitely delayed growth and development.

TREATMENT Thyroid tablets by mouth

[29]Pollack, H.: Nutritional adequacy of the diabetic diet. J. Am. Diabetes A., 2:497, 1953.

[30]Jackson, R. L.: Nutritional management of children with diabetes. J.A.M.A., *168*:42, 1958.

[31]Marble, A.: Diet for diabetic child. J.A.M.A., *177*:886, 1961.

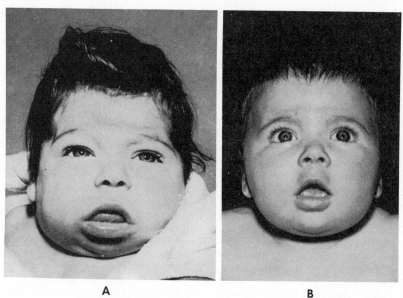

A   **B**

Figure 36–9   Cretinism. Congenitally hypothyroid infant at 6 months of age. Infant fed poorly in neonatal period and was constipated; had persistent nasal discharge and large tongue; very lethargic, no social smile and no head control. *A*, Note puffy face, dull expression, hirsute forehead. Serum cholesterol 172 mg. per 100 ml., alkaline phosphatase 4.8 Bodansky units, negligible uptake to radioiodine. Osseous development that of newborn. *B*, Four months after treatment with U.S.P. thyroid. Note decreased puffiness of face, decreased hirsutism of forehead and alert appearance. (From DiGeorge and Warkany in Nelson: Textbook of Pediatrics, W. B. Saunders Co., 7th ed.)

are specific. Without this therapeutic management, the course is regressive, and the physical and mental growth of the child are stunted (Figs. 28–5, 36–9, and 36–11). When medication is instituted during the first two years, the results are sometimes excellent, although a certain number remain slightly subnormal for their age. Signs of improvement may be

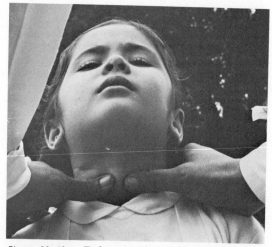

Figure 36–10   Endemic goiter. In certain provinces of Ecuador, 70 per cent of the population has been found to have goiter; in some places, the prevalence among school-children is 100 per cent as a result of iodine deficiency. In the schools of Paraguay, where this photo was taken, the children are regularly examined for symptoms of goiter. (WHO photo by Almasy.)

noted within a few weeks or months, and the dosage is regulated by checking the response to the extract. As a rule, this form of therapy is continued throughout life.

As in all patients who lack thyroid, there is a tendency toward overweight. The tissues are not firm but flabby, mottled and cool to the touch. The amount of calories in the customary diet is usually reduced in order to lose weight and maintain weight at the desired level. (See Chapter 28 for a more complete discussion of hypothyroidism.)

IMBALANCE OF BODY WEIGHT

OVERWEIGHT

Overnutrition in infants, children and adolescents in this country is becoming a matter of medical and public health concern. The child whose weight is consistently well above normal for age, height, and general development, should not be classified as "well nourished." Actually, this condition is overweight and requires investigation and treatment.

Frequently, foods are the center of interest at social gatherings. Children, especially teenagers, meet at favorite lunch counters for a soft drink, sandwich, pizza or dessert foods. The caloric equivalent of these extra snacks may well exceed energy expenditure and result in weight gain. Fortunately, many of the

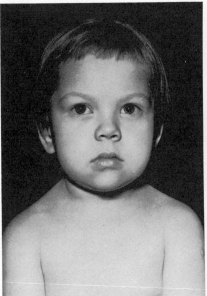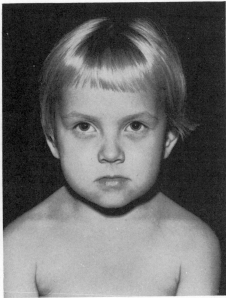

Figure 36–11 Juvenile myxedema. Acquired hypothyroidism in a girl 6 years of age. Treated with a wide variety of hematinics for refractory anemia for 3 years. Almost complete cessation of growth, constipation and sluggishness of 3 years' duration. Height age, 3 years; bone age, 4 years; sallow complexion, and immature facies with poorly developed nasal bridge. *A,* Serum cholesterol 501 mg. per 100 ml., alkaline phosphatase 1.8 Bodansky units, radioiodine uptake 7 per cent at 24 hours, PBI 2.8 micrograms per 100 ml. *B,* After therapy for 18 months. Note nasal development, increased luster and decreased pigmentation of hair and maturation of face. Height age, 5½ years; bone age, 7 years. Marked improvement in general condition. (From DiGeorge and Warkany in Nelson: Textbook of Pediatrics, W. B. Saunders Co., 7th ed.)

school lunch programs tend toward encouraging the children to make choices within the Type A pattern (p. 25). This is a step toward realistic experience in learning to make desirable choices to obtain a nutritious meal.

Heredity may be one of the factors in overweight, but too frequently parents blame family traits rather than make any attempt to correct the situation. In some cases, glandular difficulties may be responsible. But, as a rule, overeating, accompanied by a minimum amount of exercise, is the chief cause of overweight. If obesity is prevalent among family members, the entire family needs to review dietary patterns and change eating habits.

Adolescent girls are reported to have a greater prevalence of obesity than boys of corresponding age. Weight control is generally not a serious problem for normal, active, growing boys. Mayer et al. in Boston reported that obese adolescents, in general, are less active than nonobese youngsters of the same age group. It was also demonstrated that obese adolescent boys and girls both, as a group, eat less than do the nonobese. Bullen et al.[32] compared the activity of obese and nonobese

adolescent girls while engaged in sports at summer camp by motion picture sampling. The striking degree of inactivity of the obese girls appears to be a significant factor.

Unless a child is grossly obese, vigorous reducing generally is not advised. The present pattern and eating habits are evaluated and the person becomes interested in making the necessary changes to improve his dietary.

Mild overweight between the ages of 8 to 14 is often observed to be a spurt in body weight prior to a rapid gain of height and is simply a stage of development that does not last long. The weight will usually automatically adjust itself through a normal appetite and activity, providing there is no abnormal problem. Discipline is required to overcome the inclination to gorge large meals. There is a variety of wholesome foods from which the child can make a selection. Growth and development of the child demand sufficient calories to maintain weight at desired levels and protein, minerals and vitamins in the diet. The essential foods to supply these needs are milk, meat, eggs, fruits, vegetables, breads and cereals. A danger in connection with trying to reduce in a haphazard way is that a child will not get adequate nutrients, especially protein. The amount of protein ingested while losing weight should be increased. High caloric des-

[32]Bullen, B. A., et al.: Physical activity of obese and nonobese adolescent girls appraised by motion picture sampling. A. J. Clin. Nutr., *14*:211, 1964.

TABLE 36–4   BASIC MENUS FOR TEEN-AGERS*

LOW-CALORIE	HIGH-CALORIE
BREAKFAST Ready-to-eat cereal with milk Orange or orange juice Enriched or whole grain toast with butter or fortified margarine (limited) Milk (whole or fat-free)	**BREAKFAST** Ready-to-eat cereal with light cream or half n' half Orange or orange juice Eggs with ham or sausage Enriched or whole grain toast with butter or fortified margarine Jam Milk or milk beverage
LUNCH OR SUPPER Egg salad sandwich on thinly sliced whole grain bread (no butter) Sliced tomatoes Cottage cheese Milk (whole or fat-free)	**LUNCH OR SUPPER** Chicken and noodle casserole Buttered squash Cottage cheese and sliced tomato Salad dressing Hot biscuits with butter or fortified margarine Strawberry sundae Cookies Milk or milk beverage
DINNER Fruit or vegetable juice Cubed steak or lean ground beef patty Green beans with pimiento Thinly sliced bread with butter or fortified margarine (limited) Fresh, frozen or canned fruit Milk (whole or fat-free)	**DINNER** Fruit, vegetable juice or soup Cubed steak or regular ground beef patty Whipped potatoes Buttered green beans with pimiento Pineapple and banana and prune salad Salad dressing Hot bread with butter or fortified margarine Chocolate pie with pecan topping Milk or milk beverage
SNACKS Fresh fruit, carrot sticks	**SNACKS** Peanut butter and crackers Cheese and crackers

*Courtesy of Department of Home Economics Services, Kellogg Company, Battle Creek, Michigan.

serts and snacks, sweetened soft drinks, and candy between meals are discouraged. Skim milk can be substituted for whole milk. (See Chapter 29, Overweight and Underweight, for the principles involved in the dietary treatment.) See Table 36–4 for an example of a low calorie basic menu for teen-agers.

Untreated overweight in children may be the forerunner of diabetes, atherosclerosis and a number of degenerative diseases of old age. Hoffman[33] points out that the obese child is a handicapped child, both physically and emotionally. During adolescence, appearance is important, especially to girls, and those of normal weight are peppier and more popular. Normal weight is bound to bring about general improvement in health at all ages, and the sooner established, the better (Fig. 36–12).

EMOTIONAL AND SOCIAL FACTORS Understanding a child's weight problem—why he is overweight—is as important as formulating his correct diet for losing weight. The reason for the child's "hunger" must be found and replaced with satisfactions equal to that of eating. Adolescents especially have many physiological and psychological charac-

teristics[34] which must be taken into account, for at this age there is great self-concern. While girls are more concerned about their weight than boys, the markedly obese adolescent of either sex is usually self-conscious and unhappy. They are also great imitators, and here the nurse can be of invaluable help by setting a good example in her weight control. Adolescents appreciate any interest and understanding accorded their weight problem. Time spent in counseling is usually rewarding. Acceptance by the "gang" or their age group is vital as children seek group approval. The feeling that they will be more popular if not overweight is a strong motivation for changing food habits and the adoption of a satisfactory regimen in which they participate. Suggestions for change coming from the person are apt to be implemented.

Family tensions over weight must be avoided. Cooperation of parents and other members of the family is necessary to prevent frustration and increased sense of abnormality. The over-all adjustment problems require evaluation to make sure the pressures of obesity are not increased by an impossible

[33]Hoffman, R. H.: Obesity in childhood and adolescence. Am. J. Clin. Nutr., 5:1, 1957.

[34]Gallagher, J. R.: Weight control in adolescence. J. Am. Dietet. A., 40:519, 1962.

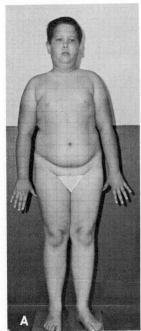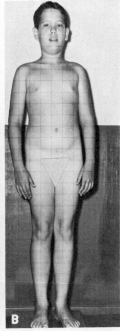

Figure 36-12   Obesity. Before and after 10 months treatment for obesity in an 11 year old boy. Weight loss was 42½ pounds. However, since there was a growth of 1½ inches during this period, the effective weight loss is calculated to be 49½ pounds. The change in facial expression is as dramatic as the weight loss, a frequent observation in these individuals. (Courtesy of Dr. R. H. Hoffman.)

regimen. Individual treatment is the keynote of management. Studies reveal overweight children tend to become overweight adults, who are the most difficult of all to lose weight. Their poor dietary habits are long established and offer great resistance to correction. They are prone to follow "crash" diets only to regain the weight lost and more. Obesity is a public health problem which can be solved only through learning on the part of individuals to avoid unwanted weight gain at any time of life.

UNDERWEIGHT

Underweight is of even greater importance than overweight. Although slimness in itself does not indicate malnutrition, if the child is more than 10 pounds below the desired optimum weight and fails to grow with regularity, a physical inventory is advised. If no disease can be demonstrated, careless eating habits and poor hygiene may be responsible.

In some instances, a scanty breakfast or no breakfast starts the day, while in others milk and other essential foods are omitted without suitable substitutes. Some children become tea or coffee addicts at an early age. Many resort to nibbling, which spoils their appetite for regular meals. Some children become so engrossed with the business of play that they eat too rapidly. Adolescent girls are often figure conscious and skip some nutritious foods in an attempt to keep slim.

The nervous, irritable child with a finicky appetite should receive attractive meals served at regular hours. A midmorning and midafternoon snack consisting of glasses of milk may prove beneficial. A diet high in all the vitamins, especially the B-complex group, usually stimulates the appetite.

The avoidance of fatigue, by restricting activity and encouraging additonal rest, is advised for some children. On the other hand, if the child is kept indoors with limited activity, plenty of fresh air and sunshine may be the solution to stimulate appetite.

The criteria to calculate the calorie needs of children are different from those of adults. The child requires extra food for growth and the activity of incessant play. In general, the food allowance for a girl 12 years old averages about 2500 kcalories per day, which is often a greater calorie requirement than that of her mother. An average adolescent boy of 15 to 16 years may use 4000 kcalories daily. Besides growing, the adolescent is extremely active. Consequently, more food is required than for adults of a corresponding size. See Table 36-4 for an example of high calorie basic menu. (Consult Chapter 29, Overweight and Underweight.)

CARDIAC DISEASES

There are a number of abnormalities of the heart which may be present at birth. Some forms are functional and disappear within months; other are serious and result in early death. Many are benefited by diet therapy and others are successfully treated by surgery.

The most common cause of acquired cardiac damage in children is rheumatic fever. See Chapter 30 for discussion of dietary treatment in heart disease.

DISEASES OF THE BLOOD AND BLOOD-FORMING ORGANS

ANEMIA

Nutritional or iron deficiency anemia is the most common form of anemia of infancy and childhood. It affects individuals of all ages, but particularly women and infants, and occurs most frequently among infants 6 to 18 months old. Most of the babies involved receive a poor supply of iron from an anemic mother, or there is fetal blood loss.[35] In recent years, evidence has accumulated[36] to indicate that sensitivity to cow's milk may cause occult loss of significant quantities of blood into the gastrointestinal tracts of some children with hypochromic microcytic anemia. Furthermore, milk is almost devoid of iron, and the anemic infant is not likely to improve unless a supplementary source is administered. In the rapidly growing infant, lack of iron in a milk diet unsupplemented by other foodstuffs is usually the cause of iron deficiency anemia. Early introduction of iron-rich supplementary foods, such as egg yolk, strained beef and liver, cereals, and certain fruits and green vegetables, is helpful. (See Appendix Table 8 for iron-rich foods.) Availability of specially prepared baby foods processed to reduce them to a semifluid form — such as meat, vegetables and fruits — makes it possible to give even the very young infants foods relatively rich in iron. In addition, many of the special infant cereals have iron added in the amounts providing 2.5 to 4 mg. to the serving ($\frac{1}{3}$ oz. or 10 gm.). See Table 11–1 for the NRC recommended allowances for iron at the various age groups.

Sisson et al.[37] report that there is an almost inevitable development of anemia and iron deficiency in the first year of life of premature infants, whose early birth limits the amount of iron they receive from the mother. In addition, the enormous increase in size during the first 2 years of life results in increased demands for hemoglobin production. Hence, there is early requirement for exogenous iron. When meat supplements were added to the infant's feedings between the second and fourth week of life, there was a marked improvement in the condition of the blood.

Lowered blood hemoglobins are not uncommon among adolescent children who consume less iron than is commonly recommended. Iron deficiency anemia (chlorosis) is not infrequently seen in girls at puberty. Growth requires additional iron and it is easy to understand how some girls become anemic when they diet to remain slim at the peak of their adolescent growth spurt. A more complete discussion of the anemias and their dietary treatment appears in Chapters 31 and 34.

LEUKEMIA

Although leukemia in children cannot yet be cured, recent studies seem to indicate that the average duration of life after diagnosis is now considerably longer than one year.[38] Leukemia is discussed in Chapter 31.

RENAL DISEASES (DISEASES OF THE KIDNEYS)

NEPHRITIS

Glomerulonephritis may appear at any age but is seen most frequently in children under 7 years of age or young adults. Clinical manifestations in severe cases may include high fever, headache, malaise, hypertension, oliguria or anuria. Cardiac failure or hypertensive encephalopathy may develop. Anemia may be present. Details of the diet treatment have been discussed in Chapter 32, Nutrition in Renal Diseases.

During the acute stage of nephritis no protein or a limited amount of protein depending upon nitrogen retention is given. The dietary treatment may at first consist chiefly of correcting the electrolyte balance and giving water orally. As the condition improves, milk and sweetened fruit juices are added. Adequate calories and the quantity of protein should be brought to a normal amount as soon as the kidneys give evidence of improvement. The appetite is usually poor and every effort should be made to have the child ingest an adequate diet. Familiar foods tempt the appetite. Unfamiliar foods are easily rejected by the child.

In chronic renal failure, protein intake may need to be reduced to the minimum necessary for growth, 1 gm. or even 0.5 gm./kg./day. Special attention must be given to sufficient calories from carbohydrate and fat, calcium, iron, and all the vitamins in an attempt to keep the body in the best possible state of nutrition for growth and development. In the event that sodium and fluids are limited, a low-sodium milk and/or a supplement (Protinal or Lonalac) low in sodium content can be used to aid in maintaining adequate protein intake. Supplemental calcium may also be indicated.

NEPHROSIS (NEPHROTIC SYNDROME)

"Pure" or lipid nephrosis is rare. Lipid nephrosis is defined as a nephrosis noted for the changes in the proteins and lipids of the blood and the accumulation of globules of cholesterol esters in the tubular epithelium of the kidneys. The etiology is unknown. The nephrotic syndrome is a general metabolic disturbance resulting in continued loss of large

[35]Woodruff, C. W.: Multiple causes of iron deficiency in infants. J.A.M.A., *167*:715, 1958.

[36]Heiner, D. C., et al.: Sensitivity to cow's milk. J.A.M.A., *189*:563, and 568, 1964.

[37]Sisson, T. R. C., et al.: Meat in the diet of premature infants. II. Influence in red cell volume and hemoglobin mass. J. Dis. Child., *95*:626, 1958.

[38]Meighan, S. S.: Leukemia in children. J.A.M.A., *190*: 578, 1964.

amounts of protein, mainly albumin, in the urine rather than a disease of the kidneys. The disease is characterized by edema, marked albuminuria, deficient secretion of urine, a decrease in the total protein content of the blood, with a relative increase in the globulin content, an increase in the lipids of the blood, and often a low basal metabolic rate. Few, if any, red cells are found in the urine. The disease is not common, occurring chiefly in children in the 2 to 4 age group. About 80% of the cases occur in persons under 15 years of age.

DIETARY TREATMENT In treatment of the nephrotic syndrome, the protein in the diet is increased to a high level (150 to 250 gm.) in an attempt to make up for the marked loss of albumin in the urine (100 to 200 ml.) and to restore depleted blood and tissues and maintain nitrogen balance. Practically, it is difficult to get a severely and chronically sick child to eat this much food. To maintain the calories at the correct level, whatever diet the child will eat, with emphasis on foods to maintain good nutrition, is encouraged. Fortunately, the appetite frequently improves spontaneously when the edemic fluid disappears.

Sodium (salt) is restricted to reverse the edematous process through diuresis. The intake is usually restricted to 500 mg. per day. Fluids are regulated to coincide with the amount of urine excreted, and to cover insensible loss. See Chapter 30 for sodium restricted diets.

Protein hydrolysates are frequently used in the early stages, especially if the patient is experiencing anorexia, nausea and vomiting. (See Chapter 26, p. 325.) However, in the presence of azotemia, protein restriction may be necessary. Supplementary protein nourishments listed in Chapter 34 (p. 510) are also recommended to increase the protein content of the diet when indicated. Tube feedings are suggested when the patient refuses solid food. (See Chapter 26, p. 384.)

DRUGS Improvement or remission of many of the evidences of the diseases have taken place with corticotropin and steroid therapy. When cortisone therapy is used, increase of potassium in the diet may be necessary (Appendix Table 9). Observations by Heymann and Hunter[39] suggest early treatment favors a satisfactory outcome.

RENAL STONES

Renal stones and nephrocalcinosis are rare conditions in childhood. Occasionally, burns, pyloric stenosis, leukemia, heavy metal poisoning, vitamin D intoxication, sarcoidosis,

and/or paralysis (or recumbence) may lead to renal calcification. See Chapter 32 for dietary treatment of nephrolithiasis. Care must be exercised to insure optimum nutrition for each age group.

DISEASES OF THE NERVOUS SYSTEM

EPILEPSY

Epilepsy rarely develops before the age of 2 years, but after the age of 6 years it is a common cause of recurrent convulsions. The dietary treatment is discussed in Chapter 33.

ALLERGY

Food allergies occur quite frequently among formula-fed infants and children. Breast milk is hypoallergenic. A child born into a family where one or both parents is allergic stands a 60 per cent chance of following suit. Cow's milk and/or eggs are common offenders for infants. Changing from cow's milk to goat's milk often solves the problem. During recent years many commercial milk substitute formulas have been made available, some with soy bean or a meat base formula, and one with amino acids. Once a satisfactory milk or milk substitute has been found, cereals such as rice or oatmeal are added. Care is taken to add one at a time in case of a sensitivity. Then single vegetable purées are tried, carrots, asparagus, spinach and beets being the least likely to cause symptoms. Fruit purées are then added, beginning with pears and apples.

The most common food allergens in children are milk, eggs, tomatoes, chocolate, cola drinks, legumes, strawberries, wheat, beef, potatoes, cinnamon, fish, pork, and corn. Wheat may be replaced by rice, oats, and corn cereals. The other foods are often more difficult to replace. Maintaining normal nutrition is somewhat of a problem in instances where the essential foods, milk, eggs and meat, must be eliminated. Careful attention must be given the individual daily diet to make certain all essential nutrients are included. (See recipes, Chap. 43.)

A child who is allergic to a specific food or foods during childhood may be desensitized and become free of the disturbance in later life. The common allergens and their treatment are discussed in Chapter 27, Nutrition in Diseases of Allergy and the Skin.

DISEASES OF THE MUSCULOSKELETAL SYSTEM

LEAD POISONING

Children with *pica,* an abnormal craving for nonfood substances, are particularly prone

---

[39]Heymann, W., and Hunter, J. L. P.: Importance of early treatment of the nephrotic syndrome. J.A.M.A., *175*:563, 1961.

to lead poisoning. Pica may result from nutritional deficiencies or from emotional disorders.

Most of the paint currently used on children's furniture and toys is free from lead. However, in many older houses and apartments, repainting at home and the construction of homemade toys and furniture lead-based paints may be used. Infants may chew their cribs and toys, or window sills, or may obtain lead from sprays used on fruits and other surfaces. When an excess amount enters the body, lead poisoning may follow. The child suffers from vomiting, irritability, loss of weight, weakness, headache, abdominal pain, insomnia and anorexia and encephalitis may occur. These children are anemic and have peripheral neuritis, muscular incoordination and joint pains. After fluid and electrolyte imbalance is corrected in acute phase the child is given milk to form insoluble salts in the intestine. Large amounts of calcium, phosphorus and vitamin D are given. Refer to Chapter 35 for further discussion of the dietary treatment.

DENTAL CARIES IN CHILDREN

A youngster has an excellent chance to develop good teeth if the expectant mother was properly nourished and received adequate calcium and vitamins. Proper nourishment with adequate calcium and vitamin D during the child's early years rates next in importance. Dentists report a sharp increase in dental caries in adolescence. Prevention of dental caries can be aided by regular brushing of the teeth with an antienzyme dentifrice, and by avoidance of sticky foods and sweets, such as cola drinks, candy and sugar.

More recently fluorides have been studied as a method of preventing tooth decay. (See Chapter 8.) If minute amounts are taken daily during the first eight years of life, the growing period when the permanent set of teeth comes through, the incidence of tooth decay has been reported to be reduced 50 per cent. Knutson and Armstrong utilized oral administration in a group of children over a 2 year period and found a marked decrease in decay formation. Dental caries is discussed in more detail in Chapter 35, Diseases of the Musculoskeletal System.

CEREBRAL PALSY

Cerebral palsy, a disturbance of muscular action caused by damage to portions of the brain, is a real challenge to nursing care in helping the child who is handicapped since birth to make use of his potential abilities. Difficulty in sucking and swallowing causes feeding problems. The spasticity of the muscles often makes eating and drinking difficult. Observations[40] on cerebral palsy children in a residential school suggest that the extent of "mouth area" involvement was closely associated with poor food intake and, correspondingly, with the general growth curve. The many problems of these individuals—food lost through dribbling due to poor function of mouth, tongue or throat and tiring easily while eating—may contribute to inadequate food intake. The nurse can not only feed the child, but she can aid in teaching him to feed himself. Dishes that will not tip over and easy-to-handle cups, glasses, and silver should be given the cerebral palsy patient, and a great deal of patience in helping him to use them should be exercised.

DIETARY TREATMENT   Many of the unfortunate children are underweight and require increased calories to meet the added expenditure of energy produced by the nature of the disease. However, calorie requirement for some spastics may be lower than for normal children. Obesity has been observed in some of these children, especially when they reach the early teens. Protein allowance should be at least the normal level due to the muscle involvement. It is suggested that the calorie requirement for athetoids with their involuntary motion is higher than for spastics who expend less energy. The diet should be adequate in all respects, with foods that are easy to handle and eat. Foods that can be held in the hand are easier to manage than those that must be eaten with fork or spoon. In feeding these patients, small amounts of food or fluids should be given at a time and time allowed between bites or drinks for muscles to relax and the nourishment to be swallowed. It is helpful with some individuals who tend to drool or expectorate to have them hyperextend the neck (head bent backward) when feeding them. Chewing is frequently a problem, and dental caries appear to be more prevalent than in the normal child. Drooling is exaggerated by citrus fruits, and ascorbic acid may have to be taken as a supplement.

Each patient will have specific problems of eating, and the achievements will be determined by the child's ability and mental capacity.

MUSCULAR DYSTROPHY

Muscular dystrophy is of unknown etiology and is considered to be a group of disorders in which the clinical features are progressive wasting and weakness of the striated muscles. It is a familial disease which generally

[40]Ruby, D. O., and Matheny, W. D.: Comments on growth of cerebral palsied children. Am. J. Dietet. A., 40:525, 1962.

has its onset in childhood. The enzymes that normally break down muscle protein become overactive, while those that normally build up the protein cannot replace it fast enough. In addition, there is a defect in creatine metabolism. Eventually there may be involvement of most of the striated muscles in the body. A child may run and play normally, but a few months later, stumble, still later become weak, have trouble getting up, and become helpless. Few such children live beyond their late teens. At present there is no specific therapy, in spite of numerous empirical remedies which have been tried, based upon the many different hypotheses of etiology. None of these has had any effect on the underlying process of the disease. The use of an anabolic steroid along with digitoxin and physical therapy has shown promise of benefiting some muscular dystrophy patients.[41] However, unless a therapy corrects the basic metabolic defect it is not the final answer to treatment.

DIETARY TREATMENT Milhorat[42] recommends a varied diet of good quality, preferably high in protein content. Intensive nutritional support is needed in the very early stages in an attempt to arrest the wasting and to prolong remissions. For the patient whose muscular disability makes it difficult to feed himself, aids for self-feeding have been designed (p. 326). The nurse can be of invaluable help in the general treatment of the patient by teaching him how to use the feeding aids and encouraging him to use them, thus keeping the muscles in use in an attempt to prevent the muscular atrophy caused by disuse.

---

[41]Dowben, R. M.: Treatment of muscular dystrophy with steroids. New England J. Med., *268*:912, 1962.

[42]Milhorat, A. T.: *In* Wohl, M. G.: Long-Term Illness, Philadelphia, W. B. Saunders Company, 1959, pp. 457–459.

PROBLEMS AND SUGGESTED TOPICS FOR DISCUSSION

1. Observe the eating habits of the children in your hospital. What considerations should be observed in feeding the sick child?
2. Is it essential to maintain adequate nutrition in a child with an acute febrile disease such as measles? Explain. In rheumatic fever? Explain.
3. If possible, observe an infant who is suffering with pyloric stenosis. Follow the eating program and evaluate food intake for a day or two. Compare the diet with the accepted nutritional standard allowances for the same age. Observe if any vomiting occurs and estimate the food lost.
4. Why is diarrhea so prevalent in the lesser developed countries? What is being done to improve the condition?
5. Study the feeding program prescribed for patients with celiac disease in your hospital. Compare the diets with the dietary treatment discussed in this text.
6. Plan a diet with a diabetic child in your children's ward. Determine what he needs to know about food

and meal planning. Involve him in planning his dietary regimen on the basis of family meals.
7. (a) Counsel an obese adolescent on how to lose weight following an adequate dietary regimen, taking into consideration any emotional and social problems. Be sure the diet is nutritionally adequate for his age. Follow his weight curve.
   (b) Follow the same procedure for an underweight child in your hospital.
8. What do galactosemia and phenylketonuria have in common? Give the treatment for each. Name two other inborn errors of metabolism occurring in infancy.
9. Plan a diet for a child who is 12 years old, 10 pounds underweight, and suffering with nephrosis. What are the principles of the diet?
10. How can the nurse help a cerebral palsy patient to feed himself?
11. What are the problems and dietary treatment for muscular dystrophy?
12. In what periods in life does iron deficiency anemia usually occur? What is the dietary and related treatment?
13. List the vitamin deficiency diseases generally associated with infancy and childhood. Give dietary treatment for each.

SUGGESTED ADDITIONAL READING REFERENCES

Acosta, P. B., and Centerwall, W. R.: Phenylketonuria: Dietary management. J. Am. Dietet. A., *36*:206, 1960.

Allen, R. J., and Wilson, J. L.: Urinary phenylpyruvic acid in phenylketonuria. J.A.M.A., *188*:720, 1964.

Anonymous: Nutritional Management of Galactosemia. Mead Johnson Laboratories, Evansville, Indiana.

Anonymous: White House Conference on Food, Nutrition and Health, Final Report, 1970. Superintendent of Documents, Washington, D.C., 20402.

Bengoa, J. M., et al.: Some indications for a broad assessment of the magnitude of protein-calorie malnutrition in young children in population groups. Am. J. Clin. Nutr., 7:714, 1959.

Berry, H. K.: Inborn errors of metabolism. J. Am. Dietet. A., *49*:401, 1966.

Bullen, B. A., et al.: Attitudes towards physical activity, food and family in obese and nonobese adolescent girls. Am. J. Clin. Nutr., *12*:1, 1963.

Coursin, D. B.: Convulsive seizures in infants with pyridoxine-deficient diet. J.A.M.A., *154*:406, 1954.

Darby, W. J.: This hungry world. Am. J. Clin. Nutr., 16: 509, 1965.

di Sant'Agnese, P. A., and Jones, W. O.: The celiac syndrome (malabsorption) in pediatrics. J.A.M.A., *180*: 308, 1962.

Editorial. Pneumonia and empyema in infants and children. J.A.M.A., *175*:1097, 1961.

Editorial. The celiac syndrome. J.A.M.A., *180*:332, 1962.

Editorial. Maple syrup urine disease. J.A.M.A., *186*:147, 1963.

Editorial. Celiac disease and gluten-free diet. J.A.M.A., *186*:1015, 1963.

Editorial. Behavior in phenylketonuria. J.A.M.A., *187*:452, 1964.

Editorial. Urinary phenylpyruvic acid in phenylketonuria. J.A.M.A., *188*:748, 1964.

Etzwiler, D. D., and Sines, L. K.: Juvenile diabetes and its management. J.A.M.A., *181*:304, 1962.

Feinstein, A. R., et al.: Oral prophylaxis of recurrent rheumatic fever. J.A.M.A., *188*:489, 1964.

Fincke, M. L.: Inborn errors of metabolism. J. Am. Dietet. A., *46*:280, 1965.

Fraumeni, J. F., et al.: Diseases of hypersensitivity and childhood leukemia. J.A.M.A., *188*:459, 1964.

Gallagher, J. R.: Weight control in adolescence. J. Am. Dietet. A., *40*:519, 1962.

Getty, G., and Hollensworth, M.: Through a child's eye seeing. Nutrition Today, 2:17, 1967.

Goodman, S. I., et al.: The treatment of maple syrup urine disease. J. Pediat., 75:485, 1969.

Gordon, J. E.: Weanling diarrhea: A synergism of nutrition and infection. Nutr. Rev., 22:161, 1964.

Griggs, R. C., et al.: Environmental factors in childhood lead poisoning. J.A.M.A., 187:703, 1964.

Hammond, M. I., et al.: A nutritional study of cerebral palsied children. J. Am. Dietet. A., 49:196, 1966.

Hamwi, G. J.: Treatment of diabetes. J.A.M.A., 181:124, 1962.

Hathaway, M. L., and Sargent, D. W.: Overweight in children. J. Am. Dietet. A., 40:511, 1962.

Heymann, W., and Hunter, J. L. P.: Importance of early treatment of the nephrotic syndrome. J.A.M.A., 175:563, 1961.

Ingelfinger, F. J.: For want of an enzyme. Nutrition Today, 3:2, 1968.

Jackson, R. L.: The child with diabetes mellitus. J.A.M.A., 176:854, 1961.

Jacobziner, H., and Raybin, H. W.: Lead poisoning in infancy and young children. New York J. Med., p. 897, March 15, 1958.

Koch, R., et al.: Nutrition in the treatment of galactosemia. Am. J. Dietet. A., 43:216, 1963.

Koch, R., et al.: Nutrition in the treatment of phenylketonuria. Am. J. Dietet. A., 43:212, 1963.

Korsch, G., and Barnett, H. L.: The physician, the family and the child with nephrosis. J. Pediat., 58:707, 1961.

Lindquist, B., and Meeuwisse, G.: Diets in disaccharidase deficiency and defective monosaccharide absorption. J. Am. Dietet. A., 48:307, 1966.

Lonsdale, D., et al.: Maple syrup urine disease. Am. J. Dis. Child., 106:258, 1963.

McCarthy, M. A., et al.: Phenylalanine and tyrosine in vegetables and fruits. J. Am. Dietet. A., 52:130, 1968.

Mike, E. M.: Practical guide and dietary management of children with seizures using the ketogenic diet. Am. J. Clin. Nutr., 17:399, 1965.

Miller, G. T., et al.: Phenylalanine content of fruit. J. Am. Dietet. A., 46:43, 1965.

Orr, M. L., and Watt, B. K.: Amino acid content of food. U.S. Department of Agriculture, Home Economics Research Dept., No. 4, 1957.

Orten, J. M., and Orten, A. U.: DNA and inborn errors of metabolism. J. Am. Dietet. A., 59:331, 1971.

Pratt, E. L.: Food allergy and food intolerance in relation to the development of good eating habits. Pediatrics, 21:642, 1958.

Ravitch, M. M., and Fein, R.: The changing picture of pneumonia and empyema in infants and children. J.A.M.A., 175:1039, 1961.

Review. A screening test for phenylketonuria. Nutr. Rev., 22:196, 1964.

Review. Dietary iron in infancy. Nutr. Rev., 21:338, 1963.

Review. Gluten enteropathy. Nutr. Rev., 21:300, 1963.

Review. Histidinemia—A new inborn error of metabolism. Am. J. Dietet. A., 42:51, 1963.

Review. Phenylketonuria. Nutr. Rev., 19:264, 1961.

Review. Recent developments in muscular dystrophy research. Nutr. Rev., 22:136, 1964.

Review. The celiac syndrome (malabsorption) in pediatrics. Nutr. Rev., 21:195, 1963.

Review. Vitamin B_6-deficiency state in infants. Nutr. Rev., 19:229, 1961.

Ruby, D. O., and Matheny, W. D.: Comments on growth of cerebral palsied children. J. Am. Dietet. A., 40:525, 1962.

Scrimshaw, N. S.: Malnutrition and the health of children. J. Am. Dietet. A., 42:203, 1963.

Silver, H. K., and Finkelstein, M.: Deprivation dwarfism. J. Pediat., 70:317, 1967.

Smith, B. A., and Waisman, H. A.: Leucine equivalency system in managing branched-chain ketoaciduria. J. Am. Dietet. A., 59:342, 1971.

Soyka, L. F.: Treatment of the nephrotic syndrome in childhood. Am. J. Dis. Child., 113:693, 1967.

Sutherland, B. S., et al.: Growth and nutrition in treated phenylketonuric patients. J.A.M.A., 211:270, 1970.

Tanis, A. L.: Lead poisoning in children. Am. J. Dis. Child., 89:325, 1955.

The Clinical Team Looks at Phenylketonuria. U.S. Department of Health, Education and Welfare. Revised 1964. U.S. Government Printing Office, Washington, D.C., 20402.

Thomson, N. B., Jr., and Jewett, T. C., Jr.: Peptic ulcers in infancy and childhood. J.A.M.A., 189:539, 1964.

Udenfriend, S.: Phenylketonuria. Am. J. Clin. Nutr., 9:691, 1961.

Umbarger, B., et al.: Advances in the management of patients with phenylketonuria. J.A.M.A., 193:784, 1965.

Wilson, J. F., et al.: Milk-induced gastrointestinal bleeding in infants with hypochronic microcytic anemia. J.A.M.A., 189:568, 1964.

Woodruff, C. W.: Growth and nutrition of Lebanese children. Nutr. Rev., 23:97, 1965.

Wright, F. H.: Preventing obesity in childhood. J. Am. Dietet. A., 40:516, 1962.

Yardley, J. H., et al.: Celiac disease: A study of the jejunal epithelium before and after a gluten-free diet. New England J. Med., 267:1173, 1962.

Part Three
FOODS

This section of the book deals with foods— their composition, uses, availability, nutritional value, and digestibility. The material is arranged according to the four food groups developed by the Institute of Home Economics, United States Department of Agriculture, and used in the daily food guide: the (1) milk, (2) meat, (3) vegetable-fruit and (4) bread-cereal groups. This arrangement points out the most important contributions of the foodstuffs toward meeting daily food requirements and makes it easy to provide variety in meals from day to day. A few basic recipes are included in each group, scaled for individual practice, or for demonstration. Many recipes combine foods from two or more groups, and can be counted toward the day's total needs. Since this is not a recipe book, space does not permit including more than a few basic recipes illustrating each food group. Although the nurse is seldom, if ever, required to prepare food for a patient, her position as an interpreter of health practices, and as a teacher, requires a working knowledge of food.

Chapter 37
INTRODUCTION TO FOODS: SELECTION, PREPARATION AND SERVICE

FOOD SELECTION

When the scientific facts about the various nutrients are put into practice through the wise selection, preparation and service of foods, nutrition becomes effective. In contrast to primitive man, who gathered available food, modern man is confused by an abundance. While the appetite of primitive man may or may not have been satisfied by local grains, berries, nuts, wild game, and fish, the appetite of modern man may be satiated with foods which appeal to the individual taste.

The business of providing food has grown into a vast industry which ignores seasons and perishability through the milling of grains into flour and cereal, the canning and freezing of vegetables and fruits, the scientific collection of milk and conversion into milk products, the packaging of meat, and the manufacture of numerous varieties of ready-to-eat foods. Because the array of food is greater, the rules of nutrition are observed more closely to help man select foods which provide healthful nutrients.

THE NUTRITIONALLY ADEQUATE DAILY MEALS

During the past century, the role of each nutrient has been clarified, and foods have been classified accordingly into groups of protein foods, energy foods, mineral-rich foods, and vitamin-rich foods. From these groups of nutrients, foods are selected for meals. It is not hard to select a daily dietary that contains enough of each of the four food groups recommended—milk, meat, vegetables and fruit, bread and cereals (Fig. 2-1). A wide range of choices is available. The arrangement of meals should follow the pattern of work and living. If the work period is during the daytime, food is usually served in the morning, at noon and in the evening. If the work period covers any other hours of the day, the meals are arranged differently. The quantity of food served during the day may follow the usual three meal pattern or be altered to include between-meal nourishments.

FEEDING THE PATIENT

In the hospital, the meals and nourishments are usually prepared in the central kitchen and/or the diet kitchen (see Fig. 37-1).

Because the service of the three daily meals and between-meal nourishments are often highlights of the day and looked forward to by the patient, the nurse should attempt to make mealtime a pleasant experience. A comfortable room temperature, free of drafts, a comfortable eating position in bed or on a chair located away from unpleasant sights, and pleasant conversation or music encourage good food intake. Most patients prefer to wash hands and face before eating and to eat from a table free of other objects (Fig. 37-2).

The arrangement of the tray should reflect thoughtfulness and consideration of the patient's needs and wishes. The china, glassware and silver on the tray are in a convenient location and within the reach of patient. Independence should be encouraged in the patient who requires assistance in

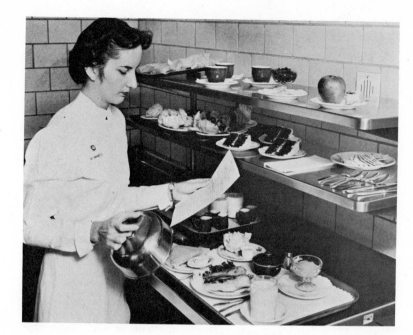

Figure 37–1   In the hospital a dietitian is frequently responsible for checking the tray as shown here. Sometimes this is the duty of the nurse, especially the nurse on private duty.

Figure 37–2   The nurse or dietitian can do much to improve appetite and food intake.

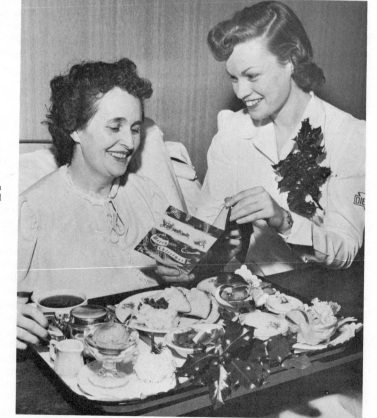

eating. The nurse can accomplish this by having the patient specify the sequence of foods eaten and having him participate in eating even if this means only holding his bread.

A patient's attitude toward his illness and hospitalization is reflected frequently in the rejection of meals or the prescribed dietary. Other reasons for poor acceptance of hospital meals may be due to unfamiliar foods, eating schedule and improper food temperatures. By giving the patient an opportunity to express himself and by accepting the patient's attitudes, the nurse can help the patient overcome his feelings and improve food acceptance. Food acceptance is also improved when self-selection of menus is encouraged and when the patient is given an explanation of why a particular diet is prescribed. Problems with food acceptance that the nurse can not handle should be communicated to the dietary department.

MEAL PLANNING

What a patient considers to be a good meal will depend upon who he is and where he lives. If a patient participates in the planning or selection of his meals, he will incorporate the factors that meet his expectation for a good meal. Refer to Chapter 13 for a review of geographic and cultural dietary variations. To ensure adequate nutrition each meal should contain a complete protein or the essential amino acids through mutual supplementation and adequate calories. Other foods can be added to provide other essential nutrients and meet individual preferences. Refer to Chapter 11, An Adequate Diet.

The pleasing contrast of colors of food can stimulate the appetite and taste buds. "It looks good enough to eat" is the praise awarded a carefully arranged tray which considers the colors of food. The addition of a slice of tomato and a sprig of parsley furnishes color and relieves the monotony of white food on a white plate.

Contrast of textures is equally important to many people. Perhaps one of the reasons why a patient tires of either a liquid diet or soft diet is the monotony of the sameness in food textures. Contrasting liquid, soft, solid and crunchy textures of food invites variety. For example, creamed potatoes are not generally enjoyed when served with creamed vegetables and ice cream.

A contrast in the temperature of foods is often desirable. If a meal is composed of cold foods, it may be prefaced with a hot soup. A cold dessert and cold salad offer contrast to hot dishes. It is also desirable to serve cold food in chilled dishes and hot food in hot dishes.

FOOD PREPARATION

Cookery standards are variable and seem to be related to the person's interest and like for foods. Food preparation procedures are usually related to nutrition principles; for example, vegetables are cooked quickly in covered saucepans and in small quantities of water to retain vitamin and mineral content.

Organization of the foods to be prepared for a meal is essential. First, all foods and ingredients needed should be checked and assembled. Next, the order of preparation should be planned so that all foods or dishes will be ready to serve at the proper time. Start with the dish that takes the longest time to prepare, or those that can be made ahead of time, and follow up with the others in the order of time it takes to prepare. Know the degree of temperature and time needed to cook a food before starting the preparation, and plan accordingly.

Careless service can spoil the appetite although the food is properly prepared. If the patient is expected to enjoy his meals, the standards for cookery and food service deserve recognition and respect. The haphazard thoughtless arrangement of plates on a tray may not encourage the finicky appetite, and may be repulsive to the hearty eater. Cleanliness and neatness are important aspects of any good food service (Fig. 37–3).

ABBREVIATIONS

Along with the specialized vocabulary which is employed in the medical, dietetic and nursing fields, there are acceptable forms of abbreviations. Here is a list of abbreviations commonly used.

aa: Gr. *ana;* of each
a.c.: L. *ante cibum;* before meals
ad., add: L. *adde, addatur,* or *addantur;* add or added
ad. lib.: L. *ad libitum;* at pleasure, as desired
aq.: L. *aqua;* water
aq. dest.: L. *aqua destillata;* distilled water
b.i.d., bis in d.: L. *bis in die;* twice a day
c̄.: L. *cum;* with
c.: cup
cc.: cubic centimeter
Cent.; cent.; C.: centigrade
cm.: centimeter
dilut.: L. *dilutus;* dilute
div.: L. *divide;* divide
fac.: make
gm.: gram
gr.: L. *granum;* grain
gtt.: L. *guttae;* drops
h.s.: L. *hora somni;* at hour of sleep, 8 P.M.
kcal.: kilocalorie
kg.: kilogram
kJ.: kilojoule
lb.: pound
mcg.: microgram
mEq.: milliequivalent

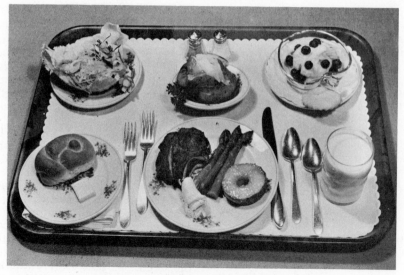

Figure 37–3   A neat and attractive dinner tray.

mg.: milligram
mil. or ml.: milliliter
oz.: ounce
p.r.n.: L. *pro re nata;* may be repeated according to instructions
pt.: pint
pulv.: L. *pulvis;* powder
q.d.: L. *quaque die;* every day
Q.I.D., q.i.d.: L. *quater in die:* four times daily
q. 3h.: every three hours
q.s.: L. *quantum satis;* a sufficient quantity
qt.: quart
s.: L. *sine;* without
sol.: solution
ss.: L. *semis;* half
stat.: L. *statim;* immediately
t., tsp.: teaspoon
T., tbsp.: tablespoon
t.i.d.: L. *ter in die;* three times a day

THE METRIC SYSTEM AND EQUIVALENTS

To measure ingredients, a standardized system has been established which is interpreted on an international basis. However, in our country we also employ another set of measure and weight. In the field of dietetics, both systems are employed. The following tables give the quantities of the measures besides stating equivalents. With this information it is possible to calculate in either system of measure and weight.

LEVEL MEASURES AND WEIGHTS

60 drops	=	1 teaspoon
		5 cc.
		5 grams
4 saltspoons	=	1 teaspoon
		5 grams

3 teaspoons	=	1 tablespoon
		15 cc.
		15 grams
1 dessert spoon	=	10 cc.
2 tablespoons	=	30 cc.
		30 grams
		1 ounce (fluid)
4 tablespoons	=	¼ cup
		60 cc.
		60 grams
8 tablespoons	=	½ cup
		120 cc.
		120 grams
16 tablespoons	=	1 cup
		240 grams
		250 ml. or mil. (fluid)
		8 ounces (fluid)
		½ pound
2 cups	=	1 pint
		480 grams
		500 ml. or mil. (fluid)
		16 ounces (fluid)
		1 pound
4 cups	=	2 pints
		1 quart
		1000 or 960 cc.
		1000 ml. or mil. (fluid)
		1 kilogram
		2.2 pounds
4 quarts	=	1 gallon
8 quarts	=	1 peck
2 gallons	=	1 peck
4 pecks	=	1 bushel
8 gallons	=	1 bushel

HOUSEHOLD MEASUREMENT EQUIVALENTS IN GRAMS

For easy computing purposes, the cubic centimeter

(cc.) is considered equivalent to 1 gram:

1 cc. = 1 gram

For easy computing purposes, one ounce equals 30 grams or 30 cubic centimeters.

1 quart	=	960 grams
1 pint	=	480 grams
1 cup	=	240 grams
½ cup	=	120 grams
1 soup cup	=	120 grams
1 glass (8 ounces)	=	240 grams
½ glass (4 ounces)	=	120 grams
1 orange juice glass	=	100 to 120 grams
1 tablespoon	=	15 grams
1 teaspoon	=	5 grams

GALLONS TO LITERS
1 =	3.785
2 =	7.57
3 =	11.36
4 =	15.14
5 =	18.93
6 =	22.71
7 =	26.50
8 =	30.28
9 =	34.07

LITERS TO GALLONS
1 =	0.264
2 =	0.53
3 =	0.79
4 =	1.06
5 =	1.32
6 =	1.59
7 =	1.85
8 =	2.11
9 =	2.38

COMPARISON OF AVOIRDUPOIS AND METRIC WEIGHTS

OUNCES TO GRAMS
1 =	28.35
2 =	56.70
3 =	85.05
4 =	113.40
5 =	141.75
6 =	170.10
7 =	198.45
8 =	226.80
9 =	255.15

GRAMS TO OUNCES
1 =	0.035
2 =	0.07
3 =	0.11
4 =	0.14
5 =	0.18
6 =	0.21
7 =	0.25
8 =	0.28
9 =	0.32

POUNDS TO KILOGRAMS
1 =	0.454
2 =	0.91
3 =	1.36
4 =	1.81
5 =	2.27
6 =	2.72
7 =	3.18
8 =	3.63
9 =	4.08

KILOGRAMS TO POUNDS
1 =	2.205
2 =	4.41
3 =	6.61
4 =	8.82
5 =	11.02
6 =	13.23
7 =	15.43
8 =	17.64
9 =	19.84

HOUSEHOLD WEIGHTS AND MEASURES

It is helpful to know the yield of certain quantities of food. For that reason the following table of weights and measures of food is useful.

To conclude the set of weights and measures, those used to measure volume and weight and avoirdupois measures for dry and liquid ingredients are given.

1	pound of butter	=	2 cups
1	square of chocolate	=	1 ounce
1	ounce of chocolate	=	¼ cup cocoa
8	average eggs	=	1 cup
8	to 10 egg whites	=	1 cup
12	to 14 egg yolks	=	1 cup
4	cups sifted all purpose flour	=	1 pound
4½	cups sifted cake flour	=	1 pound
2	cups granulated sugar	=	1 pound
2⅔	cups confectioner's sugar	=	1 pound
2⅔	cups brown sugar	=	1 pound
1	pound of walnuts or pecans in shell	=	½ pound shelled

COMPARISON OF UNITED STATES AND METRIC LIQUID MEASURE

OUNCES (FLUID) TO MILLILITERS
1 =	29.573
2 =	59.15
3 =	88.72
4 =	118.30
5 =	147.87
6 =	177.44
7 =	207.02
8 =	236.59
9 =	266.16

MILLILITERS TO OUNCES (FLUID)
1 =	0.034
2 =	0.07
3 =	0.10
4 =	0.14
5 =	0.17
6 =	0.20
7 =	0.24
8 =	0.27
9 =	0.31

QUARTS TO LITERS
1 =	0.946
2 =	1.89
3 =	2.84
4 =	3.79
5 =	4.73
6 =	5.68
7 =	6.62
8 =	7.57
9 =	8.52

LITERS TO QUARTS
1 =	1.057
2 =	2.11
3 =	3.17
4 =	4.23
5 =	5.28
6 =	6.34
7 =	7.40
8 =	8.45
9 =	9.51

MEASURES OF VOLUME
1 bushel	=	4 pecks
1 peck	=	8 quarts
1 gallon	=	4 quarts
1 quart	=	2 pints (946.4 milliliters)
1 pint	=	2 cups
1 cup	=	16 tablespoons (2 gills, 8 fluid ounces, 237 mililiters)
1 tablespoon	=	3 teaspoons (½ fluid ounce)
1 teaspoon	=	5 milliliters
1 liter	=	1000 milliliters (1.06 quarts)

MEASURES OF WEIGHT
1 gram	=	0.035 ounce
1 kilogram	=	2.21 pounds
1 ounce	=	28.35 grams
1 pound	=	453.6 grams

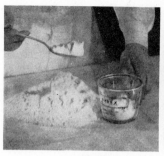 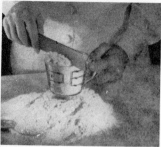

A   B

Figure 37–4 How to measure dry ingredients such as flour. *A,* Spoon sifted flour lightly into a dry measuring cup, heaping it up. *B,* Level off cup with straight-edged knife. Don't shake cup. (From Betty Crocker's Picture Cook Book. General Mills, Minneapolis, Minn.)

AVOIRDUPOIS MEASURE
(TO WEIGH OR MEASURE HEAVY
AND COARSE ARTICLES)

DRY MEASURE

16 drams (drs.)	=	1 ounce (oz.)
16 ounces (oz.)	=	1 pound (lb.)
7000 grains (gr.)	=	1 pound
25 pounds (lb.)	=	1 quarter (qr.)
4 quarters (qr.)	=	100 weight (cwt.)
20 hundredweight (cwt.)	=	1 Ton (T.)

LIQUID MEASURE

2 pints	=	1 quart (57¾ cubic inches)
4 quarts	=	1 gallon (231 cubic inches)
8 gallons	=	1 bushel (2150.42 cubic inches; a cylinder which measures 18½ inches [diameter] by 8 inches [deep])

HOW TO USE A RECIPE

A standard recipe is the result of experimental testing, and when directions are accurately followed as to measurement of ingredients and method of combining, a desirable product is assured. This includes the following points:

1. Read the recipe carefully and plan the procedure of work before starting.

2. If the product is to be baked, preheat the oven to correct temperature. Do not waste fuel by turning heat on too soon. If food is to be cooked on top of the stove, use temperature directed. Never try to hurry a product by increasing the temperature above that directed in the recipe.

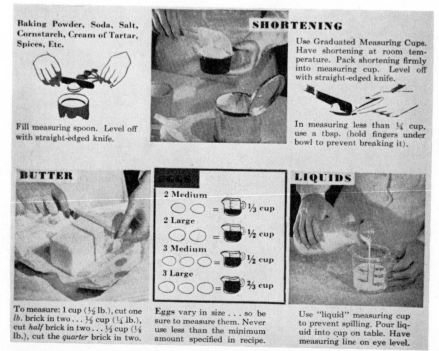

Baking Powder, Soda, Salt, Cornstarch, Cream of Tartar, Spices, Etc.

Fill measuring spoon. Level off with straight-edged knife.

SHORTENING

Use Graduated Measuring Cups. Have shortening at room temperature. Pack shortening firmly into measuring cup. Level off with straight-edged knife.

In measuring less than ¼ cup, use a tbsp. (hold fingers under bowl to prevent breaking it).

BUTTER

To measure: 1 cup (½ lb.), cut one lb. brick in two . . . ½ cup (¼ lb.), cut *half* brick in two . . . ½ cup (⅛ lb.), cut the *quarter* brick in two.

2 Medium	= ⅓ cup
2 Large	= ½ cup
3 Medium	= ½ cup
3 Large	= ⅔ cup

Eggs vary in size . . . so be sure to measure them. Never use less than the minimum amount specified in recipe.

LIQUIDS

Use "liquid" measuring cup to prevent spilling. Pour liquid into cup on table. Have measuring line on eye level.

Figure 37–5 How to measure shortening, butter, eggs and liquids. (From Betty Crocker's Picture Cook Book. General Mills, Minneapolis, Minn.)

SUBSTITUTES FOR INGREDIENTS

FOR THESE	YOU MAY USE THESE
1 whole egg, for thickening or baking	2 egg yolks. Or 2½ tablespoons sifted dried whole egg plus 2½ tablespoons water.
1 cup butter or margarine for shortening	⅞ cup lard, or rendered fat, with ½ teaspoon salt. Or 1 cup hydrogenated fat (cooking fat sold under brand name) with ½ teaspoon salt.
1 square (ounce) chocolate	3 tablespoons cocoa plus 1 tablespoon fat.
1 teaspoon sulfate-phosphate baking powder	1½ teaspoons phosphate baking powder. Or 2 teaspoons tartrate baking powder.
1 cup buttermilk or sour milk, for baking	1 cup sweet milk mixed with one of the following: 1 tablespoon vinegar. Or 1 tablespoon lemon juice. Or 1¾ teaspoons cream of tartar.
1 cup fluid whole milk	½ cup evaporated milk plus ½ cup water. Or 1 cup reconstituted dry whole milk. Or 1 cup reconstituted nonfat dry milk plus 2½ teaspoons butter or margarine. (To reconstitute dry milk follow directions on the package.)
1 cup fluid skim milk	1 cup reconstituted nonfat dry milk prepared according to directions on the package.
1 tablespoon flour, for thickening	½ tablespoon cornstarch, potato starch, rice starch, or arrowroot starch. Or 2 teaspoons quick cooking tapioca.
1 cup cake flour, for baking	⅞ cup all-purpose flour.
1 cup all-purpose flour, for baking breads	Up to ½ cup bran, whole-wheat flour, or cornmeal plus enough all-purpose flour to fill cup.

3. Assemble all ingredients to be used.
4. Choose and assemble utensils, considering size of mixing bowls and pans to fit the recipe.
5. Use standard measuring cups and measuring spoons.
6. Accurate measurement is essential to successful food preparation. All measurements are *level*. When the recipe calls for dry, liquid, and fat ingredients, measure in the order given, thereby using only one cup. (Figs. 37–4 and 37–5).
7. When substitution of one ingredient for another is necessary, the above may be used.

Not every person likes the same finished product. As skill is gained in the basic cookery procedures, more freedom can be taken in experimenting with new flavors and textures.

SUGGESTED ADDITIONAL READING REFERENCES

Conserving the Nutritive Values in Foods. Home and Garden Bulletin No. 90, U.S. Department of Agriculture, Washington, D.C.

Family Fare. (Food management and recipes.) Home and Garden Bulletin No. 1, U.S. Department of Agriculture, Washington, D.C.

Money-saving Main Dishes. Home and Garden Bulletin No. 43, U.S. Department of Agriculture, Washington, D.C.

Stumpf, G. L.: Improving quality foods. J. Am. Dietet. A., 39:22, 1961.

The Food We Eat. Miscellaneous Pub. No. 870, U.S. Department of Agriculture, Washington, D.C.

Chapter 38
GROUP I: MILK GROUP

MILK PRODUCTS IN GENERAL

SOME MILK FOR EVERYONE DAILY

Children
    Under 9 years of age—2 to 3 cups (1 pt. or more)

9 to 12 years of age—3 or more cups (3/4 qt. or more)

Teen-agers
    4 or more cups (1 qt. or more)

Adults
    2 or more cups (1 pt. or more)

The use of milk from cattle goes back to antiquity. It is mentioned in the Bible at least 50 times, and there is evidence of the common use of milk, cheese and butter in Egyptian, Greek and Roman civilizations. A 5000 year old frieze, unearthed in the Euphrates valley, portrays men seated on low stools milking cows. Marco Polo reported in the 13th century that the Asians used dairy products.

Cultures that failed to domesticate animals were handicapped; their people were not so healthy and mothers had to nurse children for two or three years because there was no substitute. The Spanish conquerors brought cattle to the new world, but our present stock is said to have come from European animals imported during the 17th century.

CALCIUM EQUIVALENTS

On the basis of calcium content, cheese and ice cream can replace the milk recommended for a day. On the basis of the calcium they provide, the following are alternates for 1 cup (8 oz.) of milk:

1⅓ ounces Cheddar, American or Swiss cheese
16 ounces cream cheese
1⅓ cups cottage cheese
1⅔ cups ice cream
3 cups milk sherbet
1 cup baked custard
1 cup nonfat milk
1 cup buttermilk
½ cup undiluted evaporated milk
¼ cup dried nonfat milk powder
¼ cup dried whole milk powder

MILK BEVERAGES

Probably the most common use of milk is as a drink. It is also the basic ingredient in making many good tasting, nutritious beverages.

Cow's milk is generally the milk of choice, although milk from other animals, such as the goat, is consumed in some countries where cows are scarce. The kinds of milk used are whole, skim, evaporated, condensed, dried whole and dried skim (nonfat solids), which are described in Chapter 12, Food Economics.

COMPOSITION OF MILK Milk is a yellowish white liquid emulsion containing a high quality protein (mainly casein with small amounts of lactalbumin and lactoglobulin), fat (cream), carbohydrate (lactose or milk sugar), the minerals calcium and phosphorus, the vitamins riboflavin, niacin, vitamin A, and (when the milk is fortified) vitamin D.

The composition of milk varies to some degree with the breed of cattle, the season of the year and with the feed of the animal. However, the milk purchased in the market is a mixture from different breeds and maintains a fairly constant average. Local and state regulations adjust the required butterfat and solids content. The average composition of cow's milk is given in Chapter 16, page 253.

NUTRITIONAL VALUE AND DIGESTIBILITY The value of milk in the dietary for all age levels has been repeatedly emphasized throughout this text. It furnishes about a hundred nutrients but is outstanding in importance for calcium, riboflavin and protein. Three-fourths of the calcium, nearly one-half of the riboflavin, and one-fourth of the protein in the country's food supply come from milk. If milk is omitted or sparingly used in the diet, it is difficult to meet the requirement for calcium and riboflavin. Surveys indicate that growing children and teen-agers, as well as adults, do not get enough milk in their diets. A study of four species of growing animals (Fig. 38–1) demonstrates that a combination of the foods recommended in the typical dietary pattern does not support

Approximate figures showing calories in milk and milk products

	QUANTITY	KCALORIES
Fresh fluid whole milk	1 cup (½ pint)	160
Fresh fluid skim milk	1 cup	90
Buttermilk (nonfat)	1 cup	90
Half-and-half	1 cup	325
Chocolate-flavored milk drink	1 cup	190
Cocoa	1 cup	235
Malted milk beverage	1 cup	280
Evaporated milk, diluted with equal water	1 cup	173
Nonfat dry milk	4 tablespoons (¼ cup)	63
Ice cream	1 slice (⅛ of qt. brick)	145
Ice milk	½ cup	143
Cheddar cheese	1-inch cube	70
Cottage cheese, creamed	½ cup	120
Cottage cheese, uncreamed	½ cup	98

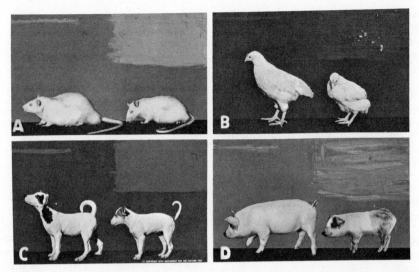

Figure 38–1   A, These rats are male siblings of the same age. They were the same size when 3 weeks old. B, These chickens are female siblings of the same age. They were the same size when 10 days old. C, These dogs are female siblings of the same age. They were the same size when 4 weeks old. D, These pigs are female siblings of the same age. They were the same size when 3 weeks old. In each case the larger animal had milk added to its food; the smaller animal received no milk. (Courtesy Dairy Council Digests, National Dairy Council, 111 North Canal Street, Chicago, Illinois 60606.)

normal growth unless milk is included in adequate amounts.

A pint of milk in the diet for the adult yields approximately 320 kcalories, while a quart will furnish 640 kcalories. If calories must be kept down, skim milk can be used to supply all the nutrients in whole milk except fat and vitamin A. One pint of skimmed milk has 180 kcalories.

If calories are to be increased in the diet, ingredients such as cocoa, chocolate, ice cream and malted milk can be added to milk. For example, one pint of malted milk beverage contains approximately 560 kcalories.

The protein in milk, casein, is of highest quality and is particularly suitable for use by the body in building muscle tissue. It contains all the amino acids needed for body building and repair of tissue. The carbohydrate is in the form of lactose, a disaccharide which is not so sweet as cane sugar, making it particularly suitable for the diet of the sick. Lactose does not ferment readily and does not cause gastric disturbances, as do some sugars. The minerals found in milk, especially calcium and phosphorus, are essential for the structure of bones and teeth for individuals of all ages, especially infants and children. The amount of iron in milk is small, but it is in a form readily used by the body. Milk is a dependable source of vitamin A, thiamin, niacin and riboflavin. Some vitamin C is present but not in adequate quantities. Natural milk does not contain adequate vitamin D to prevent rickets and produce normal growth and tooth develop-

ment, but it is especially adaptable for fortification with this vitamin. The Council on Foods and Nutrition recommends fortification of milk as a public health measure and, currently, a high proportion of bottled milk—and practically all evaporated milk—is fortified. The fat (cream) in milk is in an emulsified form which contains vitamin A and is easily digested and well tolerated.

MILK IN THE DAILY DIET   In the amounts recommended, milk contributes more protein to the diet than any other single food. When milk is omitted from the diet, the protein requirement of the child can be met only if special and expert planning is carried out. The mineral and vitamin contributions are equally important.

Adults, especially senior citizens, often feel it is not a necessary food for them. The objection that it is fattening, or not liked, can be met by encouraging the use of skim milk in reducing diets, and incorporating milk in dishes especially enjoyed if milk is not liked as a beverage. Milk can be taken in the form of cheese, used in creamed soups, in creamed dishes, baked products, vegetables, milk desserts and in beverages made with milk.

MAKING MILK SAFE   Most milk is pasteurized, a process described in Chapter 12. Pasteurized milk has been heated to destroy pathogenic bacteria, and then cooled rapidly, making it safe to drink. In addition to being pasteurized, milk may also be homogenized (Chapter 12), a process which reduces the size of the cream particles. As a result, the cream does not rise to the top of the milk but stays suspended. Certified milk is not pasteurized but must meet standards of cleanliness (Chapter 12). Federal, state and local public health service legislation protects the public milk supply.

To protect the nutritive value of milk after it reaches the consumer, the rule of "3 C's and a D" should be followed: That is, keep it clean, cold, covered and dark.

If milk is not pasteurized, a home-type pasteurizer can be used, or it can be heated until it comes to a boil. The latter is a stronger heat treatment than pasteurization; it does change the flavor, destroys all or most of the vitamin C content and some of the thiamin, but renders the milk safe to drink.

BUYER'S INFORMATION   Fresh whole or skim milk is purchased pasteurized. If the milk is "raw" it is home pasteurized before being consumed. Evaporated milk is purchased either in tall cans (14½ ounces by weight or 12 fluid ounces) containing 1⅔ cups, or small "baby" cans (6 ounces by weight or 5⅓ fluid ounces) containing ⅔ of a cup. Dried milk is sold in powdered form and packaged in cartons of different sizes. Dry milk costs less than other milk and can be used in place of other milk.

COOKERY SUGGESTIONS   1. Use only very clean utensils when preparing milk beverages.

2. Heat milk over hot or boiling water. If placed directly over low heat, be sure to watch carefully to prevent scorching or overcooking.

3. Select fresh milk or quality evaporated milk or dried milk. Always store fresh milk and opened containers of evaporated milk in a refrigerator.

4. Blend milk carefully and thoroughly with other ingredients. The usual procedure is to pour milk into or add to the other ingredients.

5. Serve milk beverages at desired temperature of hot or cold.

6. If milk beverages are not to be served immediately, they are stored in the refrigerator.

7. Keep dry milk in a cool, dry place.

8. Refrigerate dry milk after mixing with water.

9. Do not freeze dry milk.

Banana Milk Shake

1 banana
1 teaspoon sugar, if desired
1 cup cold milk
   Procedure: 1. Slice the peeled ripe banana into a bowl or blender. Add sugar and milk. 2. Beat with a rotary beater until smooth or whip in blender. 3. Serve immediately in a tall beverage glass.
   Yield: 1 serving. (See Fig. 38–2.)

Eggnog

1 egg
1 tablespoon sugar
1 tablespoon brandy, sherry or port, if desired
⅛ teaspoon salt
¾ cup milk
   Procedure: 1. Break egg into a bowl and add sugar and salt. Beat with a rotary beater until creamy. 2. Add milk and continue beating. 3. If desired, add brandy or wine for flavor. 4. Serve immediately in a tall beverage glass.
   Yield: 1 serving

COCOA AND CHOCOLATE

The dried cocoa beans or seeds are imported from Central and South America.

Chocolate has a higher fat content, while cocoa has cornstarch incorporated into the defatted powdered form. Theobromine, a substance similar to caffeine, is the stimulating substance present in cocoa and chocolate.

Cocoa

1 teaspoon cocoa
1½ teaspoons sugar
   Few grains of salt
¼ cup boiling water
1 cup milk
¼ teaspoon vanilla
   Procedure: 1. Mix cocoa, sugar and salt in saucepan. Stir in boiling water, place over heat and boil 1 minute. 2. Add milk and heat, but do not boil. Whip with a rotary beater to prevent scum. Add vanilla. Serve immediately.
   Yield: 1 serving

Hot Chocolate

½ square unsweetened chocolate
1 tablespoon sugar
¼ cup water
¾ cup milk
   Procedure: 1. Cut chocolate into small pieces and put in small saucepan or top of small size double boiler. Place over hot water to melt chocolate. 2. Stir in sugar and water. Boil 1 minute over direct heat. 3. Add milk, stirring continuously. Place over hot water and beat mixture with rotary beater to prevent formation of scum. When heated, serve immediately.
   Yield: 1 serving

MALTED MILK

The malted milk added to flavor a beverage is a dried and condensed mixture of milk, malt and wheat which has had the fiber eliminated). Malt is defined as germinated grain, usually sprouted barley, in which the enzyme diastase has changed the starch molecules to maltose. The nutritive value of the malted milk beverage is high. Sometimes ice cream is whipped into the beverage or added as a float.

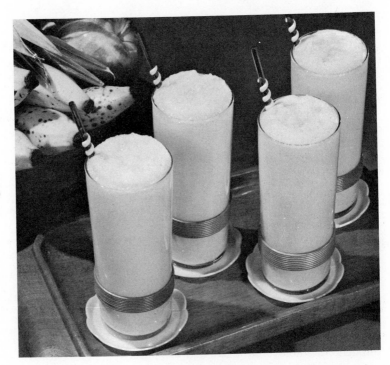

Figure 38–2   Banana milk shake.
(Courtesy of United Fruit Company.)

Malted Milk

2 tablespoons malted milk
1 cup milk
1 tablespoon cocoa syrup *or*
2 tablespoons crushed berries or fruit
  Procedure: 1. Measure malted milk into bowl, and gradually stir in cold milk. 2. Add flavoring. 3. Beat smooth with rotary beater. 4. Serve in tall beverage glass topped with whipped cream or ice cream.
  Yield: 1 serving
  Variation: Add crushed fruits such as strawberries, raspberries, peaches, cherries, prunes, bananas, pineapple, and apricot instead of syrup flavorings.

WHITE SAUCE

White sauce is a useful base for making different cream style dishes. Thin white sauce is blended with purée or strained vegetables to make creamed soups; a medium white sauce is blended with pieces of meat, fish, fowl, or eggs and vegetables to make creamed dishes; a thick white sauce is used as the base for soufflés, and a very thick white sauce is blended with other ingredients to make croquettes. To make a white sauce, milk or some other liquid is thickened with flour or some cereal product to the desired consistency.

COOKERY SUGGESTIONS   1. The purpose of the white sauce influences the proportion of fat to flour to liquid.

2. The melted butter and flour are blended thoroughly to make a smooth sauce.

3. The liquid is added slowly to the blended fat and flour to prevent lumping.

4. The sauce is cooked slowly at a low temperature to prevent scorching.

5. The sauce is seasoned with salt and pepper and, if desired, some herbs or spices, such as paprika or curry, are added for a piquant flavor. Celery salt and garlic salt are substitutes for table salt.

6. White sauce is seldom served alone but is incorporated into a cream style soup, blended with other food into creamed dishes, used as a base to make soufflé, and used as the binder to make croquettes.

Thin White Sauce

1 tablespoon butter or margarine
1 tablespoon flour
1 cup milk
¼ teaspoon salt
  Pepper or paprika, if desired
  Procedure: 1. Melt the butter in a saucepan over low heat. Stir in the flour and salt, using a wooden spoon, and blend thoroughly. 2. Add milk slowly, stirring continuously. Cook sauce for 2 to 3 minutes over low heat, or until thick. Add pepper or paprika, if desired. The sauce is ready to blend with puréed vegetables to make cream soups.
  Yield: 1 cup of sauce

Medium White Sauce

Follow the same procedure, using the proportions of 2 tablespoons butter, 2 tablespoons flour, 1 cup milk, and ¼ teaspoon salt.

Thick White Sauce

Follow the same procedure, using the proportions of 3 tablespoons butter, 3 tablespoons flour, 1 cup milk, and ¼ teaspoon salt.

Very Thick White Sauce

Follow the same procedure, using the proportions of 4 tablespoons butter, 4 tablespoons flour, 1 cup milk, and ¼ teaspoon salt.

White Sauce without Fat

To make a white sauce with no fat use 1 to 4 tablespoons flour for each cup of skim or whole milk used. Add flour to milk in a jar or can. Add about ¼ teaspoon salt for each cup of milk. Cover tightly and shake until well blended and smooth. Pour mixture into a saucepan. Heat slowly, stirring constantly, until thickened.

This white sauce can be used by the patient who needs to reduce the fat in his dietary.

CREAM SOUPS

Cream soups are a blend of vegetable purées or mixtures of chopped, diced or minced vegetables and meat, fish or poultry.

Basic Cream of Vegetable Soup

1 tablespoon butter or margarine
1 tablespoon flour
1 cup milk, fresh or diluted evaporated
¼ cup strained or puréed vegetables
    (cooked or canned asparagus, beets, carrots, peas, string beans, spinach, or tomatoes)
¼ teaspoon salt, if allowed
    Procedure: 1. Melt butter or margarine in saucepan. Stir in flour and cook for 1 minute. 2. Slowly stir in milk and continue stirring while sauce cooks about 2 minutes. 3. Heat vegetable purée and stir slowly into white sauce. Add salt if permitted. Continue heating soup until of desired serving temperature.
    Yield: 1 serving

Oyster Stew

4 oysters in own juice
1 cup milk
1 tablespoon butter
    Salt and pepper
    Procedure: 1. Heat oysters in top part of double boiler over boiling water. 2. When oysters are hot, pour in milk, and heat to boiling temperature. 3. Add butter and seasoning. Serve immediately.
    Yield: 1 serving

Fish Chowder

¼ pound haddock
1 medium size potato
½ cup water
1 slice onion
⅓ cup evaporated milk
½ tablespoon butter
    Salt and pepper
    Procedure: 1. Wash haddock, pat dry between paper towels, and cut fish into small pieces. 2. Peel potato, cut in small pieces, and boil 5 minutes in water in saucepan. Add slice of onion and fish. Cook together about 5 minutes until fish is tender. 3. Add the milk, butter, and seasoning. Heat to desired temperature. Serve.
    Yield: 1 serving

MILK IN SIMPLE DESSERTS

Desserts bring milk to the table in simple and easy to digest ways. Milk sherbets, ice cream, custards (baked or soft) and puddings (bread, cornstarch, junket, rice, and Bavarian cream) belong on the list. (See Figure 38–3.)

Baked Custard

⅔ cup hot milk
1 egg
1 tablespoon sugar
    Few grains salt and nutmeg

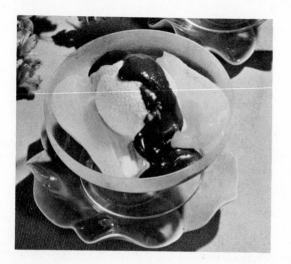

Figure 38–3   Pear sundae with chocolate mint sauce makes an attractive ice cream dessert variation. (Courtesy of American Can Company.)

Procedure: 1. Heat milk in upper part of double boiler over boiling water. 2. Beat egg in bowl, using rotary beater. Beat in sugar and salt. Stir hot milk into egg mixture. Pour into custard cup and sprinkle nutmeg over top. 3. Place custard cup in pan of hot water and bake in moderate oven (350° F.) about 30 minutes or until firm. If no custard clings to a silver knife inserted in the custard, it is baked sufficiently. 4. Remove cup from pan and serve warm or cold directly from cup or unmolded.

Yield: 1 serving

Milk Rennin Pudding

½ rennin tablet
2 teaspoons cold water
1 cup lukewarm milk
1 tablespoon sugar
¼ teaspoon vanilla

Procedure: 1. Crush rennin tablet in bowl and add the cold water. 2. Stir sugar and vanilla into lukewarm milk. Stir in dissolved rennin. Pour immediately into individual serving dishes. Allow to stand at room temperature until set. Then chill until serving time.

Yield: 2 servings

CHEESE

The tasty dishes prepared with the ingredients milk, eggs and cheese are sometimes called meat alternates. They can be interchanged in the menu with meat dishes because of the similarity in nutrients, particularly animal or complete proteins. Some cheeses are noted for their distinctive flavors, and are chiefly used for garnishing to add zest and flavor to other foods (the grated hard Parmesan) or for eating alone (the sweet Swiss and brick, or the salty bleu and Gouda) or with fruit. Cheese is also useful as flavoring for salad dressing and many sauces, or may be the major ingredient of salad (cottage cheese), dessert (cheese cake) or filling for sandwiches. Cheeses are stored in the refrigerator, the strongly flavored double wrapped to avoid contamination of other foods.

BUYERS' INFORMATION *Cheeses are classified* into categories of soft, semihard and hard cheeses. Cottage, cream cheese, and Neufchatel are unripened soft cheeses. Camembert and Brie are soft cheeses which are ripened by molds; Limburger and Liederkranz are soft cheeses ripened by bacteria. Gorgonzola, Roquefort, bleu cheese, and Stilton are semihard cheeses ripened by molds, and brick and Muenster are semihard cheeses ripened by bacteria. Among the hard cheeses without air or "gas" holes are the Cheddar, Edam and Gouda varieties, and those with holes are the Swiss, Gruyère and Parmesan. Skim milk is the basis for longhorn and cottage cheese, while Cheddar cheese is made from whole milk. A combination of milk and cream is blended into cream cheese. The domestic cheeses are usually less expensive than the imported varieties. See Table 38-1 for information about various cheeses and their uses.

COMPOSITION Cheese of the Cheddar type contains about 25 per cent protein, 32 per cent fat, 2 per cent lactose (milk sugar), minerals (especially calcium and phosphorus), vitamins (especially vitamin A and riboflavin), and 40 per cent water. It retains most of the calcium, phosphorus and iron of milk. Except for cottage cheese, it is high in fat and consequently a rich source of vitamin A, containing approximately 1700 I.U. per ounce. There is considerable variation in water and fat content, depending upon whether made from whole or skim milk.

NUTRITIVE VALUE The type of milk used in the manufacture of cheese reflects the nutritive qualities of the cheese. For example, protein, calcium and vitamin B factors are contributed by the whole milk of Cheddar cheese.

Cheese is not equal in food value to the milk from which it is made, since some of the protein (lactalbumin), lactose, certain mineral salts (some calcium), and a portion of the vitamins are separated out and left in the whey. The casein of milk is the main constituent of cheese. It has a high biologic value in protein and calcium content, making it a valuable food. Europeans use cheese as a substantial portion of the diet, and it is suggested that the proverbial vigor of the pastoral peoples of Asia and the Balkans is partly due to their consumption of large quantities of this food.

In general, it takes about ½ pound of Cheddar cheese to give about the same amount of protein as a pound of meat containing a moderate amount of bone and fat. Cottage cheese is less concentrated than

SUGGESTED CHEESE AND FRUIT COMBINATIONS*

Blue or Roquefort	Apples or pears, especially Anjou and Bosc pears.
Brick	Tokay grapes
Camembert	Apples, pears, and tart plums.
Cheddar	Tart apples or melon slices.
Edam or Gouda	Apples, orange sections, or pineapple spears.
Muenster or Swiss	Apples, seedless grapes, or orange sections.
Provolone	Sweet Bartlett pears.

*Cheese in Family Meals. Home and Garden Bulletin, No. 112, U.S. Department of Agriculture, June, 1966.

TABLE 38-1 GUIDE TO NATURAL CHEESES

KIND	CHARACTERISTICS	USES
American	See Cheddar	See Cheddar.
Bel Paese (Bel Pah-A-say.)	Mild, sweet flavor; light, creamy yellow interior; slate gray surface; soft to medium firm, creamy texture.	Appetizers, sandwiches, desserts, and snacks.
Blue	Tangy, piquant flavor; semisoft, pasty, sometimes crumbly texture; white interior marbled or streaked with blue veins of mold; resembles Roquefort.	Appetizers, salads and salad dressings, desserts, and snacks.
Brick	Mild to moderately sharp flavor; semisoft to medium firm, elastic texture; creamy white-to-yellow interior; brownish exterior.	Appetizers, sandwiches, desserts, and snacks.
Brie (Bree.)	Mild to pungent flavor; soft, smooth texture; creamy yellow interior; edible thin brown and white crust.	Appetizers, sandwiches, desserts, and snacks.
Caciocavallo (Ca-cheo-ca-VAL-lo.)	Piquant, somewhat salty flavor – similar to Provolone, but not smoked; smooth, very firm texture; light or white interior; clay or tan colored surface.	Snacks and desserts. Suitable for grating and cooking when fully cured.
Camembert (KAM-em-bear.)	Distinctive mild to tangy flavor; soft, smooth texture – almost fluid when fully ripened; creamy yellow interior; edible thin white or gray-white crust.	Appetizers, desserts, and snacks.
Cheddar (often called American)	Mild to very sharp flavor; smooth texture, firm to crumbly; light cream to orange.	Appetizers, main dishes, sauces, soups, sandwiches, salads, desserts, and snacks.
Colby	Mild to mellow flavor, similar to Cheddar; softer body and more open texture than Cheddar; light cream to orange.	Sandwiches and snacks.
Cottage	Mild, slightly acid flavor; soft, open texture with tender curds of varying size; white to creamy white.	Appetizers, salads, used in some cheesecakes.
Cream	Delicate, slightly acid flavor; soft, smooth texture; white.	Appetizers, salads, sandwiches, desserts, snacks.
Edam	Mellow, nutlike, sometimes salty flavor; rather firm, rubbery texture; creamy yellow or medium yellow-orange interior; surface coated with red wax; usually shaped like a flattened ball.	Appetizers, salads, sandwiches, sauces, desserts, and snacks.
Gjetost[1] (YET-ost.)	Sweetish, caramel flavor; firm, buttery consistency; golden brown.	Desserts and snacks
Gorgonzola (Gor-gon-ZO-la.)	Tangy, rich, spicy flavor; semisoft, pasty, sometimes crumbly texture; creamy white interior, mottled or streaked with blue-green veins of mold; clay colored surface.	Appetizers, salads, desserts, and snacks.
Gouda (GOO-da.)	Mellow, nutlike, often slightly acid flavor; semisoft to firm, smooth texture, often containing small holes; creamy yellow or medium yellow-orange interior; usually has red wax coating; usually shaped like a flattened ball.	Appetizers, salads, sandwiches, sauces, desserts, and snacks.
Gruyere (Grew-YARE.)	Nutlike, salty flavor, similar to Swiss, but sharper; firm, smooth texture with small holes or eyes; light yellow.	Appetizers, desserts, and snacks.
Liederkranz (LEE-der-krontz.)	Robust flavor, similar to very mild Limburger; soft, smooth texture; creamy yellow interior; russet surface.	Appetizers, desserts, and snacks.
Limburger	Highly pungent, very strong flavor and aroma; soft, smooth texture that usually contains small irregular openings; creamy white interior; reddish yellow surface.	Appetizers, desserts, and snacks.
Mozzarella (also called Scamorza). (Mottza-REL-la.)	Delicate, mild flavor; slightly firm, plastic texture; creamy white.	Main dishes, such as pizza or lasagna, sandwiches, and snacks.
Muenster (MUN-stir.)	Mild to mellow flavor; semisoft texture with numerous small openings; creamy white interior; yellowish tan surface.	Appetizers, sandwiches, desserts, and snacks.
Mysost (MEWS-ost.)	Sweetish, caramel flavor; firm, buttery consistency; light brown.	Desserts and snacks.
Neufchatal (New-sha-TEL.)	Mild, acid flavor; soft, smooth texture similar to cream cheese but lower in fat; white.	Salads, sandwiches, desserts, and snacks.
Parmesan	Sharp, distinctive flavor; very hard, granular texture; yellowish white.	Grated for seasoning.
Port du Salut (Pore du sa-LOO.)	Mellow to robust flavor similar to Gouda; semisoft, smooth elastic texture; creamy white or yellow.	Appetizers, desserts, and snacks.
Provolone (Pro-vo-LO-na.)	Mellow to sharp flavor, smoky and salty; firm, smooth texture; cuts without crumbling; light creamy yellow; light brown or golden yellow surface.	Appetizers, main dishes, sandwiches, desserts, and snacks.

[1]Imported; not manufactured in the United States.

Table continued on opposite page.

TABLE 38-1   GUIDE TO NATURAL CHEESES *(Continued)*

KIND	CHARACTERISTICS	USES
Ricotta............................ (Ri-COT-ah.)	Mild, sweet, nutlike flavor; soft, moist texture with loose curds (fresh Ricotta) or dry and suitable for grating; white.	Salads, main dishes such as lasagna and ravioli, and desserts.
Romano	Very sharp, piquant flavor; very hard, granular texture; yellowish white interior; greenish black surface.	Seasoning and general table use; when cured a year it is suitable for grating.
Roquefort[1]	Sharp, peppery, piquant flavor; semisoft, pasty, sometimes crumbly texture; white interior streaked with blue-green veins of mold.	Appetizers, salads and salad dressings, desserts, and snacks.
Sap Sago[1]	Sharp, pungent, cloverlike flavor; very hard texture suitable for grating; light green or sage green.	Grated for seasoning.
Stilton............................	Piquant flavor, milder than Gorgonzola or Roquefort; open, flaky texture; creamy white interior streaked with blue-green veins of mold; wrinkled, melon-like rind.	Appetizers, salads, desserts, and snacks.
Swiss (also called Emmentaler).	Mild, sweet, nutlike flavor; firm, smooth, elastic body with large round eyes; light yellow.	Sandwiches, salads, and snacks.

[1]Imported; not manufactured in the United States.
From U.S. Department of Agriculture: Cheese in family meals, A Guide for Consumers. Home and Garden Bulletin No. 112, Washington, D.C., U.S. Government Printing Office, 1966.

Cheddar cheese, with about four-fifths as much protein per pound.

DIGESTIBILITY   Cheese is easily digested, being rich in easily assimilated fat, and in protein of high biologic value. In "ripened" cheese, the protein has been partially digested by bacterial action and made more soluble in the process.

Cheese Souffle

1 tablespoon butter
1 tablespoon flour
⅓ cup scalded milk
¼ teaspoon salt
2 tablespoons grated cheese
1 egg yolk, beaten light
1 egg white, beaten stiff

Procedure: 1. Melt butter in saucepan over low heat. Stir in flour using wooden spoon. Pour in milk slowly and cook sauce 2 minutes, stirring continuously. *2.* Add salt and cheese, and remove saucepan from heat. Stir several spoonfuls of sauce into beaten egg yolk and then stir into remaining sauce. Cool. (See Fig. 38-4). *3.* Fold in stiffly beaten white. Pour mixture in buttered baking dish. Bake 30 minutes in slow oven (325° F.). Serve immediately.
Yield: 1 serving

Macaroni and Cheese

⅓ cup macaroni, broken in 1-inch pieces
1 cup boiling water
½ teaspoon salt
⅓ cup evaporated milk
⅓ cup processed cheese
2 tablespoons buttered bread crumbs

Procedure: 1. Cook macaroni in boiling salted water until tender or about 15 minutes. Drain in strainer, and pour warm water over macaroni to rinse. *2.* Scald milk over boiling water. Add cheese, cut in small pieces, and cook 5 minutes or until cheese is just melted, stirring continuously with wooden spoon. *3.* Arrange alternate layers of cooked macaroni and cheese sauce in buttered baking dish. Sprinkle buttered crumbs over top. Bake about 30 minutes in moderate oven (350° F.). Serve hot.
Yield: 1 serving

SUGGESTED ADDITIONAL READING REFERENCES

See Appendix General Reference List, Part III.

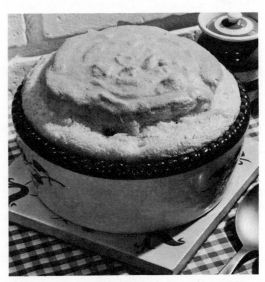

Figure 38-4   A puffy, delicate cheese soufflé is just out of the oven—to be served immediately. (Courtesy of Campbell Soup Company.)

Chapter 39
GROUP II: MEAT GROUP

Two or more servings from this group are suggested daily. These may consist of meats (beef, veal, pork, lamb), poultry, fish, or eggs. Dry beans, dry peas and nuts may be used as alternates.

MEAT

Meat is a popular high quality protein food which satisfies the appetite and taste of many people. Roasts, steaks, and chops are the most popular cuts of meat and the increased demand seems to put such cuts of meat in the higher price range. Most of the parts of the animal are equally nutritious, although the muscular sections are tougher because of the muscle cells and connective tissue. Therefore, different methods of cooking are employed: dry heat for tender roasts, steaks, and chops, and moist heat for the tougher cuts.

Meat is universally liked and widely used in the United States. It has been the backbone in the diet of man since the beginning of time. The cave man devoured deer and wild boar which were brought back from the hunt. In medieval times the great feasts consisted chiefly of meat, and food in general was referred to merely as "meat." In pioneer days, meat was plentiful and used as the basic food in the menu. Since foods had to be raised or hunted, there was small variety from which to choose, and meat was served three times a day. The early settlers in this country did heavy physical labor. Meat had the satisfying flavor and stick-to-the-ribs quality needed by hungry people. With the gradual increase in population and variety of foods available as time went on, meat became scarce. Today it is one of the most expensive items on the menu. In general, the lower the income, the less meat consumed.

Beef is the most popular meat eaten in this country, and there is a wide range of cuts (Fig. 39-1) and quality.

KINDS OF MEAT The kinds of meat are *beef* from cattle, *veal* from calf, *pork* from hog, and *lamb* (young) and *mutton* (mature) from sheep.

A cut of meat from the market includes muscle tissue, connective tissue, fat, and bone. Edible glands and organs, such as liver, heart, kidney, brains and tongue are classified as glandular or *variety* meat.

NUTRITIVE VALUE Meat is classified as a protein food with a variable amount of fat. A study by Leverton and Odell[1] of the nutritive value of cooked beef, lamb, veal and pork was made to serve as a guide in the planning and calculation of dietaries. It was suggested that extremely lean portions average 32 per cent protein and 8 per cent fat; and lean-plus-marble portions contain 28 per cent protein and 16 per cent fat. These figures are of special value in the diet of limited fat content.

Yellow connective tissue consists chiefly of the protein, *elastin,* and cooking does not make it tender. White connective tissue consists chiefly of the protein, *collagen,* and cooking does make it tender and soft.

The age of the animal, the amount and character of connective tissues, and the deposits of fat are factors which influence the tenderness of meat.

Meat is considered a rich source of the minerals iron and phosphorus and contains a variable amount of calcium. *Glycogen* is the type of carbohydrate found in meat. It changes to lactic acid, the non-nitrogenous extractive. The nitrogenous extractives give meat its distinctive flavor. They are the end-products of protein metabolism, such as creatine, creatinine, purines, and other products.

The hemoglobin present in the tissues and muscles gives the pink or red color to meat.

[1]Leverton, R. M., and Odell, G. V.: The Nutritive Value of Meat. Miscellaneous Publication MP-49, Oklahoma Ag. Experiment Station, Oklahoma State University, June, 1959.

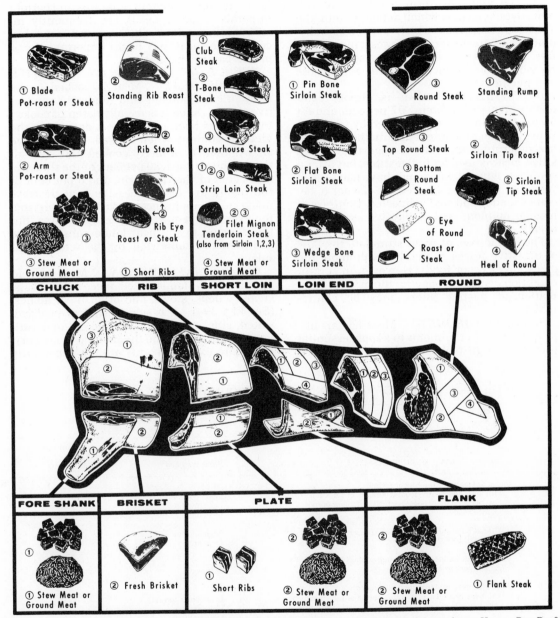

Figure 39–1   Beef chart. (From Consumer and Marketing Service, U.S. Department of Agriculture: How to Buy Beef Roasts. Home and Garden Bulletin No. 146, Washington, D.C., U.S. Government Printing Office, 1968.

The action of enzymes, alkalies, acids, and heat on meat forms new products, such as *hematin* formed by heat, the grayish brown color of well-done meat.

Vitamin A in the fat of beef and liver, and factors of the vitamin B-complex are the vitamins abundant in meat.

The enzymes or ferments in meat are proteolytic enzymes which act on protein, the amylolytic enzymes which act on carbohydrates, and the lipolytic enzymes which act on fats. The proteolytic enzymes assist in the ripening process, increasing the tenderness and juiciness.

DIGESTIBILITY   Meat is almost completely digested—proteins 97 per cent and fat 96 per cent—and is well utilized by the body. However, the fat content and method of cooking determine the rate of digestion. Fresh killed meat is usually indigestible, but after a few days, when the enzymes have had time to "age" or ripen the connective tissue, it becomes tender and easily digested. Contrary to popular opinion, veal is digested as easily as beef.

The extractives of meat stimulate the flow of digestive juices, which helps promote the digestion of other foods. However, in certain conditions such as peptic ulcer, the stimulation of gastric juices may be contraindicated.

PLACE IN THE DIET   Meat has an important place in the menu to supply essential protein of high biologic value, the minerals phosphorus and iron, and B-complex vitamins. The protein of meat can be compared with that of fish, poultry, eggs, and milk.

Meat, or equivalents such as poultry and fish, is included at least once in each day's menus, and is usually the main dish for dinner. The use of organs should be encouraged for their protein content, vitamins and certain minerals. Protein needs are frequently increased in various illnesses and convalescence, and meat may be an important therapeutic part of the diet.

EFFECT OF COOKING ON NUTRITIVE VALUE OF MEAT   Meat is cooked to destroy microorganisms and tenderize connective tissue. Since it is usually eaten in cooked form, it has been necessary to determine the vitamin content when cooked. Studies have shown that, if properly cooked and with all the drippings used, 30 per cent of the thiamin, 5 per cent of the riboflavin, and 5 per cent of the niacin are lost. Excessive heat destroys many nutrients in meat. Roasting and frying, for example, require high temperatures, but the damage to the heat labile substances is counteracted somewhat by the retention of juices.

BUYERS' INFORMATION   Meat is sold cut into the standardized pieces for roasts, steaks, chops, stews, and other meat dishes. (See Fig. 39–1.) It is sold fresh, frozen, dried, salted, smoked, or canned. The cut and variety of meat determine the method of cookery. The more expensive cuts are not necessarily

TABLE 39–1   YIELD OF COOKED MEAT PER POUND OF RAW MEAT*

MEAT AS PURCHASED	MEAT AFTER COOKING (less drippings)	
	Parts Weighed	Approximate Weight of Cooked Parts per Pound of Raw Meat
Chops or steaks for broiling or frying:		*Ounces*
With bone and relatively large amount of fat, such as: pork or lamb chops; beef rib, sirloin, or porterhouse steaks.	Lean, bone, fat	10–12
	Lean and fat	7–10
	Lean only	5–7
Without bone and with very little fat, such as round of beef; veal steaks	Lean and fat	12–13
	Lean only	9–12
Ground meat for broiling or frying, such as beef, lamb or pork patties		9–13
	Patties	
Roasts for oven cooking (no liquid added):		
With bone and relatively large amount of fat, such as beef rib, loin, chuck; lamb shoulder, leg; pork, fresh or cured	Lean, bone and fat	10–12
	Lean and fat	8–10
	Lean only	6–9
Without bone	Lean and fat	10–12
	Lean only	7–10
Cuts for pot-roasting, simmering, braising, stewing:		
With bone and relatively large amount of fat, such as beef chuck, pork shoulder	Lean, bone and fat	10–11
	Lean and fat	8–9
	Lean only	6–8
Without bone and with relatively small amount of fat, such as: trimmed beef; veal	Lean with adhering fat	9–11

*Taken from "Nutritive Value of Foods," Home and Garden Bulletin No. 72, U.S. Department of Agriculture, Washington, D.C., 1970.

higher in food value than less expensive cuts. The organs, such as liver and kidney are examples of high food value at low cost.

Characteristics of high quality beef are: the lean meat is light red, appears velvety and is veined liberally with fat; the bones are red; and the fat is flaky and white.

Two purple stamps usually appear on retail cuts of meat: the United States Department of Agriculture stamp indicates the grades: U.S. Choice, U.S. Good, and U.S. Commercial; and a round stamp indicates that the meat has been inspected and passed as wholesome food.

The amount of meat to buy per serving: ½ to 1 pound if the meat has much bone or gristle; ⅓ to ½ pound if the meat has medium amounts of bone; ¼ to ⅓ pound if the meat has little bone; and ⅕ to ¼ pound if the meat has no bone. Table 39–1 can be used as a guide to the amount of raw meat to buy in order to have a given amount of cooked meat to serve.

CARE AND STORAGE   Meat and poultry should be bought at clean, well-kept grocery stores. It should be taken home and immediately refrigerated or frozen to prevent spoilage. Figure 39–2 lists the temperatures which retard bacteria growth as well as the temperatures which allow bacteria to multiply. *Fresh meat* should be stored uncovered or loosely covered in the coldest part of the refrigerator. The meat should not be washed. A slight drying on the surface of the meat actually in-

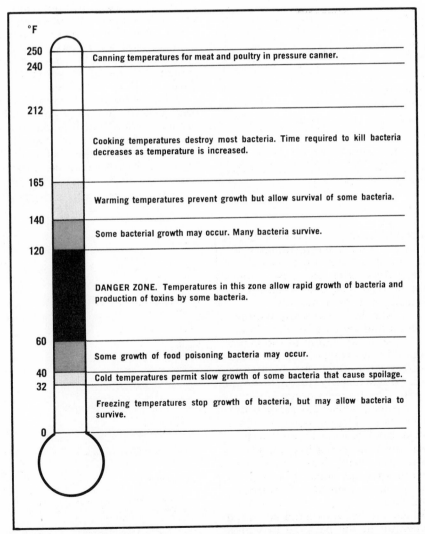

Figure 39-2   Temperatures for control of bacteria. (From Consumer and Marketing Service, U.S. Department of Agriculture: Inspection, Labeling and Care of Meat and Poultry, A Consumer Education Guide. Home and Garden Bulletin No. 416, Washington, D.C., U.S. Government Printing Office, 1971.

TABLE 39–2 MEAT STORAGE

| PRODUCT | STORAGE PERIOD (To Maintain its Quality) | |
	Refrigerator 35° to 40° F. Days	Freezer 0° F. Months
FRESH MEATS		
Roasts (Beef and Lamb)	3 to 5	8 to 12
Roasts (Pork and Veal)	3 to 5	4 to 8
Steaks (Beef)	3 to 5	8 to 12
Chops (Lamb and Pork)	3 to 5	3 to 4
Ground and Stew Meats	1 to 2	2 to 3
Variety Meats	1 to 2	3 to 4
Sausage (Pork)	1 to 2	1 to 2
PROCESSED MEATS		
Bacon	7	1
Frankfurters	7	½
Ham (Whole)	7	1 to 2
Ham (Half)	3 to 5	1 to 2
Ham (Slices)	3	1 to 2
Luncheon Meats	3 to 5	Freezing
Sausage (Smoked)	7	not
Sausage (Dry and Semi-Dry)	14 to 21	recommended
COOKED MEATS		
Cooked Meats and Meat Dishes	1 to 2	2 to 3
Gravy and Meat Broth	1 to 2	2 to 3
FRESH POULTRY		
Chicken and Turkey	1 to 2	12
Duck and Goose	1 to 2	6
Giblets	1 to 2	3
COOKED POULTRY		
Pieces (Covered with Broth)	1 to 2	6
Pieces (Not Covered)	1 to 2	1
Cooked Poultry Dishes	1 to 2	6
Fried Chicken	1 to 2	4

From Consumer and Marketing Service, U.S. Department of Agriculture: Inspection, Labeling and Care of Meat and Poultry, A consumer education guide. Agriculture Handbook No. 416, Washington, D.C., U.S. Government Printing Office, 1971.

creases its keeping quality. With the exception of smoked meats, such as ham, frankfurters, bacon, and sausage, fresh meat is cooked within a few days after purchase unless frozen. Ground fresh meat and organ meats (liver and brains) spoil more quickly.

Frozen meat should be carefully wrapped to exclude all air and stored at 0° F. or lower. Pre-wrapped fresh meat bought at the supermarket should be re-wrapped in moisture-tight, vapor-resistant (airtight) wrapping. When meat is bought already frozen, it should be hard-frozen. The frozen storage compartment of the average household refrigerator, unless it is a separate freezer, is not designed to freeze meat quickly or for long storage.

Refreezing meat is not a recommended practice. When refreezing may seem necessary to prevent spoilage, some loss in juiciness and flavor can be expected. To refreeze, first cook the meat.

Cured and *smoked meats* should be stored in the refrigerator in the package in which they are purchased. These include modern type hams, large canned hams, bacon, and boneless shoulder butts. Refrigeration is essential since the keeping quality of these mildly cured meats resembles more nearly the keeping quality of fresh pork.

Cooked meat should be stored in as large pieces as possible, covered, in the refrigerator. Covering prevents further drying of the meat, which has lost some moisture in cooking. See Table 39–2 for more information on storage of meats.

COOKERY SUGGESTIONS 1. The cut and quality or tenderness of meat determine the cookery method. Broiling, pan-frying and roasting are methods used for tender meat. Pot-roasting, braising or simmering are methods to cook less tender cuts.

2. Tender meats are cooked with dry heat (roasting, broiling and pan broiling) at temperature just high enough to produce crisp brown exterior and only long enough to be palatable because collagen changes quickly to gelatin, and other proteins coagulate quickly.

3. Less tender meats are cooked with moist heat for longer periods at lower temperature because it takes a longer time to break down collagen in the larger amount of connective tissue.

4. The temperatures should be low to moderate and the length of cooking long enough to melt fat and distribute flavor through meat and prevent shrinkage. Sometimes basting helps to distribute flavor of melted fat through meat. Table 39–3 includes internal tempera-

TABLE 39–3 MEAT COOKING CHART

| PRODUCT | INTERNAL TEMPERATURE WHEN DONE |
	°F
FRESH BEEF	
Rare	140
Medium	160
Well Done	170
FRESH VEAL	170
FRESH LAMB	
Medium	170
Well Done	180
FRESH PORK	170
CURED PORK (Cook-Before-Eating)	
Ham	160
Shoulder	170
Canadian Bacon	160
CURED PORK (Fully Cooked)	
Ham	140
POULTRY	
Turkey	180–185
Boneless Roasts	170–175
Stuffing	165

From Consumer and Marketing Service, U.S. Department of Agriculture.: Inspection, Labeling and Care of Meat and Poultry, a consumer education guide. Agriculture Handbook No. 416, Washington, D.C., U.S. Government Printing Office, 1971.

tures indicating when meat and poultry are cooked thoroughly.

5. Less tender cuts of meat are soaked in wine-vinegar, sour milk or cooked in tomato juice to hasten the change of collagen to gelatin.

6. Less tender cuts of meat are pounded to break muscle fibers.

7. Before cooking, excessive fat and heavy skin are removed from meat.

8. The "doneness" of meat is controlled by length of cooking and temperature. Pork and veal are cooked well done for easier digestion and appetizing appearance. Pork must be well cooked (white inside) to avoid any possibility of transmitting trichinae, which causes trichinosis.

9. Liver is cooked quickly because of the small amount of connective tissue. Fat is added to improve flavor because liver has little natural fat.

10. Broiled bacon is drained on absorbent paper.

11. A longer cooking period with added water increases loss of vitamins and minerals.

12. Thin cuts of meats are salted after browning because salt tends to remove extractives and juices. Salt and seasonings are added to roasts at the beginning of the cooking period.

13. Meat is served immediately after it is cooked to prevent overcooking from imprisoned hot juices, or it is eaten cold.

14. Frozen meats may be thawed before cooking, or cooked without thawing first. To cook chops and steaks without thawing, allow 2 to 15 minutes longer than usual, depending upon thickness. Thaw meats in the refrigerator. For faster defrosting, place meat or poultry in watertight wrapper in cold water or in closed double bag at room temperature. The wrappings keep the surface of the product cool while it defrosts, thus protecting against bacteria growth.

15. Heat leftovers thoroughly. Bring broth and gravy to a full rolling boil and allow to boil for several minutes to destroy bacteria.

Pan-Broiled Beef Patty

Procedure: 1. Heat a small heavy frying pan very hot over direct heat. Add ½ teaspoon bacon drippings. 2. Shape ground beef into patty and place in frying pan. Brown quickly on both sides. Season, then reduce heat and cook slowly on both sides. 3. It takes about 10 minutes to pan-broil patty which is ½ to ¾ inch thick. 4. Place broiled patty on dinner plate and serve immediately.

Pan-Broiled Scraped Beef Patty

Procedure: 1. Using a tablespoon, scrape a piece of round steak to free from the connective tissue. 2. Season with salt and form into a patty. 3. Pan-broil lightly and serve immediately.

POULTRY

Meat from poultry is a favorite food to include in dietaries. The psychological role is as important as the nutritive value. Roast chicken, turkey, goose, or duck is associated with feast days, holidays, family get-togethers, and company meals. The many different kinds and classes of poultry, as well as the many different methods of preparation offer variety for the main dish the year round.

NUTRITIVE VALUE   Like other meats, poultry has protein of high quality and is a good source of iron, phosphorus, and the B-complex vitamins, especially niacin. The fat varies with the kind, age and quality of the bird. In addition, the dark meat is slightly higher in fat content than the white meat. Contrary to popular opinion, there is no difference in the nutritive qualities of white and dark meat, except that white meat contains more nicotinic acid.

DIGESTIBILITY   The high coefficient of digestibility, as well as rapidity and ease of digestion, makes poultry a valuable addition to the menu. Since the white meat contains a little less connective tissue and fat than the dark meat, it is slightly easier to digest. Duck and goose are comparatively high in fat. Broilers and fryers, being younger, have less fat than the older roasters and stewing birds. Turkey can be classed with the latter.

BUYERS' INFORMATION   Many factors should be considered when buying poultry.

Kinds of Poultry   Chicken, turkey, duck, and goose are the kinds of poultry most commonly eaten and, of these, chicken is by far the most plentiful and popular. Less common and more expensive birds enjoyed are Cornish game hen, guinea hen and squab (pigeon).

Class   Poultry classes within each kind are based on age, weight and sex, and therefore are related to tenderness and suitable methods of cooking. A plump young chicken (usually 9 to 12 weeks of age), selected for broiling, weighs not over 2½ pounds. The weight of a frying chicken averages 2½ to 3½ pounds, and a roasting chicken (usually 3 to 5 months of age) averages 3 to 6 pounds. Capons (castrated male birds), de luxe in quality, usually under 8 months of age, weigh 6 to 9 pounds, ready-to-cook weight. They are exceptionally meaty, and the flesh is juicy, tender, unusually fine in flavor. A capon is usually roasted. Fowls or stewing chickens are mature birds (usually more than 10 months of age) and their weights are variable.

Turkeys are classed as fryers or roasters. Ducks weigh 4 pounds or under for the small size and 5 pounds or more for the large size. Ducks are usually marketed young as ducklings. Geese weigh 8 pounds or under for the

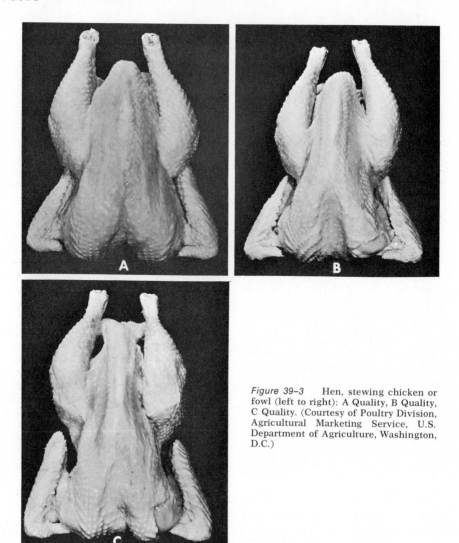

Figure 39–3   Hen, stewing chicken or
fowl (left to right): A Quality, B Quality,
C Quality. (Courtesy of Poultry Division,
Agricultural Marketing Service, U.S.
Department of Agriculture, Washington,
D.C.)

small size and 10 pounds or more for the large size. Squabs and guineas are sold in some markets.

Style of Processing   Most poultry is currently marketed ready-to-cook (whole or parts), although live and dressed birds are still available in some markets. Dressed and ready-to-cook poultry is sold fresh chilled, cold storage, or quick frozen. Cold storage poultry is kept in refrigerated storage for a minimum of 60 days. Dressed poultry indicates that the bird has been bled and the feathers removed, but the head, feet and internal organs remain. The ready-to-cook (eviscerated) poultry has been bled, feathers removed and picked, and internal organs, head, feet, and oil sac removed.

Government Standards   Some poultry is labeled to show government inspection and gradings, some to show inspection only, and some is neither graded nor inspected. The bird that carries an official grade mark has been examined for quality and then assigned a U.S. Grade A, B, or C, according to Government standards. (See Fig. 39–3.) The inspection mark refers to the bird's wholesomeness or fitness for food.

The best quality poultry show these characteristics: full-fleshed and meaty breast and legs, well-distributed fat, and skin with few blemishes and pinfeathers. Young chickens and turkeys have smooth, tender skin, soft tender meat, and a flexible breastbone. An older chicken or turkey, suitable for stewing or braising, has coarser skin and a firm breastbone.

The number of servings obtained from poultry is dependent upon the kind, weight, age, sex, grade, and method of cooking. A rough guide of the amount of dressed weight

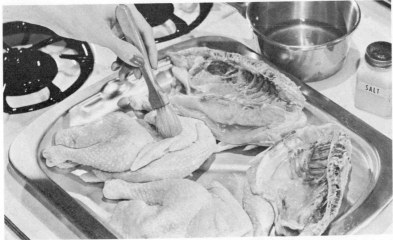

Figure 39–4 Broiling—brush with fat, and season. Start broiling with skin side down. Broiler is being used without rack. (Courtesy of Poultry and Egg National Board.)

poultry to buy per serving: ¼ to ½ chicken for broiling; ¾ to 1 pound chicken for frying and roasting; ⅓ to ¾ pound chicken for stewing; 1 to 1¼ pounds of duck; ¾ to 1 pound of goose; and ⅔ to ¾ pound of turkey. Ready-to-cook weight of poultry to buy per serving: ¼ to ½ chicken for broiling; about ½ pound of chicken for frying, roasting, and stewing; about 1 pound of duck; about ⅔ pound of goose; and about ¾ pound of turkey.

The meat of chicken and turkey is sold frozen or canned, and whole small chickens are canned commerically.

COOKERY SUGGESTIONS 1. The method of cookery depends on the bird's age, weight, quality, and amount of fat. For broiling, frying or roasting, plump young birds are best. To braise, stew or steam, either the old or lean young birds are selected.

2. The desirable cooking temperature regardless of method or quality of poultry is always low to moderate. See Table 39–3.

3. Poultry should not be overcooked.

4. Poultry is roasted uncovered at low to moderate temperatures.

5. Poultry is fried uncovered at low to moderate temperatures.

6. Frozen poultry is thawed just before cooking. If unthawed, allow 1½ times the usual cooking period.

7. Ready-to-cook poultry needs no special preparation other than removing a few pinfeathers, washing and drying the bird.

Broiled Chicken

1 young chicken, ready to cook,
   weight 1½ to 2¼ pounds
Melted fat

½ teaspoon salt
¼ teaspoon poultry seasoning
   Few grains of pepper
2 tablespoons flour

Procedure: 1. Split chicken in half, cutting along the backbone, and then into quarters by cutting through the breastbone. Break joints. Cut off tips of wings. 2. Brush melted fat on both sides of chicken, and season (Fig. 39–4). 3. Preheat the broiler and brush melted fat on broiler rack. Arrange chicken on the rack, skin side down. Replace broiler under heat. During the broiling process, turn the chicken several times to brown evenly. Baste with melted fat or drippings. Broil until chicken is well done, about 35 to 45 minutes. 4. After the chicken is browned on the broiler, it can be put into a moderate oven (350° F.) and baked until tender.

Yield: 2 to 4 servings

Creamed Chicken

½ tablespoon butter
2 tablespoons chopped celery
½ teaspoon chopped onion
1 teaspoon chopped green pepper
1 tablespoon flour
⅓ cup chicken broth
¼ cup milk
½ cup diced canned or cooked chicken
¼ teaspoon salt
   Few grains of paprika

Procedure: 1. Melt the butter in a frying pan. Add the celery, onion and green pepper and cook about 5 minutes. Stir the flour into fat and vegetable mixture. 2. Stir in chicken broth and milk and cook sauce to a smooth con-

FISH

Fish is a high quality protein food classified into categories of fresh water fish (caught in fresh water lakes, rivers and streams), salt water fish and shellfish.

COMPOSITION Fish and shellfish contain about 19 per cent protein similar in amino

TABLE 39–4   APPROXIMATE COMPOSITION AND ENERGY CONTENT OF SOME FISH AND SHELLFISH FOODS

FISH	PROTEIN *Per cent*	FAT *Per cent*	ENERGY *Kcal./100 gm.*
Cod steaks, broiled	29	5	170
Crab, steamed	17	2	93
Fish filet, smoked	19	1	90
Salmon, broiled	27	7	182
Salmon, pink, canned	21	6	141
Flounder, baked	30	8	202
Lobster, boiled	19	2	95
Oysters, Eastern, raw	8	2	66
Scallops, steamed	23	1	112
Sardines, canned in oil, drained	24	11	203
Shrimp, boiled	24	1	116

acid composition to that found in muscle meats. The fat content varies from 1 to 20 per cent, depending upon the species and the season of the year. (See Table 39–4 and Appendix Table 1.)

NUTRITIVE VALUE   Fish contains protein of high biologic value, essential minerals, vitamins and fats. In general, the nutritive value of fish is similar to that of beef, except that shellfish and salt water fish are rich in iodine and fluorine plus appreciable amounts of cobalt and, for that reason, make a valuable contribution to the dietary. Fish is also a satisfactory source of magnesium, phosphorus, iron, and copper. The iron content of fish is lower than that found in meat, but calcium is about equal. Shellfish generally have higher calcium and iodine content than fish.

A serving of fat fish, such as salmon or mackerel, will supply about 10 per cent of the daily allowance of vitamin A and all of the vitamin D. The natural oil found in canned fish should be used, since it too is a valuable source of these vitamins. An average serving of either fat or lean fish will supply about 10 per cent of the thiamin, 15 per cent of the riboflavin, and 50 per cent of the niacin required daily.

Fish and shellfish have high levels of polyunsaturated fatty acids, which lends to their use in certain dietary regimens. However, the cholesterol content of fish muscle is similar to meat and poultry (50 to 70 mg. cholesterol per 100 gm. tissue). Shellfish are low in fat but relatively rich in cholesterol. (See Appendix Table 4.)

DIGESTIBILITY   Fish and shellfish are excellent sources of easily digestible proteins of high nutritional value. Actual tests have shown that from 85 to 95 per cent of the protein are assimilable. Oyster stew (Chapter 38) is an especially suitable dish since it is easily digested, highly nutritious and easy to eat. Some individuals are allergic to shellfish, and occasionally to other fish.

USE IN THE DIET   Although 160 varie-

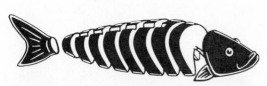

Figure 39–5   Steaks. Steaks are cross-section slices of the larger sizes of dressed fish. They are ready to cook as purchased, except for dividing the very largest into serving-size portions. A cross section of the backbone is usually the only bone in the steak. (Courtesy of U.S. Department of Interior, Fish and Wildlife Service.)

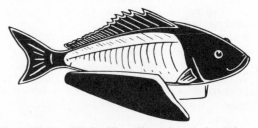

Figure 39–6   Single fillet. The sides of the fish, cut lengthwise away from the backbone are called fillets. They are practically boneless and require no preparation for cooking. Sometimes the skin, with the scales removed, is left on the fillets; others are skinned. A fillet cut from one side of a fish is called a single fillet. This is the type of fillet most generally seen in the market. (Courtesy of U.S. Department of Interior, Fish and Wildlife Service.)

TABLE 39-5   A GUIDE FOR BUYING FISH

SPECIES	FAT OR LEAN	USUAL MARKET RANGE OF ROUND FISH IN POUNDS	USUAL MARKET FORMS	MAIN PRODUCTION AREAS*	MAIN MARKET AREAS*
Salt Water:					
Bluefish	Lean	1 –7	Whole and drawn	Middle and South Atlantic	Middle and South Atlantic
Butterfish	Fat	¼–1	Whole and dressed	North and Middle Atlantic	North and Middle Atlantic
Cod	Lean	3 –20	Drawn, dressed, steaks, and fillets	North Atlantic; North Pacific	Entire United States
Croaker	Lean	½–2½	Whole, dressed, and fillets	Middle and South Atlantic	Middle and South Atlantic; Gulf
Flounder	Lean	¼–5	Whole, dressed, and fillets	Middle and South Atlantic	Entire United States
Grouper	Lean	5 –15	Whole, drawn, dressed, steaks, and fillets	South Atlantic; Gulf	South Atlantic; Gulf
Haddock	Lean	1½–7	Drawn and fillets	North Atlantic	Entire United States
Hake	Lean	2 –5	Whole, drawn, dressed, and fillets	North and Middle Atlantic	North and Middle Atlantic; Midwest
Halibut	Lean	8 –75	Dressed and steaks	Pacific	Entire United States
Herring, sea	Fat	¼–1	Whole	North Atlantic; North Pacific	North Atlantic; Pacific
Lingcod	Lean	5 –20	Dressed, steaks, and fillets	Pacific	Pacific
Mackerel	Fat	¾–3	Whole, drawn, and fillets	North and Middle Atlantic; Calif.	North and Middle Atlantic; California
Mullet	Lean	½–3	Whole	South Atlantic; Gulf	Middle and South Atlantic; Gulf; Midwest
Pollock	Lean	3 –14	Drawn, dressed, steaks, and fillets	North Atlantic	Entire United States, except Pacific
Rockfish	Lean	2 –5	Dressed and fillets	Pacific	Pacific and Midwest; Gulf
Rosefish	Lean	½–1¼	Fillets	North Atlantic	Entire United States
Salmon	Fat	3 –30	Drawn, dressed, steaks, and fillets	Pacific	Entire United States
Scup (Porgy)	Lean	½–2	Whole and dressed	North and Middle Atlantic	Middle and South Atlantic; Pacific
Sea bass	Lean	¼–4	Whole, dressed, and fillets	Middle and South Atlantic; California	Middle and South Atlantic; Gulf
Sea trout	Lean	1 –6	Whole, drawn, dressed, and fillets	Middle and South Atlantic; Gulf	North, Middle and South Atlantic; Pacific
Shad	Fat	1½–7	Whole, drawn, and fillets	Middle and South Atlantic; Pacific	Middle and South Atlantic; Gulf
Snapper, red	Lean	2 –15	Drawn, dressed, steaks, and fillets	South Atlantic; Gulf	Middle and South Atlantic; Gulf
Spot	Fat	1 –4	Whole, drawn, dressed, and fillets	South Atlantic; Gulf	Middle and South Atlantic
Spanish mackerel	Lean	¼–1¼	Whole and dressed	Middle and South Atlantic	Middle and South Atlantic
Whiting	Lean	½–1½	Whole, drawn, dressed, and fillets	North and Middle Atlantic	Entire United States, except Pacific
Fresh Water:					
Buffalofish	Lean	5 –15	Whole, drawn, dressed, and steaks	Mississippi Valley	Midwest
Carp	Lean	2 –8	Whole and fillets	Lakes and rivers	Midwest; Middle Atlantic
Catfish	Fat	1 –10	Whole, dressed, and skinned	Lakes and rivers	Middle and South Atlantic; Midwest; Gulf
Lake herring	Lean	⅓–1	Whole, drawn, and fillets	Great Lakes	Midwest
Lake trout	Fat	1½–10	Drawn, dressed, and fillets	Lakes and rivers	Midwest
Sheepshead	Lean	½–3	Whole, drawn, dressed, and fillets	Lakes and rivers	Midwest
Suckers	Lean	½–4	Whole, drawn, dressed, and fillets	Lakes and rivers	Midwest
Whitefish	Fat	2 –6	Whole, drawn, dressed, and fillets	Great Lakes	Midwest
Yellow perch	Lean	½–1	Whole and fillets	Great Lakes, lakes and rivers	Midwest
Yellow pike	Lean	1½–10	Whole, dressed, and fillets	Great Lakes and lakes	Midwest
Shellfish:					
Clams	Lean	5 –15	In the shell, shucked	All coastal areas	Entire United States
Crabs	Lean	2 –8	Live, cooked meat	All coastal areas	Entire United States, except Midwest
Lobsters	Lean	1 –10	Live, cooked meat	North and Middle Atlantic	North and Middle Atlantic; Midwest
Oysters	Lean		In the shell, shucked	All coastal areas	Entire United States
Shrimp	Lean		Headless, cooked meat	South Atlantic; Gulf and Pacific	Entire United States

* North Atlantic area includes the coastal states from Maine to Connecticut; Middle Atlantic area, New York to Virginia; South Atlantic area, North Carolina to Florida; Gulf area, Alabama to Texas; Pacific area, Washington to California (North Pacific, Washington, Oregon, and Alaska); and Midwest area, Central and Inland states. From Basic Fish Cookery, U.S. Department of the Interior, Fish and Wildlife Service.

ties of fish are sold in the United States, less than 10 species are popular. The Scandinavians are particularly fond of fish.

Fish is not so popular as meat, and in some localities fresh fish is not readily available. However, most forms of fish are frequently less expensive than comparable sources of protein such as meat and poultry, and more per capita consumption should be encouraged. Fish lends interesting flavor and variety to meal planning. Shellfish is generally more expensive than other types of fish.

BUYERS' INFORMATION   Fish is sold fresh, frozen, salted, dried, and canned.

Certain varieties of fresh fish are more economical when plentiful during specific seasons of the year. When buying whole fresh fish, look for these signs of freshness: eyes are bright, clear and bulging; gills are reddish-pink and free from slime; scales are tight to the skin, bright, and shiny; the flesh is firm and elastic; and the odor is fresh. Fresh fish are marketed (1) whole or round (internal organs, scales, head, tail, and fins removed in home before cooking), (2) drawn (whole or round fish sold after internal organs are removed) (3) dressed or pan dressed (whole or round fish sold after internal organs and scales are removed), (4) steaks are cross-section slices of the larger dressed fish and ready to cook as purchased (Fig. 39–5), and (5) fillets are the meaty sides of the fish, cut lengthwise away from the bone, require no preparation for cooking and there is no waste

(Fig. 39–6). Here are the suggested amounts to buy per serving: 1 pound whole or round fish; ½ pound large dressed fish; and ⅓ pound steaks and fillets. (See Table 39–5).

Smoked, dried, and salted fish are sold either whole (such as herring or small white fish) or in slices (such as codfish).

Frozen fish consist of steaks and fillets which are quick frozen and packaged.

Canned fish include tuna, salmon, sardines, and other varieties. Some manufacturers are canning fish with less oil for the dietetic market.

The popular varieties of shellfish include oysters, clams, shrimps, crabs, and lobsters.

CARE OF FISH AND SHELLFISH   Cold storage is a common method of preventing spoilage. See Chapter 14 for food spoilage, preservation, and public health control of fish and shellfish and Figure 39–2.

COOKERY SUGGESTIONS   1. Fish is cooked only until tender, when the flesh is easily flaked. Because fish has very little connective tissue, it cooks very quickly.

2. The fat content determines how fish is cooked. *Fat fish,* such as salmon, shad, mackerel, lake trout, and whitefish, are preferred for baking and broiling.

3. Cod, flounder, haddock, pike, rosefish, sea bass, striped bass, perch, and carp are examples of *lean fish* which are poached or boiled. However, lean fish may be baked or broiled if basted with melted butter or fat during the cooking process.

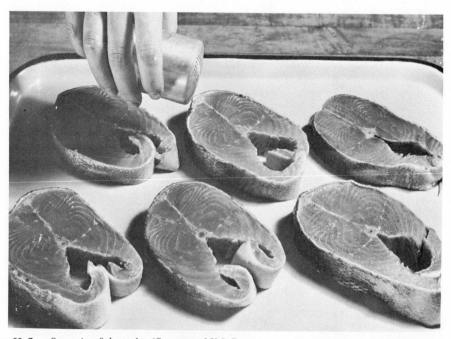

Figure 39–7   Seasoning fish steaks. (Courtesy of U.S. Department of Interior, Fish and Wildlife Service.)

4. If fish is purchased in packaged form, it should not be washed before cooking because dipping in water softens the flesh.

5. Fish is cut into serving portions before cooking, because fish is not carved (except for broiled, planked or baked whole fish).

6. Frozen fish is usually defrosted in the refrigerator before it is baked, broiled or fried. Fish is never refrozen after it thaws.

7. The oil from canned fish is used as the fat in the white sauce for creamed tuna or baked salmon loaf.

8. Suggested timetable for roasting fish:

Whole fish (approximately 1 to 4 pounds) baked 30 to 45 minutes in hot oven, 400° F.

Fish fillet (approximately 1 to 3 pounds) baked 30 minutes in moderate oven, 350° F.

Poached Fish (Boiled Fish)

¼ pound fish fillet
2 teaspoons salt
1 pint boiling water
  Procedure: 1. Tie the fish fillet in a square of double cheesecloth or parchment paper. Place in saucepan containing boiling salted water. 2. Reduce heat and cook slowly about 10 minutes. 3. Remove from boiling water onto plate, cut string, and carefully remove cheesecloth or parchment paper. Serve immediately.
  Yield: 1 serving

Broiled Fish

¼ pound fish fillet or steak
  Salt and pepper
1 tablespoon melted butter
  Procedure: 1. Preheat broiler. Sprinkle salt and pepper over fillet or steak (Fig. 39–7) and place on small pan or metal foil. Brush melted butter over fish. 2. Place pan or foil with fish on broiler under heat. Broil one side of fish 5 to 8 minutes or until brown. Baste with melted butter. Turn fish, baste over side with melted butter, and broil until brown. 3. Place broiled fish on warmed plate and serve immediately.
  Yield: 1 serving

EGGS

COMPOSITION   The average hen's egg, without shell, weighs 50 grams. The fat and protein are about equally divided, with 13 per cent protein and 12 per cent fat. The egg yolk contains half of the protein, all of the fat, minerals (except sulfur) and vitamins (except riboflavin). The egg white contains the other half of the proteins and riboflavin, and part of the sulfur. One egg yields an *average* of 80 kcalories, of which 64 are from the yolk and only 16 from the white. The composition of *averages* of hens' eggs is given in Table 39–6.

NUTRITIVE VALUE   Eggs are a good source of complete, high quality protein, easily assimilated unsaturated fats, iron, copper, phosphorus, vitamin A, riboflavin, vitamin B_{12}, and vitamin D, and they provide some calcium (chiefly in the shell), pantothenic acid, and thiamin (Table 39–6). All the nutritive substances, minerals and vitamins necessary for the development of the chick are furnished by the egg and can be compared in food value with milk and meat. The yolk contains most of the mineral and vitamin activity of whole egg. Eggs lack vitamin C and are a poor source of niacin. Egg protein contains somewhat higher amounts of the sulfur amino acids (methionine and cystine) than does meat. Egg yolk is relatively high in cholesterol (Appendix Table 4).

Some sections of the country favor brown eggs, while other localities prefer eggs with white shells. The color of the shell depends upon the breed of the fowl. The color of the shell does not affect the nutritive value of the egg nor the flavor. Neither is it a guide to yolk color. The color of the egg yolk may vary from

TABLE 39–6   AVERAGE PERCENTAGE COMPOSITION OF FRESH HENS' EGGS*†

		WHOLE EGG	EGG WHITE	EGG YOLK
Water		73.7	87.6	51.1
Protein		12.9	10.9	16
Fat		11.5	Trace	30.6
Carbohydrate		0.9	0.8	0.6
Calcium (mg.)	MINERALS	54	9	141
Phosphorus (mg.)		205	15	569
Iron (mg.)		2.3	0.1	5.5
Vitamin A (I.U.)	VITAMINS	1180	0	3400
Thiamine (mg.)		0.11	Trace	0.22
Riboflavin (mg.)		0.30	0.27	0.44
Niacin (mg.)		.1	.1	.1
Ascorbic acid (mg.)		0	0	0

  * The composition of 1 egg would be approximately ½ of whole egg figures.
  † Adapted from Composition of Foods—Raw, Processed, Prepared. Agriculture Handbook No. 8, U. S. Department of Agriculture, 1963.

light to deep yellow. Yolk color is influenced by heredity and diet but does not necessarily affect flavor and nutritive value. The food ration of the hen tends to affect the flavor of the egg and color of the yolk, and to influence the vitamin content, especially vitamin A.

PLACE IN THE DAILY DIET   Eggs may be served in innumerable ways for breakfast, as a main dish for luncheon or dinner, or they can be combined with other foods in the preparation of beverages, bread, cake, desserts, salads, salad dressings, sandwiches, sauces, vegetables and countless other dishes. The recommendation of one egg a day is believed beneficial for all.

If a dislike is exhibited toward eggs, the flavor and quality of the tasted product may have been inferior. Fresh eggs are used for table service as poached, coddled, scrambled, baked, omelet, and in custards. Cold storage eggs are used in cooking and baking where the flavor of the ingredients helps to mask the taste of "held" eggs. Frozen eggs and dried or dehydrated eggs can be used in baked goods.

Eggs are useful in cooking and baking. When air is whipped into whole egg, egg yolk, or egg white, the role of leavening agent comes into play. Eggs are used to thicken liquids (custards), to bind ingredients (sauces), to clarify (consommé), and to act as an emulsifying agent (mayonnaise).

DIGESTIBILITY   Eggs are easily digested and almost completely utilized. The fat in the yolk is of superior quality, and in a finely emulsified form similar to that of milk. Methods of cooking eggs affect their digestibility to some degree but do not affect their total utilization.

BUYERS' INFORMATION   U.S. weight classes for consumer grades for shell eggs are:

Jumbo
    30 ounces/net minimum weight/dozen
Extra large
    27 ounces/net minimum weight/dozen
Large
    24 ounces/net minimum weight/dozen
Medium
    21 ounces/net minimum weight/dozen
Small (pullet)
    18 ounces/net minimum weight/dozen

The large and medium size eggs are the most common size on the market. Small eggs are usually more plentiful in the late summer and fall months. The size does not affect the quality but does affect price. Weight for weight the nutritive value is the same for small and large eggs of equal quality.

The retail grades for shell eggs are: U.S. Grade AA, U.S. Grade A, U.S. Grade B, and U.S. Grade C. Factors to determine the grade are: (1) cleanliness and soundness of shell,

(2) size of the air cell, and (3) the condition of the yolk and white which are judged by candling. Retail cartons of officially graded eggs carry a certificate stating grade and size, and the date of grading. (See Fig. 12–1.)

STORAGE   Proper refrigeration helps to maintain the original quality of eggs. Eggs may be stored commercially for several months at temperatures as low as 32° F.

COOKERY SUGGESTIONS   1. Eggs are cooked or baked slowly at low temperatures to prevent discoloration, curdling, and tough, elastic consistency. Excessive use of heat, especially dry heat, is detrimental to the availability of amino acids, particularly the amino acid lysine. Too rapid cooking at high temperatures toughens the protein and may cause discoloration (the greenish color of overcooked eggs).

2. The length of the cooking period is governed by the coagulation of the protein and the desired thickness or thinness.

3. If eggs are used as a leavening agent, then the beating of air into whole eggs, yolk or whites must be swift and sufficient. It is just as important to avoid underbeating of eggs as overbeating. If eggs are beaten too long, they tend to make the product dry. The quality of an omelet is dependent upon this factor.

4. Beaten eggs are folded carefully into a mixture, to prevent loss of air. Egg whites at room temperature beat better than cold egg whites.

"Three Minute" Egg

Place egg of room temperature in saucepan containing just enough water to cover the egg. Place pan over heat and bring water slowly to boiling point. Reduce heat and keep water just below boiling point. Cook 3 minutes. Remove egg from pan and serve immediately. This is a soft-cooked egg.

Poached Egg

If an egg poacher is available use it. Otherwise fill a frying pan or low saucepan three-fourths full of boiling water. If salt is permitted, it is added to the water. Arrange buttered muffin ring or circular cooky cutter without handle in boiling water. Break egg carefully out of shell into saucer and slide egg into muffin ring. The water is supposed to cover the egg, but the water is not to boil after putting in egg. When the white is firm, carefully remove egg with a skimmer, or pour off water and lift egg out of pan to toast on plate. Serve immediately (Fig. 39–8).

French (Plain) Omelet

2 eggs
2 tablespoons milk or cream
¼ teaspoon salt
    Pepper
1 tablespoon butter or margarine

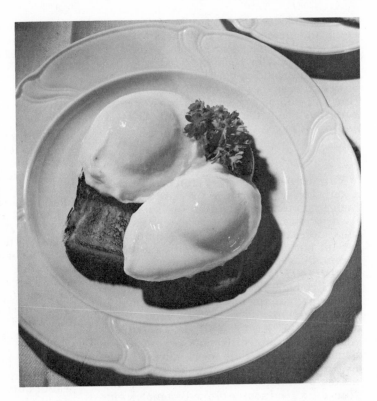

Figure 39–8 Poached eggs on toast make a nutritious meal. (Courtesy of Poultry and Egg National Board.)

Procedure: 1. Break eggs out of shells into bowl and beat slightly with whisk or beater. Add milk or cream and seasonings. 2. Melt butter in hot, heavy frying pan of medium size. When butter is melted pour in beaten egg mixture. The edges of the omelet are lifted with a spatula to allow the uncooked part to run underneath. The omelet should be made quickly. 3. Fold and remove to hot plate. Serve. (Fig. 39–9.)

Yield: 1 serving

MEAT ALTERNATES

When meat is limited, other foods – macaroni, noodles, spaghetti, rice or legumes (dried peas, beans, lentils) – can be combined with it. This is known as mutual supplementation and the prepared foods are known as meat-extending dishes. (See Chapter 6.) Meat

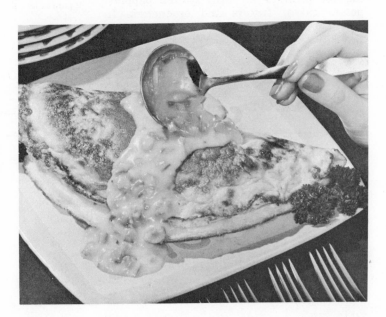

Figure 39–9 Omelet can be used plain for breakfast or with vegetables or tomato sauce for luncheon or supper. (Photo courtesy of Better Homes & Gardens.)

loaf, extended with dried milk, oats, wheat germ, and grated carrots and bound with egg, is an excellent source of protein. Dried skim milk, split peas or beans flavored with ham bone (or any kind of bone), furnishes protein as desirable as that in expensive lamb chops. One half cup of cooked dried peas or beans furnishes about the same amount of protein as 1 oz. of meat.

NUTS

Nuts are defined as a dry fruit consisting of a kernel in a shell. Since they are generally high in protein and fat, they are sometimes used as meat alternates or extenders. The nuts most commonly used are peanuts (and peanut butter), almonds, filberts, chestnuts, walnuts, cashews and Brazil nuts.

COMPOSITION   Except for the chestnut which is high in carbohydrate and low in protein and fat, the nuts are generally high in fat and protein. (See Table 39-7.)

NUTRITIVE VALUE AND DIGESTIBILITY Although the protein of nuts is not equal in quality to that of milk, eggs, cheese, meat, fish and poultry, it is of good quality and makes a valuable contribution to the diet. Nuts are a good source of the B-complex vitamins thiamin, riboflavin and niacin, and of the minerals iron, copper, phosphorus and manganese. They also contain varying amounts of calcium, depending upon the variety of nut. Since nuts are high in fat (except chestnuts), they digest slowly. Chopped nuts and nut spreads, such as peanut butter, are more easily utilized.

USE IN THE DIET   Nuts are used as meat alternates and extenders, such as stuffing for poultry, nut loaf, stuffed peppers, potato cakes, fritters and croquettes. In whole or chopped form they are also used as an ingredient in cakes, cookies, pies and various dessert dishes; and as a spread for sandwiches in the form of peanut butter.

LEGUMES

Dry beans, peas and lentils are nutritious, low cost foods that can be used in combination with other foods to provide good quality protein. There are many varieties of legumes including lima beans, split peas, lentils, red kidney beans, pinto beans and black-eye peas, chick peas and many beans.

NUTRITIVE VALUE   Legumes supply important quantities of protein, iron, thiamin and riboflavin and are low in fat. One cup of cooked legumes supplies about 290 kcalories and 31 per cent of the protein, 42 per cent of the iron, 26 per cent of the thiamin and 13 per cent of the riboflavin needed by an adult male.

BUYERS' INFORMATION   Beans, peas and lentils should have a bright uniform color, be free of visible defects and be of uniform size. Store tightly covered in a cool, dry place. To compare the relative cost of legumes, nuts, peanut butter, and meat, quotations of prices can be obtained from a retail store. The computed figure is inserted in the designated space:

4 ounces ground round steak
at ....cents a pound $..........................
4 ounces beef steak
at ....cents a pound $..........................
4 ounces liver (beef)
at ....cents a pound $..........................
2 ounces lentils
at ....cents a pound $..........................

TABLE 39-7   AVERAGE PER CENT COMPOSITION OF SOME COMMON NUTS

KIND OF NUTS	WATER %	PROTEIN %	FAT %	CARBOHYDRATE %	KCALORIES PER 100 GRAMS
Almonds, dried	5	19	54	20	598
Brazil nuts	5	14	67	11	654
Butternuts	4	24	61	8	629
Cashew nuts	5	17	46	29	561
Chestnuts, fresh	53	3	2	42	194
Chestnuts, dried	8	7	4	79	377
Filberts (hazelnuts)	6	13	62	17	634
Hickory nuts	3	13	69	13	673
Peanuts, roasted	2	26	49	21	582
Pecans	3	9	71	15	687
Pistachio nuts	5	19	54	19	594
Walnuts, black	3	21	59	15	628
Walnuts, English	4	15	64	16	651

2 ounces dried beans
    at ....cents a pound $..........................
2 ounces dried peas
    at ....cents a pound $..........................
2 ounces peanut butter
    at ....cents a pound $..........................
2 ounces almonds
    at ....cents a pound $..........................
2 ounces brazil nuts
    at ....cents a pound $..........................
2 ounces fresh chestnuts
    at ....cents a pound $..........................

COOKERY SUGGESTIONS   1. Dried peas, beans, and lentils are washed preferably soaked in a small quantity of water before cooking to allow reabsorption of water withdrawn during the drying process. A fast and effective way to soak legumes is to start by boiling them in water for two minutes.

2. The soaked legumes are cooked at low heat for a long period. The water used to soak legumes is used as part of the cooking water. Legumes may be cooked in the pressure cooker when directions of the manufacturer are followed.

3. The proportions given in the recipe are followed to maintain tested texture and flavor.

4. Beans, peas and lentils expand when cooking. One cup of dried beans yields 2 to 2¾ cups of cooked beans.

Bean Loaf with Tomato Sauce

1 cup cooked navy beans
⅓ cup bread cubes
1 egg, beaten
    Salt, pepper and celery salt
½ cup canned tomatoes
    Procedure: 1. Mash the cooked beans in a mixing bowl. Stir in the bread cubes and egg. Add seasoning. 2. Shape mixture into loaf and place in loaf pan or baking dish. Pour canned tomatoes over loaf. 3. Bake about 30 minutes in a moderate oven (350° F.). Remove from pan, slice and serve hot.
    Yield: 2 servings

Peanut-potato Cakes

1½ cups chopped salted peanuts
2¼ cups seasoned mashed potatoes (white or sweet)
2 tablespoons chopped parsley
1 egg, beaten
    Pepper or 2 or 3 drops tabasco sauce, if desired
    Flour
    Fat or drippings for frying
    Procedure: 1. Combine peanuts, potatoes, and parsley and stir in the seasoning and half of the egg. Shape into eight flat cakes. 2. Dip cakes in rest of egg, then in flour. Brown in hot fat. Cakes may be dipped in fine crumbs instead of flour if desired.
    Yield: 4 servings
    Variations: Use finely chopped pimento, green pepper, celery, or onion in place of parsley.

SUGGESTED ADDITIONAL READING REFERENCES

See Appendix General References, Part III.

Chapter 40
GROUP III: VEGETABLE– FRUIT GROUP

Four or more servings from the vegetable–fruit group are recommended daily. These should include citrus fruit or other fruit or vegetable rich in ascorbic acid, a dark green or deep yellow vegetable for vitamin A (at least every other day), and other vegetables and fruits, including potatoes.

VEGETABLES

Vegetables play an important part in the general diet and cooked vegetables appear in most of the modified diets. The abundant assortment of vegetables contributes variety to the meals. The modern retail supermarket displays a widely varied collection of fresh fruits and vegetables for the consumer's selection (Fig. 40–1). What to choose from the displays of so many different kinds of fruits and vegetables is often a difficult decision. Family nationality and locality influence the preferences for specific vegetables; for example, the Irish enjoy the white potato and people from the southern states like sweet potatoes.

Yellow vegetables provide vitamin A and

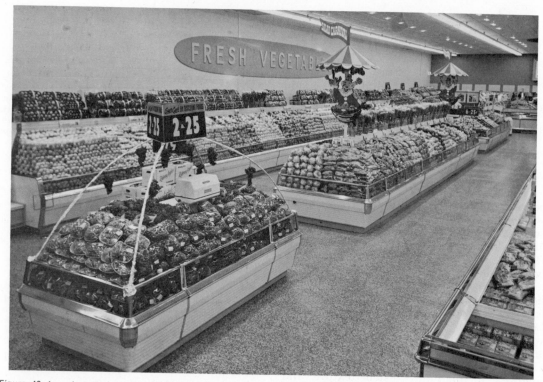

Figure 40-1   A typical display of fruits and vegetables as found in the super markets throughout the United States. (Courtesy of Progressive Grocer magazine.)

green vegetables furnish iron and vitamin A, while all of the vegetables are good sources of minerals and vitamins.

Appetizing and palatable vegetables depend upon the selection of quality produce and the careful adherence to proper food preparation techniques. Overcooked, woody in texture, and soggy vegetables are not appetizing and are usually refused. Rapid transportation facilities and the canning and freezing processes have largely eliminated the regional and seasonal factors of availability. Sources of supply vary with the changing seasons and with crop development in many divergent producing areas. Vegetables are usually lowest in price in any given market area when the local supply is most abundant. Scarcity or abundance of a commodity regulates the price more often than any other factor. Many families obtain fresh vegetables from a garden planted in the back yard. Home food freezers and refrigerators with space for storing frozen food have changed buying habits. However, the fresh vegetable flavor remains the criterion for judging frozen vegetables and canned vegetables.

CLASSIFICATION AS TO NUTRITIVE VALUE   Vegetables may be classified according to the part of the plant used for food, and according to nutritive value. Vegetables and parts of vegetables vary in nutritive value.

Green Leafy Vegetables   Lettuce, romaine, chicory, escarole, endive, cabbage, collards, Chinese cabbage and all greens are examples. They are most valuable for minerals, vitamins and cellulose; they are important sources of the minerals calcium and iron, of the vitamins A, K, and riboflavin, and are valuable sources of ascorbic acid. The young tender growing leaves contain more ascorbic acid than the mature plants. The green outer leaves of lettuce and cabbage are much richer than the white inner leaves in vitamin A, calcium, and iron. The thinner and greener the leaf, the richer in nutritive value. Green leafy vegetables are generally low in calories.

Flowering Vegetables   Broccoli and cauliflower are the two most commonly used flowering vegetables. Broccoli, being greener, rates higher in nutritive value than cauliflower and is a good source of the minerals iron and phosphorus and vitamin A, ascorbic acid and riboflavin. The outer leaves of cauliflower and broccoli are much higher in nutritive value than the flower buds and should be cooked or used in salad.

Seed Vegetables   Peas, beans, and lentils are classified as seed vegetables or legumes. The more mature legumes provide protein (incomplete), are frequently supplemented with complete protein foods, such as milk, eggs, meat or cheese, and may be used as a main dish. They are valuable for phosphorus, iron, and thiamin.

Root Vegetables   Carrots, beets, turnips, and white and sweet potatoes are examples. The yellow root vegetables are rich sources of vitamin A. The deeper the yellow color, the greater the content. Root vegetables in general are good sources of thiamin. White potatoes (modified underground stems) contain some ascorbic acid. Though not a rich source, when properly prepared and used in quantity they add materially to the total day's allowance.

Stem or Stalk Vegetables   Celery and asparagus are examples of stem vegetables. They contain minerals and vitamins in proportion to the green color, similar to that found in green leafy vegetables.

Fruit Vegetables   The tomato and pepper are the outstanding vegetables which are the fruit of the plant. Both are rich in ascorbic acid. Other fruit vegetables are cucumbers, squash, pumpkin, and eggplant. Remember, the deeper the green and yellow color, the greater the vitamin A content.

Bulb Vegetables   The onion is the outstanding bulb vegetable, and is a fair source of ascorbic acid.

COMPOSITION OF VEGETABLES   In general, the fresh, raw product contains more vitamins and minerals than the processed product. All vegetables have a high water content and vary in composition, even in a specific food, depending upon the species, conditions of growth and method of cooking. Vegetables are composed chiefly of carbohydrates. The carbohydrate content, in general, ranges from 3 per cent—as found in the leafy and stem vegetables—to 27 per cent in sweet potatoes. The root and seed vegetables are among the richest in carbohydrate content. With the exception of legumes, vegetables contain very little protein, averaging from 1 to 3 per cent. There is little or no fat in vegetables.

DIGESTIBILITY   The high value of fresh vegetables in keeping the digestive tract functioning normally has been mentioned previously. The bulky, fibrous foods, in contrast with highly refined concentrated foods, are essential for good digestion and elimination. Adequate bulk makes laxatives generally unnecessary.

There are some conditions, such as diarrhea, peptic ulcers, and ulcerative colitis (Chapters 23, 24), in which the use of bulky vegetables and roughage may be restricted or must be avoided. Furthermore, in conditions such as gallbladder (Chapter 25) and cardiac disease (Chapter 30) certain vegetables, commonly termed "gas forming," may cause distress, and discretion must be used. However, the normal individual can digest vegetables with ease.

PLACE IN THE DIET   Of the protective foods that should be eaten every day, vegetables occupy three places: (1) leafy dark green or deep yellow; (2) citrus fruits, tomato or any raw fruit or vegetable which is rich in vitamin C; (3) other vegetable and fruit, including potatoes, to total 4 or more servings. At least one of these should be eaten raw, or incorporated into salad, sandwiches or juices. The principal contributions of vegetables to good nutrition are minerals, vitamins and bulk as outlined in this chapter and throughout the text. Also, they add appetizing texture, color, and flavor to the diet.

BUYERS' INFORMATION   Supply, demand, and distribution are factors which influence the price of produce. (See Chapter 12, Food Economics, for production, marketing, and distribution of vegetables.) Although *practice* is the best teacher in the selection of fresh vegetables, here are some suggested criteria for judging:

Selecting the fresh and avoiding the shriveled, wilted or decayed is the best rule to follow. Freshness, state of ripeness, firmness, unblemished, without spoilage are some of the guiding factors. Best quality and price are available at the peak of the season.

When the average size of serving is ½ cup, one pound of vegetables (as purchased) yields the following number of servings:

Asparagus	= 4 servings	
Beans, lima (in pod)	= 2	"
Beans, snap	= 6	"
Beets, diced	= 4	"
Broccoli	= 3	"
Brussels sprouts	= 5	"
Cabbage, raw and shredded	= 7	"
Cabbage, cooked	= 4	"
Carrots, raw and shredded	= 8	"
Carrot, cooked	= 5	"
Cauliflower	= 3	"
Celery, cooked	= 3	"
Collards	= 2	"
Corn, cut off cob	= 2	(in husk)
Eggplant	= 4 servings	
Greens and kale	= 4	"
Onions	= 4	"
Peas (in pod)	= 2	"
Potatoes	= 4	"
Spinach	= 3	"
Squash	= 2	"
Sweet Potatoes	= 3	"
Turnips	= 4	"

CANNED VEGETABLES   Commercially canned vegetables offer a large variety of products to choose from the year round, helping to keep the food budget down when certain vegetables are out of season. They are cooked and ready to eat, thus saving time and assuring no waste. The vegetables used for canning are especially grown for that purpose, picked at just the right point of maturity, vacuum sealed and subjected to pressure heat in the briefest possible time after harvesting. The process used in industrial canning does not affect the food value of carbohydrate, protein and fat, and most of the vitamin and mineral nutritive values are retained. Quality canned vegetables are preferable for plain-cooked dishes, salads, or serving "as is." Second quality may do for combination dishes such as stews, casserole dishes, soups, or when wholeness or color are not so important.

For those who count calories, limit the sodium and/or potassium intake, or are diabetic, there is an increasing number of dietetic-pack canned vegetables.

When the average serving is ½ cup, the yield from canned vegetables is:

8 ounce can	= 2 servings
No. 1 tall can (16 ounces)	= 4 "
No. 303 can (16 ounces)	= 4 "
No. 2 can (20 ounces)	= 5 "
No. 2½ can (29 ounces)	= 6-7 "
No. 3 cylinder (46 ounces)	= 11 "

FROZEN VEGETABLES   Frozen vegetables are becoming increasingly popular and are available the year round. They are ready to cook and, therefore, save labor and time in preparation. The nutritive value is usually equal to that of the fresh product. The best of the crop is harvested at the peak of quality and rapidly frozen within a few hours. Only solid-frozen packages should be selected, never those that are soft and starting to thaw. Refreezing after thawing lowers quality.

Three ½ cup servings constitute the average yield from the family-size package of frozen vegetables.

DRIED VEGETABLES   Besides fresh, frozen, and canned, vegetables are also available in dried and dehydrated forms. The process of drying is discussed in Chapter 14 under Food Preservation. Legumes are the most popular dried foods, used as supplementary protein foods. Other foods such as soups and seasonings (onion, garlic, parsley) are found on the market. They take little storage space and have a definite place in the menu.

COOKERY SUGGESTIONS   1. Cook vegetables quickly (just until tender) in a minimum amount of water (just enough water to prevent scorching), in a covered pan, and serve immediately (Table 40–1). In this respect, steaming and pressure cooking have advantages over boiling. The iron content of broccoli, for example, diminishes 50 per cent after 20 minutes of boiling. Adding bicarbonate of soda to the water softens the fiber

TABLE 40–1   TIME TABLE FOR BOILING VEGETABLES
(Variety, Age and Size Influence Cooking Period)

	(FRESH) MINUTES	(FROZEN) MINUTES
Asparagus, whole	10 to 20	5 to 10
Beans, lima	20 to 30	6 to 10
Beans, snap, 1-inch pieces	12 to 16	12 to 18
Beets, young, whole	30 to 45	
Broccoli, separated into stalks	10 to 15	5 to 8
Brussels sprouts	15 to 20	4 to 9
Cabbage, shredded	3 to 10	
Cabbage, quartered	10 to 15	
Carrots, whole	15 to 25	
Cauliflower, separated into stalks	8 to 15	
Cauliflower, whole	20 to 30	
Celery, cut into pieces	15 to 20	
Collards, whole	10 to 20	
Corn, on the cob	5 to 15	
Greens, beet (young)	5 to 15	6 to 12
Greens, dandelion	10 to 20	
Greens, kale	10 to 25	8 to 12
Greens, turnip	10 to 30	
Kohlrabi, sliced	20 to 25	
Okra, whole or sliced	10 to 15	
Onions, halves or whole	20 to 40	
Parsnips, whole	20 to 40	
Peas	8 to 20	5 to 10
Potatoes, halves or whole	25 to 45	
Rutabagas, pared, cut into pieces	20 to 30	
Squash, summer, sliced	10 to 20	
Squash, winter, cut into pieces	20 to 40	
Spinach, whole	3 to 10	4 to 6
Sweet potatoes, whole	25 to 35	
Swiss chard	10 to 20	
Tomatoes, cut into wedges	7 to 15	
Turnips, cut into pieces	15 to 20	

and retains the color of green vegetables but encourages mineral and vitamin loss. Vegetables deteriorate quickly in vitamin value if exposed to air while cooking or in too long cooking periods. The nutritional content also suffers when vegetables are allowed to stand in the open or are warmed over. This is especially true of the ascorbic acid content of vegetables. Gordon and Noble[1] analyzed ascorbic acid values following three methods

---

[1]Gordon, J., and Noble, I.: "Waterless" vs. boiling water cooking of vegetables. J. Am. Dietet. A., 44:378, 1964.

of cooking vegetables: the pressure saucepan, the "waterless" saucepan, covered with boiling water. The percentage retention of ascorbic acid was highest with the pressure saucepan. The "waterless" saucepan ranked second (except for broccoli and Brussels sprouts).

2. Use liquid remaining from cooked and canned vegetables to flavor soups, sauces, and gravies.

3. Cook potatoes without peeling to retain more nutrients.

4. Peel or scrape sparingly any vegetables. The dark outer leaves of cabbage, head lettuce, and other greens are rich in iron, calcium, and vitamins.

5. Vegetables are boiled, steamed, broiled, baked or roasted, and fried. The type of diet influences the selection of the cookery method.

6. To prepare vegetables for the cooking process, vegetables are washed to remove dirt, sand and insects. They are scraped or peeled to remove skin. Any tough or woody parts are removed. Vegetables are cut into slices, thin strips (julienne), cubes, quarters, or halves. The uncooked vegetable is always stored in the refrigerator to preserve freshness and crispness. The cleaned whole vegetable is stored in protective transparent bags or special pans in the refrigerator and cut to size just before the cooking process.

7. To strain or purée vegetables, the tender cooked vegetable is pressed through a food mill or sieve.

8. The seasonings and sauces used to flavor cooked vegetables include herbs, pepper, celery salt, onion salt, paprika, butter, margarine, oil, bacon drippings, sour or sweet cream, white sauce, special sauces, buttered crumbs, and grated cheese.

Frozen vegetables should be cooked according to the directions on the package. They should be kept frozen *solid* until ready to use; they do not need to be thawed before cooking. If they have thawed, they should *not* be refrozen.

Commerically canned vegetables are already cooked so need only to be reheated. To reheat: (1) drain the liquid into a saucepan, (2) boil liquid quickly to reduce the amount about one-half, (3) add the vegetables and heat quickly, (4) season and add butter, cream sauce or dressing, as desired. If preferred, instead of reducing the liquid, use it in sauce, soup, gravy or vegetable cocktail. Do not throw it away; it contains valuable nutrients. Cream style corn, tomatoes, squash, and such vegetables are not drained.

Home canned vegetables are heated to a rolling boil and boiled at least 10 minutes to destroy harmful organisms. Home canned spinach and corn are boiled 20 minutes.

To cook vegetables in a pressure cooker, the manufacturer's directions should be followed precisely. Overcooking for a few seconds can lower the quality of the vegetable.

Dried vegetables such as peas, beans, and lentils are usually soaked before they are cooked. Follow directions on package.

SERVICE   Cooked vegetables are served hot and as soon as possible following the cooking process to prevent vitamin loss.

Panned Vegetable Greens

1 pint shredded spinach *or*
1 cup shredded cabbage, kale or collards
¼ teaspoon salt
½ tablespoon butter or drippings
   Procedure: 1. Shred cabbage, kale, collards, or spinach. 2. Melt butter or drippings in a heavy frying pan. Add shredded vegetable and sprinkle salt over vegetable. Put cover on pan to hold in steam. 3. Place frying pan over low heat and cook until tender, stirring vegetables occasionally to prevent sticking. Cabbage cooks tender in 5 to 10 minutes; other greens take a little longer cooking period.
   Yield: 1 serving

Scalloped Potatoes

¾ cup peeled, sliced potato
      (1 medium size potato)
¼ to ⅓ cup milk
¼ teaspoon salt
1 teaspoon flour
1 teaspoon butter
   Procedure: 1. Arrange layer of peeled, sliced potato in buttered baking dish. 2. Sprinkle half of the salt and flour over potatoes, and use half of the butter to dot over the potatoes. Repeat process. Pour enough milk over potatoes to reach the top layer. 3. Bake in moderate oven (350° F.) about 1 hour or until potatoes test tender. Serve immediately.
   Yield: 1 serving

VEGETABLE SEASONINGS

Boiled vegetables can be made more attractive to the palate by skillful seasoning. Following are a few hints:

1. When cooking peas, add a few mint leaves.

2. When cooking lima beans, add a small pinch of an herb or spice to the water.

3. When cooking snap beans or summer squash, add a tablespoon or two of minced onion, green pepper, or parsley.

4. Use flavorful fats such as meat drippings, butter, margarine, or salad oil—with lemon juice, horse-radish, or garlic added.

5. Add crispy bits of fried bacon to greens such as spinach.

6. A dressing made with a little vinegar and sugar heated together, with or without a few tablespoons of cream, is delicious on snap beans or cabbage.

VEGETABLE SAUCES

A sauce added to boiled vegetables gives a nice flavor and texture change. Combine the hot vegetable and hot sauce lightly just before serving. One-half cup of sauce is about right for 2 servings of vegetable. Always use the vegetable cooking liquid, if any, in the sauce.

White Sauce

See Chapter 38.

Hollandaise Sauce

¼ pound butter or fortified margarine
　Dash cayenne
　Salt
½ tablespoon lemon juice
1 egg yolk
Procedure: 1. Place butter in top of double boiler off the heat. Beat with rotary beater until creamy. Blend in cayenne and salt. 2. Beat in lemon juice, a few drops at a time. 3. Add egg yolk. Beat until fluffy. 4. Heat over hot, not boiling, water a few minutes until glossy, stirring constantly. Water should not touch top pan. 5. Spoon over hot asparagus or other vegetable. Serve immediately.
Yield: 2 to 3 servings (Fig. 40–2)

Mustard Sauce

Procedure: 1. Stir 1 teaspoon prepared mustard into ½ cup medium white sauce (Chapter 38) after cooking. 2. Very good with greens, snap beans, and cabbage.
Yield: 2 servings

Cheese Sauce

Procedure: 1. Prepare ½ cup thin white sauce (Chapter 38). 2. Add ¼ to ½ cup grated cheese. 3. Remove from heat and stir until cheese is melted. 4. Good with spinach or other greens.
Yield: 2 servings

Egg Sauce

Procedure: 1. Prepare ½ cup thin white sauce (Chapter 38). 2. Stir in ½ teaspoon lemon juice and ½ chopped hard-cooked egg just before serving. 3. Especially good with greens and Brussels sprouts.
Yield: 2 servings

SALADS

Although Caesar never knew the present-day Romaine Caesar Salad that bears his name, it was the Romans who introduced salad to the world. The plebs, or commoners, dipped *cichorium* (chicory) and *lactuca* (lettuce) in salt, and so from *sal* (salt) came salad.

PREPARATION SUGGESTIONS 1. The pieces of meat, poultry or fish used in salads are free of bone, gristle, and skin.

2. The gelatin base of a salad is tender and firm, not runny or rubbery.

3. To avoid discoloration, vegetables and fruits are cut with stainless steel knives. Cut pieces of fruits are covered with tart citrus juice to prevent fruits from turning brown.

4. To keep salad greens crisp, wash and dry them thoroughly, and then place them in a towel or special hydrator or plastic bag, and store in the refrigerator.

5. Salads are kept chilled in the refrigerator until serving time.

6. Lettuce and salad greens are shredded with scissors or torn into pieces.

7. Salad garnishes include radish roses (outside rosy skin partially peeled to form petals), carrots julienne or stick (raw carrots cut into match-thin strips), and celery curls (pieces of celery split partially into thin strips and chilled in ice water, which curls the cut strips).

SUGGESTED COMBINATIONS OF VEGETABLES FOR SALAD 1. Grated raw carrot, diced celery, and cucumber slices.

2. Raw spinach, endive or lettuce, with tomato wedges.

3. Sliced raw cauliflowerets, chopped green peppers, diced celery, and thin strips of pimiento or red peppers.

4. Shredded cabbage and cucumber cubes blended with thin strips of celery.

5. Cubed canned beets and thinly sliced celery combined with canned tiny sweet onions.

6. Canned whole kernel corn and canned French style string beans combined with slices of sweet pickle and thinly sliced onion rings.

SUGGESTED COMBINATIONS OF FRUITS AND VEGETABLES FOR SALAD 1. Shredded raw carrots and diced apples combined with raisins.

2. Sliced or ground raw cranberries and diced celery and apple combined with orange sections cut into pieces.

3. Canned pineapple cubes and thin cucumber slices blended.

4. Sliced avocado and grapefruit sections cut into pieces, combined with thin slices or wedges of tomato.

5. Canned crushed pineapple and orange sections cut into pieces and combined with shredded cabbage.

SALAD DRESSINGS

Salad dressings may be made at home or purchased ready made. They are stored in the refrigerator in air tight containers. The unique flavor of herbs and spices adds the piquant touch to salad dressings, and the combinations may be individualized.

Homemade salad dressings are blended carefully, the egg acting as the emulsifying

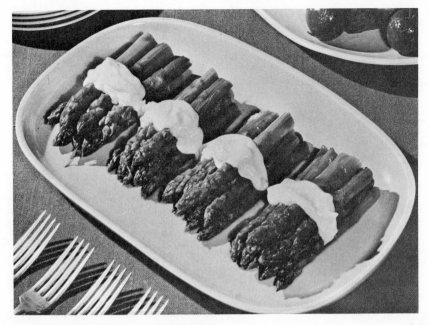

Figure 40–2   Asparagus with hollandaise sauce. (Photo courtesy of Better Homes & Gardens.)

agent and the beating breaking the ingredients into the droplets that are necessary to form an emulsion.

Mineral oil inhibits the absorption of the fat-soluble vitamins A, D, E, and K and is not recommended as a substitute for salad oil to reduce calories. Lemon juice or wine vinegar is a good substitute.

French Dressing

1/8 teaspoon salt
  Few grains of pepper, paprika and dry mustard
1/8 teaspoon sugar
 1 tablespoon vinegar or lemon juice
 2 tablespoons olive oil or salad oil
  Procedure: 1. Measure ingredients into small covered glass jar or bottle with cover. Chill in refrigerator. 2. Before using, shake bottle thoroughly for 1 minute.

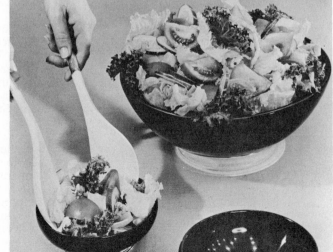

Figure 40–3   Tossed green salad. (Photo courtesy of Better Homes & Gardens.)

Variations: 1. Mix with catsup and chopped olives for green salad. 2. Add a few sprigs of crushed mint for fruit salad. 3. Add curry powder and onion juice to serve on meat salad.
Yield: 1 serving

Cooked Salad Dressing

1 egg yolk
1½ tablespoons vinegar
3 tablespoons milk
½ tablespoon butter
¼ teaspoon salt
¼ teaspoon sugar
¼ teaspoon dry mustard
    Few grains of paprika and celery salt
Procedure: 1. Blend together egg yolk and vinegar in upper part of small double boiler using wooden spoon. Stir in milk, butter, salt, sugar, dry mustard, paprika, and celery salt. 2. Cook over boiling water until mixture is thick, stirring continuously. 3. Pour into bowl or jar and cool before using.
Yield: 1 serving

VEGETABLE SALADS

Tossed Green Salad

Mustard greens
Swiss chard
Collards
Chicory
Dandelion greens
Chopped chives
Chopped dill
Tomatoes
Procedure: Wash greens well under running water. Dry on paper towels. Arrange in a salad bowl. Garnish with chives, dill, and tomato sections if desired. Add French dressing, tossing until leaves are coated but not soaked. Other suggested greens are head lettuce, water cress, spinach, parsley, beet tops or celery tops, Belgian endive, escarole, sorrel and romaine. (See Fig. 40–3.)

Cole Slaw

3 tablespoons evaporated milk,
    chilled icy cold
1 tablespoon vinegar
⅛ teaspoon salt
    Few grains of pepper
⅛ teaspoon dry mustard
½ cup shredded raw cabbage
Procedure: 1. Measure icy-cold evaporated milk into mixing bowl and whip with a rotary beater. Beat in vinegar, salt, pepper, and mustard. 2. Pour dressing over shredded cabbage in salad bowl. Serve.
Yield: 1 serving

Herbed Cottage Cheese Salad

½ pound dry cottage cheese
¼ pint sour cream
½ tablespoon minced fresh chives
½ tablespoon minced fresh dill
½ tablespoon minced fresh basil
½ tablespoon minced fresh tarragon
½ teaspoon grated onion
½ diced cucumber

½ diced green pepper
¼ teaspoon freshly ground pepper
½ teaspoon salt
Procedure: Combine all ingredients. Arrange on a bed of greens. Dressing is optional. Suggested greens: Italian parsley, leaf lettuce.
Yield: 2–4 servings

Fruit Salad

1 slice canned pineapple
1 banana
2 tablespoons cottage cheese
Lettuce
Fruit salad dressing
Procedure: 1. Put lettuce on salad plate. Arrange slice of pineapple on lettuce. Slice banana and place slices around the pineapple. 2. Fill hole in pineapple slice with cottage cheese. Pour dressing over cottage cheese and fruit.
Yield: 1 serving

FRUIT

Modern methods of transportation and refrigeration make it possible to have fresh fruits all year round. Consumption of citrus fruits has increased several times in the last century. Even so, clinical studies reveal that many children and adults do not get enough ascorbic acid, often due to lack of knowledge as to source and nutritive value rather than because of cost or availability.

COMPOSITION   Fruits provide energy value through the carbohydrate content, protective vitamins and minerals, and cellulose. They contain very little protein and are practically fat free. Two exceptions to the fat rule are avocados and olives, both of which contain appreciable amounts of fat. Fruits vary widely in their carbohydrate content. The caloric value of fresh and reconstructed dried fruit is comparatively low. Dried fruit, as such, and fruits canned or frozen with sugar have increased calories, depending upon the ingredients used in processing.

NUTRITIVE VALUE   All fresh fruits contribute some ascorbic acid, but the citrus fruits are outstanding as a source of this vitamin. For example, one medium size orange will furnish the normal adult daily requirement. Strawberries and cantaloupe are good sources, while apples and peaches are fair sources. However, a fair source can be taken in sufficient quantity to contribute substantially to the diet. (See Chapter 9, Vitamins, for comparative values of ascorbic acid in fruit.)

Most fruits also supply varying amounts of vitamins A and the B-complex. The yellow fruits, such as peaches, cantaloupe, apricots, and prunes, are good sources of the A vitamin, whereas plums and dried fruits (which have not been treated with sulfur dioxide) are the best sources of thiamin.

Fruits contribute appreciable amounts of the minerals iron and calcium. Among the fruits richest in iron are dried fruits of all kinds, apricots, peaches, bananas, grapes, and berries. Calcium is found in small amounts in the citrus fruits (the whole fruit containing double the amount contained in equal amount of the juice) strawberries, and dried figs. Sodium, magnesium, and potassium, which account for the alkaline ash of fruits when metabolized in the body, are also present in varying amounts in most fruits. This is an important therapeutic measure in conditions such as the presence of certain kidney stones and diseases. (See Chapter 32.)

Careful preparation, storage, and service are essential procedures to retain the maximum value of vitamins and minerals. There is some loss of nutritive value in the process of cooking, drying or canning, but losses are not so great as at one time supposed. The frozen foods compare favorably in vitamin content with fresh foods. See the section on Food Preservation in Chapter 14 for details of vitamin losses in processed foods. Bruising, cutting, and allowing fruit and fruit juice to be exposed to the air cause considerable loss of ascorbic acid.

DIGESTIBILITY   Ripe fruits are easily digested, the sugar content (glucose and fructose) being in the form ready for absorption. Emphasis should be on *ripeness* since the sugar in green fruits is not fully devel-oped and is, therefore, difficult to digest. For example, bananas are high in starch when green, but when ripe the starch changes to thoroughly digestible sugars. In some conditions fruits are tolerated better cooked than raw.

Fruits, like vegetables, contain indigestible cellulose which furnishes bulk necessary for good elimination. Of course, in certain conditions, cellulose is to be avoided. (See Chapters 23 and 24.) Prunes and figs are especially valuable as mild laxatives.

PLACE IN THE DAILY DIET   Fresh fruits are particularly important in the daily diet for the ascorbic acid content. Fruits offer appetite appeal through attractive color, texture, and flavor.

BUYERS' INFORMATION   When selecting fresh fruits, those with no disfigurements or just a few removable blemishes are picked, while the shriveled, wilted and decayed fruit are rejected.

Bananas are usually purchased by the hand (5 or 6 bananas attached to stem) and by weight, and the color indicates degree of ripeness. The skin of a fully ripened banana shows brown flecks and no green tips.

Among the citrus fruits the markings on the peel or the color of the peel do not influence the quality. Those with smooth thin skins usually indicate juice content. Those which are heavy for size are preferred.

The following list indicates the number of

FOOD	UNIT	APPROX. SERVINGS	FOOD	UNIT	APPROX. SERVINGS
Apples			Peaches		
Fresh	lb.	3	Fresh	lb.	4
Canned, sauce	16 oz.	4	Canned	29 oz.	7
Canned, slices	20 oz.	5	Frozen	12 oz.	3
Dried Slices	lb.	16	Dried	lb.	8
Apricots			Pears		
Fresh	lb.	6	Fresh	lb.	3
Canned	29 oz.	7	Canned	29 oz.	7
Dried	lb.	8	Dried	lb.	8
Bananas			Pineapple		
Fresh	lb.	3	Fresh	lb.	3
Blueberries			Canned, chunks	20 oz.	5
Fresh	pt.	6	Canned, juice	46 oz.	12
Canned	15 oz.	4	Frozen, chunks	lb.	4
Cherries			Plums		
Fresh	lb.	4	Fresh	lb.	4
Canned	20 oz.	5	Canned	29 oz.	7
Frozen	lb.	4	Prunes		
Cranberries			Dried	lb.	10
Fresh	lb.	12	Raspberries		
Canned	16 oz.	8	Fresh	pt.	4
Fruit Cocktail			Canned	16 oz.	4
Canned	16 oz.	4	Frozen	12 oz.	3
Grapefruit			Rhubarb		
Fresh	one	2	Fresh	lb.	4
Canned, segments	16 oz.	4	Frozen	lb.	4
Canned, juice	46 oz.	12	Raisins		
Oranges			Dried	lb.	10
Fresh, juice	½ doz. med.	4	Strawberries		
Canned, juice	46 oz.	12	Fresh	pt.	2
Frozen, juice	6 oz.	6	Frozen	12 oz.	3

servings obtainable from typical purchase units of fruits and juices. Cost per serving can easily be computed by dividing the cost of the fruit item by the number of servings.

PREPARATION SUGGESTIONS 1. To conserve nutrients, fruits are peeled thinly.

2. *Citrus fruits* are peeled before serving or the pulp is loosened from the skin. The membrane is usually removed.

3. *Juice* is extracted from fruit just before serving. Fruit juice should not be allowed to stand long after extraction or after opening the can. If fruit juices (fresh or canned) are stored in the refrigerator, they are put in covered containers to reduce oxidation and loss of vitamin C. Fresh fruit is chilled in the refrigerator before extraction of the juice.

4. *Citrus juice* is sprinkled over peeled fresh fruits which discolor quickly, such as apples, bananas, peaches, and pears, to reduce amounts of discoloration.

5. *Fruits* are cooked slowly and no longer than necessary. Fresh fruits are usually cooked without additional sugar. Lemon juice and grated lemon rind seem to enhance the flavor.

6. *Dried fruits* are softened and reconstituted in water and then cooked in the same water. They should be kept dry in a tightly covered container at room temperature, preferably not over 70°F. In warm, humid weather, store in the refrigerator.

7. *Canned fruits* are usually chilled before removal from the container. Choose the high-est quality for salads and "as is" desserts. Second quality may do for fruit puddings, or when wholeness and color are not so important.

8. *Frozen fruits* are thawed before serving. Thawed fruits cannot be refrozen.

Fruit Cup

1 small orange
2 tablespoons canned pineapple cubes
  Three fresh strawberries or cherries
  Sprig of fresh mint
  Procedure: 1. Peel orange and divide into sections. Arrange sections in glass dessert cup. Place pineapple cubes in center. Chill in refrigerator. 2. Just before serving, top with strawberries or cherries and mint sprig.
  Yield: 1 serving

Baked Banana

1 firm banana
½ tablespoon melted butter or margarine
  Salt
  Procedure: 1. Peel banana. Place in well greased baking dish. 2. Brush well with butter or margarine and sprinkle lightly with salt. 3. Bake in moderate oven (375° F.) 15 to 18 minutes, or until banana is tender—easily pierced with a fork. Serve hot as a vegetable, or as a dessert with cream, syrup or a hot fruit sauce. *Important: When browning is desired, place the baked banana under broiler flame for 1 to 2 minutes.*
  Yield: 1 serving

SUGGESTED ADDITIONAL READING REFERENCES

See Appendix General References, Part III.

Chapter 41
GROUP IV: BREAD–CEREAL GROUP

Cereal derives its name from the mythological Roman goddess of grains and harvest, Ceres, and furnishes the bulk of the world's food supply. Cereal grains are the source of many food items which are included in normal and modified dietaries. Examples are bread, crackers, cooked cereals, ready-to-eat cereals, macaroni, spaghetti, noodles, rice and barley or rice soup.

TYPES OF CEREAL GRAINS Each nationality has an attachment to certain grains, dependent upon the agricultural conditions of the country. (See Chapter 13, Geographic and Cultural Dietary Variations.) In this country, the cereal grains used most frequently include barley, corn, oats, rice, rye, and wheat. Manufacturers and bakers use cereal grains to produce commercial breads, crackers, biscuits, macaroni, spaghetti, and noodles.

CEREALS AND FLOUR

COMPOSITION   Cereal grains furnish an average of 75 per cent carbohydrate, 10 to 15 per cent protein, and 2 per cent fat. A cereal grain consists of three parts: the inner germ, which is protected by the endosperm, and the outer bran layer, as shown in Fig. 4–7, Chapter 4. The *germ* is the heart or embryo of the grain, which sprouts when the seed is planted. It is one of the best sources of thiamin and vitamin E, and it contains protein of high quality, other B-complex vitamins, fat, minerals (especially iron), and carbohydrate. The *endosperm* makes up by far the largest part of the grain, or approximately 85 per cent, and is chiefly carbohydrate, with some protein in the form of gluten. The *bran*, or outer layer, is chiefly cellulose plus the B-complex vitamins and minerals, especially iron.

NUTRITIVE VALUE   In Chapter 4 the nutritive value of carbohydrates from grain sources was discussed. Cereal and cereal products furnish approximately 50 per cent of the calories for the people of the world. Whole-grain cereals, or those enriched with vitamins and minerals or restored to whole-grain value, provide significant amounts of iron, thiamin, riboflavin, and niacin.

The protein of the germ is a complete protein, but since this is the portion of the grain that spoils first, it is removed in the refining process. The protein in the endosperm is not of such high quality, but contributes significantly to the total daily protein requirement. For example, when milk is used with or added to cereals and cereal products such as breakfast cereal and in bread making, the endosperm proteins complement the protein amino acids and become important and economical sources of protein.

The vitamin and mineral content of cereal grain products is dependent upon the amount of germ, endosperm, and bran present. Whole grains include the three parts, while highly refined cereal grain products contain only the endosperm. Enriched and restored cereal products and flours have had returned the vitamins and minerals that were removed

TABLE 41–1   INGREDIENTS OF FLOUR
(Required Ingredients per Pound of Flour)

	MINIMUM	MAXIMUM
Thiamin	2.0 mg.	2.5 mg.
Riboflavin	1.2 mg.	1.5 mg.
Niacin	16.0 mg.	20.0 mg.
Iron	13.0 mg.	16.5 mg.
	(Optional Ingredients per Pound of Flour)	
Calcium	500.0 mg.	650.0 mg.
Vitamin D	250 U.S.P. units	1000 U.S.P. units

TABLE 41–2   REVIEW OF ENRICHMENT REQUIREMENTS FOR CENTRAL GRAIN FOODS IN THE UNITED STATES*
(All Figures Represent Milligrams per Pound)

PRODUCT	THIAMINE (B₁) Min.	THIAMINE (B₁) Max.	RIBOFLAVIN (B₂) Min.	RIBOFLAVIN (B₂) Max.	NIACIN Min.	NIACIN Max.	IRON Min.	IRON Max.
Enriched bread or other *baked* products	1.1	1.8	0.7	1.6	10.0	15.0	8.0	12.5
Enriched flour[1]	2.0	2.5	1.2	1.5	16.0	20.0	13.0	16.5
Enriched farina	2.0	2.5	1.2	1.5	16.0	20.0	13.0	†
Enriched macaroni & noodle Products[2]	4.0	5.0	1.7	2.2	27.0	34.0	13.0	16.5
Enriched corn meals	2.0	3.0	1.2	1.8	16.0	24.0	13.0	26.0
Enriched corn grits[3]	2.0	3.0	1.2	1.8	16.0	24.0	13.0	26.0
Enriched Milled white rice[4]	2.0	4.0	1.2‡	2.4‡	16.0	32.0	13.0	26.0

* Courtesy of Hoffmann-La Roche Inc., Nutley, New Jersey.

† No maximum level established.

‡ The requirement for vitamin B₂ is optional pending further study and public hearings because of certain technical difficulties encountered in the application of this vitamin.

[1] In enriched self-rising flour, calcium is also required between limits of 500-1500 mg. per pound.

[2] Levels allow for 30–50% losses in kitchen procedure.

[3] Levels must not fall below 85% of minimum figures after a specific test described in the Federal Standards of Identity.

[4] The Standards state that the rice, after a rinsing test, must contain at least 85% of the minimum vitamin levels. The Governments of Puerto Rico and the Philippines also require this rinsing test. If the method of enrichment does not permit this rinsing requirement to be met, consumer size packages must bear the statement, "Do not rinse before or drain after cooking." Rice enriched by the Roche method will meet the rinsing test. The South Carolina law does not require a rinsing test on packages less than 50 pounds, as the rice in small packages is presumed to be sufficiently clean.

The maximum and minimum levels shown above for enriched bread, enriched flour, enriched farina, enriched macaroni, spaghetti and noodle products, enriched corn meal and corn grits and enriched rice are in accordance with Federal Standards of Identity or State laws. Act No. 183 of the Government of Puerto Rico requires the use of enriched flour for all products made wholly or in part of flour, including crackers, etc.

during the milling process, namely, thiamin, riboflavin, niacin and iron. See Table 41-1 for the minimum and maximum levels of flour enrichment and Table 41-2 for enrichment levels of other grain products.

DIGESTIBILITY   Cereals, cereal products and bread are easily and readily digested, making them an important food in normal and in many therapeutic diets.

USE IN THE DIET   Cereals have a wide use in the diet. They are economical foods that lend themselves to many uses. The food value is about the same for each type of grain whether cooked or ready-to-eat, and variety in the diet can be gained by alternation. Cereals are also incorporated into many foods or dishes, such as cakes, cookies and pastry. Cereal products, namely rice, noodles, macaroni and spaghetti, are frequently used as a basis for casserole dishes.

BUYERS' INFORMATION   There are four different types of wheat flour. (1) Whole wheat flour, graham flour, and entire wheat flour are synonymous. (2) Flour, white flour, wheat flour, and plain flour are synonymous terms, and the flour may be either bleached or unbleached. (3) Self-rising flour contains the correct proportions of leavening agent and salt. (4) Enriched flour is white flour with added vitamins and minerals. More recently, presifted flour has been added to the grocery shelf. However, the current trend is towards cooking and baking without sifted flour.[1] (To convert a recipe calling for

[1]Matthews, R. H., and Batcher, O. M.: Sifted versus Unsifted Flour, J. Home Ec. 55:123, 1963.

sifted to unsifted flour, spoon unsifted flour into a dry measuring cup, level it off, and remove 2 level tablespoons.)

CLASSIFICATION OF FLOURS   Flours are identified by the following classification: (1) Macaroni flours are made from durum wheats, high in protein content. (2) Bread flours are milled from blends of hard spring and hard winter wheats, bleached or unbleached. (3) General purpose or all-purpose family flours are milled from hard wheats (northern areas) and soft wheats (southern areas). (4) Pastry flours are milled usually from soft wheats. (5) Cake flours are milled from soft wheats. Other flours are buckwheat flour, corn flour (a by-product of making corn meal), cottonseed flour, lima bean flour, peanut flour, potato flour, soya flour (full-fat and low-fat), rice flour, and rye flour.

CEREAL GRAIN PRODUCTS   A variety of products are manufactured and processed from cereal grains. Corn meal, cornstarch, and hominy (pearl, lye, granulated, and grits) are processed from corn. Oatmeal or rolled oats, both the regular and quick-cooking, are processed from oats. The varieties of rice include coated (white) or uncoated (brown) long, medium and short grains, rice bran, rice polish, and wild rice. Soya grits are obtained from the soybean plant. Pearl and quick-cooking are the varieties of tapioca. Crushed wheat, cracked wheat, farina, macaroni and noodle products are processed from wheat. Table 41-2 reviews the enrichment requirements for cereal grain foods in the United States.

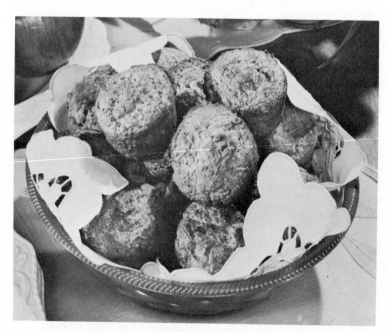

Figure 41-1   Bran muffins. (Courtesy of Kellogg Company.)

COOKERY SUGGESTIONS   1. Cereals are cooked to soften the fiber of the grain and to burst the starch granules, which aids in the digestion of the carbohydrate besides improving the flavor and appearance.

2. When cereals are used as a thickening agent, the cooking process is prolonged enough to allow the starch granules to burst.

3. To prevent lumping, fine flours and meals are mixed with cold water into a thin paste before stirring into a heated liquid.

4. Coarse cereals are poured slowly into boiling water and the stirring is continuous.

5. Cereals are cooked either in a double boiler for a longer period or over direct heat for a shorter period.

6. The usual proportions are:

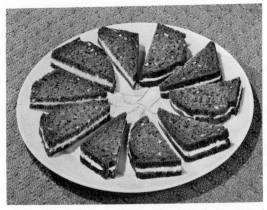

Figure 41–2   Date-nut bread with cream cheese sandwiches. (Courtesy of Kraft Foods Company.)

⅓ cup rolled oats to 1 cup liquid
2½ tablespoons corn meal to 1 cup liquid
2½ tablespoons cream of wheat to 1 cup liquid
2½ tablespoons farina to 1 cup liquid
¼ cup rice to 1 cup liquid
¼ cup whole wheat cereal to 1 cup liquid

Oatmeal

⅓ cup rolled oats
1 cup boiling water
¼ teaspoon salt

Procedure: 1. Measure boiling water into upper part of double boiler and place over heat. Stir in slowly the rolled oats and cook 3 minutes, stirring continuously. *2.* Add salt. Remove from heat and replace over lower part of double boiler. Place double boiler over heat so water in lower part boils gently. Cover and let cereal cook for an hour or more. (If the *quick-cooking* variety of rolled oats is used, the cooking time is lessened, and the cereal is cooked over direct heat for a few minutes.) *3.* Serve hot in warmed cereal dish.

Yield: 1 serving

Strained Oatmeal

Strain cooked oatmeal through sieve into warmed cereal dish and serve hot.

Oatmeal Gruel

2 tablespoons rolled oats
1 cup boiling water
¼ teaspoon salt

Procedure: 1. Measure boiling water into upper part of double boiler and place directly over heat. Stir in slowly the rolled oats and cook 3 minutes, stirring continuously. *2.* Add salt and remove from heat. Replace over lower part of double boiler. Place double boiler over heat so water in lower part boils gently. Cover and let cereal cook for 1½ hours. *3.* Strain through sieve into warmed cereal dish. Serve hot.

Yield: 1 serving

See Chapter 38 for Macaroni and Cheese.

BREAD

Down through the ages bread has held its place as man's most precious food, the "staff of life." Loaves of bread were made as far back as the Stone Age. By the time of the Pharaohs, bread making had become big business. Every village had its public ovens and every man of wealth his private baker. During the twelfth century in England, class distinction was based on breads. The bakers who made rye bread for the poor were called "brown bakers," while those who made white bread for the wealthy were known as "white bakers." Every country developed its own specialties. For example, Germany is associated with pumpernickel, which earned its name in the seventeenth century when coarse peasant loaves were nicknamed "pompernickel" ("lout" or "booby"), which eventually became pumpernickel. In France, a three-foot-long flûte of bread is seen in every woman's market bag. In Italy, crisp breadsticks and festive panetone are favorites; in Sweden, the delicate limpa; in Scotland, the honest scone. In America, we have inherited all these and have developed some characteristic varieties, too. (See Fig. 13–1.)

Milk Toast

2 slices enriched bread
1 cup milk
1 tablespoon butter or margarine
¼ teaspoon sugar
  Salt

Procedure: 1. Heat milk in upper part of double boiler. *2.* Toast bread in automatic toaster or on broiler. Cut into fourths. *3.* Add sugar and butter to milk and pour the hot milk into serving pitcher. Put toast pieces in soup bowl and place on tray, accompanied by pitcher of hot milk. Serve immediately.

Yield: 1 serving

Baking Powder Biscuits

1 cup flour
2 teaspoons baking powder
1/2 teaspoon salt
2 tablespoons shortening
1 egg
1/3 cup milk, approximately

Procedure: 1. Measure and sift dry ingredients into a mixing bowl. 2. Cut in shortening using either two knives or pastry blender. 3. Beat egg and milk and stir into mixture using knife. Toss the soft dough on floured board, and pat to 3/4 inch thickness. Cut into 2-inch squares or shape with biscuit cutter. Arrange on buttered cooky sheet and bake about 12 minutes in hot oven (450° F.). Serve immediately.

Yield: 6 biscuits

Bran Muffins

1/2 cup bran
3/8 cup milk
1/2 egg
2 tablespoons soft shortening
1/2 cup sifted flour
1 1/4 teaspoons baking powder
1/4 teaspoon salt
2 tablespoons sugar

Procedure: 1. Combine bran and milk in a mixing bowl; let stand until most of moisture is taken up. Add egg and shortening and beat well. 2. Measure and sift flour, baking powder, salt and sugar; add to first mixture, stirring only until combined. 3. Drop spoonfuls of batter into buttered muffin tins and bake 25 minutes in hot oven (400° F.). Serve immediately.

Yield: 5 to 6 muffins (Fig. 41-1)

Egg Salad Sandwich

1 finely chopped, hard-cooked egg
1 tablespoon minced ripe olives
1/4 teaspoon salt
　Dash pepper
1/2 teaspoon prepared mustard
1 tablespoon mayonnaise

Procedure: 1. Mix the ingredients together. 2. Lightly butter 2 slices enriched white or whole wheat bread. 3. Spread 1 slice with the filling and top with the second slice. 4. Toast under broiler flame or in electric sandwich toaster and trim edges. Cut into 2, 3 or 4 triangles.

Yield: 1 sandwich

Date-Nut Bread with Cream Cheese
(See Fig. 41-2)

2 slices date-nut bread
　Cream cheese
　Butter or fortified margarine

Procedure: 1. Butter lightly 2 slices date-nut bread. 2. Spread generously with cream cheese and put slices together. 3. Cut into 2, 3 or 4 triangles (Fig. 41-2). 4. Serve with celery curls and radishes.

Yield: 1 sandwich

SUGGESTED ADDITIONAL READING REFERENCES

See Appendix General References, Part III.

Chapter 42
SEASONINGS: CONDIMENTS, SPICES, HERBS AND OTHER FLAVORINGS

Seasoning is frequently termed the soul of cooking. The greater the skill in the art of seasoning, the better the cook. While seasonings do not add food value to the diet, they often make a dish which has been unacceptable a desirable food. The main purpose in seasoning foods is to make the product more palatable. Seasonings can do this in several ways: (1) by intensifying the basic flavor of a food; (2) by blending flavors into a more pleasing composite flavor; (3) by changing a flavor or combination of basic flavors to something quite different. Use imagination when adding that extra salt and pepper to cooked vegetables. Experiment by adding garlic or onion salt, monosodium glutamate, or some herbs when the diet prescription permits. Season and serve with a flair. Even the sodium-restricted diets can be made palatable by using allowed spices, herbs, and other seasonings. In general, seasonings include condiments, spices, herbs and other flavorings. It is difficult to draw a line on what should be grouped under each term. They all overlap, and can be grouped together roughly as "seasoning."

CONDIMENTS

Salt (sodium chloride) is by far the most commonly used seasoning and is also an essential body mineral. When used in moderation, it gives zest to and brings out the natural flavor of otherwise tasteless food. However, care should be taken not to use excess amounts which mask the natural food flavor and blunt the appetite.

Pepper ranks next to salt as the most common seasoning. It comes in two forms, white and black. Both come from the dried berries of the same tropical vine. The difference is in processing. For white pepper, the outer dark surface of the tiny berries is rubbed off and only the inside is used. White pepper is chiefly valued for its light hue. In creamy sauces, pale soups and such it leaves none of the dark specks that black pepper does. Also, it is somewhat less pungent than black pepper.

Cayenne pepper and *paprika* are members of the pepper family. Cayenne is a pungent chili pepper used in sauces, meat and egg dishes, and seafood. Paprika is a mild member of the pepper family, usually sprinkled on or used to add color and flavor to canapes, gravies, salad dressings, certain vegetables, fish, and meats.

SPICES

Among the more common spices used to add flavor are cinnamon, ginger, cloves, allspice (resembles blend of cinnamon, nutmeg, and cloves), mace (flavor similar to nutmeg), and aniseed (licorice-like flavor). Table 42–1 lists the more common spices with their sources and uses.

MISCELLANEOUS SEASONINGS

Among the miscellaneous seasonings are such favorites as onion salt, celery salt, curry powder, bay leaf, rosemary, whole cloves, and poultry seasoning (fragrant herbs combined with sage).

MONOSODIUM GLUTAMATE

Monosodium glutamate intensifies taste rather than adding some of its own. It is a fine white powder derived from vegetable protein. Orientals have used it for centuries; in fact it is sometimes called "Chinese powder."

Use monosodium glutamate with chicken and poultry; it probably does more for chicken than for any other food. It also is effective with meat (particularly in overcoming the astringency of beef liver), fish, stews, gravies, soups, vegetables (blots out raw starch taste of potatoes). Condensed and dried soups probably would be unmarketable without it. Add about the same amount of monosodium glutamate as you do salt; if a recipe calls for a half teaspoon salt, use an equal measure of this seasoning. Tests show that meats, poultry, and vegetables frozen with monosodium glutamate retain quality better than when frozen without it. As yet, however, there is nothing to prove that this seasoning benefits fruits or desserts.

HERBS

The nurse wondering what herbs to use might start out with the ones shown in Figure 42–1. Herbs do wonders for flavoring and seasoning foods. Go slowly at first and use only a small amount. For best results use a teaspoonful of fresh herbs to a quarter teaspoonful of the dried varieties.

Oregano, imported from Italy and Mexico, is good in or on green salads, tomatoes, cheese dishes, lasagna, omelets, spaghetti sauces, lamb, pork, beef, beef soup, stews and meat balls.

Marjoram is of the mint family from France and Chile, and should be used sparingly in or on vegetables such as carrots, greens, asparagus, lima beans, and squash; cheese, egg, and chicken dishes; roast lamb, meat pies, hash, stews, stuffings, fish or vegetable sauces.

Tarragon is a leaf with anise flavor, good added to steaks, chops, chicken, fish, vinegar, French dressing, green salad, duckling, egg dishes, sauces, tomato dishes, vegetables such as beets, greens, peas, and mushrooms.

Dill is good added to potato dishes (salad or boiled), cream or cottage cheese mixtures (canapés), fish, fish sauces, gravies, pickles, cucumbers, lamb, vegetable salads, spaghetti, and tomato dishes.

Basil is an herb from west Europe, which is good cooked with or sprinkled on tomato dishes (especially good), eggplant, salads, green beans, peas, potatoes, squash, meats (especially ham and lamb chops), stew, sausage, eggs, poultry, sauces, salad dressings, soups, and spaghetti.

Thyme is especially good in chowder, stuffings, tomatoes, eggplant, carrots, peas, stews, fish and cheese dishes, on breads, veal, and pork. *Sage* is less subtle and may be substituted for thyme.

TABLE 42–1   SPICES—SOURCES AND USES*

NAME	DESCRIPTION AND SOURCE	USES
Allspice (spice)	Dried berry of the pimento tree, grown in West Indies. Named Allspice because flavor resembles blend of cinnamon, nutmeg and cloves.	Whole, for pickling, spicing meats, seasoning gravies and boiling fish. Ground, for boiled foods, cakes, puddings and relishes.
Caraway seed (spice)	Dried seeds of plant grown in Northern Europe, notably Holland.	In rye bread, sauerkraut, new cabbage, on pork, liver and kidney before cooking. In cream and other mild cheeses.
Cayenne (spice)	Ground small hot red pepper. Grown in Africa.	With meats, fish, sauces and egg dishes.
Celery Seed (spice)	A small, dried, ripe, seed-like fruit of celery. Grown in many countries, including France, India, Holland, and the United States.	For fish, potato salad, tomato dishes and tomato soup. Used in pickling and salad dressing. Excellent for Irish stews. Gives variety to hamburgers.
Chili powder (blend)	Ground chili peppers (grown in Mexico, California, Carolinas and Louisiana) and blended spices. Two varieties: mild or hot.	For such Mexican dishes as chili con carne. Good in shell fish and oyster cocktail sauces; for boiled and scrambled eggs, gravy and stew seasoning, canned corn.
Cinnamon (spice)	Dried aromatic bark of cinnamon tree. Major source, Ceylon.	Whole, pieces of bark, in pickling, preserving and stewed fruits. Ground, in baked goods and to season mincemeat.
Cloves (spice)	Nail-shaped flower bud of the clove tree. Imported from Dutch East Indies, Madagascar and Zanzibar.	Whole, for roast ham garnish, pickling, preserving, spiced syrups and drinks. Ground, for baked goods, puddings and stews.
Curry powder (blend)	Blend of many spices, originating in India.	For curried meat, fish, eggs and chicken. Curry sauce. French dressing, scalloped tomatoes, and clam and fish chowder.
Ginger (spice)	Root stalk of plant grown mainly in Jamaica, West Africa, India and the Orient.	Ground, in cakes, puddings, pumpkin pie and cookies. Whole, *fresh* root, is used in many oriental dishes. Many canned fruits benefit by a dash of ginger, especially canned pears. Used in preserved, candied or crystallized, and dried forms.
Mace (spice)	Part of nutmeg between shell and outer husk, orange-red in color; flavor resembles nutmeg. From East and West Indies.	Blades used in pickling, preserving and fish sauces. Used ground in pound cake, doughnuts, yellow dishes, chocolate dishes and oyster stew. Use sparingly.
Mustard (spice)	Seed of mustard plant grown in England and other areas.	Dry ground mustard used as flavoring for sauces and gravy. Prepared mustard, blended with other spices and vinegar, used in salad dressing, with ham, frankfurters and cheese.
Nutmeg (spice)	Kernel of a fruit of that name, grown in Dutch East Indies and British West Indies.	Whole, to be grated as needed. Ground, used in baked goods, sauces and puddings. Good sprinkled over certain vegetables, such as cauliflower. Merges well with spinach. Topping for eggnog and custards. Favorite spice for doughnuts.
Paprika (spice)	Ground sweet red pepper grown chiefly in Spain and Hungary.	For color and mild flavor in, and sprinkled on, fish, shell fish and salad dressing. Used lavishly as a garnish, also served with sweet corn on the cob. Mixed with butter to make paprika butter.
Pepper (spice)	Most generally used of all spices. A small round berry picked before ripe; grows on a climbing vine. Grown in Dutch East Indies and India. White pepper is the mature berry with hull removed.	Whole, (black and white) used in pickling, soups and meats. Ground, (black and white) used in meat sauces, gravies, vegetables and egg dishes.
Poppy seed (spice)	Tiny seeds of poppy plant imported from Holland. About 900,000 seed to the pound.	Whole, as topping for breads, rolls, and cookies. Oil used in salad dressings and margarine.

* Adapted from U.S. Department of the Navy publication, Navsanda P-277.

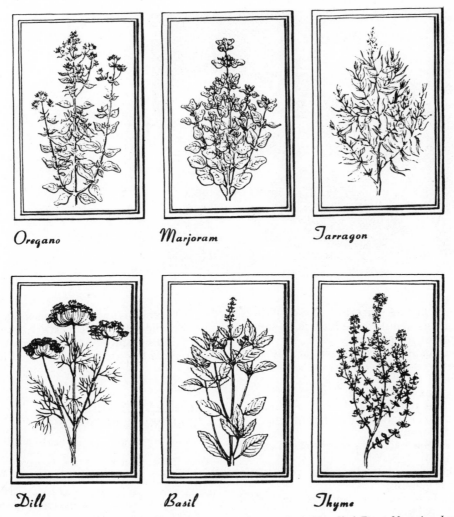

Oregano   *Marjoram*   *Tarragon*

Dill   *Basil*   *Thyme*

Figure 42-1   Some of the more popular herbs used in adding flavor to food. (New York Times Magazine, June 5, 1955.)

FRESH PLANT FLAVORINGS

For fresh flavoring, onions, garlic clove, parsley, shallots, mint, sage, dill, and chives are among the more staple and commonly used plants.

DESSERT FLAVORINGS

Flavorings are most often thought of in connection with desserts, cakes, cookies, or foods that are enhanced by the addition of extracts to lend a pleasing flavor. Vanilla, almond, and fruit extracts are the ones most frequently used. Do not limit the use to one or two flavors. Try new ones, or combine flavors such as vanilla and almond, lemon and orange. Coffee and chocolate are also used as flavorings.

BUYING AND STORAGE INFORMATION

When buying a spice or herb, make a note of the purchase date on the label and six months later discard the product if it has not been used. For by that time it will have lost its true bouquet and taste. Buy in small amounts. Keep away from heat (do not put a spice shelf over a stove), as heat promotes drying and staling. So does air; hence, a tightly covered container is a must. Shaker tops are approved provided openings are closed after the spice has been used. Prepared mustard, incidentally, best retains flavor if refrigerated.

No matter what precautions are taken, spices start to lose savor (through evaporation of volatile oils) as soon as they are ground.

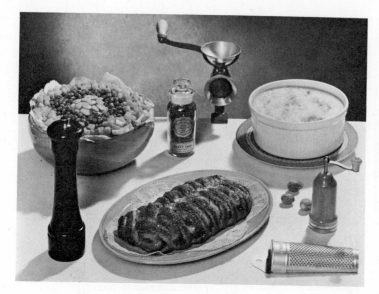

Figure 42–2   Grinding spices at home insures full aroma and flavor. The pepper mill at left is indispensable with salads and other dishes. The grinder at rear crushes poppy seeds for cake fillings. The grater and grinder at lower right are for nutmegs; fresh-ground nutmeg is especially delicious on custard. (New York Times Magazine, June 5, 1955.)

COOKERY SUGGESTIONS   1. Seasonings and flavorings should be added to enhance, not overpower food flavors.

2. When using dried herbs for the first time, start by adding ¼ teaspoonful to a dish that makes 4 servings.

Add to food as follows:

Stew and soups: Add during last hour.
Meat loaf, hamburger, and stuffing: Add when mixing.
Roasts: Sprinkle over roast toward end of roasting.
Steaks and chops: Sprinkle over while meat is cooking.
Vegetables, sauces, and gravies: Add while cooking.

Vegetable juices, salad dressings, cheese: Add and refrigerate mixture a few hours.

3. Grinding spices or herbs for immediate use insures full aroma and flavor (Fig. 42–2).

SUGGESTED ADDITIONAL READING REFERENCES

Good seasoning is always in good taste. Modern Hospital, *100*:136, 1963.

Savory Herbs. Culture and Use. Farmers' Bulletin No. 1977, U.S. Department of Agriculture, Washington 25, D.C.

Wright, E. G., Everson, A. M., and Johnson, D.: Do spices increase acceptability of therapeutic diets?, J. Am. Dietet. A., *33*:895, 1957.

Chapter 43
THERAPEUTIC DIET RECIPES AND COOKERY SUGGESTIONS

Patients with modifications of their usual dietaries often find it difficult to achieve variety and interest in menus. Food preparation becomes a real problem. Recipes in this chapter are presented to suggest ways in which foods included in the diet prescription can be combined in recipes for everyday meals.

LOW CALORIE, LOW FAT RECIPES

Following are some recipes low in calories and low in fat. These recipes can frequently be fitted into a diet prescription to give variety and interest to the menu. Nutrition as well as calorie value of foods must be considered. Those foods which contain little or no value other than fat or carbohydrate (foods such as fats, oils, sugar and flour) are limited or omitted. Lean meat, poultry, non-oily fish, eggs, skim milk, cottage cheese, low calorie fruits and vegetables are the basic foods used. The calories are determined by the ingredients used.

ARTIFICIAL NON-NUTRITIVE SWEET-ENERS   Foods prepared without the calories or carbohydrate of sugar can be made palatable by substituting saccharin, which is a widely used sweetening agent.

Saccharin may be added to beverages and foods that do not require cooking. Cooking processes often produce a bitter taste and saccharin should be added toward the end of the cooking cycle, or immediately after it. Saccharin products are available in four forms: a soluble powder pressed into a tablet; a soluble granule; an insoluble powder which is combined with a dispersing agent into a soluble tablet; and a liquid solution. Each tablet or granule is roughly equal to 1 teaspoonful of sugar in sweetening power. The sweetening power of ¼ grain of saccharin is equivalent to about 1 teaspoonful of sugar. A bitter aftertaste may develop if used in excess.

BEVERAGES   Coffee and tea, iced or hot, have no calorie value. A non-calorie sweetener may be used if desired. Milk or cream used in beverages must be counted in the day's total calorie intake.

Cocoa

¼ grain saccharin
1 teaspoon cocoa
  Few grains salt
¼ cup boiling water
1 cup milk (skim may be used to reduce fat and calories still further)
¼ teaspoon vanilla

Procedure: 1. Mash saccharin and dissolve in 2 tablespoons of milk. 2. Combine cocoa, salt and water in saucepan, bring to boil and cook 2 minutes, stirring constantly. 3. Add milk and dissolved saccharin; heat in the top of double boiler over simmering water. 4. Beat with rotary beater before serving hot. 5. Add vanilla.

Yield: 1 serving (80 kcalories using skim milk)

Lemonade

¼ grain saccharin
2 tablespoons lemon juice
  Water
  Ice, as desired

Procedure: 1. Place saccharin, or solution, in lemon juice. 2. Add 6 ounces (or enough to make 8 ounces) of water. 3. Add ice, as desired. Garnish with a slice of lemon.
Yield: 1 serving (about 5 kcalories)

SOUPS   Clear broth made from meat stock with fat removed, canned bouillon or consommé, or bouillon cubes have little or no food value. These may be eaten hot or in jellied form.

Tomato juice or low calorie vegetables (Chapter 28, Diabetic Exchange Lists) may be used in the broth to make a vegetable soup without adding appreciably to the calorie value. Instead of clear broth, skim milk may be used as a base to make a vegetable-milk soup for variety in the menu without adding appreciable amounts of calories.

MEAT, POULTRY, AND MEAT ALTER-NATES   Meats cooked for the family can be used for those restricting their intake of calories if the fat is trimmed off or not eaten. Pork, ham, sausage, duck and goose contain more fat than meats such as beef, lamb and poultry. The latter meats may be preferred when a choice is possible. Chicken and turkey are comparatively low in fat. Uncreamed cottage cheese can be a low calorie meat alternate. Other cheeses can be used for flavoring in the preparation of certain dishes.

Broiling, boiling and roasting are methods of meat cookery preferred by individuals to restrict calories. Cooking on a rack allows the fat to drain off. Excess fat may be trimmed away from a roast (oven or pot) after it has been sliced and before it is served. Pan-broiled meats should not be allowed to cook in accumulated fat, but the fat should be poured off while cooking. See Chapter 39, cuts of meat, buying information and methods of preparation.

Pan-Broiled Liver

4 thin slices liver (½ pound)
2 teaspoons shortening or bacon fat
½ teaspoon salt
  Few grains pepper

Procedure: 1. Place liver in pan and cover with boiling water. Cover and let stand for 12 minutes. Drain. 2. Melt shortening in skillet. 3. Season liver and cook for 1 minute on each side.
Yield: 4 servings

Stuffed Peppers

4 small green peppers
¾ cup lean ground beef
1½ teaspoons shortening
2 tablespoons finely cut onion
3 tablespoons finely cut celery
⅓ cup bread crumbs
⅓ cup drained, canned tomatoes
½ teaspoon salt

Procedure: 1. Remove top and seeds from green peppers. 2. Cover with boiling water; cook for 5 minutes. Drain.

3. Brown meat in hot shortening. Add onion, celery, crumbs, tomatoes, and salt. 4. Stuff peppers with meat mixture. 5. Stand peppers upright in baking dish containing 1 inch of hot water. Cover. 6. Bake in moderately slow (350° F.) oven for 1 hour.

Yield: 4 servings

Cheese Soufflé

1 tablespoon shortening
2 tablespoons flour
1/2 teaspoon salt
  Few grains pepper
2/3 cup skim milk
2/3 cup grated American cheese, or 2 ounces diced, processed variety
2 eggs, separated

Procedure: 1. Melt shortening. Stir in flour, salt, and pepper. Stir in milk and cook over low heat until mixture thickens. 2. Add grated cheese and stir until melted. 3. Stir into slightly beaten egg yolks. 4. Fold in stiffly beaten egg whites. 5. Pour into a quart, ungreased baking dish or individual ramekins. Set into pan of hot water. 6. Bake in slow (325° F.) oven for 1 hour, or until knife, when inserted in center, comes out clean. Serve at once.

Yield: 4 servings

Variations: For Tuna Fish Soufflé substitute 2/3 cup flaked or grated tuna fish for the cheese.

For Tongue Soufflé substitute 1/2 cup ground or finely cut cooked or canned, smoked tongue for the cheese.

For Vegetable Soufflé substitute 1/2 cup strained, cooked or canned, carrots, spinach or asparagus for the cheese.

FISH can be classified as to fat content. (See Tables 39–4, 39–5.) The high fat fish (higher in calories) are bonito, mackerel, salmon, herring, shad, and white-fish. Fish low in fat content (lower in calories) are cod, bass, flounder, haddock, pike, brook trout and shellfish such as lobster, crabs, clams, shrimp and oysters.

Poaching, broiling and baking are the best methods of preparation when limiting calories. See Chapter 39 for methods of preparation. Fish can also be used in gelatin salads, or in aspic, which need no dressing.

Tuna fish is available in canned form, free from oil, and sold as Dietetic Tuna, low in calories and suitable for salads or to eat as such.

Jellied Fish Salad

1 tablespoon unflavored gelatin
1/4 cup cold water
1/2 teaspoon salt
1/2 teaspoon celery seed
1/4 cup vinegar
1/4 cup water
2 eggs, beaten
2 cups flaked cooked or canned fish without oil

Procedure: 1. Soften gelatin on top of 1/4 cup cold water. 2. Add seasonings, vinegar, and 1/4 water to eggs. 3. Cook over boiling water until thickened, stirring constantly. 4. Add gelatin and stir until it is dissolved. 5. Add fish and mix thoroughly. 6. Pour into individual molds or large ring mold and chill.

Yield: 4 servings

Tomato Aspic Seafood Salad

Aspic

2 tablespoons plain gelatin
1/2 cup cold water
2 1/2 cups tomato juice
1 teaspoon chopped onion
1/2 teaspoon salt
1/2 teaspoon celery salt
1 Sucaryl tablet
2 tablespoons vinegar

Salad

1 cup Dietetic Tuna Fish, flaked
1 cup diced celery
1 cup diced 3% vegetable (Appendix Table 4)
1/4 teaspoon salt
  Dash of white pepper
1/4 cup low calorie salad dressing
1 tablespoon lemon juice
  Grapefruit sections
  Water cress

Procedure for Aspic: 1. Soften gelatin in cold water. 2. Combine tomato juice, onion, salt, celery salt, Sucaryl, and vinegar in saucepan; bring to boiling point. Add to gelatin, stirring until gelatin is dissolved. 3. Strain mixture and pour into a 1-quart ring mold. Chill until firm.

Procedure for Salad: 1. Lightly toss together tuna fish, celery, 3% vegetable, salt and pepper. 2. Combine salad dressing and lemon juice. Add to tuna fish mixture and blend carefully. 3. Unmold aspic and fill center of ring with tuna fish salad. 4. Arrange garnish of grapefruit sections and water cress around outer edge of aspic ring.

Yield: 6 servings

Variations: Lobster, shrimp or chicken may be substituted for tuna.

EGGS are frequently served poached, soft or hard cooked to limit calories. Following is a recipe for scrambled eggs, low in calories, to add variety to the diet.

Scrambled Eggs

4 eggs
1/4 cup skim milk
1/4 teaspoon salt
  Few grains pepper

Procedure: 1. Beat eggs slightly in top of double boiler. 2. Stir in milk, salt and pepper. 3. Cook over boiling water, stirring constantly until eggs are firm – about 5 minutes. Serve at once.

Yield: 4 servings

VEGETABLES The Diabetic Exchanges in Chapter 28 group vegetables and fruits according to their calorie value. These exchanges are a good guide to selection of vegetables and fruits for their calorie value. Care must be taken in the preparation in order to preserve flavor and nutritive value. Since butter, oil, sauces or margarine may be omitted or limited when restricting calories, special care is given to seasoning. (See Chapter 42, Seasonings.) Directions for cooking vegetables are given in Chapter 40.

Harvard Beets

1 cup cooked or canned beets
2½ Saccharin tablets
2 tablespoons water
½ tablespoon cornstarch
¼ teaspoon salt
2 tablespoons cider vinegar

Procedure: 1. Dice or slice beets. 2. Mash Sucaryl tablets and dissolve in water. 3. Combine cornstarch, salt, vinegar and dissolved Sucaryl tablets; cook over low heat until thickened, stirring constantly. 4. Add beets, heat until beets are hot. Serve at once.

Yield: 2 servings

Savory Stewed Tomatoes

1 no. 2 can (1 lb., 4 oz.) or 2¼ cups fresh cooked tomatoes
1 tablespoon minced green pepper
2 tablespoons grated onion
4 whole cloves
½ teaspoon curry powder
  Salt and pepper

Procedure: 1. Combine all ingredients. 2. Simmer 5 minutes.

Yield: 5 servings (½ cup equals 1 vegetable serving)

SALADS made with salad greens, tomato, cottage cheese, fruit, and gelatin base add an attractive appearance, bulk, and valuable nutrients to a low calorie or low fat dietary regimen.

SALAD DRESSINGS made with oil may contribute to excessive calorie intake of overweight individuals. Lemon juice, vinegar, a dab of uncreamed cottage cheese, or a little yogurt can be used often in place of a regular salad dressing to limit calories. An oilless dressing such as is given here is flavorful and enjoyed by many.

Low Calorie Salad Dressing

½ teaspoon gelatin
1 tablespoon water
¼ cup boiling water
½ teaspoon Sucaryl solution, or 3 saccharin tablets (¼ grain each)
1 teaspoon salt
1 teaspoon grated lemon rind
½ cup lemon juice
¼ teaspoon onion juice
¼ teaspoon paprika
⅛ teaspoon curry powder
1 pinch black pepper
1 pinch cayenne pepper

Procedure: 1. In a half-pint jar soften gelatin in the tablespoon of water. 2. Add boiling water, sweetening and salt. Stir till dissolved. 3. Add remaining ingredients. Shake well. Chill.

Yield: About 1 cup

Cole Slaw

⅓ cup shredded cabbage
2 tablespoons low calorie salad dressing
¼ cup shredded carrot
1 tablespoon finely cut celery
1 teaspoon finely cut parsley

Procedure: 1. Combine all ingredients well. 2. Chill before serving.

Yield: 1 serving

DESSERTS that are low in calories are fresh fruits or fruits cooked, frozen or canned without the addition of sugar. Variety can be had by using gelatin and noncalorie sweeteners to prepare jellied desserts. Skim milk, in fresh or dried form, can also be used to prepare simple puddings and custards. Following are a few recipe suggestions when calories are limited. Left-over servings can be refrigerated and varied by serving with different fruits or fruit juices as sauces.

Fruit Gelatin

1 envelope unflavored gelatin
¼ cup water
5 saccharin tablets
2 cups unsweetened fruit juice
2 tablespoons lemon juice

Procedure: 1. Soften gelatin in cold water for 5 minutes. 2. Mash saccharin tablets and dissolve in 1 tablespoon of the fruit juice. (Use any unsweetened fruit juice suitable for a fruit gelatin.) 3. Add to remaining fruit and lemon juices. 4. Dissolve gelatin over hot water; add to fruit juices; blend. 5. Pour into individual molds. Chill.

Yield: 4 servings

Coffee-Almond Whip

1 teaspoon unflavored gelatin
2 tablespoons cold water
3 saccharin tablets (¼ grain each)
½ cup hot coffee
⅛ teaspoon nutmeg
¼ teaspoon almond extract

Procedure: 1. Sprinkle gelatin over cold water; let stand 5 minutes. Add boiling coffee; stir until dissolved. 2. Add remaining ingredients. Chill until mixture begins to set. 3. Beat until fluffy with rotary beater. Chill until firm.

Yield: 1 serving

Baked Custard

3 saccharin tablets (¼ grain each)
1 tablespoon warm water
1 egg, well beaten
¾ cup milk or skim milk
½ teaspoon vanilla extract
  Nutmeg

Procedure: 1. Dissolve saccharin tablets in water; combine with remaining ingredients, except nutmeg. 2. Pour into large custard cup; sprinkle with nutmeg. 3. Place in shallow pan of hot water. Bake in moderate (350° F.) oven for 50 minutes, or until knife inserted near edge of custard comes out clean.

Yield: 1 serving

FAT-CONTROLLED RECIPES

In the treatment of atherosclerosis, the current trend is to modify the fat, calories and/or carbohydrate intake. Following are a few recipes using polyunsaturated vegetable oils such as corn oil, safflower oil, and cottonseed oil.[1] A number of good recipe books have been put out by the various manufacturers of vegetable oils and special shortenings. These books are generally available without charge.

Oven Barbecued Chicken

1 frying chicken (2½ to 3 pounds), cut into serving pieces
¼ cup water
¾ cup vinegar
3 tablespoons vegetable oil
½ cup chili sauce or catsup
3 tablespoons Worcestershire sauce
1 teaspoon dry mustard
1½ teaspoons salt
½ teaspoon pepper
2 tablespoons chopped onion (optional)

Procedure: Preheat oven to 350° (moderate). Combine all ingredients except chicken in saucepan, place over heat, and simmer for 5 to 10 minutes. Place chicken, skin side up, in large baking pan. Pour half of the barbecue sauce over chicken and bake, uncovered, for about 45-60 minutes. Baste with remaining barbecue sauce every 15 minutes during cooking. Dieter should remove skin from chicken.

Yield: 4 servings
(1 serving = 2 teaspoons oil)

Fish Skillet

1 pound fish fillets or steaks
3 tablespoons vegetable oil
1 onion, chopped
3 tablespoons chopped green pepper (optional)
2 tablespoons chopped parsley
2 medium tomatoes, cut in pieces, or
    1 8-ounce can stewed tomatoes
½ cup water or tomato juice
½ teaspoon salt
½ teaspoon basil or oregano (optional)
    Dash pepper

Procedure: If fish is frozen, thaw it enough to separate pieces. Heat oil in skillet. Add chopped onion, green pepper, and parsley, and cook until onion is golden, about 5 minutes. Add tomatoes, water or tomato juice, and seasonings; cook until tomatoes are soft. Add fish. Cover and cook gently about 10 minutes, or until fish is done.

Yield: 4 servings
(1 serving = 2 teaspoons oil)

Muffins

2 cups sifted all-purpose flour
½ teaspoon salt
2½ teaspoons baking powder
3 tablespoons sugar
1 egg
1 cup skim milk
¼ cup vegetable oil or special margarine or shortening, melted

Procedure: Preheat oven to 400-425° (hot). Grease muffin tin lightly with oil. Sift flour, salt, baking powder,

and sugar together into a mixing bowl. Add the egg, milk, and oil or melted shortening. Stir quickly and only until ingredients are barely blended. Do *not* beat. Fill muffin tins ⅔ full. Bake 20 to 25 minutes. (For nut muffins, add ½ cup coarsely chopped walnuts to the milk.)

Yield: 12 muffins
(1 muffin = 1 teaspoon oil or fat)

Pineapple Mold

1 package lime or strawberry flavored gelatin
1 cup hot water
1 cup canned pineapple juice
⅛ teaspoon salt
1 egg white

Procedure: Dissolve gelatin in hot water. Add the pineapple juice and salt. Chill until slightly thickened. Place in bowl of ice and water. Add the egg white, and whip with egg beater until fluffy and thick. Pile lightly in sherbet glasses. Chill until firm.

Yield: 6 servings

Sugar Cookies

2 cups all-purpose flour, sifted
2 teaspoons baking powder
½ teaspoon salt
¼ teaspoon nutmeg
2 eggs
⅔ cup oil
1 teaspoon vanilla
¾ cup sugar

Procedure: Preheat oven to 400° (hot). Sift together flour, baking powder, salt, and nutmeg. In a large bowl, beat eggs. Stir in oil and vanilla. Blend in sugar. Stir flour mixture into egg mixture. Drop by teaspoonfuls 2 inches apart on an ungreased cookie or baking sheet. Flatten each cookie with oiled glass dipped in sugar. Bake 8 to 10 minutes until a delicate brown. Remove immediately from baking sheet.

Yield: About 60 cookies
(2 cookies = 1 teaspoon oil)

DIABETIC RECIPES

Nearly all diabetic meals may be planned around the family menu with little if any extra preparation. However, the number and size of the servings may be different. The following recipes are based on the food exchange lists[2] described in Chapter 28, Metabolic Disorders Related to Nutrition. They are designed to show how foods can be combined to add variety and interest to the diet. See page 405 for beverages, soups, condiments, and foods allowed as desired. Non-nutritive sweeteners that the diabetic can use are described on page 601.

---

[1]From "Planning Fat-Controlled Meals for 1200 and 1800 Calories." American Heart Association, 44 East 23 Street, New York, N.Y. 10010.

[2]Meal Planning with Exchange Lists. Prepared by committees of the American Diabetes Association, Inc., and The American Dietetic Association, in cooperation with the Chronic Disease Program, Public Health Service, Department of Health, Education and Welfare.

SOUP

Fish Chowder

1 teaspoon fat
½ small onion, chopped
1 small potato, sliced
¼ or ½ cup cooked fish (1 or 2 oz.)
1 cup milk
    Salt and pepper
    Procedure: 1. Cook fish in salted water. 2. Melt fat in saucepan; brown the onion. 3. Add cooked fish, sliced potato, ½ cup water in which fish was cooked. 4. Cover and cook for 15 minutes until potatoes are tender. 5. Add milk and seasonings.
    Yield: 1 serving (1 serving *equals* 1 fat exchange and 1 bread exchange and 1 or 2 meat exchanges and 1 cup milk)
    (From Meal Planning with Exchange Lists, p. 405.)

Vegetable Soup

1 cup meat stock, or bouillon cube
    and 1 cup water
½ cup mixed vegetables: carrots and peas
½ small onion, chopped
¼ cup cabbage, shredded
1 stalk celery, diced
¼ cup tomato juice
    Salt and pepper
    Procedure: 1. Prepare vegetables and add to broth. 2. Boil together until vegetables are just tender, about 20 minutes.
    Yield: 1 serving (1 serving *equals* 1 vegetable from List 2B)
    (From Meal Planning with Exchange Lists, pp. 402–403.)

MEAT, POULTRY AND FISH

Meat Stew

1 teaspoon fat
½ cup mixed vegetables, list 2B
    (carrots, peas and onions)
2–3 ounces meat, cubed
1 small potato
    Salt and pepper to taste
    Procedure: 1. Brown meat in fat. 2. Add 1 cup water, salt and pepper, and a few celery leaves for seasoning. Simmer slowly, until meat is tender. 3. Add vegetables, List 2B, and any additional vegetables from List 2A, if desired. 4. Cut potato into quarters, and add. 5. Cook for 30 minutes, or until vegetables are done.
    Yield: 1 serving (1 serving *equals* 2 or 3 meat exchanges and 1 bread exchange and 1 serving vegetables from List 2B and 1 fat exchange)
    (From Meal Planning with Exchange Lists, p. 405.)

Salmon Cakes

2 ounces canned salmon
½ cup mashed potatoes
¼ teaspoon salt
    Pepper
½ teaspoon grated onion
5 small stuffed olives, sliced
2 teaspoons butter
    Procedure: 1. Combine all ingredients, except butter; shape into 2 cakes. 2. Brown in butter. Serve hot.

Yield: 1 serving (1 serving *equals* 2 meat exchanges, 1 bread exchange, 3 fat exchanges)

Baked Chicken and Rice

½ cup cooked rice
¼ or ½ cup diced chicken (1–2 oz.)
¼ cup clear broth
    Salt and pepper
    Procedure: 1. Combine ingredients and place in dish. Bake in a moderate oven until brown.
    Yield: 1 serving (1 serving *equals* 1 bread exchange and 1 or 2 meat exchanges)
    Variations: Chopped parsley, onions, celery, mushrooms, green pepper, pimento or tomatoes may be added for variety, if desired. In place of rice you may use noodles or spaghetti. For the chicken you may use any type of meat or fish, such as lamb, ham, tuna or shrimp.
    (From Meal Planning with Exchange Lists, p. 404.)

Cheese Fondue

1 egg
1 cup milk
    Salt
    Pepper
1 slice bread, cubed
¼ cup cheese, diced (1 oz.)
    Chopped parsley
    Chopped onion
    Procedure: 1. Beat the egg; add milk bread, cheese and seasonings. 2. Bake in moderate (350° F.) oven until firm in the center, about 20 or 30 minutes.
    Yield: 1 serving (1 serving *equals* 1 bread exchange, 2 meat exchanges and 1 cup milk)
    Variations: In place of cheese ¼ cup (1 oz.) of chopped ham, chicken, tuna fish or salmon may be used.
    (From Meal Planning with Exchange Lists, pp. 402–404.)

Noodle Bake

2 ounces Cheddar cheese, cubed
¼ cup milk
½ cup cooked or drained canned green beans
½ cup cooked noodles
    Salt and pepper
    Paprika
    Procedure: 1. Melt cheese in milk in small saucepan over low heat; blend until smooth. 2. Combine with beans, noodles, salt and pepper. 3. Place in individual casserole; sprinkle with paprika. 4. Bake in moderate (350° F.) oven 20 minutes, or until brown.
    Yield: 1 serving (1 serving *equals* 2 meat exchanges, 1 serving vegetable from List 2A, 1 bread exchange, and ¼ cup milk)
    Variation: Macaroni, rice or spaghetti may be substituted for noodles.

VEGETABLES

Pickled Beets

2½ cups cooked or canned beets, sliced
⅓ cup vinegar
½ teaspoon salt
4 whole cloves
1 bay leaf
4 saccharin tablets (¼ grain each)

Procedure: 1. Drain liquid from beets into saucepan; add remaining ingredients and bring to boil. 2. Pour over beets. Chill about 6 hours before serving. 3. Serve cold or reheat.

Yield: 5 servings (½ cup *equals* 1 serving vegetable from List 2B)

SALADS AND SALAD DRESSING

Chicken and Mushroom Salad

2 ounces cooked or canned chicken, diced
½ cup cooked or drained canned mushrooms, stems and pieces
½ cup diced celery
2 teaspoons mayonnaise
½ teaspoon lemon juice or vinegar
  Salt and pepper
  Lettuce
Procedure: 1. Combine all ingredients, except lettuce; toss lightly. 2. Serve on lettuce.

Yield: 1 serving (1 serving *equals* 2 meat exchanges, 2 fat exchanges, 2 vegetable List 2A servings)

Variations: Shrimp, tuna, salmon or turkey may be substituted for the chicken.

Potato Salad A

½ cup cooked potato, diced
  Salt and pepper
  Chopped onion, as desired
  Chopped green pepper, as desired
1 or 2 tablespoons zero salad dressing (see below)
  Chopped celery, as desired
  Chopped parsley, as desired
Procedure: Combine all ingredients. Serve.

Yield: 1 serving (1 serving *equals* 1 bread exchange)
(From Meal Planning with Exchange Lists, p. 404.)

Potato Salad B

Same ingredients as above, except that 1 teaspoon of mayonnaise may be used in place of zero salad dressing.
Procedure: Same as above.

Yield: 1 serving (1 serving *equals* 1 fat exchange and 1 bread exchange)
(From Meal Planning with Exchange Lists, p. 404.)

Potato Salad C

1 hard cooked egg, sliced, may be added to recipe for Potato Salad A or B.
Procedure: Same as for Potato Salad A and B.

Yield: 1 serving (1 serving *equals* 1 bread exchange, 1 meat exchange and 1 fat exchange, *if desired*)

Variation: ¼ cup (1 oz.) diced ham, bologna or frankfurter, or 5 small shrimp may be used in place of egg.
(From Meal Planning with Exchange Lists, p. 404.)

Mixed Vegetable Salad

(May be used in any amount)

Any combinations of vegetables from List 2A (p. 402) may be used such as:
  1. Lettuce, cucumber, celery, green pepper.
  2. Chicory, tomato, radish.
  3. Lettuce, parsley, raw cauliflower, tomato.
  4. Escarole, tomato, cucumber.
  5. Cabbage, celery, green pepper.
  6. Lettuce, water cress, cucumber.
  7. Lettuce, raw spinach, radish.
Procedure: Salad may be combined with zero salad dressing, French dressing, or mayonnaise, depending upon fat allowed in your meal plan.
(From Meal Planning with Exchange Lists, p. 402.)

Zero Salad Dressing

½ cup tomato juice
2 tablespoons lemon juice or vinegar
  Chopped parsley, if desired
  Horseradish, if desired
1 tablespoon onion, finely chopped
  Salt and pepper
  Chopped green pepper, if desired
  Mustard, if desired
Procedure: 1. Combine ingredients in a jar with a tightly fitted top. 2. Shake well before using.

Yield: May be used in any amount.
(From Meal Planning with Exchange Lists, p. 405.)

DESSERTS

Fresh Fruit Cup

Any fruits in List 3 (p. 403) may be combined to make a fruit cup.

½ cup of mixed fruits equals 1 serving.

Example:
  Orange, grapefruit, pineapple.
  Apple, grapefruit, strawberries.
  Peach, orange, blackberries.
  Grapes, orange, melon.
  Melon, grapefruit, banana.
(From Meal Planning with Exchange Lists, p. 403.)

Fruit Cocktail Whip

1 teaspoon unflavored gelatin
2 tablespoons cold water
½ cup boiling water
3 saccharin tablets (¼ grain each)
1 fruit exchange
1 tablespoon lemon juice
Procedure: 1. Sprinkle gelatin over cold water; let stand 5 minutes. 2. Add boiling water; stir until dissolved. 3. Add lemon juice and saccharin. Chill until mixture begins to set. 4. Beat with rotary beater until fluffy; fold in fruit cocktail. Chill until firm.

Yield: 1 serving or 1 fruit exchange

Variation: For jellied fruit salad, omit beating if preferred.

Ginger Pear Halves

½ cup liquid drained from pears (Dietetic Packed)
1 saccharin tablet (¼ grain)
¼ teaspoon ginger
2 pear halves, drained
Procedure: 1. Combine all ingredients except pear halves; heat to boiling. 2. Add pear halves. Cover and let stand in hot liquid for at least a half hour. Serve hot or chilled.

Yield: 1 serving or 1 fruit exchange

Lemon Gelatin

1 teaspoon unflavored gelatin
2 tablespoons cold water
1 tablespoon lemon juice
½ cup water

Procedure: 1. Put cold water in top of double boiler, add gelatin, let stand 10 minutes at room temperature. Place pan over boiling water to dissolve gelatin. 2. If desired, add ¼ grain saccharin. 3. Remove from stove. 4. Add lemon juice and ½ cup water. Chill.

Yield: 1 serving (may be used in any amount)

Variation: To make *Coffee Gelatin,* omit lemon juice and use ½ cup coffee in place of ½ cup water.

(From Meal Planning with Exchange Lists, p. 405.)

Orange Gelatin

Follow recipe for lemon gelatin, but use ½ cup orange juice in place of water.

Yield: 1 serving (1 serving *equals* 1 fruit exchange)
(From Meal Planning with Exchange Lists, p. 403.)

Fruit Gelatin — I

Follow recipe for lemon gelatin, and 1 serving of any fruit from List 3 (p. 403) may be added, such as ½ small banana. 1 serving *equals* 1 fruit from List 3.
(From Meal Planning with Exchange Lists, p. 403.)

Fruit Gelatin — II

Follow recipe for orange gelatin, and add 1 serving of any fruit from List 3 (p. 403). 1 serving *equals* 2 fruits from list 3.
(From Meal Planning with Exchange Lists, p. 403.)

Fruit Ice

½ cup orange juce, or ⅓ cup
   pineapple juice
1 tablespoon lemon juice
1 egg white
½ cup water

Procedure: 1. Combine fruit juice and water and freeze. Stir mixture often while freezing. 2. When almost hard, fold in 1 stiffly beaten egg white. 3. Place in individual mold; allow to set.

Yield: 1 serving (1 serving *equals* 1 fruit from List 3)
(From Meal Planning with Exchange Lists, p. 403.)

Floating Island

½ cup milk
1 egg
¼ teaspoon vanilla
   Artificial sweetener, if desired

Procedure: 1. Heat the milk in upper part of double boiler over boiling water. 2. Beat the egg yolk in bowl, using rotary beater. 3. Pour the hot milk over the yolk, mix well and pour back into top part of the double boiler. 4. Stir mixture constantly until it begins to thicken, about 10 minutes. 5. Remove from heat; add vanilla and artificial sweetener, if used. 6. Beat egg white stiff. This may be done in advance of the preparation of the custard and placed in the refrigerator to chill. 7. When ready to serve the custard, place in glass dish and top with beaten egg white. If desired, it may be placed under the broiler for a few seconds to brown.

Yield: 1 serving (1 serving *equals* ½ milk exchange and 1 meat exchange)

Cocktail

Soda water
1 maraschino cherry
Juice of ½ lime
Artificial sweetener, if desired

Procedure: 1. Mix the lime juice with a glass of soda water. 2. Garnish with a maraschino cherry. (This may be used only as a garnish and not eaten.) Sweeten with saccharin or Sucaryl as desired.

Yield: 1 serving (1 serving equals ½ fruit exchange, *if cherry is eaten*)

SODIUM-RESTRICTED RECIPES

Sodium restriction may be accomplished in part by eliminating the use of salt as a seasoning. In addition, foods that do not normally contain significant amounts may be selected. Sodium in foods must be calculated as part of the total sodium allowance. (See Appendix Table 9 for sodium content of foods.) For example, eggs and milk are sodium-rich foods, and when used in a recipe are considered as part of the daily ration. There now are a growing number of processed and manufactured foods, such as meats, vegetables, cereals, and milk, especially developed for individuals on sodium-restricted programs. All labels should be read carefully to determine whether salt (sodium) has been added during the processing or manufacture, since the sodium content, or the statement that the food is sodium-free, is printed thereon. Breads, crackers, cake and a convenient variety of other low sodium foods are also available.

Herbs, spices, and seasonings have been found to enhance the food flavor when salt is not used as a seasoning. Following are suggestions to make food more palatable without adding significant amounts of sodium to the diet. These flavoring aids may be used in unrestricted amounts:

Allspice	Mace
Almond extract	Maple extract
Anise	Marjoram
Basil	Mint
Bay leaf	Mustard, dry
Caraway	Nutmeg
Cardamon	Onion juice
Chives	Orange extract
Cinnamon	Orange peel
Cloves	Oregano
Cocoa (not	Paprika
Dutch process)	Parsley
Coriander	Pepper, black,
Curry	red or white
Dill	Peppermint
Fennel	extract
Garlic	Pimento
Ginger	Poppyseed
Horseradish	Poultry seasoning
(not prepared)	Rosemary
Leeks	Saccharin
Lemon juice	Saffron
or extract	Sage

Savory	Tarragon
Sesame	Thyme
Sugar, brown (in small amounts	Turmeric
small amounts	Vanilla extract
Sugar, white	Wine

Some flavor combinations for cooked meats, fish, eggs, and vegetables are suggested in the following list:

Beef—dry mustard, marjoram, nutmeg, onion, sage, thyme, pepper, bay leaf, grape jelly.
Pork—onion, garlic, sage; with applesauce, spiced apples.
Lamb—mint, garlic, rosemary, curry; with broiled pineapple rings.
Veal—bay leaf, ginger, marjoram, curry, current jelly, spiced apricots.
Chicken—paprika, mushroom, thyme, sage, parsley, cranberry sauce.
Fish—dry mustard, paprika, curry, bay leaf, lemon juice, mushrooms.
Eggs—pepper, green pepper, mushrooms, dry mustard, paprika, curry, jelly or pineapple omelet.
Asparagus—lemon juice.
Beans, green—marjoram, lemon juice, nutmeg, unsalted French dressing, dill seed.
Broccoli—lemon juice.
Cabbage—mustard dressing, dill seed, unsalted butter with lemon and sugar.
Carrots—parsley, unsalted butter, mint, nutmeg; glazed with butter and sugar.
Cauliflower—nutmeg.
Corn—green pepper, tomatoes.
Peas—mint, mushroom, parsley, onion.
Potatoes—parsley, unsalted butter, mace, chopped green pepper, onion; baked, French fried.
Squash—ginger, mace.
Sweet potatoes—candied or glazed with cinnamon or nutmeg; escalloped with apples, sugar.
Tomatoes—basil.

Salt-free cooked cereals gain in appeal when they are served with honey or a fresh fruit topping. Fried mush with jelly or marmalade provides variety.

A small amount of sugar added to vegetables during the cooking period helps to bring out the natural flavor of the food.

Following are additional suggestions arranged according to the seasoning:

Allspice—ground meats, stews, tomatoes, peaches.
Almond extract—puddings, custards, fruits.
Basil—eggs, fish, lamb, ground meats, liver, stews, salads, soup, sauces, fish cocktails.
Bay leaves—meats, stews, poultry, soups, tomatoes.
Caraway seeds—meats, stews, soups, salads, breads, cabbage, asparagus, noodles.
Chives—salads, eggs, sauces, soups, meat dishes, vegetables.
Cider vinegar—salads, vegetables, sauces.
Cinnamon—fruits (especially apples), breads, pie crust.
Curry powder—meats (especially lamb), chicken, fish, tomatoes, tomato soup.
Dill—fish and lamb sauces, soups, tomatoes, salads, macaroni.
Garlic (not garlic salt)—meats, soups, salads, vegetables, tomatoes.
Ginger—chicken, fruits.
Lemon juice—meats, fish, poultry, salads, vegetables.

Mace—hot breads.
Mustard (dry)—ground meats, salads, sauces.
Nutmeg—fruits, cottage cheese, pie crust, potatoes.
Onion (not onion salt)—meats, vegetables, salads.
Paprika—meats, fish, stews, sauces, soups, vegetables.
Parsley—meats, fish, soups, salads, sauces, vegetables.
Peppermint extract—puddings, fruits.
Pimento—salads, vegetables, casserole dishes.
Rosemary—chicken, veal, meat loaf, beef, pork, sauces, stuffings, potatoes, peas, lima beans.
Sage—meats, stews, biscuits, tomatoes, green beans.
Savory—salads, egg dishes, pork, ground meats, soup, green beans, squash, tomatoes, lima beans, peas.
Thyme—eggs, meats (especially veal, pork), sauces, soups, onions, peas, tomatoes, salads.
Turmeric—meats, eggs, fish, sauces, rice.

SALT SUBSTITUTES   Salt substitutes are available for use in place of salt. These should be used with the recommendation of the physician. They usually contain potassium chloride, glutamic acid, tricalcium phosphate and flavor enhancing monopotassium glutamate.

SODIUM EXTRACTION   Simple extraction of various normally high sodium foods with water for 24 hours has been found to remove from 26 to 93 per cent of the sodium.[3] Use approximately ten volumes of water to a piece of meat or fish, or a supply of vegetables, and place in the refrigerator overnight. Pour off water just before mealtime and cook. Common fresh vegetables that need to undergo this process are celery, carrots, spinach, beets, and kale. Most vegetables and fruits are low in sodium, and can be consumed in their natural state. Raw meats and fish also are permitted when prepared in this manner. Eggs can be provided in the menu if they are hard boiled and shelled before soaking. Spices, herbs, and seasonings, as well as salt substitutes (if allowed), may be added to give flavor.

There is some loss of water-soluble vitamins, and supplements are usually prescribed. By using moderate amounts of normally high sodium foods, treated as described above, and combining them with foods naturally low in sodium content, a varied and palatable diet can be achieved.

Considerable sodium may be extracted from salted meats such as ham, ham hocks, bacon and fat back by the following process. Cover with water, boil 3–5 minutes, and discard the water. This process is known as "freshening meat" in some cultures.

---

[3]Beychok, M. E., et al.: Practical methods for preparing diets low in sodium and high in protein. Am. J. Clin. Nutr. 4:254, 1956.

Tuna and Mushrooms on Macaroni

2 tablespoons flour
2 teaspoons unsalted butter
1 cup milk
1 teaspoon grated onion
  Dash of white pepper
2 teaspoons chopped pimento
3 ounces canned "Dietetic Packed" tuna
½ cup drained canned "Dietetic Packed" mushrooms
½ cup hot cooked macaroni
  Procedure: 1. Blend flour with butter and part of milk to make smooth paste; add remaining milk, onion, pepper and pimento. *2.* Cook in small saucepan over low heat until thickened, stirring constantly. *3.* Add tuna and mushrooms. *4.* Heat thoroughly. Serve over macaroni.
  Yield: 1 serving

Herb Green Beans

1 cup cooked unsalted, or "Dietetic Packed" canned green beans
1 teaspoon chopped chives or onions
2 teaspoons unsalted butter
  Dash of thyme
  Dash of pepper
  Dash of sugar
  Procedure: 1. Drain liquid from beans into small saucepan. *2.* Boil quickly until liquid is reduced to about ⅓ cup. *3.* Add beans, butter and seasonings; heat thoroughly.
  Yield: 1–2 servings

Curried Corn

1 cup whole kernel corn, cooked or "Dietetic Packed"
1 tablespoon chopped pimento
⅛–¼ teaspoon curry powder
  Dash of pepper
1 teaspoon unsalted butter
  Procedure: 1. Drain liquid from corn into small saucepan. *2.* Boil quickly until liquid is reduced to about ⅓ cup (if canned). *3.* Add corn, pimento, butter and seasonings. *4.* Heat thoroughly; toss lightly.
  Yield: 1–2 servings

Low Sodium Mayonnaise

1 egg yolk
½ teaspoon dry mustard
1 teaspoon sugar
2 tablespoons lemon juice or cider vinegar
1 cup salad oil (corn or cottonseed)
  Procedure: 1. Beat together egg yolk, mustard, sugar and 1 tablespoon lemon juice. *2.* Add salad oil very slowly, beating constantly. *3.* Beat in remaining tablespoon lemon juice. Chill in refrigerator.
  Yield: 1 cup

Low Sodium French Dressing

½ cup salad oil (corn or cottonseed)
¼ cup cider vinegar
¼ cup water
2 teaspoons sugar
1 teaspoon dry mustard
½ teaspoon paprika
  Dash of pepper
  Procedure: Combine all ingredients; beat well with rotary beater, or shake well in jar with tight-fitting cover.
  Yield: 1 cup

Spiced Applesauce

½ cup "Dietetic Packed" canned applesauce
2 teaspoons honey
⅛ teaspoon nutmeg
  Dash of cinnamon
  Dash of ginger
  Procedure: Combine all ingredients; heat thoroughly. Serve hot or cold.
  Yield: 1 serving

ALLERGY RECIPES

Wheat, milk, and eggs are the foods which most frequently cause distress or allergic symptoms. Since these are basic foods used in the daily dietary, careful planning and preparation are necessary to provide adequate nutrition. Some individuals may be allergic to one offender, while others may have symptoms from two, all three, or even additional ones. (Review Chapter 27, Nutrition in Diseases of Allergy and the Skin.)

Patients sensitive to fresh milk may be able to tolerate one of the other forms, such as dried, evaporated, boiled or cultured. It is advisable to try these before eliminating milk entirely from the diet. When all forms of milk produce allergy symptoms, water may be substituted for milk in a standard recipe. However, in such cases, the physician will usually supplement the diet with riboflavin and calcium to maintain adequate nutrition.

When egg is the offender, egg dishes, baked products, desserts, some bread, and all foods prepared with egg must be eliminated.

Persons sensitive to wheat alone may use foods made from the other grains. Cornstarch can replace flour in thickening sauces and gravies, using half as much. Prepared or ready-to-eat cereals such as cornflakes and rice cereals can be rolled and broken up into fine pieces to use in place of bread crumbs and in the preparation of dishes. Ry-Krisp, or a similar product, is suggested as a possible form of bread, since it contains only natural whole grain rye, salt, and water. Patients must be cautioned concerning the use of bread. For example, a bread sold as "rye bread" usually contains wheat flour as well as rye, making it unsuitable for use by an individual sensitive to wheat. The same precaution must be taken concerning milk and eggs.

SUBSTITUTES FOR 1 CUP WHEAT FLOUR[4]

½ cup barley flour
1 cup corn flour
¾ cup cornmeal (coarse)
1 scant cup corn meal (fine)

---

[4]Allergy Recipes, The American Dietetic Association, 620 North Michigan Avenue, Chicago, Illinois, 60611.

⁵⁄₈ cup potato flour
⁷⁄₈ cup rice flour
1¼ cups rye flour
1 cup rye meal
1⅓ cups ground rolled oats

COMBINATIONS OF FLOUR TO BE SUBSTITUTED FOR 1 CUP WHEAT FLOUR[4]

A combination of flours often produces a more palatable product than a single flour when substituted for wheat flour.

(1) Rye flour	½ cup
Potato flour	½ cup
(2) Rye flour	⅔ cup
Potato flour	⅓ cup
(3) Rice flour	⅝ cup (10 tbsps.)
Rye flour	⅓ cup
(4) Soy flour	1 cup
Potato starch flour	¾ cup

WHEAT-, MILK-, AND EGG-FREE RECIPES

Rye Bread

1⅓ cups water
2 teaspoons salt
3 tablespoons sugar
4 tablespoons fat
1½ cakes of compressed yeast or
2 tablespoons active dry yeast
5 cups rye flour

Procedure: 1. Soften the yeast in ⅓ cup lukewarm water. Add 1 tsp. sugar. 2. Measure the remaining water, the salt, sugar and softened fat into a bowl; add dissolved yeast mixture. 3. Pour half of the flour into this liquid mixture and beat until well blended. 4. Add the remaining flour, kneading on floured board until dough is smooth and will spring back when pressed lightly with finger (about 200 strokes). 5. Let rise until double in bulk, (about 1 hour) at 80° F. 7. Knead about 100 times and place in 2 small loaf pans which have been greased only on the bottom. This amount can best be separated into two small loaves and shaped before placing into the pans. 8. Let rise again until double, (about 30 minutes) at 80° F. 9. Bake 10–15 minutes at 425° F. until brown. Continue to bake 25–35 minutes at 350° F. until done.
Yield: 2 small loaves
(From Allergy Recipes, p. 5.)

Steamed Brown Bread

1 cup rye flour
1 cup corn meal
¼ teaspoon baking soda
1 teaspoon salt
1 cup quick oatmeal
¾ cup molasses
1 cup water

Procedure: 1. Sift the rye flour, corn meal, soda, and salt together. 2. Add the oatmeal and mix thoroughly. 3. Add the molasses and water; stir until well mixed. 4. Fill greased molds not more than ⅔ full. 5. Grease covers before placing on molds. 6. Steam 3½ hours. Remove covers and dry in oven 15 minutes. Bread may be baked at 375° F. about 1 hour.
Yield: 3 10-oz. can loaves
(From Allergy Recipes, p. 6.)

---

[4]Allergy Recipes, The American Dietetic Association, 620 North Michigan Avenue, Chicago, Illinois, 60611.

Banana Rye Bread

2 cakes or packages yeast
¼ cup lukewarm water
1 tablespoon salt
1½ tablespoons sugar
3 tablespoons melted vegetable shortening
2¼ cups mashed fully ripe bananas (5 to 6 bananas)
5¼ to 6 cups rye flour

Procedure: 1. Dissolve yeast in lukewarm water. 2. Mix together salt, sugar, shortening and bananas. 3. Add half the flour and beat until smooth. 4. Beat in the dissolved yeast. 5. Add remaining flour gradually and mix well. 6. Turn dough out onto a floured board. Knead about 8 minutes, adding just enough additional rye flour to prevent sticking. Place dough in a lightly greased bowl. 7. Cover and let rise in a warm place until double in bulk (about 2 hours). 8. Turn out onto floured board and knead lightly about 2 minutes. Shape dough into 2 loaves. 9. Place in lightly greased bread pans (8 × 4 × 3 inches). Cover with damp towel and let rise again until double in size (about 1 hour). 10. Bake 5–10 minutes at 425° F. until crust begins to brown. Continue to bake 35–40 minutes at 350° F. until done.
Yield: 2 loaves
(From The United Fruit Company.)

Oatmeal and Rice Muffins

¾ cup rice flour
3 tablespoons ground oatmeal
1 tablespoon baking powder
½ teaspoon salt
1 tablespoon fat, melted
½ cup water (or enough to make thin batter)
3 tablespoons raisins

Procedure: 1. Grind oatmeal in a meat grinder using a medium coarse blade. 2. Sift rice flour, baking powder and salt together; mix with ground oatmeal. 3. Combine water with fat. 4. Add liquid to dry ingredients and stir just enough to dampen the flour mixture; add raisins, combine. 5. Fill greased muffin pans ⅔ full. 6. Bake in hot oven (400° F.) about 30 minutes.
Yield: 6 large muffins
(From Allergy Recipes, p. 7.)

Corn Pone

¼ cup corn meal
⅓ teaspoon salt
½ cup boiling water

Procedure: 1. Sift corn meal and salt together. 2. Add boiling water to make a firm mixture. 3. Shape into thin cakes, place in pan well greased with bacon fat or other shortening and bake in hot (400° F.) oven 15 to 20 minutes.
Yield: 4 small cakes
(From Allergy Diets. 13th ed. St. Louis, The Ralston Purina Company.)

Meat or Poultry Stuffing

2 dozen Ry-Krisp wafers
¾ cup hot meat stock or water
¼ cup shortening
¼ cup finely cut green pepper
2 tablespoons finely cut onion
¼ cup finely cut celery
2 tablespoons finely cut parsley
¼ teaspoon sage
⅛ teaspoon pepper

Procedure: 1. Break Ry-Krisp wafers into small pieces, then soak in hot stock. 2. Add remaining ingredients and mix well.

Yield: Sufficient quantity for stuffing a 3-lb. chicken, flank steak or breast of veal.
(From Allergy Diets. 13th ed.)

Spice Cake

1 cup brown sugar
1¼ cups water
1 cup raisins, seedless
2 ounces citron, cut fine
⅓ cup fat
½ teaspoon salt
1 teaspoon nutmeg
1 teaspoon cinnamon
1 cup corn meal, fine
1 cup rye flour
4 teaspoons baking powder
Procedure: 1. Boil sugar, water, fruit, fat, and salt together in a saucepan for 3 minutes. 2. When cool add the spices, baking powder, corn meal, and flour which have been sifted together. 3. Mix thoroughly and bake in a greased loaf pan at 375° F. for 45 minutes.
Yield: 1 loaf cake
(From Allergy Recipes, p. 9.)

Ry-Krisp Crumb Crust

12 Ry-Krisp wafers
¼ cup sugar
⅓ cup shortening
Procedure: 1. Roll Ry-Krisp wafers into fine crumbs. There should be 1 cup crumbs. 2. Fold in sugar. 3. Add melted shortening and mix thoroughly. 4. With back of spoon press crumbs on bottom and sides of greased deep 9-inch pie pan. 5. Chill thoroughly. Fill with a fruit or gelatin filling.
Yield: 6–8 servings
(From Allergy Diets. 13th ed.)

WHEAT- AND MILK-FREE RECIPES

Bacon-Barley Puffs

6 slices bacon
2 cups pearl barley, cooked
1 egg, beaten
¼ teaspoon salt
¼ teaspoon pepper
1 tablespoon parsley, minced
Procedure: 1. Line muffin pans with strips of bacon. 2. Combine the remaining ingredients, fill muffin pans ⅔ full, and bake at 400° F. for 30 minutes.
Yield: 6 servings
(From Allergy Recipes, p. 42.)

Chinese Chews

5 tablespoons rice flour
1 teaspoon baking powder
1 egg, well beaten
½ cup sugar
⅛ teaspoon salt
½ cup chopped dates
½ cup chopped nuts
Procedure: 1. Sift flour and baking powder. 2. Beat egg, add sugar and salt. 3. Combine egg mixture with flour and baking powder. 4. Add dates and nuts. 5. Bake in loaf pan at 325° F. for 30 minutes. 6. While hot, cut into bars 1½ inches wide and 3 inches long. Roll in powdered sugar.
Yield: 10 cookies
(From Allergy Recipes, p. 38.)

WHEAT- AND EGG-FREE RECIPES

Rye Flour and Soybean Flour Biscuits

2 cups rye flour
1 cup soy flour
4 tablespoons fat
2 tablespoons baking powder
1 teaspoon salt
1¼ cups (approximately) milk
Procedure: 1. Sift dry ingredients together; cut in the fat. 2. Add the milk slowly and when a soft dough is formed, place on bread board floured with rye flour and knead. 3. Pat into a sheet about ½ inch thick; cut into small rounds with biscuit cutter. 4. Place on a biscuit sheet and bake at 450° F. for about 12 minutes.
Yield: 12 large biscuits
Variation: Rice flour may be substituted for rye flour in this recipe.
(From Allergy Recipes, p. 20.)

Green Peppers Stuffed with Hominy

6 strips bacon
3 cups hominy, cooked
1 teaspoon salt
¼ teaspoon pepper
1 tablespoon parsley, minced
6 peppers, green
2 tablespoons cheese, grated
Procedure: 1. Mince bacon and cook until crisp and brown. 2. Add the cooked hominy, salt, pepper, and parsley and sauté for approximately 10 minutes. 3. Cut tops from peppers and remove seeds and the white membrane. 4. Parboil peppers in salted water for 5 minutes. 5. Stuff the peppers with the hominy mixture, sprinkle with grated cheese. 6. Bake at 375° F. for 25–30 minutes.
Yield: 6 servings
(From Allergy Recipes, p. 32.)

Orange Custard

3 tablespoons cornstarch
⅓ cup sugar
⅛ teaspoon salt
1 cup orange juice
1 teaspoon grated orange rind
1 cup evaporated milk
Procedure: 1. Mix thoroughly cornstarch, sugar, salt. 2. Add ¼ cup milk; blend until smooth. 3. Heat remaining milk in double boiler. 4. Add cornstarch mixture; cook until it begins to thicken. 5. Add orange juice and grated rind; cook until thick, stirring constantly to avoid lumping. Cover and cook 20 minutes. 6. Turn into cold, wet molds and chill.
Yield: 4 servings
(From Allergy Diets. 13th ed.)

WHEAT-FREE RECIPES

Batter Bread

2 cups corn meal, uncooked
5 teaspoons baking powder
1½ teaspoons salt
2 eggs, beaten
1 cup rice, cooked
2¼ cups milk
4 tablespoons melted fat
Procedure: 1. Sift together the corn meal, baking powder, and salt; mix with rice. 2. Combine eggs, fat, and milk, and add this to the first mixture; beat until smooth. 3.

Pour batter into two well-greased 8-inch square pans and bake at 425° F. for approximately 30 minutes.

Yield: 16 servings
(From Allergy Recipes, p. 46.)

Rye Muffins

1 cup rye flour, coarse
1/4 teaspoon salt
2 teaspoons baking powder
2 tablespoons sugar
1 egg
1/2 cup milk
2 teaspoons fat, melted

Procedure: 1. Sift dry ingredients. 2. Combine beaten egg, milk, melted fat. 3. Add to dry ingredients; stir just enough to combine. (Mixture has a rough appearance.) 4. Fill greased muffin pans 2/3 full, handling the batter as little as possible. 5. Bake at 400° F. for about 25 minutes.

Yield: 6 medium-sized muffins
(From Allergy Recipes, p. 47.)

Oatmeal Drop Cookies

6 tablespoons butter or margarine
1/2 cup sugar
1 egg
2 tablespoons milk, sour
1/2 teaspoon baking soda
3/4 cup rye flour
1/2 teaspoon cinnamon
1 1/2 cups oatmeal
3/4 cup raisins
1/4 cup chopped nuts

Procedure: 1. Cream butter and sugar. 2. Add beaten egg. 3. Add sour milk. 4. Add the soda, flour, and cinnamon which have been sifted together. 5. Add oatmeal, raisins, and nuts. 6. Drop from a teaspoon on a baking sheet buttered or covered with wax paper. 7. Bake at 350° F. for 25 minutes.

Yield: 24 cookies
(From Allergy Recipes, p. 53.)

Hominy Grits with Eggs

1/2 cup hominy grits
3 cups boiling water
1 teaspoon salt
5 or 6 eggs
1/2 cup grated cheese
Salt, pepper, paprika

Procedure: 1. Slowly add the grits to the boiling salted water; cook directly over the heat until thickened; cook in double boiler for one hour. 2. Fill a shallow baking dish with hominy grits; make hollows or wells in the grits. 3. Drop a raw egg into each hollow. 4. Sprinkle with salt, pepper, grated cheese, and paprika. 5. Bake in a moderate oven (375° F.) for 20 to 25 minutes.

Yield: 6 servings
(From Allergy Recipes, p. 58.)

Welsh Rabbit

1 tablespoon butter or margarine
2 teaspoons rice flour
1/8 teaspoon salt
1/4 cup cream
1/4 cup milk
2 tablespoons grated American cheese
1/2 egg, well beaten
Paprika (if allowed)

Procedure: 1. Melt fat, add flour and salt. 2. Slowly add milk and cream; stir until thickened. 3. Add grated cheese, cooking over boiling water until cheese is melted. 4. Stir small amount of hot mixture into beaten egg, then pour back into remaining mixture and cook until mixture is smooth. 5. Add paprika, if desired. 6. Serve on toasted Ry-Krisp or rye wafer.

Yield: 1 serving
(From Allergy Recipes, p. 59.)

Indian Pudding

1 quart milk
1/3 cup corn meal
1/2 cup raisins
1/2 teaspoon cinnamon
1/2 cup brown sugar or 1/2 cup corn syrup or honey
1/2 teaspoon salt
1/2 teaspoon ginger
2 eggs

Procedure: 1. Scald milk in double boiler. Add corn meal and cook 30 minutes. Add other ingredients, except beaten eggs. 2. Stir small amount of hot mixture into eggs, before adding them. Mix well. 3. Pour into a baking dish and bake in a slow oven (350° F.) for one hour. 4. Serve with a pineapple or peach lemon sauce. Hard sauces may be used; may be topped with whipped cream and pineapple cubes or raisins.

Yield: 8 servings
(From Allergy Recipes, p. 56.)

EGG-FREE RECIPES

Eggless Mayonnaise

1/4 teaspoon salt
1/4 teaspoon paprika
1/4 teaspoon dry mustard
Few grains pepper
3 tablespoons evaporated milk
1/2 cup salad oil
4 teaspoons lemon juice

Procedure: 1. Mix salt, paprika, mustard, and pepper together in bowl. 2. Stir in milk. 3. Beat in salad oil gradually. 4. Stir in lemon juice. Keep in refrigerator in covered jar.

Yield: 3/4 cup
(From Allergy Diets. 13th ed.)

Apple Tapioca

2 medium-sized apples (1/2 lb.)
2 cups boiling water
1 1/2 tablespoons lemon juice
2 tablespoons butter
3/4 cup brown sugar, lightly packed
1/3 cup quick-cooking tapioca
1/2 teaspoon salt
1/8 teaspoon nutmeg
1/8 teaspoon cinnamon

Procedure: 1. Pare, core and slice apples. Put into greased 8-inch baking dish. 2. Add boiling water, lemon juice, and 1 1/2 tablespoons of the butter. Cover. 3. Bake in moderately slow oven (350° F.) 25 minutes, or until apples are almost tender. 4. Remove cover; stir in mixture of 1/2 cup of the sugar, the tapioca, salt, spices. Mix thoroughly. 5. Bake, uncovered, 5 minutes; then stir mixture well. 6. Sprinkle top with remaining sugar and dot with remaining 1/2 tablespoon butter. 7. Bake 10 minutes, or until tapioca is clear. Serve warm or cold.

Yield: 4 servings
(From Allergy Diets, 13th ed.)

LOW-GLUTEN DIET RECIPES
(Wheat-, Rye-, and Oat-free)

The following recipes[5] are free from cereal proteins, except those found in rice and corn, and are used in the low-gluten diet (frequently termed "gluten-free"). See Allergy Recipes for other suitable recipes.

Southern Corn Muffins

1 cup boiling water
1 cup white corn meal
½ cup milk
½ teaspoon salt
2 teaspoons baking powder
1 tablespoon soft butter or margarine
1 egg, well beaten
Procedure: Pour boiling water over corn meal. Beat in milk, salt, baking powder, butter, and egg. Pour into very well greased glass muffin cups. Bake 25 to 30 min. in a 475° F. oven. Serve hot.
Yield: 9 medium-size muffins

Crisp Corn Pone

1 teaspoon bacon drippings
½ cup boiling water
½ cup corn meal
½ teaspoon salt
1 tablespoon sugar
Procedure: Add shortening to boiling water. Stir in corn meal, salt, and sugar and stir over low heat until mixture thickens. Spread mixture on well greased 9-in. pie pan. Dot with butter or margarine. Bake in 450° F. oven for 20 min. Place under preheated broiler about 5 min. until lightly browned. Cut in pie-shaped pieces and serve with butter.

Rice Flour Bread

1 cup unsifted rice flour
½ teaspoon salt
3 teaspoons baking powder
4 tablespoons sugar
2 egg yolks
4 tablespoons vegetable shortening
½ cup milk
2 egg whites, well beaten
1 ripe medium banana
Procedure: Combine and sift flour, baking powder, and salt. Cream softened shortening; then cream with sugar until well blended. Stir in unbeaten egg yolks. Add flour alternately with the milk, beating after each addition. Fold in the well beaten egg whites. Mash banana well and fold into mixture. Spread batter into well greased 8 by 4 by 3 in. loaf pan. Bake in preheated oven at 325° F. about 45 min. until crumb is dry when tested with tooth pick. If a browner loaf is desired, temperature may be raised to 450° F. for the last 5 min. of baking. Remove bread from oven. Let stand 5 min. Loosen loaf with spatula and turn out on rack. Cool before slicing.

Rice Flour Muffins

1 cup unsifted rice flour
½ teaspoon salt

3 teaspoons baking powder
¼ cup vegetable shortening
¼ cup sugar
2 egg yolks
¾ cup milk
2 egg whites, well beaten
½ teaspoon vanilla, lemon, or almond flavoring
Procedure: Sift rice flour, baking powder, and salt together twice. Cream softened shortening, add sugar, and cream together. Stir in egg yolks. Add flour mixture alternately with milk, beating after each addition. Fold in well beaten (but not dry) egg whites. Spoon into a well greased muffin tin. Bake 30 min. in a 325° F. oven or until lightly browned.
Yield: 6 muffins

Rice Flour Sponge Cake

2 eggs separated
⅓ cup sugar
¼ cup rice flour, sifted twice before measuring
1 teaspoon lemon juice
grated rind of ¼ lemon
Dash of salt
Procedure: Sift rice flour, sugar, and salt together. Beat egg yolks until thick and lemon colored. Add lemon juice and rind to egg yolks. Beat egg whites until stiff but not dry. Fold egg yolk mixture and flour mixture alternately in small amounts into beaten egg whites with rubber spatula. Pour into a small loaf pan lined with wax paper. Bake at 350° F. for 25 to 30 min.

Rice Flour Brownies

2 squares (2 oz.) unsweetened chocolate
½ cup shortening (margarine)
1 cup sugar
2 eggs
⅔ cup rice flour, sifted twice before measuring
½ teaspoon baking powder
½ teaspoon salt
½ cup chopped nuts
Procedure: Melt chocolate and shortening in double boiler over hot water. Remove pan from hot water and beat in sugar and eggs. Sift rice flour, baking powder, and salt together and stir into chocolate mixture. Add nuts and mix. Spread into a greased 8-in. square pan. Allow mixture to stand ½ hr. before baking. Bake in a 350° F. oven for 30 to 35 min. When done, slight imprint is left when top is touched. Cool slightly; cut into squares.
Yield: 16 2-in. squares

GALACTOSE-FREE RECIPES

The preparation of food for the galactose-free diet must be done without the use of milk and all dairy products. Other foods that can yield galactose when digested, and hence must be avoided, are cocoa, chocolate, beets, peas, lima beans, liver, sweetbreads, and brains.

Following are recipes taken with permission from the "Parent's Guide for the Galactose-Free Diet" prepared by The Bureau of Public Health Nutrition of the California State Department of Public Health, 2151 Berkeley Way, Berkeley, California.

---

[5]Sleisenger, M. H., et al.: A Wheat-, rye-, and oat-free diet. J. Am. Dietet. A., 33:1139, 1957.

Lemon Chiffon Dessert

2 egg yolks
1 cup sugar
$\frac{1}{2}$ teaspoon salt
$\frac{1}{2}$ cup lemon juice
1 teaspoon grated lemon rind
2 teaspoons gelatin softened in $\frac{1}{4}$ cup cold water
2 egg whites
    Procedure: Beat egg yolks, add $\frac{1}{2}$ cup sugar, salt and lemon juice. Cook and stir in double boiler until thick. Add gelatin and stir until it dissolves. Cool. When beginning to set, beat egg whites until stiff, add remaining sugar. Fold into mixture. Chill.
    Yield: 4 servings

Pineapple Muffins

1 slightly beaten egg
1 cup canned unsweetened pineapple juice
$\frac{1}{4}$ cup melted shortening
2 cups flour
$\frac{1}{2}$ teaspoon salt
4 teaspoons baking powder
$\frac{1}{4}$ cup sugar
    Procedure: Beat egg and pineapple juice; add shortening. Add flour sifted with salt, baking powder, and $\frac{1}{4}$ cup sugar; stir just until moistened. Fill greased muffin pans $\frac{2}{3}$ full. Sprinkle with 2 tablespoons sugar mixed with orange peel. Bake in hot oven (400°) 25 minutes.
    Yield: 2 muffins

Brown Betty

2 cups bread crumbs (milk-free)
3 tablespoons melted milk-free margarine
3 or 4 medium-sized apples
1 tablespoon lemon juice
$\frac{1}{2}$ teaspoon grated lemon peel
$\frac{1}{2}$ cup brown or granulated sugar
$\frac{1}{3}$ cup hot water
    Procedure: Combine crumbs and milk-free margarine; stir over low heat until lightly browned. Place $\frac{1}{3}$ in greased baking dish. Pare, core, and slice apples; arrange half in layer over crumbs. Sprinkle with half the lemon juice, lemon peel and sugar. Add second layer of crumbs and remaining apples, lemon juice, peel and sugar. Cover with remaining crumbs. Pour water over mixture. Bake in moderately hot oven (375°) until apples are tender, 30 to 40 minutes. Serve warm.
    Yield: 6 servings

Oatmeal Cookies

$\frac{3}{4}$ cup shortening
1 cup brown sugar
$\frac{1}{2}$ cup sugar
1 egg
$\frac{1}{4}$ cup water
1 teaspoon vanilla
1 cup flour
1 teaspoon salt
$\frac{1}{2}$ teaspoon soda
3 cups oatmeal
    Procedure: Combine first six ingredients and mix well. Add flour, salt and soda. Beat. Mix in oatmeal. Drop by teaspoonsful on ungreased cookie sheet. Bake at 350°, 12 to 15 minutes.
    Yield: About 4 dozen cookies

Ice Box Cookies

1 cup shortening
2 cups brown sugar
2 eggs
1 cup chopped walnuts
3 cups flour
1 teaspoon vanilla
1 teaspoon salt
1 teaspoon baking powder
$\frac{1}{2}$ teaspoon soda
    Procedure: Cream shortening and sugar. Add vanilla and eggs one at a time. Add nuts and flour mixed with baking powder and soda and beat well. Divide into rolls. Wrap in wax paper and store in refrigerator. Slice thin and bake in 350° oven. Bake 8 to 10 minutes.
    Yield: About 6 dozen cookies

Orange Delight Cake

$\frac{3}{4}$ cup shortening
$1\frac{1}{2}$ cups sugar
3 beaten egg yolks
$2\frac{1}{4}$ cups cake flour
$\frac{1}{2}$ teaspoon salt
$3\frac{1}{2}$ teaspoons baking powder
$\frac{3}{4}$ cup cold water
$\frac{1}{4}$ cup orange juice
1 tablespoon grated orange peel
3 stiffly beaten egg whites
    Procedure: Thoroughly cream shortening and sugar; add egg yolks and beat well. Add sifted dry ingredients alternately with water, orange juice and orange peel. Fold in egg whites. Bake in 2 waxed paper-lined 9-inch layer cake pans in moderate oven (350°) 30 to 35 minutes. Put together with Orange Filling. Frost with orange frosting, if desired.

Orange Filling

    Procedure: Mix 1 cup sugar, $\frac{1}{4}$ cup cornstarch and $\frac{1}{2}$ teaspoon salt; add $1\frac{1}{2}$ tablespoons lemon juice, 1 cup chopped orange segments, and 2 tablespoons grated orange peel. Cook in double boiler until thick. Remove from heat and add 2 tablespoons of milk-free margarine. Cool.

LOW PHENYLALANINE RECIPES

Low phenylalanine diets are based on foods that provide amino acids with little phenylalanine. Many foods usually made with milk can be made with a modified casein hydrolysate such as Lofenalac.[6]

Following are recipes taken with permission from "The Low Phenylalanine Diet," prepared by The Bureau of Public Health Nutrition of the California State Department of Public Health, 2151 Berkeley Way, Berkeley, California.

Ice Cream (Chocolate)

1 cup Lofenalac (dry)
$\frac{1}{2}$ cup water
5 tablespoons sugar
10 oz. Rich's topping

---

[6] Reproduced with permission of the Dietary Service and Department of Pediatrics, Loma Linda University, Los Angeles.

2 tablespoons Hershey's chocolate sauce
Procedure: Blend dry Lofenalac with water, sugar and chocolate sauce. Set mixture in freezer for 15 minutes or until slightly firm. Fold in Rich's topping with chocolate mixture. Place in pan and freeze until firm.
Yield: Approximately 5 ⅔ cup servings

Nutrients per serving (⅔ cup):
Protein	4.9 gm.
Calories	199
Phenylalanine	30 mg.
Fat	5.7 gm.
CHO	33.1 gm.

Ice Cream (Strawberry)

1 cup Lofenalac (dry)
½ cup water
4 tablespoons sugar
10 oz. Rich's Topping
1 tablespoon frozen strawberries
1 drop red food coloring
Procedure: Follow the mixing instructions as indicated for chocolate ice cream.
Yield: Approximately 5 ⅔ cup servings

Nutrients per serving (⅔ cup):
Protein	4.8 gm.
Calories	179
Phenylalanine	27 mg.
Fat	5.6 gm.
CHO	28.2 gm.

Biscuits or Shortcake

1 cup sifted cake flour (superfine)
1½ teaspoon baking powder
½ teaspoon salt
2 tablespoons oil
⅓ cup cold water
Procedure: Sift together flour, baking powder and salt. Combine oil and water. Pour slowly over entire surface of flour mixture. Mix with fork until soft dough is formed. Shape lightly with hands to make a round ball. Place on wax paper and knead lightly until smooth. Roll between 2 squares of wax paper and cut with 1½ inch cutter. Place on ungreased baking sheet. Bake in 450° F. oven 10-12 minutes. (Light buckwheat flour, light rye flour, or pastry flour may be substituted for the cake flour.)
Yield: 12 small biscuits

Nutrients per biscuit:
Protein	0.6 gm.
Calories	43.5
Phenylalanine	31 mg.
Fat	1.9 gm.
CHO	6.0 gm.

Lemon Pudding

9 tablespoons Lofenalac (dry)
1¼ cup boiling water
½ cup sugar
2 tablespoons cornstarch
⅛ teaspoon salt
1 tablespoon oil
1 teaspoon grated lemon rind
3 tablespoons lemon juice
Procedure: Mix Lofenalac and boiling water together with rotary beater until well blended. Combine sugar, cornstarch, and salt, and mix with liquid Lofenalac. Cook in double boiler until thickened. Add oil, lemon rind, and juice. Stir until well blended. Remove from heat and cool.
Yield: 3 ½ cup servings

Nutrients per serving (approximately ½ cup):
Protein	4.5 gm.
Calories	327.9
Phenylalanine	28.0 mg.
Fat	9.9 gm.
CHO	55.2 gm.

Chocolate Pudding

9 tablespoons Lofenalac (dry)
1½ cups boiling water
½ ounce chocolate, unsweetened
½ cup sugar
2 tablespoons cornstarch
⅛ teaspoon salt
1 tablespoon oil
1 teaspoon vanilla
Procedure: Mix Lofenalac and boiling water together with rotary beater until well blended. Place in double boiler. Add unsweetened chocolate to liquid Lofenalac. Heat until chocolate melts. Combine sugar, cornstarch, and salt, then mix with Lofenalac-chocolate mixture and cook until thickened. Add oil and vanilla and stir until well blended.
Yield: 3 ½ cup servings

Nutrients per serving (approximately ½ cup):
Protein	4.5 gm.
Calories	335.3
Phenylalanine	29.6 mg.
Fat	10.9 gm.
CHO	54.8 gm.

Tapioca Pudding

1 cup boiling water
2½ tablespoons quick-cooking tapioca
¼ cup sugar
⅛ teaspoon salt
6 tablespoons Lofenalac (dry)
½ teaspoon vanilla
Procedure: Stir water slowly into tapioca. Add sugar, salt, and Lofenalac. Mix until thoroughly blended. Cook over boiling water 12 minutes or until clear, stirring frequently. Cool. Add vanilla. Chill.
Yield: 2 servings.
Variations: Peach: Before chilling, stir in 2½ tablespoons junior peaches. Pineapple: Before chilling, stir in ¼ cup drained crushed pineapple.

Nutrients per serving (approximately ½ cup):
	Vanilla	Peach	Pineapple
Protein	4.5 gm.	4.5 gm.	4.5 gm.
Calories	273.5	312.5	312.5
Phenylalanine	22.5 mg.	32.7 mg.	34.2 mg.
Fat	5.1 gm.	5.1 gm.	5.1 gm.
CHO	52.4 gm.	61.9 gm.	61.9 gm.

Vanilla Pudding and Banana Pudding

11 tablespoons Lofenalac (dry)
1½ cups boiling water
½ cup sugar
2 tablespoons cornstarch
⅛ teaspoon salt
1 tablespoon oil
2 teaspoons vanilla
1 teaspoon lemon juice
Procedure: Mix Lofenalac and boiling water together with rotary beater until well blended. Combine sugar, cornstarch, and salt; mix with Lofenalac. Cook in double boiler until thickened. Add oil, vanilla, and lemon juice. Stir until well blended. Remove from heat and cool.

Yield: 3 ½ cup servings

Variation: Banana: Follow above recipe substituting 1 teaspoon banana flavor and 2 tablespoons mashed banana for the vanilla.

Nutrients per serving (approximately ½ cup):

	Vanilla	Banana
Protein	5.2 gm.	5.7 gm.
Calories	349.2	353.6
Phenylalanine	29.0 mg.	31.0 mg.
Fat	10.8 gm.	10.8 gm.
CHO	57.8 gm.	58.4 gm.

Commercial Pudding Mixes

Various pudding mixes on the market which require cooking may be used by substituting double strength (8 tablespoons to 1 cup water) Lofenalac in place of the milk ordinarily used. A ½-cup serving gives 30 mg. of phenylalanine. These mixes should not contain gelatin, flour, milk or eggs.

Plain Cake

4 tablespoons fat (oil or margarine)
½ cup sugar
½ cup plus 1 tablespoon Lofenalac, liquid
1 cup cake flour
3 teaspoons baking powder
¼ teaspoon salt
½ teaspoon vanilla

Procedure: Sift dry ingredients together. Cream fat, add sugar, mix well. Add liquid, dry ingredients and vanilla. Bake in greased pan (9″ × 9″ × 2″) or muffin pans at 375° for 25 to 30 minutes.

Yield: 12 cupcakes.

Nutrients per cup cake or 1/12 of cake:

Protein	1.1 gm.
Calories	117
Phenylalanine	30 mg.
Fat	5.4 gm.
CHO	16.4 gm.

Rice Flour Cookies

½ cup cornstarch
½ cup confectioner's sugar
1 cup rice flour, white
¼ teaspoon salt
1 cup butter or oil
¼ teaspoon vanilla

Procedure: Sift together cornstarch, sugar, flour and salt. Blend room temperature butter (or oil) into dry ingredients with fork until a soft ball is formed. Shape into small balls with hands. Place on ungreased baking sheet about 1½ inches apart. Flatten cookies with fork. Bake in 300° F. oven for 20 to 25 minutes.

Yield: about 2 dozen small cookies.

Nutrients per cookie:

Protein	0.3 gm.
Calories	74.2
Phenylalanine	14.7 mg.
Fat	5.0 gm.
CHO	7.0 gm.

(If oil is used, phenylalanine content is slightly decreased.)

Lemon Sauce

½ cup sugar
1½ tablespoons cornstarch
¼ teaspoon salt
5 tablespoons Lofenalac (dry)
1½ cups boiling water
2 tablespoons oil
3 tablespoons lemon juice
2 teaspoons grated lemon rind

Procedure: Mix together sugar, cornstarch, salt and dry Lofenalac. Gradually add water to above ingredients. Cook over medium heat, stirring constantly until sauce thickens and comes to boil. Boil 2 minutes. Remove from heat and add oil, lemon juice, and lemon rind.

Yield: About 2 cups (use as topping for puddings)

Nutrients per serving (2 tbsp.):

Protein	0.5 gm.
Calories	57.5
Phenylalanine	3.1 mg.
Fat	2.3 gm.
CHO	8.7 gm.

White Sauce

3 tablespoons oil
2 tablespoons cornstarch
1 teaspoon salt
½ cup Lofenalac (dry)
2 cups warm water

Procedure: Place oil in saucepan. Add cornstarch and salt and blend well. Mix together Lofenalac and water using rotary beater to blend well. Add to oil-cornstarch-salt mixture and cook until thickened.

Yield: About 2 cups white sauce.

Variation: Two tablespoons of chopped parsley may be added for variety. White sauce is useful in preparation of a variety of creamed vegetables, etc.

Nutrients per serving (2 tbsp.):

Protein	0.7 gm.
Calories	48.7
Phenylalanine	4.0 mg.
Fat	3.5 gm.
CHO	3.6 gm.

HIGH PROTEIN RECIPES

The need for additional dietary protein in certain disease states and conditions has received increased recognition. Following are some concentrated supplementary agents to increase the protein intake.

Protein supplements such as dry skim milk, dried egg (whole or white) and commercial preparations can be added in varying amounts to fruit juice, milk and soups, to increase protein consumption in an easy-to-take form. Many patients, who find it difficult or impossible to eat solid food, can be easily induced to consume 25 gm. of protein, or more, in a beverage flavored to taste and served hot or cold. As shown in Table 43–1, protein supplements having low sodium content are now available for use in sodium-restricted diets.

Macaroni and Cheese with Casec

1 package macaroni
1 heaping tablespoon butter
½ cup Casec
1 egg
⅓ pound cheese, fairly sharp
1 cup milk

TABLE 43–1   APPROXIMATE VALUES OF SOME PROTEIN SUPPLEMENTS COMMONLY USED

SUPPLEMENT	PROTEIN %	FAT %	CARBO-HYDRATE %
Alacta	32.5	8.0	46.3
Amigens	75.0	—	—
Aminoids	43.3	—	43.0
Brewer's yeast	50.0	—	40.0
Casec	88.0	2.0	—
Dryco	31.0	7.7	45.5
Klim	26.2	27.5	37.5
Kralex*	13.2	0.11	7.7
Lonalac*	27.0	28.0	38.0
Meritene	33.0	0.2	58.4
Metracal	30	9	50
Nutramigen	15	15	54
Peanut flour	55.0	?	?
Powdered egg, whole	47.0	42.0	3.0
Powdered skim milk	35.6	1.0	52.0
Powdered whole milk	27.3	26.0	35.8
Protenum	42.0	2.0	46.0
Protinal*			
Provimalt	57.0	1.0	26.1
Sobee	32.0	20.0	38.0
Soy flour	50.0	—	50.0
Sustagen	23.5	3.5	66.5

*Low in sodium content.

Procedure: 1. Cook macaroni as directed on package. While it is still hot, stir in butter, Casec beaten into milk, and well beaten egg. Mix well. 2. Stir in cheese, cut fine. 3. Pour into greased casserole, and bake in oven (425° F.) until brown on top.

Yield: 4 servings; protein, 27 gm. per serving.

DESSERTS

Baked Custard

¹/₂ cup milk
1 egg
2 tablespoons skim milk powder
1 teaspoon sugar
  Few drops vanilla
  Nutmeg
  Procedure: 1. Beat egg and add sugar and skim milk powder. Mix well. 2. Stir in hot milk and vanilla. 3. Pour into custard cup and sprinkle with nutmeg. 4. Bake according to directions for baked custard (p. 569).
  Yield: 1 serving; protein, 12 gm.

Tapioca Cream

1¹/₂ tablespoons tapioca (minute)
  2 cups milk, scalded
  2 eggs, separated
  3 tablespoons sugar
  1 teaspoon vanilla
  4 tablespoons vanilla Dietene
  Procedure: 1. Scald milk in double boiler. 2. Separate eggs and beat yolks slightly. 3. Blend sugar and Dietene into egg yolks. 4. Add the minute tapioca and blend well. 5. Add the scalded milk. 6. Return to double boiler and cook over slow heat, stirring constantly until mixture thickens and coats the spoon. 7. Remove from heat and cool. 8. When cool, add vanilla and fold in stiffly beaten egg whites. 9. Divide into four equal portions.

Yield: 4 servings; protein, 11 gm. per serving.
(From Suggested Recipes and Formulas for High Protein Diets, p. 7.)

SUGGESTED WAYS TO USE PROTEIN SUPPLEMENTS

1. Include in meat, egg, and cheese dishes.
2. Add to gravies, sauces, and salad dressings used with meat and vegetables.
3. Stir into cooked cereals, mashed potatoes, squash, etc.
4. Mix with milk, eggs, and flavorings in beverages to be served hot or cold.
5. Incorporate in custards and other simple desserts.

The recipes which follow may be used as a guide in combining protein supplements with other ingredients. The various drug and chemical companies, manufacturers of protein supplements, have additional suggestions and recipes in pamphlets which accompany their products.

BEVERAGES

Special Casec Chocolate Milk

8 ounces milk
2 eggs
2 tablespoons sugar
4 tablespoons Casec
1 scoop vanilla ice cream
1 tablespoon cocoa
1 teaspoon vanilla
2 teaspoons lactose
  Procedure: Add milk slowly to Casec to make a smooth paste. Beat in the eggs, sugar, lactose, ice cream, and vanilla.
  Yield: 1 serving; protein, 43 gm.

Casec Chocolate Milk

5 ounces milk
4 tablespoons Casec
1 ounce chocolate syrup
¹/₂ teaspoon vanilla
  Procedure: Add milk slowly to Casec to make a smooth paste. Add syrup and vanilla. Mix thoroughly.
  Yield: 1 serving; protein, 22 gm.

Eggnog with Casec

3 ounces milk
2 tablespoons sugar
1 egg
3 level tablespoons, packed, Casec
  Nutmeg and vanilla
  Procedure: 1. Beat egg thoroughly with rotary beater or in blender; beat in sugar and Casec. 2. Add milk and vanilla; beat well. 3. Pour in glass, top with nutmeg. Serve very cold.
  Yield: 1 serving; protein, 21 gm.

Banana Skimmed Milk Drink

¹/₂ medium banana
6 ounces skim milk
1 level tablespoon, packed, Casec
1 teaspoon sugar

Procedure: 1. Dissolve Casec and sugar in skim milk.
2. Mash banana with fork and beat into skim milk mixture
with egg beater or in blender.
Yield: 1 serving; protein, 11 gm.

OTHER FORTIFIED BEVERAGES

To supply additional nutrients and protective substances, milk can be fortified with
additional sugar, syrup, proteins (such as
egg, dry milk, or undiluted evaporated milk),
protein hydrolysates, and vitamins.

COOKERY SUGGESTIONS 1. If cane
sugar is added, dissolve in cold liquid before
blending with other ingredients.

2. If glucose is added, dissolve in warm
liquid before blending with other ingredients.
The amount of sweetening is calculated on a
percentage basis and according to the diet
prescription.

3. If lactose is added, dissolve in hot
liquid before blending with other ingredients.

4. If Dextri-maltose is added, dissolve in
hot liquid before blending with other ingredients.

5. Powdered milk is mixed with dry ingredients, and then the cold liquid is stirred in.

6. Evaporated milk is used undiluted and
the procedure given in the recipe followed.

7. Whole egg, egg yolk, or egg white is
beaten before blending with other ingredients.

8. Brewer's yeast is sprinkled over the top
of milk and then the mixture is beaten with
a rotary beater.

9. The protein hydrolysates are added according to the directions on the package.

10. If instant breakfast mixes or other
mixes are used, follow directions on package.

Koumyss

1 quart whole milk
1½ tablespoons sugar
⅕ compressed yeast cake
¼ cup boiled water cooled to lukewarm
Procedure: 1. Scald milk in saucepan or double boiler
and then reduce the temperature of milk to 80° F. 2. Stir
in sugar. Dissolve yeast in warm water. Add dissolved
yeast to milk. 3. In the meantime wash and sterilize 4 or
more bottles fitted with corks or patent stoppers. Pour
milk into bottles filling to within two inches from top.
Cork and tie string around each cork to hold firmly to
bottle. Shake bottles. Place the bottles in a warm place
for six hours, then store in the refrigerator and serve
when needed.

Peptonized Milk

½ cup boiled water
1 peptonizing powder:
    5 grains pancreatin and
    15 grains sodium bicarbonate
2 cups milk
Procedure: 1. Mix peptonizing powder in boiled water.
Pour into a sterilized one-quart jar which is fitted with a
cover. 2. Add milk and mix thoroughly. Adjust cover
tightly and shake jar. 3. Set the jar in a warm water bath,

115° F., for 10 minutes. 4. Remove the jar from water
bath and refrigerate immediately. Serve when needed.

Albumen Beverage

1 egg white
½ cup water
1 teaspoon strained lemon juice, if desired
Procedure: 1. Whip together egg white and water using
a rotary beater. 2. Add lemon juice, if desired. 3. Strain into
beverage glass. Serve immediately.
Yield: 1 serving

Milk Albumen Beverage

1 egg white
½ cup milk
Procedure: 1. Whip together egg white and milk using
a rotary beater. 2. Strain into a beverage glass. Serve
immediately.
Yield: 1 serving

MAIN DISHES

Baked Soybeans

1 cup precooked soybeans
½ cup tomato sauce
½ cup onions
1 teaspoon salt
½ teaspoon pepper
¼ pound salt pork
Procedure: 1. Pour tomato sauce over precooked beans;
add onions, salt and pepper. 2. Lay strips of salt pork over
beans and bake for one hour in a moderate oven.
Yield: 1 serving; protein, 15 gm.
(From Suggested Recipes and Formulas for High Protein
Diets. Diet Therapy Section, 1944–45, page 9, The American Dietetic Association, 620 North Michigan Ave.,
Chicago, Illinois, 60611.)

Beef Patty

3 ounces ground round steak
2 level tablespoons, packed, skim milk powder
Salt and pepper
Procedure: 1. Combine ingredients and form into a
patty. 2. Broil as directed for pan-broiled beef patty (p. 573).
Yield: 1 serving; protein, 25 gm.

Scrambled Eggs

2 eggs
¼ cup milk
2 level tablespoons, packed, Casec
2 tablespoons green pepper, cut fine
¼ small onion, cut fine
Salt and pepper
Procedure: 1. Beat Casec into milk with rotary beater.
2. Combine remaining ingredients; beat lightly. 3. Pour
into greased pan, and cook slowly over low heat, stirring
constantly.
Yield: 1 serving; protein, 23 gm.

Meat Loaf with Casec

1 pound lean ground beef, round or chuck
1 cup Casec
12 thin crackers, rolled fine
1 medium onion, finely chopped

1 teaspoon sage
2 teaspoons Worcestershire sauce
1 tablespoon ketchup
1 teaspoon salt
¼ teaspoon chili powder
    Black pepper, as desired
1 cup water
Procedure: 1. Mix meat and Casec thoroughly. 2. Add all other ingredients except water, and mix well. 3, Add water. Shape into loaf. 4. Bake in open greased pan for 1 to 1½ hours at 350° F.
    Yield: 6 servings; protein, 27 gm. per serving.
    Procedure: 1. Dissolve Casec and sugar in skim milk. 2. Mash banana with fork and beat into skim milk mixture with egg beater or in blender.
    Yield: 1 serving; protein, 11 gm.

LOW PROTEIN BREAD RECIPES

The following recipes are low in protein and sodium. They are used in dietaries limited in protein and in sodium to provide calories and variety.

YEAST-LEAVENED, LOW-PROTEIN, LOW-ELECTROLYTE BREAD*

RECIPE FOR HOME PREPARATION

INGREDIENT	WEIGHT	MEASURE
Yeast, active dry (Fleisch- mann's)	4 gm.	1½ tsp.
Sugar, granulated	25 gm.	2 Tbsp.
Water, distilled	480 gm.	2 c.
Methyl cellulose (Dow Chemical Methocel 4,000 cps. HG65)	5 gm.	3 tsp.
Margarine, unsalted (fat portion only) (Fleisch- mann's)	120 gm.	⅔ c.
Wheat starch (Cellu, Chicago Dietetic Supply House)	630 gm.	4⅔ c.

PROCEDURE:
    1. Add yeast and ½ tsp. sugar to 2 Tbsp. water (105°F.). Let stand for 10 min.
    2. Melt margarine, then heat to rapid boil (for easy separation of fat and milky sediment). Cool to 100°F. Separate fat and sediment and discard sediment.
    3. Heat remaining water to boiling; add methyl cellulose and blend with wire whip. Pour into mixing bowl and cool to 115°F. or until it begins to form colloidal solution. Stir frequently.
    4. Add wheat starch and remaining sugar; blend with spoon.
    5. Add margarine fat and blend.
    6. Add yeast mixture and blend with electric mixer at low speed for 6 to 8 min. Guide batter into beaters and scrape sides and bottom of mixing bowl with rubber spatula.
    7. Divide batter into two 8 by 4 by 2¼ in. loaf pans greased with liquid margarine fat. Smooth top of batter and spread 2 tsp. liquid margarine evenly over top.
    8. Cover pans with foil and let rise in warm (90°F.) place for approximately 1½ to 2 hr., or until batter reaches top edge of pan. Remove foil.

*J. Am. Dietet. A., 56:522, 1970.

    9. Place in oven preheated to 350°F. Bake for 5 min.; turn temperature to 525°F.; bake for 25 min.
    10. Remove pans from oven; remove bread from pans and cool on wire rack.
    Yield: 2 loaves

LOW PROTEIN BREAD*

1 tbsp. sugar	1 tsp. salt
1¼ cups warm water (100°F.)	2¾ cups DPP Wheat Starch
1 pkg. dry active yeast	¼ cup hydrogenated shortening
3 tbsp. sugar	
½ tsp. double-acting baking powder	

Grease loaf pan, 9 × 5 × 2¾″ or 8½ × 4½ × 2⅝″; set aside. Place 1 tbsp. sugar and water in a large mixer bowl. Add yeast and stir until dissolved; let stand 5 minutes. Add dry ingredients and shortening. Beat at low speed, scraping sides of bowl until ingredients are moistened; then beat 1 minute at high speed, scraping sides of bowl with rubber spatula. Pour into greased loaf pan. Cover with towel and let stand at room temperature for 30 minutes. Heat oven to 425°. Bake 25 to 30 minutes or until golden brown. **Yield: approximately 27 slices (³⁄₈″ thick).** Weight per slice: Approximately 23 gm.

Important!! Add 1 to 2 tbsp. water if bread mixture is like biscuit dough. Add 1 or 2 tbsp. DPP Wheat Starch if bread mixture is like pancake batter.

LOW SODIUM, LOW PROTEIN BREAD

Use recipe above except omit the salt and baking powder.

PER SLICE	REGULAR	LOW SODIUM
Calories	80	80
Pro., gm.	.2	.2
CHO., gm.	15	15
Na, mg.	95	7
K, mg.	7	8
Phenylalanine, mg.	9	

NOTE: A few drops of yellow food color enhance the appearance of this bread.

GINGERBREAD†

½ cup soft butter	1 tsp. soda
2 tbsp. sugar	1 tsp. ginger
¾ cup mild molasses	1 tsp. cinnamon
2¼ cups DPP Wheat Starch	2 tbsp. boiling water

Heat oven to 325°. Grease and dust with DPP Wheat Starch a square pan, 9 × 9 × 1¾″. Thoroughly mix butter, sugar and molasses. Blend in dry ingredients and beat until smooth. Add water and beat until smooth. Spread into pan. Bake 40–45 minutes. Serve while still warm. **Yield: 16 servings.**

LOW SODIUM GINGERBREAD

Use recipe above except for the butter. Substitute **unsalted** butter for the regular butter.

---

*Dietetic Paygel-P Wheat Starch, General Mills.
    †*Ibid.*

Serve Lemon Pudding as a topping, if desired.

PER PIECE	REGULAR	LOW SODIUM
Calories	169	169
Pro., gm.	.1	.1
CHO., gm.	30	30
Na, mg.	150	81
K, mg.	145	144
Phenylalanine, mg.	5.7	

Na, mg.	124	9	113	10
K, mg.	10	170	19	260
Phenylal- anine, mg.	23.5		63.1	

CRUNCHY HERB TOAST

Heat oven to 500°.

Cut Low Protein Bread into slices about ⅜″ thick. Place bread slices on baking sheet and put in oven for 3 minutes or until bread is dry but not brown. Remove from oven. Turn bread slice over and spread with butter; then sprinkle with a favorite herb or seasoning. Toast in oven for 4 minutes or until browned.

Suggested herbs and seasonings: onion powder, garlic powder, toasted sesame seed, poppy seed, dill weed, anise seed, caraway seed.

BLUEBERRY MUFFINS*

¼ cup butter	¾ cup plus 2 tbsp. DPP
½ cup sugar	Wheat Starch
3 tbsp. water	1 egg white, stiffly beaten
½ tsp. vanilla	½ cup blueberries,
2 tsp. double-acting	thawed and drained
baking powder	or fresh

Heat oven to 375°. Cream butter and sugar. Add water and vanilla. Add dry ingredients and mix thoroughly. Fold in beaten egg white and then gently fold in blueberries. Pour batter into greased muffin pans. Bake 20 minutes. **Yield: 12 muffins.**

LOW SODIUM BLUEBERRY MUFFINS

Use recipe above except substitute **unsalted** butter and **sodium free** baking powder for regular butter and baking powder.

CORNMEAL MUFFINS

1 cup boiling water	3 tsp. double-acting
1 cup cornmeal	baking powder
¼ cup melted hydro-	or 4½ tsp. sodium-free
genated shortening	baking powder
¼ cup sugar	1 egg white,
1 cup DPP Wheat Starch	stiffly beaten

Heat oven to 400°. Add boiling water to cornmeal and let stand 15 minutes. Add shortening, sugar, DPP Wheat Starch and baking powder and beat. Fold in egg white. Drop batter into paper cups or greased muffin pans. Bake 20 minutes. **Yield: 12 muffins.**

	BLUEBERRY		CORNMEAL	
PER MUFFIN	REGULAR	LOW SODIUM	REGULAR	LOW SODIUM
Calories	109	109	147	147
Pro., gm.	.4	.4	1.3	1.3
CHO., gm.	18.9	18.9	24.5	24.5

*Dietetic Paygel-P Wheat Starch, General Mills.

REFERENCES

Allergy Diets. Ralston Purina Company.

Allergy Recipes. 1969, The American Dietetic Association, 620 North Michigan Avenue, Chicago, Illinois, 60611.

Behrman, Deaconess M.: A Cookbook for Diabetics. American Diabetes Association, Inc., 18 East 48th Street, New York, N.Y.

Cavanna, E., and Welton, J.: Gourmet Cookery for a Low Fat Diet. Englewood Cliffs, N. J. Prentice-Hall, Inc. Revised 1961.

Cellu Products. The Chicago Dietetic Supply House, 1750 West VanBuren Street, Chicago, Ill.

Conrad, M. L.: Allergy Cooking. New York, Thomas Y. Crowell Company, 1955.

Council on Foods and Nutrition: Artificial Sweeteners. J.A.M.A., 160:875, 1956.

Dietetic Paygel-P Wheat Starch, General Mills, Inc., Nutrition Service Department 5, Minneapolis, Minn. 55440.

Field, F.: Gourmet Cooking for Cardiac Diets. New York, Collier Books, 1962.

Hasker, R. R.: The Cook Book for Low Sodium Diet. Boston, Massachusetts Heart Association, 1955.

High Protein Recipes. Mead Johnson and Company, Evansville, Ind.

Jolliffe, N., Family Circle's Reducing Diet Guide. New York, Simon and Schuster, Inc., 1955.

Keyes, A., and Keyes, M.: Eat Well and Stay Well. Garden City, N.Y., Doubleday and Company, Inc., 1959.

Low Gluten Diet with Recipes. Department of Dietetics, University Hospital, University of Michigan, Ann Arbor, Michigan (50 cents).

Meal Planning with Exchange Lists. New York, American Diabetes Association, Inc., 18 East 48th Street, New York. The American Dietetic Association, 620 North Michigan Ave., Chicago (25 cents).

Nilson, B.: Cooking for Special Diets. Baltimore, Penguin Books, Inc., 1964.

Parent's Guide for the Galactose-free Diet. California State Department of Public Health, 2151 Berkeley Way, Berkeley, California.

Payne, A. S., and Callahan, D.: The Low Sodium—Fat Controlled Cookbook. Boston, Little, Brown and Company, 1960.

Planning Fat Controlled Meals for Unrestricted Calories; Planning Fat Controlled Meals for 1200 and 1800 Calories. Available from local Heart Association or from the American Heart Association, 44 East 23rd Street, New York 10010, New York.

Revell, D.: Cholesterol Control Cookery. New York, Carelton Publishing Company, 1961.

Rosenthal, S.: Live High on a Low Fat Diet. Philadelphia, J. B. Lippincott Company, 1962.

Sleisenger, M. H., et al.: A Wheat, Rye and Oat Free Diet. American Dietetic Association, 620 North Michigan Avenue, Chicago (15 cents).

Stead, E. S., and Warren, G. K.: Low-Fat Cookery. New York, McGraw-Hill Book Co., 1959.

Strachan, C. B.: The Diabetic's Cookbook. Houston, Texas. The Medical Arts Publishing Foundation, 1955.

Swank, R. L., and Grimsgaard, A.: Low Fat Diet. Reasons, Rules and Recipes. Eugene, Oregon, University of Oregon Books, 1959.

The Low Phenylalanine Diet. State of California Department of Public Health, 2151 Berkeley Way, Berkeley, California.

Waldo, M.: Cooking for Your Heart and Health. New York, G. P. Putnam's Sons, 1961.

West, B. M.: Diabetic Menus, Meals and Recipes. Garden City, N.Y. Doubleday and Company, Inc., 1959.

APPENDIX

GENERAL REFERENCES

PART I. BOOKS

Anderson, L., and Browe, J. H.: Nutrition and Family Health Service. Philadelphia, W. B. Saunders Company, 1960.

Beaton, G., and McHenry, E. (eds.): Nutrition: A Comprehensive Treatise. New York, Academic Press, 1964–1966.

Bogert, L. J.: Nutrition and Physical Fitness. 8th ed. Philadelphia, W. B. Saunders Company, 1966.

Bondy, P. K.: Diseases of Metabolism. 6th ed. Philadelphia, W. B. Saunders Company, 1969.

Brennan, R.: Nutrition. Dubuque, Iowa, Wm. C. Brown Company, 1967.

Burgess, A., (ed.): Malnutrition and Food Habits. New York, Macmillan Company, 1962.

Burton, B. R. (ed.): The Heinz Handbook of Nutrition. 2nd ed. New York, McGraw-Hill Book Company, Inc., 1965.

Church, C. F., and Church, H. N.: Food Values of Portions Commonly Used. 11th ed. Philadelphia, J. B. Lippincott Company, 1970.

Composition of Foods – Raw, Processed, Prepared. Agriculture Handbook No. 8, U.S. Department of Agriculture, Washington, D.C., 1963.

Deutsch, R. M.: The Nuts Among the Berries. Revised edition. New York, Ballantine Books, Inc., 1967.

———: The Family Guide to Better Food and Better Health. Des Moines, Iowa, Meredith Company, 1971.

Donahoe, V.: Diabetic Cooking Made Easy. Minneapolis, Education for Health, Inc., 1965.

Duncan, G. G.: A Modern Pilgrim's Progress for Diabetics. 2nd ed. Philadelphia, W. B. Saunders Company, 1967.

Eppright, E., Pattison, M., and Barbour, H.: Teaching Nutrition. 2nd ed. Ames, Iowa; The Iowa State University Press, 1963.

Fleck, H., and Munves, E. D.: Everybody's Book of Modern Diet and Nutrition. 2nd ed. New York, Dell Publishing Company, 1959.

———, ———: Introduction to Nutrition. 2nd ed. New York, The Macmillan Company, 1971.

Fomon, S. J.: Infant Nutrition. Philadelphia, W. B. Saunders Company, 1967.

Food, The Yearbook of Agriculture, 1959. U.S. Department of Agriculture, Washington, D.C.

Godshall, F. R.: Nutrition in Elementary School. New York, Harper and Bros., 1958.

Goldsmith, G. A.: Nutritional Diagnosis. Springfield, Illinois, Charles C Thomas, 1959.

Goodhart, R., and Wohl, M.: Manual of Clinical Nutrition. Philadelphia, Lea and Febiger, 1968.

Gutherie, H.: Introductory Nutrition. 2nd ed. St. Louis, Missouri, The C. V. Mosby Company, 1971.

Guyton, A. C.: Textbook of Medical Physiology. 4th ed. Philadelphia, W. B. Saunders Company, 1971.

Hayes, J. (ed.): Food For Us All. Yearbook of Agriculture, U.S. Department of Agriculture, Washington, D.C., 1969.

Holt, L. E., Jr., and McIntosh, R.: Holt Pediatrics. 13th ed. New York, Appleton-Century-Crofts, Inc., 1961.

Jelliffe, D. B.: Child Nutrition in Developing Countries. Public Health Service Publication No. 1822, Washington, D.C., U.S. Government Printing Office.

Jolliffe, N. (ed.): Handbook of Clinical Nutrition. 2nd ed. New York, Paul B. Hoeber Medical Book Division, Harper & Brothers, 1962.

King, C. G.: Food for Family Fitness. New York, The Nutrition Foundation, Inc., 1962.

Klinger, J. L., et al.: Mealtime Manual for the Aged and Handicapped. New York, Simon and Schuster Inc., 1970.

Leverton, R. N.: Food Becomes You. 3rd ed. Ames, Iowa, Iowa State University Press, 1965.

Lowenberg, M., et al.: Food and Man. New York, John Wiley & Sons, Inc., 1968.

Maddox, G.: Slim Down, Shape Up Diets for Teenagers. New York, Avon Book Division, Hearst Corp., 1963.

Marlow, D. R.: Textbook of Pediatric Nursing. 3rd ed. Philadelphia, W. B. Saunders Company, 1969.

Martin, E. A.: Nutrition Education in Action – A Guide for Teachers. New York, Holt, Rinehart and Winston, 1963.

———: Nutrition in Action, 2nd ed. New York, Holt, Rinehart and Winston, 1965.

———: Robert's Nutrition Work with Children. Chicago, University of Chicago Press, 1967.

Mayo Clinic Diet Manual. 4th ed. (The Committee on Dietetics of the Mayo Clinic.) Philadelphia, W. B. Saunders Company, 1971.

Mazur, A., and Harrow, B.: Textbook of Biochemistry. 10th ed. Philadelphia, W. B. Saunders Company, 1971.

McCollum, E. V.: A History of Nutrition. Boston, Houghton Mifflin Company, 1957.

McGilvery, R. W.: Biochemistry – A Functional Approach. Philadelphia, W. B. Saunders Company, 1970.

McHenry, E. W.: Basic Nutrition. 2nd ed. Philadelphia, J. B. Lippincott Company, 1963.

McHenry, W. F.: Foods Without Fads. Philadelphia, J. B. Lippincott Company, 1960.

McWilliams, M.: Nutrition for the Growing Years. New York, John Wiley and Sons, Inc., 1967.

Milner, M. (ed.): Protein-Enriched Cereal Foods for World Needs. St. Paul, Minnesota, Association of American Cereal Chemists, 1969.

Mitchell, H., et al.: Cooper's Nutrition in Health and Disease. 15 ed. Philadelphia, J. B. Lippincott Company, 1968.

———: Recommended and Nonrecommended Nutrition Books for Lay Readers. Massachusetts Dept. of Public Health, 1964.

National Research Council Committee on Maternal Nutrition: Maternal Nutrition and the Course of Pregnancy. Food and Nutrition Board, National Academy of Sciences, Washington, D.C., 1970.

Orr, M. L.: Pantothenic Acid, Vitamin B_6 and Vitamin B_{12} in Foods. Home Economics Research Report No. 36, Agricultural Research Service, U.S. Department of Agriculture, 1969.

Peyton, A. B.: Practical Nutrition. Philadelphia, J. B. Lippincott Company, 1962.

Pike, R., and Brown, M.: Nutrition: An Integrated Approach. New York, John Wiley and Sons, Inc., 1967.

Present Knowledge in Nutrition. 3rd ed. New York, Nutrition Reviews Editorial Staff and Advisory Board, The Nutrition Foundation, Inc., 1967.

Recommended Dietary Allowances. 7th revised ed. Washington, D.C., Food and Nutrition Board, National Academy of Sciences-National Research Council, Publication No. 1694, 1968.

Robinson, C.: Proudfit-Robinson's Normal and Therapeutic Nutrition. 11th ed. New York, The Macmillan Company, 1967.

Robinson, C.: Basic Nutrition and Diet Therapy. 2nd ed. New York, The Macmillan Company, 1970.

Schmitt, C.: Diabetes for Diabetics. Miami, Florida, Diabetes Press of America, 1968.

Scrimshaw, N., and Gordon, J., (eds.): Malnutrition, Learning and Behavior. Cambridge, Massachusetts, Massachusetts Institute of Technology Press, 1967.

Sense, E.: Clinical Studies in Nutrition. Philadelphia, J. B. Lippincott Company, 1960.

Shearman, C. W.: Diets Are for People. New York, Appleton-Century-Crofts, Inc., 1963.

Simoons, F. J.: Eat Not This Flesh. Madison, University of Wisconsin Press, 1961.

Smith, R. L.: The Health Hucksters. New York, Thomas Y. Crowell Company, 1960.

Turner, D.: Handbook of Diet Therapy. 5th ed. Chicago, University of Chicago Press, 1970.

Williams, R. D.: Alcoholism: The Nutritional Approach. Austin, Texas, University of Texas Press, 1959.

Williams, R. D.: You Are Extraordinary. New York, John Wiley and Sons, Inc., 1967.

Williams, R. H.: Textbook of Endocrinology. 4th ed. Philadelphia, W. B. Saunders Company, 1968.

Williams, R. J.: Biochemical Individuality. New York, John Wiley and Sons, Inc., 1956.

Williams, S. R.: Nutrition and Diet Therapy. St. Louis, The C. V. Mosby Company, 1969.

Wilson, E. D., Fisher, K. H., and Fuqua, M. E.: Principles of Nutrition. 2nd ed. New York, John Wiley and Sons, Inc., 1967.

Wohl, M. G., and Goodhart, R. S.: Modern Nutrition in Health and Disease—Dietotherapy. 3rd ed. Philadelphia, Lea and Febiger, 1964.

————: The Problem of Changing Food Habits. Washington, D.C., National Academy of Sciences, National Research Council. Bulleton No. 108, October, 1943.

————: Manual for the Study of Food Habits. Washington, D.C., National Academy of Sciences, National Research Council. Bulletin No. 11, January, 1945.

————: Control of Malnutrition in Man. New York, American Public Health Association, Inc., 1960.

————: Report by UNICEF: Children of the Developing Countries. Cleveland, The World Publishing Company, 1963.

————: Family Food Plans. Revised edition. Hyattsville, Maryland, Agricultural Research Service Consumer and Food Economics Research Division, U.S. Department of Agriculture, 1964.

————: Western Hemisphere Nutrition Conference. Chicago, American Medical Association, 1965.

————: Obesity and Health: A Sourcebook of Current Information for Professional Health Personnel. Arlington, Virginia, U.S. Public Health Service, National Center for Chronic Disease Control, 1966.

Young, J.: The Medical Messiahs: A Social History of Health Quackery in Twentieth Century America. Princeton, New Jersey, Princeton University Press, 1967.

————: Hearings before the Select Committee on Nutrition and Human Needs of the United States Senate, Washington, D.C., 1968, 1969, 1970, 1971.

————: White House Conference on Food, Nutrition and Health. Washington, D.C., U.S. Government Printing Office, 1970.

————: Western Hemisphere Nutrition Conference, Chicago, American Medical Association, 1971.

PART II. JOURNALS

American Journal of Nursing
American Journal of Public Health
Borden's Review of Nutrition Research
Dairy Council Digest
Journal of the American Dietetic Association
Journal of Nutrition Education
Nursing Outlook
Nutrition Review
Nutrition Today
The American Journal of Clinical Nutrition
Today's Health
World Health

PART III. RELIABLE RESOURCES FOR NUTRITION INFORMATION AND VISUAL AID

American Can Company, 730 Park Avenue, New York 10017.

American Diabetes Association, 18 E. 48th Street, New York 10017.

American Dietetic Association, 620 N. Michigan Avenue, Chicago, Illinois 60611.

American Heart Association, 44 E. 23rd Street, New York 10010.

American Home Economics Association, 1600 20th Street N. W., Washington, D.C. 20009.

American Institute of Baking, Consumer Service Department, 400 E. Ontario Street, Chicago, Illinois 60611

Borden Company, 350 Madison Avenue, New York 10017.

Cereal Institute, Inc., 135 South LaSalle Street, Chicago, Illinois 60603.

Cooperative Extension Work in Agriculture and Home Economics, Cooperative Extension Services of States. (Contact the services of the State in which you reside.)

Council on Food and Nutrition, American Medical Association, 535 N. Dearborn Street, Chicago, Illinois 60610.

Evaporated Milk Association, 228 North LaSalle Street, Chicago, Illinois 60601.

Extension Service, Department of Home Economics, State Colleges and Universities.

Federal Trade Commission, Bureau of Investigation, Office of Chief Project Attorney, Washington, D.C. 20580.

Fish and Wildlife Service, U.S. Department of Interior, Washington, D.C. 20240.

Food and Nutrition Board, National Research Council, 2101 Constitution Avenue, Washington, D.C. 20237.

Food and Nutrition News, National Live Stock and Meat Board, Chicago, Illinois 60603.

Food and Nutrition Section, American Public Health Association, 1790 Broadway, New York, New York 10019.

General Foods Corporation, 250 North Street, White Plains, New York 10602.

General Mills, Inc., 9200 Wayzata Blvd., Minneapolis, Minnesota 55426.

Gerber Products, Department of Nutrition, Fremont, Michigan 49412.

Home Economics Department, Campbell Soup Company, 385 Memorial Avenue, Camden, New Jersey 08103.

John Hancock Life Insurance Company, 200 Berkley Street, Boston, Massachusetts, 02117.

Metropolitan Life Insurance Company, Health and Welfare Division, 1 Madison Avenue, New York, New York 10010.

National Dairy Council, 111 North Canal Street, Chicago, Illinois 60606.

Nutrition Committee News, U.S. Department of Agriculture, Washington, D.C. 20250.

Nutrition Foundation, Inc., 99 Park Avenue, New York 10016.

Nutrition News, National Dairy Council, Chicago, Illinois.

Nutrition Today, Enloe, Stalvey and Associates, Inc., 1140 Connecticut Avenue N.W., Washington, D.C. 20036. Slides: Gastrointestinal Absorption; Where Old Age Begins; Intestinal Malabsorption; Iron Metabolism; How to Diagnose Nutritional Deficiencies in Daily Practice; Stress; On Just Being Sick; How the Body Uses Water; What Should A Pregnant Woman Eat; Treating the Alcoholic; The Child With Diabetes; The Stomach.

Poultry and Egg National Board, 250 West 57th Street, New York, New York 10010.

State Department of Health, Nutrition Division.

United Fresh Fruit and Vegetable Association, Washington, D.C.

U.S. Department of Agriculture, Institute of Home Economics, Washington, D.C. 20250.

U.S. Department of Health, Education and Welfare, Food and Drug Administration, Health Services, Children's Bureau, Washington, D.C. 20204.

APPENDIX TABLE 1   NUTRITIVE VALUES OF THE EDIBLE PART OF FOODS[1]*

[Dashes in the columns for nutrients show that no suitable value could be found although there is reason to believe that a measurable amount of the nutrient may be present]

Food, approximate measure, and weight (in grams)	Water	Food energy	Protein	Fat	Fatty acids			Carbohydrate	Calcium	Iron	Vitamin A value	Thiamin	Riboflavin	Niacin	Ascorbic acid
					Saturated (total)	Unsaturated Oleic	Linoleic								
	Grams	Per cent	Calories	Grams	Grams	Grams	Grams	Grams	Grams	Milligrams	Milligrams	International units	Milligrams	Milligrams	Milligrams	Milligrams

MILK, CHEESE, CREAM, IMITATION CREAM; RELATED PRODUCTS

Food, approximate measure, and weight	Grams	Water (Per cent)	Food energy (Calories)	Protein (Grams)	Fat (Grams)	Saturated (total) (Grams)	Unsaturated Oleic (Grams)	Linoleic (Grams)	Carbohydrate (Grams)	Calcium (Milligrams)	Iron (Milligrams)	Vitamin A value (Int. units)	Thiamin (Milligrams)	Riboflavin (Milligrams)	Niacin (Milligrams)	Ascorbic acid (Milligrams)
Milk:																
Fluid:																
1 Whole, 3.5% fat---- 1 cup----	244	87	160	9	9	5	3	Trace	12	288	0.1	350	0.07	0.41	0.2	2
2 Nonfat (skim)------ 1 cup----	245	90	90	9	Trace				12	296	.1	10	.09	.44	.2	2
3 Partly skimmed, 2% nonfat milk solids added. 1 cup----	246	87	145	10	5	3	2	Trace	15	352	.1	200	.10	.52	.2	2
Canned, concentrated, undiluted:																
4 Evaporated, unsweetened. 1 cup----	252	74	345	18	20	11	7	1	24	635	.3	810	.10	.86	.5	3
5 Condensed, sweetened. 1 cup----	306	27	980	25	27	15	9	1	166	802	.3	1,100	.24	1.16	.6	3
Dry, nonfat instant:																
6 Low-density (1⅓ cups needed for reconstitution to 1 qt.). 1 cup----	68	4	245	24	Trace				35	879	.4	[1]120	.24	1.21	.6	5
7 High-density (⅞ cup 1 cup needed for reconstitution to 1 qt.).	104	4	375	37	1				54	1,345	.6	[1]30	.36	1.85	.9	7
Buttermilk:																
8 Fluid, cultured, made from skim milk. 1 cup----	245	90	90	9	Trace				12	296	.1	10	.10	.44	.2	2
9 Dried, packaged------ 1 cup----	120	3	465	41	6	3	2	Trace	60	1,498	.7	260	.31	2.06	1.1	----
Cheese:																
Natural:																
Blue or Roquefort type:																
10 Ounce-------- 1 oz.----	28	40	105	6	9	5	3	Trace	1	89	.1	350	.01	.17	.3	0
11 Cubic inch------ 1 cu. in.----	17	40	65	4	5	3	2	Trace	Trace	54	.1	210	.01	.11	.2	0

[1] Value applies to unfortified product; value for fortified low-density product would be 1500 I.U. and the fortified high-density product would be 2290 I.U.

*Reprinted from Nutritive Value of Foods, U.S. Dept. of Agriculture, Home and Garden Bulletin No. 72, 1970.

APPENDIX TABLE 1 NUTRITIVE VALUES OF THE EDIBLE PART OF FOODS* (Continued)

[Dashes in the columns for nutrients show that no suitable value could be found although there is reason to believe that a measurable amount of the nutrient may be present]

	Food, approximate measure, and weight (in grams)	Water	Food energy	Protein	Fat	Fatty acids			Carbohydrate	Calcium	Iron	Vitamin A value	Thiamin	Riboflavin	Niacin	Ascorbic acid
						Saturated (total)	Unsaturated Oleic	Unsaturated Linoleic								
		Percent	Calories	Grams	Grams	Grams	Grams	Grams	Grams	Milligrams	Milligrams	International units	Milligrams	Milligrams	Milligrams	Milligrams
	MILK, CHEESE, CREAM, IMITATION CREAM; RELATED PRODUCTS—Con.															
	Cheese—Continued															
	Natural—Continued															
12	Camembert, packaged in 4-oz. pkg. with 3 wedges per pkg. 1 wedge----- 38	52	115	7	9	5	3	Trace	1	40	0.2	380	0.02	0.29	0.3	0
	Cheddar:															
13	Ounce----------- 1 oz----------- 28	37	115	7	9	5	3	Trace	1	213	.3	370	.01	.13	Trace	0
14	Cubic inch------- 1 cu. in.------ 17	37	70	4	6	3	2	Trace	Trace	129	.2	230	.01	.08	Trace	0
	Cottage, large or small curd:															
	Creamed:															
15	Package of 12-oz., net wt. 1 pkg.------- 340	78	360	46	14	8	5	Trace	10	320	1.0	580	.10	.85	.3	0
16	Cup, curd pressed down. 1 cup------ 245	78	260	33	10	6	3	Trace	7	230	.7	420	.07	.61	.2	0
	Uncreamed:															
17	Package of 12-oz., net wt. 1 pkg.------- 340	79	290	58	1	1	Trace	Trace	9	306	1.4	30	.10	.95	.3	0
18	Cup, curd pressed down. 1 cup------ 200	79	170	34	1	Trace	Trace	Trace	5	180	.8	20	.06	.56	.2	0
	Cream:															
19	Package of 8-oz., net wt. 1 pkg.------- 227	51	850	18	86	48	28	3	5	141	.5	3,500	.05	.54	.2	0
20	Package of 3-oz., net wt. 1 pkg.------- 85	51	320	7	32	18	11	1	2	53	.2	1,310	.02	.20	.1	0
21	Cubic inch------- 1 cu. in.------ 16	51	60	1	6	3	2	Trace	Trace	10	Trace	250	Trace	.04	Trace	0
	Parmesan, grated:															
22	Cup, pressed down. 1 cup------ 140	17	655	60	43	24	14	1	5	1,893	.7	1,760	.03	1.22	.3	0
23	Tablespoon------ 1 tbsp.----- 5	17	25	2	2	1	Trace	Trace	Trace	68	Trace	60	Trace	.04	Trace	0
24	Ounce----------- 1 oz----------- 28	17	130	12	9	5	3	Trace	1	383	.1	360	.01	.25	.1	0
	Swiss:															
25	Ounce----------- 1 oz----------- 28	39	105	8	8	4	3	Trace	1	262	.3	320	Trace	.11	Trace	0
26	Cubic inch------- 1 cu. in.------ 15	39	55	4	4	2	1	Trace	Trace	139	.1	170	Trace	.06	Trace	0

No.	Food	Measure	Grams	Water (%)	Food energy	Protein (g)	Fat (g)	Saturated	Oleic	Linoleic	Carbohydrate (g)	Calcium (mg)	Iron (mg)	Vitamin A (I.U.)	Thiamin (mg)	Riboflavin (mg)	Niacin (mg)	Ascorbic acid (mg)
	Pasteurized processed cheese:																	
	American:																	
27	Ounce	1 oz.	28	40	105	7	9	5	3	Trace	1	198	.3	350	.01	.12	Trace	0
28	Cubic inch	1 cu. in.	18	40	65	4	5	3	2	Trace	Trace	122	.2	210	Trace	.07	Trace	0
	Swiss:																	
29	Ounce	1 oz.	28	40	100	8	8	4	3	Trace	1	251	.3	310	Trace	.11	Trace	0
30	Cubic inch	1 cu. in.	18	40	65	5	5	3	2	Trace	Trace	159	.2	200	Trace	.07	Trace	0
	Pasteurized process cheese food, American:																	
31	Tablespoon	1 tbsp.	14	43	45	3	3	2	1	Trace	1	80	.1	140	Trace	.08	Trace	0
32	Cubic inch	1 cu. in.	18	43	60	4	4	2	1	Trace	1	100	.1	170	Trace	.10	Trace	0
33	Pasteurized process cheese spread, American.	1 oz.	28	49	80	5	6	3	2	Trace	2	160	.2	250	Trace	.15	Trace	0
	Cream:																	
34	Half-and-half (cream and milk).	1 cup	242	80	325	8	28	15	9	1	11	261	.1	1,160	.07	.39	.1	2
35		1 tbsp.	15	80	20	1	2	1	1	Trace	1	16	Trace	70	Trace	.02	Trace	Trace
36	Light, coffee or table	1 cup	240	72	505	7	49	27	16	1	10	245	.1	2,020	.07	.36	.1	2
37		1 tbsp.	15	72	30	1	3	2	1	Trace	1	15	Trace	180	Trace	.02	Trace	Trace
38	Sour	1 cup	230	72	485	7	47	26	16	1	10	235	.1	1,930	.07	.35	.1	2
39		1 tbsp.	12	72	25	Trace	2	1	1	Trace	1	12	Trace	100	Trace	.02	Trace	Trace
40	Whipped topping (pressurized).	1 cup	60	62	155	2	14	8	5	Trace	6	67	---	570	---	.04	---	---
41	Whipping, unwhipped (volume about double when whipped):	1 tbsp.	3	62	10	Trace	1	Trace	Trace	Trace	Trace	3	---	30	---	Trace	---	---
42	Light	1 cup	239	62	715	6	75	41	25	2	9	203	.1	3,060	.05	.29	.1	2
43		1 tbsp.	15	62	45	Trace	5	3	2	Trace	1	13	Trace	190	Trace	.02	Trace	Trace
44	Heavy	1 cup	238	57	840	5	90	50	30	3	7	179	.1	3,670	.05	.26	.1	2
45		1 tbsp.	15	57	55	Trace	6	3	2	Trace	1	11	Trace	230	Trace	.02	Trace	Trace
	Imitation cream products (made with vegetable fat):																	
	Creamers:																	
46	Powdered	1 cup	94	2	505	4	33	31	1	0	52	21	.6	²200	---	Trace	Trace	---
47		1 tsp.	2	2	10	Trace	1	Trace	Trace	0	1	1	Trace	²Trace	---	---	---	---
48	Liquid (frozen)	1 cup	245	77	345	3	27	25	1	0	25	29	---	²100	0	0	---	0
49		1 tbsp.	15	77	20	Trace	2	1	Trace	0	2	2	---	²10	0	0	---	0
50	Sour dressing (imitation sour cream) made with nonfat dry milk.	1 cup	235	72	440	9	38	35	1	Trace	17	277	.1	10	.07	.38	.2	1
51		1 tbsp.	12	72	20	Trace	2	2	Trace	Trace	1	14	Trace	Trace	Trace	Trace	Trace	Trace
	Whipped topping:																	
52		1 cup	70	61	190	1	17	15	1	0	9	5	---	²340	0	0	---	0
53	Pressurized	1 tbsp.	4	61	10	Trace	1	1	Trace	0	Trace	Trace	---	²20	0	0	---	0

² Contributed largely from beta-carotene used for coloring.

APPENDIX TABLE 1   NUTRITIVE VALUES OF THE EDIBLE PART OF FOODS* (Continued)

[Dashes in the columns for nutrients show that no suitable value could be found although there is reason to believe that a measurable amount of the nutrient may be present]

	Food, approximate measure, and weight (in grams)		Water	Food energy	Protein	Fat	Fatty acids			Carbohydrate	Calcium	Iron	Vitamin A value	Thiamin	Riboflavin	Niacin	Ascorbic acid
							Saturated (total)	Unsaturated									
								Oleic	Linoleic								
		Grams	Percent	Calories	Grams	Grams	Grams	Grams	Grams	Grams	Milligrams	Milligrams	International units	Milligrams	Milligrams	Milligrams	Milligrams
	MILK, CHEESE, CREAM, IMITATION CREAM; RELATED PRODUCTS—Con.																
	Whipped topping—Continued																
54	Frozen ———— 1 cup ————	75	52	230	1	20	18	Trace	0	15	5	—	[2]2,560	—	0	—	—
55	1 tbsp ————	4	52	10	Trace	1	1	Trace	0	1	Trace	—	[2]230	—	0	—	—
56	Powdered, made with whole milk. 1 cup ————	75	58	175	3	12	10	1	Trace	15	62	Trace	[2]330	.02	.08	.1	Trace
57	1 tbsp ————	4	58	10	Trace	1	1	Trace	Trace	1	3	Trace	[2]20	Trace	Trace	Trace	Trace
	Milk beverages:																
58	Cocoa, homemade ———— 1 cup ————	250	79	245	10	12	7	4	Trace	27	295	1.0	400	.10	.45	.5	3
59	Chocolate-flavored drink made with skim milk and 2% added butterfat. 1 cup ————	250	83	190	8	6	3	2	Trace	27	270	.5	210	.10	.40	.3	3
	Malted milk:																
60	Dry powder, approx. 1 oz., 3 heaping teaspoons per ounce.	28	3	115	4	2	—	—	—	20	82	.6	290	.09	.15	.1	0
61	Beverage ———— 1 cup ————	235	78	245	11	10	—	—	—	28	317	.7	590	.14	.49	.2	2
	Milk desserts:																
62	Custard, baked ———— 1 cup ————	265	77	305	14	15	7	5	1	29	297	1.1	930	.11	.50	.3	1
	Ice cream:																
63	Regular (approx. 10% fat). ½ gal ————	1,064	63	2,055	48	113	62	37	3	221	1,553	.5	4,680	.43	2.23	1.1	11
64	1 cup ————	133	63	255	6	14	8	5	Trace	28	194	.1	590	.05	.28	.1	1
65	3 fl. oz. cup——	50	63	95	2	5	3	2	Trace	10	73	Trace	220	.02	.11	.1	1
66	Rich (approx. 16% fat). ½ gal ————	1,188	63	2,635	31	191	105	63	6	214	927	.2	7,840	.24	1.31	1.2	12
67	1 cup ————	148	63	330	4	24	13	8	1	27	115	Trace	980	.03	.16	.1	1
	Ice milk:																
68	Hardened ———— ½ gal ————	1,048	67	1,595	50	53	29	17	2	235	1,635	1.0	2,200	.52	2.31	1.0	10
69	1 cup ————	131	67	200	6	7	4	2	Trace	29	204	.1	280	.07	.29	.1	1
70	Soft-serve ———— 1 cup ————	175	67	265	8	9	5	3	Trace	39	273	.2	370	.09	.39	.2	2

No.	Food	Measure	Grams	Water (%)	Calories	Protein	Fat	Sat. fat	Oleic	Linoleic	Carb.	Calcium	Iron	Vit. A	Thiamine	Riboflavin	Niacin	Ascorbic
71	Yoghurt: Made from partially skimmed milk.	1 cup	245	89	125	8	4	2	1	Trace	13	294	.1	170	.10	.44	.2	2
72	Made from whole milk.	1 cup	245	88	150	7	8	5	3	Trace	12	272	.1	340	.07	.39	.2	2
	EGGS																	
	Eggs, large, 24 ounces per dozen: Raw or cooked in shell or with nothing added:																	
73	Whole, without shell.	1 egg	50	74	80	6	6	2	3	Trace	Trace	27	1.1	590	.05	.15	Trace	0
74	White of egg.	1 white	33	88	15	4	Trace	---	---	---	Trace	3	Trace	0	Trace	.09	Trace	0
75	Yolk of egg.	1 yolk	17	51	60	3	5	2	2	Trace	Trace	24	.9	580	.04	.07	Trace	0
76	Scrambled with milk and fat.	1 egg	64	72	110	7	8	3	3	Trace	1	51	1.1	690	.05	.18	Trace	0
	MEAT, POULTRY, FISH, SHELLFISH; RELATED PRODUCTS																	
77	Bacon, (20 slices per lb. raw), broiled or fried, crisp.	2 slices	15	8	90	5	8	3	4	1	1	2	.5	0	.08	.05	.8	---
	Beef,[3] cooked: Cuts braised, simmered, or pot-roasted:																	
78	Lean and fat.	3 ounces	85	53	245	23	16	8	7	Trace	0	10	2.9	30	.04	.18	3.5	---
79	Lean only.	2.5 ounces	72	62	140	22	5	2	2	Trace	0	10	2.7	10	.04	.16	3.3	---
	Hamburger (ground beef), broiled:																	
80	Lean.	3 ounces	85	60	185	23	10	5	4	Trace	0	10	3.0	20	.08	.20	5.1	---
81	Regular.	3 ounces	85	54	245	21	17	8	8	Trace	0	9	2.7	30	.07	.18	4.6	---
	Roast, oven-cooked, no liquid added: Relatively fat, such as rib:																	
82	Lean and fat.	3 ounces	85	40	375	17	34	16	15	1	0	8	2.2	70	.05	.13	3.1	---
83	Lean only.	1.8 ounces	51	57	125	14	7	3	3	Trace	0	6	1.8	10	.04	.11	2.6	---
	Relatively lean, such as heel of round:																	
84	Lean and fat.	3 ounces	85	62	165	25	7	3	3	Trace	0	11	3.2	10	.06	.19	4.5	---
85	Lean only.	2.7 ounces	78	65	125	24	3	1	1	Trace	0	10	3.0	Trace	.06	.18	4.3	---
	Steak, broiled: Relatively fat, such as sirloin:																	
86	Lean and fat.	3 ounces	85	44	330	20	27	13	12	1	0	9	2.5	50	.05	.16	4.0	---
87	Lean only.	2.0 ounces	56	59	115	18	4	2	2	Trace	0	7	2.2	10	.05	.14	3.6	---
	Relatively lean, such as round:																	
88	Lean and fat.	3 ounces	85	55	220	24	13	6	6	Trace	0	10	3.0	20	.07	.19	4.8	---
89	Lean only.	2.4 ounces	68	61	130	21	4	2	2	Trace	0	9	2.5	10	.06	.16	4.1	---
	Beef, canned:																	
90	Corned beef.	3 ounces	85	59	185	22	10	5	4	Trace	0	17	3.7	20	.01	.20	2.9	---
91	Corned beef hash.	3 ounces	85	67	155	7	10	5	4	Trace	9	11	1.7	---	.01	.08	1.8	---
92	Beef, dried or chipped.	2 ounces	57	48	115	19	4	2	2	Trace	0	11	2.9	---	.04	.18	2.2	---
93	Beef and vegetable stew.	1 cup	235	82	210	15	10	5	5	Trace	15	28	2.8	2,310	.13	.17	4.4	15

[2] Contributed largely from beta-carotene used for coloring.

[3] Outer layer of fat on the cut was removed to within approximately ½-inch of the lean. Deposits of fat within the cut were not removed.

APPENDIX TABLE 1 NUTRITIVE VALUES OF THE EDIBLE PART OF FOODS* (Continued)

[Dashes in the columns for nutrients show that no suitable value could be found although there is reason to believe that a measurable amount of the nutrient may be present]

	Food, approximate measure, and weight (in grams)		Water	Food energy	Protein	Fat	Fatty acids			Carbohydrate	Calcium	Iron	Vitamin A value	Thiamin	Riboflavin	Niacin	Ascorbic acid
							Saturated (total)	Unsaturated Oleic	Linoleic								
		Grams	Percent	Calories	Grams	Grams	Grams	Grams	Grams	Grams	Milligrams	Milligrams	International units	Milligrams	Milligrams	Milligrams	Milligrams
	MEAT, POULTRY, FISH, SHELLFISH; RELATED PRODUCTS—Continued																
94	Beef potpie, baked, 4¼-inch diam., weight before baking about 8 ounces.	1 pie — 227	55	560	23	33	9	20	2	43	32	4.1	1,860	0.25	0.27	4.5	7
	Chicken, cooked:																
95	Flesh only, broiled	3 ounces — 85	71	115	20	3	1	1	1	0	8	1.4	80	.05	.16	7.4	—
	Breast, fried, ½ breast:																
96	With bone	3.3 ounces — 94	58	155	25	5	1	2	1	1	9	1.3	70	.04	.17	11.2	—
97	Flesh and skin only	2.7 ounces — 76	58	155	25	5	1	2	1	1	9	1.3	70	.04	.17	11.2	—
	Drumstick, fried:																
98	With bone	2.1 ounces — 59	55	90	12	4	1	2	1	Trace	6	.9	50	.03	.15	2.7	—
99	Flesh and skin only	1.3 ounces — 38	55	90	12	4	1	2	1	Trace	6	.9	50	.03	.15	2.7	—
100	Chicken, canned, boneless	3 ounces — 85	65	170	18	10	3	4	2	0	18	1.3	200	.03	.11	3.7	3
101	Chicken potpie, baked, 4¼-inch diam., weight before baking about 8 ounces.	1 pie — 227	57	535	23	31	10	15	3	42	68	3.0	3,020	.25	.26	4.1	5
	Chili con carne, canned:																
102	With beans	1 cup — 250	72	335	19	15	7	7	Trace	30	80	4.2	150	.08	.18	3.2	—
103	Without beans	1 cup — 255	67	510	26	38	18	17	1	15	97	3.6	380	.05	.31	5.6	—
104	Heart, beef, lean, braised	3 ounces — 85	61	160	27	5	—	—	—	1	5	5.0	20	.21	1.04	6.5	1
	Lamb,³ cooked:																
105	Chop, thick, with bone, broiled.	1 chop, 4.8 ounces. — 137	47	400	25	33	18	12	1	0	10	1.5	—	.14	.25	5.6	—
106	Lean and fat	4.0 ounces — 112	47	400	25	33	18	12	1	0	10	1.5	—	.14	.25	5.6	—
107	Lean only	2.6 ounces — 74	62	140	21	6	3	2	Trace	0	9	1.5	—	.11	.20	4.5	—
	Leg, roasted:																
108	Lean and fat	3 ounces — 85	54	235	22	16	9	6	Trace	0	9	1.4	—	.13	.23	4.7	—
109	Lean only	2.5 ounces — 71	62	130	20	5	3	2	Trace	0	9	1.4	—	.12	.21	4.4	—
	Shoulder, roasted:																
110	Lean and fat	3 ounces — 85	50	285	18	23	13	8	1	0	9	1.0	—	.11	.20	4.0	—
111	Lean only	2.3 ounces — 64	61	130	17	6	3	2	Trace	0	8	1.0	—	.10	.18	3.7	—

No.	Food, approximate measure, and weight	Grams	Water (pct)	Food energy (cal.)	Protein (g)	Fat (g)	Saturated (g)	Oleic (g)	Linoleic (g)	Carbohydrate (g)	Calcium (mg)	Iron (mg)	Vitamin A (I.U.)	Thiamine (mg)	Riboflavin (mg)	Niacin (mg)	Ascorbic acid (mg)
112	Liver, beef, fried — 2 ounces	57	57	130	15	6	—	—	—	3	6	5.0	30,280	.15	2.37	9.4	15
	Pork, cured, cooked:																
113	Ham, light cure, lean and fat, roasted. — 3 ounces	85	54	245	18	19	7	8	2	0	8	2.2	0	.40	.16	3.1	—
	Luncheon meat:																
114	Boiled ham, sliced — 2 ounces	57	59	135	11	10	4	4	1	0	6	1.6	0	.25	.09	1.5	—
115	Canned, spiced or unspiced. — 2 ounces	57	55	165	8	14	5	6	1	1	5	1.2	0	.18	.12	1.6	—
	Pork, fresh,[3] cooked:																
116	Chop, thick, with bone. — 1 chop, 3.5 ounces.	98	42	260	16	21	8	9	2	0	8	2.2	0	.63	.18	3.8	—
117	Lean and fat — 2.3 ounces	66	42	260	16	21	8	9	2	0	8	2.2	0	.63	.18	3.8	—
118	Lean only — 1.7 ounces	48	53	130	15	7	2	3	1	0	7	1.9	0	.54	.16	3.3	—
	Roast, oven-cooked, no liquid added:																
119	Lean and fat — 3 ounces	85	46	310	21	24	9	10	2	0	9	2.7	0	.78	.22	4.7	—
120	Lean only — 2.4 ounces	68	55	175	20	10	3	4	1	0	9	2.6	0	.73	.21	4.4	—
	Cuts, simmered:																
121	Lean and fat — 3 ounces	85	46	320	20	26	9	11	2	0	8	2.5	0	.46	.21	4.1	—
122	Lean only — 2.2 ounces	63	60	135	18	6	2	3	1	0	8	2.3	0	.42	.19	3.7	—
	Sausage:																
123	Bologna, slice, 3-in. diam. by 1/8 inch. — 2 slices	26	56	80	3	7	—	—	—	Trace	2	.5	—	.04	.06	.7	—
124	Braunschweiger, slice 2-in. diam. by 1/4 inch. — 2 slices	20	53	65	3	5	—	—	—	Trace	2	1.2	1,310	.03	.29	1.6	—
125	Deviled ham, canned — 1 tbsp.	13	51	45	2	4	2	2	Trace	0	1	.3	—	.02	.01	.2	—
126	Frankfurter, heated (8 per lb. purchased pkg.). — 1 frank	56	57	170	7	15	—	—	—	1	3	.8	—	.08	.11	1.4	—
127	Pork links, cooked (16 links per lb. raw). — 2 links	26	35	125	5	11	4	5	1	Trace	2	.6	0	.21	.09	1.0	—
128	Salami, dry type — 1 oz.	28	30	130	7	11	—	—	—	Trace	4	1.0	—	.10	.07	1.5	—
129	Salami, cooked — 1 oz.	28	51	90	5	7	—	—	—	Trace	3	.7	—	.07	.07	1.2	—
130	Vienna, canned (7 sausages per 5-oz. can). — 1 sausage	16	63	40	2	3	—	—	—	Trace	1	.3	—	.01	.02	.4	—
	Veal, medium fat, cooked, bone removed:																
131	Cutlet — 3 oz.	85	60	185	23	9	5	4	Trace	0	9	2.7	—	.06	.21	4.6	—
132	Roast — 3 oz.	85	55	230	23	14	7	6	Trace	0	10	2.9	—	.11	.26	6.6	—
	Fish and shellfish:																
133	Bluefish, baked with table fat. — 3 oz.	85	68	135	22	4	—	—	—	0	25	.6	40	.09	.08	1.6	—
	Clams:																
134	Raw, meat only — 3 oz.	85	82	65	11	1	—	—	—	2	59	5.2	90	.08	.15	1.1	8
135	Canned, solids and liquid. — 3 oz.	85	86	45	7	1	—	—	—	2	47	3.5	—	.01	.09	.9	—
136	Crabmeat, canned — 3 oz.	85	77	85	15	2	—	—	—	1	38	.7	—	.07	.07	1.6	—

[3] Outer layer of fat on the cut was removed to within approximately 1/2-inch of the lean. Deposits of fat within the cut were not removed.

APPENDIX TABLE 1   NUTRITIVE VALUES OF THE EDIBLE PART OF FOODS* (Continued)

[Dashes in the columns for nutrients show that no suitable value could be found although there is reason to believe that a measurable amount of the nutrient may be present]

	Food, approximate measure, and weight (in grams)	Water	Food energy	Protein	Fat	Fatty acids Saturated (total)	Unsaturated Oleic	Unsaturated Linoleic	Carbohydrate	Calcium	Iron	Vitamin A value	Thiamin	Riboflavin	Niacin	Ascorbic acid
		Percent	Calories	Grams	Grams	Grams	Grams	Grams	Grams	Milligrams	Milligrams	International units	Milligrams	Milligrams	Milligrams	Milligrams
	MEAT, POULTRY, FISH, SHELLFISH; RELATED PRODUCTS—Continued															
	Fish and shellfish—Continued															
137	Fish sticks, breaded, cooked, frozen; stick 3¾ by 1 by ½ inch. 10 sticks or 8 oz. pkg. *Grams* 227	66	400	38	20	5	4	10	15	25	0.9		0.09	0.16	3.6	
138	Haddock, breaded, fried 3 oz 85	66	140	17	5	1	3	Trace	5	34	1.0		.03	.06	2.7	2
139	Ocean perch, breaded, fried. 3 oz 85	59	195	16	11				6	28	1.1		.08	.09	1.5	
140	Oysters, raw, meat only (13-19 med. selects). 1 cup 240	85	160	20	4				8	226	13.2	740	.33	.43	6.0	
141	Salmon, pink, canned 3 oz 85	71	120	17	5	1	1	Trace	0	⁴167	.7	60	.03	.16	6.8	
142	Sardines, Atlantic, canned in oil, drained solids. 3 oz 85	62	175	20	9				0	372	2.5	190	.02	.17	4.6	
143	Shad, baked with table fat and bacon. 3 oz 85	64	170	20	10				0	20	.5	20	.11	.22	7.3	
144	Shrimp, canned, meat. 3 oz 85	70	100	21	1				1	98	2.6	50	.01	.03	1.5	
145	Swordfish, broiled with butter or margarine. 3 oz 85	65	150	24	5				0	23	1.1	1,750	.03	.04	9.3	
146	Tuna, canned in oil, drained solids. 3 oz 85	61	170	24	7	2	1	1	0	7	1.6	70	.04	.10	10.1	
	MATURE DRY BEANS AND PEAS, NUTS, PEANUTS; RELATED PRODUCTS															
147	Almonds, shelled, whole kernels. 1 cup 142	5	850	26	77	6	52	15	28	332	6.7	0	.34	1.31	5.0	Trace
	Beans, dry: Common varieties as Great Northern, navy, and others: Cooked, drained:															
148	Great Northern 1 cup 180	69	210	14	1				38	90	4.9	0	.25	.13	1.3	0

149	Navy (pea)	1 cup	190	69	225	15	1	--	--	--	40	95	5.1	0	.27	.13	1.3	0
	Canned, solids and liquid:																	
	White with—																	
150	Frankfurters (sliced)	1 cup	255	71	365	19	18	--	--	--	32	94	4.8	330	.18	.15	3.3	Trace
151	Pork and tomato sauce.	1 cup	255	71	310	16	7	2	3	1	49	138	4.6	330	.20	.08	1.5	5
152	Pork and sweet sauce.	1 cup	255	66	385	16	12	4	5	1	54	161	5.9	--	.15	.10	1.3	--
153	Red kidney	1 cup	255	76	230	15	1	--	--	--	42	74	4.6	10	.13	.10	1.5	--
154	Lima, cooked, drained.	1 cup	190	64	260	16	1	--	--	--	49	55	5.9	--	.25	.11	1.3	--
155	Cashew nuts, roasted	1 cup	140	5	785	24	64	11	45	4	41	53	5.3	140	.60	.35	2.5	--
	Coconut, fresh, meat only:																	
156	Pieces, approx. 2 by 2 by ½ inch.	1 piece	45	51	155	2	16	14	1	Trace	4	6	.8	0	.02	.01	.2	1
157	Shredded or grated, firmly packed.	1 cup	130	51	450	5	46	39	3	Trace	12	17	2.2	0	.07	.03	.7	4
158	Cowpeas or blackeye peas, dry, cooked.	1 cup	248	80	190	13	1	--	--	--	34	42	3.2	20	.41	.11	1.1	Trace
159	Peanuts, roasted, salted, halves.	1 cup	144	2	840	37	72	16	31	21	27	107	3.0	--	.46	.19	24.7	0
160	Peanut butter	1 tbsp	16	2	95	4	8	2	4	2	3	9	.3	--	.02	.02	2.4	0
161	Peas, split, dry, cooked	1 cup	250	70	290	20	1	--	--	--	52	28	4.2	100	.37	.22	2.2	--
162	Pecans, halves	1 cup	108	3	740	10	77	5	48	15	16	79	2.6	140	.93	.14	1.0	2
163	Walnuts, black or native, chopped.	1 cup	126	3	790	26	75	4	26	36	19	Trace	7.6	380	.28	.14	.9	--

VEGETABLES AND VEGETABLE PRODUCTS

	Asparagus, green:																	
	Cooked, drained:																	
164	Spears, ½-in. diam. at base.	4 spears	60	94	10	1	Trace				2	13	.4	540	.10	.11	.8	16
165	Pieces, 1½ to 2-in. lengths.	1 cup	145	94	30	3	Trace				5	30	.9	1,310	.23	.26	2.0	38
166	Canned, solids and liquid.	1 cup	244	94	45	5	1				7	44	4.1	1,240	.15	.22	2.0	37
	Beans:																	
167	Lima, immature seeds, cooked, drained.	1 cup	170	71	190	13	1				34	80	4.3	480	.31	.17	2.2	29
	Snap:																	
	Green:																	
168	Cooked, drained	1 cup	125	92	30	2	Trace				7	63	.8	680	.09	.11	.6	15
169	Canned, solids and liquid.	1 cup	239	94	45	2	Trace				10	81	2.9	690	.07	.10	.7	10

[4] If bones are discarded, value will be greatly reduced.

APPENDIX TABLE 1   NUTRITIVE VALUES OF THE EDIBLE PART OF FOODS* (Continued)

[Dashes in the columns for nutrients show that no suitable value could be found although there is reason to believe that a measurable amount of the nutrient may be present]

	Food, approximate measure, and weight (in grams)	Water	Food energy	Protein	Fat	Fatty acids			Carbohydrate	Calcium	Iron	Vitamin A value	Thiamin	Riboflavin	Niacin	Ascorbic acid
						Saturated (total)	Unsaturated Oleic	Unsaturated Linoleic								
		Percent	Calories	Grams	Grams	Grams	Grams	Grams	Grams	Milligrams	Milligrams	International units	Milligrams	Milligrams	Milligrams	Milligrams
	VEGETABLES AND VEGETABLE PRODUCTS—Continued															
	Beans—Continued															
	Snap—Continued															
	Yellow or wax:															
170	Cooked, drained... 1 cup — 125	93	30	2	Trace	---	---	---	6	63	0.8	290	0.09	0.11	0.6	16
171	Canned, solids and liquid. 1 cup — 239	94	45	2	1	---	---	---	10	81	2.9	140	.07	.10	.7	12
172	Sprouted mung beans, cooked, drained. 1 cup — 125	91	35	4	Trace				7	21	1.1	30	.11	.13	.9	8
	Beets:															
	Cooked, drained, peeled:															
173	Whole beets, 2-in. diam. 2 beets — 100	91	30	1	Trace				7	14	.5	20	.03	.04	.3	6
174	Diced or sliced 1 cup — 170	91	55	2	Trace				12	24	.9	30	.05	.07	.5	10
175	Canned, solids and liquid. 1 cup — 246	90	85	2	Trace				19	34	1.5	20	.02	.05	.2	7
176	Beet greens, leaves and stems, cooked, drained. 1 cup — 145	94	25	3	Trace				5	144	2.8	7,400	.10	.22	.4	22
	Blackeye peas. See Cowpeas.															
	Broccoli, cooked, drained:															
177	Whole stalks, medium size. 1 stalk — 180	91	45	6	1				8	158	1.4	4,500	.16	.36	1.4	162
178	Stalks cut into ½-in. pieces. 1 cup — 155	91	40	5	1				7	136	1.2	3,880	.14	.31	1.2	140
179	Chopped, yield from 10-oz. frozen pkg. 1⅜ cups — 250	92	65	7	1				12	135	1.8	6,500	.15	.30	1.3	143
180	Brussels sprouts, 7–8 sprouts (1¼ to 1½ in. diam.) per cup, cooked. 1 cup — 155	88	55	7	1				10	50	1.7	810	.12	.22	1.2	135
	Cabbage:															
	Common varieties:															

No.	Food	Measure																
181	Raw: Coarsely shredded or sliced.	1 cup	70	92	15	1	Trace	----	----	----	4	34	.3	90	.04	.04	.2	33
182	Finely shredded or chopped.	1 cup	90	92	20	1	Trace	----	----	----	5	44	.4	120	.05	.05	.3	42
183	Cooked.	1 cup	145	94	30	2	Trace	----	----	----	6	64	.4	190	.06	.06	.4	48
184	Red, raw, coarsely shredded.	1 cup	70	90	20	1	Trace	----	----	----	5	29	.6	30	.06	.04	.3	43
185	Savoy, raw, coarsely shredded.	1 cup	70	92	15	2	Trace	----	----	----	3	47	.6	140	.04	.06	.2	39
186	Cabbage, celery or Chinese, raw, cut in 1-in. pieces.	1 cup	75	95	10	1	Trace	----	----	----	2	32	.5	110	.04	.03	.5	19
187	Cabbage, spoon (or pakchoy), cooked.	1 cup	170	95	25	2	Trace	----	----	----	4	252	1.0	5,270	.07	.14	1.2	26
	Carrots: Raw:																	
188	Whole, 5½ by 1 inch, 1 carrot (25 thin strips).		50	88	20	1	Trace	----	----	----	5	18	.4	5,500	.03	.03	.3	4
189	Grated.	1 cup	110	88	45	1	Trace	----	----	----	11	41	.8	12,100	.06	.06	.7	9
190	Cooked, diced.	1 cup	145	91	45	1	Trace	----	----	----	10	48	.9	15,220	.08	.07	.7	9
191	Canned, strained or chopped (baby food).	1 ounce	28	92	10	Trace	Trace	----	----	----	2	7	.1	3,690	.01	.01	.1	1
192	Cauliflower, cooked, flowerbuds.	1 cup	120	93	25	3	Trace	----	----	----	5	25	.8	70	.11	.10	.7	66
193	Celery, raw: Stalk, large outer, 8 by about 1½ inches, at root end.	1 stalk	40	94	5	Trace	Trace	----	----	----	2	16	.1	100	.01	.01	.1	4
194	Pieces, diced.	1 cup	100	94	15	1	Trace	----	----	----	4	39	.3	240	.03	.03	.3	9
195	Collards, cooked.	1 cup	190	91	55	5	1	----	----	----	9	289	1.1	10,260	.27	.37	2.4	87
196	Corn, sweet: Cooked, ear 5 by 1¾ inches.[5]	1 ear	140	74	70	3	1	----	----	----	16	2	.5	[6]310	.09	.08	1.0	7
197	Canned, solids and liquid.	1 cup	256	81	170	5	2	----	----	----	40	10	1.0	[6]690	.07	.12	2.3	13
198	Cowpeas, cooked, immature seeds.	1 cup	160	72	175	13	1	----	----	----	29	38	3.4	560	.49	.18	2.3	28
	Cucumbers, 10-ounce; 7½ by about 2 inches:																	
199	Raw, pared.	1 cucumber	207	96	30	1	Trace	----	----	----	7	35	.6	Trace	.07	.09	.4	23
200	Raw, pared, center slice ⅛-inch thick.	6 slices	50	96	5	Trace	Trace	----	----	----	2	8	.2	Trace	.02	.02	.1	6
201	Dandelion greens, cooked.	1 cup	180	90	60	4	1	----	----	----	12	252	3.2	21,060	.24	.29	----	32

[5] Measure and weight apply to entire vegetable or fruit including parts not usually eaten.

[6] Based on yellow varieties; white varieties contain only a trace of cryptoxanthin and carotenes, the pigments in corn that have biological activity.

APPENDIX TABLE 1   NUTRITIVE VALUES OF THE EDIBLE PART OF FOODS* (Continued)

[Dashes in the columns for nutrients show that no suitable value could be found although there is reason to believe that a measurable amount of the nutrient may be present]

	Food, approximate measure, and weight (in grams)	Water	Food energy	Protein	Fat	Fatty acids Saturated (total)	Unsaturated Oleic	Unsaturated Linoleic	Carbohydrate	Calcium	Iron	Vitamin A value	Thiamin	Riboflavin	Niacin	Ascorbic acid
		Percent	Calories	Grams	Grams	Grams	Grams	Grams	Grams	Milligrams	Milligrams	International units	Milligrams	Milligrams	Milligrams	Milligrams
	VEGETABLES AND VEGETABLE PRODUCTS—Continued															
202	Endive, curly (including escarole). 2 ounces ---- 57	93	10	1	Trace	---	---	---	2	46	1.0	1,870	0.04	0.08	0.3	6
203	Kale, leaves including stems, cooked. 1 cup ------ 110	91	30	4	.1	---	---	---	4	147	1.3	8,140	---	---	---	68
	Lettuce, raw:															
204	Butterhead, as Boston types; head, 4-inch diameter. 1 head ------ 220	95	30	3	Trace	---	---	---	6	77	4.4	2,130	.14	.13	.6	18
205	Crisphead, as Iceberg; 1 head, 4¾-inch diameter. 454	96	60	4	Trace	---	---	---	13	91	2.3	1,500	.29	.27	1.3	29
206	Looseleaf, or bunching varieties, leaves. 2 large ----- 50	94	10	1	Trace	---	---	---	2	34	.7	950	.03	.04	.2	9
207	Mushrooms, canned, solids and liquid. 1 cup ------ 244	93	40	5	Trace	---	---	---	6	15	1.2	Trace	.04	.60	4.8	4
208	Mustard greens, cooked. 1 cup ------ 140	93	35	3	1	---	---	---	6	193	2.5	8,120	.11	.19	.9	68
209	Okra, cooked, pod 3 by ⅝ inch. 8 pods ----- 85	91	25	2	Trace	---	---	---	5	78	.4	420	.11	.15	.8	17
	Onions:															
	Mature:															
210	Raw, onion 2½-inch diameter. 1 onion ----- 110	89	40	2	Trace	---	---	---	10	30	.6	40	.04	.04	.2	11
211	Cooked. 1 cup ------ 210	92	60	3	Trace	---	---	---	14	50	.8	80	.06	.06	.4	14
212	Young green, small, without tops. 6 onions ---- 50	88	20	1	Trace	---	---	---	5	20	.3	Trace	.02	.02	.2	12
213	Parsley, raw, chopped. 1 tablespoon ---- 4	85	Trace	Trace	Trace	---	---	---	Trace	8	.2	340	Trace	.01	Trace	7
214	Parsnips, cooked. 1 cup ------ 155	82	100	2	1	---	---	---	23	70	.9	50	.11	.12	.2	16
	Peas, green:															
215	Cooked. 1 cup ------ 160	82	115	9	1	---	---	---	19	37	2.9	860	.44	.17	3.7	33
216	Canned, solids and liquid. 1 cup ------ 249	83	165	9	1	---	---	---	31	50	4.2	1,120	.23	.13	2.2	22

No.	Food	Measure	Grams	Water	Food energy	Protein	Fat	Saturated	Oleic	Linoleic	Carbohydrate	Calcium	Iron	Vitamin A	Thiamin	Riboflavin	Niacin	Ascorbic acid
217	Canned, strained (baby food).	1 ounce	28	86	15	1	Trace	—	—	—	3	3	.4	140	.02	.02	.4	3
218	Peppers, hot, red, without seeds, dried (ground chili powder, added seasonings).	1 tablespoon	15	8	50	2	2	—	—	—	8	40	2.3	9,750	.03	.17	1.3	2
	Peppers, sweet:																	
	Raw, about 5 per pound:																		
219	Green pod without stem and seeds.	1 pod	74	93	15	1	Trace	—	—	—	4	7	.5	310	.06	.06	.4	94
220	Cooked, boiled, drained	1 pod	73	95	15	1	Trace	—	—	—	3	7	.4	310	.05	.05	.4	70
	Potatoes, medium (about 3 per pound raw):																		
221	Baked, peeled after baking.	1 potato	99	75	90	3	Trace	—	—	—	21	9	.7	Trace	.10	.04	1.7	20
	Boiled:																		
222	Peeled after boiling	1 potato	136	80	105	3	Trace	—	—	—	23	10	.8	Trace	.13	.05	2.0	22
223	Peeled before boiling	1 potato	122	83	80	2	Trace	—	—	—	18	7	.6	Trace	.11	.04	1.4	20
	French-fried, piece 2 by ½ by ½ inch:																		
224	Cooked in deep fat	10 pieces	57	45	155	2	7	2	2	4	20	9	.7	Trace	.07	.04	1.8	12
225	Frozen, heated	10 pieces	57	53	125	2	5	1	1	2	19	5	1.0	Trace	.08	.01	1.5	12
	Mashed:																		
226	Milk added	1 cup	195	83	125	4	1	—	—	—	25	47	.8	50	.16	.10	2.0	19
227	Milk and butter added.	1 cup	195	80	185	4	8	3	4	Trace	24	47	.8	330	.16	.10	1.9	18
228	Potato chips, medium, 2-inch diameter.	10 chips	20	2	115	1	8	2	2	4	10	8	.4	Trace	.04	.01	1.0	3
229	Pumpkin, canned	1 cup	228	90	75	2	1	—	—	—	18	57	.9	14,590	.07	.12	1.3	12
230	Radishes, raw, small, without tops.	4 radishes	40	94	5	Trace	Trace	—	—	—	1	12	.4	Trace	.01	.01	.1	10
231	Sauerkraut, canned, solids and liquid.	1 cup	235	93	45	2	Trace	—	—	—	9	85	1.2	120	.07	.09	.4	33
	Spinach:																		
232	Cooked	1 cup	180	92	40	5	1	—	—	—	6	167	4.0	14,580	.13	.25	1.0	50
233	Canned, drained solids	1 cup	180	91	45	5	1	—	—	—	6	212	4.7	14,400	.03	.21	.6	24
	Squash:																		
	Cooked:																		
234	Summer, diced	1 cup	210	96	30	2	Trace	—	—	—	7	52	.8	820	.10	.16	1.6	21
235	Winter, baked, mashed.	1 cup	205	81	130	4	1	—	—	—	32	57	1.6	8,610	.10	.27	1.4	27
	Sweetpotatoes:																		
	Cooked, medium, 5 by 2 inches, weight raw about 6 ounces:																		
236	Baked, peeled after baking.	1 sweetpotato	110	64	155	2	1	—	—	—	36	44	1.0	8,910	.10	.07	.7	24
237	Boiled, peeled after boiling.	1 sweetpotato	147	71	170	2	1	—	—	—	39	47	1.0	11,610	.13	.09	.9	25

APPENDIX TABLE 1 NUTRITIVE VALUES OF THE EDIBLE PART OF FOODS* (Continued)

[Dashes in the columns for nutrients show that no suitable value could be found although there is reason to believe that a measurable amount of the nutrient may be present]

	Food, approximate measure, and weight (in grams)	Water	Food energy	Protein	Fat	Fatty acids			Carbohydrate	Calcium	Iron	Vitamin A value	Thiamin	Riboflavin	Niacin	Ascorbic acid
						Saturated (total)	Unsaturated Oleic	Unsaturated Linoleic								
		Per cent	Calories	Grams	Grams	Grams	Grams	Grams	Grams	Milligrams	Milligrams	International units	Milligrams	Milligrams	Milligrams	Milligrams
	VEGETABLES AND VEGETABLE PRODUCTS—Continued															
	Sweetpotatoes—Continued															
238	Candied, 3½ by 2¼ inches. 1 sweetpotato. 175	60	295	2	6	2	3	1	60	65	1.6	11,030	0.10	0.08	0.8	17
239	Canned, vacuum or solid pack. 1 cup. 218	72	235	4	Trace				54	54	1.7	17,000	.10	.10	1.4	30
	Tomatoes:															
240	Raw, approx. 3-in. diam. 2⅛ in. high; wt., 7 oz. 1 tomato. 200	94	40	2	Trace				9	24	.9	1,640	.11	.07	1.3	[7] 42
241	Canned, solids and liquid. 1 cup. 241	94	50	2	1				10	14	1.2	2,170	.12	.07	1.7	41
	Tomato catsup:															
242	Cup. 1 cup. 273	69	290	6	1				69	60	2.2	3,820	.25	.19	4.4	41
243	Tablespoon. 1 tbsp. 15	69	15	Trace	Trace				4	3	.1	210	.01	.01	.2	2
	Tomato juice, canned:															
244	Cup. 1 cup. 243	94	45	2	Trace				10	17	2.2	1,940	.12	.07	1.9	39
245	Glass (6 fl. oz.). 1 glass. 182	94	35	2	Trace				8	13	1.6	1,460	.09	.05	1.5	29
246	Turnips, cooked, diced. 1 cup. 155	94	35	1	Trace				8	54	.6	Trace	.06	.08	.5	34
247	Turnip greens, cooked. 1 cup. 145	94	30	3	Trace				5	252	1.5	8,270	.15	.33	.7	68
	FRUITS AND FRUIT PRODUCTS															
248	Apples, raw (about 3 per lb.).[5] 1 apple. 150	85	70	Trace	Trace				18	8	.4	50	.04	.02	.1	3
249	Apple juice, bottled or canned. 1 cup. 248	88	120	Trace	Trace				30	15	1.5	---	.02	.05	.2	2
	Applesauce, canned:															
250	Sweetened. 1 cup. 255	76	230	1	Trace				61	10	1.3	100	.05	.03	.1	[8] 3
251	Unsweetened or artificially sweetened. 1 cup. 244	88	100	1	Trace				26	10	1.2	100	.05	.02	.1	[8] 2

No.	Food, approximate measure, and weight		grams	Water (%)	Food energy (cal.)	Protein (g)	Fat (g)	Saturated fatty acids (total) (g)	Unsaturated Oleic (g)	Unsaturated Linoleic (g)	Carbohydrate (g)	Calcium (mg)	Iron (mg)	Vitamin A (I.U.)	Thiamine (mg)	Riboflavin (mg)	Niacin (mg)	Ascorbic acid (mg)
	Apricots:																	
252	Raw (about 12 per lb.)[5]	3 apricots	114	85	55	1	Trace				14	18	.5	2,890	.03	.04	.7	10
253	Canned in heavy sirup	1 cup	259	77	220	2	Trace				57	28	.8	4,510	.05	.06	.9	10
254	Dried, uncooked (40 halves per cup).	1 cup	150	25	390	8	1				100	100	8.2	16,350	.02	.23	4.9	19
255	Cooked, unsweetened, fruit and liquid.	1 cup	285	76	240	5	1				62	63	5.1	8,550	.01	.13	2.8	8
256	Apricot nectar, canned	1 cup	251	85	140	1	Trace				37	23	.5	2,380	.03	.03	.5	[8]8
257	Avocados, whole fruit, raw:[5] California (mid- and late-winter; diam. 3⅛ in.).	1 avocado	284	74	370	5	37	7	17	5	13	22	1.3	630	.24	.43	3.5	30
258	Florida (late summer, fall; diam. 3⅝ in.).	1 avocado	454	78	390	4	33	7	15	4	27	30	1.8	880	.33	.61	4.9	43
259	Bananas, raw, medium size.[5]	1 banana	175	76	100	1	Trace				26	10	.8	230	.06	.07	.8	12
260	Banana flakes	1 cup	100	3	340	4	1				89	32	2.8	760	.18	.24	2.8	7
261	Blackberries, raw	1 cup	144	84	85	2	1				19	46	1.3	290	.05	.06	.5	30
262	Blueberries, raw	1 cup	140	83	85	1	1				21	21	1.4	140	.04	.08	.6	20
263	Cantaloups, raw; medium; 5-inch diameter about 1⅔ pounds.[5]	½ melon	385	91	60	1	Trace				14	27	.8	[9]6,540	.08	.06	1.2	63
264	Cherries, canned, red, sour, pitted, water pack.	1 cup	244	88	105	2	Trace				26	37	.7	1,660	.07	.05	.5	[10]40
265	Cranberry juice cocktail, canned.	1 cup	250	83	165	Trace	Trace				42	13	.8	Trace	.03	.03	.1	5
266	Cranberry sauce, sweetened, canned, strained.	1 cup	277	62	330	Trace	1				85	14	.5	50	.02	.02	.1	5
267	Dates, pitted, cut	1 cup	178	22	490	4	1				130	105	5.3	90	.16	.17	3.9	0
268	Figs, dried, large, 2 by 1 in.	1 fig	21	23	60	1	Trace				15	26	.6	20	.02	.02	.1	0
269	Fruit cocktail, canned, in heavy sirup.	1 cup	256	80	195	1	Trace				50	23	1.0	360	.05	.03	1.3	5

[5] Measure and weight apply to entire vegetable or fruit including parts not usually eaten.

[7] Year-round average. Samples marketed from November through May, average 20 milligrams per 200-gram tomato; from June through October, around 52 milligrams.

[8] This is the amount from the fruit. Additional ascorbic acid may be added by the manufacturer. Refer to the label for this information.

[9] Value for varieties with orange-colored flesh; value for varieties with green flesh would be about 540 I.U.

[10] Value listed is based on products with label stating 30 milligrams per 6 fl. oz. serving.

APPENDIX TABLE 1   NUTRITIVE VALUES OF THE EDIBLE PART OF FOODS* (Continued)

[Dashes in the columns for nutrients show that no suitable value could be found although there is reason to believe that a measurable amount of the nutrient may be present]

	Food, approximate measure, and weight (in grams)	Water	Food energy	Protein	Fat	Fatty acids Saturated (total)	Fatty acids Unsaturated Oleic	Fatty acids Unsaturated Linoleic	Carbohydrate	Calcium	Iron	Vitamin A value	Thiamin	Riboflavin	Niacin	Ascorbic acid
		Grams · Percent	Calories	Grams	Grams	Grams	Grams	Grams	Grams	Milligrams	Milligrams	International units	Milligrams	Milligrams	Milligrams	Milligrams
	FRUITS AND FRUIT PRODUCTS—Con.															
	Grapefruit:															
270	Raw, medium, 3¾-in. diam.[5] White ½ grapefruit	241 · 89	45	1	Trace	---	---	---	12	19	0.5	10	0.05	0.02	0.2	44
271	Pink or red ½ grapefruit	241 · 89	50	1	Trace	---	---	---	13	20	0.5	540	0.05	0.02	0.2	44
272	Canned, sirup pack 1 cup	254 · 81	180	2	Trace	---	---	---	45	33	.8	30	.08	.05	.5	76
	Grapefruit juice:															
273	Fresh 1 cup	246 · 90	95	1	Trace	---	---	---	23	22	.5	(11)	.09	.04	.4	92
	Canned, white:															
274	Unsweetened 1 cup	247 · 89	100	1	Trace	---	---	---	24	20	1.0	20	.07	.04	.4	84
275	Sweetened 1 cup	250 · 86	130	1	Trace	---	---	---	32	20	1.0	20	.07	.04	.4	78
	Frozen, concentrate, unsweetened:															
276	Undiluted, can, 6 fluid ounces 1 can	207 · 62	300	4	1	---	---	---	72	70	.8	60	.29	.12	1.4	286
277	Diluted with 3 parts water, by volume 1 cup	247 · 89	100	1	Trace	---	---	---	24	25	.2	20	.10	.04	.5	96
278	Dehydrated crystals 4 oz	113 · 1	410	6	1	---	---	---	102	100	1.2	80	.40	.20	2.0	396
279	Prepared with water 1 cup (1 pound yields about 1 gallon)	247 · 90	100	1	Trace	---	---	---	24	22	.2	20	.10	.05	.5	91
	Grapes, raw:[5]															
280	American type (slip skin) 1 cup	153 · 82	65	1	1	---	---	---	15	15	.4	100	.05	.03	.2	3
281	European type (adherent skin) 1 cup	160 · 81	95	1	Trace	---	---	---	25	17	.6	140	.07	.04	.4	6
	Grapejuice:															
282	Canned or bottled 1 cup	253 · 88	165	1	Trace	---	---	---	42	28	.8	---	.10	.05	.5	Trace
	Frozen concentrate, sweetened:															
283	Undiluted, can, 6 fluid ounces 1 can	216 · 53	395	1	Trace	---	---	---	100	22	.9	40	.13	.22	1.5	(12)

No.	Food, approximate measure	Measure	Grams	Water (%)	Food energy	Protein	Fat		Carbohydrate	Calcium	Iron	Vitamin A	Thiamine	Riboflavin	Niacin	Ascorbic acid
284	Diluted with 3 parts water, by volume.	1 cup	250	86	135	1	Trace	---	33	8	.3	10	.05	.08	.5	[12]
285	Grapejuice drink, canned	1 cup	250	86	135	Trace	1	---	35	8	.3	---	.03	.03	.3	[12]
286	Lemons, raw, 2⅛-in. diam., size 165.[5] Used for juice.	1 lemon	110	90	20	1	Trace	---	6	19	.4	10	.03	.01	.1	39
287	Lemon juice, raw	1 cup	244	91	60	1	Trace	---	20	17	.5	50	.07	.02	.2	112
	Lemonade concentrate:															
288	Frozen, 6 fl. oz. per can.	1 can	219	48	430	Trace	Trace	---	112	9	.4	40	.04	.07	.7	66
289	Diluted with 4⅓ parts water, by volume.	1 cup	248	88	110	Trace	Trace	---	28	2	Trace	Trace	Trace	.02	.2	17
	Lime juice:															
290	Fresh	1 cup	246	90	65	1	Trace	---	22	22	.5	20	.05	.02	.2	79
291	Canned, unsweetened	1 cup	246	90	65	1	Trace	---	22	22	.5	20	.05	.02	.2	52
	Limeade concentrate, frozen:															
292	Undiluted, can, 6 fluid ounces.	1 can	218	50	410	Trace	Trace	---	108	11	.2	Trace	.02	.02	.2	26
293	Diluted with 4⅓ parts water, by volume.	1 cup	247	90	100	Trace	Trace	---	27	2	Trace	Trace	Trace	Trace	Trace	5
294	Oranges, raw, 2⅝-in. diam., all commercial, varieties.[5]	1 orange	180	86	65	1	Trace	---	16	54	.5	260	.13	.05	.5	66
295	Orange juice, fresh, all varieties.	1 cup	248	88	110	2	1	---	26	27	.5	500	.22	.07	1.0	124
296	Canned, unsweetened	1 cup	249	87	120	2	Trace	---	28	25	1.0	500	.17	.05	.7	100
	Frozen concentrate:															
297	Undiluted, can, 6 fluid ounces.	1 can	213	55	360	5	Trace	---	87	75	.9	1,620	.68	.11	2.8	360
298	Diluted with 3 parts water, by volume.	1 cup	249	87	120	2	Trace	---	29	25	.2	550	.22	.02	1.0	120
299	Dehydrated crystals	4 oz.	113	1	430	6	2	---	100	95	1.9	1,900	.76	.24	3.3	408
300	Prepared with water (1 pound yields about 1 gallon).	1 cup	248	88	115	2	1	---	27	25	.5	500	.20	.07	1.0	109
301	Orange-apricot juice drink	1 cup	249	87	125	1	Trace	---	32	12	.2	1,440	.05	.02	.5	[10]40

[5] Measure and weight apply to entire vegetable or fruit including parts not usually eaten.

[10] Value listed is based on product with label stating 30 milligrams per 6 fl. oz. serving.

[11] For white-fleshed varieties value is about 20 I.U. per cup; for red-fleshed varieties, 1,080 I.U. per cup.

[12] Present only if added by the manufacturer. Refer to the label for this information.

APPENDIX TABLE 1   NUTRITIVE VALUES OF THE EDIBLE PART OF FOODS* (Continued)

[Dashes in the columns for nutrients show that no suitable value could be found although there is reason to believe that a measurable amount of the nutrient may be present]

	Food, approximate measure, and weight (in grams)	Water	Food energy	Pro-tein	Fat	Fatty acids Satu-rated (total)	Fatty acids Unsaturated Oleic	Fatty acids Unsaturated Lin-oleic	Carbo-hy-drate	Cal-cium	Iron	Vita-min A value	Thia-min	Ribo-flavin	Niacin	Ascor-bic acid
		Grams	Per-cent	Calo-ries	Grams	Grams	Grams	Grams	Grams	Grams	Milli-grams	Milli-grams	Inter-national units	Milli-grams	Milli-grams	Milli-grams	Milli-grams

FRUITS AND FRUIT PRODUCTS—Con.

Orange and grapefruit juice:
Frozen concentrate:

	Food, approximate measure, and weight	Grams	Water Per-cent	Food energy Calories	Pro-tein Grams	Fat Grams	Satu-rated (total) Grams	Oleic Grams	Lin-oleic Grams	Carbo-hydrate Grams	Cal-cium Milli-grams	Iron Milli-grams	Vita-min A value Inter-national units	Thia-min Milli-grams	Ribo-flavin Milli-grams	Niacin Milli-grams	Ascor-bic acid Milli-grams
302	Undiluted, can, 6 fluid ounces. 1 can	210	59	330	4	1	-	-	-	78	61	0.8	800	0.48	0.06	2.3	302
303	Diluted with 3 parts water, by volume. 1 cup	248	88	110	1	Trace	-	-	-	26	20	.2	270	.16	.02	.8	102
304	Papayas, raw, ½-inch cubes. 1 cup	182	89	70	1	Trace				18	36	.5	3,190	.07	.08	.5	102
	Peaches: Raw:																
305	Whole, medium, 2-inch diameter, about 4 per pound.[5] 1 peach	114	89	35	1	Trace				10	9	.5	[13]1,320	.02	.05	1.0	7
306	Sliced 1 cup	168	89	65	1	Trace				16	15	.8	[13]2,230	.03	.08	1.6	12
	Canned, yellow-fleshed, solids and liquid: Sirup pack, heavy:																
307	Halves or slices 1 cup	257	79	200	1	Trace				52	10	.8	1,100	.02	.06	1.4	7
308	Water pack 1 cup	245	91	75	1	Trace				20	10	.7	1,100	.02	.06	1.4	7
309	Dried, uncooked 1 cup	160	25	420	5	1				109	77	9.6	6,240	.02	.31	8.5	28
310	Cooked, unsweetened, 10-12 halves and juice. 1 cup	270	77	220	3	1				58	41	5.1	3,290	.01	.15	4.2	6
	Frozen:																
311	Carton, 12 ounces, not thawed. 1 carton	340	76	300	1	Trace				77	14	1.7	2,210	.03	.14	2.4	[14]135
	Pears:																
312	Raw, 3 by 2½-inch diameter.[5] 1 pear	182	83	100	1	1				25	13	.5	30	.04	.07	.2	7
	Canned, solids and liquid: Sirup pack, heavy:																
313	Halves or slices 1 cup	255	80	195	1	1				50	13	.5	Trace	.03	.05	.3	4

No.	Food, approximate measure, and weight	Measure	Grams	Water (%)	Food energy (cal.)	Protein (g)	Fat (g)	Carbohydrate (g)	Calcium (mg)	Iron (mg)	Vit. A (I.U.)	Thiamine (mg)	Riboflavin (mg)	Niacin (mg)	Ascorbic acid (mg)
	Pineapple:														
314	Raw, diced	1 cup	140	85	75	1	Trace	19	24	.7	100	.12	.04	.3	24
	Canned, heavy sirup pack, solids and liquid:														
315	Crushed	1 cup	260	80	195	1	Trace	50	29	.8	120	.20	.06	.5	17
316	Sliced, slices and juice.	2 small or 1 large	122	80	90	Trace	Trace	24	13	.4	50	.09	.03	.2	8
317	Pineapple juice, canned	1 cup	249	86	135	1	Trace	34	37	.7	120	.12	.04	.5	[8]22
	Plums, all except prunes:														
318	Raw, 2-inch diameter, 1 plum, about 2 ounces.[5]	1 plum	60	87	25	Trace	Trace	7	7	.3	140	.02	.02	.3	3
	Canned, sirup pack (Italian prunes):														
319	Plums (with pits) and juice.[5]	1 cup	256	77	205	1	Trace	53	22	2.2	2,970	.05	.05	.9	4
	Prunes, dried, "softenized", medium:														
320	Uncooked.[5]	4 prunes	32	28	70	1	Trace	18	14	1.1	440	.02	.04	.4	1
321	Cooked, unsweetened, 17–18 prunes and ⅓ cup liquid.[5]	1 cup	270	66	295	2	1	78	60	4.5	1,860	.08	.18	1.7	2
322	Prune juice, canned or bottled.	1 cup	256	80	200	1	Trace	49	36	10.5	------	.03	.03	1.0	[8]5
	Raisins, seedless:														
323	Packaged, ½ oz. or 1½ tbsp. per pkg.	1 pkg	14	18	40	Trace	Trace	11	9	.5	Trace	.02	.01	.1	Trace
324	Cup, pressed down	1 cup	165	18	480	4	Trace	128	102	5.8	30	.18	.13	.8	2
	Raspberries, red:														
325	Raw	1 cup	123	84	70	1	1	17	27	1.1	160	.04	.11	1.1	31
326	Frozen, 10-ounce carton, not thawed.	1 carton	284	74	275	2	1	70	37	1.7	200	.06	.17	1.7	59
327	Rhubarb, cooked, sugar added.	1 cup	272	63	385	1	Trace	98	212	1.6	220	.06	.15	.7	17
	Strawberries:														
328	Raw, capped	1 cup	149	90	55	1	1	13	31	1.5	90	.04	.10	1.0	88
329	Frozen, 10-ounce carton, not thawed.	1 carton	284	71	310	1	1	79	40	2.0	90	.06	.17	1.5	150
330	Tangerines, raw, medium, 1 tangerine, 2⅜-in. diam., size 176.[5]	1 tangerine	116	87	40	1	Trace	10	34	.3	360	.05	.02	.1	27
331	Tangerine juice, canned, sweetened.	1 cup	249	87	125	1	1	30	45	.5	1,050	.15	.05	.2	55
332	Watermelon, raw, wedge, 4 by 8 inches (⅙ of 10 by 16-inch melon, about 2 pounds with rind).[5]	1 wedge	925	93	115	2	1	27	30	2.1	2,510	.13	.13	.7	30

[5] Measure and weight apply to entire vegetable or fruit including parts not usually eaten.

[8] This is the amount from the fruit. Additional ascorbic acid may be added by the manufacturer. Refer to the label for this information.

[13] Based on yellow-fleshed varieties; for white-fleshed varieties value is about 50 I.U. per 114-gram peach and 80 I.U. per cup of sliced peaches.

[14] This value includes ascorbic acid added by manufacturer.

APPENDIX TABLE 1 NUTRITIVE VALUES OF THE EDIBLE PART OF FOODS* (Continued)

[Dashes in the columns for nutrients show that no suitable value could be found although there is reason to believe that a measurable amount of the nutrient may be present]

No.	Food, approximate measure, and weight		Water	Food energy	Pro-tein	Fat	Fatty acids			Carbo-hy-drate	Cal-cium	Iron	Vita-min A value	Thia-min	Ribo-flavin	Niacin	Ascor-bic acid
							Satu-rated (total)	Unsaturated									
								Oleic	Lin-oleic								
		Grams	Percent	Calo-ries	Grams	Grams	Grams	Grams	Grams	Grams	Milli-grams	Milli-grams	Inter-national units	Milli-grams	Milli-grams	Milli-grams	Milli-grams
	GRAIN PRODUCTS																
	Bagel, 3-in. diam.:																
333	Egg — 1 bagel	55	32	165	6	2	—	1	1	28	9	1.2	30	0.14	0.10	1.2	0
334	Water — 1 bagel	55	29	165	6	2	—	1	1	30	8	1.2	0	.15	.11	1.4	0
335	Barley, pearled, light, uncooked. 1 cup	200	11	700	16	2	Trace	1	1	158	32	4.0	0	.24	.10	6.2	0
336	Biscuits, baking powder from home recipe with enriched flour, 2-in. diam. 1 biscuit	28	27	105	2	5	1	2	1	13	34	.4	Trace	.06	.06	.1	Trace
337	Biscuits, baking powder from mix, 2-in. diam. 1 biscuit	28	28	90	2	3	1	1	1	15	19	.6	Trace	.08	.07	.6	Trace
338	Bran flakes (40% bran), added thiamin and iron. 1 cup	35	3	105	4	1				28	25	12.3	0	.14	.06	2.2	0
339	Bran flakes with raisins, added thiamin and iron. 1 cup	50	7	145	4	1				40	28	13.5	Trace	.16	.07	2.7	0
	Breads:																
340	Boston brown bread, slice 3 by ¾ in. 1 slice	48	45	100	3	1				22	43	.9	0	.05	.03	.6	0
	Cracked-wheat bread:																
341	Loaf, 1 lb. 1 loaf	454	35	1,190	40	10	2	5	2	236	399	5.0	Trace	.53	.41	5.9	Trace
342	Slice, 18 slices per loaf. 1 slice	25	35	65	2	1				13	22	.3	Trace	.03	.02	.3	Trace
	French or vienna bread:																
343	Enriched, 1 lb. loaf. 1 loaf	454	31	1,315	41	14	3	8	2	251	195	10.0	Trace	1.27	1.00	11.3	Trace
344	Unenriched, 1 lb. loaf. 1 loaf	454	31	1,315	41	14	3	8	2	251	195	3.2	Trace	.36	.36	3.6	Trace
	Italian bread:																
345	Enriched, 1 lb. loaf. 1 loaf	454	32	1,250	41	4	Trace	1	2	256	77	10.0	0	1.32	.91	11.8	0
346	Unenriched, 1 lb. loaf. 1 loaf	454	32	1,250	41	4	Trace	1	2	256	77	3.2	0	.41	.27	3.6	0
	Raisin bread:																
347	Loaf, 1 lb. 1 loaf	454	35	1,190	30	13	3	8	2	243	322	5.9	Trace	.23	.41	3.2	Trace

No.	Food	Amount	Grams	Water (%)	Food energy	Protein (g)	Fat (g)	Saturated (g)	Oleic (g)	Linoleic (g)	Carbohydrate (g)	Calcium (mg)	Iron (mg)	Vitamin A	Thiamin (mg)	Riboflavin (mg)	Niacin (mg)	Ascorbic acid
348	Slice, 18 slices per loaf.	1 slice	25	35	65	2	1	—	—	—	13	18	.3	Trace	.01	.02	.2	Trace
	Rye bread:																	
	American, light (⅓ rye, ⅔ wheat):																	
349	Loaf, 1 lb.	1 loaf	454	36	1,100	41	5	—	—	—	236	340	7.3	0	.82	.32	6.4	0
350	Slice, 18 slices per loaf.	1 slice	25	36	60	2	Trace	—	—	—	13	19	.4	0	.05	.02	.4	0
351	Pumpernickel, loaf, 1 lb.	1 loaf	454	34	1,115	41	5	—	—	—	241	381	10.9	0	1.04	.64	5.4	0
	White bread, enriched:[15]																	
	Soft-crumb type:																	
352	Loaf, 1 lb.	1 loaf	454	36	1,225	39	15	3	8	2	229	381	11.3	Trace	1.13	.95	10.9	Trace
353	Slice, 18 slices per loaf.	1 slice	25	36	70	2	1	—	—	—	13	21	.6	Trace	.06	.05	.6	Trace
354	Slice, toasted.	1 slice	22	25	70	2	1	—	—	—	13	21	.6	Trace	.06	.05	.6	Trace
355	Slice, 22 slices per loaf.	1 slice	20	36	55	2	1	—	—	—	10	17	.5	Trace	.05	.04	.5	Trace
356	Slice, toasted.	1 slice	17	25	55	2	1	—	—	—	10	17	.5	Trace	.05	.04	.5	Trace
357	Loaf, 1½ lbs.	1 loaf	680	36	1,835	59	22	5	12	3	343	571	17.0	Trace	1.70	1.43	16.3	Trace
358	Slice, 24 slices per loaf.	1 slice	28	36	75	2	1	—	—	—	14	24	.7	Trace	.07	.06	.7	Trace
359	Slice, toasted.	1 slice	24	25	75	2	1	—	—	—	14	24	.7	Trace	.07	.06	.7	Trace
360	Slice, 28 slices per loaf.	1 slice	24	36	65	2	1	—	—	—	12	20	.6	Trace	.06	.05	.6	Trace
361	Slice, toasted.	1 slice	21	25	65	2	1	—	—	—	12	20	.6	Trace	.06	.05	.6	Trace
	Firm-crumb type:																	
362	Loaf, 1 lb.	1 loaf	454	35	1,245	41	17	4	10	2	228	435	11.3	Trace	1.22	.91	10.9	Trace
363	Slice, 20 slices per loaf.	1 slice	23	35	65	2	1	—	—	—	12	22	.6	Trace	.06	.05	.6	Trace
364	Slice, toasted.	1 slice	20	24	65	2	1	—	—	—	12	22	.6	Trace	.06	.05	.6	Trace
365	Loaf, 2 lbs.	1 loaf	907	35	2,495	82	34	8	20	4	455	871	22.7	Trace	2.45	1.81	21.8	Trace
366	Slice, 34 slices per loaf.	1 slice	27	35	75	2	1	—	—	—	14	26	.7	Trace	.07	.05	.6	Trace
367	Slice, toasted.	1 slice	23	24	75	2	1	—	—	—	14	26	.7	Trace	.07	.05	.6	Trace
	Whole-wheat bread, soft-crumb type:																	
368	Loaf, 1 lb.	1 loaf	454	36	1,095	41	12	2	6	2	224	381	13.6	Trace	1.36	.45	12.7	Trace
369	Slice, 16 slices per loaf.	1 slice	28	36	65	3	1	—	—	—	14	24	.8	Trace	.09	.03	.8	Trace
370	Slice, toasted.	1 slice	24	24	65	3	1	—	—	—	14	24	.8	Trace	.09	.03	.8	Trace

[15] Values for iron, thiamin, riboflavin, and niacin per pound of unenriched white bread would be as follows:

	Iron Milligrams	Thiamin Milligrams	Riboflavin Milligrams	Niacin Milligrams
Soft crumb	3.2	.31	.39	5.0
Firm crumb	3.2	.32	.59	4.1

APPENDIX TABLE 1   NUTRITIVE VALUES OF THE EDIBLE PART OF FOODS* (Continued)

[Dashes in the columns for nutrients show that no suitable value could be found although there is reason to believe that a measurable amount of the nutrient may be present]

	Food, approximate measure, and weight (in grams)	Water	Food energy	Protein	Fat	Fatty acids Saturated (total)	Unsaturated Oleic	Unsaturated Linoleic	Carbohydrate	Calcium	Iron	Vitamin A value	Thiamin	Riboflavin	Niacin	Ascorbic acid
		Grams	Percent	Calories	Grams	Grams	Grams	Grams	Grams	Grams	Milligrams	Milligrams	International units	Milligrams	Milligrams	Milligrams	Milligrams
	GRAIN PRODUCTS—Continued																
	Bread—Continued																
	Whole-wheat bread, firm-crumb type:																
371	Loaf, 1 lb_____ 1 loaf_____	454	36	1,100	48	14	3	6	3	216	449	13.6	Trace	1.18	0.54	12.7	Trace
372	Slice, 18 slices per loaf. 1 slice_____	25	36	60	3	1				12	25	.8	Trace	.06	.03	.7	Trace
373	Slice, toasted_____ 1 slice_____	21	24	60	3	1				12	25	.8	Trace	.06	.03	.7	Trace
374	Breadcrumbs, dry, grated. 1 cup_____	100	6	390	13	5	1	2	1	73	122	3.6	Trace	.22	.30	3.5	Trace
375	Buckwheat flour, light, sifted. 1 cup_____	98	12	340	6	1				78	11	1.0	0	.08	.04	.4	0
376	Bulgur, canned, seasoned. 1 cup_____	135	56	245	8	4				44	27	1.9	0	.08	.05	4.1	0
	Cakes made from cake mixes:																
	Angelfood:																
377	Whole cake_____ 1 cake_____	635	34	1,645	36	1				377	603	1.9	0	.03	.70	.6	0
378	Piece, 1/12 of 10-in. diam. cake. 1 piece_____	53	34	135	3	Trace				32	50	.2	0	Trace	.06	.1	0
	Cupcakes, small, 2½ in. diam.:																
379	Without icing_____ 1 cupcake_____	25	26	90	1	3	1	1	1	14	40	.1	40	.01	.03	.1	Trace
380	With chocolate icing. 1 cupcake_____	36	22	130	2	5	2	2	1	21	47	.3	60	.01	.04	.1	Trace
	Devil's food, 2-layer, with chocolate icing:																
381	Whole cake_____ 1 cake_____	1,107	24	3,755	49	136	54	58	16	645	653	8.9	1,660	.33	.89	3.3	1
382	Piece, 1/16 of 9-in. diam. cake. 1 piece_____	69	24	235	3	9	3	4	1	40	41	.6	100	.02	.06	.2	Trace
383	Cupcake, small, 2½ in. diam. 1 cupcake_____	35	24	120	2	4	1	2	Trace	20	21	.3	50	.01	.03	.1	Trace
	Gingerbread:																
384	Whole cake_____ 1 cake_____	570	37	1,575	18	39	10	19	9	291	513	9.1	Trace	.17	.51	4.6	2
385	Piece, 1/9 of 8-in. square cake. 1 piece_____	63	37	175	2	4	1	2	1	32	57	1.0	Trace	.02	.06	.5	Trace
	White, 2-layer, with chocolate icing:																
386	Whole cake_____ 1 cake_____	1,140	21	4,000	45	122	45	54	17	716	1,129	5.7	680	.23	.91	2.3	2

No.	Food, approximate measure	Measure	Grams	Water (%)	Food energy	Protein	Fat	Saturated fatty acids	Oleic	Linoleic	Carbohydrate	Calcium	Iron	Vitamin A	Thiamin	Riboflavin	Niacin	Ascorbic acid
387	Piece, 1/16 of 9-in. diam. cake.	1 piece	71	21	250	3	8	3	3	1	45	70	.4	40	.01	.06	.1	Trace
	Cakes made from home recipes:[16]																	
388	Boston cream pie; piece 1/12 of 8-in. diam.	1 piece	69	35	210	4	6	2	3	1	34	46	.3	140	.02	.08	.1	Trace
	Fruitcake, dark, made with enriched flour:																	
389	Loaf, 1-lb.	1 loaf	454	18	1,720	22	69	15	37	13	271	327	11.8	540	.59	.64	3.6	2
390	Slice, 1/30 of 8-in. loaf.	1 slice	15	18	55	1	2	Trace	1	Trace	9	11	.4	20	.02	.02	.1	Trace
	Plain sheet cake: Without icing:																	
391	Whole cake	1 cake	777	25	2,830	35	108	30	52	21	434	497	3.1	1,320	.16	.70	1.6	2
392	Piece, 1/9 of 9-in. square cake.	1 piece	86	25	315	4	12	3	6	2	48	55	.3	150	.02	.08	.2	Trace
393	With boiled white icing, piece, 1/9 of 9-in. square cake.	1 piece	114	23	400	4	12	3	6	2	71	56	.3	150	.02	.08	.2	Trace
	Pound:																	
394	Loaf, 8½ by 3½ by 3 in.	1 loaf	514	17	2,430	29	152	34	68	17	242	108	4.1	1,440	.15	.46	1.0	0
395	Slice, ½-in. thick.	1 slice	30	17	140	2	9	2	4	1	14	6	.2	80	.01	.03	.1	0
	Sponge:																	
396	Whole cake	1 cake	790	32	2,345	60	45	14	20	4	427	237	9.5	3,560	.40	1.11	1.6	Trace
397	Piece, 1/12 of 10-in. diam. cake.	1 piece	66	32	195	5	4	1	2	Trace	36	20	.8	300	.03	.09	.1	Trace
	Yellow, 2-layer, without icing:																	
398	Whole cake	1 cake	870	24	3,160	39	111	31	53	22	506	618	3.5	1,310	.17	.70	1.7	2
399	Piece, 1/16 of 9-in. diam. cake.	1 piece	54	24	200	2	7	2	3	1	32	39	.2	80	.01	.04	.1	Trace
	Yellow, 2-layer, with chocolate icing:																	
400	Whole cake	1 cake	1,203	21	4,390	51	156	55	69	23	727	818	7.2	1,920	.24	.96	2.4	Trace
401	Piece, 1/16 of 9-in. diam. cake.	1 piece	75	21	275	3	10	3	4	1	45	51	.5	120	.02	.06	.2	Trace
	Cake icings. See Sugars, Sweets. Cookies: Brownies with nuts:																	
402	Made from home recipe with enriched flour.	1 brownie	20	10	95	1	6	1	3	1	10	8	.4	40	.04	.02	.1	Trace
403	Made from mix.	1 brownie	20	11	85	1	4	1	2	1	13	9	.4	20	.03	.02	.1	Trace

[16] Unenriched cake flour used unless otherwise specified.

APPENDIX TABLE 1   NUTRITIVE VALUES OF THE EDIBLE PART OF FOODS* (Continued)

[Dashes in the columns for nutrients show that no suitable value could be found although there is reason to believe that a measurable amount of the nutrient may be present]

	Food, approximate measure, and weight (in grams)		Water	Food energy	Pro-tein	Fat	Fatty acids			Carbo-hy-drate	Cal-cium	Iron	Vita-min A value	Thia-min	Ribo-flavin	Niacin	Ascor-bic acid
							Satu-rated (total)	Unsaturated									
								Oleic	Lin-oleic								
		Grams	Per cent	Calo-ries	Grams	Grams	Grams	Grams	Grams	Grams	Milli-grams	Milli-grams	Inter-national units	Milli-grams	Milli-grams	Milli-grams	Milli-grams
	GRAIN PRODUCTS—Continued																
	Cookies—Continued																
	Chocolate chip:																
404	Made from home recipe with en-riched flour. 1 cookie	10	3	50	1	3	1	1	1	6	4	0.2	10	0.01	0.01	0.1	Trace
405	Commercial 1 cookie	10	3	50	1	2	1	1	Trace	7	4	.2	10	Trace	Trace	Trace	Trace
406	Fig bars, commercial 1 cookie	14	14	50	1	1				11	11	.2	20	Trace	.01	.1	Trace
407	Sandwich, chocolate or vanilla, commercial. 1 cookie	10	2	50	1	2	1	1	Trace	7	2	.1	0	Trace	Trace	.1	0
	Corn flakes, added nutrients:																
408	Plain 1 cup	25	4	100	2	Trace				21	4	.4	0	.11	.02	.5	0
409	Sugar-covered 1 cup	40	2	155	2	Trace				36	5	.4	0	.16	.02	.8	0
	Corn (hominy) grits, degermed, cooked:																
410	Enriched 1 cup	245	87	125	3	Trace				27	2	.7	[17] 150	.10	.07	1.0	0
411	Unenriched 1 cup	245	87	125	3	Trace				27	2	.2	[17] 150	.05	.02	.5	0
	Cornmeal:																
412	Whole-ground, unbolted, dry. 1 cup	122	12	435	11	5	1	2	2	90	24	2.9	[17] 620	.46	.13	2.4	0
413	Bolted (nearly whole-grain) dry. 1 cup	122	12	440	11	4	Trace	1	2	91	21	2.2	[17] 590	.37	.10	2.3	0
	Degermed, enriched:																
414	Dry form 1 cup	138	12	500	11	2				108	8	4.0	[17] 610	.61	.36	4.8	0
415	Cooked 1 cup	240	88	120	3	1				26	2	1.0	[17] 140	.14	.10	1.2	0
	Degermed, unenriched:																
416	Dry form 1 cup	138	12	500	11	2				108	8	1.5	[17] 610	.19	.07	1.4	0
417	Cooked 1 cup	240	88	120	3	1				26	2	.5	[17] 140	.05	.02	.2	0
418	Corn muffins, made with enriched de-germed cornmeal and enriched flour; muffin 2⅜-in. diam. 1 muffin	40	33	125	3	4	2	2	Trace	19	42	.7	[17] 120	.08	.09	.6	Trace

No.	Food	Measure	Weight (g)	Water (%)	Food energy	Protein (g)	Fat (g)	Saturated (g)	Oleic (g)	Linoleic (g)	Carbohydrate (g)	Calcium (mg)	Iron (mg)	Vitamin A	Thiamin (mg)	Riboflavin (mg)	Niacin (mg)	Ascorbic acid (mg)
419	Corn muffins, made with mix, egg, and milk; muffin 2⅜-in. diam.	1 muffin	40	30	130	3	4	1	2	1	20	96	.6	100	.07	.08	.6	Trace
420	Corn, puffed, presweetened, added nutrients.	1 cup	30	2	115	2	Trace	----	----	----	27	3	.5	0	.13	.05	.6	0
421	Corn, shredded, added nutrients.	1 cup	25	3	100	2	Trace	----	----	----	22	1	.6	0	.11	.05	.5	0
	Crackers:																	
422	Graham, 2½-in. square	4 crackers	28	6	110	2	3	----	----	----	21	11	.4	0	.01	.06	.4	0
423	Saltines	4 crackers	11	4	50	1	1	----	----	----	8	2	.1	0	Trace	Trace	.1	0
	Danish pastry, plain (without fruit or nuts):																	
424	Packaged ring, 12 ounces.	1 ring	340	22	1,435	25	80	24	37	15	155	170	3.1	1,050	.24	.51	2.7	Trace
425	Round piece, approx. 4¼-in. diam. by 1 in.	1 pastry	65	22	275	5	15	5	7	3	30	33	.6	200	.05	.10	.5	Trace
426	Ounce	1 oz.	28	22	120	2	7	2	3	1	13	14	.3	90	.02	.04	.2	Trace
427	Doughnuts, cake type	1 doughnut	32	24	125	1	6	1	4	Trace	16	13	[18].4	30	[18].05	[18].05	[18].4	Trace
428	Farina, quick-cooking, enriched, cooked.	1 cup	245	89	105	3	Trace	----	----	----	22	147	[19].7	0	[19].12	[19].07	[19]1.0	0
	Macaroni, cooked:																	
	Enriched:																	
429	Cooked, firm stage (undergoes additional cooking in a food mixture).	1 cup	130	64	190	6	1	----	----	----	39	14	[19]1.4	0	[19].23	[19].14	[19]1.8	0
430	Cooked until tender	1 cup	140	72	155	5	1	----	----	----	32	8	[19]1.3	0	[19].20	[19].11	[19]1.5	0
	Unenriched:																	
431	Cooked, firm stage (undergoes additional cooking in a food mixture).	1 cup	130	64	190	6	1	----	----	----	39	14	.7	0	.03	.03	.5	0
432	Cooked until tender	1 cup	140	72	155	5	1	----	----	----	32	11	.6	0	.01	.01	.4	0
433	Macaroni (enriched) and cheese, baked.	1 cup	200	58	430	17	22	10	9	2	40	362	1.8	860	.20	.40	1.8	Trace
434	Canned	1 cup	240	80	230	9	10	4	3	1	26	199	1.0	260	.12	.24	1.0	Trace
435	Muffins, with enriched white flour; muffin, 3-inch diam.	1 muffin	40	38	120	3	4	1	2	1	17	42	.6	40	.07	.09	.6	Trace
	Noodles (egg noodles), cooked:																	
436	Enriched	1 cup	160	70	200	7	2	1	1	Trace	37	16	[19]1.4	110	[19].22	[19].13	[19]1.9	0
437	Unenriched	1 cup	160	70	200	7	2	1	1	Trace	37	16	1.0	110	.05	.03	.6	0

[17] This value is based on product made from yellow varieties of corn; white varieties contain only a trace.

[18] Based on product made with enriched flour. With unenriched flour, approximate values per doughnut are: Iron, 0.2 milligram; thiamin, 0.01 milligram; riboflavin, 0.03 milligram; niacin, 0.2 milligram.

[19] Iron, thiamin, riboflavin, and niacin are based on the minimum levels of enrichment specified in standards of identity promulgated under the Federal Food, Drug, and Cosmetic Act.

APPENDIX TABLE 1 NUTRITIVE VALUES OF THE EDIBLE PART OF FOODS* (Continued)

[Dashes in the columns for nutrients show that no suitable value could be found although there is reason to believe that a measurable amount of the nutrient may be present]

	Food, approximate measure, and weight (in grams)	Water	Food energy	Pro-tein	Fat	Fatty acids Satu-rated (total)	Fatty acids Unsaturated Oleic	Fatty acids Unsaturated Lin-oleic	Carbo-hy-drate	Cal-cium	Iron	Vita-min A value	Thia-min	Ribo-flavin	Niacin	Ascor-bic acid
		Per-cent	Calo-ries	Grams	Grams	Grams	Grams	Grams	Grams	Milli-grams	Milli-grams	Inter-national units	Milli-grams	Milli-grams	Milli-grams	Milli-grams
	GRAIN PRODUCTS—Continued															
438	Oats (with or without corn) puffed, added nutrients. 1 cup — 25 g	3	100	3	1	—	—	—	19	44	1.2	0	0.24	0.04	0.5	0
439	Oatmeal or rolled oats, cooked. 1 cup — 240 g	87	130	5	2	—	—	1	23	22	1.4	0	.19	.05	.2	0
	Pancakes, 4-inch diam.:															
440	Wheat, enriched flour (home recipe). 1 cake — 27 g	50	60	2	2	Trace	1	Trace	9	27	.4	30	.05	.06	.4	Trace
441	Buckwheat (made from mix with egg and milk). 1 cake — 27 g	58	55	2	2	1	1	Trace	6	59	.4	60	.03	.04	.2	Trace
442	Plain or buttermilk (made from mix with egg and milk). 1 cake — 27 g	51	60	2	2	1	1	Trace	9	58	.3	70	.04	.06	.2	Trace
	Pie (piecrust made with unenriched flour): Sector, 4-in., ⅐ of 9-in. diam. pie:															
443	Apple (2-crust). 1 sector — 135 g	48	350	3	15	4	7	3	51	11	.4	40	.03	.03	.5	1
444	Butterscotch (1-crust). 1 sector — 130 g	45	350	6	14	5	6	2	50	98	1.2	340	.04	.13	.3	Trace
445	Cherry (2-crust). 1 sector — 135 g	47	350	4	15	4	7	3	52	19	.4	590	.03	.03	.7	Trace
446	Custard (1-crust). 1 sector — 130 g	58	285	8	14	5	6	2	30	125	.8	300	.07	.21	.4	0
447	Lemon meringue (1-crust). 1 sector — 120 g	47	305	4	12	4	6	2	45	17	.6	200	.04	.10	.2	4
448	Mince (2-crust). 1 sector — 135 g	43	365	3	16	4	8	3	56	38	1.4	Trace	.09	.05	.5	1
449	Pecan (1-crust). 1 sector — 118 g	20	490	6	27	4	16	5	60	55	3.3	190	.19	.08	.4	Trace
450	Pineapple chiffon (1-crust). 1 sector — 93 g	41	265	6	11	3	5	2	36	22	.8	320	.04	.08	.4	1
451	Pumpkin (1-crust). 1 sector — 130 g	59	275	5	15	5	6	2	32	66	.7	3,210	.04	.13	.7	Trace
	Piecrust, baked shell for pie made with:															
452	Enriched flour. 1 shell — 180 g	15	900	11	60	16	28	12	79	25	3.1	0	.36	.25	3.2	0
453	Unenriched flour. 1 shell — 180 g	15	900	11	60	16	28	12	79	25	.9	0	.05	.05	.9	0

No.	Food, approximate measure, and weight																
454	Piecrust mix including stick form: Package, 10-oz., for double crust. 1 pkg.	284	9	1,480	20	93	23	46	21	141	131	1.4	0	.11	.11	2.0	0
455	Pizza (cheese) 5½-in. sector; ⅛ of 14-in. diam. pie. 1 sector	75	45	185	7	6	2	3	Trace	27	107	.7	290	.04	.12	.7	4
	Popcorn, popped:																
456	Plain, large kernel 1 cup	6	4	25	1	Trace	—	—	—	5	1	.2	—	—	.01	.1	0
457	With oil and salt 1 cup	9	3	40	1	2	—	—	—	5	1	.2	—	—	.01	.2	0
458	Sugar coated 1 cup	35	4	135	2	1	—	—	—	30	2	.5	—	—	.02	.4	0
	Pretzels:																
459	Dutch, twisted 1 pretzel	16	5	60	2	1	—	—	—	12	4	.2	0	Trace	Trace	.1	0
460	Thin, twisted 1 pretzel	6	5	25	1	Trace	—	—	—	5	1	.1	0	Trace	Trace	Trace	0
461	Stick, small, 2¼ inches 10 sticks	3	5	10	Trace	Trace	—	—	—	2	1	Trace	0	Trace	Trace	Trace	0
462	Stick, regular, 3⅛ inches 5 sticks	3	5	10	Trace	Trace	—	—	—	2	1	Trace	0	Trace	Trace	Trace	0
	Rice, white: Enriched:																
463	Raw 1 cup	185	12	670	12	1	—	—	—	149	44	[20]5.4	0	[20].81	[20].06	[20]6.5	0
464	Cooked 1 cup	205	73	225	4	Trace	—	—	—	50	21	[20]1.8	0	[20].23	[20].02	[20]2.1	0
465	Instant, ready-to-serve 1 cup	165	73	180	4	Trace	—	—	—	40	5	[20]1.3	0	[20].21	[20]—	[20]1.7	0
466	Unenriched, cooked 1 cup	205	73	225	4	Trace	—	—	—	50	21	.4	0	.04	.02	.8	0
467	Parboiled, cooked 1 cup	175	73	185	4	Trace	—	—	—	41	33	[20]1.4	0	[20].19	[20]—	[20]2.1	0
468	Rice, puffed, added nutrients 1 cup	15	4	60	1	Trace	—	—	—	13	3	.3	0	.07	.01	.7	0
	Rolls, enriched: Cloverleaf or pan:																
469	Home recipe 1 roll	35	26	120	3	3	1	1	1	20	16	.7	30	.09	.09	.8	Trace
470	Commercial 1 roll	28	31	85	2	2	Trace	1	Trace	15	21	.5	Trace	.08	.05	.6	Trace
471	Frankfurter or hamburger 1 roll	40	31	120	3	2	1	1	1	21	30	.8	Trace	.11	.07	.9	Trace
472	Hard, round or rectangular 1 roll	50	25	155	5	2	Trace	1	Trace	30	24	1.2	Trace	.13	.12	1.4	Trace
473	Rye wafers, whole-grain, 1⅞ by 3½ inches 2 wafers	13	6	45	2	Trace	—	—	—	10	7	.5	0	.04	.03	.2	0
474	Spaghetti, cooked, tender stage, enriched 1 cup	140	72	155	5	1	—	—	—	32	11	[19]1.3	0	[19].20	[19].11	[19]1.5	0

[19] Iron, thiamin, riboflavin, and niacin are based on the minimum levels of enrichment specified in standards of identity promulgated under the Federal Food, Drug, and Cosmetic Act.

[20] Iron, thiamin, and niacin are based on the minimum levels of enrichment specified in standards of identity promulgated under the Federal Food, Drug, and Cosmetic Act. Riboflavin is based on unenriched rice. When the minimum level of enrichment for riboflavin specified in the standards of identity becomes effective the value will be 0.12 milligram per cup of parboiled rice and of white rice.

APPENDIX TABLE 1   NUTRITIVE VALUES OF THE EDIBLE PART OF FOODS* (Continued)

[Dashes show that no basis could be found for imputing a value although there was some reason to believe that a measurable amount of the constituent might be present]

	Food, approximate measure, and weight (in grams)	Water	Food energy	Protein	Fat	Fatty acids Saturated (total)	Unsaturated Oleic	Unsaturated Linoleic	Carbohydrate	Calcium	Iron	Vitamin A value	Thiamin	Riboflavin	Niacin	Ascorbic acid
		Grams	Per cent	Calories	Grams	Grams	Grams	Grams	Grams	Grams	Milligrams	Milligrams	International units	Milligrams	Milligrams	Milligrams	Milligrams
	GRAIN PRODUCTS—Continued																
	Spaghetti with meat balls, and tomato sauce:																
475	Home recipe --- 1 cup ---	248	70	330	19	12	4	6	1	39	124	3.7	1,590	0.25	0.30	4.0	22
476	Canned --- 1 cup ---	250	78	260	12	10	2	3	4	28	53	3.3	1,000	.15	.18	2.3	5
	Spaghetti in tomato sauce with cheese:																
477	Home recipe --- 1 cup ---	250	77	260	9	9	2	5	1	37	80	2.3	1,080	.25	.18	2.3	13
478	Canned --- 1 cup ---	250	80	190	6	2	1	1	1	38	40	2.8	930	.35	.28	4.5	10
479	Waffles, with enriched flour, 7-in. diam. --- 1 waffle ---	75	41	210	7	7	2	4	1	28	85	1.3	250	.13	.19	1.0	Trace
480	Waffles, made from mix, enriched, egg and milk added, 7-in. diam. --- 1 waffle ---	75	42	205	7	8	3	3	1	27	179	1.0	170	.11	.17	.7	Trace
481	Wheat, puffed, added nutrients. --- 1 cup ---	15	3	55	2	Trace	---	---	---	12	4	.6	0	.08	.03	1.2	0
482	Wheat, shredded, plain --- 1 biscuit ---	25	7	90	2	1	---	---	---	20	11	.9	0	.06	.03	1.1	0
483	Wheat flakes, added nutrients. --- 1 cup ---	30	4	105	3	Trace	---	---	---	24	12	1.3	0	.19	.04	1.5	0
	Wheat flours:																
484	Whole-wheat, from hard wheats, stirred. --- 1 cup ---	120	12	400	16	2	Trace	1	1	85	49	4.0	0	.66	.14	5.2	0
	All-purpose or family flour, enriched:																
485	Sifted --- 1 cup ---	115	12	420	12	1	---	---	---	88	18	[193]3.3	0	[193].51	[19].30	[194]4.0	0
486	Unsifted --- 1 cup ---	125	12	455	13	1	---	---	---	95	20	[193]3.6	0	[193].55	[19].33	[194]4.4	0
487	Self-rising, enriched --- 1 cup ---	125	12	440	12	1	---	---	---	93	331	[193]3.6	0	[193].55	[19].33	[194]4.4	0
488	Cake or pastry flour, sifted. --- 1 cup ---	96	12	350	7	1	---	---	---	76	16	.5	0	.03	.03	.7	0
	FATS, OILS																
	Butter:																
	Regular, 4 sticks per pound:																
489	Stick --- ½ cup ---	113	16	810	1	92	51	30	3	1	23	0	[213]3,750	---	---	---	0

No.	Food, approximate measure	Measure	Grams	Water (%)	Food energy	Protein	Fat	Saturated	Oleic	Linoleic	Carbohydrate	Calcium	Iron	Vitamin A	Thiamin	Riboflavin	Niacin	Ascorbic acid
490	Tablespoon (approx. 1/8 stick)	1 tbsp	14	16	100	Trace	12	6	4	Trace	Trace	3	0	[21]470	---	---	---	0
491	Pat (1-in. sq. 1/3-in. high; 90 per lb.)	1 pat	5	16	35	Trace	4	2	1	Trace	Trace	1	0	[21]170	---	---	---	0
	Whipped, 6 sticks or 2, 8-oz. containers per pound:																	
492	Stick	1/2 cup	76	16	540	1	61	34	20	2	1	15	0	[21]2,500	---	---	---	0
493	Tablespoon (approx. 1/8 stick)	1 tbsp	9	16	65	Trace	8	4	3	Trace	Trace	2	0	[21]310	---	---	---	0
494	Pat (1 1/4-in. sq. 1/3-in. high; 120 per lb.)	1 pat	4	16	25	Trace	3	2	1	Trace	Trace	1	0	[21]130	---	---	---	0
	Fats, cooking:																	
495	Lard	1 cup	205	0	1,850	0	205	78	94	20	0	0	0	0	0	0	0	0
496		1 tbsp	13	0	115	0	13	5	6	1	0	0	0	0	0	0	0	0
497	Vegetable fats	1 cup	200	0	1,770	0	200	50	100	44	0	0	0	---	0	0	0	0
498		1 tbsp	13	0	110	0	13	3	6	3	0	0	0	---	0	0	0	0
	Margarine:																	
	Regular, 4 sticks per pound:																		
499	Stick	1/2 cup	113	16	815	1	92	17	46	25	1	23	0	[22]3,750	---	---	---	0
500	Tablespoon (approx. 1/8 stick)	1 tbsp	14	16	100	Trace	12	2	6	3	Trace	3	0	[22]470	---	---	---	0
501	Pat (1-in. sq. 1/3-in. high; 90 per lb.)	1 pat	5	16	35	Trace	4	1	2	1	Trace	1	0	[22]170	---	---	---	0
	Whipped, 6 sticks per pound:																		
502	Stick	1/2 cup	76	16	545	1	61	11	31	17	1	15	0	[22]2,500	---	---	---	0
	Soft, 2 8-oz. tubs per pound:																		
503	Tub	1 tub	227	16	1,635	1	184	34	68	68	1	45	0	[22]7,500	---	---	---	0
504	Tablespoon	1 tbsp	14	16	100	Trace	11	2	4	4	Trace	3	0	[22]470	---	---	---	0
	Oils, salad or cooking:																		
505	Corn	1 cup	220	0	1,945	0	220	22	62	117	0	0	0	0	0	0	0	0
506		1 tbsp	14	0	125	0	14	1	4	7	0	0	0	0	0	0	0	0
507	Cottonseed	1 cup	220	0	1,945	0	220	55	46	110	0	0	0	0	0	0	0	0
508		1 tbsp	14	0	125	0	14	4	3	7	0	0	0	0	0	0	0	0
509	Olive	1 cup	220	0	1,945	0	220	24	167	15	0	0	0	0	0	0	0	0
510		1 tbsp	14	0	125	0	14	2	11	1	0	0	0	0	0	0	0	0
511	Peanut	1 cup	220	0	1,945	0	220	40	103	64	0	0	0	0	0	0	0	0
512		1 tbsp	14	0	125	0	14	3	7	4	0	0	0	0	0	0	0	0
513	Safflower	1 cup	220	0	1,945	0	220	18	37	165	0	0	0	0	0	0	0	0
514		1 tbsp	14	0	125	0	14	1	2	10	0	0	0	0	0	0	0	0
515	Soybean	1 cup	220	0	1,945	0	220	33	44	114	0	0	0	0	0	0	0	0
516		1 tbsp	14	0	125	0	14	2	3	7	0	0	0	0	0	0	0	0

[19] Iron, thiamin, riboflavin, and niacin are based on the minimum levels of enrichment specified in standards of identity promulgated under the Federal Food, Drug, and Cosmetic Act.

[21] Year-round average.

[22] Based on the average vitamin A content of fortified margarine. Federal specifications for fortified margarine require a minimum of 15,000 I.U. of vitamin A per pound.

APPENDIX TABLE 1   NUTRITIVE VALUES OF THE EDIBLE PART OF FOODS* (Continued)

[Dashes in the columns for nutrients show that no suitable value could be found although there is reason to believe that a measurable amount of the nutrient may be present]

Food, approximate measure, and weight (in grams)		Water	Food energy	Protein	Fat	Fatty acids			Carbohydrate	Calcium	Iron	Vitamin A value	Thiamin	Riboflavin	Niacin	Ascorbic acid
						Saturated (total)	Unsaturated Oleic	Unsaturated Linoleic								
	Grams	Per cent	Calories	Grams	Grams	Grams	Grams	Grams	Grams	Milligrams	Milligrams	International units	Milligrams	Milligrams	Milligrams	Milligrams
FATS, OILS—Continued																
Salad dressings:																
517 Blue cheese------- 1 tbsp.-------	15	32	75	1	8	2	2	4	1	12	Trace	30	Trace	0.02	Trace	Trace
Commercial, mayonnaise type:																
518 Regular------- 1 tbsp.-------	15	41	65	Trace	6	1	1	3	2	2	Trace	30	Trace	Trace	Trace	---
519 Special dietary, low-calorie. 1 tbsp.-------	16	81	20	Trace	2	Trace	Trace	1	1	3	Trace	40	Trace	Trace	Trace	---
French:																
520 Regular------- 1 tbsp.-------	16	39	65	Trace	6	1	1	3	3	2	.1	---	---	---	---	---
521 Special dietary, low-fat with artificial sweeteners. 1 tbsp.-------	15	95	Trace	Trace	Trace	---			Trace	2	.1	---	---	---	---	---
522 Home cooked, boiled----- 1 tbsp.-----	16	68	25	1	2	1	1	Trace	2	14	.1	80	.01	.03	Trace	Trace
523 Mayonnaise----- 1 tbsp.-----	14	15	100	Trace	11	2	2	6	Trace	3	.1	40	Trace	.01	Trace	---
524 Thousand island----- 1 tbsp.-----	16	32	80	Trace	8	1	2	4	3	2	.1	50	Trace	Trace	Trace	Trace
SUGARS, SWEETS																
Cake icings:																
525 Chocolate made with milk and table fat. 1 cup-----	275	14	1,035	9	38	21	14	1	185	165	3.3	580	.06	.28	.6	1
526 Coconut (with boiled icing). 1 cup-----	166	15	605	3	13	11	1	Trace	124	10	.8	0	.02	.07	.3	0
527 Creamy fudge from mix with water only. 1 cup-----	245	15	830	7	16	5	8	3	183	96	2.7	Trace	.05	.20	.7	Trace
528 White, boiled------- 1 cup-----	94	18	300	1	0	---			76	2	Trace	0	Trace	.03	Trace	0
Candy:																
529 Caramels, plain or chocolate. 1 oz-------	28	8	115	1	3	2	1	Trace	22	42	.4	Trace	.01	.05	.1	Trace
530 Chocolate, milk, plain-- 1 oz-------	28	1	145	2	9	5	3	Trace	16	65	.3	80	.02	.10	.1	Trace
531 Chocolate-coated peanuts. 1 oz-------	28	1	160	5	12	3	6	2	11	33	.4	Trace	.10	.05	2.1	Trace

No.	Food	Measure	Grams	Water (%)	Food energy (cal)	Protein (g)	Fat (g)	Saturated fat (g)	Oleic (g)	Linoleic (g)	Carbohydrate (g)	Calcium (mg)	Iron (mg)	Vitamin A (I.U.)	Thiamin (mg)	Riboflavin (mg)	Niacin (mg)	Ascorbic acid (mg)
532	Fondant; mints, uncoated; candy corn.	1 oz.	28	8	105	Trace	1	---	---	---	25	4	.3	0	0	Trace	Trace	0
533	Fudge, plain.	1 oz.	28	8	115	1	4	---	---	---	21	22	.3	Trace	.01	.03	.1	Trace
534	Gum drops.	1 oz.	28	12	100	Trace	Trace	---	---	---	25	2	.1	0	0	Trace	Trace	0
535	Hard.	1 oz.	28	1	110	0	Trace	---	---	---	28	6	.5	0	0	0	0	0
536	Marshmallows.	1 oz.	28	17	90	1	Trace	---	---	---	23	5	.5	0	0	Trace	Trace	0
	Chocolate-flavored sirup or topping:																	
537	Thin type.	1 fl. oz.	38	32	90	1	1	Trace	Trace	Trace	24	6	.6	Trace	.01	.03	.2	0
538	Fudge type.	1 fl. oz.	38	25	125	2	5	3	2	Trace	20	48	.5	60	.02	.08	.2	Trace
	Chocolate-flavored beverage powder (approx. 4 heaping teaspoons per oz.):																	
539	With nonfat dry milk.	1 oz.	28	2	100	5	1	Trace	Trace	---	20	167	.5	10	.04	.21	.2	1
540	Without nonfat dry milk.	1 oz.	28	1	100	1	1	Trace	Trace	---	25	9	.6	---	.01	.03	.1	0
541	Honey, strained or extracted.	1 tbsp.	21	17	65	Trace	0				17	1	.1	0	Trace	.01	.1	Trace
542	Jams and preserves.	1 tbsp.	20	29	55	Trace	Trace				14	4	.2	Trace	Trace	.01	Trace	Trace
543	Jellies.	1 tbsp.	18	29	50	Trace	Trace				13	4	.3	Trace	Trace	.01	Trace	1
	Molasses, cane:																	
544	Light (first extraction).	1 tbsp.	20	24	50	---	---				13	33	.9	---	.01	.01	Trace	---
545	Blackstrap (third extraction).	1 tbsp.	20	24	45	---	---				11	137	3.2	---	.02	.04	.4	---
	Sirups:																	
546	Sorghum.	1 tbsp.	21	23	55	---	---				14	35	2.6	---	---	.02	Trace	0
547	Table blends, chiefly corn, light and dark.	1 tbsp.	21	24	60	0	0				15	9	.8	---	---	0	0	0
	Sugars:																	
548	Brown, firm packed.	1 cup.	220	2	820	0	0				212	187	7.5	0	.02	.07	.4	0
	White:																	
549	Granulated.	1 cup.	200	Trace	770	0	0				199	0	.2	0	0	0	0	0
550	Granulated.	1 tbsp.	11	Trace	40	0	0				11	0	Trace	0	0	0	0	0
551	Powdered, stirred before measuring.	1 cup.	120	Trace	460	0	0				119	0	.1	0	0	0	0	0
	MISCELLANEOUS ITEMS																	
552	Barbecue sauce.	1 cup.	250	81	230	4	17	2	5	9	20	53	2.0	900	.03	.03	.8	13
	Beverages, alcoholic:																	
553	Beer.	12 fl. oz.	360	92	150	1	0				14	18	Trace	---	.01	.11	2.2	---
	Gin, rum, vodka, whiskey:																	
554	80-proof.	1½ fl. oz. jigger.	42	67	100	---	---				Trace	---	---	---	---	---	---	---
555	86-proof.	1½ fl. oz. jigger.	42	64	105	---	---				Trace	---	---	---	---	---	---	---
556	90-proof.	1½ fl. oz. jigger.	42	62	110	---	---				Trace	---	---	---	---	---	---	---

APPENDIX TABLE 1   NUTRITIVE VALUES OF THE EDIBLE PART OF FOODS* (Continued)

[Dashes in the columns for nutrients show that no suitable value could be found although there is reason to believe that a measurable amount of the nutrient may be present]

	Food, approximate measure, and weight (in grams)	Water	Food energy	Protein	Fat	Fatty acids — Saturated (total)	Fatty acids — Unsaturated Oleic	Fatty acids — Unsaturated Linoleic	Carbohydrate	Calcium	Iron	Vitamin A value	Thiamin	Riboflavin	Niacin	Ascorbic acid
		Grams / Percent	Calories	Grams	Grams	Grams	Grams	Grams	Grams	Milligrams	Milligrams	International units	Milligrams	Milligrams	Milligrams	Milligrams
	MISCELLANEOUS ITEMS—Continued															
	Beverages, alcoholic—Continued															
	Gin, rum, vodka, whiskey—Con.															
557	94-proof 1½ fl. oz. jigger.	42 / 60	115	—	0				Trace							
558	100-proof 1½ fl. oz. jigger.	42 / 58	125	—	0				Trace							
	Wines:															
559	Dessert 3½ fl. oz. glass.	103 / 77	140	Trace	0				8	8	—		.01	.02	.2	—
560	Table 3½ fl. oz. glass.	102 / 86	85	Trace	0				4	9	.4		Trace	.01	.1	—
	Beverages, carbonated, sweetened, nonalcoholic:															
561	Carbonated water 12 fl. oz.	366 / 92	115	0	0				29	—	—	0	0	0	0	0
562	Cola type 12 fl. oz.	369 / 90	145	0	0				37	—	—	0	0	0	0	0
563	Fruit-flavored sodas and Tom Collins mixes. 12 fl. oz.	372 / 88	170	0	0				45	—	—	0	0	0	0	0
564	Ginger ale 12 fl. oz.	366 / 92	115	0	0				29	—	—	0	0	0	0	0
565	Root beer 12 fl. oz.	370 / 90	150	0	0				39	—	—	0	0	0	0	0
566	Bouillon cubes, approx. ½ in. 1 cube.	4 / 4	5	1	Trace				Trace							
	Chocolate:															
567	Bitter or baking 1 oz.	28 / 2	145	3	15	8	6	Trace	8	22	1.9	20	.01	.07	.4	0
568	Semi-sweet, small pieces. 1 cup.	170 / 1	860	7	61	34	22	1	97	51	4.4	30	.02	.14	.9	0
	Gelatin:															
569	Plain, dry powder in envelope. 1 envelope.	7 / 13	25	6	Trace				0							
570	Dessert powder, 3-oz. package. 1 pkg.	85 / 2	315	8	0				75							
571	Gelatin dessert, prepared with water. 1 cup.	240 / 84	140	4	0				34							

No.	Food, approximate measure	Measure	Grams	Water (%)	Food energy (cal.)	Protein (g)	Fat (g)	Sat. fat (g)	Oleic (g)	Linoleic (g)	Carbohydrate (g)	Calcium (mg)	Iron (mg)	Vit. A (I.U.)	Thiamine (mg)	Riboflavin (mg)	Niacin (mg)	Ascorbic acid (mg)
	Olives, pickled:																	
572	Green	4 medium or 3 extra large or 2 giant.	16	78	15	Trace	2	Trace	2	Trace	Trace	8	.2	40	—	—	—	—
573	Ripe: Mission	3 small or 2 large.	10	73	15	Trace	2	Trace	2	Trace	Trace	9	.1	10	Trace	Trace	—	—
	Pickles, cucumber:																	
574	Dill, medium, whole, 3¾ in. long, 1¼ in. diam.	1 pickle	65	93	10	1	Trace				1	17	.7	70	Trace	.01	Trace	4
575	Fresh, sliced, 1½ in. diam., ¼ in. thick.	2 slices	15	79	10	Trace	Trace				3	5	.3	20	Trace	Trace	Trace	1
576	Sweet, gherkin, small, whole, approx. 2½ in. long, ¾ in. diam.	1 pickle	15	61	20	Trace	Trace				6	2	.2	10	Trace	Trace	Trace	1
577	Relish, finely chopped, sweet.	1 tbsp.	15	63	20	Trace	Trace				5	3	.1	—	—	—	—	—
	Popcorn. See Grain Products.																	
578	Popsicle, 3 fl. oz. size	1 popsicle	95	80	70	0	0	0	0	0	18	0	Trace	0	0	0	0	0
	Pudding, home recipe with starch base:																	
579	Chocolate	1 cup	260	66	385	8	12	7	4	Trace	67	250	1.3	390	.05	.36	.3	1
580	Vanilla (blanc mange)	1 cup	255	76	285	9	10	5	3	Trace	41	298	Trace	410	.08	.41	.3	2
581	Pudding mix, dry form, 4-oz. package.	1 pkg.	113	2	410	3	2	1	1	Trace	103	23	1.8	Trace	.02	.08	.5	0
582	Sherbet	1 cup	193	67	260	2	2				59	31	Trace	120	.02	.06	Trace	4
	Soups: Canned, condensed, ready-to-serve: Prepared with an equal volume of milk:																	
583	Cream of chicken	1 cup	245	85	180	7	10	3	3	3	15	172	.5	610	.05	.27	.7	2
584	Cream of mushroom	1 cup	245	83	215	7	14	4	4	5	16	191	.5	250	.05	.34	.7	1
585	Tomato	1 cup	250	84	175	7	7	3	2	3	23	168	.8	1,200	.10	.25	1.3	15
	Prepared with an equal volume of water:																	
586	Bean with pork	1 cup	250	84	170	8	6	1	2	2	22	63	2.3	650	.13	.08	1.0	3
587	Beef broth, bouillon consomme.	1 cup	240	96	30	5	0				3	Trace	.5	Trace	Trace	.02	1.2	—
588	Beef noodle	1 cup	240	93	70	4	3	1	1	1	7	7	1.0	50	.05	.07	1.0	Trace
589	Clam chowder, Manhattan type (with tomatoes, without milk).	1 cup	245	92	80	2	3				12	34	1.0	880	.02	.02	1.0	—
590	Cream of chicken	1 cup	240	92	95	3	6	1	2	3	8	24	.5	410	.02	.05	.5	Trace
591	Cream of mushroom	1 cup	240	90	135	2	10	1	3	5	10	41	.5	70	.02	.12	.7	Trace
592	Minestrone	1 cup	245	90	105	5	3				14	37	1.0	2,350	.07	.05	1.0	—

APPENDIX TABLE 1   NUTRITIVE VALUES OF THE EDIBLE PART OF FOODS* (Continued)

[Dashes in the columns for nutrients show that no suitable value could be found although there is reason to believe that a measurable amount of the nutrient may be present]

	Food, approximate measure, and weight (in grams)	Water	Food energy	Protein	Fat	Saturated (total)	Unsaturated Oleic	Unsaturated Linoleic	Carbohydrate	Calcium	Iron	Vitamin A value	Thiamin	Riboflavin	Niacin	Ascorbic acid
		Percent	Calories	Grams	Grams	Grams	Grams	Grams	Grams	Milligrams	Milligrams	International units	Milligrams	Milligrams	Milligrams	Milligrams
	MISCELLANEOUS ITEMS—Continued															
	Soups—Continued															
	Canned, condensed, ready-to-serve—Con.															
	Prepared with an equal volume of water—Con.															
593	Split pea 1 cup 245	85	145	9	3	1	2	Trace	21	29	1.5	440	0.25	0.15	1.5	1
594	Tomato 1 cup 245	90	90	2	3	Trace	1	1	16	15	.7	1,000	.05	.05	1.2	12
595	Vegetable beef 1 cup 245	92	80	5	2	---	---	---	10	12	.7	2,700	.05	.05	1.0	---
596	Vegetarian 1 cup 245	92	80	2	2	---	---	---	13	20	1.0	2,940	.05	.05	1.0	---
	Dehydrated, dry form:															
597	Chicken noodle (2-oz. package). 1 pkg 57	6	220	8	6	2	3	1	33	34	1.4	190	.30	.15	2.4	3
598	Onion mix (1½-oz. package). 1 pkg 43	3	150	6	5	1	2	1	23	42	.6	30	.05	.03	.3	6
599	Tomato vegetable with noodles (2½-oz. pkg.). 1 pkg 71	4	245	6	6	2	3	1	45	33	1.4	1,700	.21	.13	1.8	18
	Frozen, condensed:															
	Clam chowder, New England type (with milk, without tomatoes):															
600	Prepared with equal volume of milk. 1 cup 245	83	210	9	12	---	---	---	16	240	1.0	250	.07	.29	.5	Trace
601	Prepared with equal volume of water. 1 cup 240	89	130	4	8	---	---	---	11	91	1.0	50	.05	.10	.5	---
	Cream of potato:															
602	Prepared with equal volume of milk. 1 cup 245	83	185	8	10	5	3	Trace	18	208	1.0	590	.10	.27	.5	Trace
603	Prepared with equal volume of water. 1 cup 240	90	105	3	5	3	2	Trace	12	58	1.0	410	.05	.05	.5	---

No.	Food, approximate measure	Weight (g)	Water (%)	Food energy (cal.)	Protein (g)	Fat (g)	Saturated (g)	Oleic (g)	Linoleic (g)	Carbohydrate (g)	Calcium (mg)	Iron (mg)	Vit. A (I.U.)	Thiamine (mg)	Riboflavin (mg)	Niacin (mg)	Ascorbic acid (mg)
604	Cream of shrimp: Prepared with equal volume of milk.	1 cup	245	82	245	9	16	----	----	----	15	189	.5	290	.07	.27	.5	Trace
605	Prepared with equal volume of water.	1 cup	240	88	160	5	12	----	----	----	8	38	.5	120	.05	.05	.5	----
606	Oyster stew: Prepared with equal volume of milk.	1 cup	240	83	200	10	12	----	----	----	14	305	1.4	410	.12	.41	.5	Trace
607	Prepared with equal volume of water.	1 cup	240	90	120	6	8	----	----	----	8	158	1.4	240	.07	.19	.5	----
608	Tapioca, dry, quick-cooking.	1 cup	152	13	535	1	Trace	----	----	----	131	15	.6	0	0	0	0	0
	Tapioca desserts:																	
609	Apple	1 cup	250	70	295	1	Trace	----	----	----	74	8	.5	30	Trace	Trace	Trace	Trace
610	Cream pudding	1 cup	165	72	220	8	8	4	3	Trace	28	173	.7	480	.07	.30	.2	2
611	Tartar sauce	1 tbsp	14	34	75	Trace	8	1	1	4	1	3	.1	30	Trace	Trace	Trace	Trace
612	Vinegar	1 tbsp	15	94	Trace	Trace	0	----	----	----	1	1	.1	0				----
613	White sauce, medium	1 cup	250	73	405	10	31	16	10	1	22	288	.5	1,150	.10	.43	.5	2
	Yeast:																	
614	Baker's, dry, active	1 pkg.	7	5	20	3	Trace				3	3	1.1	Trace	.16	.38	2.6	Trace
615	Brewer's, dry	1 tbsp	8	5	25	3	Trace				3	17	1.4	Trace	1.25	.34	3.0	Trace
	Yoghurt. See Milk, Cheese, Cream, Imitation Cream.																	

APPENDIX TABLE 2   FOOD COMPOSITION TABLE FOR SHORT METHOD OF DIETARY ANALYSIS (3RD REVISION)

Food and Approximate Measure	Weight, gm	Food Energy, Cal.	Protein, gm	Fat, gm	Carbohydrate, gm	Calcium, mg	Iron, mg	Vitamin A Value, IU	Thiamine, mg	Riboflavin, mg	Niacin, mg	Ascorbic Acid, mg
Milk, cheese, cream; related products												
Cheese: blue, cheddar (1 cu in., 17 gm), cheddar process (1 oz), Swiss (1 oz)	30	105	6	9	1	165	0.2	345	0.01	0.12	trace	0
cottage (from skim) creamed (½ c)	115	120	16	5	3	105	0.4	190	0.04	0.28	0.1	0
Cream: half-and-half (cream and milk) (2 tbsp)	30	40	1	4	2	30	trace	145	0.01	0.04	trace	trace
For light whipping add 1 pat butter												
Milk: whole (3.5% fat) (1 c)	245	160	9	9	12	285	0.1	350	0.08	0.42	0.1	2
fluid, nonfat (skim) and buttermilk (from skim)	245	90	9	trace	13	300	trace	—	0.10	0.44	0.2	2
milk beverages, (1 c) cocoa, chocolate drink made with skim milk. For malted milk add 4 tbsp half-and-half (270 gm)	245	210	8	8	26	280	0.6	300	0.09	0.43	0.3	trace
milk desserts, custard (1 c) 248 gm, ice cream (8 fl oz) 142 gm		290	8	17	29	210	0.4	785	0.07	0.34	0.1	1
cornstarch pudding (248 gm), ice milk (1 c) 187 gm		280	9	10	40	290	0.1	390	0.08	0.41	0.3	2
White sauce, med (½ c)	130	215	5	16	12	150	0.2	610	0.06	0.22	0.3	trace
Egg: 1 large	50	80	6	6	trace	25	1.2	590	0.06	0.15	trace	0
Meat, poultry, fish, shellfish, related products												
Beef, lamb, veal: lean and fat, cooked, inc. corned beef (3 oz) (all cuts)	85	245	22	16	0	10	2.9	25	0.06	0.19	4.2	0
lean only, cooked; dried beef (2 + oz) (all cuts)	65	140	20	5	0	10	2.4	10	0.05	0.16	3.4	0
Beef, relatively fat, such as steak and rib, cooked (3 oz)	85	350	18	30	0	10	2.4	60	0.05	0.14	3.5	0
Liver: beef, fried (2 oz)	55	130	15	6	3	5	5.0	30,280	0.15	2.37	9.4	15
Pork, lean & fat, cooked (3 oz) (all cuts)	85	325	20	24	0	10	2.6	0	0.62	0.20	4.2	0
lean only, cooked (2 + oz) (all cuts)	60	150	18	8	0	5	2.2	0	0.57	0.19	3.2	0
ham, light cure, lean & fat, roasted (3 oz)	85	245	18	19	0	10	2.2	0	0.40	0.16	3.1	0
Luncheon meats: bologna (2 sl), pork sausage, cooked (2 oz), frankfurter (1), bacon, broiled or fried crisp (3 sl)		185	9	16	—	5	1.3	—	0.21	0.12	1.7	0
Poultry												
chicken: flesh only, broiled (3 oz)	85	115	20	3	0	10	1.4	80	0.05	0.16	7.4	0
fried (2 + oz)	75	170	24	6	1	10	1.6	85	0.05	0.23	8.3	0
turkey, light & dark, roasted (3 oz)	85	160	27	5	0	—	1.5	—	0.03	0.15	6.5	0
Fish and shellfish												
salmon (3 oz) (canned)	85	130	17	5	0	165	0.7	60	0.03	0.16	6.8	0
fish sticks, breaded, cooked (3–4)	75	130	13	7	5	10	0.3	—	0.03	0.05	1.2	0
mackerel, halibut, cooked; blue fish, haddock, herring, perch, shad, cooked (3 oz)	85	175	19	10	0	10	0.8	515	0.08	0.15	6.8	0
clams, canned; crab meat, canned; lobster; oyster, raw; scallop; shrimp, canned (tuna canned in oil, 20 gm)	85	160	19	8	2	20	1.0	60	0.06	0.11	4.4	0
raw; scallop; shrimp, canned	85	75	14	1	2	65	2.5	65	0.10	0.08	1.5	0
Mature dry beans and peas, nuts, peanuts, related products												
Beans: white with pork & tomato, canned (1 c) red (128 gm), Lima (96 gm), cowpeas (125 gm), cooked (½ c)	260	320	16	7	50	140	4.7	340	0.20	0.08	1.5	5
cooked (½ c)		125	8	—	25	35	2.5	5	0.13	0.06	0.7	—

Nuts: almonds (12), cashews (8), peanuts (1 tbsp), peanut butter (1 tbsp), pecans (12), English walnuts (2 tbsp), coconut (¼ c)	15	95	3	8	4	15	0.5	5	0.05	0.04	0.9	—
Vegetables and vegetable products												
Asparagus, cooked, cut spears (⅔ c)	115	25	3	trace	4	25	0.7	1,055	0.19	0.20	1.6	30
Beans: green (½ c) cooked 60 gm; canned 120 gm		15	1	trace	3	30	0.4	340	0.04	0.06	0.3	8
Lima, immature, cooked (½ c)	80	90	6	1	16	40	2.0	225	0.14	0.08	1.0	14
Broccoli spears, cooked (⅔ c)	100	25	3	trace	4	90	0.8	2,500	0.09	0.20	0.8	90
Brussels sprouts, cooked (⅔ c)	85	30	3	trace	5	30	1.0	450	0.07	0.12	0.7	75
Cabbage (110 gm); cauliflower, cooked (80 gm); and sauerkraut, canned (150 gm) (reduce ascorbic acid value by one-third for kraut) (⅔ c)		20	1	trace	4	35	0.5	80	0.05	0.05	0.3	37
Carrots, cooked (⅔ c)	95	30	1	trace	7	30	0.6	10,145	0.05	0.05	0.5	6
Corn, 1 ear, cooked (140 gm); canned (130 gm) (½ c)		75	2	trace	18	5	0.4	315	0.06	0.06	1.1	6
Leafy greens: collards (125 gm), dandelions (120 gm), kale (75 gm), mustard (95 gm), spinach (120 gm), turnip (100 gm cooked, 150 gm canned) (⅔ c cooked and canned) (reduce ascorbic acid one-half for canned)		30	3	trace	5	175	1.8	8,570	0.11	0.18	0.8	45
Peas, green (½ c)	80	60	4	1	10	20	1.4	430	0.22	0.09	1.8	16
Potatoes-baked, boiled (100 gm), 10 pc French fried (55 gm) (for fried, add 1 tbsp cooking oil)		85	3	trace	30	10	0.7	trace	0.08	0.04	1.5	16
Pumpkin, canned (½ c)	115	40	1	1	9	30	0.5	7,295	0.03	0.06	0.6	6
Squash, winter, canned (½ c)	100	65	2	1	16	30	0.8	4,305	0.05	0.14	0.7	14
Sweetpotato, canned (½ c)	110	120	2	—	27	25	0.8	8,500	0.05	0.05	0.7	15
Tomato, 1 raw, ⅔ c canned, ⅔ c juice	150	35	2	trace	7	14	0.8	1,350	0.10	0.06	1.0	29
Tomato catsup (2 tbsp)	35	30	1	trace	8	10	0.2	480	0.04	0.02	0.6	6
Other, cooked (beets, mushrooms, onions, turnips) (½ c)	95	25	1	—	5	20	0.5	15	0.02	0.10	0.7	7
Others commonly served raw, cabbage (½ c, 50 gm), celery (3 sm stalks, 40 gm), cucumber (¼ med, 50 gm), green pepper (½, 30 gm), radishes (5, 40 gm)		10	trace	trace	2	15	0.3	100	0.03	0.03	0.2	20
carrots, raw (½ carrot)	25	10	trace	trace	2	10	0.2	2,750	0.02	0.02	0.2	2
lettuce leaves (2 lg)	50	10	1	trace	2	34	0.7	950	0.03	0.04	0.2	9
Fruits and fruit products												
Cantaloup (½ med)	385	60	1	trace	14	25	0.8	6,540	0.08	0.06	1.2	63
Citrus and strawberries: orange (1), grapefruit (½), juice (½ c), strawberries (½ c), lemon (1), tangerine (1)		50	1	—	13	25	0.4	165	0.08	0.03	0.3	55
Yellow, fresh: apricots (3), peach (2 med); canned fruit and juice (½ c) or dried, cooked, unsweetened: apricot, peaches (½ c)		85	—	—	22	10	1.1	1,005	0.01	0.05	1.0	5
Other, dried: dates, pitted (4), figs (2), raisins (¼ c)	40	120	1	—	31	35	1.4	20	0.04	0.04	0.5	—
Other, fresh: apple (1), banana (1), figs (3), pear (1)		80	—	—	21	15	0.5	140	0.04	0.03	0.2	6
Fruit pie: to 1 serving fruit add 1 tbsp flour, 2 tbsp sugar, 1 tbsp fat												

APPENDIX TABLE 2   FOOD COMPOSITION TABLE FOR SHORT METHOD OF DIETARY ANALYSIS (3RD REVISION) (Continued)

Food and Approximate Measure	Weight, gm	Food Energy, Cal.	Protein, gm	Fat, gm	Carbohydrate, gm	Calcium, mg	Iron, mg	Vitamin A Value, IU	Thiamine, mg	Riboflavin, mg	Niacin, mg	Ascorbic Acid, mg
Grain products												
Enriched and whole grain: bread (1 sl, 23 gm), biscuit (½), cooked cereals (⅔ c), prepared cereals (1 oz), Graham crackers (2 lg), macaroni, noodles, spaghetti (½ c, cooked), pancake (1, 27 gm), roll (½), waffle (½, 38 gm)		65	2	1	16	20	0.6	10	0.09	0.05	0.7	—
Unenriched: bread (1 sl, 23 gm), cooked cereal (⅔ c), macaroni, noodles, spaghetti (½ c), popcorn (½ c), pretzel sticks, small (15), roll (½)		65	2	1	16	10	0.3	5	0.02	0.02	0.3	—
Desserts												
Cake, plain (1 pc), doughnut (1). For iced cake or doughnut add value for sugar (1 tbsp). For chocolate cake add chocolate (30 gm)	45	145	2	5	24	30	0.4	65	0.02	0.05	0.2	—
Cookies, plain (1)	25	120	1	5	18	10	0.2	20	0.01	0.01	0.1	—
Pie crust, single crust (¼ shell)	20	95	1	6	8	3	0.3	0	0.04	0.03	0.3	—
Flour, white, enriched (1 tbsp)	7	25	1	trace	5	1	0.2	0	0.03	0.02	0.2	0
Fats and Oils												
Butter, margarine (1 pat, ½ tbsp)	7	50	trace	6	trace	1	0	230	—	—	—	0
Fats and oils, cooking (1 tbsp), French dressing (2 tbsp)	14	125	0	14	0	0	0	0	0	0	0	0
Salad dressing, mayonnaise type (1 tbsp)	15	80	trace	9	1	2	0.1	45	trace	trace	trace	0
Sugars, sweets												
Candy, plain (½ oz), jam and jelly (1 tbsp), sirup (1 tbsp), gelatin dessert, plain (½ c), beverages, carbonated (1 c)		60	0	0	14	3	0.1	trace	trace	trace	trace	trace
Chocolate fudge (1 oz), chocolate sirup (3 tbsp)		125	1	2	30	15	0.6	10	trace	0.02	0.1	trace
Molasses (1 tbsp), caramel (½ oz)		40	trace	trace	8	20	0.3	trace	trace	trace	trace	trace
Sugar (1 tbsp)	12	45	0	0	12	0	trace	0	0	0	0	0
Miscellaneous												
Chocolate, bitter (1 oz)	30	145	3	15	8	20	1.9	20	0.01	0.07	0.4	0
Sherbet (½ c)	96	130	1	1	30	15	trace	55	0.01	0.03	trace	2
Soups: bean, pea (green) (1 c)		150	7	4	22	50	1.6	495	0.09	0.06	1.0	4
noodle, beef, chicken (1 c)		65	4	2	7	10	0.7	50	0.03	0.04	0.9	trace
clam chowder, minestrone, tomato, vegetable (1 c)		90	3	2	14	25	0.9	1,880	0.05	0.04	1.1	3

The use of the short method of dietary analysis reduces the time required to compute the nutritive value of a diet. In the evaluation of a mixed dietary using this method the accuracy approximates that of computations using the conventional food table.

The values in Table A-7 were computed chiefly from the figures compiled by Watt and Merrill in Agriculture Handbook 8, *Composition of Foods—Raw, Processed, Prepared*, revised 1963.

Courtesy of Leichsenring and Wilson, *J. Am. Dietet. Assoc.* Nov., 1965.

APPENDIX TABLE 3 CALORIE VALUES OF BEVERAGES AND SNACK FOODS

FOOD	WEIGHT (gm.)	APPROXIMATE MEASURE	KCALORIES	FOOD	WEIGHT (gm.)	APPROXIMATE MEASURE	KCALORIES
Beverages				Doughnut, cake type,			
Carbonated, cola type	369	1 bottle, 12 ounces	145	plain	32	1 average	125
Malted milk	235	1 regular (1 cup)	245	Doughnut, jelly	65	1 average	226
Chocolate milk				Doughnut, raised	30	1 average	120
(made with skim milk)	250	1 cup	190				
Cocoa	250	1 cup	245	**Fruits**			
soda, vanilla ice cream	242	1 regular	60	Apple	150	1 medium, 2½ in. diameter	70
				Banana	100	1 medium, 6 by 1½ in.	85
Beverages, alcoholic				Grapes, European type	160	1 cup	95
Beer	360	1 bottle, 12 ounces	150	Orange	180	1 medium, 2⅝ in.	65
Brandy	30	1 brandy glass	75			diameter	
Gin	43	1 jigger	107	Pear	182	1 medium, 3 by 2½ in.	100
Liqueurs (average)	20	1 cordial glass	165			diameter	
Martini		1 cocktail glass	145				
Manhattan		1 cocktail glass	165	**Miscellaneous**			
Rum	43	1 jigger	105	Hamburger and bun	96	1 average	334
Whiskey	43	1 jigger	107	Ice cream, vanilla	62	3-ounce container	95
Wine, port	100	1 wine glass	160	Sherbet	96	½ cup	130
Wine, sauterne	100	1 wine glass	85	Jams, jellies,			
				marmalades, preserves	21	1 tablespoon	55
Cake				Syrup, blended	21	1 tablespoon	60
Angel food	53	1 piece	135	Waffles	75	1 waffle, 4½ by 5½ by	210
Cupcake, chocolate, iced	36	1 cake, 2¾ in.	130			½ inch	
		diameter					
Fruit cake	30	1 piece, 2 by 2 by ½ in.	110	**Nuts**			
				Mixed, shelled	15	8 to 12	94
Candy and Popcorn				Peanut butter	16	1 tablespoon	95
Butterscotch	15	3 pieces	60	Peanuts, shelled,			
Candy bar, plain	28	1 bar	145	roasted	144	1 cup	840
Caramels	28	3 medium	115				
Choc. coated peanuts	28	1 ounce	160	**Pie**			
Fudge	28	1 piece	115	Apple	135	4-inch sector	350
Peanut brittle	30	1 ounce	128	Cherry	135	4-inch sector	350
Popcorn with oil added	9	1 cup	40	Custard	130	4-inch sector	285
				Lemon meringue	120	4-inch sector	305
Cheese				Mince	135	4-inch sector	365
Camembert	38	1 wedge	115	Pumpkin	130	4-inch sector	275
Cheddar	28	1 ounce	115				
Cream	28	1 ounce	106	**Potato chips**			
Swiss (domestic)	28	1 ounce	100	Potato chips	20	10 chips, 2 inches in	115
						diameter	
Cookies							
Brownies, made with				**Sandwiches**			
mix	20	1 piece	85	Bacon, lettuce, tomato	148	1 sandwich	282
Cookies, plain and		1 cooky, 3 in.		Egg salad	138	1 sandwich	279
assorted	25	diameter	120	Ham	81	1 sandwich	281
				Liverwurst	91	1 sandwich	251
Crackers				Peanut butter	83	1 sandwich	328
Cheese	18	5 crackers	86				
Graham	14	2 medium	55	**Soups, commercial canned**			
Saltines	11	4 crackers	50	Bean with pork	250	1 cup	170
Rye	26	4 crackers	85	Beef noodle	250	1 cup	70
				Chicken noodle	198	1 cup	51
Dessert type cream puff				Cream (mushroom)	241	1 cup	215
and doughnuts				Tomato	198	1 cup	73
Cream puff – custard				Vegetable with beef			
filling	100	1 average	233	broth	241	1 cup	80

APPENDIX TABLE 4   FATTY ACID AND CHOLESTEROL CONTENT OF FOODS*

Food	Approximate amount	Weight gm	Total fat gm	Saturated fat gm	Unsaturated fatty acids		Choles-terol mg
					Oleic gm	Linoleic gm	
Meat Group							
Beef	1 oz	30	7.5	3.6	3.3	Trace	27
Veal	1 oz	30	3.6	1.8	1.5	Trace	27
Lamb	1 oz	30	6.3	3.6	2.4	Trace	27
Pork, ham	1 oz	30	7.8	3.0	3.3	Trace	27
Liver	1 oz	30	1.5	0.4	Trace	Trace	75
Beef, dried	2 slices	20	1.2	0.6	0.6	...	18
Pork sausage	2 links	40	17.6	6.4	7.6	1.6	45
Cold cuts	1 slice	45	9.7	2.4	2.7	0.6	30
Frankfurters	1	50	17.4	9.0	8.0	0.4	50
Fowl	1 oz	30	3.6	1.2	1.2	0.6	23
Eggs	1	50	6.0	2.0	2.5	0.5	253
Fish	1 oz	30	2.7	0.5	1.7	0.5	21
Salmon and tuna	1/4 cup	30	5.1	1.4	1.5	1.2	...
Shellfish	1 oz	30	1.9	0.6	1.0	0.3	45
Cheese	1 oz	30	9.0	5.1	3.0	...	45
Cottage cheese	1/4 cup	50	2.1	1.0	0.5	...	5
Peanut butter	2 T	30	15.0	2.7	7.5	4.2	...
Peanuts	25	25	12.0	2.5	5.0	3.2	...
Fat Group							
Avocado	1/8	30	5.1	0.9	2.4	0.6	...
Bacon	1 strip	5	2.6	0.9	1.0	0.3	5
Butter	1 tsp	5	4.0	2.3	1.2	...	12
Margarine	1 tsp	5	4.0	1.1	2.5	0.4	...
Special margarine	1 tsp	5	4.0	0.6	2.3	1.1	...
Coconut oil	1 tsp	5	5.0	4.4	0.5	0.1	...
Corn oil	1 tsp	5	5.0	0.5	1.8	2.7	...
Cottonseed oil	1 tsp	5	5.0	1.3	1.2	2.5	...
Olive oil	1 tsp	5	5.0	0.6	4.0	0.4	...
Peanut oil	1 tsp	5	5.0	0.9	1.6	1.5	...
Safflower oil	1 tsp	5	5.0	0.4	1.0	3.6	...
Sesame oil	1 tsp	5	5.0	0.9	1.0	2.1	...
Soybean oil	1 tsp	5	5.0	0.8	1.6	2.6	...
Vegetable fat	1 tsp	5	5.0	1.0	2.6	0.4	...
Half and half	2 T	30	3.6	1.8	1.8	...	12
Cream substitute, dried	1 T	2	0.5	0.3	0.2	...	
Whipping cream	1 T	15	5.6	3.2	2.2	0.2	18
Cream cheese	1 T	15	5.3	3.0	2.2	0.1	18
Mayonnaise	1 tsp	5	4.0	0.7	1.3	2.0	8
French dressing	1 T	15	5.0	1.1	1.1	3.0	...
Nuts							
Almonds	5	6	3.5	0.3	2.5	0.7	...
Pecans	4	5	3.6	0.3	2.6	0.7	...
Walnuts	5	10	6.5	0.4	2.0	4.0	...
Olives	3	30	4.2	0.6	3.0	0.3	...

APPENDIX TABLE 4   FATTY ACID AND CHOLESTEROL CONTENT OF FOODS* (Continued)

Food	Approximate amount	Weight gm	Total fat gm	Saturated fat gm	Unsaturated fatty acids		Choles- terol mg
					Oleic gm	Linoleic gm	
Milk Group							
Milk, whole	1 cup	240	8.5	4.9	3.6	...	27
2% milk	1 cup	240	4.9	2.4	2.5	...	15
Skim milk	1 cup	240	...	...	...	...	7
Cocoa (skim milk)	1 cup	240	1.9	0.7	1.2	...	...
Chocolate milk	1 cup	240	8.5	2.5	6.0	...	...
Bread Group							
Bread	1 slice	25	0.8	0.3	0.5	...	...
Biscuit	1	35	6.5	2.3	3.4	0.8	17
Muffin	1	35	3.5	0.7	2.4	0.4	16
Cornbread	1 (1 1/2″ cube)	35	4.0	1.4	2.1	0.4	16
Roll	1	28	1.3	0.3	0.7	0.3	...
Pancake	1 (4″ diam)	45	3.2	0.9	1.9	0.4	38
Waffle	1	35	3.4	1.0	2.1	0.4	28
Sweet roll	1	35	8.2	2.4	5.1	0.7	25
French toast	1 slice	65	8.1	3.9	3.4	0.8	130
Doughnut	1	30	6.0	1.3	4.4	0.3	27
Cereal, cooked	2/3 cup	140	1.4	...	1.4	0.3	...
Crackers (saltines)	6	20	2.4	0.6	1.4	...	...
Popcorn (unbuttered)	1 cup	15	0.7	0.1	0.2	0.4	...
Potatoes							
Potato chips	1–oz bag	30	12.0	3.0	4.0	6.0	...
French fried							
In corn oil	10	50	6.2	0.4	2.3	3.5	...
In hydroge- nated fat	10	50	6.2	1.6	4.0	0.6	...
Mashed potato	1/2 cup	100	4.3	2.0	2.3	...	...
Soup, cream	1/2 cup	100	4.2	1.0	2.2	1.0	9
Dessert							
Ice milk	1/2 cup	75	2.5	1.5	...	...	5
Ice cream	1/2 cup	75	9.0	5.0	3.9	...	43
Sherbet	1/3 cup	50	0.6	0.4	0.2	...	...
Low fat cookies	5	15	1.8	0.3	...	...	...
Cake	1 piece	50	14.0	2.0	...	0.5	45
Fruit pie	1/6 pie (9″)	160	15.0	4.0	9.5	1.4	11
Miscellaneous							
Gravy	1/4 cup	60	13.8	6.8	6.6	0.4	18
White sauce	1/4 cup	60	8.2	4.6	3.6	...	29
Coconut	1 oz	28	10.9	9.5	1.4	...	...
Chocolate sauce	1 oz	30	3.8	2.0	1.8	...	...

*From Mayo Clinic Diet Manual, 4th Ed. Philadelphia, W. B. Saunders Co., 1971.

APPENDIX TABLE 5   NATURAL FATS AND OILS*
(Composition* and Chemical/Physical Properties)

ACID commonly refd. to: predominant specie	G.C. Common Designation	Babassu	Butter Fat (1)	Cocoa Butter	Coconut	Corn	Cotton-Seed	Lard (1)	Olive	Palm	Palm Kernel	Peanut	Safflower	High Oleic Safflower	Sesame (USA)	Sorghum	Soybean	Sunflower	Tallow-beef	Tallow-mutton
CAPRYLIC	C8:0	7	1.5	–	8	–	–	–	–	–	4	–	–	–	–	–	–	–	–	–
CAPRIC	C10:0	5	3	–	7	–	–	–	–	–	4	–	–	–	–	–	–	–	–	–
LAURIC	C12:0	45	4	–	48	–	–	–	–	–	50	–	–	–	–	–	–	–	–	–
MYRISTIC	C14:0	15	12	0.5	18	0.2	0.9	3	–	1	16	0.1	–	–	–	–	–	–	2	1
PALMITIC	C16:0	9	25	25	8.5	12	23.5	23	14	46	8	11	8	5	9	12	11	8	35	21
STEARIC	C18:0	3	9	35	2.3	2.2	2.5	13	2.5	4	2.5	3	3	1.2	5	1	4	3	16	30
OLEIC	C18:1	13	32	37.5	6	27	18	46	68	38	12	46	13	84	42	31	25	20	44	43
LINOLEIC	C18:2	2	–	2	2	57	54	14	13	10	3	31	75	10	43	53	50	67.8	2	5
ARACHIDIC	C20:0	0.1	1	–	–	0.3	0.3	0.2	0.4	0.4	0.1	1.5	trace	trace	trace	0.1	0.4	0.5	0.4	–
LINOLENIC	C18:3	–	–	–	–	1	–	1	0.7	0.3	0.1	1.5	1	trace	0.5	2	8	0.5	–	–
GADOLEIC	C20:1	–	–	–	–	–	–	–	–	–	–	–	–	–	–	–	–	–	–	–
BEHENIC	C22:0	–	–	–	–	–	–	–	0.2	–	–	3.5	–	–	–	–	0.3	0.2	–	–
IODINE NO. (WIJS) TYPICAL		16	30	40	9	125	110	73	85	50	17	98	132	93	110	115	130	130	40	40
IODINE NO. (WIJS) RANGE		15-19	25-35	35-43	8-12	120-128	105-116	65-80	80-88	45-55	16-20	90-110	127-140	90-100	100-120	105-120	125-140	120-140	35-50	35-46
SAPONIFICATION VALUE RANGE		247-250	216-240	190-200	254-262	189-193	189-198	190-198	188-196	196-200	244-255	180-195	190-194	185-195	188-195	188-195	188-194	188-195	193-195	192-197

*By Gas – Liquid Chromatography (100% fatty acid basis)

(1) Wide variation in composition normally encountered.

*Adapted from Food Engineering, May, 1970, p. 99.

APPENDIX TABLE 6 AMINO ACID CONTENT OF FOODS. 100 GRAMS. EDIBLE PORTION*

ITEM, PROTEIN CONTENT, AND NITROGEN CONVERSION FACTOR	TRYPTO-PHAN	THREO-NINE	ISO-LEUCINE	LEUCINE	LYSINE	SULFUR CONTAINING			PHENYL-ALANINE	TYRO-SINE	VALINE	ARGININE	HISTIDINE
						Meth-ionine	Cystine	Total					
	Gm.	Gm.	Gm.	Gm.	Gm.	Gm.	Gm.	Gm.	Gm.	Gm.	Gm.	Gm.	Gm.
Milk; Milk Products:													
Milk (Protein, N x 6.38):													
Cow:													
Fluid, whole and nonfat (3.5% protein).....	0.049	0.161	0.223	0.344	0.272	0.086	0.031	0.117	0.170	0.178	0.240	0.128	0.092
Canned:													
Evaporated, unsweetened (7.0% protein).	.099	.323	.447	.688	.545	.171	.063	.234	.340	.357	.481	.256	.185
Condensed, sweetened (8.1% protein).....	.114	.374	.518	.796	.631	.198	.072	.271	.393	.413	.557	.296	.214
Dried:													
Whole (25.8% protein)........	.364	1.191	1.648	2.535	2.009	.632	.231	.863	1.251	1.316	1.774	.944	.680
Nonfat (35.6% protein).......	.502	1.641	2.271	3.493	2.768	.870	.318	1.188	1.724	1.814	2.444	1.300	.937
Goat (3.3% protein).......	.039	.217	.087	.278	.312	.065	.027	.055	.121		.139	.174	.068
Human (1.4% protein).......	.023	.062	.075	.124	.090	.028		.055	.060	.071	.086	.055	.030
Indian buffalo (4.2% protein).......	.059	.212	.204	.420	.331	.112	.058	.170	.177		.255	.136	.086
Milk Products:													
Buttermilk (3.5% protein, N x 6.38).........	.038	.165	.219	.348	.291	.082	.032	.114	.186	.137	.262	.168	.099
Casein (100.0% protein, N x 6.29)............	1.335	4.277	6.550	10.048	8.013	3.084	.382	3.466	5.389	5.819	7.393	4.070	3.021
Cheese (protein, N x 6.38):													
Blue mold (21.5% protein).....	.293	.799	1.449	2.096	1.577	.559	.121	.680	1.153	1.028	1.543	.785	.701
Camembert (17.5% protein).....	.239	.650	1.179	1.706	1.284	.455	.099	.554	.938	.837	1.256	.639	.571
Cheddar (25.0% protein).....	.341	.929	1.685	2.437	1.834	.650	.141	.791	1.340	1.195	1.794	.913	.815
Cheddar processed (23.2% protein).....	.316	.862	1.563	2.262	1.702	.604	.131	.735	1.244	1.109	1.665	.847	.756
Cheese foods, cheddar (20.5% protein).....	.280	.761	1.382	1.998	1.504	.533	.116	.649	1.099	.980	1.472	.749	.668
Cottage (17.0% protein).....	.179	.794	.989	1.826	1.428	.469	.147	.616	.917	.917	.978	.802	.549
Cream cheese (9.0% protein).....	.080	.408	.519	.923	.721	.229	.085	.314	.547	.408	.538	.313	.278
Limburger (21.2% protein).....	.289	.788	1.429	2.067	1.555	.552	.120	.672	1.136	1.014	1.522	.774	.691
Parmesan (36.0% protein).....	.491	1.337	2.426	3.510	2.641	.937	.203	1.140	1.930	1.721	2.584	1.315	1.174
Swiss (27.5% protein).....	.375	1.021	1.853	2.681	2.017	.715	.155	.870	1.474	1.315	1.974	1.004	.896
Swiss processed (26.4% protein).....	.360	.981	1.779	2.574	1.937	.687	.149	.836	1.415	1.262	1.895	.964	.861
Lactalbumin (100.0% protein, N x 6.49).......	2.203	5.239	6.209	12.342	9.060	2.250	3.405	5.655	4.360	3.806	5.686	3.498	1.911
Whey (Protein, N x 6.49):													
Fluid (0.9% protein).....	.010	.048	.052	.074	.055	.013	.018	.031	.023	.009	.045	.017	.011
Dried (12.7% protein).....	.147	.677	.734	1.043	.769	.188	.250	.438	.323	.131	.640	.235	.159

*Adapted from the more comprehensive Table 2 compiled by M. L. Orr and B. K. Watt in "Amino Acid Content of Foods," Home Economics Research Report No. 4, 1968, U.S. Dept. of Agriculture. For sale by the Supt. of Documents, U.S. Gov't. Printing Office, Washington, D.C., 45 cents.

APPENDIX TABLE 6   AMINO ACID CONTENT OF FOODS, 100 GRAMS, EDIBLE PORTION (Continued)

ITEM, PROTEIN CONTENT, AND NITROGEN CONVERSION FACTOR	TRYPTOPHAN	THREONINE	ISO-LEUCINE	LEUCINE	LYSINE	SULFUR CONTAINING			PHENYL-ALANINE	TYROSINE	VALINE	ARGININE	HISTIDINE
						Methionine	Cystine	Total					
	Gm.	Gm.	Gm.	Gm.	Gm.	Gm.	Gm.	Gm.	Gm.	Gm.	Gm.	Gm.	Gm.
Eggs, Chicken (Protein, N x 6.25):													
Fresh or stored:													
Whole (12.8% protein)	0.211	0.637	0.850	1.126	0.819	0.401	0.299	0.700	0.739	0.551	0.950	0.840	0.307
Whites (10.8% protein)	.164	.477	.698	.950	.648	.420	.263	.683	.689	.449	.842	.634	.233
Yolks (16.3% protein)	.235	.827	.996	1.372	1.074	.417	.274	.691	.717	.756	1.121	1.132	.368
Dried:													
Whole (46.8% protein)	.771	2.329	3.108	4.118	2.995	1.468	1.093	2.561	2.703	2.014	3.474	3.070	1.123
Whites (85.9% protein)	1.306	3.793	5.553	7.559	5.154	3.340	2.089	5.429	5.484	3.573	6.693	5.044	1.855
Yolks (31.2% protein)	.449	1.582	1.907	2.626	2.057	.799	.524	1.323	1.373	1.448	2.147	2.167	.704
Meat; Poultry; Fish and Shellfish; Their Products:													
Meat (Protein, N x 6.25):													
Beef carcass or side:													
Thin (18.8% protein)	.220	.830	.984	1.540	1.642	.466	.238	.704	.773	.638	1.044	1.212	.653
Medium fat (17.5% protein)	.204	.773	.916	1.434	1.529	.434	.221	.655	.720	.594	.972	1.128	.608
Fat (16.3% protein)	.190	.720	.853	1.335	1.424	.404	.206	.610	.670	.553	.905	1.051	.566
Very fat (13.7% protein)	.160	.605	.717	1.122	1.197	.340	.173	.513	.563	.465	.761	.883	.476
Medium fat, trimmed to retail basis (18.2% protein)	.213	.804	.952	1.491	1.590	.451	.230	.681	.748	.617	1.010	1.174	.632
Beef cuts, medium fat:													
Chuck (18.6% protein)	.217	.821	.973	1.524	1.625	.461	.235	.696	.765	.631	1.033	1.199	.646
Flank (19.9% protein)	.232	.879	1.041	1.630	1.738	.494	.252	.746	.818	.675	1.105	1.283	.691
Hamburger (16.0% protein)	.187	.707	.837	1.311	1.398	.397	.202	.599	.658	.543	.888	1.032	.556
Porterhouse (16.4% protein)	.192	.724	.858	1.343	1.433	.407	.207	.614	.674	.556	.911	1.057	.569
Rib roast (17.4% protein)	.203	.768	.910	1.425	1.520	.432	.220	.652	.715	.590	.966	1.122	.604
Round (19.5% protein)	.228	.861	1.020	1.597	1.704	.484	.246	.730	.802	.661	1.083	1.257	.677
Rump (16.2% protein)	.189	.715	.848	1.327	1.415	.402	.205	.607	.666	.550	.899	1.045	.562
Sirloin (17.3% protein)	.202	.764	.905	1.417	1.511	.429	.219	.648	.711	.587	.960	1.116	.601
Beef, canned (25.0% protein)	.292	1.104	1.308	2.048	2.184	.620	.316	.936	1.028	.848	1.388	1.612	.868
Beef, dried or chipped (34.3% protein)	.401	1.515	1.795	2.810	2.996	.851	.434	1.285	1.410	1.163	1.904	2.212	1.191
Lamb carcass or side:													
Thin (17.1% protein)	.222	.782	.886	1.324	1.384	.410	.224	.634	.695	.594	.843	1.114	.476
Medium fat (15.7% protein)	.203	.718	.814	1.216	1.271	.377	.206	.583	.638	.545	.774	1.022	.437
Fat (13.0% protein)	.168	.595	.674	1.007	1.052	.312	.171	.483	.528	.451	.641	.847	.362
Lamb cuts, medium fat:													
Leg (18.0% protein)	.233	.824	.933	1.394	1.457	.432	.236	.668	.732	.625	.887	1.172	.501
Rib (14.9% protein)	.193	.682	.772	1.154	1.206	.358	.195	.553	.606	.517	.734	.970	.415
Shoulder (15.6% protein)	.202	.714	8.09	1.208	1.263	.374	.205	.579	.634	.542	.769	1.016	.434

Meat; Poultry; Fish and Shellfish; Their Products—Continued

Meat (Protein, N x 6.25)—Continued

	Gm.	Gm.	Gm.	Gm.	Gm.	Gm.	Gm.	Gm.	Gm.	Gm.	Gm.	Gm.	Gm.
Pork, packer's carcass or side:													
Thin (14.1% protein)	0.183	0.654	0.724	1.038	1.157	0.352	0.165	0.517	0.555	0.503	0.733	0.864	0.487
Medium fat (11.9% protein)	.154	.552	.611	.876	.977	.297	.139	.436	.468	.425	.619	.729	.411
Fat (9.8% protein)	.127	.455	.503	.721	.804	.245	.114	.359	.386	.350	.510	.601	.339
Pork cuts, medium fat, fresh:													
Ham (15.2% protein)	.197	.705	.781	1.119	1.248	.379	.178	.557	.598	.542	.790	.931	.525
Loin (16.4% protein)	.213	.761	.842	1.207	1.346	.409	.192	.601	.646	.585	.853	1.005	.567
Miscellaneous lean cuts (14.5% protein)	.188	.673	.745	1.067	1.190	.362	.169	.531	.571	.517	.754	.889	.501
Pork, cured:													
Bacon, medium fat (9.1% protein)	.095	.306	.399	.728	.587	.141	.106	.247	.434	.234	.434	.622	.246
Fat back or salt pork (3.9% protein)	.006	.141	.110	.367	.317	.055	.043	.098	.157	.052	.168	.379	.035
Ham (16.9% protein)	.162	.692	.841	1.306	1.420	.411	.273	.684	.646	.652	.879	1.068	.544
Luncheon meat:													
Boiled ham (22.8% protein)	.219	.934	1.135	1.762	1.915	.554	.368	.923	.872	.879	1.186	1.441	.733
Canned, spiced (14.9% protein)	.143	.610	.741	1.151	1.252	.362	.241	.603	.570	.575	.775	.942	.479
Rabbit, domesticated, flesh only (21.0% protein)		1.021	1.082	1.636	1.818	.541		.793			1.021	1.176	.474
Veal, carcass or side:													
Thin (19.7% protein)	.258	.854	1.040	1.444	1.645	.451	.233	.684	.801	.709	1.018	1.283	.634
Medium fat (19.1% protein)	.251	.828	1.008	1.400	1.595	.437	.226	.663	.776	.688	.987	1.244	.614
Fat (18.5% protein)	.243	.802	.977	1.356	1.545	.423	.219	.642	.752	.666	.956	1.205	.595
Veal cuts, medium fat:													
Round (19.5% protein)	.256	.846	1.030	1.429	1.629	.446	.231	.677	.792	.702	1.008	1.270	.627
Shoulder (19.4% protein)	.255	.841	1.024	1.422	1.620	.444	.230	.674	.788	.698	1.003	1.263	.624
Stew meat (18.3% protein)	.240	.793	.966	1.341	1.528	.419	.217	.636	.744	.659	.946	1.192	.589
Poultry (Protein, N x 6.25):													
Chicken, flesh only:													
Broilers or fryers (20.6% protein)	.250	.877	1.088	1.490	1.810	.537	.277	.814	.811	.725	1.012	1.302	.593
Hens (21.3% protein)	.259	.907	1.125	1.540	1.871	.556	.286	.842	.838	.750	1.046	1.346	.613
Ducks, domesticated, flesh only (21.4% protein)		.935	1.109	1.657	1.842	.531			.842		1.027	1.301	.486
Turkey, flesh only (24.0% protein)		1.014	1.260	1.836	2.173	.664	.330	.994	.960		1.187	1.513	.649
Fish and Shellfish (Protein, N x 6.25):													
Blue fish (20.5% protein)	.203	.889	1.040	1.548	1.797	.597	.276	.873	.761	.554	1.092	1.155	
Cod:													
Fresh (16.5% protein)	.164	.715	.837	1.246	1.447	.480	.222	.702	.612	.446	.879	.929	
Dried (81.8% protein)	.811	3.547	4.149	6.178	7.172	2.383	1.099	3.481	3.036	2.212	4.358	4.607	

APPENDIX TABLE 6   AMINO ACID CONTENT OF FOODS, 100 GRAMS, EDIBLE PORTION (Continued)

ITEM, PROTEIN CONTENT, AND NITROGEN CONVERSION FACTOR	TRYPTO-PHAN	THREO-NINE	ISO-LEUCINE	LEUCINE	LYSINE	SULFUR CONTAINING			PHENYL-ALANINE	TYRO-SINE	VALINE	ARGININE	HISTIDINE
						Meth-ionine	Cystine	Total					
	Gm.	Gm.	Gm.	Gm.	Gm.	Gm.	Gm.	Gm.	Gm.	Gm.	Gm.	Gm.	Gm.
Meat; Poultry; Fish and Shellfish; Their Products— Continued													
Fish and Shellfish (Protein, N x 6.25)—Continued													
Croaker (17.8% protein)	0.177	0.772	0.903	1.344	1.561	0.518	0.239	0.757	0.661	0.481	0.948	1.002	—
Eel (18.6% protein)	.185	.806	.943	1.405	1.631	.542	.250	.792	.690	.503	.991	1.048	—
Flounder (14.9% protein)	.148	.646	.756	1.125	1.306	.434	.200	.634	.553	.403	.794	.839	—
Haddock (18.2% protein)	.181	.789	.923	1.374	1.596	.530	.245	.775	.676	.492	.970	1.025	—
Halibut (18.6% protein)	.185	.806	.943	1.405	1.631	.542	.250	.792	.690	.503	.991	1.048	—
Herring:													
Atlantic (18.3% protein)	.182	.793	.928	1.382	1.605	.533	.246	.779	.679	.495	.975	1.031	—
Lake (18.5% protein)	.184	.802	.938	1.397	1.622	.539	.249	.788	.687	.500	.986	1.042	—
Pacific (16.6% protein)	.165	.720	.842	1.254	1.455	.483	.223	.706	.616	.449	.884	.935	—
Mackerel:													
Raw, common Atlantic (18.7% protein)	.186	.811	.948	1.412	1.640	.545	.251	.796	.694	.506	.996	1.053	—
Canned, solids and liquid:													
Atlantic (19.3% protein)	.191	.837	.979	1.458	1.692	.562	.259	.821	.716	.522	1.028	1.087	—
Pacific (21.1% protein)	.209	.915	1.070	1.593	1.850	.614	.284	.898	.783	.571	1.124	1.188	—
Salmon:													
Raw, Pacific (Chinook or King) (17.4% protein)	.173	.754	.883	1.314	1.526	.507	.234	.741	.646	.470	.927	.980	—
Canned, solids and liquid (Sockeye or red) (20.2% protein)	.200	.876	1.025	1.526	1.771	.588	.271	.859	.750	.546	1.076	1.138	—
Sardines, canned, solids and liquid:													
Atlantic type (21.1% protein)	.209	.915	1.070	1.593	1.850	.614	.284	.898	.783	.571	1.124	1.188	—
Pacific type (17.7% protein)	.176	.767	.898	1.337	1.552	.515	.238	.753	.657	.479	.943	.997	—
Shrimp, canned, solids and liquid (18.7% protein)	.186	.811	.948	1.412	1.640	.545	.251	.796	.694	.506	.996	1.053	—
Products from Meat, Poultry, and Fish (Protein, N x 6.25):													
Brains (10.4% protein)	.138	.494	.504	.845	.760	.220	.145	.365	.506	.433	.536	.614	0.278
Chitterlings (8.6% protein)	.094	.398	.308	.457	.670	.193	.109	.302	.359	.228	.462	1.406	.169
Fish flour (76.0% protein)	.754	4.378	4.232	6.189	7.381	2.019			2.845		3.916	5.204	1.289
Gelatin (85.6% protein, N x 5.55)	.006	1.912	1.357	2.930	4.226	.787	.077	.864	2.036	.401	2.421	7.866	.771
Gizzard, chicken (23.1% protein)	.207	1.072	1.094	1.689	1.567	.554	.218	.772	.968	.680	1.116	1.741	.480
Heart:													
Beef or pork (16.9% protein)	.219	.776	.857	1.509	1.387	.403	.168	.571	.765	.627	.973	1.068	.433
Chicken (20.5% protein)	.266	.941	1.040	1.830	1.683	.489	.203	.692	.928	.761	1.181	1.296	.525

	Gm.	Gm.	Gm.	Gm.	Gm.	Gm.	Gm.	Gm.	Gm.	Gm.	Gm.	Gm.	Gm.
Meat; Poultry; Fish and Shellfish; Their Products—Continued													
Products from Meat, Poultry, and Fish (Protein N x 6.25)—Continued													
Kidney:													
Beef (15.0% protein)	0.221	0.665	0.730	1.301	1.087	0.307	0.182	0.489	0.706	0.557	0.876	0.934	0.377
Pork (16.3% protein)	.240	.722	.793	1.414	1.181	.334	.198	.532	.767	.605	.952	1.015	.409
Sheep (16.6% protein)	.244	.736	.807	1.440	1.203	.340	.202	.542	.781	.616	.969	1.033	.417
Liver:													
Beef or pork (19.7% protein)	.296	.936	1.031	1.819	1.475	.463	.243	.706	.993	.738	1.239	1.201	.523
Calf (19.0% protein)	.286	.903	.994	1.754	1.423	.447	.234	.681	.958	.711	1.195	1.158	.505
Chicken (22.1% protein)	.332	1.050	1.156	2.040	1.655	.520	.272	.792	1.114	.827	1.390	1.347	.587
Sheep or lamb (21.0% protein)	.316	.998	1.099	1.939	1.572	.494	.259	.753	1.058	.786	1.320	1.280	.558
Pancreas:													
Beef (13.5% protein)	.175	.626	.683	1.054	.996	.244	—	—	.562	.590	.724	.771	.266
Pork (14.5% protein)	.188	.673	.733	1.132	1.070	.262	—	—	.603	.633	.777	.828	.285
Pork and beef, canned (14.3% protein)	.151	.618	.730	1.190	1.345	.327	.261	.588	.579	.570	.810	1.050	.460
Potted meat (16.1% protein)	.149	.662	.641	1.203	1.061	.361	—	—	.641	—	.943	1.002	.322
Sausage:													
Bologna (14.8% protein)	.126	.606	.718	1.061	1.191	.313	.185	.498	.540	.481	.744	1.028	.398
Braunschweiger (15.4% protein)	.172	.668	.754	1.291	1.200	.320	.187	.507	.700	.471	.956	.954	.458
Frankfurters (14.2% protein)	.120	.582	.688	1.018	1.143	.300	.177	.477	.518	.461	.713	.986	.382
Head cheese (15.0% protein)	.079	.418	.509	.946	.907	.250	.209	.459	.569	.569	.617	1.075	.278
Liverwurst (16.7% protein)	.187	.724	.818	1.400	1.301	.347	.203	.550	.759	.510	1.037	1.034	.497
Pork, links or bulk, raw (10.8% protein)	.092	.442	.524	.774	.869	.228	.135	.363	.394	.351	.543	.750	.290
Pork, bulk, canned (15.4% protein)	.131	.631	.747	1.104	1.239	.325	.192	.517	.562	.500	.774	1.069	.414
Salami (23.9% protein)	.203	.979	1.159	1.713	1.923	.505	.298	.803	.872	.776	1.201	1.660	.642
Vienna sausage, canned (15.8% protein)	.134	.647	.766	1.133	1.272	.334	.197	.531	.576	.513	.794	1.097	.425
Tongue:													
Beef (16.4% protein)	.197	.708	.792	1.286	1.364	.357	.207	.564	.661	.548	.840	1.065	.412
Pork (16.8% protein)	.202	.726	.812	1.317	1.398	.366	.212	.578	.677	.562	.860	1.091	.422
Veal and pork loaf, canned (17.2% protein)	.198	.627	.859	1.236	1.258	.418	.209	.627	.619	.468	.958	.916	.388
Legumes (Dry Seed); Common Nuts; Other Nuts and Dry Seeds; Their Products:													
Legume Seeds and Their Products:													
Beans (Phaseolus vulgaris) (N x 6.25):													
Pinto and red Mexican (23.0% protein)	.213	.997	1.306	1.976	1.708	.232	.228	.460	1.270	.887	1.395	1.384	.655

APPENDIX TABLE 6 AMINO ACID CONTENT OF FOODS, 100 GRAMS, EDIBLE PORTION (Continued)

ITEM, PROTEIN CONTENT, AND NITROGEN CONVERSION FACTOR	TRYPTO-PHAN	THREO-NINE	ISO-LEUCINE	LEUCINE	LYSINE	SULFUR CONTAINING			PHENYL-ALANINE	TYRO-SINE	VALINE	ARGININE	HISTIDINE
						Meth-ionine	Cystine	Total					
	Gm.	Gm.	Gm.	Gm.	Gm.	Gm.	Gm.	Gm.	Gm.	Gm.	Gm.	Gm.	Gm.
Legumes (Dry Seed); Common Nuts; Other Nuts and Dry Seeds; Their Products—Continued													
Legume Seeds and Their Products—Continued													
Beans (Phaseolus vulgaris) (N x 6.25)—Continued													
Red kidney:													
Raw (23.1% protein)	0.214	1.002	1.312	1.985	1.715	0.233	0.229	0.462	1.275	0.891	1.401	1.390	0.658
Canned, solids and liquid (5.7% protein)	.053	.247	.324	.490	.423	.057	.057	.114	.315	.220	.346	.343	.162
Other common beans including navy, peabean, white marrow:													
Raw (21.4% protein)	.199	.928	1.216	1.839	1.589	.216	.212	.428	1.181	.825	1.298	1.287	.609
Baked with pork, canned (5.8% protein)	.057	.274	.291	.486	.354	.059	.018	.077	.333	.165	.312	.251	.186
Black gram, raw (23.6% protein, N x 6.25)	.242	.801	1.390	2.062	1.510	.332	.287	.619	1.242	.551	1.450	1.552	.559
Broadbeans, raw (25.4% protein, N x 6.25)	.236	.829	1.593	2.211	1.426	.106	.179	.285	1.057	.687	1.276	1.780	.748
Chickpeas (20.8% protein, N x 6.25)	.170	.739	1.195	1.538	1.434	.276	.296	.572	1.012	.692	1.025	1.551	.559
Cowpeas (22.9% protein, N x 6.25)	.220	.901	1.110	1.715	1.491	.352	.297	.649	1.198	.678	1.293	1.473	.692
Dolichos, twinflower (21.6% protein, N x 6.25)	.221	.836	1.448	1.707	1.700	.294	.480	.774	1.486	.560	1.286	1.230	.650
Lentils, whole (25.0% protein, N x 6.25)	.216	.896	1.316	1.760	1.528	.180	.204	.384	1.104	.664	1.360	1.908	.548
Lima beans (20.7% protein, N x 6.25)	.195	.980	1.199	1.722	1.378	.331	.311	.642	1.222	.543	1.298	1.315	.669
Lupine (32.3% protein, N x 6.25)		1.101	1.618	1.964	1.447	.114			1.271		1.328	2.718	.811
Moth beans (24.4% protein, N x 6.25)	.164		1.093	1.484	1.202	.191	.109	.300	1.003	1.245	.695		.722
Mung beans (24.4% protein, N x 6.25)	.180	.765	1.351	2.202	1.667	.265	.152	.417	1.167	.390	1.444	1.370	.543
Peanuts (26.9% protein, N x 5.46)	.340	.828	1.266	1.872	1.099	.271	.463	.734	1.557	1.104	1.532	3.296	.749
Peanut flour (51.2% protein, N x 5.46)	.647	1.575	2.410	3.563	2.091	.516	.881	1.397	2.963	2.100	2.916	6.273	1.425
Peanut butter (26.1% protein, N x 5.46)	.330	.803	1.228	1.816	1.066	.263	.449	.712	1.510	1.071	1.487	3.198	.727
Peas (Pisum sativum) (N x 6.25):													
Entire seeds (23.8% protein)	.251	.918	1.340	1.969	1.744	.286	.308	.594	1.200	.960	1.333	2.102	.651
Split (24.5% protein)	.259	.945	1.380	2.027	1.795	.294	.318	.612	1.235	.988	1.372	2.164	.670
Pigeonpeas, without seed coat (21.9% protein, N x 6.25)	.119	.834	1.346	1.717	1.580	.256	.308	.564	1.875	.725	1.153	1.489	.617
Soybeans, whole (34.9% protein, N x 5.71)	.526	1.504	2.054	2.946	2.414	.513	.678	1.191	1.889	1.216	2.005	2.763	.911
Soybean flour, flakes, and grits (protein, N x 5.71):													
Low fat (44.7% protein)	.673	1.926	2.630	3.773	3.092	.658	.869	1.527	2.419	1.558	2.568	3.538	1.166
Medium fat (42.5% protein)	.640	1.831	2.501	3.588	2.940	.625	.826	1.451	2.300	1.481	2.441	3.364	1.109
Full fat (35.9% protein)	.541	1.547	2.112	3.030	2.483	.528	.698	1.226	1.943	1.251	2.062	2.842	.937
Soybean curd (7.0% protein, N x 5.71)						.081	.091	.172					
Soybean milk (3.4% protein, N x 5.71)	.051	.176	.175	.305	.269	.054	.071	.125	.195	.193	.186	.302	.121
Vetch (28.8% protein, N x 6.25)	.203	.899	2.198	2.290	1.898	.346	.336	.682	1.014	.369	1.442	2.249	.659

Legumes (Dry Seed); Common Nuts; Other Nuts and Dry Seeds; Their Products:—Continued

	Gm.	Gm.	Gm.	Gm.	Gm.	Gm.	Gm.	Gm.	Gm.	Gm.	Gm.	Gm.	Gm.
Common Nuts and Their Products:													
Almonds (18.6% protein, N x 5.18)	0.176	0.610	0.873	1.454	0.582	0.259	0.377	0.636	1.146	0.618	1.124	2.729	0.517
Brazil nuts (14.4% protein, N x 5.46)	.187	.422	.593	1.129	.443	.941	.504	1.445	.617	.483	.823	2.247	.367
Cashews (18.5% protein, N x 5.30)	.471	.737	1.222	1.522	.792	.353	.527	.880	.946	.712	1.592	2.098	.415
Coconut (3.4% protein, N x 5.30)	.033	.129	.180	.269	.152	.071	.062	.133	.174	.101	.212	.486	.069
Coconut meal (20.3% protein, N x 5.30)	.199	.770	1.076	1.605	.908	.421	.372	.793	1.038	.605	1.268	2.899	.414
Filberts (12.7% protein, N x 5.30)	.211	.415	.853	.939	.417	.139	.165	.304	.537	.434	.934	2.171	.288
Peanuts. See Legumes.													
Pecans (9.4% protein, N x 5.30)	.138	.389	.553	.773	.435	.153	.216	.369	.564	.316	.525	1.185	.273
Walnuts (English or Persian) (15.0% protein, N x 5.30)	.175	.589	.767	1.228	.441	.306	.320	.626	.767	.583	.974	2.287	.405
Other Nuts and Seeds and Their Products (Protein, N x 5.30):													
Acorns (10.4% protein)	.126	.434	.561	.808	.636	.139	.184	.323	.473	——	.718	.722	.251
Amaranth (14.6% protein)	.149	.832	.882	1.209	1.074	.372	.521	.893	1.141	.617	.849	1.747	.441
Balsampear seed meal (41.9% protein)					1.265		.142		2.609	——	.927	5.914	.917
Breadnuttree, Ramon (9.6% protein)	.261	.373	.543	1.041	.418	.056			.453	2.011	4.510	.884	.147
Chinese tallow tree-nut flour (57.6% protein)	.837	2.174	3.510	4.347	1.587	.924	.696	1.620	2.847			10.031	1.587
Chocolatetree, Nicaragua (38.5% protein)	.588	1.496	2.092	3.952	2.223	.276	.814	1.500	2.630	1.365	2.404	4.220	.683
Cottonseed flour and meal (42.3% protein)	.591	1.764	1.884	2.945	2.139	.686			2.610		2.458	5.603	1.325
Earpodtree, Guanacaste (34.1% protein)	.444	1.165	2.213	4.581	1.930	.360			1.325	——	1.570	2.857	1.004
Leadtree (24.1% protein)	.191	.828	1.651	1.787	1.164	.055			.855	——	.864	2.410	.564
Pumpkin seed (30.9% protein)	.560	.933	1.737	2.437	1.411	.577		——	1.749	——	1.679	4.810	.711
Safflower seed meal (42.1% protein)	.675	1.462	1.914	2.740	1.525	.731		——	2.605	——	2.446	4.623	.985
Sesame:													
Seed (19.3% protein)	.331	.707	.951	1.679	.583	.637	.495	1.132	1.457	.951	.885	1.992	.441
Meal (33.4% protein)	.573	1.223	1.645	2.905	1.008	1.103	.857	1.960	2.521	1.645	1.531	3.447	.763
Sunflower:													
Kernel (23.0% protein)	.343	.911	1.276	1.736	.868	.443	.464	.907	1.220	.647	1.354	2.370	.586
Meal (39.5% protein)	.589	1.565	2.191	2.981	1.491	.760	.797	1.557	2.094	1.110	2.325	4.069	1.006
Grains and Their Products:													
Barley (12.8% protein, N x 5.83)	.160	.433	.545	.889	.433	.184	.257	.441	.661	.466	.643	.659	.239
Bread, white (4% nonfat dry milk, flour basis) (8.5% protein, N x 5.70)	.091	.282	.429	.668	.225	.142	.200	.342	.465	.243	.435	.340	.192

APPENDIX TABLE 6 AMINO ACID CONTENT OF FOODS, 100 GRAMS, EDIBLE PORTION (Continued)

ITEM, PROTEIN CONTENT, AND NITROGEN CONVERSION FACTOR	TRYPTO-PHAN	THREO-NINE	ISO-LEUCINE	LEUCINE	LYSINE	SULFUR CONTAINING			PHENYL-ALANINE	TYRO-SINE	VALINE	ARGININE	HISTIDINE
						Meth-ionine	Cystine	Total					
	Gm.	Gm.	Gm.	Gm.	Gm.	Gm.	Gm.	Gm.	Gm.	Gm.	Gm.	Gm.	Gm.
Grains and Their Products—Continued													
Buckwheat flour:													
Dark (11.7% protein, N x 6.25)	0.165	0.461	0.440	0.683	0.687	0.206	0.228	0.434	0.442	0.240	0.607	0.930	0.256
Light (6.4% protein, N x 6.25)	.090	.252	.241	.374	.376	.113	.125	.238	.242	.131	.332	.509	.140
Cañihua (14.7% protein, N x 6.25)	.118	.706	1.000	.851	.882	.263	.162	.425	.529	.294	.677	1.162	.367
Cereal combinations:													
Corn and soy grits (18.0% protein, N x 6.25)	.161	.792	.841	1.656	.772	.271	.311	.582	.832	.562	1.054	.982	.472
Infant food, precooked, mixed cereals with non-fat dry milk and yeast (19.4% protein, N x 6.25)	.118					.310	.137	.447	.543	.447		.447	.233
Oat-corn-rye mixture, puffed (14.5% protein, N x 5.83)	.172	.545	.841	1.368	.343	.388	.234	.622	.933	.622	.900	.776	.326
Corn, field (10.0% protein, N x 6.25)	.061	.398	.462	1.296	.288	.186	.130	.316	.454	.611	.510	.352	.206
Corn flour (7.8% protein, N x 6.25)	.047	.311	.361	1.011	.225	.145	.101	.246	.354	.477	.398	.275	.161
Corn grits (8.7% protein, N x 6.25)	.053	.347	.402	1.128	.251	.161	.113	.274	.395	.532	.444	.306	.180
Cornmeal:													
Whole ground (9.2% protein, N x 6.25)	.056	.367	.425	1.192	.265	.171	.119	.290	.418	.562	.470	.324	.190
Degermed (7.9% protein, N x 6.25)	.048	.315	.365	1.024	.228	.147	.102	.249	.359	.483	.403	.278	.163
Corn products:													
Flakes (8.1% protein, N x 6.25)	.052	.275	.306	1.047	.154	.135	.152	.157	.354	.283	.386	.231	.226
Germ (14.5% protein, N x 6.25)	.144	.622	.578	1.030	.791	.232	.130	.362	.483	.343	.789	1.134	.464
Gluten (10.0% protein, N x 6.25)	.059	.344	.443	1.563	.179	.282	.141	.423	.558	.582	.512	.322	.200
Hominy (8.7% protein, N x 6.25)	.084	.316	.349	.810	.358	.099			.333	.331	.398	.444	.203
Masa (2.8% protein, N x 6.25)	.010				.103	.108	.030	.138					
Pozol (5.9% protein, N x 6.25)	.042	.336	.304	.591	.234	.087			.254		.267	.197	.122
Tortilla (5.8% protein, N x 6.25)	.031	.235	.345	.939	.145	.111			.252		.304	.223	.128
Zein (16.1% protein, N x 6.25)	.010	.495	.822	3.184		.281	.162	.443	1.664	.981	.654	.286	.216
Job's tears (13.8% protein, N x 5.83)	.066	.620	1.065	3.506	.362	.459	.265	.724	.703			.518	.317
Millets:													
Foxtail millet (9.7% protein, N x 5.83)	.103	.323	7.90	1.737	.218	.291			.697		.717	.374	.218
Little millet (7.2% protein, N x 5.83)	.047	.262	.517	.841	.138	.178			.370		.471	.363	.147
Pearlmillet (11.4% protein, N x 5.83)	.248	.456	.635	1.746	.383	.270	.152	.422	.506		.682	.524	.240
Ragimillet (6.2% protein, N x 5.83)	.085	.270	.398	.620	.202	.270	.187	.457	.263		.473	.100	.079
Oatmeal and rolled oats (14.2% protein, N x 5.83)	.183	.470	.733	1.065	.521	.209	.309	.518	.758	.524	.845	.935	.261
Quinoa (11.0% protein, N x 6.25)	.120	.523	.722	.781	.729	.278	.107	.385	.394	.253	.447	.820	.297
Rice:													
Brown (7.5% protein, N x 5.95)	.081	.294	.352	.646	.296	.135	.102	.237	.377	.343	.524	.432	.126
White and converted (7.6% protein, N x 5.95)	.082	.298	.356	.655	.300	.137	.103	.240	.382	.347	.531	.438	.128

ITEM, PROTEIN CONTENT, AND NITROGEN CONVERSION FACTOR	TRYPTO-PHAN	THREO-NINE	ISO-LEUCINE	LEUCINE	LYSINE	SULFUR CONTAINING			PLENYL-ALANINE	TYRO-SINE	VALINE	ARGININE	HISTIDINE
						Meth-ionine	Cystine	Total					
	Gm.	Gm.	Gm.	Gm.	Gm.	Gm.	Gm.	Gm.	Gm.	Gm.	Gm.	Gm.	Gm.
Fruits (Protein, N x 6.25):													
Abiu (1.7% protein).............	0.028				0.085	0.013							
Avocados (1.3% protein).........	.014				.074	.012				0.031			
Bananas, ripe:													
Common (1.2% protein).........	.018				.055	.011				0.031			
Dwarf (1.2% protein)...........	.012				.049	.004							
Dates (2.2% protein)............	.061	0.061	0.074	0.077	.065	.027			0.063		0.094	0.049	0.049
Grapefruit (0.5% protein)........	.001				.006	.000							
Guavas, common (1.0% protein)...	.010				.030	.010							
Limes (0.8% protein)............	.003				.015	.002							
Mamey (0.5% protein)...........	.006				.040	.007							
Mangos (0.7% protein)..........	.014				.093	.008							
Muskmelons (0.6% protein)......	.001				.015	.002							
Oranges, sweet (0.9% protein)....	.003				.024	.003							
Orange juice (0.8% protein)......	.003				.021	.002							
Oranges, mandarin including tangerines (0.8% protein)........	.005				.028	.004							
Papayas (0.6% protein)..........	.012				.038	.002	0.016	0.021	.049				
Pineapple (0.4% protein).........	.005	.027	.056	.059	.009	.001					.065	.045	
Plantain or baking banana (1.1% protein)........................	.010				.050	.005							
Soursop (1.0% protein)..........	.011				.060	.007							
Sugarapple (1.8% protein).......	.009				.071	.008							
Vegetables:													
Immature Seeds (Protein, N x 6.25):													
Corn, sweet, white or yellow:													
Raw (3.7% protein)...........	.023	.151	.137	.407	.137	.072	.062	.134	.207	.124	.231	.174	.095
Canned, solids and liquid (2.0% protein)...	.012	.082	.074	.220	.074	.039	.033	.072	.112	.067	.125	.094	.052
Cowpeas (9.4% protein).........	.099	.353	.465	.653	.617	.131			.523		.513	.615	.310
Lima beans:													
Raw (7.5% protein)...........	.097	.338	.460	.605	.474	.080	.083	.163	.389	.259	.485	.454	.247
Canned, solids and liquid (3.8% protein).....	.049	.171	.233	.306	.240	.041	.042	.083	.197	.131	.246	.230	.125
Peas:													
Raw (6.7% protein)...........	.056	.245	.308	.418	.316	.054	.073	.127	.257	.163	.274	.595	.109
Canned, solids and liquid (3.4% protein).....	.028	.125	.156	.212	.160	.027	.037	.064	.131	.083	.139	.302	.055

APPENDIX TABLE 6   AMINO ACID CONTENT OF FOODS, 100 GRAMS, EDIBLE PORTION (Continued)

	Gm.	Gm.	Gm.	Gm.	Gm.	Gm.	Gm.	Gm.	Gm.	Gm.	Gm.	Gm.	Gm.
Grains and Their Products—Continued													
Rice products:													
Flakes or puffed (5.9% protein, N x 5.95).....	0.046	2.177			0.056		0.044		0.286	0.124		0.137	0.137
Germ (14.2% protein, N x 5.95)........	.270		.630	.838	1.707	.420	.169	.589	.750	.929	.938	1.559	.430
Rye (12.1% protein, N x 5.83)........	.137	.448	.515	.813	.494	.191	.241	.432	.571	.390	.631	.591	.276
Rye flour:													
Light (9.4% protein, N x 5.83).....	.106	.348	.400	.632	.384	.148	.187	.335	.443	.303	.490	.459	.214
Medium (11.4% protein, N x 5.83).....	.129	.422	.485	.766	.465	.180	.227	.407	.538	.368	.594	.557	.260
Sorghum (11.0% protein, N x 6.25).....	.123	.394	.598	1.767	.299	.190	.183	.373	.547	.303	.628	.417	.211
Teosinte (22.0% protein, N x 6.25).....	.049				.348	.496	.183						
Wheat, whole grain:													
Hard red spring (14.0% protein, N x 5.83).....	.173	.403	.607	.939	.384	.214	.307	.521	.691	.523	.648	.670	.286
Hard red winter (12.3% protein, N x 5.83).....	.152	.354	.534	.825	.338	.188	.270	.458	.608	.460	.570	.589	.251
Soft red winter (10.2% protein, N x 5.83).....	.126	.294	.443	.684	.280	.156	.224	.380	.504	.382	.472	.488	.208
White (9.4% protein, N x 5.83).....	.116	.271	.408	.630	.258	.143	.206	.349	.464	.351	.435	.450	.192
Durum (12.7% protein, N x 5.83).....	.157	.366	.551	.852	.348	.194	.279	.473	.627	.475	.588	.608	.259
Wheat flour:													
Whole grain (13.3% protein, N x 5.83)........	.164	.383	.577	.892	.365	.203	.292	.495	.657	.497	.616	.636	.271
Intermediate extraction (12.0% protein, N x 5.70)........		.392	.619	.924	.356	.198	.320	.518	.732	.335	.583	.549	.286
White (10.5% protein, N x 5.70).....	.129	.302	.483	.809	.239	.138	.210	.348	.577	.359	.453	.466	.210
Wheat products:													
Bran (12.0% protein, N x 6.31)............	.196	.342	.485	.717	.491	.145	.270	.415	.434	.259	.552	.742	.280
Burghul (12.4% protein, N x 5.83).....	.070				.430	.300	.319	.619					
Farina (10.9% protein, N x 5.70).....	.124	.356	.496	.891	.199	.143	.184	.327	.579	.447		.424	.268
Flakes (10.8% protein, N x 5.70).....	.121				.360	.127	.191	.318	.478	.311	.572	.559	.231
Germ (25.2% protein, N x 5.80).....	.265	1.343	1.177	1.708	1.534	.404	.287	.691	.908	.882	1.364	1.825	.687
Gluten, commercial (80.0% protein, N x 5.70).....	.856	2.119	3.677	5.993	1.530	1.389	1.726	3.115	4.351	2.596	3.789	3.481	1.825
Gluten flour (41.4% protein, N x 5.70).....	.443	1.097	1.903	3.101	.792	.719	.893	1.612	2.252	1.344	1.961	1.801	.944
Macaroni or spaghetti (12.8% protein, N x 5.70).....	.150	.499	.642	.849	.413	.193	.243	.436	.669	.422	.728	.582	.303
Noodles, contain egg solids (12.6% protein, N x 5.70).....	.133	.533	.621	.834	.411	.212	.245	.457	.610	.312	.745	.621	.301
Shredded wheat (10.1% protein, N x 5.83).....	.085	.405	.449	.684	.331	.139	.204	.343	.481	.236	.577	.523	.236
Whole wheat with added germ (12.8% protein, N x 5.83).....	.136				.466		.246		.755	.481		.742	.371

Vegetables—Continued

Leafy Vegetables, Raw (Protein, N x 6.25):

	Gm.	Gm.	Gm.	Gm.	Gm.	Gm.	Gm.	Gm.	Gm.	Gm.	Gm.	Gm.	Gm.
Amaranth (3.5% protein)	0.038	0.056	0.164	0.206	0.141	0.025	0.024	0.049	0.096	0.105	0.136	0.134	0.069
Beet greens (2.0% protein)	.024	.076	.084	.129	.108	.034			.116		.101	.083	.026
Brussels sprouts (4.4% protein)	.044	.153	.186	.194	.197	.046		.041	.148	.030	.193	.279	.106
Cabbage (1.4% protein)	.011	.039	.040	.057	.066	.013	.028		.030		.043	.105	.025
Chard (1.4% protein)	.014	.058	.060	.076	.055	.004				.040	.055	.035	.018
Chicory (1.6% protein)	.024				.052	.016	.006	.022		.151	.195	.258	.024
Collards (3.9% protein)	.055	.114	.121	.218	.202	.046	.059	.105	.124		.184	.202	.087
Kale (3.9% protein)	.042	.139	.133	.252	.121	.035	.036	.071	.158				.062
Lettuce (1.2% protein)	.012				.070	.004				.121	.108	.167	.041
Mustard greens (2.3% protein)	.037	.060	.075	.062	.111	.024	.035	.059	.074				
Parsley, curly garden (2.5% protein)	.050				.160	.012							
Spinach (2.3% protein)	.037	.102	.107	.176	.142	.039	.046	.085	.099	.073	.126	.116	.049
Turnip greens (2.9% protein)	.045	.125	.107	.207	.129	.052	.045	.097	.146	.105	.149	.167	.051
Watercress (1.7% protein)	.028	.084	.076	.131	.091	.010			.062	.036	.084	.053	.034

Starchy Roots and Tubers (Protein, N x 6.25):

	Gm.	Gm.	Gm.	Gm.	Gm.	Gm.	Gm.	Gm.	Gm.	Gm.	Gm.	Gm.	Gm.
Apio arracacia (1.2% protein)	.008				.042	.003							
Cassava: Flour (1.6% protein)	.021	.044	.045	.066	.066	.010	.018	.028	.045	.030	.049	.159	.025
Cassava: Root (1.1% protein)	.014	.030	.031	.045	.045	.007	.012	.019	.031	.021	.033	.110	.017
Potatoes: Raw (2.0% protein)	.021	.079	.088	.100	.107	.025	.019	.044	.088	.036	.107	.099	.029
Potatoes: Canned, solids and liquid (1.7% protein)	.018	.067	.075	.085	.091	.021	.016	.037	.075	.030	.091	.084	.024
Potatoes: Flour (7.1% protein)	.076	.279	.311	.353	.378	.089	.068	.157	.314	.127	.379	.350	.102
Sweetpotatoes (Ipomaea batatas): Raw (1.8% protein)	.031	.085	.087	.103	.085	.033	.029	.062	.100	.081	.135	.094	.036
Sweetpotatoes: Dehydrated (5.0% protein)	.087	.235	.241	.286	.236	.093	.080	.173	.278	.225	.374	.261	.099
Taro (1.9% protein)	.035	.089	.099	.169	.110	.021			.099		.114	.118	.032
Yam (Dioscorea spp.) (2.1% protein)	.035	——	——	——	.110	.034	——	——	——	——	——	——	——
Yautia malanga (1.7% protein)	.023	——	——	——	.067	.016	——	——	——	——	——	——	——

Other Vegetables (Protein, N x 6.25):

	Gm.	Gm.	Gm.	Gm.	Gm.	Gm.	Gm.	Gm.	Gm.	Gm.	Gm.	Gm.	Gm.
Asparagus: Raw (2.2% protein)	.027	.066	.080	.096	.103	.032			.069		.106	.123	.036
Asparagus: Canned, solids and liquid (1.9% protein)	.023	.057	.069	.083	.089	.027			.060		.092	.106	.031

APPENDIX TABLE 6   AMINO ACID CONTENT OF FOODS, 100 GRAMS, EDIBLE PORTION *(Continued)*

ITEM, PROTEIN CONTENT, AND NITROGEN CONVERSION FACTOR	TRYPTOPHAN	THREONINE	ISO-LEUCINE	LEUCINE	LYSINE	SULFUR CONTAINING			PHENYLALANINE	TYROSINE	VALINE	ARGININE	HISTIDINE
						Methionine	Cystine	Total					
	Gm.	Gm.	Gm.	Gm.	Gm.	Gm.	Gm.	Gm.	Gm.	Gm.	Gm.	Gm.	Gm.
Vegetables—Continued													
Other Vegetables (Protein, N x 6.25)—Continued													
Beans, snap:													
Raw (2.4% protein)	0.033	0.091	0.109	0.139	0.126	0.035	0.024	0.059	0.057	0.050	0.115	0.101	0.045
Canned, solids and liquid (1.0% protein)	.014	.038	.045	.058	.052	.014	.010	.024	.024	.021	.048	.042	.019
Beets:													
Raw (1.6% protein)	.014	.034	.051	.055	.086	.006			.027		.049	.028	.022
Canned, solids and liquid (0.9% protein)	.008	.019	.029	.031	.048	.003			.015		.028	.016	.012
Broccoli (3.3% protein)	.037	.122	.126	.163	.147	.050			.119		.170	.192	.063
Carrots:													
Raw (1.2% protein)	.010	.043	.046	.065	.052	.010	.029	.039	.042	.020	.056	.041	.017
Canned, solids and liquid (0.5% protein)	.004	.018	.019	.027	.022	.004	.012	.016	.018	.008	.023	.017	.007
Cauliflower (2.4% protein)	.033	.102	.104	.162	.134	.047			.075	.034	.144	.110	.048
Celery (1.3% protein)	.012				.021	.015	.006	.021		.016			
Chayote (0.6% protein)	.008				.038	.001							
Cowpeas, yardlong, immature pod (3.4% protein)	.034				.203	.021							
Cucumbers (0.7% protein)	.005	.019	.022	.030	.031	.007			.016		.024	.053	.001
Cushaw (1.5% protein)	.014				.044	.008							
Eggplant (1.1% protein)	.010	.038	.056	.068	.030	.006			.048		.065	.037	.019
Mallow (3.7% protein)	.144	.155		.259	.155	.030			.166		.181	.189	.063
Mushrooms:													
(Agaricus campestris)[1]	.006	.156	.532	.281	.088	.167			.018		.378	.235	.027
(Lactarius spp.)[2]	.006		.201	.139		.021				.079	.116	.021	
Okra (1.8% protein)	.018	.066	.069	.101	.076	.022	.017	.039	.065	.046	.091	.093	.030
Onions, mature (1.4% protein)	.021	.022	.021	.037	.064	.013			.039		.031	.180	.014
Peppers (1.2% protein)	.009	.050	.046	.046	.051	.016			.055		.033	.024	.014
Pricklypears (1.1% protein)	.009	.053	.044	.057	.044	.008			.059		.041	.032	.016
Pumpkin (1.2% protein)	.016	.028	.044	.063	.058	.011			.032		.045	.043	.019
Radishes (1.2% protein)	.005	.059			.034	.002				.016	.030		
Seepweed (2.6% protein)	.027	.089	.113	.152	.089	.013			.116		.091	.062	.036
Soybean sprouts (6.2% protein)		.159	.225	.265	.211	.045			.186		.225	.225	.133
Squash, summer (0.6% protein)	.005	.014	.019	.027	.023	.008			.016		.022	.027	.009

[1] Total nitrogen is 0.58%. This is equivalent to 2.4% protein on the basis that ⅔ of the nitrogen is protein nitrogen. If total nitrogen is used for the calculation, the protein content is 3.6%.

[2] Total nitrogen is 0.69%. This is equivalent to 2.9% protein on the basis that ⅔ of the nitrogen is protein nitrogen. If total nitrogen is used for the calculation, the protein content is 4.3%.

Vegetables—Continued
Other Vegetable (Protein, N x 6.25)—Continued

	Gm.	Gm.	Gm.	Gm.	Gm.	Gm.	Gm.	Gm.	Gm.	Gm.	Gm.	Gm.	Gm.
Tomatoes and cherry tomatoes (1.0% protein)..	0.009	0.033	0.029	0.041	0.042	0.007	—	—	0.028	0.014	0.028	0.029	0.015
Turnips (1.1% protein)............	—	—	.020	—	.057	.012	—	—	.020	.029	—	—	—
Waxgourd, Chinese (0.4% protein)........	.002	—	—	—	.009	.003	—	—	—	—	—	—	—
Miscellaneous Food Items:													
Vegetable patty or steak (principally wheat protein) (15% protein, N x 5.70)........	.142	.411	.884	1.079	.321	.253	—	—	.811	.580	.705	.597	.321
Yeast:													
Baker's, compressed (3, N x 6.25)........	.122	.655	.655	1.151	.914	.248	0.120	0.368	.607	1.902	.840	.536	.353
Brewer's, dried (4, N x 6.25)........	.710	2.353	2.398	3.226	3.300	.836	.548	1.384	1.902	—	2.723	2.250	1.251
Primary, dried:													
(Saccharomyces cerevisiae) (4, N x 6.25).....	.636	2.353	2.708	3.300	3.337	.851	.444	1.295	1.813	2.472	2.553	1.931	1.103
(Torulopsis utilis) (4, N x 6.25)........	.636	2.331	3.323	3.707	3.648	.710	.422	1.132	2.361	2.464	2.901	3.337	1.251

3 Total nitrogen is 2.1%. This is equivalent to 10.6% protein on the basis that 4/5 of the nitrogen is protein nitrogen. If total nitrogen is used for the calculation, the protein content is 13.1%.

4 Total nitrogen is 7.4%. This is equivalent to 36.9% protein on the basis that 4/5 of the nitrogen is protein nitrogen. If total nitrogen is used for the calculation, the protein content is 46.1%.

APPENDIX TABLE 7   FOODS HIGH IN CALCIUM*
(More Than 25 Milligrams Calcium per Serving)

Food	Approximate amount	Weight gm	Calcium mg
Meat Group			
Egg	1	50	27
Fish			
Salmon (with bones)	1 oz	30	51
Sardines	1 oz	30	115
Clams	1 oz	30	29
Oysters	1 oz	30	31
Shrimp	1 oz	30	35
Cheese			
Cheddar	1 oz	30	218
Cheese foods	1 oz	30	160
Cheese spread	1 oz	30	158
Cottage cheese	1/4 cup	50	53
Fat			
Cream			
Half and half	2 T	30	32
Sour	2 T	30	31
Bread Group			
Bread			
Biscuit	2″ diameter	35	42
Muffin	2″ diameter	35	36
Cornbread	1 1/2 cube	35	36
Pancake	4″ diameter	45	45
Waffle	1/2 square	35	39
Beans, dry (canned or cooked)	1/2 cup	90	45
Lima beans	1/2 cup	100	42
Parsnips	2/3 cup	100	45
Milk			
Whole	1 cup	240	288
Evaporated whole milk	1/2 cup	120	302
Powdered whole milk	1/2 cup	30	252
Buttermilk	1 cup	240	296
Skim milk	1 cup	240	298
Powdered skim milk, dry	1/4 cup	30	367

APPENDIX TABLE 7   FOODS HIGH IN CALCIUM* *(Continued)*

Food	Approximate amount	Weight *gm*	Calcium *mg*
Fruit			
Blackberries	3/4 cup	100	32
Orange	1 medium	100	41
Raspberries	3/4 cup	100	30
Rhubarb	1 cup	100	96
Tangerine	2 small	100	40
Vegetable A, cooked			
Beans, green or wax	1/2 cup	100	50
Beet greens	1/2 cup	100	99
Broccoli	1/2 cup	100	88
Cabbage	1/2 cup	100	49
Cabbage, Chinese	1/2 cup	100	43
Celery	1/2 cup	100	39
Chard	1/2 cup	100	73
Collards	1/2 cup	100	188
Cress	1/2 cup	100	81
Dandelion greens	1/2 cup	100	140
Mustard greens	1/2 cup	100	138
Sauerkraut	1/2 cup	100	36
Spinach	1/2 cup	100	93
Squash, summer	1/2 cup	100	25
Turnip greens	1/2 cup	100	184
Turnips	1/2 cup	100	35
Vegetable B, cooked			
Artichokes	1/2 cup	100	51
Brussels sprouts	1/2 cup	100	32
Carrots	1/2 cup	100	33
Kale	1/2 cup	100	187
Kohlrabi	1/2 cup	100	33
Leeks, raw	3–4	100	52
Okra	1/2 cup	100	92
Pumpkin	1/2 cup	100	25
Rutabagas	1/2 cup	100	59
Squash, winter	1/2 cup	100	28
Dessert			
Cake, white	1 piece	50	32
Custard, baked	1/3 cup	100	112
Ice cream	1/2 cup	75	110
Ice milk	1/2 cup	75	118
Pie, cream	1/6 of 9″ pie	160	120
Pudding	1/2 cup	100	117
Sherbet	1/3 cup	50	25

*From Mayo Clinic Diet Manual, 4th Ed. Philadelphia, W. B. Saunders Co., 1971.

APPENDIX TABLE 8   FOODS HIGH IN IRON*

FOOD	AVERAGE SERVING		IRON, MG.	
	Weight Gm.	Approximate Measure	Per Serving	Per 100 Gm.
Almonds	15	12–15	0.7	4.4
Apricots, dried	30	5 halves	1.5	4.9
Bacon, cooked	25	4–5 slices	0.8	3.3
Beans, dried	30 (dry)	½ cup (cooked)	2.1	6.9
Lima, dried	30 (dry)	½ cup (cooked)	2.3	7.5
Beef, rib roast, cooked	60	2 ounces	1.8	3.0
Corned, medium fat	60	2 ounces	2.6	4.3
Dried	30	1 ounce	1.5	5.1
Beet greens, cooked	75	½ cup	2.4	3.2
Bologna	30	1 slice	0.7	2.2
Bran flakes, 40 per cent	15	½ cup	0.8	5.1
Brazil nuts	15	2 medium	0.5	3.4
Breaded, whole wheat	25	1 slice	0.6	2.2
Cashews	15	6–8	0.8	5.0
Chard	75	½ cup	1.9	2.5
Chocolate, bitter	30	1 square	1.3	4.4
Sweetened, plain	30	1 square	0.8	2.8
Clams	60	2 ounces	4.2	7.0
Cocoa	7	1 tablespoon	0.8	11.6
Coconut, fresh	15	½ ounce	0.3	2.0
Dried	15	2 tablespoons	0.5	3.6
Cornmeal, degermed, enriched	15 (dry)	½ cup (cooked)	0.4	2.9
Cress, garden	10	5–8 sprigs	0.3	2.9
Currants, dried	30	2 tablespoons	0.8	2.7
Dandelion greens	75	½ cup	2.3	3.1
Dates	30	3–4	0.6	2.1
Egg, whole	50	1	1.4	2.7
Yolk	20	1	1.4	7.2
Figs, dried	30	2 small	0.9	3.0
Flour, all-purpose, enriched	15	2 tablespoons	0.4	2.9
Flour, whole wheat	15	2 tablespoons	0.5	3.3
Ham, smoked	60	2 ounces	1.7	2.9
Hazelnuts	15	10–12	0.6	4.1
Heart, beef	60	2 ounces	2.8	4.6
Kale	75	¾ cup	1.7	2.2
Kidney, beef	60	2 ounces	4.7	7.9
Lamb, leg	60	2 ounces	1.9	3.1
Lentils, dry	30 (dry)	½ cup (cooked)	2.2	7.4
Liver, beef	60	2 ounces	4.7	7.8
Liver sausage	30	1 slice	1.6	5.4
Molasses, light	20	1 tablespoon	0.9	4.3
Oatmeal	15 (dry)	½ cup (cooked)	0.7	4.5
Oysters, raw	60	2 ounces	3.4	5.6
Parsley	10	10 small sprigs	0.4	4.3
Peaches, dried	30	3 halves	1.9	6.9
Peas, dry	30 (dry)	½ cup (cooked)	1.4	4.7
Pecans	15	12 halves	0.4	2.4
Popcorn	15	1 cup, popped	0.4	2.7
Pork loin, cooked	60	2 ounces	1.8	3.0
Pork sausage	60	2 ounces	1.4	2.3
Prunes, dried	30	4 prunes	1.2	3.9
Raisins, dried	50	5 tablespoons	1.7	3.3
Rice, brown	15 (dry)	½ cup (cooked)	0.3	2.0
Rye, whole meal	15	1 tablespoon	0.6	3.7
Sardines	60	2 ounces	1.6	2.7
Shrimp, canned	60	2 ounces	1.9	3.1

APPENDIX TABLE 8   FOODS HIGH IN IRON *(Continued)*

FOOD	AVERAGE SERVING		IRON, MG.	
	Weight Gm.	Approximate Measure	Per Serving	Per 100 Gm.
Syrup, table blends	20	1 tablespoon	0.8	4.1
Soybeans, dried	25	2 tablespoons	2.0	8.0
Flour, medium fat	15	3 tablespoons	2.0	13.0
Spinach, cooked	75	½ cup	1.5	2.0
Sugar, brown	15	1 tablespoon	0.4	2.6
Tongue, beef	60	2 ounces	1.7	2.8
Turkey	60	2 ounces	2.3	3.8
Turnip greens	75	½ cup	1.8	2.4
Veal roast, cooked	60	2 ounces	2.2	3.6
Walnuts	15	8 to 15 halves	0.3	2.1
Wheat flakes	15	½ cup	0.5	3.0
Shredded, plain	30	1 biscuit	1.1	3.5
Whole meal	15	½ cup (cooked)	0.5	3.4
Yeast, compressed	30	1 ounce	1.5	4.9
Dried brewer's	15	2 tablespoons	2.7	18.2

*From Mayo Clinic Diet Manual. 3rd Ed. Philadelphia, W. B. Saunders Company, 1961, pp. 188–189.

APPENDIX TABLE 9   SODIUM AND POTASSIUM CONTENT OF FOODS*

Food	Approximate amount	Weight gm	Sodium mEq	Potassium mEq
Meat				
Meat (cooked)				
Beef	1 ounce	30	0.8	2.8
Ham	1 ounce	30	14.3	2.6
Lamb	1 ounce	30	0.9	2.2
Pork	1 ounce	30	0.9	3.0
Veal	1 ounce	30	1.0	3.8
Liver	1 ounce	30	2.4	3.2
Sausage, pork	2 links	40	16.5	2.8
Beef, dried	2 slices	20	37.0	1.0
Cold cuts	1 slice	45	25.0	2.7
Frankfurters	1	50	24.0	3.0
Fowl				
Chicken	1 ounce	30	1.0	3.0
Goose	1 ounce	30	1.6	4.6
Duck	1 ounce	30	1.0	2.2
Turkey	1 ounce	30	1.2	2.8
Egg	1	50	2.7	1.8
Fish	1 ounce	30	1.0	2.5
Salmon				
Fresh	1/4 cup	30	0.6	2.3
Canned	1/4 cup	30	4.6	2.6
Tuna				
Fresh	1/4 cup	30	0.5	2.2
Canned	1/4 cup	30	10.4	2.3
Sardines	3 medium	35	12.5	4.5
Shellfish				
Clams	5 small	50	2.6	2.3
Lobster	1 small tail	40	3.7	1.8
Oysters	5 small	70	2.1	1.5
Scallops	1 large	50	5.7	6.0
Shrimp	5 small	30	1.8	1.7
Cheese				
Cheese, American or Cheddar type	1 slice	30	9.1	0.6
Cheese foods	1 slice	30	15.0	0.8
Cheese spreads	2 tablespoons	30	15.0	0.8
Cottage cheese	1/4 cup	50	5.0	1.1
Peanut butter	2 tablespoons	30	7.8	5.0
Peanuts, unsalted	25	25	...	4.5
Fat				
Avocado	1/8	30	...	4.6
Bacon	1 slice	5	2.2	0.6
Butter or magarine	1 teaspoon	5	2.2	...
Cooking fat	1 teaspoon	5	...	...

*From Mayo Clinic Diet Manual, 4th ed. Philadelphia, W. B. Saunders Co., 1971.

APPENDIX TABLE 9   SODIUM AND POTASSIUM CONTENT OF FOODS* *(Continued)*

Food	Approximate amount	Weight *gm*	Sodium *mEq*	Potassium *mEq*
Cream				
Half and half	2 tablespoons	30	0.6	1.0
Sour	2 tablespoons	30	0.4	...
Whipped	1 tablespoon	15	0.3	1.0
Cream cheese	1 tablespoon	15	1.7	...
Mayonnaise	1 teaspoon	5	1.3	...
Nuts				
Almonds, slivered	5 (2 teaspoons)	6	...	0.8
Pecans	4 halves	5	...	0.8
Walnuts	5 halves	10	...	1.0
Oil, salad	1 teaspoon	5	...	...
Olives, green	3 medium	30	31.3	0.4
Bread				
Bread	1 slice	25	5.5	0.7
Biscuit	1 (2″ diameter)	35	9.6	0.7
Muffin	1 (2″ diameter)	35	7.3	1.2
Cornbread	1 (1 1/2″ cube)	35	11.3	1.7
Roll	1 (2″ diameter)	25	5.5	0.6
Bun	1	30	6.6	0.7
Pancake	1 (4″ diameter)	45	8.8	1.1
Waffle	1/2 square	35	8.5	1.0
Cereals				
Cooked	2/3 cup	140	8.7	2.0
Dry, flake	2/3 cup	20	8.7	0.6
Dry, puffed	1 1/2 cups	20	...	1.5
Shredded wheat	1 biscuit	20	...	2.2
Crackers				
Graham	3	20	5.8	2.0
Melba toast	4	20	5.5	0.7
Oyster	20	20	9.6	0.6
Ritz	6	20	9.5	0.5
Rye-Krisp	3	30	11.5	3.0
Saltines	6	20	9.6	0.6
Soda	3	20	9.6	0.6
Dessert				
Commercial gelatin	1/2 cup	100	2.2	...
Ice cream	1/2 cup	75	2.0	3.0
Sherbet	1/3 cup	50	...	...
Angel food cake	1 1/2″ × 1 1/2″	25	3.0	0.6
Sponge cake	1 1/2″ × 1 1/2″	25	1.8	0.6
Vanilla wafers	5	15	1.7	...
Flour products				
Cornstarch	2 tablespoons	15	...	...
Macaroni	1/4 cup	50	...	0.8
Noodles	1/4 cup	50	...	0.6
Rice	1/4 cup	50	...	0.9
Spaghetti	1/4 cup	50	...	0.8
Tapioca	2 tablespoons	15	...	...

APPENDIX TABLE 9   SODIUM AND POTASSIUM CONTENT OF FOODS* *(Continued)*

Food	Approximate amount	Weight gm	Sodium mEq	Potassium mEq
Milk				
Whole milk	1 cup	240	5.2	8.8
Evaporated whole milk	1/2 cup	120	6.0	9.2
Powdered whole milk	1/4 cup	30	5.2	10.0
Buttermilk	1 cup	240	13.6	8.5
Skim milk	1 cup	240	5.2	8.8
Powdered skim milk	1/4 cup	30	6.9	13.5
Fruit				
Figs				
Canned	1/2 cup	120	...	4.6
Dried	1 small	15	...	2.5
Fresh	1 large	60	...	3.0
Fruit cocktail	1/2 cup	120	...	5.0
Grapes				
Canned	1/3 cup	80	...	2.2
Fresh	15	80	...	3.2
Juice				
Bottled	1/4 cup	60	...	2.8
Frozen	1/3 cup	80	...	2.4
Grapefruit				
Fresh	1/2 medium	120	...	3.6
Juice	1/2 cup	120	...	4.1
Sections	3/4 cup	150	...	5.1
Mandarin orange	3/4 cup	200	...	6.5
Mango	1/2 small	70	...	3.4
Melon				
Cantaloupe	1/2 small	200	...	13.0
Honeydew	1/4 medium	200	...	13.0
Watermelon	1/2 slice	200	...	5.0
Nectarine	1 medium	80	...	6.0
Orange				
Fresh	1 medium	100	...	5.1
Juice	1/2 cup	120	...	5.7
Sections	1/2 cup	100	...	5.1
Papaya	1/2 cup	120	...	7.0
Peach				
Canned	1/2 cup	120	...	4.0
Dried	2 halves	20	...	5.0
Fresh	1 medium	120	...	6.2
Nectar	1/2 cup	120	...	2.4
Pear				
Canned	1/2 cup	120	...	2.5
Dried	2 halves	20	...	3.0
Fresh	1 small	80	...	2.6
Nectar	1/3 cup	80	...	0.9
Pineapple				
Canned	1/2 cup	120	...	3.0
Fresh	1/2 cup	80	...	3.0
Juice	1/3 cup	80	...	3.0

APPENDIX TABLE 9   SODIUM AND POTASSIUM CONTENT OF FOODS* *(Continued)*

Food	Approximate amount	Weight *gm*	Sodium *mEq*	Potassium *mEq*
Plums				
Canned	1/2 cup	120	...	4.5
Fresh	2 medium	80	...	4.1
Prunes	2 medium	15	...	2.6
Juice	1/4 cup	60	...	3.6
Raisins	1 tablespoon	15	...	2.9
Rhubarb	1/2 cup	100	...	6.5
Tangerines				
Fresh	2 small	100	...	3.2
Juice	1/2 cup	120	...	5.5
Sections	1/2 cup	100	...	3.2

*Value for products without added salt.
†Estimated average based on addition of salt, approximately 0.6% of the finished product.
From Mayo Clinic Diet Manual. 4th Ed. Philadelphia, W. B. Saunders Company, 1971.

TO CONVERT MILLIGRAMS TO MILLIEQUIVALENTS

1. Divide milligrams by atomic weight

Example: 1,000 mg sodium $= \dfrac{1,000}{23} = 43.5$ mEq sodium

Mineral	Atomic weight
Sodium	23
Potassium	39

TO CONVERT SPECIFIC WEIGHT OF SODIUM TO SODIUM CHLORIDE

1. Multiply by 2.54

Example: 1,000 mg sodium $= 1,000 \times 2.54 = 2,540$ mg sodium chloride (2.5 gm)

TO CONVERT SPECIFIC WEIGHT OF SODIUM CHLORIDE TO SODIUM

1. Multiply by 0.393

Example: 2.5 gm sodium chloride $= 2.5 \times 0.393 = 1,000$ mg sodium

Milligrams	Sodium Values Milliequivalents	Grams of Sodium Chloride
500	21.8	1.3
1,000	43.5	2.5
1,500	75.3	3.8
2,000	87.0	5.0

APPENDIX TABLE 10   EXCESS OF ACIDITY OR ALKALINITY IN FOODS[1]

(Neutral Foods)

Butter	Lard	Sugar, white
Candy, plain	Oil, olive and salad	Tapioca
Coffee	Postum	Tea
Cornstarch		

Foods with Acid Ash

FOOD	SIZE OF SERVING		NORMAL ACID, CC.	
	Weight Gm.	Approximate Measure	Per Serving	Per 100 Gm.
Bread				
White	25	1 slice	1.2	4.8
Whole Wheat	25	1 slice	1.5	6.1
Rye	25	1 slice	1.3	5.2
Cake, plain	75	1 piece	1.7	2.3
Cereal				
Cornflakes	15	½ cup	0.3	2.1
Farina	15 (dry)	½ cup (cooked)	1.4	9.6
Macaroni	15 (dry)	½ cup (cooked)	1.8	12.0
Oatmeal	15 (dry)	½ cup (cooked)	2.0	13.1
Puffed wheat	15	1 cup	1.6	10.8
Puffed rice	15	1 cup	1.4	9.0
Rice	15 (dry)	½ cup (cooked)	1.2	7.8
Shredded wheat	15	½ biscuit	1.8	12.2
Fat, mayonnaise	15	1 tablespoon	0.3	2.3
Fruit				
Cranberries	100	½ cup	+	+
Plums	100	½ cup	+	+
Prunes	100	½ cup	+	+
Meat				
Bacon	30	5 strips	5.9	19.6
Beef, roast	60	2 ounces	10.6	17.7
Cheese, Cheddar	30	1 ounce	1.7	5.5
Cheese, cottage	70	2 heaping tablespoons	3.2	4.5
Chicken	60	2 ounces	10.7	17.8
Eggs	50	1	7.7	15.4
Fish, halibut	60	2 ounces	12.4	20.7
Ham	60	2 ounces	9.1	15.2
Lamb	60	2 ounces	11.1	18.5
Pork	60	2 ounces	9.8	16.3
Veal	60	2 ounces	11.3	18.8
Nuts				
Brazil nuts	15	2 medium	1.7	11.0
Peanut butter	15	1 tablespoon	0.7	4.7
Peanuts	15	16–17 nuts	0.9	6.0
Walnuts, English	15	4–8 nuts	1.3	8.4
Vegetables				
Corn	100	½ cup	3.6	3.6
Lentils, dried	30	½ cup (cooked)	1.8	6.0

[1] From Mayo Clinic Diet Manual. 3rd ed. Philadelphia, W. B. Saunders Company, 1961, pp. 182–184.

APPENDIX TABLE 10   EXCESS OF ACIDITY OR ALKALINITY IN FOODS[1]
(Continued)
(Neutral Foods)
Foods with Alkaline Ash

FOOD	SIZE OF SERVING Weight Gm.	SIZE OF SERVING Approximate Measure	NORMAL BASE, CC. Per Serving	NORMAL BASE, CC. Per 100 Gm.
Cream	75	⅓ cup	0.8	1.0
Fruit				
Apple	100	1 small	3.8	3.8
Apricots, raw	100	2–3	6.8	6.8
Apricots, dried	30	4–6 halves	10.9	36.3
Banana	100	1 small	7.9	7.9
Blackberries, raw	100	⅝ cup	5.0	5.0
Blueberries, raw	100	⅝ cup	2.7	2.7
Cantaloupe	150	½ melon	9.0	6.0
Cherries, fresh	100	15 large	7.0	7.0
Currants, fresh	100	¾ cup	7.5	7.5
Dates, dried	30	3–4	2.9	9.7
Figs, dried	30	2 small	10.8	36.0
Gooseberries	100	⅔ cup	4.1	4.1
Grapefruit	100	½ medium	6.0	6.0
Grapes	100	1 bunch	6.0	6.0
Lemon	30	1 ounce	1.2	4.0
Lime	30	1 ounce	1.2	4.0
Loganberries	100	⅔ cup	5.0	5.0
Mango	100	1 small	5.0	5.0
Nectarines	100	2 small	6.2	6.2
Olives, green. and ripe	30	3 medium	6.5	21.5
Orange	100	1 small	5.0	5.0
Peach, raw	100	1 medium	7.0	7.0
Pear, raw	100	1 medium	3.3	3.3
Persimmon	100	1 medium	7.5	7.5
Pineapple, raw	100	½ cup	6.5	6.5
Pineapple juice	200	1 cup, scant	6.0	3.0
Raisins	30	3 tablespoons	4.5	15.0
Raspberries, black and red	100	¾ cup	6 0	6.0
Strawberries	100	10 large	3.5	3.5
Tangerine	100	1 large	5.5	5.5
Watermelon	600	1 slice	22 8	3.8
Ice cream	70	⅓ cup	0.5	0.7
Jam	20	1 rounded teaspoon	0.7	3.3
Milk	240	½ pint	4.8	2.0
Nuts				
Almonds	15	12–15 nuts	1.8	12.0
Chestnuts	15	2 large	1.5	10.0
Coconut, fresh	15	1 piece	0.6	4.0
Sweets				
Molasses, medium	20	1 tablespoon	7.0	35.0
Vegetables				
Asparagus	75	6–8 tips	2.3	3.0
Beans, baked	100	½ cup	2.8	2.8
Beans, lima	75	⅓ cup	9.8	13.1
Beans, navy, pea	30	½ cup (cooked)	5.4	18.0
Beans, snap	75	⅓ cup	2.5	3.3
Beets	75	⅓ cup	7.9	10.5
Beet greens	75	⅓ cup	20.3	27.0
Broccoli	75	½ cup	3.0	4.0

APPENDIX TABLE 10   EXCESS OF ACIDITY OR ALKALINITY IN FOODS[1] *(Continued)*

(Neutral Foods)

| FOOD | SIZE OF SERVING | | NORMAL BASE, CC. | |
	Weight Gm.	*Approximate Measure*	*Per Serving*	*Per 100 Gm.*
Vegetables (continued)				
Cabbage, cooked	75	⅓ cup	3.3	4.4
Carrots	75	½ cup	5.2	6.9
Cauliflower	75	½ cup	1.5	2.0
Celery	30	3 strips	2.5	8.4
Chard, Swiss	75	½ cup	12.0	16.0
Cucumber	50	½ medium	4.0	8.0
Dandelion greens	75	⅓ cup	14.7	19.6
Eggplant	75	⅓ cup	3.0	4.0
Endive, curly	50	10 leaves	4.5	9.0
Kale	75	⅓ cup	7.4	9.8
Kohlrabi	75	⅓ cup	8.3	11.1
Lettuce	50	5 leaves	3.0	6.0
Mushrooms	75	⅓ cup	2.3	3.1
Okra	75	⅓ cup	2.0	2.6
Onions	75	⅓ cup	0.1	0.1
Parsnips	75	⅓ cup	6.0	8.0
Peas	75	⅓ cup	0.7	0.9
Peppers	30	3 strips	0.6	2.0
Potato, white	100	1 small	9.0	9.0
Potato, baked	100	1 small	10.6	10.6
Potato, mashed	100	½ cup	9.6	9.6
Pumpkin	75	⅓ cup	5.9	7.8
Radish	50	5	1.5	3.0
Rutabagas	75	⅓ cup	6.4	8.5
Salsify	75	½ cup	2.2	2.9
Sauerkraut	75	½ cup	4.3	5.7
Squash, summer	75	⅓ cup	0.8	1.0
Squash, winter	75	⅓ cup	2.3	3.0
Sweet potato	100	1 small	6.0	6.0
Tomatoes or juice	75	½ large or ⅓ cup	3.8	5.0
Turnip greens	75	⅓ cup	1.7	2.3
Turnip	75	⅓ cup	1.7	2.3
Water cress	50	10 leaves	4.0	8.0

APPENDIX TABLE 11   COMMON CARBOHYDRATES IN FOODS PER 100 GM. EDIBLE PORTION*

FOOD	MONO-SACCHARIDES		REDUC-ING SUGARS*	DISACCHARIDES			POLYSACCHARIDES					
	Fructose	Glucose		Lactose	Maltose	Sucrose	Cellulose	Dextrins	Hemi-cellulose	Pectin	Pento-sans	Starch
						Fruits						
	gm.	gm.	gm.	gm.	gm.	gm.	gm.	gm.	gm.	gm.	gm.	gm.
Agave juice	17.0		19.0	†								
Apple	5.0	1.7	8.3			3.1	0.4		0.7	0.6		0.6
Apple juice			8.0			4.2						
Apricots	0.4	1.9				5.5	0.8		1.2	1.0		
Banana												
Yellow green			5.0			5.1						8.8
Yellow			8.4			8.9						1.9
Flecked	3.5	4.5				11.9						1.2
Powder			32.6			33.2		9.6				7.8
Blackberries	2.9	3.2				0.2						
Blueberry juice, com- mercial			9.6			0.2						
Boysenberries			5.3			1.1				0.3		
Breadfruit												
Hawaiian			1.8			7.7						
Samoan			4.9			9.7						
Cherries												
Eating	7.2	4.7	12.5			0.1				0.3		
Cooking	6.1	5.5	11.6			0.1						
Cranberries	0.7	2.7				0.1						
Currants												
Black	3.7	2.4				0.6						
Red	1.9	2.3				0.2						
White	2.6	3.0										
Dates												
Invert sugar, seedling type	23.9	24.9				0.3						
Deglet Noor			16.2			45.4						
Egyptian			35.8			48.5						3.0
Figs, Kadota												
Fresh	8.2	9.6				0.9						0.1
Dried	30.9	42.0				0.1						0.3
Gooseberries	4.1	4.4				0.7						
Grapes												
Black	7.3	8.2										
Concord	4.3	4.8	9.5			0.2						
Malaga			22.2			0.2						
White	8.0	8.1										
Grapefruit	1.2	2.0				2.9					1.3	
Guava			4.4			1.9						
Lemon												
Edible portion			1.3			0.2				3.0	0.7	
Whole	1.4	1.4				0.4						
Juice	0.9	0.5				0.1						
Peel			3.4			0.1						
Loganberries	1.3	1.9				0.2						
Loquat												
Champagne		12.0				0.8						
Thales		9.0				0.9						
Mango			3.4			11.6						0.3
Melon												
Cantaloupe	0.9	1.2	2.3			4.4				0.3		
Cassaba,												
Vine ripened			2.8			6.2						
Picked green			3.2			3.9						
Honeydew												
Vine ripened			3.3			7.4						
Picked green			3.6			3.3						
Yellow	1.5	2.1				1.4						
Mulberries	3.6	4.4										
Orange												
Valencia (Calif.)	2.3	2.4	4.7			4.2						
Composite values	1.8	2.5	5.0			4.6	0.3		0.3	1.3	0.3	
Juice												
Fresh	2.4	2.4	5.1			4.7						
Frozen, reconstituted			4.6			3.2						

*From: Hardinge, M. G., et al.: Carbohydrate in foods. J. Am. Dietet. A. 46:197, 1965.

APPENDIX TABLE 11   COMMON CARBOHYDRATES IN FOODS PER 100 GM. EDIBLE PORTION* (Continued)

FOOD	MONO-SACCHARIDES Fructose	Glucose	REDUC-ING SUGARS*	DISACCHARIDES Lactose	Maltose	Sucrose	POLYSACCHARIDES Cellu-lose	Dextrins	Hemi-Cellu-lose	Pectin	Pento-sans	Starch
	gm.	gm.	gm.	gm.	gm.	gm.	gm.	gm.	gm.	gm.	gm.	gm.
FRUITS, continued												
Palmyra palm, tender kernel	1.5	3.2				0.4						
Papaw (*Asimina triloba*) (North America)			5.9			2.7						
Papaya (*Carica papaya*) (tropics)			9.0			0.5						
Pashion fruit juice	3.6	3.6				3.8						1.8
Peaches	1.6	1.5	3.1			6.6		0.7		0.7		
Pears												
Anjou			7.6			1.9				0.7		
Bartlett	5.0	2.5	8.0			1.5				0.6		
Bosc	6.5	2.6				1.7				0.6		
Persimmon			17.7									
Pineapple												
Ripened on plant	1.4	2.3	4.2			7.9						
Picked green			1.3			2.4						
Plums												
Damson	3.4	5.2	8.4			1.0						
Green Gage	4.0	5.5				2.9						
Italian prunes			4.6			5.4				0.9		
Sweet	2.9	4.5	7.4			4.4		0.5		1.0	0.1	
Sour	1.3	3.5				1.5				1.0		
Pomegranate			'12.0			0.6						
Prunes, uncooked	15.0	30.0	47.0			2.0	2.8		10.7	0.9	2.0	0.7
Raisins, Thompson seedless			70.0							1.0		
Raspberries	2.4	2.3	5.0			1.0				0.8		
Sapote	3.8	4.2		0.7								
Strawberries												
Ripe	2.3	2.6				1.4						
Medium ripe			3.8			0.3						
Tangerine			4.8			9.0						
Tomatoes	1.2	1.6	3.4				0.2		0.3	0.3		
Canned			3.0			0.3						
Seedless pulp			6.5			0.4	0.4			0.5		
Watermelon												
Flesh red and firm, ripe			3.8			4.0				0.1		
Red, mealy, overripe			3.0			4.9				0.1		
Vegetables												
Asparagus, raw			1.2						0.3			
Bamboo shoots			0.5			0.2	1.2					
Beans												
Lima												
Canned						1.4						
Fresh						1.4						
Snap, fresh			1.7			0.5	0.5	0.3	1.0	0.5	1.2	2.0
Beets, sugar						12.9	0.9		0.8			
Broccoli							0.9		0.9		0.9	1.3
Brussel Sprouts							1.1		1.5			
Cabbage, raw			3.4			0.3	0.8		1.0			
Carrots, raw			5.8			1.7	1.0		1.7	0.9		
Cauliflower		2.8				0.3	0.7		0.6			
Celery												
Fresh			0.3			0.3						
Hearts			1.7			0.2						
Corn												
Fresh		0.5				0.3	0.6	0.1	0.9		1.3	14.5
Bran									77.1		4.0	
Cucumber			2.5			0.1						
Eggplant			2.1			0.6			0.5			
Lettuce			1.4			0.2	0.4		0.6			
Licorice root		1.4				3.2						22.0
Mushrooms, fresh			0.1		0.9				0.7			2.5
Onions, raw			5.4			2.9			0.3	0.6		
Parsnips, fresh						3.5						7.0
Peas, green						5.5	1.1		2.2			4.1

APPENDIX TABLE 11   COMMON CARBOHYDRATES IN FOODS PER 100 GM. EDIBLE PORTION* *(Continued)*

FOOD	MONO-SACCHARIDES		REDUC-ING SUGARS*	DISACCHARIDES			POLYSACCHARIDES					
	Fructose	Glucose		Lactose	Maltose	Sucrose	Cellu-lose	Dextrins	Hemi-Cellu-lose	Pectin	Pento-sans	Starch
VEGETABLES, continued												
	gm.	gm.	gm.	gm.	gm.	gm.	gm.	gm.	gm.	gm.	gm.	gm.
Potatoes, white	0.1	0.1	0.8			0.1	0.4		0.3			17.0
Pumpkin			2.2			0.6			0.5			0.1
Radishes			3.1			0.3			0.3	0.4		
Rutabagas		5.0				1.3					0.8	
Spinach			0.2				0.4		0.8			
Squash												
Butternut	0.2	0.1				0.4						2.6
Blue Hubbard	1.2	1.1				0.4	0.7					4.8
Golden Crookneck			2.8			1.0						
Sweet potato												
Raw	0.3	0.4	0.8		1.6	4.1	0.6		1.4	2.2		16.5
Baked			14.5			7.2						4.0
Mature Dry Legumes												
Beans												
Mung												
Black gram						1.6						
Green gram						1.8						
Navy							3.1	3.7	6.4		8.2	35.2
Soy			**1.6**			7.2	2.6	1.4	6.6		4.0	1.9
Cow pea						1.5	5.4		4.8			
Garbanzo (chick peas)						2.4						
Garden pea (*Pisum sativum*)‡						6.7	5.0		5.1			38.0
Horse gram (*Dolichos biflorus*)						2.7						
Lentils						2.1						28.5
Pigeon pea (red gram)						1.6						
Soybean												
Flour						6.8						
Meal						6.8						
Milk and Milk Products												
Buttermilk												
Dry				39.9								
Fluid, genuine and cultured				5.0								
Casein		**0.1**		4.9								
Ice cream (14.5% cream)				3.6		16.6						
Milk												
Ass				6.0								
Cow				4.9								
Dried												
Skim				52.0								
Whole				38.1								
Fluid												
Skim				5.0								
Whole				4.9								
Sweetened, condensed				14.1		43.5						
Ewe				4.9								
Goat				4.7								
Human												
Colostrum				5.3								
Mature				6.9								
Whey				4.9								
Yogurt				3.8								
Nuts and Nut Products												
Almonds, blanched			0.2			2.3					2.1	
Chestnuts			2.2			3.6					1.2	18.0
Virginia			1.2			8.1		0.3			2.8	18.6
French			3.3			3.6					2.5	33.1
Coconut milk, ripe						2.6						
Copra meal, dried	1.2	1.2				14.3	15.6	0.6			2.2	0.9
Macadamia nut			0.3			5.5						

APPENDIX TABLE 11   COMMON CARBOHYDRATES IN FOODS PER 100 GM. EDIBLE PORTION* (Continued)

FOOD	MONO-SACCHARIDES		REDUC-ING SUGARS*	DISACCHARIDES			POLYSACCHARIDES					
	Fructose	Glucose		Lactose	Maltose	Sucrose	Cellu-lose	Dextrins	Hemi-cellu-lose	Pectin	Pento-sans	Starch
Nuts and Nut Products, continued												
	gm.	gm.	gm.	gm.	gm.	gm.	gm.	gm.	gm.	gm.	gm.	gm.
Peanuts			0.2			4.5	2.4	2.5	3.8			4.0
Peanut butter			0.9									5.9
Pecans						1.1					0.2	
Cereals and Cereal Products												
Barley												
Grain, hulled							2.6		6.0		8.5	62.0
Flour						3.1					1.2	69.0
Corn, yellow							4.5		4.9		6.2	62.0
Flaxseed							1.8		5.2			
Millet grain									0.9		6.5	56.0
Oats, hulled											6.4	56.4
Rice												
Bran			1.4			10.6	11.4		7.0		7.4	
Brown, raw			0.1			0.8		2.1			2.1	69.7
Polished, raw		2.0	trace#			0.4	0.3	0.9			1.8	72.9
Polish			0.7								3.8	
Rye												
Grain							3.8		5.6		6.8	57.0
Flour											4.1	71.4
Sorghum grain											2.5	70.2
Soya-wheat (cereal)											3.3	46.4
Wheat												
Germ, defatted						8.3					6.2	
Grain			2.0			1.5	2.0	2.5	5.8		6.6	59.0
Flour, patent			2.0		0.1	0.2		5.5			2.1	68.8
Spices and Condiments												
Allspice (pimenta)			18.0			3.0						
Cassia			23.3									
Cinnamon			19.3									
Cloves			9.0									2.7
Nutmeg			17.2									14.6
Pepper, black			38.6									34.2
Sirups and Other Sweets												
Corn sirup		21.2			26.4			34.7				
High conversion		33.0			23.0			19.0				
Medium conversion		26.0			21.0			23.0				
Corn sugar		87.5			3.5			0.5				
Chocolate, sweet dry						56.4						
Golden sirup			37.5			31.0						
Honey	40.5	34.2				1.9		1.5				
Invert sugar			74.0			6.0						
Jellies, pectin						40-65						
Royal jelly	11.3	9.8				0.9						
Jellies, starch						25-60						7=12
Maple sirup			1.5			62.9						
Milk chocolate				8.1		43.0						
Molasses	8.0	8.8				53.6						
Blackstrap	6.8	6.8	26.9			36.9						
Sorghum sirup			27.0			36.0						
Miscellaneous												
Beer			1.5					2.8			0.3	
Cacao beans, raw, Arriba	0.6	0.5	1.1			1.9						
Carob bean												
Pod			11.2			23.2						
Pod and seeds			11.1			19.4				1.4		
Soy sauce	0.9											

*Mainly monosaccharides plus the disaccharides, maltose and lactose.
†Blanks indicate lack of acceptable data.
‡Also known as Alaska pea, field pea, and common pea.
#Trace = less than 0.05 gm.

APPENDIX TABLE 12   INORGANIC ELEMENTS IN COMMON FOODS*

(Milligrams per 100 Gram Food)

mg./100 gm.

FOOD	DESCRIPTION	PHOS-PHORUS	POTAS-SIUM	CAL-CIUM	MAGNE-SIUM	SODIUM	ALUMI-NUM	BARIUM	IRON	STRON-TIUM	BORON	COPPER	ZINC	MANGA-NESE	CHRO-MIUM
Beverages and Dietary Concentrates															
Chocolate sirup		88	183	15	64	57	<0.2	0.17	1.4	0.13	0.3	0.43	1.1	0.23	<0.06
Coffee															
Instant	dry	367	1,103	156	380	56	<1.0	0.36	5.5	0.16	1.6	0.28	1.2	2.1	0.79
Ground	dry	119	2,045	98	179	<1.0	1.1	0.32	3.1	0.61	0.79	1.3	0.36	1.5	0.06
Beverage	brewed	2.4	65	7	6.7	0.86	0.04	0.008	<0.02	<0.004	0.016	<0.004	0.042	0.014	<0.012
Cocoa	dry	526	1,990	100	442	89	4.5	1.2	8	1.7	2.2	5	5.4	2.5	0.06
Drinking and cooking water		0.5	2.0	8.8	4.5	3.8	<0.02	<0.004	0.011	<0.002	0.0035	<0.002	0.015	<0.004	<0.006
Meritene, plain flavor	dry	664	2,020	846	89	588	1.9	0.11	12	0.38	0.37	0.09	3.3	<0.04	<0.06
Sustagen, imitation vanilla flavor	dry	425	750	663	58	285	1.6	0.056	1.02	0.28	0.26	0.085	2.9	0.04	<0.06
Tea, orange pekoe															
Bag	dry	277	1,795	465	192	37	128	2.7	33	1.3	2.6	4.8	5.4	71	0.3
Beverage	steeped	<0.5	9.3	7.3	4.2	0.7	0.28	<0.004	<0.01	0.002	0.002	0.007	0.037	0.22	<0.006
Breads, Cereal Products, Crackers, and Pastas															
Bread															
Rye	enriched, 4% nonfat milk solids; calcium propionate added	145	183	96	42	873	<0.2	0.062	1.5	0.3	0.042	0.17	1.2	0.5	<0.06
White		105	154	128	25	863	0.3	0.051	1.9	0.31	0.069	0.11	0.75	0.25	<0.06
Whole wheat		192	176	74	59	752	0.54	0.11	3.8	0.15	0.048	0.17	1.7	1.2	<0.06
Bran flakes, 40%		483	730	34	175	923	<0.2	0.39	15	0.15	0.23	0.64	3.9	4.1	<0.06
Cheerios		359	353	147	106	1,150	0.47	0.13	3.9	0.18	0.13	0.34	3	2.7	<0.06
Corn flakes		31	111	<10	8.7	1,000	<0.2	0.04	1.4	0.024	<0.02	0.023	0.13	<0.04	<0.06
Crackers															
Graham		80	100	12	18	725	<0.2	0.11	0.55	0.066	<0.02	0.04	0.76	0.43	<0.06
Saltines		85	100	15	18	1,335	<0.2	0.04	1.7	0.14	<0.02	0.09	0.7	0.39	<0.06
Egg noodles	uncooked	242	266	31	74	30	<0.2	0.16	4.6	0.06	0.105	0.17	2.2	0.78	<0.06
Macaroni	uncooked	181	233	15	50	5.7	<0.2	0.11	3.1	0.024	0.063	0.13	1.6	0.5	<0.06
Oatmeal, rolled oats (quick)	uncooked	368	390	39	128	4.7	<0.2	0.11	3.7	0.024	0.13	0.022	3.4	3.7	<0.06
Puffed Rice		154	229	15	40	6.7	<0.2	<0.04	0.21	<0.02	0.15	0.17	1.3	1.5	<0.06
Quick Cream of Wheat															
Enriched	uncooked	1,028	388	1,010	41	345	2.5	0.2	84	0.55	0.65	0.12	2.2	1.1	0.3
Regular	uncooked	441	149	403	17	267	0.8	0.15	34	0.16	0.2	0.11	1.1	0.58	<0.06
Rice Krispies		102	89	<10	30	1,100	<0.2	0.04	2.2	0.024	0.024	0.085	1.4	0.99	<0.06
Rice, white	uncooked	120	89	14	28	25	1.4	<0.04	0.27	<0.02	0.024	<0.02	1.8	1.5	<0.06
Shredded Wheat		355	390	26	109	4.7	<0.2	0.22	2.7	0.024	0.24	0.17	3.2	2.9	<0.06
Spaghetti	uncooked	169	183	18	61	4.7	<0.2	0.11	2.4	0.066	0.069	0.068	1.7	0.54	<0.06
Wheaties		297	390	30	89	1,400	<0.2	0.14	3.0	0.15	0.048	0.34	2.4	1.5	<0.06

*From Gormican, A.: Inorganic elements in foods used in hospital menus. J. Am. Dietet. A., 56:397, 1970.

APPENDIX TABLE 12 INORGANIC ELEMENTS IN COMMON FOODS* (Continued)

(Milligrams per 100 Gram Food)

mg./100 gm.

FOOD	DESCRIPTION	PHOSPHORUS	POTASSIUM	CALCIUM	MAGNESIUM	SODIUM	ALUMINUM	BARIUM	IRON	STRONTIUM	BORON	COPPER	ZINC	MANGANESE	CHROMIUM
Eggs and Dairy Products															
Cheese															
American		795	167	545	20	1,770	69.5	0.12	0.63	0.29	0.24	0.11	4.1	<0.4	0.17
Cottage	creamed	159	89	74	5.5	444	<0.2	<0.04	<0.1	<0.02	<0.02	<0.02	0.4	<0.04	0.06
Swiss		530	180	843	34	297	1.9	0.22	0.46	0.26	0.13	0.11	4.6	<0.04	0.06
Eggs															
Whole		191	100	48	9.8	147	0.14	0.76	2.1	0.02	0.063	0.053	1.8	<0.02	0.052
White		10	140	3.6	9.9	180	<0.05	<0.01	<0.025	0.024	0.013	0.005	0.009	<0.01	<0.015
Yolk		255	89	72	4.0	20	<0.1	0.058	2.1	0.027	0.066	0.01	1.5	<0.02	0.03
Milk															
Nonfat solids		710	1,940	991	94	561	1.7	<0.08	<0.2	0.24	0.29	<0.04	4.4	<0.08	<0.16
Fluid Whole	3.5% butterfat; vitamin D enriched, 400 U.S.P. units/qt.)	85	145	105	9	50	0.2	<0.01	0.028	0.022	0.028	0.005	0.43	<0.01	<0.015
Skim	0% butterfat; 2,000 U.S.P. units vitamin A and 400 U.S.P. units vitamin D added/qt.	82	170	108	9.2	56	0.2	<0.01	0.027	0.017	0.029	0.005	0.46	<0.01	<0.015
Buttermilk	Grade A, cultured	75	190	98	8.4	238	0.2	<0.01	0.028	0.028	0.027	<0.005	0.37	<0.01	<0.015
Ice cream	vanilla	96	210	120	12	87	0.26	<0.01	0.037	0.033	0.033	0.005	0.53	<0.01	<0.015
Sherbet	orange	46	90	59	6.7	39	0.14	<0.01	0.067	0.019	0.053	0.022	0.24	<0.01	<0.015
Fruits and Fruit Juices															
Apple															
Raw	with peel	6.9	95	7.1	4.8	0.5	<0.05	0.075	2.0	0.008	0.37	0.014	0.012	0.035	<0.015
Juice	canned	4.2	85	3.1	3.2	2.2	0.08	<0.002	0.4	<0.001	0.12	0.023	0.043	0.21	<0.006
Sauce	canned, drained	5.6	70	2.9	2.0	16	<0.05	<0.01	0.24	<0.005	0.19	0.01	0.013	<0.01	<0.015
Apricots	canned, drained	16	170	8.3	6.4	22	<0.05	<0.01	0.23	0.063	0.58	0.041	0.085	0.13	<0.015
Banana	ripe	17	405	<2.5	26	2.9	0.26	<0.01	0.17	0.024	0.074	0.11	0.15	0.15	<0.015
Blueberries	water-pack, drained	14	45	6.2	3.8	0.9	0.26	0.014	9.2	<0.005	0.12	0.027	0.085	0.15	<0.015
Cantaloupe		10	295	9	8.4	33	<0.05	<0.01	0.6	0.05	0.24	0.014	0.14	<0.01	<0.015
Cherries, Royal Anne	canned, drained	20	155	12	8.4	1.2	<0.05	0.029	1.7	0.041	0.57	0.061	0.11	0.029	<0.015
Grapes															
Fresh	with peel	29	230	12	5.8	<0.5	<0.05	<0.05	1.1	0.064	0.45	0.035	0.035	0.065	<0.015
Juice	canned	10.3	125	4.8	7.3	2.2	0.11	0.023	0.15	0.017	0.23	0.009	0.04	0.36	<0.006
Grapefruit Juice	canned	11	125	7	7.7	2.2	<0.04	<0.008	0.27	0.13	0.026	0.008	0.03	<0.008	<0.012
Grapefruit Sections															
Fresh	skinless	23	170	18	12	<0.5	<0.05	<0.01	0.17	0.071	0.15	0.041	0.10	<0.01	<0.015
Canned	drained	10	100	20	7.2	3.6	<0.05	<0.01	0.35	0.61	0.059	0.014	0.04	<0.01	<0.015

APPENDIX TABLE 12 INORGANIC ELEMENTS IN COMMON FOODS* (Continued)

(Milligrams per 100 Gram Food)

mg./100 gm.

FOOD	DESCRIPTION	PHOS-PHORUS	POTAS-SIUM	CAL-CIUM	MAGNE-SIUM	SODIUM	ALUMI-NUM	BARIUM	IRON	STRON-TIUM	BORON	COPPER	ZINC	MANGA-NESE	CHRO-MIUM
Fruit and Fruit Juices—Concluded															
Orange Juice	frozen, re-constituted	10.2	185	10	8.2	1.8	<0.04	<0.008	0.042	0.011	0.055	0.0075	0.015	<0.008	0.012
Sections	skinless	14	135	6.2	6.7	<0.4	<0.04	<0.003	0.042	0.019	0.18	0.004	0.02	<0.008	<0.012
Pineapple															
Crushed	canned, drained	6.9	95	16	14	3.6	<0.05	0.014	0.2	0.17	0.085	0.15	0.08	1.16	<0.015
Juice	canned	6.9	145	11	11	0.9	<0.04	0.008	0.119	0.025	0.067	0.04	0.07	0.99	<0.012
Peach, cling	canned, drained	12	100	<2.5	3.8	1.6	<0.05	<0.01	1.0	<0.005	0.28	0.041	0.05	<0.01	<0.015
Pear	canned, drained	6.9	73	3.6	3.8	9.0	<0.05	0.047	0.04	0.026	0.15	0.041	0.055	<0.01	<0.015
Prunes															
Cooked		35	340	28	24	3.6	0.62	0.064	1.3	0.19	0.71	0.25	0.33	0.078	<0.015
Juice	canned	8.3	170	5.1	5.8	1.3	<0.04	0.014	0.35	0.025	0.28	0.018	0.12	0.02	<0.012
Watermelon		5.6	95	14	10.2	1.6	<0.05	0.022	0.25	0.014	0.108	0.017	0.085	0.026	<0.015
Meat, Poultry, Fish, and Shellfish															
Beef, fresh, uncooked															
Flank	U. S. Good	148	365	<5	16	73	<0.1	<0.02	1.4	<0.01	<0.01	0.02	3.6	<0.02	<0.03
Ground	U. S. Cutter	182	350	<5	17	65	<0.1	<0.02	2.6	0.012	0.034	0.061	3.4	<0.02	<0.03
Liver		355	323	<10	8.2	77	<0.2	<0.04	2.9	<0.02	0.054	4.6	4.2	0.17	0.06
Round	U. S. Good	160	285	<5	16	63	<0.1	<0.02	2	0.012	0.044	0.045	3	<0.02	<0.03
Rump	U. S. Good	172	370	<5	18	67	<0.1	<0.02	2.1	<0.01	<0.01	0.077	3.3	<0.02	<0.03
Sirloin	U. S. Good, medium fat	159	395	<5	16	53	<0.1	<0.02	1.4	<0.01	<0.21	0.042	3.1	<0.02	<0.03
Tenderloin	U. S. Prime	153	330	<5	16	55	<0.1	<0.02	1.5	<0.01	<0.01	0.012	2.5	<0.02	<0.03
Lamb, fresh, uncooked															
Chop	medium fat	145	325	6.8	16	83	<0.1	<0.02	1.3	<0.01	<0.01	0.045	2.4	<0.02	<0.03
Leg	medium fat	159	350	<5	17	107	<0.1	<0.02	1	<0.01	<0.01	0.063	3.2	<0.02	<0.03
Luncheon meat, big bologna		77	148	8.5	8.9	2,275	<0.1	<0.02	1.6	0.078	<0.01	0.02	1.5	<0.02	<0.03
Pork, fresh, uncooked															
Bacon	medium fat	131	122	<10	6.9	979	<0.2	<0.04	0.81	0.1	<0.02	0.023	1.4	<0.04	<0.06
Ham	cured	217	350	10	14	2,505	<0.1	<0.02	0.71	0.081	0.024	0.034	1.7	<0.02	<0.03
Liver		366	296	<10	14	118	<0.2	<0.04	3.8	<0.02	0.069	0.55	6.7	0.23	<0.06
Loin	medium fat	141	300	<5	15	35	<0.1	<0.02	0.8	<0.01	<0.01	0.011	1.4	<0.02	0.93
Veal, fresh, uncooked															
Round	medium fat	136	245	7.4	11	124	<0.1	<0.02	1.5	<0.01	0.01	0.043	2.3	<0.02	<0.03
Steak	medium fat	160	295	<5	15	92	<0.1	<0.02	0.8	<0.01	<0.01	0.052	2.9	<0.02	<0.03
Poultry, uncooked															
Chicken, roaster															
Dark meat		137	240	7.4	16	81	<0.1	<0.02	1.1	0.011	0.014	0.02	1.5	<0.02	<0.03
White meat		152	225	8.7	17	49	<0.1	<0.02	0.8	<0.01	0.024	0.011	0.59	<0.02	<0.03
Turkey, roaster															
Dark meat		175	330	<5	17	69	<0.1	<0.02	1.5	<0.01	0.024	0.037	2.4	<0.02	<0.03
White meat		185	235	<5	20	48	<0.1	<0.02	0.73	0.012	0.024	0.037	1.8	<0.02	<0.03

APPENDIX TABLE 12   INORGANIC ELEMENTS IN COMMON FOODS* (Continued)

(Milligrams per 100 Gram Food)

mg./100 gm.

FOOD	DESCRIPTION	PHOS-PHORUS	POTAS-SIUM	CAL-CIUM	MAGNE-SIUM	SODIUM	ALUMI-NUM	BARIUM	IRON	STRON-TIUM	BORON	COPPER	ZINC	MANGA-NESE	CHRO-MIUM
Meat, Poultry, Fish, and Shellfish—Concluded															
Fish and shell fish															
Crab	canned, salted	147	265	25	41	500	<0.1	<0.02	0.48	0.37	0.01	0.27	3.6	<0.02	<0.03
Haddock	uncooked, frozen	164	370	10	24	202	<0.1	<0.02	1.4	0.031	0.021	0.011	0.32	<0.02	<0.03
Salmon, Sockeye	canned, salt-free	312	400	272	29	51	0.82	<0.02	1.4	1.0	0.064	0.076	1.1	<0.02	<0.03
Shrimp	canned, salted	141	163	18	23	2,300	<0.1	<0.02	1.6	0.17	0.022	0.17	1.9	<0.02	<0.03
Sole	uncooked, frozen	110	220	25	44	397	<0.1	0.02	0.33	0.2	0.062	0.011	0.31	<0.02	<0.03
Tuna	canned, salt-free, water pack	184	330	<5	23	44	<0.1	<0.02	3.2	<0.01	0.054	0.011	0.44	<0.02	<0.03
Nuts															
Peanuts	smooth	314	790	34	172	602	<0.2	<0.04	1.8	0.127	0.03	0.61	2.9	1.9	<0.06
Butter	salted, blanched	326	830	36	160	324	<0.2	0.21	1.2	0.14	1.7	0.43	2.9	1.5	<0.06
Pecans	unsalted	281	368	76	110	11	<0.2	0.67	1.7	0.36	0.76	1.1	4.1	1.5	<0.06
Walnuts	unsalted	337	530	103	144	6.4	0.2	0.072	4.2	<0.02	<0.059	1.4	3.2	2.1	<0.06
Sugars and Flours															
Sugar															
Brown		<5	640	68	62	44	<0.2	<0.04	1.8	0.127	0.03	<0.02	0.029	<0.04	<0.06
Powdered		<5	<20	<10	<1	1.4	<0.2	<0.04	<0.1	<0.02	<0.02	<0.02	<0.02	<0.04	<0.06
White		5	<20	<10	<1	1.2	<0.2	<0.04	<0.1	<0.02	<0.02	<0.02	<0.02	<0.04	<0.06
Flour	bleached, enriched	121	117	14	27	6.1	<0.2	0.072	4.2	<0.02	0.059	0.13	0.93	0.4	<0.06
Vegetables															
Asparagus spears	frozen, uncooked	91	300	32	14	3.3	<0.1	<0.02	2.1	0.012	0.26	0.21	0.76	0.18	<0.03
Beans															
Baked with pork		85	240	50	28	427	<0.1	<0.02	2.5	0.073	0.18	0.17	1.7	0.2	<0.06
Green	frozen, uncooked	30	148	38	21	0.9	<0.1	0.16	1.5	0.2	0.19	0.04	0.31	0.27	<0.06
Lima, baby	frozen, uncooked	116	560	34	57	136	<0.1	0.031	2.6	0.31	0.31	0.18	0.77	0.54	<0.06
Wax	canned, salt-free, drained	20	90	40	11	7	0.28	0.11	3.5	0.065	0.064	0.02	0.23	0.21	<0.06
Beets	canned, salt-free, drained	22	148	13	23	69	<0.1	0.26	1	0.14	0.14	0.2	0.3	0.082	<0.03
Broccoli	frozen, uncooked	52	220	34	15	25	<0.1	<0.02	0.75	0.101	0.16	0.011	0.27	0.056	<0.03
Brussels sprouts	frozen, uncooked	65	475	29	21	14	<0.1	<0.02	1.5	0.075	0.23	0.011	0.37	0.11	<0.03
Cabbage	uncooked	31	199	46	16	6.9	<0.1	<0.02	2.4	0.023	0.34	0.06	0.14	0.063	<0.03
Carrots	uncooked	36	315	28	9.4	109	<0.1	0.052	1.6	0.2	0.21	0.011	0.12	<0.02	<0.03
Cauliflower	frozen, uncooked	66	310	18	14	12	<0.1	<0.02	1.4	0.068	0.17	0.011	0.46	0.16	<0.03
Celery	fresh	20	245	23	8.7	87	<0.1	<0.02	1.1	0.069	0.14	<0.01	0.065	<0.02	<0.03
Corn, whole kernel	canned, salt-free, drained	44	117	<5	11	<0.5	<0.1	<0.02	0.26	<0.01	0.021	0.011	0.33	<0.02	<0.03
Cucumber		13	148	18	10	0.7	<0.1	<0.02	0.59	0.12	0.044	<0.01	0.1	0.056	<0.03
Lettuce		31	139	22	12	7.6	<0.1	0.02	0.53	0.078	0.082	0.037	0.25	0.069	<0.03
Mushrooms, stems and pieces	canned	66	98	13	6.5	355	0.4	<0.02	2.3	0.067	<0.01	0.26	1.1	0.033	<0.03
Onions	fresh, mature	33	141	22	10.1	2.2	<0.1	0.053	0.75	0.2	0.17	0.097	0.11	0.078	<0.03

APPENDIX TABLE 12   INORGANIC ELEMENTS IN COMMON FOODS* (Continued)

(Milligrams per 100 Gram Food)

Vegetables—Concluded — mg./100 gm.

FOOD	DESCRIPTION	PHOSPHORUS	POTASSIUM	CALCIUM	MAGNESIUM	SODIUM	ALUMINUM	BARIUM	IRON	STRONTIUM	BORON	COPPER	ZINC	MANGANESE	CHROMIUM
Peas	canned, salt-free, drained	71	118	23	22	5.4	<0.1	<0.02	1.2	0.012	0.16	0.13	1.3	0.11	<0.03
Potato															
Fresh	uncooked	44	280	6.7	14	1.45	<0.1	<0.02	0.58	0.012	0.052	0.052	0.2	0.042	<0.03
Instant	uncooked	179	625	66	68	124	<0.2	0.056	0.97	0.18	0.26	0.17	0.56	0.16	<0.06
Pumpkin	canned	38	176	36	18	0.7	0.26	0.053	16	0.056	0.27	0.054	0.19	0.11	<0.03
Spinach	frozen, uncooked	40	575	139	104	140	2.2	0.04	3.3	0.48	0.33	0.083	0.37	0.56	<0.03
Squash	frozen, cooked	28	172	32	26	0.9	0.34	0.082	1.1	0.15	0.2	0.14	0.3	0.096	<0.03
Sweet potatoes	canned	22	164	22	18	16	<0.1	0.22	0.47	0.23	0.08	0.063	0.16	0.62	<0.03
Tomato															
Fresh		13	178	<5	4.3	1.45	<0.1	<0.02	0.53	0.012	0.014	<0.01	0.046	<0.02	<0.03
Juice	canned, salt-free	8.3	250	2.9	4.1	2.2	<0.04	<0.008	0.053	<0.004	0.023	<0.004	0.065	0.013	<0.012

Analyzed values for inorganic elements in representative hospital menus

mg./day

MENU	PHOSPHORUS*	POTASSIUM	CALCIUM*	MAGNESIUM*	SODIUM	ALUMINUM	BARIUM	IRON	STRONTIUM	BORON	COPPER	ZINC	MANGANESE	CHROMIUM
General														
Summer	1,486	3,942	1,304	294	5,912	6.974	<0.303	7.6	1.243	1.577	0.425	13.34	0.88	<0.455
Winter	2,041	4,881	1,390	385	7,158	5.324	<0.592	9.2	1.893	1.154	0.296	14.49	1.78	<0.887
Mechanical soft														
Summer	1,153	3,436	1,031	226	4,221	5.644	<0.245	6.6	0.810	1.055	0.466	12.52	0.66	<0.368
Winter	1,591	4,473	1,291	330	4,263	9.006	0.721	11.1	0.360	0.600	0.600	16.81	1.38	<0.901
Low (1 gm.)-sodium														
Summer	1,180	3,934	1,124	250	1,377	3.934	0.337	9.0	0.871	1.461	0.731	12.08	0.76	<0.422
Winter	1,323	3,737	986	311	960	<2.595	0.519	12.2	0.260	0.467	<0.260	18.43	1.43	<0.779
40-gm. protein														
Summer	776	2,209	716	191	3,343	<1.990	<0.398	3.6	0.856	0.935	<0.199	7.56	0.40	<0.597
Winter	635	1,813	505	142	1,420	1.869	0.374	5.2	0.262	0.561	0.187	6.36	0.38	<0.561
1,000-calorie														
Summer	1,179	3,237	1,064	277	3,491	4.393	0.324	16.2	0.948	1.272	0.532	16.65	0.95	<0.347
Winter	1,231	2,904	999	200	4,251	<2.323	0.465	6.0	0.372	0.465	0.232	11.38	0.47	<0.697
1,500-calorie														
Summer	909	2,751	765	220	3,755	3.349	0.431	13.2	0.622	0.789	0.455	13.40	1.24	<0.359
Winter	1,224	3,492	867	219	5,327	4.843	0.510	6.6	0.357	0.510	0.255	12.24	1.17	<0.765
Giovanetti†	846	1,481	1,058	134	150	634.5	0.752	25.9	1.105	0.917	<0.235	<3.29	0.85	<0.705
20-gm. protein (no salt added)†	430	1,328	359	110	323	<1.795	<0.359	2.3	<0.180	0.539	<0.180	1.98	<0.36	<0.539
Full liquid†	1,354	3,745	1,815	242	3,832	4.033	<0.288	2.9	0.807	0.951	0.288	8.64	1.18	<0.432
Clear liquid†	<21	736	57	57	2,618	2.290	<0.164	1.1	<0.082	0.164	0.082	0.33	0.92	<0.245
Estimated daily intake of Americans (1, 13)	800–1,200	2,000–6,000	800–1,200	300–450	2,300–6,900	36.4	16.0	15.0	2.0	10.0	2.0	12.0	5.0	0.06

*A daily allowance is recommended by Food and Nutrition Board (1).
†Winter menu only.

APPENDIX TABLE 13   DESIRABLE WEIGHTS FOR MEN

*(Ages 25 and Over)**

HEIGHT (WITH SHOES, 1-INCH HEELS)		WEIGHT IN POUNDS ACCORDING TO FRAME (IN INDOOR CLOTHING)		
		Small Frame	*Medium Frame*	*Large Frame*
Feet	Inches			
5	2	112–120	118–129	126–141
5	3	115–123	121–133	129–144
5	4	118–126	124–136	132–148
5	5	121–129	127–139	135–152
5	6	124–133	130–143	138–156
5	7	128–137	134–147	142–161
5	8	132–141	138–152	147–166
5	9	136–145	142–156	151–170
5	10	140–150	146–160	155–174
5	11	144–154	150–165	159–179
6	0	148–158	154–170	164–184
6	1	152–162	158–175	168–189
6	2	156–167	162–180	173–194
6	3	160–171	167–185	178–199
6	4	164–175	172–190	182–204

*Courtesy of the Metropolitan Life Insurance Company, New York, N.Y. Derived from data of the 1969 Build and Blood Pressure Study, Society of Actuaries.

APPENDIX TABLE 14   DESIRABLE WEIGHTS FOR WOMEN

*(Ages 25 and Over)**

HEIGHT (WITH SHOES, 2-INCH HEELS)		WEIGHT IN POUNDS ACCORDING TO FRAME (IN INDOOR CLOTHING)		
		Small Frame	*Medium Frame*	*Large Frame*
Feet	Inches			
4	10	92– 98	96–107	104–119
4	11	94–101	98–110	106–122
5	0	96–104	101–113	109–125
5	1	99–107	104–116	112–128
5	2	102–110	107–119	115–131
5	3	105–113	110–122	118–134
5	4	108–116	113–126	121–138
5	5	111–119	116–130	125–142
5	6	114–123	120–135	129–146
5	7	118–127	124–139	133–150
5	8	122–131	128–143	137–154
5	9	126–135	132–147	141–158
5	10	130–140	136–151	145–163
5	11	134–144	140–155	149–168
6	0	138–148	144–159	153–173

*Note: for girls between 18 and 25, subtract 1 pound for each year under 25. Courtesy of the Metropolitan Life Insurance Company, New York, N.Y. Derived from data of the 1959 Build and Blood Pressure Study, Society of Actuaries.

APPENDIX TABLE 15   HEIGHT-WEIGHT-AGE TABLE FOR BOYS OF SCHOOL AGE*

(Weight is Expressed in Pounds)

HT. INS.	5 YRS.	6 YRS.	7 YRS.	8 YRS.	9 YRS.	10 YRS.	11 YRS.	12 YRS.	13 YRS.	14 YRS.	15 YRS. •	16 YRS.	17 YRS.	18 YRS.	19 YRS.	HT. INS.
38	34	34														38
39	35	35														39
40	36	36														40
41	38	38	38													41
42	39	39	39													42
43	41	41	41	41												43
44	44	44	44	44												44
45	46	46	46	46	46											45
46	47	48	48	48	48											46
47	49	50	50	50	50	50										47
48		52	53	53	53	53										48
49		55	55	55	55	55	55									49
50		57	58	58	58	58	58	58								50
51			61	61	61	61	61	61								51
52			63	64	64	64	64	64	64							52
53			66	67	67	67	67	68	68							53
54				70	70	70	70	71	71	72						54
55				72	72	73	73	74	74	74						55
56				75	76	77	77	78	78	78	80					56
57					79	80	81	81	82	83	83					57
58					83	84	84	85	85	86	87					58
59						87	88	89	89	90	90	90				59
60						91	92	92	93	94	95	96				60
61							95	96	97	99	100	103	106			61
62							100	101	102	103	104	107	111	116		62
63							105	106	107	108	110	113	118	123	127	63
64								109	111	113	115	117	121	126	130	64
65								114	117	118	120	122	127	131	134	65
66									119	122	125	128	132	136	139	66
67									124	128	130	134	136	139	142	67
68										134	134	137	141	143	147	68
69										137	139	143	146	149	152	69
70										143	144	145	148	151	155	70
71										148	150	151	152	154	159	71
72											153	155	156	158	163	72
73											157	160	162	164	167	73
74											160	164	168	170	171	74

The following percentages of net weight have been added for clothing (shoes and sweaters not included): 35 to 64 pounds: 3.5 per cent; 64 pounds and over: 2.0 per cent.

*From material prepared by Bird T. Baldwin, Ph.D., Iowa Child Welfare Research Station, State University of Iowa, and Thomas D. Wood, M.D., Columbia University, New York.

APPENDIX TABLE 16   HEIGHT-WEIGHT-AGE TABLE FOR GIRLS OF SCHOOL AGE*

(Weight is Expressed in Pounds)

HT INS.	5 YRS.	6 YRS.	7 YRS.	8 YRS.	9 YRS.	10 YRS.	11 YRS.	12 YRS.	13 YRS.	14 YRS.	15 YRS.	16 YRS.	17 YRS.	18 YRS.	HT. INS.
38	33	33													38
39	34	34													39
40	36	36	36												40
41	37	37	37												41
42	39	39	39												42
43	41	41	41	41											43
44	42	42	42	42											44
45	45	45	45	45	45										45
46	47	47	48	48											46
47	49	50	50	50	50	50									47
48		52	52	52	52	53									48
49		54	54	55	55	56	56								49
50		56	56	57	58	59	61	62							50
51			59	60	61	61	63	65							51
52			63	64	64	64	65	67							52
53			66	67	67	68	68	69	71						53
54				69	70	70	71	71	73						54
55				72	74	74	74	75	77	78					55
56					76	78	78	79	81	83					56
57					80	82	82	82	84	88	92				57
58						84	86	86	88	93	96	101			58
59						87	90	90	92	96	100	103	104		59
60						91	95	95	97	101	105	108	109	111	60
61						99	100	101	101	105	108	112	113	116	61
62							104	105	106	109	113	115	117	118	62
63								110	110	112	116	117	119	120	63
64								114	115	117	119	120	122	123	64
65								118	120	121	122	123	125	126	65
66									124	124	125	128	129	130	66
67									128	130	131	133	133	135	67
68									131	133	135	136	138	138	68
69										135	137	138	140	142	69
70										136	138	140	142	144	70
71										138	140	142	144	145	71

The following percentages of net weight have been added for clothing (shoes and sweaters not included): 35 to 65 pounds: 3.0 per cent; 66 to 82 pounds: 2.5 per cent; 83 pounds and over: 2 per cent.

*From material prepared by Bird T. Baldwin, Ph.D., Iowa Child Welfare Research Station, State University of Iowa, and Thomas D. Wood, M.D., Columbia University, New York.

INDEX

Page numbers in *italics* indicate illustrations.
Page numbers followed by (t) indicate tables.